Clinical Pain Management
Practical Applications and Procedures

Series editors

Andrew S C Rice MB BS MD FRCA
Senior Lecturer in Pain Research, Department of
Anaesthetics, Faculty of Medicine, Imperial College,
Chelsea & Westminster Hospital Campus, London,
UK

Carol A Warfield MD
Edward Lowenstein Professor of Anesthesia,
Harvard Medical School; Chairman, Department of
Anesthesia and Critical Care, Beth Israel Deaconess
Medical Center, Boston, Massachusetts, USA

Douglas Justins MB BS FRCA
Pain Management Centre, St Thomas' Hospital,
London, UK

Christopher Eccleston PhD
Director, Pain Management Unit, University of
Bath & The Royal National Hospital for Rheumatic
Diseases, Bath, UK

Acute Pain
Edited by David J Rowbotham and
Pamela E Macintyre

Chronic Pain
Edited by Troels S Jensen, Peter R Wilson, and
Andrew S C Rice

Cancer Pain
Edited by Nigel Sykes, Marie T Fallon, and
Richard B Patt

Practical Applications and Procedures
Edited by Harald Breivik, William Campbell, and
Christopher Eccleston

Clinical Pain Management

Practical Applications and Procedures

Edited by

Harald Breivik MD DMedSci FRCA (elected)
Professor of Anaesthesiology, Department of
Anaesthesiology, Rikshospitalet University Clinic,
Oslo, Norway

William Campbell MD PhD FRCA FFARCSI Dip Pain Med
Consultant in Anaesthesia and Pain Medicine, Ulster
Hospital Dundonald, Belfast, UK

and

Christopher Eccleston
Director, Pain Management Unit, University of Bath &
The Royal National Hospital for Rheumatic Diseases,
Bath, UK

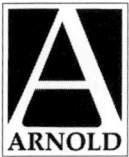

A member of the Hodder Headline Group
LONDON

First published in Great Britain in 2003 by
Arnold, a member of the Hodder Headline Group,
338 Euston Road, London NW1 3BH

http://www.arnoldpublishers.com

Distributed in the United States of America by
Oxford University Press Inc.,
198 Madison Avenue, New York, NY10016
Oxford is a registered trademark of Oxford University Press

Whilst the advice and information in this book are believed to
be true and accurate at the date of going to press, neither the
authors nor the publisher can accept any legal responsibility
or liability for any errors or omissions that may be made. In
particular (but without limiting the generality of the preceding
disclaimer) every effort has been made to check drug dosages;
however it is still possible that errors have been missed.
Furthermore, dosage schedules are constantly being revised
and new side-effects recognized. For these reasons the reader
is strongly urged to consult the drug companies' printed
instructions before administering any of the drugs recommended
in this book.

British Library Cataloguing in Publication Data
A catalogue record for this book is available from the British
Library

Library of Congress Cataloging-in-Publication Data
A catalog record for this book is available from the Library of
Congress

ISBN 0 340 80995 7 (Practical Applications and Procedures)

ISBN 0 340 73153 2 (2-vol set: Acute Pain/Practical Applications
and Procedures)

ISBN 0 340 73154 0 (2-vol set: Chronic Pain/Practical
Applications and Procedures)

ISBN 0 340 73152 4 (2-vol set: Cancer Pain/Practical Applications
and Procedures)

ISBN 0 340 70635 X (4-vol set: Acute Pain/Chronic Pain/Cancer
Pain/Practical Applications and Procedures)

1 2 3 4 5 6 7 8 9 10

Commissioning Editor: Joanna Koster
Development Editor: Sarah Burrows
Production Editor: James Rabson
Production Controller: Martin Kerans
Project Manager: Lindsey Williams
Cover Designer: Terry Griffiths

Typeset in 10 on 12 pt Minion by Prepress Projects Ltd, Perth

Printed and bound in the UK by The Bath Press

Contents

Contributors   ix

Series preface   xiii

Introduction to Clinical Pain Management: Practical Applications and Procedures   xv

Cross-references, evidence scoring, and reference annotation   xvii

PART I   **PRINCIPLES OF MEASUREMENT AND DIAGNOSIS**

1   **Selecting and applying pain measures**
Amanda C de C Williams   3

2   **Practical methods for pain intensity measurements**
William I Campbell   15

3   **Sensory testing and clinical neurophysiology**
Ellen Jørum and Lars Arendt-Nielsen   27

4   **Pharmacological diagnostic tests**
Andrew P Baranowski   39

5   **Nerve blocks in pain diagnosis**
Robert A Boas   49

PART II   **PHARMACOLOGICAL THERAPIES**

6   **Opioid analgesics**
Michael L Tran and Carol Warfield   59

7   **Treatment protocols for opioids in chronic nonmalignant pain**
Harald Breivik   77

8   **Subcutaneous drug infusions for the control of cancer pain**
Ivan F Trotman and Faeqa Hami   85

9   **Antidepressants, antiepileptics, and antiarrhythmic drugs**
Søren H Sindrup and Flemming W Bach   101

PART III   **PSYCHOLOGICAL TECHNIQUES**

10   **Self-regulation skills training for adults, including relaxation**
David Spiegel   113

11   **Biofeedback**
Frank Andrasik and Herta Flor   121

12   **Attentional regulation for adults with chronic pain**
Elizabeth Elliott and Chris Eccleston   135

13   **Hypnosis, biofeedback, and self-regulation skills for children in pain**
Leora Kuttner and Timothy Culbert   147

14   **Graded exposure *in vivo* for pain-related fear**
Johan W S Vlaeyen, Jeroen de Jong, Peter H T G Heuts, and Geert Crombez   163

PART IV   PHYSICAL THERAPY AND REHABILITATION PROTOCOLS

15   **Physiotherapy**
Anne Elisabeth Ljunggren and Jan Magnus Bjordal   179

16   **Manual medicine**
Somayaji Ramamurthy and Philip E Greenman   189

PART V   INTERVENTIONS

17   **Peripheral nerve blocks: practical aspects**
David Hill   197

18   **Sympathetic blocks**
Harald Breivik   233

19   **Neurolytic blocks**
Étienne de Médicis and Oscar A de Leon-Casasola   247

20   **Intra-articular injections**
John Etherington and Simon Paul   255

21   **Facet (zygapophyseal) joint injections and medial branch blocks**
Ron Cooper   269

22   **Botulinum toxin injections**
Lauren C Seeberger and Christopher F O'Brien   277

23   **Long-term intrathecal and intracisternal treatment of malignant and nonmalignant pain using external pumps**
Petre V Nitescu, Lennart K Appelgren (deceased), and Ioan A Curelaru   285

24   **Long-term epidural treatment of refractory malignant and nonmalignant pain using internal and external pumps**
Andrew Lawson and Olga Siemaszko   307

25   **Cryoanalgesia**
Thomas A Edell and Somayaji Ramamurthy   319

26   **Radiofrequency lesioning**
Ben J P Crul and Maarten Van Kleef   327

PART VI   STIMULATION ANALGESIA

27   **Transcutaneous electrical nerve stimulation**
Timothy P Nash   343

28   **Acupuncture**
Cynthia M Kahn and Jonathan Ammen   355

29   **Spinal cord stimulation**
      John R Wedley   381

PART VII   PATIENT-CONTROLLED ANALGESIA

30   **Intravenous and subcutaneous patient-controlled analgesia: practical points and protocols**
      Richard Barrett   393

31   **Alternative opioid PCA delivery systems – transcutaneous, nasal, and others**
      Gunnvald Kvarstein   401

PART VIII   EPIDURAL AND SPINAL ANALGESIA – PROTOCOLS AND CHARTS

32   **Epidural analgesia for acute pain, including patient-controlled epidural analgesia**
      Harald Breivik   409

33   **Epidural steroid injections for back pain and sciatica**
      Edward Walsh   417

PART IX   PEDIATRIC TECHNIQUES

34   **Procedures for pediatric pain management**
      Richard Howard   431

PART X   CLINICAL TRIALS

35   **Clinical trials: acute and chronic pain**
      Audun Stubhaug   449

36   **Clinical trials: dental pain**
      Else K Breivik   461

37   **Clinical trials: cancer pain**
      Ulf E Kongsgaard   469

38   **Clinical experimental pharmacological protocols: how to evaluate the use of a new drug**
      Märta Segerdahl   483

39   **Techniques of systematic reviews and meta-analysis in pain research**
      Anna D Oldman and Lesley A Smith   495

PART XI   OTHER ISSUES

40   **The expert medicolegal report**
      Peter J D Evans   509

      Index   517

      Cumulative index to Clinical Pain Management   539

Contributors

Jonathan B Ammen LicAc MEd
Pain Management Center, Symmes Hospital, Arlington, MA, USA

Frank Andrasik PhD
Senior Research Scientist and Professor of Psychology, Institute for Human and Machine Cognition, University of West Florida, Pensacola, FL, USA

Lennart K Appelgren (deceased)
Formerly Associate Professor of Anesthesiology, Gothenburg University, and Senior Consultant, Department of Anaesthesia and Intensive Care, Sahlgrenska University Hospital, Gothenburg, Sweden

Lars Arendt-Nielsen
Professor, Center for Sensory–Motor Interaction, Laboratory for Experimental Pain Research, Aalborg University, Aalborg, Denmark

Flemming W Bach MD
Consultant Neurologist, Department of Neurology, Aarhus University Hospital, Aarhus, Denmark

Andrew P Baranowski MBBS FRCA BSc (Hons) MD
Consultant in Pain Management, The Pain Management Department, University College London Hospitals, The National Hospital for Neurology and Neurosurgery, London, UK

Richard Barrett MB BS FRCA
Consultant Anaesthetist, Salisbury District Hospital, Salisbury, UK

Jan Magnus Björdal PT MSc
Specialist in Rehabilitation (Orthopaedics/Rheumatology) and Research Fellow, Bergen University College, Bergen, Norway

Robert A Boas MB BCh FANZCA FRCA
Anaesthesia Associates, Takapuna, Auckland, New Zealand

Harald Breivik MD DMSc FRCA
Professor of Anaesthesiology, Department of Anaesthesiology, Rikshospitalet University Clinic, Oslo, Norway

Else K Breivik DDS PhD
Department of Oral Surgery and Oral Medicine, Faculty of Dentistry, University of Oslo, Oslo, Norway

William I Campbell MD PhD FRCA FFARCSI
Consultant in Anaesthesia and Pain Medicine, Ulster Hospital, Newtownards, Belfast, UK

Ron Cooper MD FFARCSI DRCOG DPMed RCSI
Consultant in Anaesthesia and Pain Medicine, Causeway Hospital, Coleraine, UK

Geert Crombez PhD
Professor of Health Psychology, Faculty of Psychology and Educational Sciences, Ghent University, Ghent, Belgium

Ben J P Crul MD PhD
Professor of Pain Management and Head, Pain Centre, Department of Anesthesiology, University Hospital, Nijmegen, The Netherlands

Timothy Culbert MD FAAP
Assistant Professor of Clinical Pediatrics, Behavioral Pediatrics Program, Department of Pediatrics, University of Minnesota, and Medical Director, Integrative Medicine and Cultural Care, Children's Hospitals and Clinics, Minneapolis, MN, USA

Ioan A Curelaru MD PhD
Retired Associate Professor of Anaesthesiology, Gothenburg University, and Senior Consultant and Former Director of Pain Section, Sahlgrenska University Hospital, Gothenburg, Sweden

Jeroen De Jong
Rehabilitation Centre "Hoensbroeck," Hoensbroek, The Netherlands

Oscar A de Leon-Casasola MD
Professor of Anesthesiology and Vice-Chair for Clinical Affairs, Department of Anesthesiology, University at Buffalo, and Chief, Pain Medicine, Roswell Park Cancer Institute, SUNY-Buffalo School of Medicine, Buffalo, NY, USA

Étienne de Médicis MSc MD FRCP(C)
Assistant Professor, Département d'Anesthésiologie-Réanimation, Centre Hospitalier Universitaire de Sherbrooke, Fleurimont, Québec, Canada

Christopher Eccleston PhD
Pain Management Unit, University of Bath, Claverton Down, Bath, UK

Thomas A Edell MD Major USAF MC
Assistant Professor of Anesthesiology, Uniformed Services
University of the Health Sciences, and Director, Pain
Medicine, Wilford Hall Medical Center, Lackland AFB, TX,
USA

Elizabeth Elliott BA (Hons) MCCP MAPs
Independent Licensee, Integrity Coaching Group,
Cleveland, Australia

John Etherington MSc FRCP
Consultant in Rheumatology and Rehabilitation, Defence
Services Medical Rehabilitation Centre, Epsom, UK

Peter J D Evans MB BS FRCA
Consultant Anaesthetist and Director, Pain Management
Centre, Department of Anaesthetics, Charing Cross
Hospital, London, UK

Herta Flor PhD
Department of Clinical and Cognitive Neuroscience,
University of Heidelberg, Central Institute of Mental
Health, Mannheim, Germany

Philip E Greenman DO FAAO
Emeritus Professor, Department of Osteopathic
Manipulative Medicine, Emeritus Professor, Department
of Physical Medicine and Rehabilitation, and Emeritus
Senior Associate Dean, Michigan State University, College
of Osteopathic Medicine, East Lansing, MI, USA

Faeqa Hami MB DA MRCP(UK)
Consultant in Palliative Medicine, South Bucks NHS Trust,
Wycombe Hospital, High Wycombe, UK

Peter H T G Heuts
Rehabilitation Centre "Hoensbroeck," Hoensbroek, The
Netherlands

Richard Howard BSc FRCA
Consultant in Anaesthesia and Pain Management,
Department of Anaesthesia, Great Ormond Street Hospital
for Children NHS Trust, London, UK

Ellen Jørum MD PhD
Specialist in Neurology and Clinical Neurophysiology and
Consultant in Clinical Neurophysiology, Department of
Neurology, The National Hospital, Oslo, Norway

Cynthia M Kahn MD
Pain Management Center, Winchester Hospital,
Winchester, MA, USA

Ulf E Kongsgaard MD PhD
Professor and Chairman, Department of Anaesthesia
and Intensive Care, The Norwegian Radium Hospital,
Montebello, Oslo, Norway

Leora Kuttner PhD
Clinical Professor, Department of Paediatrics, University
of British Columbia, B.C. Children's Hospital, Vancouver,
BC, Canada

Gunnvald Kvarstein MD
Department of Anaesthesiology, The National Hospital,
Oslo, Norway

Andrew Lawson FFARCSI FRCA FANZCA
Consultant in Anaesthesia and Pain Management, Magill
Department of Anaesthesia, Intensive Care and Pain
Management, Chelsea and Westminster Hospital, London,
UK

Anne Elisabeth Ljunggren PhD
Professor, Section of Physiotherapy Science, University of
Bergen, Bergen, Norway

Timothy P Nash MBBS FRCA DObst RCOG
Honorary Senior Lecturer and Honorary Director of
Pain Studies, Department of Neuroscience, University of
Liverpool, and Consultant Pain Physician, Walton Centre
for Neurology and Neurosurgery, Liverpool, UK

Petre V Nitescu MD PhD
Associate Professor of Anaesthesiology and Intensive
Care, Gothenburg University, and Senior Consultant and
Director of Pain Section, Sahlgrenska University Hospital,
Gothenburg, Sweden

Christopher O'Brien MD
Vice President Medical Affairs, Elan Biopharmaceuticals,
San Diego, CA, USA

Anna D Oldman DPhil
Post-doctoral Research Associate, Pain Research, Nuffield
Department of Anaesthetics, Oxford Radcliffe Hospital,
University of Oxford, Oxford, UK

Simon Paul BSc MRCP(UK)
Specialist Registrar in Rheumatology and Rehabilitation,
Defence Services Medical Rehabilitation Centre, Epsom,
UK

Somayaji Ramamurthy MD
Professor, Department of Anaesthesiology, University of
Texas, Health Sciences Center MC 7838, San Antonio, TX,
USA

Lauren Seeberger MD
CNI Movement Disorder Center, Colorado Neurological
Institute, Englewood, CO, USA

Märta Segerdahl MD PhD
Center for Surgical Sciences, Unit for Anaesthesia,
Karolinska Institutet, and Department of Anaesthesia and
Intensive Care, Huddinge University Hospital, Stockholm,
Sweden

Olga Siemaszko FRCA
Specialist Registrar in Pain Management, St Thomas'
Hospital, London, UK

Søren Sindrup MD
Consultant Neurologist, Department of Neurology, Odense
University Hospital, Odense, Denmark

Lesley A Smith PhD
Research Fellow, ICRF/NHS Centre for Statistics in
Medicine, Institute of Health Sciences, University of
Oxford, Oxford, UK

David Spiegel MD
Willson Professor in the School of Medicine, Associate
Chair, Department of Psychiatry and Behavioral Sciences,
Stanford University School of Medicine, Stanford, CA, USA

Audun Stubhaug MD DMSc
Department of Anaesthesiology, Rikshospitalet University
Hospital, Oslo, Norway

Michael L Tran
652 Petaluma Avenue, Suite HB, Sebastopol, CA, USA

Ivan F Trotman MD FRCP
Consultant Physician, Department of Palliative
Medicine, Michael Sobell House, Mount Vernon Hospital,
Northwood, UK

Prof. Dr Maarten van Kleef
Department of Anaesthesiology and Pain Management,
University Hospital of Maastricht, Maastricht, The
Netherlands

Johan W S Vlaeyen PhD
Associate Professor of Behavioral Medicine, Department
of Medical, Clinical and Experimental Psychology, Maastricht
University, Maastricht, The Netherlands

Edward Walsh MB BS BSc FRCA
Consultant in Pain Medicine, Pain Relief Clinic,
Southmead Hospital, Westbury-on-Trym, Bristol, UK

Carol Warfield MD
Edward Lowenstein Professor of Anesthesia, Harvard
Medical School, and Chairman, Department of Anesthesia
and Critical Care, Beth Israel Deaconess Medical Center,
Boston, MA, USA

John R Wedley MB ChB FRCA DA
Consultant in Pain Management, Guy's & St Thomas' NHS
Trust, Pain Management Centre, St Thomas' Hospital,
London, UK

Amanda C de C Williams MSc PhD CPsychol
Senior Lecturer in Clinical Health Psychology, GKT School
of Medicine and Dentistry, University of London, and
Consultant Clinical Psychologist, INPUT Pain Management
Unit, Guy's & St Thomas' Hospital NHS Trust, London, UK

Series preface

Clinical Pain Management is a brand new reference text, providing comprehensive coverage of this broad discipline for those training and practicing in pain management and related specialties. The work comprises four volumes, three covering the three major clinical disciplines of pain relief (acute, chronic, and cancer pain) accompanied by a fourth complementary volume discussing practical aspects of clinical management and clinical research that share a greater or lesser degree of communality with all three disciplines.

We believe that practice should be firmly based on the best available evidence. However, as things currently stand, a truly evidence-based textbook of pain management would be a relatively scant affair. We were anxious not to exclude discussion of clinical management strategies that are thought to represent reasonable practice by an appreciable body of clinicians, but for which there is currently a lack of evidence to either support or refute such a practice. Nevertheless, we were also concerned that the reader should be instantly aware of the quality of evidence that supports any recommendation for a clinical intervention. Therefore, we have encouraged authors to use a universal system for scoring quality of evidence. If no score is included in the text then the implication is that the supporting evidence is of very low quality.

As befits the multidisciplinary nature of modern pain management, both the authorship and editorship of *Clinical Pain Management* is drawn from a wide range of medical and paramedical clinical specialties. The team of contributors is truly international in nature, with a total of over 200 authors and editors practicing in 16 different countries. While we have attempted to ensure that each author has contributed a balanced discussion that crosses national boundaries, inevitably in a few chapters the authors' views will predominantly reflect the viewpoint as seen from a particular country or system of health care delivery.

Although the textbook of *Clinical Pain Management* is extensively referenced, we are also keen that the reader can easily identify key references. Accordingly, in the reference list at the end of each chapter important and seminal papers and key reviews are highlighted with special symbols.

Clinical Pain Management is not intended to replace the most prestigious and well-known textbook edited by Ronald Melzack and the late Patrick Wall. Instead it represents a complementary work, addressing the practical clinical aspects immediately relevant to those working on the 'factory floor' of clinical pain management rather than the equally important cutting edge of laboratory research into pain. We believe that there is a proper place for both titles on the bookshelves of pain management clinicians.

Finally, we are greatly indebted to the volume editors and chapter authors, without the considerable efforts of whom publication would not have been possible. We are also most grateful to the publishing team at Arnold, particularly the publisher, Joanna Koster, without whose Herculean efforts in holding together a team of editors and authors spanning the globe none of this would have seen the light of day. Thanks are also due to her predecessor, Annalisa Page, who was instrumental in conceiving and administering the early stages of the project, and to the production and project management teams.

Andrew S C Rice
Carol Warfield
Douglas Justins
Christopher Eccleston
London, Boston, and Bath
August 2002

Introduction to Clinical Pain Management: Practical Applications and Procedures

Despite extensive research into the origins and mechanisms of acute and chronic pain, its management remains a challenge to all involved in health care. This is partly because of our incomplete knowledge of the subject and the plasticity of the mechanisms involved. The need to educate patients and develop therapeutic means that are effective but which are well tolerated are additional problems encountered in daily practice. Each chapter in *Practical Applications and Procedures* can stand alone or work to complement the chapters in preceding volumes – *Acute Pain, Chronic Pain,* and *Cancer Pain.* Authors have been chosen as having a special interest and expertise in the practical applications they describe. They have been invited to present their work in a style that is not only comprehensive but also easy to read, with summaries of key points and evidence-based references. The editors and authors have endeavored to provide the reader with a contemporary text that utilizes our latest knowledge on the management of pain to maximize a favorable outcome.

Practical Applications and Procedures covers various forms of pain assessment in addition to a wide range of therapies that can be provided by a diverse range of health care disciplines, including practical procedures and applications in the management of acute, chronic, and cancer pain. The volume concludes with valuable chapters about clinical research methods and writing medicolegal reports.

We trust that this volume will be of value to all health care workers, regardless of their discipline, and that it will help them to keep abreast of developments and challenges in the maturing discipline of applied pain medicine.

Harald Breivik
William Campbell
Christopher Eccleston
Oslo, Belfast, and Bath

Cross-references, evidence scoring, and reference annotation

The four volumes of *Clinical Pain Management* incorporate the following special features to aid the readers' understanding and navigation of the text.

Cross-references

Cross-references to other chapters within *Clinical Pain Management* are prefixed by a code indicating the volume in which the chapter referred to is to be found. The codes are as follows:

A   Acute Pain
Ch   Chronic Pain
Ca   Cancer Pain
P   Practical Applications and Procedures

Evidence scoring

In chapters in which recommendations for surgical, medical, psychological and complementary treatment, and diagnostic tests are presented, the quality of evidence supporting authors' statements relating to clinical interventions is graded by insertion of the following symbols into the text:

***   systematic review or meta-analysis
**   one or more well designed randomized controlled trials
*   nonrandomized controlled trials, cohort study etc.

Where no * is inserted, the quality of supporting evidence, if any exists, is of low grade only (e.g. case reports, clinical experience).

Other textbooks devoted to the subject of pain include a tremendous amount of anecdotal and personal recommendations, and it is often difficult to distinguish these from those with an established evidence base. This text is thus unique in allowing the reader the opportunity to do this with confidence.

Reference annotation

The reference lists are annotated, where appropriate, to guide readers to key primary papers and major review articles as follows:

Key primary papers are indicated by a ◆
Major review articles are indicated by a ●

We hope that this feature will render extensive lists of references more useful to the reader and will help to encourage self-directed learning among both trainees and practicing physicians.

PART I

Principles of measurement and diagnosis

Selecting and applying pain measures

AMANDA C DE C WILLIAMS

Content of measures and considerations for their selection	3	Conclusion	13
Quality of measures and interpretation of their output	9	References	13

The range of possible measures associated with pain treatment can be bewildering because the effects of pain are so far reaching. Although the aims of assessment (such as diagnosis) or treatment should determine the choice of measures, and they certainly provide the basis, there is still a huge choice among pain-specific or general measurement instruments: long-established or more recently developed, broad scope or narrow focus. Eventually, the choice is often made pragmatically, guided by recommendations from fellow clinicians, availability, length, and language. During this process, important considerations may be lost. This chapter aims to help to address these considerations to enable the reader to make a more confident choice of what best suits the evaluation in hand.

The first major area is that of outcome domains: measures should be straightforward to enable results to be interpreted with reference to the aims and methods of treatment. Many evaluations of acute and chronic pain problems rely heavily or solely on pain as an outcome, even when it is acknowledged that changing pain is not the main or sole target of treatment. Some broad measures (such as quality of life) appear to promise almost a panacea to measurement problems. However, a total score can be no more than the sum of its constituent item scores, interpreted according to data on its use in the real world, with all the limitations of those data. An appreciation of the conceptual basis of any measurement domain, and of unresolved conceptual problems that are inevitably represented in measures which arise from them, engenders a critical and strong interpretation of study results.

The second major area is that of the psychometric qualities of measures, appreciation of which assists in their interpretation. Distinguishing true from error variance is like detecting the signal against a background of noise – choosing a less noisy instrument, and recognizing that in a different location (population) it may pick up different noise, provides more confident identification of the signal, such as variance due to treatment. The section on psychometric qualities of measures, which is not exhaustive but which covers the commonest areas of concern, also incorporates a short section on the definition of clinically significant change.

A comprehensive guide to measures may be found in Turk and Melzack[1] and in McDowell and Newell.[2] Many chapters in these volumes cover assessment specific to their subject areas. There is no short answer with adequate scientific credibility to the question of what is the "success rate" in a single study of a treatment for pain. Attempts at evaluation require time and effort from patients, clinicians, and researchers, and the guidelines in this chapter aim to make their investment as productive as possible by judicious choice, analysis, and interpretation of measures.

CONTENT OF MEASURES AND CONSIDERATIONS FOR THEIR SELECTION

The outcomes to be assessed are effectively determined by the aims of treatment, and may also be required by methods of treatment. However, the statement of treatment aims is often rather narrow (e.g. pain relief), leaving implicit the associated gains that are often listed as part of the rationale for trying to improve pain treatment: mood, function, activity, overall quality of life, and greater independence in health care. For this reason, it can be helpful to use a short checklist of outcome domains to ensure that relevant outcomes are covered. Most clinicians and patients embark on treatment with multiple aims, which usually, but not necessarily, consist of reductions in pain experience and health care use and improvements in activity levels, mood and well-being, and physical state. Despite mutual influence among these areas, it is not the case that improvement in one domain implies proportional improvements in all the others. So, outcome measurement requires attention to as many of these domains as there are targets of treatment. Measurement of associated variables that are not targeted by treatment but that are relevant to understanding outcome data is worth a brief reminder because it is surprisingly often overlooked. For instance, in trials of a new drug from a family with marked adverse effects on a minority of users, data on previous use and reactions among those in the trial sample is important.

Method of measurement

An important consideration is that of the sampling method used in the measures that are available. If the target of assessment is what a person feels (symptom, mood, experience), it can only be sampled by self-report. If the target of assessment is what a person does, then either self-report or direct measurement are options. Self-report is the common choice, as substantial practical obstacles may be presented by prolonged observation or there may be difficulties in obtaining independent sources of relevant information (such as work or health records). This is not a problem where the selected self-report measure is well validated, as described below. However, in some current instruments, the "gold standard" used for validation has simply been a longer established self-report measure, not infrequently developed using both concepts and psychometric methods that have been superseded as our understanding improves – perhaps a "fool's gold" standard. Behavioral measures are generally underused in the health field, not least in pain treatment where several of the major targets of pain treatment are behavioral: increased activity in general; return to work or other improvement in work activities; greater independence in health care resulting in less use of health and disability-related resources.

Domains of outcome

One of the most frequently asked questions concerning outcome of pain treatment, particularly in chronic pain, is whether there is a single, simple measure of treatment success. If there were, it would be of enormous benefit to patients, pain treatment staff, and those who fund treatment. But can pain treatment ever have a single relevant outcome? Even the briefest assessment of experimentally produced pain in healthy subjects must address the multiple dimensions of pain. So, when subjects are clinical patients, with some degree of interference by pain in their lives, a single outcome is inconceivable.

There are many possible ways of grouping possible outcomes. Below, the broad domains of biomedical variables, psychosocial variables, and behavior and function, taken from Turk and Rudy,[3] are explained. Further distinctions are made between domains derived in a meta-analysis of cognitive–behavior therapy (CBT) for chronic pain in adults[4] that are also applicable to children.

Biomedical domains

Biomedical assessment tends to be most specific to the symptom or problem, except for pain itself, and is covered throughout this textbook in sections on assessment. The critical reader may wish to investigate further some of the statements about reliability and validity and the population(s) within which those parameters were established. Interrogation of interrater (and even intrarater) reliability for reading radiographs and quantifying clinical examination findings has revealed widespread shortcomings.[5,6] Some measures – of disease processes, of performance in clinical tests, or in general use (e.g. aerobic capacity) – may show good reliability but may lack the validation and comparison data that are required to render them interpretable in pain populations, i.e. they may be poor proxies for everyday function and mobility (see Chapter Ch6). Such measures may be of interest in their own right, or they may be used to investigate what variance they explain in the overall function of the patient. In some cases, they belie the use of an outdated model that is attempting to predict pain from the extent of the physical pathology.

Pain experience incorporates multiple dimensions of pain, variously described. The simplest classification is threefold – as sensory or discriminative, affective (emotional) and cognitive, and behavioral (interference) – and spans several domains of measurement. Although not easily separable, there is good evidence[7] for attempting to do so in experimental and clinical settings. Turk and Okifuji (Chapter Ch6) illustrate this well with the example of pain report in a man with chest pain before and after he is tested who is told that he has no cardiac pathology. Although intensity may not change at all, the meaning of the pain to the individual does change and, with it, behavior, emotions, and others' responses. A single or global pain rating represents pain dimensions in unknown quantities, and probably in combinations which vary between patients and across assessment contexts, obscuring their meaning. More detailed consideration of the advantages and disadvantages of particular pain measurement techniques and instruments can be found in the chapters by Turk and Okifuji (Chapter Ch6) and Campbell (Chapter P2).

Pain relief is belatedly gaining the attention it has long deserved. By far the commonest pain relief outcome criterion is 50%, which has considerable face validity, provides a ratio scale for analysis, and has been refined to provide a cumulative measure.[8] However, the 50% criterion does not arise from studies of patients' stated goals or of changes in target behaviors in relation to pain relief, and there are indications that in relation to behavioral change it may be higher than necessary. For instance, a study that compared cancer patients' ratings of breakthrough pain and pain relief after an analgesic with their request for further analgesic[9] found that nearer 30% pain relief sufficed. Although the results of this study were interpreted conservatively, they suggest the need to examine pain relief criteria further because other variables affect patients' willingness to ask for analgesia. The results also demonstrate a more patient-based and clinically useful approach to measuring analgesic effectiveness than is often used.

It may be important to assess *other symptoms* that are inherently unpleasant and that have an impact on quality of life, such as fatigue, nausea, and numbness, particularly in chronic illness such as cancer (see Chapter Ca4) or when they occur as adverse effects of treatment. These symptoms can be measured by the same methods as pain.

Psychosocial domains

Psychosocial variables include separate, although often related, areas – affect, cognitive content and process, and coping – that cannot be represented by a single measure (see Chapters Ch6 and Ch7). What the measures share is that the latent constructs to which they refer are hypothetical, are dependent on their definitions and therefore on their theoretical origins, and represent a late conscious phase of complex nonconscious processes. Because most have heuristic value, they take on a meaning beyond the limits of their definitions and origins that confounds their interpretation (see Chapter P2). Particular examples of the overinterpretation of constructs represented by measures that have a total which can be no more than the sum of their items, answered without reference to context or consequences, are those of pain behavior and of coping, both of which are described further below. Assigning numbers to the extent of agreement with a statement or degrees of intensity of an emotion does not mean that the construct is linear and distinct from related constructs. Some of the issues of importance to patients' welfare are best addressed by sensitive open-ended questioning (see Chapter Ca5), the responses to which can at best be categorized.

Affect or emotion measured in pain studies includes constructs such as depression, anxiety, anger or more broadly distress, or negative and positive affect. The possible list of overlapping terms for emotions is a long one, and these terms tend to draw heavily on psychiatric and personality psychology models where more normal psychology, particularly cognitive psychology, probably offers more appropriate terms. Anxiety may be more helpfully construed in terms of worry[10] and specific fears:[11] depression in terms of a distress related to the impact of pain on the patient's life, negative view of the self, and

functional and physical disturbance.[12] Positive emotion (well-being, happiness) is often overlooked, although it may provide a better measurement of mood improvement than depression and anxiety measures. Patients may describe their emotions using terms such as frustration, for which there is no psychological model or measure. For this reason, simple numerical or visual analog rating scales for emotions can be appropriate (e.g. see Chapter Ca4) and are represented in some quality of life measures.

Like pain, emotions have no unequivocal referents for validation: all have – and share – correlates in overt behavior, physiology, and cortical and subcortical activity. Comparison with psychiatric diagnosis, with which the measures share a theoretical framework, is common but problematic. Anxiety and depression show systematic differences from their parent constructs in psychiatry. Generalized anxiety has proved much less relevant in experimental and clinical pain than pain-related fear, and several fear measures have recently been developed[11,13] (see also Chapters Ch6 and Ch7). In depression or depressed mood, drawing on a psychiatric model produced measures with somatic items that, unlike in psychiatric populations, are often preferentially endorsed by patients in pain. Since there is no current measure of cognitive content (such as self-blame, guilt, sense of punishment) and affective content (such as feeling sad, loss of interest, feeling hopeless) without somatic items, interpretation of measures should include a check on somatic item endorsement. In those studies where diagnosis of depressive disorder is potentially an issue, for example in trials of antidepressants, then psychiatric interview is superior to self-report measures (Chapter Ch6).

Cognitive measures are used to sample patients' thinking about pain, but without an agreed model of the mind there is no satisfactory classification. These measures can be grouped approximately into those of content, process, and coping strategies (in measures that may also sample behavioral strategies). Cognitive content covers beliefs, such as those concerning control, self-efficacy, and attribution, and some beliefs may also appear as the cognitive statements in coping lists and as the cognitive content of emotion measures. Cognitive processes, particularly biases in appraisal and interpretation such as catastrophizing, are central to cognitive theory of emotion, and there is some overlap with emotion measures. Cognitive strategies, such as distraction, are also processes, but the patient is assumed to have greater voluntary control over these; however, cognitive measures may cover both. As with emotion, effective measurement tends toward the pain specific, exemplified by the move from general locus of control, which poorly predicted patients' thinking and behavior in relation to pain, to pain-specific appraisal and self-efficacy. Careful consideration of the purpose of evaluation is needed to select measures; for general treatment studies, a way to select among the many measures on offer is to examine their validation data. Those that involve prediction of behavior, such as adherence to treatment, or prediction of change in variables that were not too closely related can be interpreted more confidently than those that provide only concurrent validation against a similar instrument.[1,2,13]

Coping as a construct requires radical overhaul. It has considerable face validity and is part of lay discourse, usually implying a positive means of managing. However, negative strategies, behavioral or cognitive, may have more important effects on the individual's life. The labels positive and negative are in themselves problematic: the efficacy of a coping strategy depends on its appropriateness to the problem and to the context and on the short- and long-term outcome (not necessarily the same) for the individual patient – information which is difficult to collect. In its place, checklists use generalizations to classify strategies, relying on characteristics that may lack empirical support, of which active/passive is the commonest. Any strategy – seeking social support, attempting distraction, using analgesics – can be effective in one set of circumstances, irrelevant in another, and disastrous in a third. Therefore, such classifications are not reliably agreed by researchers. Selection among existing coping checklists, and particularly any use of interpretative rather than descriptive subtotals, should be made with these points in mind.

Behavior and activity

This broad area of assessment can be subdivided into specific and summary measures of behavior and physical function, by observer or by self-report; into broader measures of function, disability, and quality of life that include some psychosocial content and that take as their focus the interference with a variety of roles and activities by functional deficits rather than the deficits themselves; and into behaviors that are not necessarily the target of change for the patient but that reflect societal goals and those of the referrers and funders, such as reduction of use of health and welfare resources.

Pain behavior presents particular problems as a hypothetical construct that is defined differently by different measuring instruments, almost without exception making assumptions of in/appropriateness and in/effectiveness, as is the case for measures of coping. The functions of pain behavior – including decreasing disability as well as increasing it, deliberate communication and attempts not to communicate, and pain relief – require further exploration before measures of pain behavior provide the information desired. Some observational measures can provide high reliability. Used in contexts such as medical consultation and domestic activity with the spouse, these have extended understanding, but the measures themselves cannot incorporate context or

consequences (see Chapter Ch6) and therefore serve poorly to describe treatment outcome.

Within a behavioral formulation of chronic pain, behaviors such as limping or guarding were theoretically and empirically associated with greater disability, and were therefore considered to be an appropriate target of treatment. Within a cognitive behavioral framework, and with appreciation that the association is not as straightforward as assumed, pain behavior is less appropriate as a treatment outcome measure. For instance, while walking with a stick or cane may be associated with greater disability than walking unaided, it may enable users to be more mobile and active than they would otherwise be. This may protect against greater disability as well as contributing to a better quality of life. Measurement of specific behaviors may relate to the processes of change: limping in relation to mobility, groaning in relation to communication. If those are the targets of treatment, observational pain behavior scales offer a means of measurement. Specific behaviors or functions are covered by the comments on observed physical performance in the biomedical domain: good reliability is often attainable, but validation is less satisfactorily tackled for many, requiring demonstration of a relationship with relevant everyday physical performance.

A specific component of pain behavior, for which detailed measurement usually requires videotaping and training of observers, is that of facial expression of pain. For nonverbal subjects unable to use pictorial scales, this is the only measure of pain available, and is used with infants, nonverbal children, and adults such as cognitively impaired elderly patients.[14] Pain behavior may be reported by someone other than the patient. This is particularly the case in children, for whom general behavioral scales may be used at home or in school as accessory measures of a child's distress or disturbance.[1]

Items concerning social support, including the quality of intimate relationships, are rare in pain studies other than as coping resources or pain behaviors. However, close confiding relationships promote good physical and mental health and health maintenance, and arguably should be better represented as outcomes of treatments that aim toward a more normal life through pain relief or pain management (see Chapters Ch6 and Ch7).

Quality of life and other compound measures were intended in part to address the desire for a single comprehensive measure, since overall improvement in quality of life summarizes the aims of many treatments for pain. All of the many measures in use in the pain field rely on self-report and combine different behaviors and functions that are ascribed different weightings to obtain one or more totals. Attention to content can help selection. Table 1.1 gives the number of items, response options, and an impression of the content of some of the most popular

Table 1.1 *Content of widely used measures of function and disability in pain*

Measure	Reference	Summary	Content (number of items) — More physical → More psychosocial		
Short form 36 of Medical Outcomes Study (SF-36)	15	9 separate domains rescaled 0–100; age–sex norms available	Physical functioning (10), Role physical (4), Bodily pain (2)	Social functioning (5), General health (5), Vitality (4)	Mental health (5), Role emotional (3)
Sickness Impact Profile (SIP)	16	Single total (%) or physical and psychosocial separately	Ambulation (12), Body care and movement (23), Mobility (10), Eating (9) Work (9), Home management (10)	Sleep and rest (7)	Emotional behavior (9), Alertness behavior (10), Social interaction (20), Recreation and pastimes (8), Communication (9)
Roland and Morris short SIP	17	Single total 0–24	Physical function (18)	Activity (3)	Appetite (1), Sleep (1), Irritability (1)
Nottingham Health Profile (NHP)	18	Total of domains or "profile"	Pain (8), Physical abilities (8)	Sleep (5), Energy levels (3)	Emotional reactions (9), Social isolation (5)
Multidimensional Pain Inventory (MPI/WHYMPI)	19	Domain totals as mean 0–6, or patient type	Pain and pain interference including control and mood (20) Activity (18)		Spouse response (14)
Pain Disability Index (PDI)	20	Single total 0–70	Self-care (1), Life-support activity (1)	Family/home responsibilities (1), Recreation (1), Social activity (1), Occupation (1), Sexual activity (1)	
Brief Pain Inventory (BPI)	21	Single total 0–110, or pain 0–40 and interference 0–70	Pain (4), Walking ability (1)	General activity (1), Normal work (1), Sleep (1)	Mood (1), Relationships (1), Enjoyment (1)
Oswestry Low Back Pain Disability Questionnaire	22	Single total as percentage of possible maximum	Pain intensity (6), Lifting (6), Walking (6), Sitting (6), Standing (6)	Personal care (6), Sleeping (6), Sex life (6), Traveling (6)	Social life (6)

along a rough dimension from physical to psychosocial. The wider the range of activities covered by items in the measure, the more relevant are influences other than pain and physical impairment, such as beliefs and mood, lifestyle preferences, availability of resources, and cultural norms. The more comprehensive disability questionnaires effectively rank order the various degrees of compromise of mobility, and suggest goals that are observable within the clinic setting. The narrower the range of activities included, the higher the risk of excluding some that are important to reasonable numbers of pain respondents. Consideration of content affects both selection and interpretation of the measure.

Other properties of measures that may guide choice concern the population on which the measure was developed (e.g. chronicity of the pain, specificity of the type of pain or pain site, inclusion or not of intermittent pain such as headache, the proportion working, the sex ratio, age range, and similar characteristics) and the number of response levels available: from two (yes/no) to a 10-point or 101-point (visual analog scale; VAS) rating of difficulty or frequency, depending on the extent of change expected.

Satisfaction ratings belong among psychosocial measures rather than among those of activity and function. They are the simplest form of a single outcome measure and are used extensively in the audit of treatments. They constitute a very transparent measure, are rarely adequately tested for bias arising from the context of testing, and are therefore unsuitable as the major or only outcome assessment.

Interference with social roles, such as domestic work and employment, family involvement, and community activity, is included in many compound measures. However, it is important not to assume that severe physical disability necessarily restricts family or social life or even work. Independent sources of information are available for some aspects: employment or welfare records may provide number of work days lost, welfare benefits claimed, or state-provided help with domestic and family duties. Of course, extent of state provision varies between and within countries and people differ in what they attempt to manage independently, thus making comparisons difficult.

Third-party-defined outcomes are those identified not by patients or those close to them but by treatment staff, treatment funders, and national policies. In particular, outcomes concerned with cost may override patient-defined outcomes such as extent of improvement. There are many stakeholders in the treatment of an individual patient: family members, employers, and work colleagues, as well as funders, insurance companies, and policy-makers, may subscribe to diverse and even conflicting anticipated outcomes. For instance, patients may reduce work hours or demands when the effort to maintain employment adversely affects their lives outside work. Although this change may improve their quality of life and that of

their families, reduction in work is usually seen to represent a deterioration in patients' function and is unlikely to be the goal of treatment providers. Another example is that of welfare provision, which may improve the quality of life for patients and their families but which represents a target of treatment to reduce costs to society. Other goals, although associated with health improvement, may be substantially determined by variables beyond the control of the patient or health carers: it is not uncommon for patients to reach a level of function which is compatible with work but for employers to find them poor prospects, or for the patient's skills not to match the requirements in the local job market. Setting goals of treatment such as return to work need to take this into account.

Health care resources are a particularly important outcome that may be identified by the patient and/or others. The resources can be described using a range of events from daily drug use to surgery, or from visits to primary carer to specialist-level hospital treatments. Concern over the veracity and accuracy of patients' accounts of drugs consumed and treatments undertaken can lead to an overcritical approach to an area where multiple sources of information may be examined for convergence (availability of health records permitting) and a best estimate made. Another source of reluctance to quantify post-treatment recourse to pain-related drugs and other health care may be differences within the treatment team – as there are within the pain community – about the aims of treatment: is it abstinence from all analgesics, or from all drugs prescribed for pain or mood, or restriction to nonopioids? In addition, is all further pain-related treatment undesirable, or might a patient build on treatment gains by individual physiotherapy or psychological therapy? Specifying agreed goals of treatment is essential not only for the selection of measures but also for consistent interpretation of results. Considerations similar to third-party-defined outcomes may apply: it may be that intervention with health carers rather than patients is required to achieve an outcome, e.g. less repeated unnecessary treatment, adequate postoperative analgesia, or curbing excessive opioid prescription.

Nonoutcome variables: treatment process

While considering measurement, it is worth asking whether treatment methods or processes require assessment. In general, treatment is given with confidence that it is what it claims to be, i.e. that relaxation is relaxing, that the epidural analgesic is delivered epidurally, that the drug tested in a 4-week trial is taken as directed for 4 weeks, that the no treatment control group is having no treatment. Not only does monitoring of treatment components contribute to confidence in the findings of a trial but it can also in some cases allow for substudies, e.g. of dose–response relationships, of subgroup responses, or of differences among care providers.

QUALITY OF MEASURES AND INTERPRETATION OF THEIR OUTPUT

The psychometric properties of a measure – reliability, validity, and sensitivity to change – are not unconditional qualities of the measure but describe its performance under particular conditions of population, time, and extent of change. This makes it relevant to consider the likeness of the properties to those of the study for which outcome measures are sought. Psychometric qualities of tests are established over time. Newer tests may have better established psychometric qualities; older instruments, although they have acquired a track record, may have tested to standards which are now superceded. Long clinical use is no guarantee of reliability, as is evident from the data on many clinical tests.

Reliability

Reliability describes the extent to which the instrument will give a consistent result that is minimally affected by error across content, time, and observers if they are not the subject. Reliability is calculated by the ratio of true variance to that of true variance plus error variance. The error variance, in turn, is made up of systematic error plus random error. Thus, minimizing both systematic and random error improves reliability. Some random error is inevitable, but some arises from poor wording or problematic response categories. For instance, you might ask your patients "Can you climb stairs?" and provide the responses "yes" or "no." A patient who can only climb stairs with great difficulty, or using a handrail, might on one occasion decide that this qualified as yes, and on another decide that it did not meet the questioner's expectations and answer no. The more specific the question and/or response categories, the more consistent the responses. Such concerns are beyond the needs of someone selecting among existing tests, but are covered by McDowell and Newell.[2]

Low reliability effectively wastes the efforts of measurement, and erodes confidence in the data obtained and in their interpretation. A scale with poor internal consistency can mislead. If it is measuring more than one construct, the total becomes a complex amalgam of the constructs, and change or difference between two totals could represent all sorts of processes that cannot be distinguished from one another. A scale or measure with poor test–retest reliability is responding to influences other than changes in the construct of interest. As those influences are likely to vary across assessment occasions in ways that are not observed or taken into account, their variance is misattributed to variance in the construct. This might equally obscure real change as give an illusion of change where there is none: there would be no means to identify either. A measure or observation with poor interrater reliability is likewise subject to substantial influences unrelated to the construct of interest, and usually attributable to particular characteristics or beliefs of the raters. Again, this is as likely to miss real differences as to report them mistakenly. So how good is good enough? Reliability coefficients run from 0, where all variance is error variance, to 1.0, where there is no error variance.

Internal consistency is a measure of closeness of all items to the underlying construct, and is usually expressed as Cronbach's alpha. It is improved by dropping items that have a low correlation, i.e. share little variance, with the total score and with other items. The disadvantages of high consistency are that some of the most interesting content may be lost, for example items which represented diversity within the original development population, and this limits applicability and generalizability. It also explains why some widely used tests with good reliability are rather repetitive – a fact which does not escape patients. An alpha of 0.85 may be considered acceptable.[23]

Test–retest reliability, or repeatability, effectively stability over time, is often calculated by simple correlation but better by intraclass correlation (ICC) or kappa. The ideal, assuming stability of the underlying construct, is identical scores across time in the absence of identifiable sources of change, as measured by intraclass correlation, rather than identical rank order of scores across the population, as measured by simple parametric or nonparametric correlation. Of course, people do vary across time for an infinite number of reasons. The highest test–retest reliability coefficients tend to occur where time between tests is short, not infrequently 24 or 48 h. However, change in clinical treatments often involves time spans of weeks, months, or years, and there is often no untreated control group that provides repeated assessment data. A good test–retest correlation is 0.9 or more;[2] 0.8–0.9 is often considered acceptable; for kappa, it is 0.6 or more.

Interrater reliability used to be measured by bivariate correlation, parametric or nonparametric, or by percentage agreement between raters of all possible ratings. Consensus now requires ICC or kappa, which gives a more conservative estimate by calculating actual agreement (not relative order) and discounting for chance agreement by reference to the base rate of the event of interest. Good ICC indicates high variance in ratings due to subjects and low variance due to raters; a high kappa indicates a high level of agreement between raters. Use of video allows multiple raters to observe the same subject, and can be used for calibration of raters on the same material. Iterative training with discussion of differences and, where possible, rectification of their causes can be used to attain satisfactory levels of reliability. It cannot be assumed without such procedures that raters are making the judgments intended. For both ICC and kappa, 0 represents no agreement and 1 represents perfect agreement; Dworkin and Whitney[23] suggest that an ICC below 0.8 or kappa below 0.6 is unacceptable.

Validity

Validity identifies the extent to which a test actually measures what it is intended to measure, which may be a real quality or a hypothetical construct, and does not measure instead, or as well, some unknown construct(s). A measure can be reliable but can lack a clear relationship with a construct. For instance, there are several measures of "somatization" and tests of "fibromyalgia" but there is far from universal agreement on what they tell us, even on the existence of either phenomenon. Validity is estimated by comparison of the output of the measure with its object – the real quality or construct, or as close as possible an approximation. For instance, a noninvasive and low-risk new diagnostic test can be compared with biopsy or other findings from invasive or high-risk procedures or from longer term outcome. To the extent that the data coincide, for both positive and negative results, that diagnostic test can be said to be valid in that population. Its validity in a population with a very different base rate of the event(s) of interest (disease, item content) would have to be reestablished. For instance, a self-report inventory of function developed largely on students may be heavily weighted toward certain types of social activity that are characteristic of young, independent adult life. This could cause decreasing validity with increasing age in the population to which it is applied, e.g. a fit and active 70-year-old might find little to endorse and thereby be scored as functioning poorly.

Many tests lack such a concrete "gold standard" for establishing validity. Perhaps this is because the construct poses practical difficulties for measurement, but more often it is hard to define and operationalize. Many of the constructs in everyday use – fitness, health, distress, motivation, social support – are so well understood that it is hard to recognize that there is no agreed definition or measurement. Tests are compiled from a wide pool of definitions, observations, and expert opinions on the construct, then content is narrowed until a reliable measure is achieved. The choice of referent can be difficult and controversial, as is well exemplified by "intelligence." As is also the case with intelligence, what is measured by the test (IQ) comes to be taken for the construct itself, leading to culturally inappropriate use of the tool, and attempts to locate the construct in the cortex.

Construct validity is best established by using one or more behavioral referents, but they can be difficult to identify and/or to measure. However, measures vary considerably in the extent to which they address this problem, or they have acquired validation over time by being shown to predict behavior. Those which have such data allow more confident interpretation than those without. Details of validation are usually published with the test, and are available in texts on measures.[1,2,13]

Concurrent validity is the aspect of validity that is generally the easiest to establish. The referent is an existing measure purportedly of the same construct. If scores on the new measure correlate well with scores of the same subjects on the existing measure, and this "gold standard" is itself well validated, convergent validity is established. The "gold standard," constructed, tested, and published according to norms which have been substantially improved over the intervening decades, may not be adequate or entirely appropriate but may, through the passage of time and scarcity of alternative measures, have acquired criterion status.

Divergent validity is a variant of convergent validity, obtained by demonstrating relatively poor correlation with measures of unlike constructs or those for which the new instrument might inadvertently be a proxy measure. Careful choice is needed in order that this does not become a superficial exercise. For example, it is important that a measure of coping (depending on how it is defined) is not too highly related to measures of mood, range of activities, or social desirability of self-presentation. It might, however, share more variance with measures of problem-solving and confidence.

Cutpoints are a special case of validity and are often used with little respect for their specificity to the population in which they were derived. The subject is beyond the scope of this chapter and is easily found in texts on test validity;[2,3] for the choice of test, the only information required is the base rate of the problem in the original population and the population under study. If the populations are substantially different, the structure of the measuring instrument in the new population needs to be checked. Even where the populations are similar, some caution needs to be exercised in that, depending on the consistency of items within the measurement instrument, all patients with the same score are not identical. The number of possible combinations of items for an instrument with N items is 2^N. Thus, for instance, a five-item questionnaire has 32 possible item combinations; dichotomizing responses using a cutpoint of 3 would give 16 possible combinations of items in each category.

Sensitivity to change

Sensitivity to change, or responsiveness, is related to validation and is subject to some of the same problems. It is estimated by comparing scores on the instrument before and after change with a referent that is known to indicate change, and so is a function of the measurement instrument within population parameters. Overlooking this and using it on sufficiently different populations results in floor and ceiling effects before or after treatment that can prevent calculation of change. It is increasingly tested in new measuring instruments; sometimes, establishing sensitivity to differences between a healthy group and a pain group is substituted. This can be an issue if the treatment is not expected to bring about large changes and/or if the population is not expected to achieve the healthy norm, as in many chronic pain and cancer populations. Details of testing sensitivity to change are beyond the range of this chapter, but can be found in texts on measurement.[2,23]

Estimating change or difference

Use of an unsuitable or unsatisfactory measure, or poor choice of statistical test, can obscure positive or null outcomes. Reporting an effect where none exists – type I error – is analogous to the specificity of a test; reporting no effect where one does exist – type II error – is analogous to the sensitivity of a test.[24] In clinical treatment studies, numbers are often small; therefore, the power of the tests is low and variance is often high (in a heterogeneous clinical population), raising the likelihood of a type II error. Although surprisingly common even in respectable journals, the solution is not to perform multiple tests and set a low criterion for statistical significance (increasing the likelihood of type I error), and then to select the "significant" results according to researchers' expectations. By contrast, in a large and relatively homogeneous group, a mean change in a 100-mm pain VAS of 5 mm will achieve statistical significance, but this is likely to be considerably less than patients had hoped for and clinicians intended. The substitution of statistical significance for clinical significance is unfortunate and misses the opportunity to describe the changes anticipated from treatment, which are of major interest to readers.

Clinical significance of change can be variously defined and calculated (see below). The first focuses on the return to a healthy or healthier state; the second to the meaningfulness of the change achieved; the third to the broader improvements brought about by specific treatment. The interested reader is referred to Kendall,[25] Kazdin,[24] and Jacobson *et al.*[26]

1 A criterion is set by reference to healthy norms (empirically established, as in a few self-report instruments such as the SF-36 and in many diagnostic tests, or no more than the local mean such as of work days lost through sickness); to a proportional change agreed or argued to be meaningful (such as the use of 50% pain relief or a doubling of distance walked in a specified time); or to nonoccurrence of an event characteristic of the ill population (such as no further investigations or treatments for pain, or no waking from sleep as a result of pain). The proportion of the treated population meeting this criterion (given that none did so before treatment) is reported.

2 Reliable change is calculated by reference to the standard deviation. Assuming normally distributed and not extensively overlapping healthy and dysfunctional scores, a post-treatment score that falls within two standard deviations of the healthy mean, that falls outside two standard deviations to the healthy side of the dysfunctional mean, or that falls the healthy side of the intersection of the distributions can be considered to indicate significant change.[25] Again, the proportion of the treated population meeting this criterion is reported.

3 Meaningfulness of clinical change in a specific problem, such as pain, can also be defined by the extent to which it is associated with overall change in quality of life or function.

These methods of defining clinical change can be combined, but their results do not necessarily coincide. For all three, it can be a problem that the aim of treatment in chronic and cancer pain is usually not total cure but improvement of the specific symptom or the overall quality of life. Healthy norms, where available, may therefore not be appropriate or attainable. Particularly where there is steady deterioration and the aim of treatment is to slow or halt it, quality of life may be the most suitable measure of whether treatment is worthwhile. Even in acute pain, as mentioned in Chapter P2, the absence of pain may not be a realistic endpoint, and the decision must be made on what is meaningful change. Patients are too rarely asked this question.

Inspecting raw data plots can be helpful in deciding on tests. Variability in response is of clinical interest, and planned tests are better than *post hoc* snooping of data. Figures 1.1 and 1.2 show data for 200 patients on a questionnaire that was scored between 0 and 60, where 0 represents a very poor state and 60 a very good one. The overall population had a pretreatment mean of 22 [standard deviation (s.d.) 11] and a post-treatment mean of 27 (s.d. 16), a mean gain of 5 points. This change is statistically significant ($t = 8.2$, $P < 0.0001$). It would be easy to stop at this point and conclude that treatment was successful in bringing about significant change, problematically equating clinical change (equal to half a standard deviation) with statistical significance.

However, both the pre- versus post-treatment scatterplot of data in Fig. 1.1 (in which differences appear larger the higher the pretreatment score) and the histograms in Fig. 1.2, which suggest a roughly bimodal response, invite further investigation. A median split (at 20) of the pretreatment scores shows the lower half scoring a mean of 13 (s.d. 5) pretreatment and 14 (s.d. 7) post treatment, i.e. no real change at all; the upper half scores a mean of 30 (s.d. 7) pretreatment and 38 (s.d. 12) post treatment, a change of over one standard deviation, and arguably of clinical as well as statistical significance. The implication for treatment is that the lower scorers' pretreatment needs something more to enable them to change – information which does not emerge from an overall analysis.

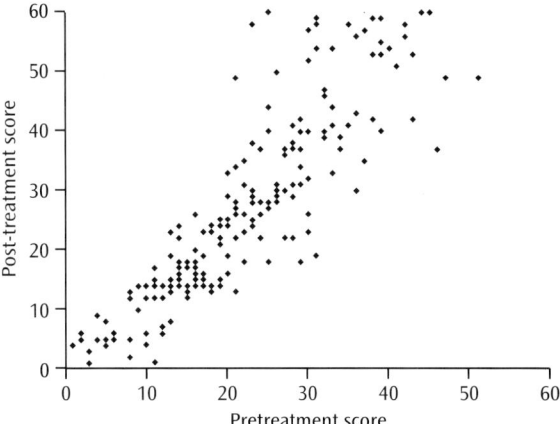

Figure 1.1 *Scatterplot of pre- versus post-treatment scores.*

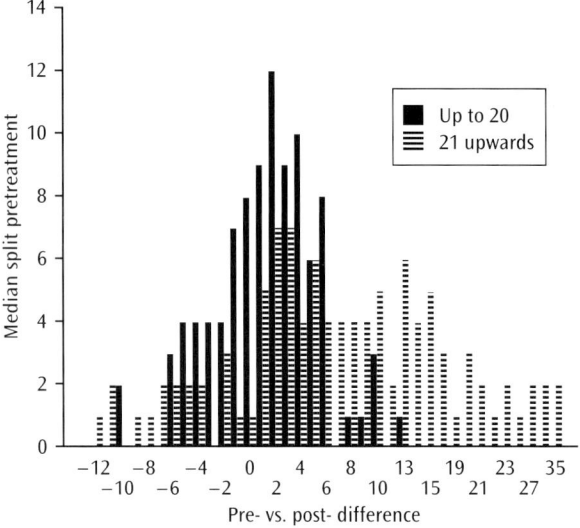

Figure 1.2 *Histogram of score change with treatment, displayed by median split of pretreatment score.*

Example

Increasing pressure for clinical services to audit their performance demands the use of measures. How should those responsible choose among the possibilities?

1 Aims of treatment are defined in general terms, such as "reducing pain, improving function," mainly by treatment staff using experience of the service and knowledge of the literature; however, patient groups, treatment facility mission statements, or local or national charters may all contribute. These aims are then operationalized in achievable terms, such as "at least 50% pain relief by discharge" and "significant reduction in disability in nonworkers, and reduction to local sickness absence norm in workers," for x% of treated patients. Particularly where patients may present relatively intractable problems, minimum expectations may be appropriate, e.g. "All patients will gain

an explanation of their pain and feel that they are believed and understood by staff," which is operationalized in terms of patients' ratings of such statements.

2 Treatment aims determine which domains require measurement, and the headings in this chapter can be used as a checklist. A pain clinic that serves mainly early referrals from primary care may focus more on rapid pain abolition or substantial reduction. It may use measures of affect and cognition to screen for patients with or at risk of developing psychological problems, and a brief measure of function to check that pain relief is accompanied by recovery of previous activity levels. A pain clinic with a large proportion of chronic pain patients, referred from other specialists, is likely to have more modest pain reduction goals and to use more extensive measures of affect, cognition, and function or disability. Its major aims will be reduction of problems in these areas, i.e. improvement in quality of life. Pain ratings would be recorded at every visit (perhaps with use of diary measures by the patient in the interim); pain relief would be rated at specific points in the evaluation of the treatment. Psychosocial and functional measures would be taken at longer intervals, or only at initial assessment and discharge; use of further primary care and specialist services would be recorded. Both clinics might sample satisfaction with a range of aspects of the service at discharge.

3 In choosing these measures, concerns of test–retest reliability and validation in settings as near as possible to everyday life will be paramount. In addition, the existence of healthy population norms, or norms of similar treated and untreated pain patients, help to set criteria for clinical significance of change.

4 Processes of treatment also require specific measures so that outcomes can be investigated adequately. Patient adherence to recommended treatment, whether pharmacotherapy, exercise, relaxation, or thought monitoring, should be sampled. Therapist adherence to treatment guidelines may also be sampled as therapists' skills can affect treatment efficacy. Data such as numbers of visits, numbers of treatments, dropout before discharge, length of time to discharge, and rereferral after discharge are relevant for service audit.

5 Most measures in use in the pain field rely on self-report, therefore attention to minimizing demand characteristics is important. This may be achieved by computerized measures where possible, or by administration in a standard fashion by staff not involved in the patient's treatment. If possible, third-party reports should be added, e.g. from employment sources or primary care physician or a family member could confirm when a patient can walk a set local distance without a stop or without a stick.

6 The package of measures, piloted on an unselected sample of patients, may prove too long or repetitive,

compromising reliability. Increasing use of computerized questionnaires and scanning of paper versions leaves the patient, rather than data entry personnel, bearing the burden of overlong assessments. However, patients' altruism should not be underestimated. For many, the assurance that the clinic uses their responses to understand better the needs of future patients and to improve services is enough to obtain full cooperation.

CONCLUSION

It is alarming that many of the treatments routinely performed on patients in pain, as in other areas of medicine, remain inadequately evaluated. It is not an easy task to evaluate the effectiveness of a treatment. Particularly when driven by concerns for continued referral and funding, or even when motivated by concern to quantify the medical, social, and psychological benefits, the task requires consideration. Most clinicians will want to answer questions such as "Is my treatment as effective as the published studies?" or "Is it making a worthwhile difference to patients and those concerned for them?" rather than seeking to compare treatments in a controlled trial or to identify sources of variance.[27] The investments made in careful formulation of the question (or questions) to be addressed, and in the judicious choice and use of measures, can bring major dividends and considerably enhance clinical practice.

REFERENCES

● 1. Turk DC, Melzack R eds. *Handbook of Pain Assessment*, 2nd edn. New York, NY: Guilford Press, 2001.

● 2. McDowell I, Newell C. *Measuring Health: a Guide to Rating Scales and Questionnaires*, 2nd edn. New York, NY: Oxford University Press, 1996.

3. Turk DC, Rudy TE. Classification logic and strategies in chronic pain. In: Turk DC, Melzack R eds. *Handbook of Pain Assessment*. New York, NY: Guilford Press, 1992: 409–28.

4. Morley SJ, Eccleston C, Williams ACdeC. Systematic review and meta-analysis of randomised controlled trials of cognitive behaviour therapy and behaviour therapy for chronic pain in adults, excluding headache. *Pain* 1999; **80:** 1–13.

● 5. Waddell G, Turk DC. Clinical assessment of low back pain. In: Turk DC, Melzack R eds. *Handbook of Pain Assessment*, 2nd edn. New York, NY: Guilford Press, 2001: 431–53.

● 6. Rudy TE, Turk DC, Brody MC. Quantification of biomedical findings in chronic pain: problems and solutions. In: Turk DC, Melzack R eds. *Handbook of Pain Assessment*. New York, NY: Guilford Press, 1992: 447–69.

7. Price DD. *Psychological Mechanisms of Pain and Analgesia*. Seattle, WA: IASP Press, 1999.

8. Moore A, Moore O, McQuay H, Gavaghan D. Deriving dichotomous outcome measures from continuous data in randomised controlled trials of analgesics: use of pain intensity and visual analogue scales. *Pain* 1997; **69:** 311–15.

9. Farrar JT, Portenoy RK, Berlin JA, *et al.* Defining the clinically important difference in pain outcome measures. *Pain* 2000; **88:** 287–94.

10. Aldrich S, Eccleston C, Crombez G. Worry about chronic pain: vigilance to threat and misdirected problem solving. *Behav Res Ther* 2000; **38:** 457–70.

11. Vlaeyen JWS, Linton SJ. Fear-avoidance and its consequences in chronic musculoskeletal pain: a state of the art. *Pain* 1999; **85:** 317–32.

12. Pincus T, Morley SJ. Cognitive processing bias in chronic pain: a review and integration. *Psychol Bull* 2001; **127:** 599–617.

● 13. Williams ACdeC. Measures of function and psychology. In: Melzack R, Wall PD eds. *Textbook of Pain*, 4th edn. Edinburgh: Churchill Livingstone, 1999: 427–44.

14. Craig KD, Prkachin KM, Grunau RVE. The facial expression of pain. In: Turk DC, Melzack R eds. *Handbook of Pain Assessment*, 2nd edn. New York, NY: Guilford Press, 2001: 153–69.

15. Ware JE, Snow KK, Kosinski M, Gandek B. *SF-36 Health Survey: Manual and Interpretation Guide*. Boston, MA: Health Institute, New England Medical Center, 1993.

16. Bergner M, Bobbitt RA, Carter WB, Gilson BS. The Sickness Impact Profile: development and final revision of a health status measure. *Med Care* 1981; **19:** 787–805.

17. Roland M, Morris R. A study of the natural history of back pain. Part I. Development of a reliable and sensitive measure of disability in low-back pain. *Spine* 1983; **8:**141–4.

18. Hunt SM, McEwen J, McKenna SP. Measuring health status: a new tool for clinicians and epidemiologists. *J R Coll Gen Pract* 1985; **35:** 185–8.

19. Kerns RD, Turk DC, Rudy TE. The West Haven–Yale Multidimensional Pain Inventory (WHYMPI) *Pain*, 1985; **23:** 345–56.

20. Tait RC, Pollard CA, Margolis RB, *et al.* The Pain Disability Index: psychometric and validity data. *Arch Phys Med Rehabil* 1987; **68:** 438–41.

21. Daut RL, Cleeland CS, Flaner RC. Development of the Wisconsin Brief Pain Questionnaire to assess pain in cancer and other diseases. *Pain* 1983; **17:** 197–210.

22. Fairbank JCT, Couper J, Davies JB, O'Brien JP. The Oswestry Low Back Pain Disability Questionnaire. *Physiotherapy* 1980; **66:** 271–3.

23. Dworkin SF, Whitney CW. Relying on objective and subjective measures of chronic pain: guidelines for use and interpretation. In: Turk DC, Melzack R eds. *Handbook of Pain Assessment*, 2nd edn. New York, NY: Guilford Press, 2001: 619–38.

24. Kazdin AE. The meanings and measurement of clinical significance. *J Consult Clin Psychol* 1999; **67:** 332–9.

25. Kendall PC. Clinical significance. *Psychol Bull* 1999; **67:** 283–4.

26. Jacobson NS, Roberts LJ, Berns SB, McGlinchey JB. Methods for defining and determining the clinical significance of treatment effects: description, application, and alternatives. *J Consult Clin Psychol* 1999; **67:** 300–7.

27. Crombie IK, Davies HTO. *Research in Health Care*. Chichester: Wiley, 1996.

2

Practical methods for pain intensity measurements

WILLIAM I CAMPBELL

Factors altering the perception of pain	15	Cancer pain	23
The memory of pain	16	Serial measures of pain	23
Scales used to rate pain intensity	16	Handling and interpreting measurement results	24
The McGill Pain Questionnaire	18	Concluding remarks	25
Assessing pain at the extremes of age	21	References	25
Chronic pain	23		

Pain is a private internal event which cannot be directly observed by others. The physiological response to nociception is invariably accompanied by an affective and reactive component, depending largely on the meaning of the pain and previous experiences. These psychological components, which are part of the pain experience, are largely responsible for its unpleasant nature and the difficulties in its assessment. There is a widely accepted view that the rating of pain should be carried out by the patient where possible, since an observer cannot accurately assess the feelings of another person and may grossly misjudge the suffering experienced. The measurement of pain intensity is essential to determine the efficacy of new analgesics compared with placebos and recognized standards. It is also valuable in the clinical situation to determine the intensity, quality, and relative effectiveness of therapy. Qualitative and temporal features of the pain also have a diagnostic value, especially in the chronic pain situation.

Pain is considered to be a construct, like depression, anxiety, and intelligence.[1] Constructs are labels which categorize related groups of observations that cannot be assessed directly but are inferred from a variety of these observations. The group of observations which make up a construct do not always exist at the same time or in each individual suffering pain. The various components which help form such a construct for pain are its intensity, quality, and affective components. Intensity may be defined as how much a pain hurts. This can be estimated rela-

tively quickly and appears to be a homogeneous dimension which is easily conveyed. The affective component of pain is much more complex to assess, anxiety frequently being associated with acute pain or depression and hopelessness if the pain is chronic.

FACTORS ALTERING THE PERCEPTION OF PAIN

It is a common belief that the intensity of pain is closely, if not directly, related to the extent of injury. This is grossly untrue since pain and suffering are more closely associated with the meaning of pain and psychological state. Anxiety is a factor often associated with heightened awareness of pain. Trait-anxiety is a personality disposition, remaining relatively stable with time. Childhood experiences in particular can influence the development of trait-anxiety of individuals, i.e. parent–child relationships centering around punishment. Those with a high trait-anxiety tend to perceive a wider range of stimulus situations as dangerous or threatening. This in turn elevates state-anxiety, which with time increases the unpleasantness of the situation. Anticipating pain induces anxiety but, if the anxiety levels are reduced through the provision of information, pain reaction and perception can be reduced in clinical and experimental situations. Recent evidence indicates that the effect of anxiety on pain perception may be mediated largely by attention.[2]** Anxiety directed at a pain stimulus increases attention to that stimulus, whereas anxiety directed away from the stimulus to an external event decreases pain sensitivity. The effects of attention and anxiety at the time of pain measurement are important, but the relationship between these variables is more complex than it was previously thought to be.

In the same way that acute pain is often associated with anxiety, chronic pain is frequently associated with depression. Many chronic pain patients acknowledge a depressed mood, but may not acknowledge a depression as such. A common mechanism may underlie both chronic pain and depression, but the exact nature of the relationship remains controversial. This relationship may explain why mood-enhancing drugs can increase pain tolerance, although not pain threshold. Depression accounts for more variance in chronic pain than do other health-related variables, and has been demonstrated to have a substantial effect on treatment response.

Clinical and laboratory investigations have frequently upheld the view that males have a higher pain tolerance than females. Recent evidence would indicate that there may be several reasons for this. Males do not rate noxious stimuli as highly as females, especially in the presence of female investigators. It is considered that males are thought to have been socialized to suppress outward signs of pain in certain circumstances and consequently underreport their pain experiences.[3]*** In addition, animal research has identified gonadotrophic hormonal differences associated with pain tolerance – females being more pain sensitive following the midcycle luteal phase. It is therefore important to test for differences in pain due to gender if the measurement is being carried out for research purposes.

Other factors which may influence the perception and therefore the assessment of pain are climatic conditions and time of day when the measurement is carried out. Patients suffering from chronic pain often have exacerbations of their symptoms as the weather changes. Many of these observations have been reflected in folklore: "aches and pains, coming rains." The most frequently reported meteorological factors which alter pain complaint are temperature and humidity. These weather conditions alter pain perception mostly in disorders involving joints, muscles, and postoperative scars. Most patients are aware of a fluctuation in pain intensity according to the time of day. Pain due to inflammatory disorders often peaks early in the morning, whereas other types of pain peak in the early afternoon or evening. Those patients who do not convey regular trends of pain intensity throughout the day also report significantly higher ratings of emotional stress. Ideally, patients should rate their pain at the same time of day. There is no control over climatic conditions, but the observer should be aware that it may affect pain scores.

Factors which may be associated with changes in pain perception

- Anxiety and attention directed towards the noxious stimulus.
- Depressed affect.
- Gender of the subject.
- Circadian variation.
- Climatic conditions.

THE MEMORY OF PAIN

The ability to remember pain is needed to create an upper anchor point for most pain intensity scales. The ability to recall acute pain intensity for up to 1 week is very accurate. After several weeks, recall is generally within 10% of its original value. Memory for the specific qualities of the pain and the patient's mood at the time of pain is less accurate than for intensity when assessed after several weeks.[4]** A high affect such as anxiety at the time of initial registration of pain is thought to interfere with recall and results in an exaggerated memory of pain intensity. Further episodes of acute pain may also interfere with accurate recall. In the chronic pain situation, the current level of pain and mood influences the accuracy of remembered pain, e.g. patients with lower levels of pain at the moment of recall tend to underestimate their past pain levels and vice versa.[5]** Attempts to assess pain by recall are therefore not recommended since they may be inaccurate both in intensity and quality – contemporary pain scores are much more appropriate and less prone to error.

Factors which influence memory for a specific painful event

- Affect at the time of nociception.
- Affect at the time of recall.
- Time between nociception and recall.
- Painful events occurring after that to be recalled.

Measurement of pain intensity should be carried out at the time of nociception, since recall is associated with unpredictable error.

SCALES USED TO RATE PAIN INTENSITY

The most frequently assessed dimension of pain is its intensity. This concept is readily understood by patients and permits the measurement of their pain intensity through the conversion of a subjective experience to a rating on a scale. The measurement should represent only the feeling which is being assessed and should be reproducible.

There are different types of pain rating scales, which may use:

- numbers – numerical rating scale;
- words – verbal rating scale;
- a line – visual analog scale;
- pictures – faces rating scale.

Numerical rating scales

Numbers are one of the most convenient ways of determining pain intensity, the scale using up to 101 points.[1] Anchor points are used at either end of the numerical rating scale (NRS), zero representing no pain and the highest number indicating the most intense pain possible. The numbers used in this situation refer to rank order, but they may also possess ratio properties, i.e. a change from 6 to 3 indicates a reduction in pain which equates to a 50% reduction in pain intensity. Numerical rating scales with a small number of points such as four or five are simple to use, but they may lack sensitivity to small changes in pain intensity. Having access to many points on these scales should increase their sensitivity, but patients do not utilize this extra capacity. One study has shown that most patients use a 101-point NRS as though pain intensity changed in steps of 10 units, i.e. they treated the scale as though there were 11 points.[6]* This is particularly likely to occur if the patient gives a verbal indication of pain intensity rather than marking the scale themselves. It seems that little information is lost by using an 11-point NRS over a 101-point scale. It has even been suggested that fewer than 11 points are necessary since there is a tendency to pick preferred numbers in the same way that children choose red sweets.[7] The number of points must not be reduced excessively, however, since sensitivity may be reduced to the extent that it is difficult to detect the mean change in an actively treated group compared with a placebo group.[8]** An 11-point NRS has been documented as being accurate, effective, and reliable in detecting small but clinically significant differences as a 0–100 VAS.[9] A clear advantage of the 11-point NRS is that it can be scored even when the patient is not physically able to use a pen or pencil on a VAS.

Verbal rating scales

A verbal rating scale (VRS) contains lists of adjectives reflecting various levels or categories of pain intensity from no pain through to the most intense pain possible. There should be a sufficient number of adjectives to permit the patient to express a graded range of pain intensities. Patients are asked to read over the list of words and choose the one best describing their pain intensity. Like the NRS, the VRS is simple and fast to use and may use four or more words, e.g. none, mild, moderate, severe.[10]** It suffers from similar problems to the NRS. The magnitude of change between any two points on the scale cannot be assumed to be the same, i.e. the extent of the difference between mild and moderate pain cannot be interpreted as the same as that between moderate and severe pain. In addition, each patient will interpret the difference between any two specific adjectives differently: the difference between mild and moderate pain may be interpreted as 10% or 30% depending on the individual. Since the gradations of pain intensity vary between adjectives, the VRS does not possess any ratio properties.[11]

A typical seven-category verbal rating scale for pain intensity would be:

- none;
- weak;
- mild;
- moderate;
- severe;
- excruciating;
- unbearable.

Visual analog scales

A visual analog scale (VAS) consists of a line labeled at either end with the extremes of the feeling to be measured. The patient is asked to indicate which point along the scale best represents their pain intensity. If there is any difficulty in understanding the concept, this may be overcome by describing the scale in terms of a thermometer indicating pain intensity, which gradually changes from no pain to worst pain possible. Optimum line length appears to be 100–150 mm. Pain intensity is scored numerically as the distance in millimeters from zero. This type of scale has the advantages of being fast, sensitive to small changes, and the data can be analyzed relatively easily. The VAS was originally employed in 1923 for educational purposes, but was not widely used for pain assessment until the 1960s. It is considered to be an excellent communication bridge between patient and observer and avoids some of the problems which arise through the use of categorical scales because the scale is continuous.

The VAS may be vertical or horizontal, with optional graduations or words throughout its length (see Fig. 2.1). Graduations, numbers, or words along the line are inappropriate because they cause clustering of results around these points, interfering with what would otherwise be an even distribution. Many would, in fact, argue that the use of any marks or words along a VAS renders it a categorical scale. Orientation of the scale is generally horizontal, with least pain to the left side. It is essential that the same type and orientation of scale is used throughout any series of measurements, otherwise the variation in measurement method may no longer render the results suitable for

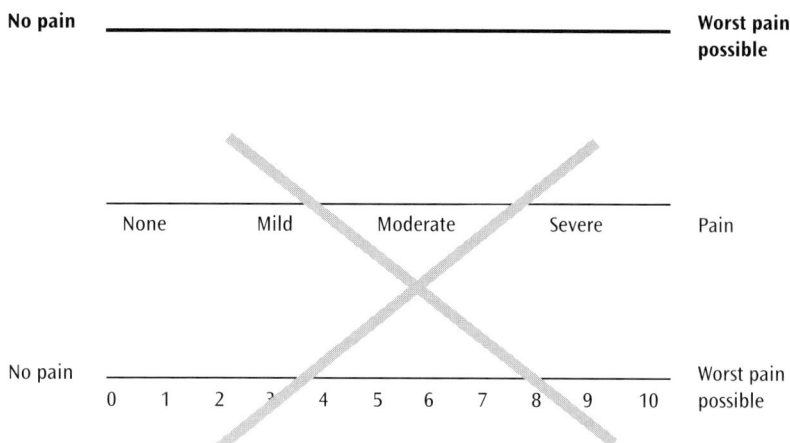

No pain _____ Worst pain possible

None   Mild   Moderate   Severe   Pain

No pain _____ Worst pain possible
0 1 2 3 4 5 6 7 8 9 10

Figure 2.1 *Different types of visual analog scale. The upper scale is the preferred type since it leads to a relatively even distribution of results along the line. Clustering of results around chosen words or preferred numbers may occur with the other two scales.*

meaningful scrutiny. A brief verbal explanation is generally more effective than written advice when instructing patients on the completion of a VAS. Care must be taken when reproducing these scales since photocopying can result in changes in the size of the scale. Although the overall change in scale size may appear insignificant, it can lead to erroneous measures, especially if some of the pain scores are small.

The VAS has been used very widely over the last few decades in research associated with all types of pain. It has been shown to be reliable, valid, and internally consistent. This consistency does not alter as a function of pain intensity or time. The VAS is considered to have ratio properties, implying that the changes throughout the scale are accepted by the patient in a continuous manner, i.e. it may be assumed that a drop in pain intensity from 50 mm to 25 mm is a 50% reduction in pain.[10] The scale is:

- valid, i.e. provided it is designed and used properly it will measure that which was intended;
- internally consistent and reliable, i.e. repeated assessments of a single pain experience over time will be identical or very similar.

Advantages of the visual analog scale

- Simple to use.
- A valid measure for pain.
- Sensitive at detecting small changes in pain.
- Has ratio properties.
- Is internally consistent and reliable.

Disadvantages of the visual analog scale

- Slow for the observer to calculate score.
- Some patients may not understand the abstract concept involved, e.g. the elderly.

Pain measurement by pictures and toys

Pictorial pain rating scales frequently use diagrams of facial expression ranging from an appearance of being content to extreme distress (see Fig. 2.2).[12]** The pictures are ranked and assigned a score. Patients are asked to indicate which picture best indicates their pain experience, the number associated with the chosen picture being the pain score. The main advantage of this type of scale over others is that the patient does not need to be literate, but in other respects it has limitations similar to an NRS or VRS.

Toys and other pictorial methods have been successfully used to assess pain intensity in children. Most of these devices are modifications of the VAS (see Fig. 2.3). Some observers prefer to use a neutral facial expression rather than one of contentment to convey the absence of pain. They therefore have the advantages of a continuously variable scale combined with the ease of communication with nonliterate patients. In its simplest form, neither the visual analog toy nor the faces scale differentiates between pain intensity and the reaction to pain. One device, however, incorporates a colored analog scale to assess intensity and a facial affective scale to assess the aversive component of pain.[13]** Test–retest data suggest that there is good rank ordering of the faces in association with pain in children.

THE McGILL PAIN QUESTIONNAIRE

Although intensity may be considered the most important component of a painful experience, it is only one of many elements which when combined create the overall feeling of pain. If several of these key elements were measured, they would convey a global impression of the patient's feelings. The McGill Pain Questionnaire (MPQ) addresses this issue by assessing several components within the one questionnaire (see Fig. 2.4).[14]*

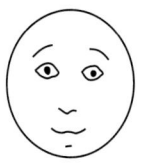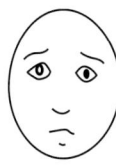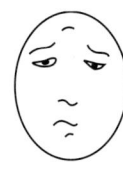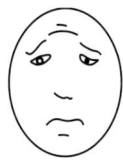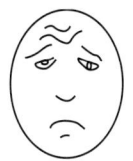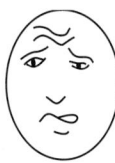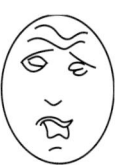

Figure 2.2 *The faces pain scale (after Bieri et al.[11]). The faces are ranked from no pain on the extreme left (pain score 0) through to severe pain on the extreme right (pain score 6).*

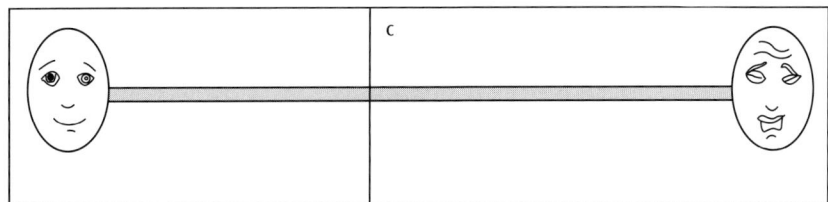

Figure 2.3 *The visual analog toy. The toy depicts two facial expressions to illustrate the extremes of pain experienced. A cursor or sliding indicator (c) is positioned by the patient between the two facial expressions to indicate current pain intensity, and the distance to the cursor is used to estimate the pain score. Some devices have a graduated scale on the reverse side of the toy, so that the score under the back of the cursor may be read off directly.*

The questionnaire consists of 78 words describing pain in sensory, affective, and evaluative terms. The sensory part of the questionnaire uses words describing the quality of the pain, e.g. throbbing, burning, or aching. These words have been arranged in groups, each with similar sensory qualities, and ranked according to their intensity. Affective words such as tiring, sickening, and frightful, together with evaluative words such as annoying and troublesome, are also arranged in groups and ranked. A miscellaneous group of sensory adjectives is included, as is a six-point VRS for pain intensity.

The questionnaire is normally completed by the patient, who marks the words which best describe their current pain. If the MPQ is completed by an observer at interview, there is a tendency to obtain different results from self-administration, using it as a pencil-and-paper test. The difference may be due to patients having the opportunity to inquire about unfamiliar words when the questionnaire is administered at interview. A numerical score for the sensory, affective, and evaluative components of pain can now be obtained by adding the scores for the ranked words chosen in each subclass. For example, if the words chosen are throbbing, burning, and dull, the respective sensory scores would be 4, 2, and 1, giving a score of 7 in that subclass. Likewise, cruel and annoying would result in scores of 3 and 1 in the affective and evaluative subclasses respectively. The pain rating index is the score derived from the sum of the values for each subclass. Although the total number of words chosen can also be used to provide a score, this is rather crude since it does not take into account the rank value of the words chosen. It may be that the questionnaire is insensitive to small changes in pain intensity, but it has the advantage of detecting the sensory qualities of pain and so has a diagnostic capacity.

- Toothache – throbbing, sharp, boring, annoying, rhythmic.
- Phantom limb pain – stabbing, cramping, burning, aching.
- Postherpetic neuralgia – sharp, tender, pulling, aching, stinging.

Some of these words will be chosen with greater frequency than others for certain pain problems, such that a pattern of words will become evident for these specific pains.

The MPQ has been used extensively to investigate all types of pain but can take 10–15 min to administer. It is a valuable tool in the clinical situation. The ratings obtained from the present pain intensity (PPI) before and after therapy indicate the response to treatment – a change of one point on the PPI often being considered clinically significant by the patient. When full use is made of the MPQ, the sensory descriptors have diagnostic value in nociceptive and neuropathic pain states, as described above. If a relatively large number of affective, compared with sensory, words are chosen, a more detailed psychological assessment is probably appropriate. Some investigators have expressed concern that subscales for the sensory, affective, and evaluative components may overlap. Despite these concerns, the predictive validity, construct validity, and the test–retest reliability have indicated the strengths of this questionnaire:

- Predictive validity – if a pain measure is valid, it should predict the future course of the pain condi-

McGill Pain Questionnaire

Patient's Name _____ Date _____ Time _____ am/pm

DATE PAIN COMMENCED _____

PR1: S _____ A _____ E _____ M _____ PRI(T) _____ PPI _____
    (1–10)   (11–15)   (16)   (17–20)   (1–20)

DATE FIRST TREATMENT _____   **DATE TREATMENT COMPLETED** _____

1 FLICKERING —
  QUIVERING
  PULSING
  THROBBING
  BEATING
  POUNDING —

2 JUMPING
  FLASHING
  SHOOTING

3 PRICKING —
  BORING —
  DRILLING —
  STABBING —
  LANCINATING —

4 SHARP
  CUTTING
  LACERATING —

5 PINCHING —
  PRESSING —
  GNAWING
  CRAMPING —
  CRUSHING —

6 TUGGING —
  PULLING —
  WRENCHING —

7 HOT —
  BURNING —
  SCALDING —
  SEARING —

8 TINGLING —
  ITCHY —
  SMARTING —
  STINGING —

9 DULL —
  SORE —
  HURTING —
  ACHING —
  HEAVY —

10 TENDER —
  TAUT —
  RASPING —
  SPLITTING —

11 TIRING —
  EXHAUSTING —

12 SICKENING
  SUFFOCATING

13 FEARFUL —
  FRIGHTFUL
  TERRIFYING

14 PUNISHING —
  GRUELLING
  CRUEL
  VICIOUS
  KILLING

15 WRETCHED —
  BLINDING

16 ANNOYING —
  TROUBLESOME —
  MISERABLE
  INTENSE
  UNBEARABLE —

17 SPREADING —
  RADIATING
  PENETRATING
  PIERCING

18 TIGHT —
  NUMB
  DRAWING —
  SQUEEZING
  TEARING —

19 COOL —
  COLD
  FREEZING

20 NAGGING —
  NAUSEATING —
  AGONIZING —
  DREADFUL —
  TORTURING —

      PPI
0 NO PAIN —
1 MILD —
2 DISCOMFORTING —
3 DISTRESSING —
4 HORRIBLE —
5 EXCRUCIATING —

BRIEF —	RHYTHMIC —	CONTINUOUS —
MOMENTARY	PERIODIC	STEADY
TRANSIENT —	INTERMITTENT —	CONSTANT —

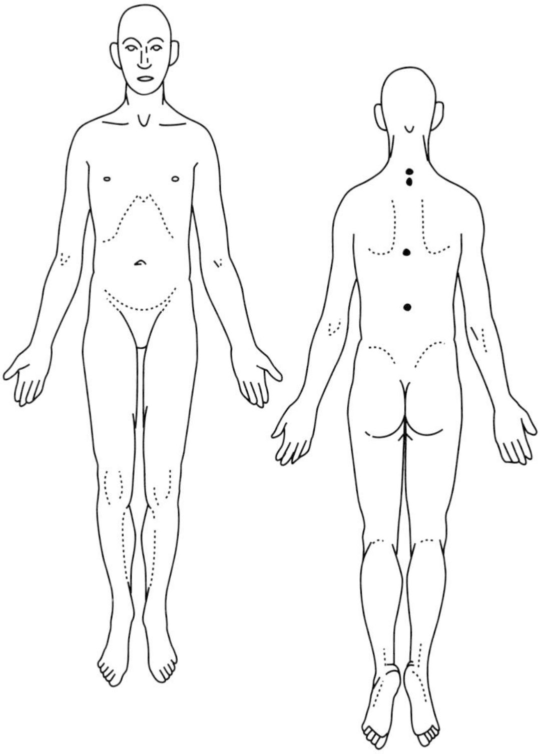

E = EXTERNAL   I = INTERNAL

COMMENTS:

tion, e.g. with postoperative pain the intensity should become less with time whereas if the pain is chronic it should remain relatively stable with time.

- Construct validity – the test should measure what it is intended to. There should not be, for example, very close correlations between pain intensity ratings and behavior ratings.
- Test–retest reliability – this is the degree to which tests at different times of the same pain agree. An *r*-value (coefficient of correlation) of 0.8 is acceptable, but 0.9 is preferable.

A more concise form of the MPQ was introduced in 1987. This short-form McGill Pain Questionnaire (SF-MPQ) consists of 15 descriptors (11 sensory and four affective), each of which is rated on an intensity scale from none (0) to severe (3) (Fig. 2.5).[15*] Three pain scores are derived from the sum of the ranked values obtained from the chosen descriptors – sensory, affective, and total. A VAS and a PPI scale are also included within the SF-MPQ. These permit sensitivity of pain intensity measurement to be combined with qualitative information within a questionnaire, which is quicker to administer than the original MPQ. The SF-MPQ has the capacity to discriminate between different acute and chronic pain syndromes. It is of value in research and in clinical situations where both qualitative and quantitative information are required quickly.

MPQ strengths

- A validated, well-tested scale which has been used to assess most types of pain.
- Determines the affective and evaluative components of pain, as well as intensity.
- Assesses the quality of pain and has some diagnostic properties.

MPQ weaknesses

- Slow to use.
- Slow for the observer to calculate the pain intensity.
- Subscales may overlap in what they assess.

ASSESSING PAIN AT THE EXTREMES OF AGE

The assessment of children's pain is a major challenge. A feeling has to be assessed, and this may have to be done for a patient who is unable to communicate readily. Pain intensity measures can be carried out using behavioral, physiological, or psychological means.[16] Infants' expressions are relatively bias-free reflections of their emotional distress in response to pain. The pattern of facial expression may change, however, following repeated noxious stimulation. Nonverbal behavior has often been regarded as being more reliable in the older child and a more objective index of their pain than their verbal descriptions. This is partly because of their limited and immature vocabulary, which will range widely according to social background, education, and previous pain experience. Unfortunately, health professionals may interpret children's behavior in differing manners – the subjectivity possibly leading to the perception that a child is anxious or emotionally disturbed rather than in pain. As the child matures, self-report measures of pain may be used, such as the faces scale, visual analog scales, or even questionnaires.[13**,15*]

As part of the aging process, degenerative changes occur at the receptor organs, such as Pacini's and Meissner's corpuscles. Peripheral nerves undergo segmental demyelination, and the degeneration which occurs within the central nervous system leads to neurotransmitter changes with altered sensory processing. The ability to tolerate deep pain is consistent throughout childhood and adolescence but declines by the age of 60 years. Tolerance to cutaneous pain becomes elevated with aging. These changes do not seem to confer many advantages, since persistent pain is a very common problem within the elderly population. Any of the pain rating scales mentioned above may be used in the elderly, but difficulties in understanding the abstract concept of visual analog scales seem to be particularly prevalent in this age group and may result in errors or the inability to obtain a pain measure from some patients. In this situation, it may therefore be more appropriate to assess pain intensity with a VRS or an NRS.

Figure 2.4 *The McGill Pain Questionnaire (courtesy of Melzack[14]). The descriptors are grouped into four categories: sensory (sections 1–10, flickering to splitting), affective (sections 11–15, tiring to blinding), evaluative (section 16, annoying to unbearable), and miscellaneous (sections 17–20, spreading to torturing). Scoring is carried out for each category by summing the rank value of each chosen word. The rank value is based on its position within each set of words, e.g. throbbing in section 1 would be given a score of 4. Scoring all sections 1–20 provides the pain rating index (PRI), whereas scoring sections 1–10 and 11–15 separately permits an estimate of the sensory and affective components of pain independently. Present pain intensity is determined from the six-point rating scale.*

SHORT-FORM McGILL PAIN QUESTIONNAIRE
RONALD MELZACK

PATIENT'S NAME: _____   DATE: _____

	NONE	MILD	MODERATE	SEVERE
THROBBING	0) _____	1) _____	2) _____	3) _____
SHOOTING	0) _____	1) _____	2) _____	3) _____
STABBING	0) _____	1) _____	2) _____	3) _____
SHARP	0) _____	1) _____	2) _____	3) _____
CRAMPING	0) _____	1) _____	2) _____	3) _____
GNAWING	0) _____	1) _____	2) _____	3) _____
HOT–BURNING	0) _____	1) _____	2) _____	3) _____
ACHING	0) _____	1) _____	2) _____	3) _____
HEAVY	0) _____	1) _____	2) _____	3) _____
TENDER	0) _____	1) _____	2) _____	3) _____
SPLITTING	0) _____	1) _____	2) _____	3) _____
TIRING–EXHAUSTING	0) _____	1) _____	2) _____	3) _____
SICKENING	0) _____	1) _____	2) _____	3) _____
FEARFUL	0) _____	1) _____	2) _____	3) _____
PUNISHING–CRUEL	0) _____	1) _____	2) _____	3) _____

NO PAIN _____ WORST POSSIBLE PAIN

PPI

0	NO PAIN	_____
1	MILD	_____
2	DISCOMFORTING	_____
3	DISTRESSING	_____
4	HORRIBLE	_____
5	EXCRUCIATING	_____

(PPI is Present Pain Intensity)

Figure 2.5 *The short-form McGill Pain Questionnaire (courtesy of Melzack[14]). The descriptors are divided into two groups: sensory (throbbing to splitting) and affective (tiring–exhausting to punishing–cruel). Scoring is carried out by summing the checked values beside the appropriate descriptor, according to the intensity of each. The provision of a visual analog scale and a present pain intensity scale permits a more direct estimation of pain intensity.*

Assessment of pain at the extremes of age

- The younger and less literate patient often finds analog scales or toys easiest to use.
- Elderly patients sometimes find visual analog scales difficult to understand and prefer scales using numbers or words.

CHRONIC PAIN

Chronic pain assessment is a complex issue. Unlike acute pain where intensity may be altered mainly by affect alone, behavior and mood can become a greater issue than the pain itself. The scales mentioned earlier can be used to measure pain intensity in chronic pain conditions, but it is important that they are interpreted with the understanding that the results may be markedly distorted by the patient's depressed mood, high expectations, or poor coping skills. If outcome of treatment is to be assessed in these patients, the measurement of pain intensity alone will therefore be inadequate.[17] A wide variety of specialized questionnaires has been developed for patients who suffer from chronic pain, and these incorporate scales to determine the patients' pain beliefs, expectations, and coping skills together with analgesic use and affective and intensity measures.[18] If pain intensity alone is to be evaluated, it is preferable to carry out a series of measures each day because the pain is likely to fluctuate in intensity during the day. As stated earlier, memory for pain is not as accurate as contemporary ratings, so the use of a "pain diary" utilizing categorical or analog scales at set times during the day is a more satisfactory way of recording pain during the day rather than estimating a daily average. Even severely ill patients can easily complete a pain diary several times each day.

CANCER PAIN

The measurement of pain in patients with cancer can be more difficult than in those with benign disease. Mood disturbance and beliefs about the meaning of the pain in relation to the illness are known to be significant predictors of perceived pain intensity. Concerns about social and spiritual matters add to the complexity. In addition to the psychological distress of the cancer patient confounding pain measurement, several differing pain problems may coexist, e.g. acute nociceptive pain due to bone or visceral carcinoma in conjunction with neuropathic pain from nerve root involvement. One must also bear in mind the pain induced by investigative and therapeutic processes, which may add to any suffering. Detailed evaluation of pain intensity in these situations is pivotal to effective therapeutic decision-making.[19] Regular pain intensity measurements of each symptomatic site will

then be necessary when titrating toward optimum analgesia, in keeping with the individual patient's needs. A full assessment of the patient with cancer would not be complete without an evaluation of all the factors which alter pain perception as well as its intensity, but this is beyond the scope of this chapter. Pain intensity measures are generally carried out by one of the scales mentioned above. The MPQ can be used during the initial assessment as it permits evaluation of various qualities of pain. This can be of diagnostic value in pain management, but its repeated administration may be deemed inappropriate. The use of a pain diary is useful in this situation and may even help some patients to cope with their pain. Patients with advanced disease often cannot complete lengthy or complex questionnaires, so the use of four- or five-point categorical scales may be the most appropriate in these circumstances, especially if administered by a trained observer.[20] The use of any pain rating scale in these circumstances should be perceived to be clinically relevant by the patient, family, and staff. Scoring by a trained observer using a four- or five-point categorical VRS may in fact be the most appropriate.

For patients suffering from persistent pain

- Any of the scales mentioned previously may be used.
- The assessment of psychological and behavioral factors often proves to be much more valuable than evaluating pain intensity alone.
- Simple forms of pain assessment are the most appropriate if the patient is seriously ill or dying.

SERIAL MEASURES OF PAIN

The measurement of pain should only be carried out at the time during which it is perceived. A single measurement is therefore like a "snapshot" of the pain intensity and may not reflect the pain experienced over a period of hours or days. A series of measurements carried out at regular time intervals can build up a better picture of the overall problem. The arithmetic sum of the scores over a set time can therefore provide an "area under the pain curve" against time value. For example, for four VAS ratings of, for instance, 75, 55, 45, and 25 at 3-hourly intervals, the sum of the VAS (SUMVAS) would be 200 over a 9-h period.

Another method is to determine the pain intensity difference (PID), at set times, from the original pain score and calculate the sum of these over a set time period (Table 2.1).

A correction factor is applied to each PID, depending on the time difference between the current rating and the previous one. This gives a corrected "time-weighted" PID, and the sum of these over the set time period provides the SPID.

Table 2.1 *Calculation of pain intensity difference (PID) over a set time period*

Time (h)	Current pain (A)	Initial pain (B)	PID (B−A)	Correction factor	Corrected PID
0.5	2	3	1	0.5	0.5
1.0	1	3	2	0.5	1.0
2.0	1	3	2	1.0	2.0
3.0	2	3	1	1.0	1.0
4.0	3	3	0	1.0	0.0
Sum of pain intensity differences (SPID)					4.5
Maximum possible SPID[a]					12.0
Percentage of maximum possible pain intensity difference rating					37.5%

a. Initial pain rating × number of hours over which ratings were recorded.

Table 2.2 *Calculation of total pain relief (TOTPAR)*

Time (h)	Current pain relief	Correction factor	Corrected score
0.5	2	0.5	1.0
1.0	3	0.5	1.5
2.0	3	1.0	3.0
3.0	2	1.0	2.0
4.0	1	1.0	1.0
TOTPAR			8.5
Maximum TOTPAR[a]			12.0
Percentage of maximum TOTPAR			70.83%

a. Maximum relief score × time in hours.

If pain relief is now assessed in a similar fashion, the total pain relief (TOTPAR) can be calculated as described in Table 2.2.[21]

HANDLING AND INTERPRETING MEASUREMENT RESULTS

Data from pain intensity measures using ranked scales such as the VRS or the NRS may not be normally distributed, in which case nonparametric tests, such as the Mann–Whitney U-test, are appropriate. The wide range of words available through the MPQ are normally assessed by nonparametric means, although Melzack originally suggested that the t-test could be used to assess differences in mean pain scores.[14]* Ratio scale data such as those derived from the VAS, although continuously variable, should also be tested by nonparametric means, such as the Wilcoxon ranked sums test or the Kruskal–Wallis one-way analysis of variance. Some statisticians suggest that arcsin or logistic transformation of the raw data lead to increased sensitivity at the extreme ends of the scale with a more normal distribution of results, thus making appropriate the use of the more powerful parametric tests such as the t-test, analysis of variance, or regression analysis.[22] Although parametric tests permit a much more flexible and powerful analysis to be carried out than the nonparametric methods, their power is reduced when data come from a non-normal distribution. Tests for nor-mal distribution of data may be easily performed using standard statistical programs such as SPSS.

Establishing sample sizes for research purposes can be a difficult problem, and it is often necessary to revert to methods using expressions assuming a normal distribution. The number of patients or subjects needed for a study will depend on the magnitude of change one wishes to detect and on the variance of the observations. This information can be derived from previously published work or a pilot study. Sample size to achieve 90% power at the 95% level of statistical significance can be estimated using the formula:

$$n > 21 \times (S/d)^2 \text{ for independent samples}$$

where S is the standard deviation of the observed data; d is the difference in the outcome measure to be detected, between individuals; and n is the number of subjects per group.[22] When observations are made on paired data, the same power and level of significance are achieved as above using the formula:

$$n > 10.5 \times (SD/d)^2 \text{ for paired samples}$$

where SD is the standard deviation of the differences within subjects; d is the difference in the outcome measure to be detected, within each individual; and n is the number of individuals, which will create pairs of observations. A power of 80% is calculated by replacing 21 with 15.8 and 10.5 with 7.9 in these formulae.

Determining the magnitude of a meaningful change is of prime importance in both the clinical and research situations. It is not only important in determining sample size but in evaluating the efficacy of treatment. Various ways of determining the change in magnitude which is considered meaningful have been proposed. These correspond to an approximate reduction in pain of 30 percent.[23]* It is best to select a homogeneous, well-defined, small group of patients to study a specific issue. The use of a large but less well-defined group of patients with many pain problems results in a study with a lot of "noise," low sensitivity, and large type II error.

CONCLUDING REMARKS

There is a variety of methods by which pain intensity can be assessed, each having its own limitations and advantages. The most appropriate method is that which permits the patient to express the intensity of their present pain experience directly on some form of rating scale. Long-term memory for pain is poor, and any measurement should be made at the time of pain perception. Some researchers would argue that when a series of pain measures are made the patient should not have access to previous scores. Currently, it is considered more appropriate to let patients have access to their previous scores because there is no need to depend on memory of the previous scores when rating either a change in pain intensity or pain relief.

Pain intensity measures are a good way to compare intrapatient treatment effects (in response to time or treatment within any one individual). However, they should not be used in their raw form for interpatient assessment. If one wishes to assess the effect of a treatment within a group of individuals, this should be expressed as a ratio change (e.g. a percentage) from the original baseline score in each individual rather than, for instance, quoting mean changes in the group in terms of millimeters on a VAS.

Ideally, one would wish to assess all of the dimensions of the pain and, currently, the simplest and most frequently used method of doing so is the MPQ. The VAS also has much to commend it in relation to sensitivity, reliability, ease of use, and its ratio properties. However, some patients have difficulties in understanding this abstract form of pain measurement, especially those at the extremes of the age. Modification of this scale through the use of a series of facial expressions may appear to overcome this problem, but may result in an assessment of affect in conjunction with pain intensity. One could argue that this is indeed appropriate since it conveys the overall feeling of suffering associated with pain. Considering the limitations of most assessment techniques and the confounding effects of extraneous factors, great care is necessary in the interpretation of any results, regardless of the scoring method used.

REFERENCES

● 1. Jensen MP, Karoly P. Self-report scales and procedures for assessing pain in adults. In: Turk DC, Melzack R eds. *Handbook of Pain Assessment*. New York, NY: The Guilford Press, 1992: 135–51.

2. Janssen SA, Arntz A. Anxiety and pain: attentional and endorphinergic influences. *Pain* 1996; **66:** 145–50.

3. Riley JL, Robinson ME, Wise EA, *et al.* Sex differences in the perception of noxious experimental stimuli: a meta-analysis. *Pain* 1998; **74:** 181–7.

4. Ekblom A, Hansson P. Pain intensity measurements in patients with acute pain receiving afferent stimulation. *J Neurol Neurosurg Psychiatry* 1988; **51:** 481–6.

5. Feine JS, Lavigne GJ, Dao TTT, *et al.* Memories of chronic pain and perceptions of relief. *Pain* 1998; **77:** 137–41.

6. Jensen MP, Turner JA, Romano JM. What is the maximum number of levels needed in pain intensity measurement? *Pain* 1994; **58:** 387–92.

● 7. Huskisson EC. Measurement of pain. *J Rheumatol* 1982;
◆ **9:** 768–9.

8. Huskisson EC, Shenfield GM, Taylor RT, Hart FD. A new look at ibuprofen. *Rheumatol Phys Med Suppl* 1970; **10** (10): 88–92.

9. Breivik EK, Bjornson GA, Skovlund E. A comparison of pain rating scales by sampling from clinical trial data. *Clin J Pain* 2000; **16:** 22–8.

10. Jensen MP, Karoly P, Braver S. The measurement of clinical pain intensity: a comparison of six methods. *Pain* 1986; **27:** 117–26.

● 10. Price DD, Harkins SW. Psychophysical approaches to pain measurement and assessment. In: Turk DC, Melzack R eds. *Handbook of Pain Assessment*. New York, NY: The Guilford Press, 1992: 111–34.

12. Bieri D, Reeve RA, Champion GD, *et al.* The Faces Pain Scale for the self-assessment of the severity of pain experienced by children: development, initial validation, and preliminary investigation for ratio scale properties. *Pain* 1990; **41:** 139–50.

13. McGrath PA, Seifert CE, Speechley KN, *et al.* A new analogue scale for assessing children's pain: an initial validation study. *Pain* 1996; **64:** 435–443.

◆ 14. Melzack R. The McGill Pain Questionnaire: major properties and scoring methods. *Pain* 1975; **1:** 277–99.

15. Melzack R. The short-form McGill Pain Questionnaire. *Pain* 1987; **30:** 191–7.

● 16. McGrath PA. An assessment of children's pain: a review
◆ of behavioral, physiological and direct scaling techniques. *Pain* 1987; **31:** 147–76.

● 17. Nilges P. Outcome measures in pain therapy. In: Zenz M ed. *Bailliere's Clinical Anaesthesiology International Practice and Research*, vol. 12. London: Bailliere Tindall, 1998: 1–18.

● 18. Williams ACdeC. Pain measurement in chronic pain
◆ management. *Pain Rev* 1995; **2:** 39–63.

● 19. Cherry NI, Portenoy RK. Cancer pain: principles of

assessment and syndromes. In: Wall PD, Melzack R eds. *Textbook of Pain*. New York, NY: Churchill Livingstone, 1994: 787–823.

● 20. Higginson IJ. Innovations in assessment: epidemiology and assessment of pain in advanced cancer. In: Jensen TS, Turner JA, Wiesenfeld-Hallin Z eds. *Proceedings of the 8th World Congress on Pain, Progress in Pain Research and Management*, vol. 8. Seattle, WA: IASP Press, 1997: 707–16.

● 21. Max MB, Laska EM. Single-dose analgesic comparisons.
◆ In: Max MB, Portenoy RK, Laska EM eds. *The Design of Analgesic Clinical Trials. Advances in Pain Research and Therapy*, vol. 18. New York, NY: Raven Press, 1991: 55–95.

◆ 22. Armitage P. *Statistical Methods in Medical Research*. Oxford: Blackwell Scientific Publications, 1977: 184–8 and 355–61.

23. Campbell WI, Patterson CC. Quantifying meaningful changes in pain. *Anaesthesia* 1998; **53:** 121–5.

3

Sensory testing and clinical neurophysiology

ELLEN JØRUM AND LARS ARENDT-NIELSEN

Neurophysiological mechanisms	27	Determination of vibratory thresholds by vibrameter	31
Somatosensory evaluation of pain	28	Determination of pressure thresholds by algometer	32
Pain conditions	28	Thermotest	32
Nociceptive pain	29	Testing for abnormal temporal summation	34
Neuropathic pain	29	Conventional neurophysiological techniques	34
Sensory qualities	30	Other neurophysiological techniques	35
Basis for sensory testing	30	Future perspective in advanced sensory testing	35
Quantitative sensory testing	31	References	37
Estimation of tactile sensibility by von Frey nylon filaments	31		

The diagnosis of neuropathic (and nociceptive pain) is in most cases based on a thorough interview and a clinical examination of the patient. In many cases, however, there is a need for further classification of a painful syndrome, and the question arises as to which testing procedures are adequate. This chapter describes the different clinical neurophysiological and sensory testing methods available and their role in the evaluation of painful syndromes. The conventional clinical neurophysiological methods such as neurography- (nerve conduction studies) and somatosensory-evoked potentials using peripheral electrical stimulation are of little value since they assess the function of the fast-conducting Aβ-fiber and dorsal column system, which does not mediate the sensation of pain. Somatosensory potentials following CO_2 laser stimulation relate to pain and nociceptive impulses projected in the spinothalamic tract, but the large interindividual variation in the amplitude of the laser-evoked potentials suggests that they may not be suitable for routine examinations in clinical practice.

Neuropathic pain is in most cases characterized by sensory abnormalities that are caused by lesions of sensory nerve fibers or sensory pathways within the central nervous system. Further diagnostic and descriptive characterization of a painful syndrome may be obtained by performing quantitative sensory testing (QST), which allows a quantitative evaluation of sensory thresholds to tactile, vibratory, pressure, and temperature stimuli. Because neuropathic pain is often characterized by dys-

functions of the sensory qualities that are mediated by thin Aδ- and C-fibers, thermotesting (quantitative evaluation of thermal thresholds), which allows testing of heat, cold, and heat and cold pain, is of special importance. Testing for allodynia/hyperalgesia to tactile and thermal stimulation as well as testing for abnormal temporal summation or "windup-like" pain is of great value in the evaluation of neuropathic pain, and may be helpful in assessing underlying pathophysiological mechanisms.

NEUROPHYSIOLOGICAL MECHANISMS

It is beyond the scope of this chapter to describe in detail the complicated pathophysiological mechanisms involved in acute and, particularly, chronic pain. The mechanisms of nociception and inflammatory and neuropathic pain are discussed in detail in Chapters A1, A2, and Ch14. To a large extent, most mechanisms are still unknown. However, it may be helpful to have some understanding of the known basic mechanisms. The sensation of acute pain is the result of activation of normal (not sensitized) nociceptors classified as Aδ- or C-nociceptors, according to the peripheral nerve fiber transmitting the neural impulses. Several classes of C-nociceptors in humans have been identified by the technique of microneurography.[1] Of special importance for pathophysiological mechanisms may be the discovery of silent nociceptors, i.e. nociceptors that are not activated by normal noxious stimuli but become active in a state of injury, particularly following inflammation.[2]

If a peripheral injury occurs, the C-nociceptors may become sensitized as a result of the effect of a large number of inflammatory substances released at the site of the injury. Sensitization of C-nociceptors may produce sensory changes that are restricted to this site. The sensory changes that are produced are, first and foremost, a lowering of the heat pain threshold or *allodynia* to heat (allodynia is defined as pain produced by a nonpainful stimulus) and, second, *hyperalgesia* to heat (hyperalgesia is defined as an increased response to a stimulus that is normally painful). It is important to note that sensory changes due to nociceptor sensitization will be detectable within the site of injury alone, and not in the surrounding tissue.

In the event of acute pain, the incoming stimuli to the spinal cord are processed normally, and the nociceptive impulses are passed over to second-order neurons and transmitted in central projection pathways. If sustained peripheral injury (or an injury to a peripheral nerve) occurs, an increased barrage of nociceptive impulses reaches the dorsal horn of the spinal cord and *central sensitization* may occur. This general term includes a complicated series of events in neurons in the dorsal horn. Windup, a cumulative increase of action potentials caused by nociceptive stimulation, is considered to be a possible first initial step that is mediated by the activation of *N*-methyl-D-aspartate (NMDA) receptors.[3] A state of central hyperexcitability is produced, which is characterized in animal experiments by allodynia to light mechanical stimulation and an increase in the size of the peripheral receptive fields of the central neurons.[4] It may not yet be possible to explain all of the clinical symptoms, findings, and sensory abnormalities in patients with chronic pain using the theory of central sensitization, but the demonstration of central hyperexcitability has had a tremendous impact on the understanding of some of the phenomena observed in patients with chronic pain. For instance, allodynia to mechanical stimulation, which is frequently encountered in neuropathic pain patients, and the increase (over time) in the extent of the areas of pain have been accredited to central hyperexcitability. Whether the occurrence of spontaneous and paroxysmal pain may be explained entirely or partly by the same mechanisms remains an unresolved question. In general, a substantial amount of research is still needed to understand fully the different aspects of clinical pain.

Traditionally, clinical pain syndromes have been treated according to the etiology of the pain (e.g. postherpetic neuralgia, painful diabetic neuropathy). Because of the current knowledge of the possible common neurophysiological mechanisms involved in different pain entities, it has recently been suggested that, instead of focusing on the different etiologies, it might be possible to assess and treat pain according to the underlying neurophysiological mechanisms involved, i.e. mechanism-based classification of pain.[5]

This opens up new perspectives for the future management of pain, and represents a huge challenge for developing test procedures that will enable us to distinguish between different mechanisms in a clinical setting.

SOMATOSENSORY EVALUATION OF PAIN

A patient's subjective estimate of the magnitude of pain intensity may be determined by means of a visual analog scale. However, for better classification and documentation of a painful syndrome, supplementary investigations are often required. The aim of this chapter is to give an overview of the available supplementary tests. The purposes of employing such tests will fall mainly into the categories of diagnostic or objective documentation of a pain condition. Ideally, the results of testing could be used as a basis for treatment algorithms. Until now, sensory testing and some clinical neurophysiological tests have been mainly used in clinical research, for classifying the different abnormalities found in painful syndromes, and in clinical pharmacological trials. However, sensory testing is increasingly employed in the clinical evaluation of pain syndromes. Procedures as well as equipment in use vary between different laboratories. To give simple recommendations and general practical guidelines for the use of such testing in a purely clinical setting is, therefore, difficult. The aim of this chapter is to give some guidelines as to when and how to perform clinical neurophysiological or sensory testing.

It will be strongly emphasized throughout the chapter that all supplementary testing must be correlated to the clinical symptoms and findings of the patient and that it is not appropriate to make a diagnosis of a painful syndrome based on the results from sensory testing or clinical neurophysiological testing alone. The chapter will focus on the methods that are currently in use, but will also present methods that are currently more experimental and are still not regarded as conventional tools in the diagnosis of pain.

PAIN CONDITIONS

Pain conditions may be categorized in many ways – one approach is to describe the pain as nociceptive or neuropathic, depending on its cause. This is a general classification disregarding the etiology of the pain. Pain can also be categorized as acute or chronic, according to whether its duration is less than or more than 3 months respectively. Most patients referred for supplementary sensory or clinical neurophysiological testing will suffer from chronic pain. The neuropathic pain condition is primarily known to produce sensory abnormalities and, thus, deserves special attention. For the clinician, it is important to note that nociceptive pain may also produce sensory changes.[6]

Visceral pain referred to the skin may show sensory abnormalities that are detectable by sensory testing,[7] as well as areas referred from muscle pain.[8] For the reader, it is important to be aware of the existence of such findings, in the sense that the usefulness of sensory assessment is not restricted to neuropathic pain conditions. The finding of sensory abnormalities in different pain types may reflect the involvement of some common neurophysiological mechanisms.

NOCICEPTIVE PAIN

Nociceptive pain derives from the activation of nociceptors alone. The nociceptors may be normal or sensitized. When cutaneous nociceptors are normal, no sensory abnormalities have been described. When nociceptors become sensitized as a result of injuries to peripheral tissues and the subsequent release of inflammatory agents, sensory changes will result.

As mentioned above, sensitization of nociceptors will result in allodynia/hyperalgesia to heat and possibly some types of mechanical stimuli within the site of injury[9,10] – changes that are detectable with sensory testing.

In contrast to cutaneous pain, muscle pain is described as aching and cramping, is difficult to localize, and has characteristic referred pain patterns. Unfortunately, knowledge of the basic aspects of muscle pain in humans is still very poor as most of the information originates from experiments using anesthetized animals. Furthermore, the data on the neurophysiology of pain have mainly been obtained from studies of cutaneous nociception. This lack of knowledge about the neural mechanisms involved in muscle pain has led to much debate and speculation about the mechanisms related to the etiology, pathogenesis, diagnosis, and treatment.

Experimental approaches to the study of muscle pain in humans are a way of increasing knowledge. This is important as the socioeconomic impact of musculoskeletal pain disorders is substantial, and new insight into the pathophysiological mechanisms can help to prevent chronicity.

Experimental methods can be used in the laboratory for basic studies (e.g. central hyperexcitability or screening of treatment procedures) and also in the clinic to characterize patients with musculoskeletal disorders (e.g. fibromyalgia).

The primary advantages of experimental approaches to assess pain sensitivity under normal and pathological conditions are:

1 The stimulus can be controlled, i.e. the pain intensity and quality do not vary over time.

2 Pain reactions to controlled stimuli can be assessed quantitatively.

3 Pain reactions can be compared quantitatively between controls and patients.

One disadvantage of experimental pain research is that the stimulus paradigm (intensity, duration, and modality) might not mimic clinical pain conditions completely.

Several experimental models have been used to induce and assess muscle pain in humans. Intramuscular (i.m.) injection of algogenic substances (bradykinin, serotonin, capsaicin, hypertonic saline), i.m. electrical stimulation, ischemia, or eccentric exercise are some examples.

Injection of hypertonic saline has been used extensively in the past because the quality of the induced pain is similar to clinical muscle pain that is localized and referred. Injections of chemical substances are, however, not suitable if the muscle pain needs to be turned on and off more rapidly. Recently, a model has been developed based on continuous intramuscular electrical stimulation in which the local and referred pain vanish immediately when the stimulation is terminated.[11]

Infusion of a variety of algogenic substances has been tested, and a combination of, for example, serotonin and bradykinin is particularly effective in causing muscular hyperalgesia to muscle pressure stimulation. It seems that the severity of the referred pain is related to the intensity and duration of the ongoing muscle pain and most likely also to the degree of central hyperexcitability.[12] In patients with chronic pain syndromes such as fibromyalgia or whiplash, the pain responses to experimental muscle pain are substantially exaggerated compared with controls.[13] Experimental models are valuable for assessing the basic aspects of muscle pain in volunteers and in patients with musculoskeletal disorders.

NEUROPATHIC PAIN

Neuropathic pain results from a lesion or a dysfunction of the nervous system (peripheral or central). One may distinguish between nociceptive neuropathic pain, which is caused by the activation of nociceptors connected to nervous tissue (e.g. cervical or lumbar radiculopathy), and the deafferentation type of neuropathic pain, which often involves mechanisms of central sensitization. It is this latter form of neuropathic pain that will be described here. A painful condition may develop immediately after injury or after a long delay, such as days, weeks, or even months. The results of sensory and, eventually, clinical neurophysiological testing need to be correlated with the patient's symptoms and clinical findings. Typically, the patient may complain of several types of pain, but there is a large interindividual variability (Table 3.1). Most patients will complain of constant pain, the quality of which may vary; commonly used descriptors include "burning," "aching,"

Table 3.1 *Characteristics of neuropathic pain*

Spontaneous pain	Burning, aching, squeezing, cutting, piercing, pricking, sore (and other descriptions)	Constant, but with possible variation in intensity
Spontaneous, paroxysmal pain	Shooting, sharp, stinging, throbbing, radiating	Duration, seconds to minutes; frequency, from 0 to several per day
Evoked pain	Pain or unpleasant sensation by stimulation of painful area (usually light touch)	

and "sore." The constant pain may vary spontaneously in intensity, but will typically be intensified by physical activity and exposure to cold. Many patients will suffer from paroxysmal pain, lasting for seconds up to minutes, within the painful area and with radiation from this area. The frequency of paroxysms may vary, from several times a day until a few times every week. The quality of the paroxysmal pain may be described as "shooting," "intense," or "sharp." Typically, the patient also complains of evoked pain, which is mostly caused by lightly touching the skin or by exposure to wind. A painful condition may develop from the time of onset, often resulting in an increase in the area of pain or an intensification of the constant pain. In most cases, neuropathic pain is accompanied by sensory abnormalities[14,15] that are related to lesions in the sensory nerve fibers or sensory pathways within the central nervous system.[16] Sensory disturbances may develop from both causes, as shown in Table 3.2.

Sensory disturbances may sometimes be detected by routine neurological sensory examination (light touch with a cotton swab or pinprick with a needle). However, hypoesthesia is often masked by allodynia to light mechanical stimulation. Nevertheless, reduced sensibility to light touch may be reported by some patients. Hyperalgesia to pinprick is often reported as a different, more painful, sensation, often with radiation and an unpleasant aftersensation.

The diagnosis of neuropathic pain may in most cases be confirmed by careful interviewing of the patient and a routine neurological examination. Further diagnostic and descriptive characterization is obtained by performing quantitative sensory training (QST), which allows, as indicated by the name, a quantitative evaluation of the different sensory qualities.

Table 3.2 *Sensory abnormalities in neuropathic pain*

Quantitative	Hypoesthesia	Hypoalgesia
	Hyperesthesia	Hyperalgesia
Qualitative	Allodynia	
	Paresthesia	
	Dysesthesia	
Spatial	Dyslocalization	
	Radiation	
Temporal	Abnormal latency	
	Abnormal aftersensation	
	Abnormal summation	

SENSORY QUALITIES

The sensation of touch, pressure, and vibration are all mechanosensitive modalities that are transmitted in large-diameter myelinated Aβ afferent neurons, spinal dorsal columns, and medial lemniscal pathways, which are accessible to testing through conventional neurophysiological techniques such as neurography and electrically induced sensory-evoked potentials.

For testing modalities such as fast pain (Aδ-fibers), dull, burning, aching pain (C-fibers), heat and heat pain (C-fibers), and cold (Aδ-fibers) and cold pain (Aδ- and C-fibers), neurography and somatosensory-evoked potentials (SEP) are of little value.

Many disorders, for example diabetic neuropathy, affect the small-diameter fibers before the large-diameter fibers, and a clinical diagnosis concerning nerve impairment can only be obtained when the large-diameter fibers start to show measurable signs of dysfunction. At that time, the thin fibers may be severely affected, with the possibility of developing severe neuropathic chronic pain. Methods to assess early impairment of the thin-fiber function are needed.

BASIS FOR SENSORY TESTING

Routine neurological sensibility testing is inadequate for a quantitative, modality-specific assessment of sensory disturbance. Sensory testing has developed in recent years as a valuable supplement to the quantitative determination of modality-specific disturbances. In general, sensory testing in humans involves a large variety of disciplines (auditory, visual, somatic, kinesthetic, etc.). In particular, sensory testing involves the standardized activation of the specific sensory pathways system and the measurement of evoked responses. The ultimate goal of advanced human sensory testing is to obtain a better understanding of mechanisms involved in sensory transduction, transmission, and perception under normal and pathophysiological conditions. Sensory testing can be applied in the laboratory for basic studies or in the clinic to characterize patients with dysfunctions affecting pain pathways. At present, there are different stimulation techniques available in the laboratory, including electrical, thermal, and mechanical techniques; however, commercially available equipment needed to apply these techniques is scarce.

To differentiate between the dysfunctions that are related to various disorders of the sensory system, it is necessary to establish a series of sensory tests with different stimulus modalities activating different pathways. The design of adequate regimes to test sensory fibers involves two separate topics:

1 standardized activation;
2 measurement and quantification of the evoked reactions.

QUANTITATIVE SENSORY TESTING

Quantitative sensory testing (QST) is used to measure the intensity of stimuli needed to produce specific sensory perceptions. Tests have been developed for the determination of sensory thresholds for tactile, vibratory, pressure, and temperature stimulation.

Various laboratories have used different approaches and paradigms, but only a few laboratories use routine QST in the evaluation of pain patients.

All quantitative sensory tests are psychophysical tests that require patients to be awake and alert, to fully understand the instructions given, and to be fully capable of cooperating during testing.

ESTIMATION OF TACTILE SENSIBILITY BY VON FREY NYLON FILAMENTS

For quantitative testing of tactile sensibility, von Frey nylon filaments are easy to use. They consist of a series of filaments of varying thickness, calibrated according to the force required to make them bend. The hairs primarily stimulate the rapidly adapting cutaneous receptors when hairs with low bending pressures are applied to the skin. One method of assessing tactile sensation is to apply the hairs in an ascending and descending order of magnitude and to record both the appearance and disappearance threshold. In neuropathic pain, tactile sensibility, as measured by von Frey hairs, may be reduced in the affected skin areas.[17] This is a typical finding that may be observed in a routine neurological examination, in which testing for tactile sensibility with a cotton swab may only give a sensation of hyperesthesia (in fact, allodynia to light mechanical stimulation) that masks an eventual reduction in tactile sensibility. Another way of assessing the tactile threshold is to determine the value of the bending force of the filament which is detected in 50% of applications. One should be aware that the nominal bending force of von Frey hairs varies with temperature and humidity, and it may be necessary to calibrate the bending force against a balance for each experimental session.[18]

The von Frey hairs increasingly excite skin nociceptors with increasing bending force, and may be used to determine tactile pain detection thresholds.

The nylon filaments have been used for the determination of allodynia/hyperalgesia to punctate stimuli in human experimental models.[19] The von Frey hairs may also be employed for mapping areas of secondary hyperalgesia to punctate stimuli (owing to central sensitization) in experimental models of pain[19] or in a clinical context.[20] It has recently been shown that secondary hyperalgesia to punctate stimuli is mediated by conduction in Aδ-nociceptive fibers,[21] in contrast to the Aβ-fiber-mediated secondary hyperalgesia to light brush.

Summary of von Frey hair testing

Indication: for quantitative testing of tactile sensibility.
How it is executed: apply the hairs in an ascending and descending order of magnitude and record both the appearance and disappearance thresholds, or determine the value of the bending force of the filament which is detected in 50% of applications:

- with increasing bending force, the von Frey hairs will excite skin nociceptors and may be used to determine tactile pain detection thresholds;
- may be used to map the area of allodynia/hyperalgesia to punctate stimuli.

Contraindications: none.
Typical findings and interpretations: reduced tactile sensibility as well as allodynia/hyperalgesia to punctate stimuli.

DETERMINATION OF VIBRATORY THRESHOLDS BY VIBRAMETER

The vibrameter (equipment for quantitative evaluation of vibratory thresholds) may be used for the evaluation of both vibratory and vibratory pain thresholds. The vibrameter determines the stimulus level needed to produce the sensation of vibration and is easily and quickly performed. The vibratory perception threshold can be determined on any point of the human body.

The determination of vibratory thresholds is primarily of value in the quantitative evaluation of vibratory sensory deficit. Hyperalgesia to vibration has been described in the evaluation of pain patients.[22] In an investigation of patients with neuralgia, it was found that the vibration frequency could be raised to 130 Hz without causing pain, in both normal volunteers and patients' uninjured areas (hands). In all patients with neuralgia, allodynia to vibration in the affected part was demonstrated.

Summary of vibrameter testing

Indication: quantitative evaluation of vibratory perception and vibratory pain thresholds.
How it is executed: the vibrameter may be applied on any point of the human body.
Contraindications: none.
Typical findings: increased vibratory threshold (reduced sensibility) and allodynia/hyperalgesia to vibration.

DETERMINATION OF PRESSURE THRESHOLDS BY ALGOMETER

The algometer is used for quantitative determination of thresholds to pressure or pinching. The measurement of pressure pain thresholds has been used in a large variety of test situations. In clinical practice, the pressure algometer is usually applied over a bony surface (for instance the tibia) or over muscles. The essence of pressure algometry is that increasing pressure is applied to the part of the body that is being investigated and the outcome is the patients' or volunteers' reaction to the pressure. The outcome measures in pressure algometry are the pain detection threshold and/or the pain tolerance threshold. Pressure rate and pressure area have been shown to be important factors for reliable results. To date, pressure algometry has, for instance, been used to assess the effects of drugs, different treatment modalities, pain thresholds in children, experimental pain in muscles, pain thresholds in populations studies, head and neck pain,[23] masseter muscle soreness, myofascial trigger points, and pain in patients with fibromyalgia.[24] The method seems to be well suited for the determination of pressure hyperalgesia in musculoskeletal disorders.

Summary of algometer testing

Indication: quantitative determination of the threshold to pressure or pinching.
How it is executed: the algometer is applied over bony surface or muscle (for pressure threshold) or is used for pinching a fold of the skin.
Contraindications: none.
Typical findings: reduced sensibility or allodynia/hyperalgesia to pressure or pinching.

THERMOTEST

Painful syndromes (mainly neuropathic pain) are often characterized by dysfunctions in the sensory qualities that are mediated by thin nerve fibers, which are not easily investigated by conventional electrophysiological testing such as neurography. Thermotest (quantitative evalua-

tion of thermal thresholds) allows the testing of qualities such as heat, cold, and heat and cold pain sensations (Fig. 3.1). It is important to note that, whereas neurography tests dysfunction of peripheral nerve fibers, the thermotest describes the status of temperature somatosensory afferents all the way from the cutaneous receptors to the brain, but it is not possible to determine the level of any lesion. There are different thermotest devices commercially available that have varying technical parameters. Testing for thermal sensory abnormalities is employed not only in the evaluation of pain patients but also in patients with thermal sensory abnormalities in general, such as thin-fiber neuropathies. Some devices are primarily designed to evaluate the sensory deficits of heat, cold, and heat pain. Prominent findings in neuropathic pain conditions are heat and cold hyperalgesia. Testing only for heat and cold functions in patients with neuropathic pain will give inconclusive results because heat and cold hyperalgesia may occur in the presence of normal heat and cold thresholds. When evaluating neuropathic pain patients, all four thermal qualities should be tested – heat, cold, heat pain, and cold pain.[25] As well as determining the threshold values, it is important to ask the patient about the quality of the sensation. Paradoxical sensations are frequently reported, most often that cold pain is perceived as heat. Heat and cold pain are often described as having a sudden onset, with radiation and aftersensations, which is valuable information in the evaluation of hyperalgesia. It is important to note that the interindividual variability in sensory abnormalities is large and may develop in both directions, as shown in Fig. 3.2.

There are two different methods of thermal sensory testing that are generally available: the two-alternative forced choice method and the method of limits. The two-alternative forced choice method implies that a stimulus at a given level of intensity is presented to the patient during only one of a pair of stimulus events and the patient has to indicate which of the stimuli is perceived. Success or failure at this level results in subsequent stimuli being

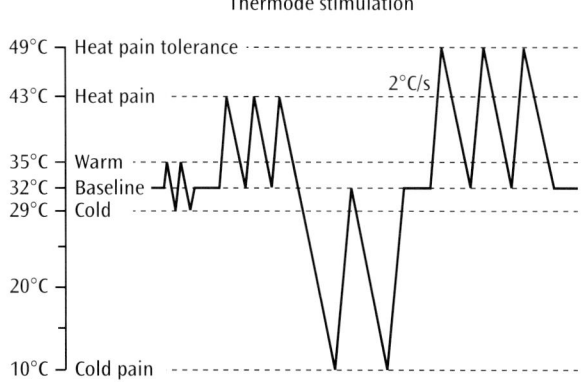

Figure 3.1 *Normal thermal thresholds measured by thermotest from a baseline of 32°C.*

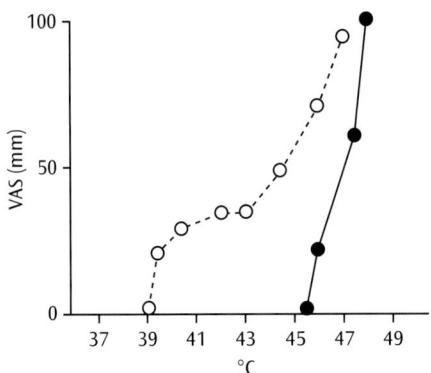
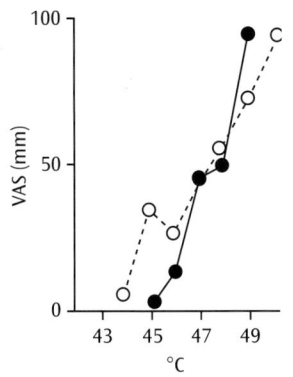

Figure 3.2 *Patterns of abnormal sensory disturbances to heat stimulation of patient with neuropathic pain. Open circles, nonaffected side; filled circles, affected side.*

delivered at lesser or greater stimulus intensities respectively.[26] The forced choice method reduces the response bias and seems therefore better suited for a psychophysical examination, but the method is time-consuming. The method has mainly been employed in the evaluation of neurological patients with sensory deficits in general and not in pain patients in particular. For the evaluation of pain patients, the method of limits, in which the intensity of stimulation is continuously increased from 0 (or from skin temperature) to the point of detection threshold, is probably the most appropriate. This is mainly because of ethical considerations as a suprathreshold stimulus may evoke severe pain, which is often sustained. For the same reason, it is desirable to use as few stimuli as possible to determine a pain threshold. The pain tolerance threshold may also be determined; however, for some patients, the detection threshold itself will represent the level of tolerance. For cold and heat detection thresholds, it is usual to use a total of 5–10 repeated tests, whereas for cold and heat pain three repeated measurements are often used.

There are many parameters that may influence the results of the testing. The baseline skin temperature is an important factor that may influence the ability to discriminate between a rise or fall in temperature. In many laboratories, the contact probe is applied at a standard temperature of 32°C, thereby reducing the interindividual variability in perception thresholds. Alternatively, the temperature of the contact probe may be set at a lower or a higher temperature. By employing a higher baseline temperature, heat thresholds would be assessed at the baseline temperature itself or at a very short interval from baseline. A lower baseline temperature would create a bias in favor of a cold threshold at a short interval from baseline. It is not recommended that the patient's skin should be warmed before testing. Another possibility is to adjust the temperature of the contact probe to be the same as the patient's skin temperature. One should be aware that, because of autonomic dysfunction in patients with complex regional pain syndromes, the skin temperature may be 1–3°C lower in the affected part. It may be difficult to compare sensory thresholds in affected and normal skin areas in these patients if the baseline temperature of the contact probe is set at different levels within the same

individual. The baseline temperature should therefore be kept constant for each individual. It is difficult to give strict recommendations regarding the choice between using a fixed baseline of 32°C or a baseline temperature adjusted to the skin temperature. However, using a fixed temperature of 32°C allows easier comparison of sensory thresholds between individuals.

The rate of stimulus rise may also influence the sensory threshold. The most commonly employed rate of temperature change is 1°C/s. Quicker rates may induce reaction time artifacts, whereas slower changes create stimuli that are too long.

Because of the influence of spatial summation of sensory modalities, the size of the contact probe may also influence the sensory thresholds, in the sense that recruitment of more receptors will lower the threshold. For practical reasons, it means that thresholds are not comparable when probes of different sizes have been employed. Surface areas may vary from 9 to 12.5 cm^2, and smaller contact probes are used to test the face or fingertip.

A major question is to decide which skin areas should be tested. For the individual evaluation of pain patients, it is recommended that the patient should serve as their own control by testing normal contralateral "mirror" areas; of course, this is not possible in bilateral disease states such as diabetic or human immunodeficiency virus (HIV)-related neuropathy. Since thermal sensibility normally varies between regions of the body (e.g. higher sensitivity in the thenar eminence than in proximal parts of the extremities or the truncus), testing of a contralateral asymptomatic skin area is often performed. However, one should be aware that because of central plasticity (central sensitization) sensory thresholds in contralateral regions may be abnormal. Therefore, in many cases, it may be recommended that sensory thresholds are tested in a third skin area as a supplementary control. Testing all four modalities in three different skin regions may be time-consuming, but in many cases it is worthwhile.

In order to prevent injuries to the skin, the maximum temperature limit is recommended to be 50°C and the minimum to be 5°C.

Once again, it is emphasized that the results of thermotesting should be correlated with the patient's symptoms and clinical findings, and that a diagnosis or an evaluation of a painful syndrome based on thermotest alone is of little value.

Summary of thermotesting

Indications: to test perception thresholds of heat and cold; to determine heat and cold pain thresholds; to detect possible qualitative abnormalities in thermal perception; to examine for possible allodynia/hyperalgesia to heat or cold.

How it is executed: thermotesting may be performed in many ways. We recommend:

- using the method of limits;
- testing all four thermal qualities;
- keeping a constant baseline temperature for each individual;
- that the maximum temperature limit is 50°C and the minimum is 5°C.

Contraindications: none (when used appropriately).
Typical findings: there are large variations in the results obtained. In patients with neuropathic pain, findings may be reduced sensibility to heat and cold as well as allodynia/hyperalgesia to thermal stimuli, especially cold.

TESTING FOR ABNORMAL TEMPORAL SUMMATION

Temporal summation of neural impulses in nociceptive nerve fibers is a physiologically important mechanism by which the sensation of pain can be intensified.[27] From clinical practice, it is well known that repetitive stimulation of a painful skin area in a patient suffering from neuropathic pain may produce an intense and long-lasting pain. This is referred to as an abnormal temporal summation (often called "windup like pain,"[17] even though no direct correlation to the windup phenomenon in the neurons of the dorsal horn that has been observed in animal studies can be confirmed). The abnormal temporal summation seen in patients may be assessed very roughly by repetitive stimulation (usually with a frequency of 2–3 Hz) of the skin by a von Frey hair, for up to 20–30 s. If the phenomenon of abnormal temporal summation is present, the patient will report the sudden onset of an intense pain within the stimulated area, often occurring within a few seconds, that is associated with the presence of aftersensation and radiation. Abnormal temporal summation may be regarded as a sign of central hyperexcitability. By measuring latency, duration of aftersensation, and area of radiation, it is possible to quantify the phenomenon. For scientific purposes, more elegant techniques are available, either by von Frey application by

standardized pressure and frequencies or by the use of electrical skin stimulation.

CONVENTIONAL NEUROPHYSIOLOGICAL TECHNIQUES

The practical details of conventional neurophysiological techniques, such as neurography or the measurement of evoked potentials, will not be given since these tests should be performed by trained clinical neurophysiologists. However, the indications for ordering such investigations will be discussed.

Neurography

Neurography is a generic term for the measurement of parameters such as conduction velocity, distal delay, motor and sensory amplitudes, and latency of late volleys such as the H- and F-wave. Nerve conduction studies play an important role in precisely delineating the extent and distribution of a peripheral nerve lesion and give some indication of nerve-root pathology (by evaluation of late reflexes). Neurography does not evaluate the function of thin nerve fibers such as Aδ-fibers that mediate cold/sharp pain nor that of C-fibers mediating the sensation of heat, heat pain, and some forms of tactile pain. The indication for neurography would be to evaluate whether there is a peripheral nerve lesion in the context of a general or polyneuropathy that is also affecting large myelinated nerve fibers. (The diagnosis of polyneuropathy cannot be excluded on basis of a normal neurography since a pure thin-fiber polyneuropathy may only be demonstrated by means of thermotesting.)

Sensory-evoked potentials

In routine neurophysiological practice, sensory-evoked potentials are measured following peripheral electrical stimulation. Unfortunately, some clinical papers assume that the evoked potentials to painful electrical stimulation represent aspects of nociceptive transmission. Based on reported evidence, it is obvious that the electrically evoked potentials that project to the dorsal columns are associated with sensory qualities such as light touch, vibration, and pressure. On the other hand, sensory-evoked potentials following CO_2 laser stimulation relate to pain and nociceptive impulses projected in the spinothalamic tract.

The potentials evoked by nonpainful and painful electrical stimulation are surprisingly similar. None of the components of the evoked potentials elicited by painful electrical stimuli can be considered as pain specific in the sense that they appear only following stimuli above the pain threshold.[28,29] The shape or amplitude of the vertex potential does not change when the intensity of the electrical stimulus exceeds the pain threshold.[29,30] This has led to the suggestion that vertex potentials evoked by nociceptive electrical stimuli are not reliable correlates for changes within the nociceptive system.[31]

The large interindividual variation in the amplitude of the laser-evoked potentials suggests that they may not be suitable for routine examinations in clinical practice. A large set of normative data based on laser-evoked potentials from normal, healthy, age- and sex-adjusted controls is essential. A statistical criterion of three standard deviations might be used to categorize sensory abnormality associated with laser-evoked potentials. In studies in which the patient and control groups serve as their own controls, for example by comparing the differences in amplitude for potentials evoked from two areas or by follow-up after surgery, measurement of laser-evoked potentials is suitable for monitoring purposes. Laser-evoked potentials can also provide useful information that is not accessible by conventional electrophysiological techniques. Laser-evoked potentials have been shown to be of value in assessing impairment of pain and temperature sensation in patients with peripheral neuropathies.[32]

A correlation between pain/temperature impairment and changes in the laser-evoked potential measurement has been found in patients with syringomyelia,[33] patients with multiple sclerosis,[34] and in neurological patients with various dissociated sensory deficits.[35] Sensory testing and clinical neurophysiology studies have indicated that patients with central pain syndromes occasionally have impairment of pain and temperature sensation. Central pain syndromes could be caused by disinhibition of spinothalamic excitability or by the reduction of spinothalamic function as a result of other central changes or disease in the brain. Casey et al.[36] found that central pain patients (cerebral or brainstem infarctions) with normal tactile sensation had significantly lower laser-evoked potentials on the affected side than on the nonaffected side. This study supports a deficit in spinothalamic tract function, but does not suggest excessive central responses to the activation of cutaneous nociceptive pathways. The laser-evoked potential may also be pathologically exaggerated.

Fibromyalgia patients show a dramatically exaggerated reaction to muscle stimulation.[37] Evoked potentials to cutaneous laser stimulation have indicated larger amplitudes in these patients than in controls.[38] The major alteration in laser-evoked potentials is found only in the late components (N170–P390). These effects suggest the presence of exogenous factors such as reduced cortical and subcortical inhibition or central hypervigilence to the nociception, probably involving the limbic midcingulate generator. However, it has been shown that hypnotically induced hyperalgesia can also increase the laser-evoked vertex potentials.[39]

OTHER NEUROPHYSIOLOGICAL TECHNIQUES

Microneurography

Microneurography is an invasive technique that was developed by Swedish neurophysiologists Hagbarth and Vallbo to make single-fiber recordings from nerve fibers in subjects who are awake. Erik Torebjörk was the first to record from single afferent C-fibers in humans in 1974.[40] Since then, he has described the human nociceptive system, both mapping the different classes of C-nociceptors[1] and describing the pathophysiology of C-nociceptors in peripheral injury.[2,9] Very few reports have been published on this technique in patients, and only one report described the peripheral mechanisms (nociceptor sensitization) in a patient with chronic pain.[41]

Microneurography is technically a very difficult and time-consuming process, often requiring repeated investigations in one subject; therefore, it is only suitable for research purposes. Since the technique is also invasive, it should only be employed by those trained in its use and following discussion of the risks of nerve injury with the patient.

FUTURE PERSPECTIVE IN ADVANCED SENSORY TESTING

It has recently been proposed[5] that pain assessment and management should be mechanism based. For this to be feasible, it is necessary to have quantitative techniques available that are capable of accurately determining which mechanisms are operative in the individual patient. This has not yet been achieved, and further concerted efforts are required to develop clinically useful techniques.

It is very important that sensory tests should be combined with the information obtained from the clinical history and examination of the patient to produce a comprehensive picture of the abnormalities in that patient, and possibly an indication of the mechanisms involved in the generation of that patient's pain.[42] A battery of sensory tests should consist of those that selectively activate the different afferent pathways – Aβ-, Aδ-, and C-fibers – and hence their respective spinocortical pathways. Clinical symptoms related to, for example, neuropathic pain can manifest themselves in many ways, and the results of sensory testing can be just as diverse. However, quantitative measures for follow-up are mandatory. As substantial plasticity can take place in the central nervous system, it is therefore important to include tests that quantitatively evaluate this aspect, e.g. tactile hyperalgesia or allodynia to touch.

In many cases, no abnormalities to a single stimulus may be measured, but when the stimulus is repeated pain is elicited. The facilitation of central summation is an example of mechanism-based assessment. In complex regional pain syndromes (reflex dystrophy or causalgia) and neuropathic pain syndromes, repetitive tactile stimuli summate and evoke pain as a result of facilitation of the central integrative mechanisms, most likely in second-order dorsal horn neurons.

Without a controlled electronic device, it can be difficult to apply repetitive tactile von Frey hair stimulation at a fixed frequency. In a number of experimental studies, a 2-Hz train of repetitive stimuli seems to be adequate to generate "windup-like" pain and aftersensations in patients with neuropathic pain. Laboratory models exist in which the frequency and stimulus duration can be adjusted electronically, and different stimulation probes can be attached.

The currently available thermode stimulators have very slow rates of temperature change (e.g. 2°C/s), therefore they are not applicable for repetitive thermal stimulation. Recently, a thermal stimulator based on heat-foil technology has been developed for repetitive thermal stimulation (Fig. 3.3). This device can provide a pulse rise time of up to 40°C/s and hence deliver pulses at, for example, 2 Hz. Another problem can arise in patients with severe allodynia to touch when the heat thresholds to thermode or heat-foil stimulation have to be measured. Applying the thermode to the skin evokes pain and hampers the determination of the heat threshold.

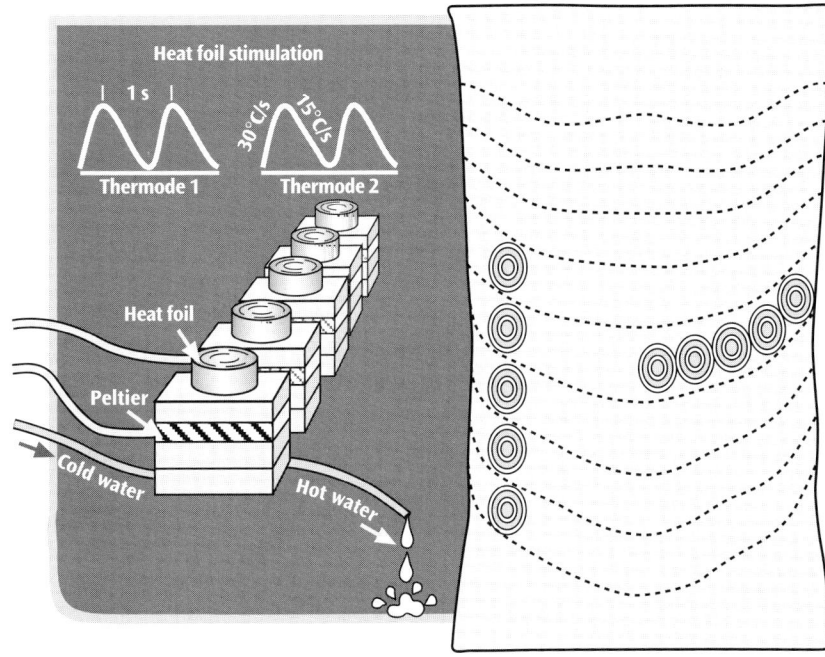

Figure 3.3 *Thermal stimulation based on heat-foil technology. The example shows how temporal summation (response to repeated stimulation) can be assessed within and between dermatomes.*

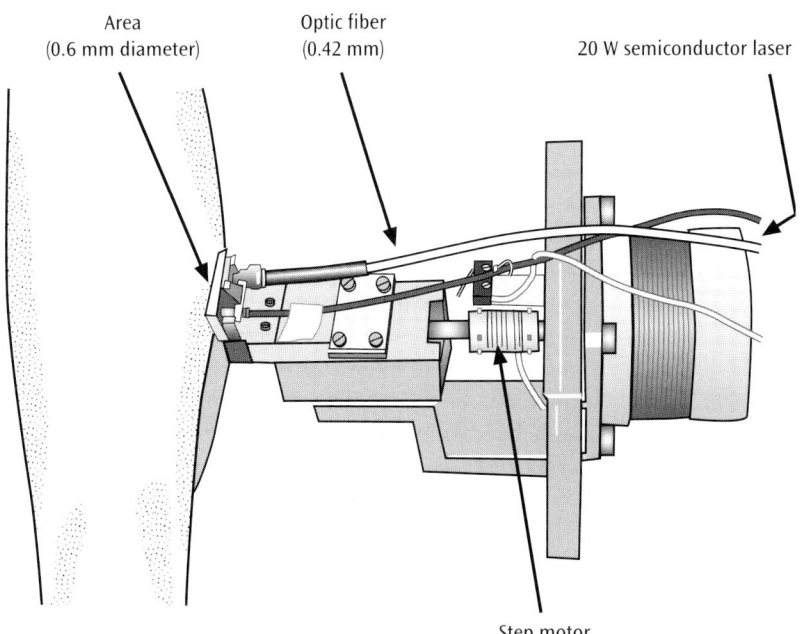

Figure 3.4 *Heat pulses can be delivered to the skin by a semiconductor laser without touching the skin. The laser selectively activates the thin nerve fibers. the dark fiber is another optical fiber used by a low-intensity laser for determining the distance to the skin. As the heat beams diverge, a step motor will constantly adjust the distance to the skin so that the diameter of the stimulated skin is constant. The heat pulse can also be used to generate brain-evoked potentials.*

In experimental pain research, high-energy laser has been used as a selective thin-fiber activator. The currently available lasers are very expensive and are complicated to operate; hence, they are not suitable for clinical routine and bedside testing. In recent years, the developments within the field of semiconductor lasers (e.g. 20 W, 970 nm) are promising, and such lasers may be available in the near future (Fig. 3.4).

Because of accessibility, cutaneous stimulation has predominantly been used in sensory testing. Most often, the abnormalities are not restricted to the skin but may also manifest in deeper structures. At a minimum, the general sensitivity of muscles should be assessed by pressure algometry or electrical stimulation.

In conclusion, quantitative sensory testing has a role to play in clinical neurophysiology, neurology, and pain management. The challenge for the future is to develop techniques to (1) assess not only the pain pathways as such but also, in more detail, the various mechanisms involved and (2) investigate pain originating not only from skin but also from deeper structures.

REFERENCES

◆ 1. Schmidt R, Schmelz M, Forster C, *et al*. Novel classes of responsive and unresponsive C nociceptors in human skin. *Neuroscience* 1995; **15**: 333–41.

◆ 2. Schmelz M, Schmidt R, Ringkamp M, *et al*. Sensitization of insensitive branches of C nociceptors in human skin. *J Physiol* 1994; **480**: 389–94.

3. Davies SN, Lodge D. Evidence for involvement of N-methyl-D-aspartate receptors in "wind-up" of class 2 neurones in the dorsal horn of the rat. *Brain Res* 1987; **424**: 402–6.

4. Woolf CJ, King AE. Dynamic alterations in the cutaneous mechanosensitive receptive fields of dorsal horn neurons in the rat spinal cord. *J Neurosci* 1990; **10**: 2717–26.

◆ 5. Woolf C, Bennett GJ, Doherty M, *et al*. Towards a mechanism-based classification of pain. *Pain* 1998; **77**: 227–9.

6. Hansson P, Lindblom U. Quantitative evaluation of sensory disturbances accompanying focal or referred nociceptive pain. In: Vecchiet L, Albe-Fessard D, Lindblom U eds. *New Trends in Referred Pain and Hyperalgesia*. Amsterdam: Elsevier Science Publishers, 1993: 251–8.

7. Vecchiet L, Giamberardino MA, Dragani L, Albe-Fessard D. Pain from renal/ureteral calculosis: evaluation of sensory thresholds in the lumbar area. *Pain* 1989; **36**: 289–95.

8. Graven-Nielsen T, Arendt-Nielsen L, Svensson P, Jensen TS. Stimulus–response functions in areas with experimentally induced referred muscle pain – a psychophysical study. *Brain Res* 1997; **744**: 121–8.

◆ 9. LaMotte RH, Thalhammer JG, Torebjörk HE, Robinson CJ. Peripheral neural mechanisms of cutaneous hyperalgesia following mild injury by heat. *J Neurosci* 1982; **2**: 765–81.

◆ 10. Kilo S, Schmelz M, Koltzenburg M, Handwerker HO. Different patterns of hyperalgesia induced by experimental inflammation in human skin. *Brain* 1994; **117**: 385–96.

11. Laursen R, Graven-Nielsen T, Jensen TS, Arendt-Nielsen L. The effect of compression and regional anaesthetic block on referred pain intensity in humans. *Pain* 1999; **80**: 257–63.

12. Babenko V, Graven-Nielsen T, Svensson P, *et al*. Experimental human muscle pain and muscular hyperalgesia induced by combinations of serotonin and bradykinin. *Pain* 1999; **8**: 21–8.

13. Sörensen J, Graven-Nielsen T, Henriksson KG, *et al*. Hyperexcitability in fibromyalgia. *J Rheumatol* 1998; **25**: 152–5.

◆ 14. Lindblom U, Verrillo RT. Sensory functions in chronic neuralgia. *J Neurol Neurosurg Psychiatry* 1979; **42**: 422–35.

◆ 15. Lindblom U. Assessment of abnormal evoked pain in neurological pain patients and its relation to spontaneous pain: a descriptive and conceptual model with some analytical results. In: Fields HL, Dubner R, Cervero F. eds. *Advances in Pain Research and Therapy*. New York, NY: Raven Press, 1985: 409–23.

◆ 16. Boivie J, Leijon G, Johansson I. Central post-stroke pain – a study of the mechanisms through analyses of the sensory abnormalities. *Pain* 1989; **37**: 173–85.

17. Eide PK, Jørum E, Stubhaug A, *et al*. Relief of postherpetic neuralgia with the N-methyl-D-aspartic acid receptor antagonist ketamine: a double-blind, crossover comparison with morphine and placebo. *Pain* 1994; **58**: 347–54.

18. Andrews K. The effect of changes in temperature and humidity on the accuracy of von Frey hairs. *J Neurosci Methods* 1993; **50**: 91–3.

19. Warncke T, Stubhaug A, Jørum E. Ketamine, an NMDA receptor antagonist, suppresses spatial and temporal properties of burn-induced secondary hyperalgesia in man: a double-blind, cross-over comparison with morphine and placebo. *Pain* 1997; **72**: 99–106.

20. Stubhaug A, Breivik H, Eide PK, *et al*. Mapping of punctate hyperalgesia around a surgical incision demonstrates that ketamine is a powerful suppressor of central sensitisation to pain following surgery. *Acta Anaesthesiol Scand* 1997; **41**: 1124–32.

21. Ziegler EA, Magerl W, Meyer RA, Treede RD. Secondary hyperalgesia to punctate mechanical stimuli. Central sensitization to A-fibre nociceptor input. *Brain* 1999; **122**: 2245–57.

22. Engkvist O, Wahren LK, Wallin G, *et al*. Effects of regional intravenous guanethidine block in posttraumatic cold intolerance in hand amputees. *J Hand Surg* 1985; **10**: 145–50.

23. Bovim G. Cervicogenic headache, migraine and tension-type headache. Pressure–pain threshold measurements. *Pain* 1992; **51:** 169–73.

24. Kosek E, Ekholm J, Hansson P. Modulation of pressure pain sensibility in fibromyalgia patients is located deep to the skin but not restricted to muscle tissue. *Pain* 1995; **63:** 335–9.

◆ 25. Verdugo R, Ochoa JL. Quantitative somatosensory thermotest. A key method for functional evaluation of small calibre afferent channels. *Brain* 1992; **115:** 1–21.

26. Dyck PJ, Karnes JL, O'Brien PC, Zimmerman IR. Detection thresholds of cutaneous sensation in humans. In: Dyck PJ, Thomas PK, Griffin J, *et al.* eds. *Peripheral Neuropathy*, 3rd edn. Philadelphia, PA: WB Saunders, 1993: 706–28.

27. Lundberg LER, Jørum E, Holm E, Torebjörk HE. Intraneural electrical stimulation of cutaneous nociceptive fibres in humans: effects of different pulse patterns on magnitude of pain. *Acta Physiol Scand* 1992; **51:** 207–19.

28. Debecker J, Desmedt JE. Les potentiels évoqués cérébraux et les potentiels de nerf sensible chez l'Homme. *Acta Neurol Psychiatr Belg* 1965; **64:** 1212–48.

29. De Broucker T, Willer JC. Etude comparative du réflexe nociceptif et des composantes tardives du potentiel évoqué somésthésique lors de stimulations du nerf sural chez l'homme normal. *Rev Electroenceph Clin Neurophysiol* 1985; **15:** 149–53.

30. Brennum J, Jensen TS. Relationship between vertex potentials and magnitude of pre-pain and pain sensations evoked by electrical skin stimuli. *Electroenceph Clin Neurophysiol* 1992; **85:** 387–90.

31. Leandri M, Campbell JA, Lahuerta J. The effect of attention on tooth-pulp evoked potentials. In: Fields HL, Dubner R, Cervero F eds. *Advances in Pain Research and Therapy*. New York, NY: Raven Press, 1985: 331–6.

◆ 32. Kakigi R, Shibasaki H, Tanaka K, *et al.* CO_2 laser-induced pain-related somatosensory evoked potentials in peripheral neuropathies: correlation between electrophysiological and histopathological findings. *Muscle Nerve* 1991; **14:** 441–50.

◆ 33. Kakigi R, Shibasaki H, Kuroda Y, *et al.* Pain-related somatosensory evoked potentials in syringomyelia. *Brain* 1991; **114:** 1871–89.

34. Kakigi R, Kuroda Y, Neshige R, *et al.* Physiological study of the spinothalamic tract conduction in multiple sclerosis. *J Clin Neurol Sci* 1992; **107:** 205–9.

● 35. Bromm B, Treede RD. Laser-evoked cerebral potentials in the assessment of cutaneous pain sensitivity in normal subjects and patients. *Rev Neurol* 1991; **147:** 625–43.

◆ 36. Casey KL, Beydoun A, Boivie J, *et al.* Laser-evoked cerebral potentials and sensory function in patients with central pain. *Pain* 1996; **64:** 485–91.

37. Sørensen J, Graven-Nielsen T, Henriksson KG, *et al.* Hyperexcitability in fibromyalgia. *J Rheumatol* 1998; **25:** 152–5.

38. Gibson SJ, Littlejohn GO, Gorman MM, *et al.* Altered heat pain threshold and cerebral event-related potentials following painful CO_2 laser stimulation in subjects with fibromyalgia syndrome. *Pain* 1994; **58:** 185–93.

39. Arendt-Nielsen L. First pain related evoked potentials to argon laser stimuli – recording and quantification. *J Neurol Neurosurg Psychiatry* 1990; **53:** 398–404.

40. Torebjörk HE. Afferent C units responding to mechanical, thermal and chemical stimuli in human non-glabrous skin. *Acta Physiol Scand* 1974; **92:** 374–90.

41. Cline MA, Ochoa JL, Torebjörk HE. Chronic hyperalgesia and warming of skin caused by sensitized C nociceptors and antidromic vasodilatation. *Brain* 1989; **112:** 621–47.

● 42. Arendt-Nielsen L. Induction and assessment of experimental pain from human skin, muscle and viscera. In: Jensen TS, Turner JA, Wiesenfeld-Hallin Z eds. *Proceedings of the 8th World Congress on Pain*. Seattle, WA: IASP Press, 1997: 393–425.

4

Pharmacological diagnostic tests

ANDREW P BARANOWSKI

Intravenous lidocaine (lignocaine)	40	Intravenous opioids	44
Intravenous phentolamine	42	References	45
Intravenous ketamine	43		

A pharmacological diagnostic test is usually a drug challenge in which a drug is administered intravenously over a relatively short period of time and titrated against a patient's pain. Different drugs are thought to act upon different pathophysiological mechanisms. Subjecting a patient to a range of drugs will help in understanding which mechanisms are important in an individual patient. Different drug groups may provide clues about treatments to which a patient may respond.

Pharmacological challenges may also be combined with quantitative sensory testing (QST) to enable alterations in sensory phenomena to be monitored. This combined approach has the potential of providing us with more information about the underlying pathophysiology than a drug challenge alone.[1] The combined approach may inform us about sensory changes that are occurring with the drug challenge independent of a reduction in pain. If a reduction in a sensory abnormality is detected by QST independent of a reduction in pain perception, it still has to be proven whether that drug group should be continued and a further agent should be added. The list of agents and their effects on different sensory abnormalities is growing.[2–5] Small doses of several different drugs may increase the chance of reducing pain with fewer side-effects. Also, several different drugs may be required to reduce all the sensory phenomena and hence the pain.

In this chapter, only intravenous drug challenges will be considered. Drug challenges may also be oral or spinal (epidural/intrathecal). In clinical practice, all drugs should be titrated against effect and side-effects.

Advantages of intravenous drug challenges

1 The effect of a potential treatment may be rapidly ascertained.

2 A number of potential treatments may be screened over a relatively short period of time.
3 "Clean" drugs with single modes of action may be used to provide very precise information about specific pathophysiological mechanisms.
4 Combining intravenous drug challenges with QST may yield information about the pathophysiological mechanisms and hence possible treatments.
5 Side-effects will be observed in a controlled environment and serious side-effects can be appropriately managed.
6 Blinding and double-blinding is possible and sometimes necessary.

Disadvantages of intravenous drug challenges

1 Side-effects may be more common as the drug is titrated up to a relatively high dose within a relatively short time. For instance, when establishing opioid sensitivity, oral medication may be titrated up over weeks with fewer side-effects than if the same plasma level were achieved during the short time frame of an intravenous drug challenge. This problem with side-effects may result in:
   a the benefit of a drug being missed;
   b the patient refusing a potentially helpful treatment because of concerns over side-effects.
2 Even within a particular drug group, different drugs may have different effects. As a consequence, using a single agent from a drug group may result in the potential benefits of another agent within that group being missed.
3 A positive result to an intravenous drug challenge does not always imply that the oral equivalent will be effective.

4 If the endpoint of the drug challenge is solely a reduction in pain, a potentially useful drug group may be missed.

5 Intravenous drug challenges are time-consuming.

6 Protocols vary from site to site and, as a result, the outcomes may be difficult to interpret.

INTRAVENOUS LIDOCAINE (LIGNOCAINE)***

Background

Nerve injury is associated with a reduction of some sodium channels and the development of novel sodium channels (downregulation of NaV1.8 and NaV1.9 sodium channels is associated with slow tetrodotoxin-resistant currents; upregulation of NaV1.3 sodium channels is associated with fast tetrodotoxin-sensitive currents). There is also a change in the distribution of these channels (cell body, dendrites, and tips of injured axons). The consequences of these changes are that injured cutaneous afferents become prone to generating more prolonged and higher frequency discharges. The refractory period is reduced. These changes in the characteristics of sodium channels are thought to underlie the mechanisms of mechanosensitivity, thermosensitivity, and chemosensitivity.[6]

Low doses of the sodium channel blocker lidocaine have been demonstrated in animal models of neuropathic pain to reduce spontaneous neuronal firing in a selective manner that does not block normal axonal firing.[7,8] Human studies have demonstrated that low plasma doses of lidocaine reduce neuropathic pain and sensory phenomena such as allodynia without an effect on nociceptive pain.[9] Nociceptive pain may be reduced with intravenous lidocaine, but only with high doses.

A positive lidocaine challenge may be followed by repeated infusions of lidocaine. Some of our patients have significant benefit from infusions for 3 months or so. A role for the oral analog mexiletine may also be defined,[10] however a positive result to intravenous (i.v.) lidocaine does not always indicate that mexiletine will work. In cancer patients, subcutaneous infusions of lidocaine may be used.[11]

Indications

An intravenous lidocaine trial is indicated in neuropathic pain and in pain where there is a suggestion of central sensitization, such as some of the visceral pains with referred muscle hyperalgesia and cutaneous hypersensitivity.[12–14] Also, some of the diffuse muscle pains such as fibromyalgia may benefit from repeated intravenous infusions.[15] Visual analog scale (VAS) scores should be greater than 5 on the day, and the pain scores should not fluctuate significantly over short periods of time.

Contraindications

- Absolute contraindications: failure to obtain patient consent and allergy to lidocaine.
- Relative contraindications: these depend on the dose and duration of infusion. Care should be taken with those patients that have a history of cardiac disease (particularly arrhythmias) or epilepsy. In such patients, the low-dose 4-hourly regimens could be considered (see below).

Doses and paradigms

Within the pain management center of the National Hospital for Neurology and Neurosurgery, London, UK, we have three different protocols:

1 *The bolus regimen*: 1 mg/kg lidocaine slow bolus (3 min); repeated after 15 min, up to three times (a maximum of 4 mg/kg over 60 min).

   a The bolus regimen can be used as a screening tool. The problem is that side-effects are common (see below). Also, the results may be debatable as the high plasma levels achieved may block different pathways to the low-dose regimen and may have a central cognitive effect associated with sedation.

   b Higher bolus doses of lidocaine have been given by other groups without complications, therefore we feel that in healthy patients the above regimen is safe:

      i Marchettini *et al.*[4] – 1.5 mg/kg as a single bolus over 60 s;

      ii Boas *et al.*[9] – 3 mg/kg over 3 min.[9] However, it must be noted that when Tucker and Boas[16] infused 3 mg/kg over 3 min toxic plasma levels in the range of 15 µg/ml were reached.

   If higher doses are used as repeated boluses, extreme care must be exercised as toxic peak levels may be reached because of accumulation.

2 *Short infusion regimen*: 3 mg/kg lidocaine over 1 h using an infusion pump.

   a Higher doses have been given by other groups:

      i Rowbotham *et al.*[17] – 5 mg/kg over 1 h, maximum 450 mg, all patients achieved plasma levels > 1 µg/ml, the maximum being 4.8 µg/ml (please see below for relevance).

      ii McQuay and Moore[18] stated that "The best documented effective dose of intravenous lidocaine was 5 mg/kg, which was well tolerated when infused over 30 minutes."

      iii In our paper,[12] we reported on an infusion of 5 mg/kg over 2 h; at 1 h, plasma levels as high as

10 μg/ml were seen (see below). Caution must therefore be exercised with higher doses.

3 *Four-hour infusion*: 2 mg/kg over 4 h by infusion pump.

   a In our paper,[12] we also reported an infusion of 1 mg/kg over 2 h. All patients achieved plasma levels > 1 μg/ml after 15 min or so, with a maximum of 2 μg/ml [± standard error of the mean (s.e.m.) 0.6] at 2 h.

   b This is a relatively safe technique and should be considered the method of choice in those patients for whom there is concern about epilepsy or cardiac disease.

   c We have extended the duration of infusion from 2 to 4 h as we feel that the longer the infusion the better the result.[12,19]

Key points

- Plasma levels of 1–2 μg/ml appear to be adequate for a reduction in neuropathic pain.
- All patients should be "nil by mouth" for the procedure. With the 4-h infusion method, we normally feed patients after 1 h of the infusion as we feel that toxicity is unlikely and our main reason for starving relates to the rare incidence of lidocaine allergy. Diabetic patients are often not starved for the 4-h 2 mg/kg infusion.
- Informed, written consent is obtained.
- It is the 4-h 2 mg/kg infusion that we routinely use on the ward for inpatients. In that case, the doctor setting up the infusion is only with the patient for the first 30 min and ward staff monitor thereafter.
- Full monitoring [electrocardiograph (EKG), blood pressure (BP), and oxygen saturation (SpO$_2$)] is instigated. In the bolus regimen, BP is measured every 5 min for the duration of the test and 30 min after the last bolus. For the infusion techniques, BP is measured every 5 min for 30 min, then every 15 min for the duration of the infusion. EKG and oxygen saturation monitoring is continuous.
- Lidocaine is diluted with saline to a volume that is easy for the pump to infuse, e.g. 60 ml.
- Pain scores [VAS, short-form McGill Pain Questionnaire (MPQ) or some alternative] should be measured every 15 min or so.
- If QST is employed, it is used before and just after the infusion.
- Following a positive response to intravenous lidocaine, some patients obtain significant benefit associated with repeated infusions of lidocaine. We currently run a nurse-led clinic where some patients return every 3 months for their intravenous lidocaine infusion.
- The correlation of benefit to the patient between oral mexiletine and intravenous lidocaine is not clear.[20] However, following a positive lidocaine infusion, it

is traditional for a patient to try oral mexiletine. The author would normally start with mexiletine 50 mg and titrate up to mexiletine 10 mg/kg/day (see within for other regimens).

Side-effects and their management

- Idiosyncratic reactions[21] are rare and are managed as for any allergic response.
- Most side-effects are dose related.[16,22] This makes the procedure very safe if performed with caution. Heart failure and increasing age may result in an accumulation of lidocaine, resulting in an increased risk of toxicity.
  - For neuropathic pain, therapeutic plasma levels appear to be 1–2 μg/ml.[12,19,20]
  - Light-headedness, feeling drunk, and sedation occur at around 4–5 μg/ml. Other minor, subjective, central nervous system (CNS) symptoms may occur, such as circumoral numbness, dizziness, and tinnitus.
  - Serious neurotoxicity is felt to occur at levels of 10–15 μg/ml, and minor CNS symptoms should warn of the risk of the more serious convulsions.
  - Cardiac side-effects due to the lidocaine, such as heart block, asystole, and negative inotropic effects, have been reported. These are usually associated with large doses of lidocaine administered over a short period of time, with children and the elderly, and with patients with severe cardiac disease. Convulsions and hypoxia may contribute to these cardiac events. Early treatment of convulsions and hypoxia may prevent cardiac complications.

Pharmaceutical considerations

Lidocaine (xylocaine) 1% is equivalent to 10 mg/ml of lidocaine.

Practical tips

Lidocaine should be diluted in saline to a volume that makes calculation of the infusion rate easy, e.g. 60 ml. Ensure that the lidocaine and saline are carefully and adequately mixed. All infusions should be labeled and used immediately.

Efficacy

Evidence shows that intravenous lidocaine is most effective for peripheral nerve injury.[18] It can also be tried for all conditions of neuropathic pain or where central sensitization may be present. Intravenous lidocaine may reduce muscular pain, such as that associated with fibromyalgia.

Key points

- Intravenous lidocaine may indicate that an oral analog of lidocaine (e.g. mexiletine) could be helpful in managing a patient's pain.
- Repeated doses of intravenous lidocaine may also be helpful for pain management.
- Intravenous lidocaine is known to be safe if used judiciously and with care.

INTRAVENOUS PHENTOLAMINE**

Background

Animal models of neuropathic pain[23,24] and the capsaicin model in humans[25] have indicated that the sympathetic nervous system may be involved in the development and maintenance of pain. Intravenous phentolamine has been shown to produce pain relief in some patients with chronic, nonacute pain.[26–29] In early studies, approximately 50% of patients with reflex sympathetic dystrophy (RSD) were thought to have sympathetically maintained pain (SMP), as determined by an intravenous phentolamine test (where the RSD was probably equivalent to complex regional pain syndrome type I).[27] Pain conditions other than the CRPSs may also exhibit sympathetic maintenance.

Interestingly, the reduction in pain associated with intravenous phentolamine may persist even after phentolamine has theoretically been eliminated from the body.[28] Also, the onset of pain relief may be hours or even days after the infusion has ended. There is a complex relationship between the results of an active infusion and a placebo infusion. Some authors are now disputing the results of intravenous phentolamine infusion trials and suggesting that the results are due to the placebo response.[30–33]

There are other ways of investigating whether or not a pain is sympathetically maintained than intravenous phentolamine. However, these other tests have their own problems. For instance, local anesthetic sympathetic trunk blocks (including stellate ganglion blockade) may block somatic afferent input. They may also be associated with significant systemic levels of the local anesthetic being achieved. Both of these may result in false-positive tests. A regional intravenous guanethidine block (with tourniquet cuff applied to the proximal part of a limb) cannot be used to investigate whether a pain is sympathetically maintained. Such blocks are often associated with the tourniquet cuff producing a pressure blockade of the Aβ afferent neurons, which would reduce the phenomenon of allodynia. Also, over a period of time, Aδ- and C-fiber acute nociceptive afferents would also be blocked by the pressure of the cuff. Finally, the procedure often involves the use of local anesthetic that would modify the pain pathways both peripherally and centrally.

Indications

Complex regional pain syndromes types I and II are the principal indications. The test may be used to investigate many other pains, including central neuropathic pain, visceral pain, and myofascial pains. VAS scores should be greater than 50 out of a 100 on the day, and the pain scores should not fluctuate significantly over short periods of time.

Contraindications

These include conditions where hypotension may be detrimental, e.g. ischemic heart disease and cerebral vascular disease. Asthma/bronchospasm may be considered a relative contraindication as intravenous propranolol may also be required. Patients who cannot lie supine should also be excluded. Care should be exercised with patients that have peripheral vascular disease.

Doses and paradigms

At our pain management center, we use a modified version of the Baltimore protocol:[34]

1. phentolamine 0.5 mg/kg over 20 min for frail patients;
2. phentolamine 1 mg/kg over 10 min for fit patients.

Key points

- All patients should be "nil by mouth" for the procedure and provide informed, written consent.
- Full monitoring is instigated (EKG, BP, SpO_2), with BP every 5 min. EKG and saturation monitoring are continuous. Monitoring should be continued until observations have returned to baseline with no postural hypotension and for at least 0.5 h after the last of the phentolamine has been infused.
- The patient lies flat during the infusion phase.
- An intravenous solution of sodium lactate intravenous compound (Hartman solution) or saline is instigated (4–8 ml/kg). The intravenous line should be long enough so that, with a three-way tap, intravenous injections may be given to a patient without the patient knowing the exact timing of injection of the individual agents.
- Pain scores (VAS, short-form MPQ or some alternative) should be measured every 5 min during the test and for 30 min after the last dose of phentolamine.

- After 15 min of the Hartman/saline infusion and measuring baseline pain scores, 1–2 mg of propranolol is given as a slow intravenous injection.
- Ten minutes after the intravenous propranolol, phentolamine is infused according to the above dose regimen.
- Significant hypotension is unusual if the patient is fit and recumbent. However, if a fall in blood pressure does occur, it is usually treated with intravenous infusions as appropriate. Care on mobilizing the patient must be exercised, in view of the risk of postural hypotension.
- QST may be combined with the phentolamine test. Cold allodynia is said to be associated with SMP,[35] and in our laboratory we have seen cold allodynia resolved with the phentolamine test.

Side-effects and their management[36]

- Propranolol may result in bradycardia and possibly cardiac failure. Peripheral vascular disease may also be exacerbated. Bronchospasm is a real risk in asthmatics.
- Phentolamine will cause significant hypotension, which can be prevented by the patient adopting a reclined posture and receiving intravenous solutions. Without propranolol, the patient will develop tachycardia.

Pharmaceutical considerations (including trade names)

Phentolamine (Rogitine, Regitine) 10 mg/ml in 1 ml ampoules. Dilute to a manageable volume with saline 0.9%.

Practical tips

Both propranolol and the saline infusion prior to phentolamine serve as a placebo as well as preventing the side-effects (hypotension and tachycardia). The injections should be given blind to the patient, hence the need for an intravenous drip extension with a three-way tap. A positive phentolamine test occurs when there is a significant fall in pain (30–50%) associated with the phentolamine and not the placebo infusion or propranolol.

Efficacy

There is still some disagreement about whether pain can be maintained by the sympathetic nervous system.[32,33] Despite this, the author feels that the test is useful and that it helps to identify a group of patients that may respond to other types of sympathetic blockade. We will continue to use the test in our pain management center until further evidence is available.

Key points

- In certain pain conditions, the pain may be maintained by the sympathetic nervous system. Blocking the sympathetic system may reduce the perceived pain.
- Transient blockade of the sympathetic system by means of an intravenous phentolamine test is a specific method of investigating whether a pain is sympathetically maintained.

INTRAVENOUS KETAMINE**

Background

The N-methyl-D-aspartate (NMDA) receptor channel complex is known to be an important channel for the development and maintenance of chronic pain. It is felt to be particularly important when there is evidence for central sensitization and opioid tolerance.[37]

Ketamine has been used as a general anesthetic for over 30 years. It has also been used as an intravenous analgesic in burns units and accident and emergency units. Ketamine is thought to act primarily at the NMDA receptor, although it may also have actions at sodium channels and at kappa and mu opioid receptors.[38]

Ketamine has been shown in animal models of neuropathic pain to reduce central sensitization and windup (see above).

Ketamine has been found to be useful in a number of chronic pain states, including peripheral neuropathies with allodynia, stump and phantom pain, central pain, and cancer-related pain with and without a neurological component.[39–43] Ketamine may be useful in opioid-resistant pain in which the ketamine may restore the opioid dose–response curve toward normal.[40,44]

Oral ketamine has a bioavailability of about 17% (see below). An intravenous infusion test dose is a quick way of establishing whether or not oral ketamine may be viable. Certain chronic pain patients, especially those with cancer pain, may be sent home on an infusion of ketamine, which may be either subcutaneous or intravenous. Ketamine is a drug which is associated with abuse potential, and great care must be exercised if a patient is to be managed at home on parenteral ketamine.

Indications

- Neuropathic pain states and patients with pain that is resistant to opioids.

- Cancer pain patients: particularly in the terminal stages and patients with head and neck cancer (airway maintenance).

Contraindications

These include hypertension, cardiac disease, and psychotic states. Swallowing problems may be a relative contraindication in view of increased salivation.

Doses and paradigms

- All patients should be "nil by mouth" for the procedure and provide informed, written consent.
- Full monitoring is instigated (EKG, BP, SpO_2), with BP checked every 5 min. EKG and saturation monitoring are continuous. Monitoring should be continued until observations have returned to baseline; normally, this would be for 1 h after the end of the infusion.
- Intravenous access is established, and a syringe driver is set up to deliver ketamine 0.15 mg/kg over 20 min. Normally, ketamine is diluted to 20 ml with saline; we use a 60-ml syringe and infuse at a rate of 60 ml/h.
- Pain scores (VAS, short-form MPQ, or some alternative) should be measured every 5 min during the test, and for 30 min after the last dose of ketamine.
- QST may be combined with the ketamine test.
- The test is terminated if:
  - the pain is abolished completely or the VAS score is less than 20/100.
  - The patient experiences dysphoria or extreme drowsiness.
  - BP becomes greater than 30% of baseline.
- The patient may be discharged 1 h after the end of the infusion providing observations have returned to normal/baseline and there are no residual central nervous system effects.
- If the patient has a significant reduction in pain and minimal side-effects, oral ketamine may be substituted. The calculation for the dose is difficult. In general, the final oral dose of ketamine is calculated by taking into account the dose infused to provide analgesia and the variable bioavailability of oral ketamine, which is between 10% and 20% of the intravenous dose. However, the usual starting dose of oral ketamine is a maximum of about 100 mg/day,[45] the final dose being arrived at by careful titration. Some patients may not even tolerate 100 mg/day.

Side-effects and their management

Tachycardia and hypertension may result in the test being abandoned. Hallucinations and psychotic states may also be a problem. These side-effects are usually curtailed by stopping the infusion, but may continue for many hours.[46] Hypersalivation may also be a problem.

Pharmaceutical considerations (including trade names)

Ketamine (Ketalar) infusions may be diluted with 5% glucose or normal saline. Note, ketamine is a general anesthetic agent, so overdose will result in an anesthetized patient!

Practical tips

A small dose of atropine or glycopyrrolate may reduce the salivation. Psychotic states may respond to midazolam.

Key points

- Ketamine is a general anesthetic. However, in lower doses it has good analgesic properties.
- Ketamine is an NMDA antagonist and appears to reduce secondary hyperalgesia by a mechanism independent of opioid antagonism.
- An intravenous drug trial of ketamine may be used to determine whether oral ketamine may be of benefit to a patient.
- Oral bioavailability is variable and care must be taken when calculating an oral dose of ketamine from an intravenous dose. Start oral ketamine judiciously.

INTRAVENOUS OPIOIDS**

Background

Opioids are well recognized as having an important role in the management of acute pain. In nonacute pain, the role of opioids is more debatable. If opioids are to be used in nonacute pain conditions, it is important that the efficacy be proven. Prescribing opioids to a patient with an opioid-insensitive pain may not only produce unnecessary side-effects but also predispose the patient to opioid addictive behavior.

Neuropathic pains *may* be insensitive to opioids, although this may be a relative phenomenon in which large doses of opioids may produce an analgesic response but side-effects are limiting.[47] Certain opioids may be more beneficial in neuropathic pains than others. For instance, methadone is thought to have NMDA receptor antagonist properties.[48] Such activity may be advantageous in the management of neuropathic pains. It must also be remembered that whereas the neuropathic component of a patient's pain may be relatively unresponsive to an opioid, the nociceptive component, frequently also present, will be responsive.

Intravenous opioid drug challenges are notoriously difficult to perform. Side-effects may interfere with the test if the opioid is administered *too quickly* and the potential benefits from the opioid may be missed. Also, there is some debate about which opioid should be used. Should a placebo also be given and should the opioid be reversed with naloxone? There is an argument that, even if the intravenous opioid test is positive, an oral opioid test must be carried out before the patient is started on prolonged oral opioid treatments.

Indication

Nonacute pains that are not responsive to other treatments.

Contraindication

- Opioid sensitivity and allergy; drug addiction.
- Relative contraindications include: a past history of drug addiction and patients with severe respiratory disease.

Doses and paradigms

- *Morphine*: the patient may need to be an inpatient. The Oxford group[47,49] have used a patient-controlled analgesia system with nurse/observer measurement of analgesia, mood, and adverse effects.
- *Alfentanyl*: in patients without previous exposure to strong opioids, we normally inject 100-µg aliquots every minute up to a maximum of 1,000 µg (10 times 100-µg aliquots). Each incremental dose is given in the absence of effect or side-effects. Higher doses may be required in patients either taking opioids or with a history of previous exposure to opioids. Higher doses may also be given in the absence of effect or side-effects.
- Intravenous access is obtained and oxygen supplementation is applied, as is full monitoring, including measurement of the patient's oxygen saturation. Falls in oxygen saturation may occur late, and monitoring of depth and frequency of respiratory effort as well as levels of consciousness is mandatory. VAS scores should be measured prior to each increment. It may be necessary to have different VAS measurements for different components of the patient's pain.
- Reversal with naloxone should be contemplated in patients not routinely on maintenance opioids. We would normally inject naloxone 100 µg intravenously every minute to a total of 400 µg in the absence of a positive response (i.e. return of VAS to baseline).

Side-effects and their management

The principal side-effect is respiratory depression. Only personnel trained in the recognition and treatment of respiratory depression should perform the procedure. Full monitoring, resuscitation equipment, and naloxone must be available.

Practical tips

As a placebo, low-dose intravenous benzodiazepine could be considered. The effects of the benzodiazepine could be reversed with flumazenil (Anexate) as a part of the test.

Key points

- Opioids may have an important role in the management of chronic pain. Some form of opioid challenge (oral or intravenous) should be instigated prior to starting regular oral opioids.
- Only an appropriately trained person, with full monitoring and resuscitation equipment available to them, should undertake the opioid challenge.
- Different opioids may have different effects and side-effects.

REFERENCES

- 1. Woolf CJ, Bennett GJ, Doherty M, *et al.* Towards a mechanism-based classification of pain? [editorial]. *Pain* 1998; **77**: 227–9.
2. Gottrup H, Hansen PO, Arendt-Nielsen L, Jensen TS. Differential effects of systemically administered ketamine and lidocaine on dynamic and static hyperalgesia induced by intradermal capsaicin in humans. *Br J Anaesth* 2000; **84**: 155–62.
3. Park KM, Max MB, Robinovitz E, *et al.* Effects of intravenous ketamine, alfentanil, or placebo on pain, pinprick hyperalgesia, and allodynia produced by intradermal capsaicin in human subjects. *Pain* 1995; **63**: 163–72.
4. Marchettini P, Lacerenza M, Marangoni C, *et al.* Lidocaine test in neuralgia. *Pain* 1992; **48**: 377–82.
5. Attal N, Nicholson B, Serra J eds. *New Directions in Neuropathic Pain: Focusing Treatment on Symptoms and Mechanisms.* Worcester: Royal Society of Medicine Press, 2000.
6. Cummins T, Dib-Hajj S, Black J, *et al.* Sodium channels as molecular targets in pain. In: Devor M, Rowbotham M, Wiesenfeld-Hallin Z eds. *Proceedings of the 9th World Congress on Pain*, vol. 8. Seattle, WA: IASP, 2000: 77–91.
7. Chabal C, Russell LC, Burchiel KJ. The effect of intravenous lidocaine, tocainide, and mexiletine on spontaneously active fibers originating in rat sciatic neuromas. *Pain* 1989; **38**: 333–8.

8. Woolf CJ, Wiesenfeld-Hallin Z. The systemic administration of local anaesthetics produces a selective depression of C-afferent fibre evoked activity in the spinal cord. *Pain* 1985; **23**: 361–74.

9. Boas RA, Covino BG, Shahnarian A. Analgesic responses to i.v. lignocaine. *Br J Anaesth* 1982; **54**: 501–5.

10. Galer BS, Harle J, Rowbotham MC. Response to intravenous lidocaine infusion predicts subsequent response to oral mexiletine: a prospective study. *J Pain Symptom Manage* 1996; **12**: 161–7.

11. Brose WG, Cousins MJ. Subcutaneous lidocaine for treatment of neuropathic cancer pain. *Pain* 1991; **45**: 145–8.

12. Baranowski AP, De Courcey J, Bonello E. A trial of intravenous lidocaine on the pain and allodynia of postherpetic neuralgia. *J Pain Symptom Manage* 1999; **17**: 429–33.

13. Ferrante FM, Paggioli J, Cherukuri S, Arthur GR. The analgesic response to intravenous lidocaine in the treatment of neuropathic pain. *Anesth Analg* 1996; **82**: 91–7.

14. Nagaro T, Shimizu C, Inoue H, *et al.* The efficacy of intravenous lidocaine on various types of neuropathic pain [in Japanese]. *Masui Jpn J Anesthesiol* 1995; **44**: 862–7.

15. Bennett MI, Tai YM, Galer BS, *et al* Intravenous lignocaine in the management of primary fibromyalgia syndrome. Response to intravenous lidocaine infusion predicts subsequent response to oral mexiletine: a prospective study. *Int J Clin Pharmacol Res* 1995; **15**: 115–19.

16. Tucker GT, Boas RA. Pharmacokinetic aspects of intravenous regional anesthesia. *Anesthesiology* 1971; **34**: 538–49.

17. Rowbotham MC, Reisner-Keller LA, Fields HL. Both intravenous lidocaine and morphine reduce the pain of postherpetic neuralgia. *Neurology* 1991; **41**: 1024–8.

18. McQuay HJ, Moore RA. Systemic local anaesthetic-type drugs in chronic pain. In: McQuay HJ, Moore RA eds. *An Evidence-based Resource for Pain Relief*. Oxford: Oxford University Press, 1999: 242–8.

19. Ferrante FM, Paggioli J, Cherukuri S, Arthur GR. The analgesic response to intravenous lidocaine in the treatment of neuropathic pain. *Anesth Analg* 1996; **82**: 91–7.

20. Galer BS, Harle J, Rowbotham MC. Response to intravenous lidocaine infusion predicts subsequent response to oral mexiletine: a prospective study. *J Pain Symptom Manage* 1996; **12**: 161–7.

21. Wallace MS, Dyck JB, Rossi SS, *et al.* Computer-controlled lidocaine infusion for the evaluation of neuropathic pain after peripheral nerve injury. The analgesic response to intravenous lidocaine in the treatment of neuropathic pain. Anaphylactic shock following intravenous administration of lignocaine. *Pain* 1996; **66**: 69–77.

22. Tucker GT, Mather LE. Clinical pharmacokinetics of local anaesthetics. *Clin Pharmacokinet* 1979; **4**: 241–78.

23. Baron R. Peripheral neuropathic pain: from mechanisms to symptoms. *Clin J Pain* 2000; **16** (Suppl. 2): S12–20.

24. Ramer MS, Thompson SW, McMahon SB. Causes and consequences of sympathetic basket formation in dorsal root ganglia. *Pain* 1999; 6 (Suppl.): S111–20.

25. Kinnman E, Nygards EB, Hansson P. Peripheral alpha-adrenoreceptors are involved in the development of capsaicin induced ongoing and stimulus evoked pain in humans. *Pain* 1997; **69**: 79–85.

26. Dellemijn PL, Fields HL, Allen RR, *et al.* The interpretation of pain relief and sensory changes following sympathetic blockade. *Brain* 1994; **117** (Part 6): 1475–87.

27. Arner S. Intravenous phentolamine test: diagnostic and prognostic use in reflex sympathetic dystrophy. *Pain* 1991; **46**: 17–22.

28. Galer BS. Peak pain relief is delayed and duration of relief is extended following intravenous phentolamine infusion. Preliminary report. *Reg Anesth* 1995; **20**: 444–7.

29. Raja SN, Treede RD, Davis KD, Campbell JN. Systemic alpha-adrenergic blockade with phentolamine: a diagnostic test for sympathetically maintained pain. *Anesthesiology* 1991; **74**: 691–8.

30. Dotson RM. Causalgia–reflex sympathetic dystrophy–sympathetically maintained pain: myth and reality. *Muscle Nerve* 1993; **16**: 1049–55.

31. Fine PG, Roberts WJ, Gillette RG, Child TR. Slowly developing placebo responses confound tests of intravenous phentolamine to determine mechanisms underlying idiopathic chronic low back pain. *Pain* 1994; **56**: 235–42.

32. Verdugo RJ, Ochoa JL. "Sympathetically maintained pain." I. Phentolamine block questions the concept [see comments]. *Neurology* 1994; **44**: 1003–10.

33. Verdugo RJ, Campero M, Ochoa JL. Phentolamine sympathetic block in painful polyneuropathies. II. Further questioning of the concept of "sympathetically maintained pain". *Neurology* 1994; **44**: 1010–14.

34. Raja SN, Turnquist JL, Meleka S, Campbell JN. Monitoring adequacy of alpha-adrenoceptor blockade following systemic phentolamine administration. *Pain* 1996; **64**: 197–204.

35. Choi Y, Yoon YW, Na HS, *et al.* Behavioral signs of ongoing pain and cold allodynia in a rat model of neuropathic pain. Effects of short-acting NMDA receptor antagonist MRZ 2/576 on morphine tolerance development in mice. *Pain* 1994; **59**: 369–76.

36. Shir Y, Cameron LB, Raja SN, Bourke DL. The safety of intravenous phentolamine administration in patients with neuropathic pain. *Anesth Analg* 1993; **76**: 1008–11.

37. Price DD, Mayer DJ, Mao J, Caruso FS. NMDA-receptor antagonists and opioid receptor interactions as related to analgesia and tolerance. *J Pain Symptom Manage*

2000; **19** (Suppl. 1): S7–11.

38. Mikkelsen S, Ilkjaer S, Brennum J, *et al*. The effect of naloxone on ketamine-induced effects on hyperalgesia and ketamine-induced side effects in humans. *Anesthesiology* 1999; **90:** 1539–45.

39. Backonja M, Arndt G, Gombar KA, *et al*. Response of chronic neuropathic pain syndromes to ketamine: a preliminary study [published erratum appears in *Pain* 1994; **58:** 433]. *Pain* 1994; **56:** 51–7.

◆ 40. Eide PK, Jorum E, Stubhaug A, *et al*. Relief of postherpetic neuralgia with the *N*-methyl-D-aspartic acid receptor antagonist ketamine: a double-blind, crossover comparison with morphine and placebo. *Pain* 1994; **58:** 347–54.

41. Eide PK, Stubhaug A, Stenehjem AE. Central dysesthesia pain after traumatic spinal cord injury is dependent on *N*-methyl-D-aspartate receptor activation. *Neurosurgery* 1995; **37:** 1080–7.

◆ 42. Graven-Nielsen T, Aspegren KS, Henriksson KG, *et al*. Ketamine reduces muscle pain, temporal summation, and referred pain in fibromyalgia patients. *Pain* 2000; **85:** 483–91.

43. Sorensen J, Bengtsson A, Backman E, *et al*. Pain analysis in patients with fibromyalgia. Effects of intravenous morphine, lidocaine, and ketamine. *Scand J Rheumatol* 1995; **24:** 360–5.

● 44. Dickenson AH. Neurophysiology of opioid poorly responsive pain. *Cancer Surv* 1994; 21: 5–16.

45. Enarson MC, Hays H, Woodroffe MA. Clinical experience with oral ketamine. *J Pain Symptom Manage* 1999; **17:** 384–6.

46. Max MB, Byas-Smith MG, Gracely RH, Bennett GJ. Intravenous infusion of the NMDA antagonist, ketamine, in chronic posttraumatic pain with allodynia: a double-blind comparison to alfentanil and placebo. *Clin Neuropharmacol* 1995; **18:** 360–8.

◆ 47. Jadad AR, Carroll D, Glynn CJ, *et al*. Morphine responsiveness of chronic pain: double-blind randomised crossover study with patient-controlled analgesia. *Lancet* 1992; **339:** 1367–71.

48. Ebert B, Thorkildsen C, Andersen S, *et al*. Opioid analgesics as noncompetitive *N*-methyl-D-aspartate (NMDA) antagonists. *Biochem Pharmacol* 1998; **56:** 553–9.

49. McQuay HJ, Jadad AR, Carroll D, *et al*. Opioid sensitivity of chronic pain: a patient-controlled analgesia method. *Anaesthesia* 1992; **47:** 757–67.

5

Nerve blocks in pain diagnosis

ROBERT A BOAS

History	49	Response patterns	52
Scope of nerve blocks in pain diagnosis	50	Response interpretation	54
Patient selection and preparation	50	Prognostic interpretation of diagnostic blocks	55
Procedural guidelines	51	Conclusions	55
Response assessments and outcome monitoring	51	References	55

The value of nerve blocks in pain diagnosis is to determine the source of pain and define anatomical correlates of clinical pain disorders.

When patients are referred with diagnoses of neck pain, low back pain, abdominal pain, or shoulder pain as the problem requiring treatment, further diagnostic evaluations, as exemplified by Bogduk,[1] have demonstrated that nerve blocks can add to both the anatomical and pathological diagnosis of many such disorders. This pertains even when extensive imaging, laboratory testing, or surgical exploration have been negative. A case will be made for greater use of diagnostic blocks in refractory or poorly defined pain disorders, seeking to bring a diverse range of procedures and their application to a set of enduring principles. In this context, two outstanding difficulties arise with the use of diagnostic local anesthetic blocks. First, these procedures require precision in their conduct. Such precision should ideally approach 100%, seeking to eliminate error in the placement and spread of local anesthetic solution. Precision equates with reproducibility, thereby promoting maximum sensitivity of diagnostic blocks.

Second, interpretation of block response is predicated on objective assessment of outcome. Multifunctional assessment and high clinical skills are needed to establish specificity of any conclusion. Validation for such interpretation still falls short of modern demands for evidence-based "best practice," which in the absence of a gold standard by which to judge the value of diagnostic blocks is reduced to one of supposedly "rational strategy" as the basis of practice. This chapter will endeavor to promote good technique in the conduct of diagnostic blocks and encourage the disciplines required in evaluating the outcome and appropriate interpretation of such blocks.

Within such advocacy lie the pitfalls of many procedurally based teachings that have difficulty in meeting the demands of balanced care and patient sensitivity while also providing treatments that have proven efficacy. Nor have there been any symposia or multicenter studies on this topic, and there is little in the way of guidelines or consensus criteria. Because of these challenges and the need to avoid dogma, an analysis of both the benefits and the pitfalls is offered in the hope of providing guidance, validity, and balance for those who use or wish to embark on the use of diagnostic blocks in their quest for better pain management.

HISTORY

Several early texts on regional anesthesia included advocacy of therapeutic blocks in the treatment of pain, some suggesting diagnostic utility for these same procedures, particularly with spinal and sympathetic blockade. Bonica combined much of this original work with that of his classic ground-breaking textbook on pain to produce an additional monograph on diagnostic and therapeutic nerve blocks that set the standard for all who followed.[2] Others have given a renewed impetus to diagnostic blocks with emphasis on sympathetic blockade,[3]*** facet joint injections,[4] and nerve blocks[5] sufficient to provide maturity, depth, and understanding to the issues involved. The reviews by Hogan and Abram[6,7]*** form the current benchmark writing on the subject. In spite of this shift to a more critical analysis, particularly within the interpretation of diagnostic blocks, much uncertainty persists in a sparse literature on the subject.

SCOPE OF NERVE BLOCKS IN PAIN DIAGNOSIS

Almost any regional pain disorder is amenable to diagnostic blocks, but modern imaging techniques have given such precision to soft-tissue and body structures that the role of nerve blocks in pain diagnosis is diminishing. Those where blocks can still be relevant are in somatic soft tissues, sites of previous injury or surgery, and in some of the complex pain disorders about the vertebral axis. One application rarely discussed but providing critical distinction is at a central spinal level, where segmental block is capable of determining the segmental or higher level of neuronal discharge that may be responsible for central pain states. Suppose a patient has severe perineal pain following rectal excision for carcinoma. If a dense saddle block spinal anesthetic to a T12 level fails to relieve pain, it could be safely assumed that the pain is arising primarily from a spinal cord level or higher. The same process can discern peripheral from central components of other chronic pain, as occurs in some complex regional pain syndrome (CRPS) disorders.

Some of the relatively simple but rewarding examples for the use of diagnostic blocks are for the diagnosis and treatment of postherniorrhaphy pain, in which entrapment of the ilioinguinal or genitofemoral nerves can cause severe and distressing groin pains. Similar scar entrapments are encountered following gynecological procedures. Other postoperative examples can involve the cutaneous branches of the cervical plexus, branches of the subcostal nerve following classical gallbladder incisions or dorsal approaches to the kidney, and breast reconstruction or even biopsy procedures. Post-thoracotomy pains can also arise because of entrapment, injury, or severance of intercostal nerves. Injury or arthroscopy surgery can create anterior knee pain with damage to the infrapatellar nerve. Direct nerve entrapment between muscle sheaths is dramatically identified and treated in cases of greater occipital nerve entrapment and in cases of lower abdominal pains with compression of the iliohypogastric nerve at the lateral edge of the rectus sheath. This condition of abdominal cutaneous nerve entrapment syndrome can yield simple and dramatic resolution of pains that have previously defied surgery and extensive imaging studies. A broad depiction of the overall utility of diagnostic blocks is presented in Table 5.1. These applications are essentially self-evident in their presentation and will not be elaborated on as they are thoroughly detailed in the review papers cited.[6]

An additional, more specific listing of procedures (Table 5.2) is indicative of the range of blocks available, encompassing most commonly described blocks and even others that are not depicted in usual textbook descriptions. Sometimes, a clinical presentation is encountered which is beyond previous experiences. Such cases may demand a more entrepreneurial approach and perhaps the deployment of skills founded on anatomical and physiological principles, rather than on a prescriptive text-based technique. Fortunately, the advent of postoperative pain services and the training requirements for pain in specialist certification have given renewed impetus and opportunity to skill acquisition in this area.

PATIENT SELECTION AND PREPARATION

Patients should have proceeded through a normal workup within the discipline appropriate to their pain disorder and have failed to obtain either a formal diagnosis or responded to standard treatments. An ability to understand and express some of the language nuances required in presenting their problem for consent and more importantly for subsequent evaluation is another criterion for patient inclusion. Their pain needs to be reasonably consistent over time and free of analgesic cover during the course of the block, and they should be willing to proceed through a series of block procedures if required. If anxiety is a problem, sedatives as for anesthesia premedication may be needed, but the use of small doses of intravenous midazolam just prior to the block itself gives amnesia and improves patient well-being.

Table 5.1 *Scope of nerve blocks*

Anatomical/structural localization of nociceptive source
Identifying the extent of sympathetic pain component
Separation of somatic from visceral pain
Separation of local disease from referred pain
Establishing nerve, dermatomal, and segmental levels of nociception
Identifying the extent and anatomical level of pain centralization
Helping to determine longer term outcome to block procedures
Determining range of motion and function testing in the absence of pain

Table 5.2 *Sites for diagnostic nerve blocks*

Trigger points and tender points in fibromyalgia and myofascial pain syndromes
Capsule, ligaments, and tendons about sites of joint pain
Intra-articular injections, and/or articular nerve supply
Scars, as indicative of postsurgical or post-traumatic nerve entrapment
Peripheral nerves involved in compression/irritation or possible neuroma formation
Paravertebral nerve block
Plexus blocks to limbs or regions of the body
Sympathetic ganglia or plexus blocks
Epidural and intrathecal blocks
Splanchnic/celiac block and hypogastric plexus block

Superficial and painful body wall disorders can be assessed in a clinic or office setting with little special preparation. Complex cases involving the vertebral column or sympathetic system require the facilities of a hospital or, for some, even a tertiary referral center. Training in behavioral and functional evaluation beyond the range of usual anesthetic experience is also important to any response analysis, ensuring a well-informed outcome assessment.

PROCEDURAL GUIDELINES

The recommendations from the International Spinal Injection Society[8] provide a standard that should meet wide acceptance. Although these apply to vertebral joint injections, they meet similar needs and disciplines as for other procedures and are recommended in their entirety. Perhaps the only point of contention lies in the use of saline injections as a means to minimize placebo-reactive interpretations giving false-positive diagnoses. A more detailed alternative approach is presented later under discussion of placebo reactivity in general. Other more basic considerations are presented in Table 5.3.

One issue deserving special mention is that of block validation. This entails more than the usual needle placement, as in regional anesthesia techniques. Several "endpoints" of success need to be ascertained, with imaging studies providing the most specific means of determining needle-point placement and, more importantly, the spread of anesthetic solution. Incorporation of contrast medium with, or in sequence with, local anesthetic gives precise limits of solution spread and allows for a hard copy of this outcome to be incorporated in the patient's record. Image-intensified portable radiograph equipment is a readily available resource for this purpose and provides an additional learning tool for even the most experienced practitioner. Unless some form of accurate monitoring is employed, failure rates of up to 40% are reported for difficult procedures, even in the best of hands. For procedures such as vertebral facet, paravertebral, sympathetic, sacroiliac, or blocks in patients with difficult anatomy, imaging assistance is critical. This approach should be considered to be as important as in orthopedic practice, which demands similar confirma-

Table 5.3 *Procedural guidelines*

Use quick onset/short-duration local anesthetic agents
Use small volume injections ± radio-opaque dye
Gentle, minimum needling pain in performance of blocks
Use clear predetermined endpoints to confirm block
Patient monitoring and care provided by nonoperator staff member
Block performed by experienced and skilled staff
Use imaging tools to aid or confirm accuracy

tion of outcome. Just as important is the availability of real-time visualization of solution spread, with the added benefit of minimizing hazardous reactions with intravascular injection. Ultimately, the development of a specific local anesthetic block effect confirms the correct functional outcome.

In terms of the conduct of the block and the equally critical clinical testing, a suggested procedural sequence is advised to facilitate achievement of relevant outcome responses.

1 Conduct a clinical examination and scoring of symptoms/signs relevant to the pain disorder just prior to the block.
2 Measure all local anesthetic block effects to ensure the procedure has been conducted specifically as intended.
3 Repeat all examination measures and scoring of modalities as for pretreatment assessments.
4 Repeat measures 1 and 3 at a time appropriate to the expected duration of action for the local anesthetic used.

RESPONSE ASSESSMENTS AND OUTCOME MONITORING

Confirmation of block success criteria should be appropriate to the procedure used. It may be necessary to assess sensory, motor, and/or sympathetic function with objective operator-independent measures, recording each in a time sequence. Subjective pain scores may need to use all of verbal pain ratings: short-form McGill Pain Questionnaire (MPQ), visual analog scales (VAS), image-scoring systems, or some of the specialized experimental scoring systems, e.g. *Handbook of Pain Assessment*.[9] Objective sensory and tenderness changes can use graphic mapping or photographs to record before and after measurements. Digital photography has added to this capability. Muscle strength, range of motion testing (both active and passive), functional mobility, and gait testing can show the impairment induced by pain and demonstrate the likely improvement with rehabilitation. Sequential documentation of an individual's signature gives visualization of changes in tremor, weakness, and coordination of the hand. Physiological measures of temperature, sweating, and blood flow changes are the domain of sympathetic block outcome measures, although other specific investigative measures are used in research settings or where more advanced resources are available.

If the perfection attained in the conduct of any block is measured by the visual accuracy of needle placement and solution spread, so then is the action of anesthetic effect measured as the degree to which the desired outcome is attained. The sensitivity of the test is born out of persistence to ensure that the desired block is successfully accomplished.

RESPONSE PATTERNS

The variability and range of factors generating response patterns are clearly more than those of direct local anesthetic action at the site of injection. These may depend on one factor, or a combination of factors, consequent to a diagnostic block, as depicted in Fig. 5.1 – the diagnostic blocks "bag of tricks."

The complexity of these responses is as diverse as pain disorders themselves, and must be recognized as critical determinants in assigning specificity to block procedures. Specificity might be considered as the ability of the anesthetic block to achieve changes in pain patterns that are due solely to the block and nothing else. Given that issues of judgment and interpretation are so critical in this context, detailed consideration is presented for each of the possible response scenarios that can account for the expected outcome. These processes may be acting synergistically, in parallel, or quite separately, as alternative explanation to the response obtained.

A range of all the possible outcome explanations is offered to help facilitate specificity in the use of diagnostic blocks:

1 Singular interruption of nociceptive generator or conduction pathways as intended.
2 Placebo response in a manner that is not well understood.
3 Systemic action of the injectate.
4 Drug spill to adjacent structures.
5 Downregulation of central nervous system (CNS) excitatory processes.
6 Unreliable patient reporting.
7 Failure from incorrect needle placement and solution spread.
8 Failure due to aberrant or alternative nociceptive pathways.
9 Observer variability.

The desired block is successful

A specific desired block and response consistent with this forms the basis of practice. The preceding content is focused on this end. In well-structured diagnostic facilities, the accuracy is likely to be high, although there is no yardstick by which to judge success other than in surgical practice, where rates over 97% are achieved. Unfortu-

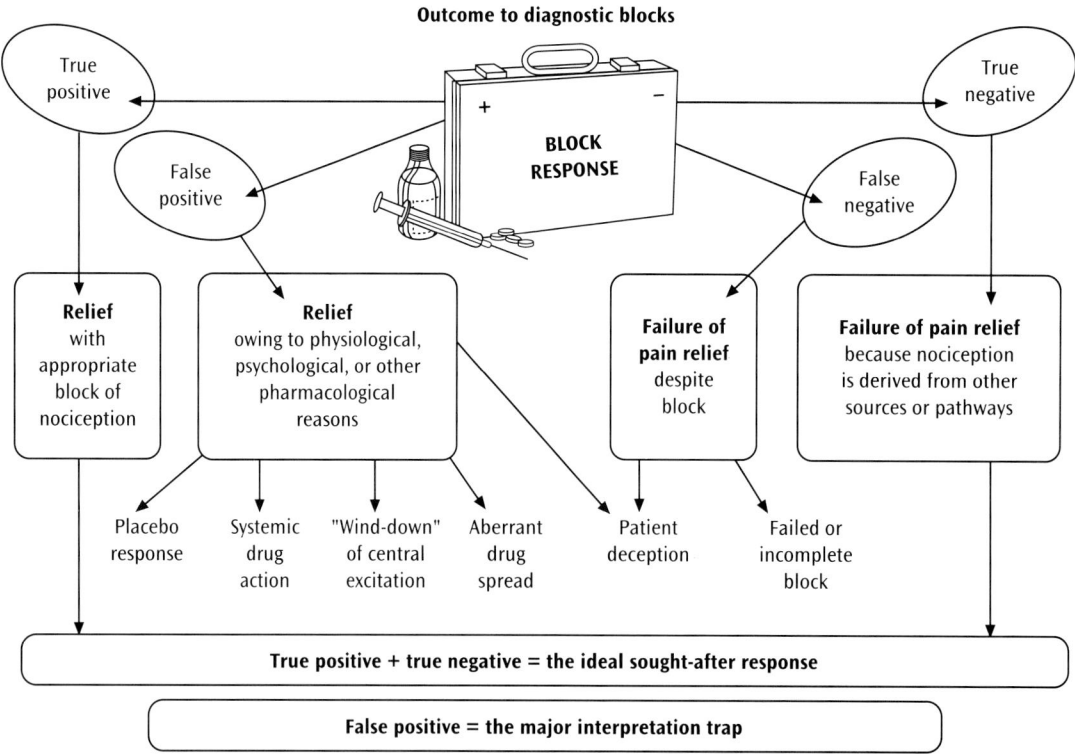

Figure 5.1 *Diagnostic block's "bag of tricks." The extent of analgesic response following diagnostic block is designated as positive or negative in respect of pain alleviation. True or false assignment is then accorded to either outcome based on the mechanistic generation of this response. These attributes confer specificity and positive predictive value to diagnostic blocks in pain medicine.*

nately, even in those with successful procedures, the final determination is compounded by erroneous assessments, as in the following presentations, to give mostly false-positive results but also some false-negative results.

Placebo responses

Placebo responses exhibit several distinctive features, which manifest in both diagnostic testing and therapeutic outcome evaluations. The critical feature of placebo responses is that they do not signify a psychological basis to the cause for pain or dysfunction. Positive placebo responses occur in 30–40% of all cases irrespective of the underlying cause for pain. As reviewed by Price,[10]*** the extent of this response can be influenced by conditioning, the intensity and milieu of the treatment/test provided by the therapist–patient relationship, and the expectancy, desire, and motivation of the patient. The response tends to be less complete, of shorter duration, and of lesser reproducibility than that for specific block responses.

Aggressive postblock testing for tenderness and sensory and functional changes will help to unmask placebo analgesic responses by revealing continued nociception and functional inhibition. This may extend to provocation testing in an attempt to reproduce pain with previously painful actions. Examples of this would be at sites of superficial scar entrapment of nerves or, very specifically, in presentations of abdominal cutaneous nerve entrapment syndromes. Such critical testing reduces the rate of misinterpretation for false-positive results. By so doing, the operator increases the specificity of the diagnostic test.

This raises the issue of double-blind testing with placebo (saline) diagnostic blocks to avoid the pitfalls of false-positive determination. Contrary to most written advice, it is suggested that the problems and variability of responses to placebo blocks probably outweigh the perceived benefits. Price[10] states that "the present limited capacity to ascertain, measure and control for placebo effects is at the heart of complex and difficult questions about therapies for pain." He contends that alternative measures of desire and expectation can serve as additional or substitute measures of placebo effect.

The reasons for claiming against the routine use of placebo blocks are:

1 It is difficult to exactly reproduce most forms of regional block, therefore the response pattern can be variable from one procedure to a repeat of the same procedure in the same patient at another time. This further confounds block assessment even outside the variability induced by placebo responses.
2 Greater value expressed in terms of block specificity may be obtained from a repeat diagnostic block using an alternative anesthetic drug with a different latency/duration profile.

3 Another means of cross-testing for specificity of response is to compare different methods for seeking the same end result. The techniques of phentolamine infusion, as proposed by Raja et al., can be compared with the response to sympathetic ganglion blocks in the evaluation of sympathetically maintained pain.[11]
4 All invasive procedures carry some degree of risk to the patient. How far can this risk be carried for low-level benefits?
5 Injection of normal saline can have physiological actions that give a positive outcome response.
6 Use of pre- and postblock testing of all measures will usually unmask placebo inhibition of pain.
7 As the specificity and sensitivity of testing with nerve blocks has not been established, there is no gold standard with which to make a comparison. Further placebo testing only compounds the difficulties of interpretation.
8 Patient motivation and expectation may not be consistent between various diagnostic blocks, altering the extent of placebo response patterns.
9 Diagnostic imaging tools have so increased anatomical and pathological diagnostic accuracy in today's medical practice that more definitive diagnostic testing can be directed to specific targets, as identified by local anesthetic blocks.

Based on these contentions, it seems that any additional discriminative value that might be derived from placebo blocks is therefore conjectural and does not have evidence-based validation.

Systemic actions of lidocaine (lignocaine)

The systemic analgesic action of lidocaine (lignocaine) is well documented,[12]*** occurring at low concentrations of 1 µg/ml plasma – levels encountered following many regional blocks. Disorders of neuropathic pain seem more sensitive to this action. There is an additional anti-inflammatory response with implications for many pain states.[13]***

Aberrant solution spread

Drug spill to adjacent structures can cause false-positive determinations in sites such as paravertebral, sympathetic, or facet joint injections. Stellate ganglion injections undertaken at the C6 level, as usually recommended, are not only anatomically incorrect but they can also result in aberrant spread, such that diagnostic blocks performed at this level are essentially useless in validating any form of sympathetic pain in the arm.[14] Despite the overwhelming evidence for this effect, there has been no apparent change in practice. Bogduk would make similar claims with respect to vertebral joint injection procedures undertaken without imaging control.[1]

Neuronal desensitization

Downregulation of second-order hyperalgesic neurons within the dorsal horn of the spinal cord is evident in animal models when nonspecific drivers of pain or mechanical stimulation are obtunded. Even injections into adjacent areas of sensory input such as referred pain sites can temporarily diminish pain, although the primary site of stimulation is still active. Perhaps the first description of this phenomenon was in 1938 by Steindler and Luck,[15] who showed that injections in the sciatic nerve well distal to the spine were able to abolish pain and physical signs of sciatica in 70% of cases with spinal stenosis. This phenomenon is also the likely explanation for the extended relief that sometimes lasts for days or weeks after nerve block even though the underlying cause is untreated.[16]

Patient misrepresentation

Patient reporting can be purposely or subconsciously deceitful. When confronted with this finding, the explanations are either that the patient was so desirous of therapy that they feign the outcome or that they are trying to please the operator, perhaps again to sustain continuation of care.

Procedural failure

Technical failures occur even in the best of hands, although precautions to avoid this have already been discussed. Innumerable texts, videos, and courses are available to those who seek improvement in their technical skills.

Abnormal conduction pathways

Less resolvable are the failures consequent to development of aberrant or alternative pathways for nerve conduction. These are more common within the sympathetic nervous system.

Operator variability

Consistency and standardization of practice are difficult to achieve, even in apparently simple determinations such as the presence of trigger points in myofascial pains. Perhaps the best approach to this problem is to ensure the same operator maintains involvement in the testing and evaluation steps, except that another practitioner or other skilled individual ideally undertakes the testing, independent from the person performing the block. Use of trainee staff in the performance of some demanding tasks is an additional source for error and begs the question as to their degree of involvement in complex tasks unless in a completely supervised role.

RESPONSE INTERPRETATION

As if the difficulties of conduct of the block itself and the subsequent outcome testing were not difficult enough, the process of interpretation of these outcome measures is again fraught with many obstacles. A thorough analysis of outcome assessment is addressed in the review by Bogduk[1]**– a "gold standard" for the topic.

Competency in the procedural aspects of diagnostic blocks requires different skills from those necessary in the subsequent interpretation of the result in the context of pain anatomy and pathophysiology. One requires technical and procedural skills, whereas the other falls into the category of judgment – a much less definable entity. The literature is replete with examples of false-positive outcomes leading to repeat spinal surgeries,[5] sometimes with dire consequences for the patient. Many of the errors are due to persistence of old concepts or ignorance of current physiology, whereas others have arisen from teachings that have not been substantiated. Some of these discarded precepts are included in Table 5.4.

Perhaps the most enduring of persisting misconceptions is the so-called "straight line" concept of pain, whereby the tissue site nociceptive signal is considered to pass through the peripheral nerve, spinal cord, and brain stem/thalamic structures to reach conscious perception in a linear relationship of signal intensity to pain severity. This Cartesian concept, and the almost universal assessment that pain relief with blocks signifies that nociception from the blocked site must be the source of pain and that short-term relief will then equate to long-term relief on permanent ablation, forms the most frequent of the misconceptions. There was an era when attempts were directed to differential nerve fiber conduction block with progressive rises or falls in concentration of local anesthetic agent. Supposed separation of sympathetic from

Table 5.4 *Common misconceptions*

Cartesian model of pain serves as the basis for pain transmission/recognition

Pain relief after block = the blocked site is the source of nociception

Short-term relief = long-term relief

Failure of relief after accurate block to painful area = nonsomatic etiology

Local anesthetic drugs only block nerve conduction

Differential fiber block is attainable with predetermined drug concentrations fine and large sensory fibers and larger non-nociceptive conduction was thought feasible. Evidence for wide overlap between individuals, between fiber types, and in variable pain states has essentially negated this concept and it is now discarded. Occasional failings arise when failure of pain relief with successful block to a painful area is assessed to imply the patient has a nonsomatic pain, usually of psychogenic origin. The dichotomy of psychogenic versus somatic causes for pain is still an enduring contention that pervades the literature, no better exemplified than the commentary by Kendall et al. and those who followed.[17,18] At other times, the relief that is attained, particularly in patients with neuropathic pains, is the result of either downregulation of hyperalgesia or the analgesic actions of systemic lidocaine rather than the peripheral local effect on nociception. Our understanding of pain physiology has improved immensely in the past 10 years. We now have a better understanding of concepts such as primary and secondary hyperalgesia, sympathetic pain, neuronal plasticity, excitatory and inhibitory transmitters, descending inhibitory control processes, spinal convergence, tissue and inflammatory pain mediators, etc. to an extent that was not envisaged when the early practitioners of diagnostic blocks were expounding their teachings. Similarly, advances in the pharmacology of analgesia are defining the receptors, ion channels, transmitters, and facilitators involved in each of the multiple nuances of pain qualitative states and responses. Each of these advances confounds the biological simplicity that we seek in trying to solve the problems confronting us clinically. No wonder we have an international society dedicated to the study of pain. Is there any other similar body in modern medicine?

PROGNOSTIC INTERPRETATION OF DIAGNOSTIC BLOCKS

The limited capacity for diagnostic block responses to accurately predict the outcome of permanent ablative procedures is one of the clear messages derived from evidence-based studies. A 1980 study by Tasker[19] of 100 consecutive cases was surprising for its time, in that it revealed during long-term follow-up that all patients failed to gain lasting benefit from permanent sympathetic ablation after positive responses to sympathetic blocks. Similarly, in 1972, Loeser[20] showed that the results of diagnostic paravertebral blocks could not be reproduced with subsequent dorsal rhizotomy. A further long-term, follow-up surgical study by North et al.,[5] again utilizing paravertebral blocks, revealed similar total failure to reproduce the same response with dorsal root ganglionectomy in the treatment of back pain. Better results were obtained in a series of well-structured studies on neck pain by Lord et al., when double-blind placebo and sequential diagnostic blocks revealed dorsal arch joints were the primary

source of pain in approximately 50% of patients with whiplash.[21,22**] Treatment of these joint-positive patients with facet denervation initially obtained high levels of relief in 24 out of 27 patients, but within 9 months pain levels had returned to 50% of pretreatment values.

Another clinical audit from Mailis et al.[23] revealed long-term benefit in only 35% of cases who underwent permanent sympathectomy for CRPS after previously responding well to sympathetic blocks.

In many pain states subjected to diagnostic blocks and ablative procedures, the subsequent recurrence or persistence of pain represents a wider etiology than just a peripheral pain generator. Chronic pain is often associated with a centralized component, which responds well to the initial diminution of a peripheral nociceptive driver but is reactivated subsequently by low-threshold or even nonspecific stimuli, causing the pain to recur within days or weeks. A case in point is evidenced by Arendt-Nielsen's group,[24**] who demonstrated a generalized neural hyperexcitability in patients suffering from chronic whiplash syndrome.

CONCLUSIONS

What might previously have been considered an art in the conduct and interpretation of diagnostic blocks in pain medicine is now a more structured process. Technical proficiency using image intensifier or imaging studies to control for block performance is no longer a luxury but rather a mandatory requirement for complex procedures. Laboratory-derived research of nociception and signal processing has changed concepts of pain physiology, placebo reactivity, and central nervous system changes in chronic pain, such that our clinical concepts of old have been quite dramatically challenged and changed. Dogma has been replaced by science, expediency replaced by precision, and response interpretation has become a behavioral science of its own. These factors have combined to give greater levels of true-positive and true-negative outcomes to assessment for diagnostic blocks, raising the positive predictive value of their use. It is likely that advances in the applied pharmacology of nociception will in time lead to even greater advances, but such is the continuing utility of current diagnostic blocks that they are commended for application in all fields of pain medicine.

REFERENCES

1. Bogduk N. Musculoskeletal pain: towards precision diagnosis. In: Jensen TS, Turner JA, Wiessenfield-Hallin Z eds. *Proceedings of the 8th World Congress on Pain.* Seattle, WA: IASP Press, 1997: 507–25.
2. Bonica JJ. *Clinical Applications of Diagnostic and Thera-*

peutic Nerve Blocks. Springfield, IL: Charles C. Thomas, 1959.

3. Boas R.A. Sympathetic nerve blocks: in search of a role. *Reg Anesth Pain Med* 1998; **23:** 292–305.

4. Dreyfuss P, Schwarzer AC, Lau P, Bogduk N. Specificity of medial branch and L5 dorsal ramus blocks. *Spine* 1997; **22:** 895–902.

5. North RB, Kidd DH, Campbell JN, Long DM. Dorsal root ganglionectomy for failed back surgery syndrome: a 5 year follow-up study. *J Neurosurg* 1991; **74:** 236–42.

● 6. Hogan QH, Abram SE. Neural blockade for diagnosis and prognosis. *Anesthesiology* 1997; **86:** 216–41.

7. Hogan QH, Abram SE. Diagnostic and prognostic neural blockade. In: Cousins MJ, Bridenbaugh PO eds. *Neural Blockade in Clinical Anesthesia and Management of Pain*. Philadelphia, PA: Lippincott Raven Publishers, 1998: 837–77.

◆ 8. Bogduk N. International Spinal Injection Society Guidelines for the performance of spinal injections procedures. *Clin J Pain* 1997; **13:** 285–302.

9. Turk DC, Melzack R eds. *Handbook of Pain Assessment*. New York, NY: Guilford Press, 1992.

● 10. Price DD. Factors that determine the magnitude and presence of placebo analgesia. In: Devor M, Rowbotham MC, Wiesenfield-Hallin Z eds. *Proceedings of the 9th World Congress on Pain. Progress in Pain Research and Management*, vol. 16. Seattle, WA: IASP Press, 2000: 1085–95.

11. Raja SN, Treede RD, Davis KD, Campbell JN. Systemic alpha-adrenergic blockade with phentolamine: a diagnostic test for sympathetically maintained pain. *Anesthesiology* 1991; **74:** 691–8.

● 12. Mao J, Chen LL. Systemic lidocaine for neuropathic pain relief. *Pain* 2000; **87:** 7–17.

13. Hollmann MW, Durieux ME. Local anesthetics and the inflammatory response. *Anesthesiology* 2000; **93:** 858–75.

14. Hogan QH, Erickson SJ, Haddox JD, Abram SE. The spread of solutions during stellate ganglion block. *Reg Anesth* 1992; **17:** 78–83.

15. Steindler A, Luck JV. Differential diagnosis of pain low in the back: allocation of the source of pain by a procaine hydrochloride method. *JAMA* 1938; **110:** 106–13.

16. Arner S, Lindblom U, Meyerson BA, Molander C. Prolonged relief of neuralgia after regional anesthetic blocks. A call for further experimental and systematic clinical studies. *Pain* 1990; **43:** 287–97.

17. Kendall N, Main CJ, Linton SJ, *et al.* Resolution of psychological distress of whiplash patients following treatment by radiofrequency neurotomy. *Pain* 1998; **78:** 223–5.

18. Gillette RD. Commentary on Thompson EN. *Pain* 2000; **85:** 523–4.

19. Tasker R. Deafferentation and causalgia In: Barica JJ ed. *Pain*. New York, NY: Raven Press, 1980; 305–29.

20. Loeser JD. Dorsal rhizotomy for the relief of chronic pain. *J Neurosurg* 1972; **36:** 745–54.

21. Lord SM, Barnsley L, Bogduk N. The utility of comparative local anesthetic blocks versus placebo controlled blocks for the diagnosis of cervical zygapophysial joint pain. *Clin J Pain* 1995; **11:** 208–13.

22. Lord SM, Barnsley L, Wallis BJ, *et al.* Percutaneous radio-frequency neurotomy for chronic cervical zygapophysial joint pain. *N Engl J Med* 1996; **335:** 1721–6.

23. Mailis A, Meindok H, Papagapiou M, Pham D. Alteration in the three-phase bone scan after sympathectomy. *Clin J Pain* 1994; **10:** 146–55, 335–9.

24. Johansen MK, Graven-Nielsen T, Olesen AS, Arendt-Nielsen L. Generalised muscle hyperalgesia in chronic whiplash syndrome. *Pain* 1999; **83:** 229–34.

PART II

Pharmacological therapies

Opioid analgesics

MICHAEL L TRAN AND CAROL WARFIELD

Terminology	59	Pharmacokinetics	65
Classifications	59	Pharmacodynamics	66
Mechanism of action	59	Individual agents	66
General pharmacological properties of opioid agonists	62	Clinical application of opioid analgesics	69
Clinical side-effects	63	Conclusion	75
Factors that may influence opioid pharmacokinetics	64	References	75
Tolerance and physical and psychological dependence	64		

Since the discovery of the pharmacological properties of opium extracted from the juice of the poppy plant in ancient times, an enormous amount of research and clinical experience in the areas of opiate receptors and opiate receptor agonists and antagonists has been undertaken. In an effort to simplify this body of knowledge, this chapter will discuss the clinical pharmacology of opioid analgesics in the context of information that is clinically relevant, practical, and relatively noncontroversial. Inadequately treated acute and chronic pain remains a major cause of suffering despite the rapid progress in the field of pharmacology.[1] Opioids provide a powerful and flexible tool with which the pain often associated with medical illnesses can be managed. In this chapter, the discussion will focus on an overview of basic considerations of opioid pharmacology and the integration of this knowledge in the general therapeutic application across various clinical settings, specifically acute pain, chronic cancer pain, chronic nonmalignant pain, and pediatric pain.

TERMINOLOGY

- *Opiates*: drugs derived from opium, including morphine, codeine, thebaine, and a variety of semisynthetic congeners derived from them.
- *Opioids*: any drug, natural or synthetic, which possesses morphine-like activity.
- *Narcotic*: Greek word for stupor. Used in a legal context to refer to any substance that can cause dependence, including opiate analgesics. The term is

no longer useful in the pharmacological and clinical context.
- *Endorphin*: referring to the three families of endogenous opioid peptides – the enkephalins, dynorphins, and β-endorphins.[2] Each family is derived from a distinct precursor polypeptide, which becomes a histologically active agent only after enzymatic cleavage.

CLASSIFICATIONS

Three classification systems were developed for describing opioids (Table 6.1):[3]

1 Weak or strong. The simplest scheme because only codeine and propoxyphene are considered weak, all others are considered strong.
2 The chemical derivation and separation of opioids into naturally occurring, semisynthetic, and synthetic compounds. There are also subgroups within each group.
3 Opioids are separated into four categories of: agonists, partial agonists, agonist–antagonists, and antagonists.

MECHANISM OF ACTION

Opioid effects are mediated by specific receptors located on cell membranes. These receptors have been identified both pre- and postsynaptically in the central nervous

Table 6.1 *Various classification systems for opioids*

Weak or strong opioids	Opium and its derivatives	Agonists and antagonists
Weak	**Natural opium alkaloids**	**Agonists**
Codeine	*Phenanthrene derivatives*	Alfentanil
Propoxyphene	Morphine	Codeine
Strong	Codeine	Diacetylmorphine
Alfentanil	Thebaine (nonanalgesic)	Fentanyl
Buprenorphine	*Benylisoquinoline derivatives (nonanalgesic)*	Ketobemidone
Butorphanol	Papaverine	Levorphanol
Diacetylmorphine	Noscapine	Meperidine
Hydromorphone	**Semisynthetic derivatives of opium alkaloids**	Methadone
Dihydrohydroxymorphinone	*Morphine derivatives*	Morphine
Oxymorphone	Diacetylmorphine	Oxycodone
Fentanyl	Dihydromorphinone	Propoxyphene
Ketobemidone	Dihydrohydroxymorphinone	Remifentanil
Levorphanol	*Thebaine derivatives*	Sufentanil
Meperidine	Buprenorphine	**Partial agonists, agonist–antagonists**
Methadone	Oxycodone	Buprenorphine
Morphine	**Synthetic compounds**	Butorphanol
Nalbuphine	*Morphinans*	Nalbuphine
Naloxone	Levorphanol	Pentazocine
Naltrexone	Nalbuphine	Ketobemidone (possibly)
Oxycodone	Naloxone	**Antagonists**
Pentazocine	Naltrexone	Cholecystokinin
Remifentanil	*Phenylheptylamines*	Naloxone
Sufentanil	Methadone	Naltrexone
	Propoxyphene	
	Phenylpiperidines	
	Alfentanil	
	Alphaprodine	
	Fentanyl	
	Ketobemidone	
	Meperidine	
	Remifentanil	
	Sufentanil	

Meperidine (pethidine).

system. In humans, peripheral opioid mechanisms have been suggested by controlled trials that demonstrated analgesia following intra-articular administration of a small dose of morphine at the time of surgery.[4,5**,6] The interaction of the opioid agonist with the receptor results in observable histological changes. The basic effect of opioids is that of neuronal inhibition either by blocking the release of neurotransmitters or by hyperpolarization of the cell by causing changes in calcium and potassium ion channels (Fig. 6.1). This physiological reaction is mediated by a second messenger system, such as the G-protein.[7,8]

Several opioid receptors are now known. As many as five receptors have been described: mu, kappa, delta, epsilon, and sigma.[9] A sixth receptor, structurally homologous to the previous opioid receptors, was discovered in 1995 and is termed opioid-like receptor (ORL). At both spinal and supraspinal levels, analgesia is mediated by interactions between opioids and multiple subtypes of these five receptors (Table 6.2).

- *Mu (μ) receptors:* mediate analgesia, euphoria, respiratory depression, and physical dependence. Mu_1 provides most of the analgesia, whereas Mu_2 receptors are responsible for most of the negative side-effects.
- *Kappa (κ) receptors:* mediate spinal analgesia, miosis, and sedation. Instead of euphoria, they can produce psychotomimetic effects (dysphoria, hallucination, and respiratory stimulation).
- *Delta (δ) receptors:* mediate analgesia, show little or no cross-tolerance with μ agonists, and could greatly potentiate morphine analgesia.
- *Sigma (σ) receptors:* produce psychotomimetic effects in humans (dysphoria, hallucination, and respiratory stimulation) and are not reversed by naloxone. This would suggest that the sigma receptors might not belong to the family of opiate receptors.[10]
- *Epsilon (ε) receptors:* described in rat models were noted to attenuate the stress response via stimulation of β-endorphin. One suggested mechanism for acupuncture's effect is its agonist effect on this receptor.

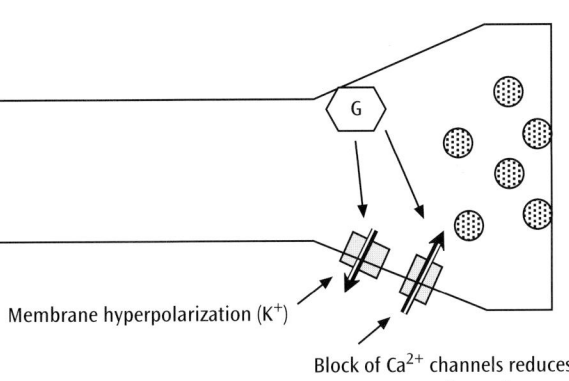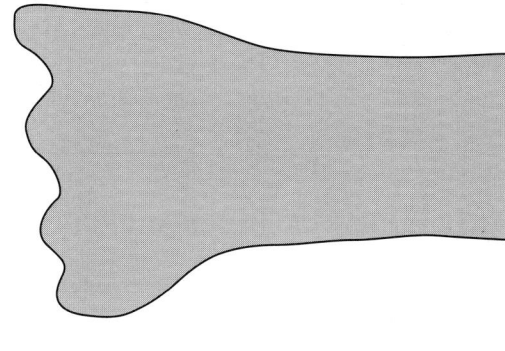

Membrane hyperpolarization (K⁺)

Block of Ca²⁺ channels reduces
neurotransmitter release

Figure 6.1 *Presynaptic opioid receptors reduce synaptic transmission via reduced neurotransmitter release through the block of Ca²⁺ channels and membrane hyperpolarization (K⁺). (Adapted with permission from ASC Rice, Faculty of Medicine, Imperial College of Science, Technology and Medicine, London, UK.)*

- *Opioid-like receptors (ORLs):* widely distributed throughout the body. ORLs have displayed little to no affinity for opioid ligands. The ORL endogenous ligand was named nociceptin and orphanin FQ by two different teams that discovered it at the same time.[11,12] The nature and role of this neuropeptide has pointed to actions at the molecular and cellular levels reminiscent of traditional opioids. However, it produces pharmacological and physiological effects that sometimes differ from, and even oppose, those of opioids.

The role of this receptor is still in doubt – many believe it has a role in nociception, learning, feeding, mobility, and potentially several other actions. From a clinical perspective, patients who experience little to no pain relief from traditional opioids and derivatives may have a problem with their ORL pathway.

A review of recent literature has shown current research has not progressed to human subjects. *In vitro* studies in animal models testing a variety of ORL ligands demonstrate a need for peptides or nonpeptide molecules that interact selectively with ORL functional sites.[13] Results of several studies point to the interaction of ago-

Table 6.2 *Opioid receptors*

Receptor	Agonists	Effects
Mu		
Mu₁	Morphine	Bradycardia
	Phenylpiperidines	Euphoria
	Phenylheptylamines	Sedation
		Supraspinal analgesia
Mu₂	Morphine	Constipation
	Phenylpiperidines	Nausea
		Physical dependence
		Pulmonary depression
Delta	Enkephalins	Pulmonary depression
		Spinal analgesia
Kappa	Butorphanol	Pulmonary depression
	Dynorphin	Sedation
	Nalbuphine	Spinal analgesia
Epsilon	β-Endorphin	Possible mechanism for acupuncture effects
Opioid-like receptor (ORL)	Nociceptin/OFQ (endogenous ligand)	Nociception
		Appetite, feeding
		Mobility
		Learning

OFQ, orphanin FQ.

nists with ORLs as having an effect on anxiety. Studies testing the effect of antagonists on ORLs indicate prevention of hyperalgesia. These studies raise the possibility of a novel class of drugs for the treatment of anxiety and chronic pain.

GENERAL PHARMACOLOGICAL PROPERTIES OF OPIOID AGONISTS

Morphine and other related opioids have widespread pharmacological effects on almost every organ and function in the human body by acting as agonists relatively selective for mu receptors. However, they can also interact with other receptors, particularly at higher doses. These interactions may be reflected in a number of clinical side-effects associated with the use of opioids.[3,7,14–16]

Central nervous system

1 *Analgesia*: the primary therapeutic application for opioids is relieving pain. They are selective in that analgesia occurs without affecting other sensory modalities, including vision, hearing, touch, or motor function.
2 *Mood alteration*: patients may occasionally experience euphoria or dysphoria from opioids. The mechanism is not clear but it may involve both dopaminergic and nondopaminergic processes.
3 *Convulsions*: morphine, methadone and D-propoxyphene, when given in high doses, can cause convulsions that are reversible with naloxone. Alternatively, normeperidine (norpethidine) and thebaine cause convulsions that are not reversible by naloxone.
4 *Temperature*: opioids can shift the equilibrium points of hypothalamic heat-regulatory mechanisms, causing slightly lower body temperature in humans; however, chronic use of opioids seems to increase body temperature.
5 *Neuroendocrine effects*: opioids at therapeutic doses cause a slight decrease in pituitary hormone levels, including luteinizing hormone (LH), follicle-stimulating hormone (FSH), adrenocorticotropic hormone (ACTH), and β-endorphins. This is a result of decreasing gonadotropin-releasing hormone and corticotropin-releasing hormone from the hypothalamus. There are reports of patients having lower sexual desire secondary to decreasing levels of testosterone.
6 *Pupils*: most opioids act on the Edinger–Westphal nucleus of the oculomotor nerve, causing pupillary constriction. Pinpoint pupils are pathognomonic for toxicity of mu agonists, however mydriasis is the hallmark of severe hypoxia.
7 *Cough*: opioids depress the cough reflex by blocking the cough center in the medulla.
8 *Nausea and emesis*: these are common side-effects of opioids produced by:
   a Direct stimulation of the chemoreceptor trigger zone in the area postrema of the medulla.
   b An increase in vestibular sensitivity so that ambulatory patients experience more frequent nausea and vomiting.

Treatments to decrease nausea and vomiting include:
   a anticholinergic drugs, e.g. scopolamine (glycopyrrolate is ineffective because it does not cross the blood–brain barrier);
   b butyrophenones, e.g. inapsine;
   c phenothiazines, e.g. prochlorperazine;
   d metoclopramide.

Cardiovascular system

1 *Heart rate and rhythm*: opioids induce bradycardia through stimulation of the central vagus nucleus. Meperidine (pethidine) is the only opioid known to cause tachycardia as a result of its vagolytic effect.
2 *Hypotension*: potential mechanisms behind morphine-induced hypotension include:
   a Histamine release.
   b Vagus-induced bradycardia.
   c Direct and indirect venous and arterial vasodilation.
   d Decreased sympathetic tone.
   e Splanchnic sequestration of blood.

Opioids should be used with caution in patients with decreased blood volume since they can aggravate hypovolemic shock. Morphine at therapeutic doses has been reported to cause death in patients with corpulmonale. Fentanyl and sufentanil are less likely to cause hemodynamic instability since they do not cause histamine release.

Gastrointestinal system

1 *Stomach*: opioids cause a decrease in the secretion of hydrochloric acid, increase in antral tone, and decrease in gastric motility, resulting in an increased gastric emptying time (up to 12 h).
2 *Small intestine*: decrease in digestion of food and biliary and pancreatic secretion. Smooth muscle tone increases and peristaltic contractions markedly decrease.

3 *Large intestine*: decreased colon contraction and increased tone further delays transit of gastrointestinal contents. Subsequently, feces lose a considerable amount of water and become dry and compacted, leading to constipation.

4 *Biliary tract*: all opioids are thought to cause a dose-dependent increase in biliary duct pressure, particularly at the sphincter of Oddi. This can be reversed fully with glucagon and naloxone, and partially with atropine and nitroglycerin.

Therefore, with the initiation of opioid therapy, provisions should be made for a regular bowel regimen, including cathartics, stool softeners, and fluids.

Genitourinary system

1 *Ureter/bladder*: ureteral contractions increase in tone, resulting in inhibition of the urinary voiding reflex. The bladder develops tolerance to these opioid effects.

2 *Uterus*: therapeutic doses of morphine may decrease uterine contraction, causing prolonged labor.

Respiratory system

1 *Chest wall rigidity*: opioid-induced muscle rigidity and stiffness, particularly in the thoracic and abdominal muscles after high-dose intravenous infusion, can impair spontaneous ventilation. The precise mechanism is unknown, however both muscle relaxants and naloxone reverse the rigidity.

2 *Respiratory depression*: opioids depress respiration primarily by a direct effect on the brainstem respiratory centers, causing a reduction in the responsiveness of such centers to carbon dioxide. All phases of respiratory activity including rate, tidal volume, and minute volume are depressed.

   a The respiratory depressant effects of opioids are potentiated with concurrent administration of other central nervous system depressants (i.e. benzodiazepines, alcohol, and anesthetics).

   b Pain and surgical stimulation counteract respiratory depression.

   c Maximum respiratory depression occurs within 5–10 min of intravenous morphine or 30–90 min of intramuscular or subcutaneous administration.

Skin

Morphine can cause the skin of the face, neck, and thorax to become flushed, presumably from histamine release causing dilation of cutaneous blood vessels. This may also be responsible for the sweating and some pruritus following systemic administration of morphine.

CLINICAL SIDE-EFFECTS

A number of side-effects are associated with the use of opioids. Some patients develop more intense side-effects than the general population, and intensity may vary with different opioids. Therefore, patients receiving opioid or opioid combination therapy should be monitored closely for complications and treated accordingly.

Central nervous system

1 Euphoria, dysphoria.

2 Suppression of cough reflex.

3 Sedation, drowsiness, confusion, unsteadiness – usually clears in 3–5 days. this may be treated by:

   a amphetamines;

   b reducing dose and increasing frequency of dose administration.

4 Multifocal myoclonus:

   a most common with large parenteral doses of meperidine (pethidine). This results from the accumulation of its active metabolite, normeperidine, which lowers seizure threshold and increases central nervous system hyperexcitability;

   b can be suppressed with intravenous anticonvulsants, for example clonazepam, or by switching to another opioid;

   c myoclonus is not reversed by naloxone.

Constipation

This is the most common and most uncomfortable side-effect for which tolerance does not develop. Therefore, at the initiation of opioid therapy, provisions should be made for a regular bowel regimen, including cathartics, stool softeners, and fluids to diminish this adverse effect.

Pruritus

Systemic administration of opiates, including morphine, is known to cause pruritus from histamine release. However, opiate administration through the neuroaxial routes including epidural and intraspinal may trigger pruritus through central effects on the spinal cord or spinal roots.[17]** Thus, antihistamine treatment may not always be effective in treating opioid-induced, centrally acting pruritus; naloxone may be a more effective alternative.

FACTORS THAT MAY INFLUENCE OPIOID PHARMACOKINETICS

Variations in opioid pharmacokinetics may be specific to age, disease, or drug interactions – leading to a clinically significant alteration in opioid response.

Age

The clearance of morphine is decreased in individuals over the age of 50; this may explain the greater sensitivity of older patients to opioids.[18]*** There is also an increase in centrally induced, adverse effects of opioids. Approaches to minimize the adverse effects of opioids in elderly patients include:

- Use of drugs with short half-lives, e.g. oxycodone, hydromorphone.
- Reduce doses and lengthen the time interval between doses.

Disease interactions

- Hepatic disease, including cirrhosis, may cause a decreased hepatic biotransformation, resulting in increased bioavailability and half-lives of parent compounds such as meperidine, pentazocine, and propoxyphene. However, the disposition of morphine and methadone is unchanged.
- Renal diseases may cause a decrease in renal clearance of pharmacologically active metabolites such as morphine-6-glucuronide, normeperidine, and norpropoxyphene, resulting in accumulation.
- One should exercise caution when administering opioids to patients with compromised respiratory reserve, e.g. obesity, chronic obstructive pulmonary disease, and kyphoscoliosis. Histamine release by opioids may trigger asthma attacks and bronchoconstriction.

Drug interactions

Drugs that induce the hepatic oxidase systems can alter the dispositions of certain opioids (Table 6.3). Phenobarbital and phenytoin increase metabolism of meperidine (pethidine), whereas phenobarbital and rifampin increase metabolism of methadone.

Severe reactions, including malignant hypertension, excitation, convulsions, hyperpyrexia, and death, have been reported following administration of meperidine (pethidine) to patients being treated with a monoamine oxidase inhibitor (MAOI). The exact mechanism is not well understood.

Tricyclic antidepressants such as amitriptyline may increase morphine levels by increasing half-life and bioavailability.[19]**

TOLERANCE AND PHYSICAL AND PSYCHOLOGICAL DEPENDENCE

Opioid tolerance

Tolerance is a normal pharmacological response to chronic opioid therapy. Tolerance is characterized by the occurrence of decreasing analgesic effects and other actions of a drug, or the need for a higher dose to maintain its effect. Tolerance develops at different rates for the various effects, including analgesia, nausea, sedation, urinary retention, and respiratory depression.

1 *Acute tolerance*: tolerance that develops very quickly, following a single or few doses over a short period of time.
2 *Chronic tolerance*: tolerance that develops over a longer period of time.
3 *Cross-tolerance*: tolerance to one drug confers tolerance to another. Cross-tolerance is incomplete, therefore patients who develop a tolerance to one drug may well obtain analgesic relief from another.

Management of opioid tolerance can involve:

- Appropriate increases in the frequency or dosage of the drug or both.
- Switching to an alternative opioid is appropriate based on the concept of incomplete cross-tolerance.
- Changing the type of opioid from one of low efficacy to one with a higher efficacy. If starting a new drug, only one-half of the equianalgesic dose of the new drug should be used as the initial starting dose, then titrated to effective analgesia.

Physical dependence

Physical dependence represents a physiological response to the effects of chronic opioid use. It can manifest as withdrawal or abstinence with sudden removal of an opioid or administration of an opioid antagonist.

Withdrawal syndrome is manifested by symptoms of increased sympathetic hyperactivity. Longer acting opioids, such as methadone or fentanyl patch, are less likely to produce withdrawal symptoms than shorter acting agents, such as morphine and hydromorphone.

1 Clinical manifestations:
  a Early: yawning, sweating, lacrimation, sneezing, agitation.
  b Late: tremor, chills, fever, tachycardia, hypertension.
2 Management of opioid withdrawal:

Table 6.3 *Drug- or age-induced alterations in opioid pharmacokinetics and/or pharmacodynamics*

Opioid	Interaction	Result
Morphine	Older than 50 years	Decreased clearance = accumulation
Morphine	Clomipramine	Increased bioavailability
Morphine	Amitriptyline	Increased bioavailability
Meperidine	Phenobarbital	Increased biotransformation = accumulation of normeperidine
Meperidine	Phenytoin	Increased biotransformation = faster elimination
Methadone/meperidine (pethidine)	Phenytoin	Increased biotransformation = faster elimination
Methadone/meperidine (pethidine)	Rifampicin	Increased biotransformation = faster elimination
Meperidine	Monoamine oxidase inhibitors	Excitation, hyperpyrexia, and convulsions
Any opioid	Alcohol or other CNS depressants	Enhanced depressant effects

Meperidine (pethidine); normeperidine (norpethidine).
CNS, central nervous system.

Table 6.4 *Pharmacokinetic and physicochemical variables for opioid analgesics*

Drug	V_c (l/kg)	V_d (l/kg)	Cl (ml/min/kg)	$T_{1/2\beta}$ (min)	Partition coefficient (octanol–water)
Morphine	0.23	2.8	15.5	134	1
Hydromorphone	0.34	4.1	22.7	15	1
Meperidine	0.6	2.6	12	180	21
Methadone	0.15	3.4	1.6	23 h	115
Levorphanol		10	10.5	11 h	
Alfentanil	0.12	0.9	7.6	94	130
Fentanyl	0.85	4.6	21	186	820
Sufentanil	0.1	2.5	11.3	149	1,750
Buprenorphine	0.2	2.8	17.2	184	10,000
Nalbuphine	0.45	4.8	23.1	222	
Butorphanol		5	38.6	159	
Dezocine		12	52	156	

V_c, central volume of distribution; V_d, volume of distribution; Cl, clearance; $T_{1/2\beta}$, elimination half-life.
Meperidine (pethidine).

a   Abstinence syndrome can be prevented by slowly tapering the dose of opioid at a daily rate of 15–20%.
b   Withdrawal can be reversed effectively by reinstituting the drug in doses at 25–40% of previous daily dose.
c   Since the syndrome is mediated by the adrenergic system, an α_2-agonist such as clonidine may also prevent its development.

Psychological dependence

Psychological dependence is another term for addiction. Addiction is a psychological and behavioral syndrome characterized by:

- Loss of control over drug use: craving for a drug for effects rather than analgesia.
- Compulsive involvement in the procurement of the drug.
- Continued use despite harm.

Issues with opioid-addicted patients:

- A history of substance abuse is a relative contrain-dication to opioid administration for nonmalignant pain.
- In the setting of acute pain, this relative contraindication must yield to the compassionate use of opioids.
- Methadone maintenance therapy for psychological dependence will induce tolerance, requiring greater than normal analgesic doses of opioid for acute pain.

Evidence suggests that the risk of addiction is extremely low in patients with no prior history of drug abuse who are prescribed opioids for a painful medical condition.[16,17] It is crucial to recognize that it is possible for patients to be physically dependent without evidence of psychological dependence.

PHARMACOKINETICS

Absorption, distribution, and elimination patterns compose the study of pharmacokinetics. The characteristics of, and partition coefficients (octanol–water) for, some commonly used opioid analgesics are summarized in Table 6.4.

- Opioids are biotransformed in the liver mainly

through the conjugation activity of microsomal enzyme systems. The main conjugation reaction in the detoxification process is glucuronide synthesis.

- Elimination is primarily through renal excretion by glomerular filtration and active tubular secretion. Minor portions are excreted by the gastrointestinal tract through bile.

PHARMACODYNAMICS

The potency, speed of onset, and duration of action of the opioids are probably the most clinically relevant pharmacodynamic measures.

- The potency of a drug used intravenously will differ from its potency when used by extravascular routes, for example oral or rectal, owing to the drug's bioavailability.
- The gradient between the concentration in blood and that in brain tissue is the most important factor in determining the speed of onset of systemic administration of opioids. Other factors such as lipid solubility and nonionized drug fraction play significant roles in the drug entering into the central nervous system.
- MEAC (minimal effective analgesic concentration) is the minimal plasma level of an opioid that can control severe pain in a particular patient. There is great intersubject variation for MEAC, yet it is fairly consistent for the general population.

INDIVIDUAL AGENTS

Naturally occurring opium alkaloids

Morphine

Morphine is the prototype and standard for comparison with other opioid analgesics. Morphine's oral bioavailability varies from 35% to 75%. Its plasma half-life is 2–3 h, while its duration of analgesia (4–6 h) limits accumulation.

Morphine is metabolized by glucuronidation into morphine 3-glucuronide (M3G) and morphine 6-glucuronide (M6G) in a 2:1 ratio. M6G is twice as potent as morphine systemically, but is approximately 100 times more potent intracerebrally; M3G is nonanalgesic.[5]

In patients with renal failure, M6G will accumulate and is responsible in part for the adverse effects experienced by this group of patients. While the data are not conclusive, it is appropriate to consider an alternative opioid for patients who experience a decrease in renal function and a concomitant increase in undesirable side-effects.

Based on single dose studies in patients with acute pain, the relative potency of intramuscular (i.m.) to oral (p.o.) morphine is 1:6. However, when patients are dosed on a regular schedule, the i.m./p.o. ratio is reduced to 1:2 or 1:3.

Sustained- and controlled-release preparations (MS Contin and Kadian) provide analgesia with a duration of 8–24 h. The preparations are not intended to increase the oral bioavailability but to permit sustained analgesia. The 12-h preparation pills should not be crushed or altered, since doing so is likely to considerably increase the amount of morphine available for absorption with some preparations, resulting in possible toxicity. However, the 24-h capsule may be opened and sprinkled over food.

Peak morphine concentration in peripheral venous plasma typically occurs at 0.5–1.0 h after ingestion of morphine solution, whereas it occurs at approximately 2.5 h for sustained release preparations.

Morphine is predominantly bound to albumin at an average bound fraction of 35% in normal patients and 20–30% in patients with severe renal and hepatic dysfunction. Hence, pathological conditions influencing albumin kinetics could predispose patients to exaggerated effects from morphine.

Codeine

Codeine is considered to be a weak opioid, generally not used for severe pain. It has good antitussive activity. It is contained in numerous analgesic combinations (liquid, tablets, and capsules). It has a high oral–parenteral potency ratio (60%). Very few opioids have such a high oral–parenteral potency ratio; levorphanol, oxycodone, and methadone also share this attribute. This phenomenon is the result of less first-pass metabolism in the liver. Approximately 10% of administered codeine is demethylated to form morphine.

Semisynthetic derivatives of morphine

1 Hydromorphone is a semisynthetic derivative of morphine that is approximately six to eight times as potent. Because of its lipid solubility, it is well absorbed from oral, rectal, or parenteral sites. The analgesic effect appears approximately 15 min after intravenous and 30 min after oral administration. It is often recommended for patients with renal failure owing to the lack of any identifiable active metabolites. It is only 8% protein bound in human serum. Mean oral bioavailability is approximately 50%.
2 Oxymorphone is a parenteral opioid with a potency of 7–10 times that of morphine. It has had a limited but important role in the management of pain in cancer patients. A rectal suppository preparation is available.
3 Diacetylmorphine (diamorphine) is formed semisynthetically by the deacetylation of morphine. When

metabolized in the body, diacetylmorphine is bio-transformed into 6-acetylmorphine and morphine. This biotransformation is quite rapid, contributing to a quicker onset of pain relief and greater potency than an equivalent amount of morphine. Diacetyl-morphine is more lipid soluble than morphine and other opiates, thus it is able to cross the blood–brain barrier within minutes. This higher solubility allows for the rapid deposition of diacetylmorphine and its metabolites in the central nervous system.[20] In addition, the high bioavailability of diacetylmorphine would allow for lower equipotent doses when infusate volume is an issue.

Semisynthetic derivatives of codeine

1 Oxycodone is a semisynthetic codeine analog. Its potency is slightly less than morphine: 10–15 mg of oxycodone is equivalent to 10 mg of morphine sub-cutaneously. It is about one-half as potent orally as parenterally. Oxycodone is widely used in combination with aspirin or acetaminophen (paracetamol) or alone.
2 Tramadol is a synthetic analog of codeine. It produces analgesia via weak mu receptor agonism in addition to inhibiting the reuptake of serotonin and norepi-nephrine. Oral bioavailability is 68%, its half-life is 5 h, but the half-life of its active metabolite is 9 h.

Synthetic compounds

1 Levorphanol is a synthetic opioid with a long half-life of 12–16 h, and a good oral–parenteral potency ratio of 1:2. Clinical reports suggest that it produces less nausea and vomiting. It can be crushed and adminis-tered effectively through a gastrostomy tube.
2 Methadone is slightly more potent than morphine. It produces less euphoria and less sedation than many other opioids. Supplied as a racemic mixture of two optical isomers, most of its activity comes from the L-isomer. Methadone has a long half-life, primar-ily because the majority of the drug is protein bound and then slowly released back to plasma as diffus-ible fraction. It also has the advantages of high bio-availability (85%) and no active metabolites. Plasma half-life averages 24 h but may range from 13 to 50 h; duration of analgesia is only 4–8 h. Drawbacks of methadone include accumulation and a longer time to reach steady state than other opioids, i.e. days for methadone versus hours for morphine. Because of this, it should be considered a second-line drug. In an opioid-naive patient, initial doses should be titrated carefully and on an as needed (*pro re nata*, p.r.n.) basis.
3 Propoxyphene is structurally related to methadone and binds primarily to mu receptors. It is prescribed mainly for mild to moderate pain. Unlike other opi-oids, it causes depression of the cardiac conduction system similar to lidocaine (lignocaine). As an anal-gesic, propoxyphene is about one-half to two-thirds as potent as codeine when taken orally. The average half-life is about 30 h. Patients with hepatic disease are at risk of propoxyphene toxicity, and there is signifi-cant first-pass metabolism. Patients with renal fail-ure develop very high blood concentrations of both propoxyphene and norpropoxyphene since neither is well removed by dialysis. Propoxyphene also inhibits carbamazepine metabolism.
4 Meperidine is a synthetic phenylpiperidine opioid analgesic. It produces less smooth muscle contrac-tion than morphine. Its oral bioavailability is 40–60%, and duration of action is about 50% less than mor-phine. Meperidine is metabolized chiefly in the liver, with a half-life of about 3 h. In patients with cirrho-sis, the bioavailability is increased to as much as 80%, clearance is one-half normal, and terminal elimina-tion half-life is doubled. Therefore, in these patients, initial parenteral doses should not be altered, but sub-sequent doses should be spaced further apart. Oral doses should be reduced by 50%. Renal elimination of meperidine is less than 10%, but it has been shown that the clearance is reduced and the half-life is pro-longed in patients with renal disease. Normeperidine, an active metabolite of meperidine, has a long half-life (15–20 h) and may accumulate in renal failure, causing central nervous system hyperactivity. This is characterized by subtle mood effects, followed by tremors, myoclonus, and occasional seizures.

Severe reaction may follow administration of meperidine to patients being treated with MAO inhibitors. Reactions include severe respiratory depression or excitation, delirium, hyperpyrexia, and convulsions.
5 Fentanyl is a synthetic opiate related to phenylpiperi-dine, approximately 80–100 times more potent than morphine. Fentanyl is highly lipophilic and has a high rate of clearance from blood, but slow removal from fatty tissues results in a half-life longer than that of morphine. Because the half-life is long, repeated doses may cause accumulation to occur and respi-ratory depression then becomes a problem. When administered orally, fentanyl has a poor bioavailabil-ity because of its high hepatic clearance, so this route is not used. However, the high lipid solubility of fen-tanyl makes buccal administration in the form of a "lollipop" possible, which is an appealing noninvasive dosing for children. Continuous blood fentanyl con-centrations can be obtained noninvasively through the use of a transdermal patch.
6 Alfentanil is less lipid soluble than fentanyl – charac-terized by rapid onset and short duration of action. Although its clearance is not as high as fentanyl, it has

a much smaller volume of distribution than fentanyl and therefore its half-life is very short. There is no difference in the elimination rate in patients with renal dysfunction.

7 Sufentanil is more lipid soluble than fentanyl, and has pharmacokinetic properties intermediate between fentanyl and alfentanil. Its clinical significance is from the higher specificity for opioid analgesic receptors and fewer peripheral effects than any of the other opioids.

   When studied in patients with renal dysfunction and those with renal transplantation, the kinetics of sufentanil were found to be similar to the kinetics in patients with normal renal function.

8 Remifentanil is structurally related to alfentanil but is 20–50 times more potent and is characterized by a rapid onset of analgesia (1–3 min). Since it has a very short half-life, a steady state is achieved shortly after starting an intravenous infusion. It has a very short duration of action (3–10 min). It is metabolized by rapid hydrolysis by nonspecific esterases. Dose reduction is not required in renal or hepatic impairment patients.

9 Ketobemidone is a synthetic derivative of meperidine and has been used widely in Europe for the past 50 years. It is a mixed receptor ligand, being both a potent mu receptor agonist and a weak, noncompetitive N-methyl-D-aspartate (NMDA) receptor antagonist. The pharmacokinetics of ketobemidone are similar to other opioid analgesics, and it has a mean elimination half-life of 2.3 h and a mean oral bioavailability of 34%. Ketobemidone undergoes first-pass metabolism to form norketobemidone, which has shown to be about five times more potent than its parent compound at NMDA receptors. Because of this unique property, it is a potential treatment for neuropathic pain that does not respond well to traditional pure agonists.

Agonist–antagonist drugs

Agonist–antagonist opioids are less efficacious than pure agonists, but they cause less respiratory depression and have lower potential for abuse. With this class of opioid, there tends to be a ceiling effect to both analgesia and respiratory suppression. They exert their analgesic actions primarily as agonists at kappa receptors, while acting as competitive antagonists at mu receptors. They have the ability to reverse opioid effects in patients who are physically dependent on pure agonists and are associated with a higher incidence of psychotomimetic effects.

1 Pentazocine has the pharmacokinetic profile of a high-clearance drug. Therefore, it has a low bioavailability after oral administration (~ 18%). It has high lipid solubility, a large volume of distribution, and a short half-life of 3–4 h.

   In patients with hepatic dysfunction, the dosing interval should be prolonged. Doses given orally should be further reduced, since a threefold increase in bioavailability occurs because of decreased first-pass metabolism. Renal dysfunction would not necessitate dose revision since there is little renal clearance and there are no known active metabolites.

2 Buprenorphine, butorphanol, and nalbuphine can be grouped together because of their many similarities, although buprenorphine is a partial agonist at the mu receptor instead of mixed agonist–antagonist.

   a When given in equianalgesic doses, each drug depresses respiration and causes nausea and vomiting to the same degree as the pure agonists.

   b There is a well-defined ceiling effect for analgesia.

   c The agents dissociate very slowly from opioid receptors, therefore there may be a need for higher than traditional doses of antagonist (e.g. naloxone).

   d All these drugs undergo significant first-pass hepatic elimination after oral administration.

Opioid antagonists

These substances have the ability to competitively displace an opioid agonist from the receptor. Naloxone and naltrexone are two opioid antagonists. They have high affinity for mu receptors and also interact with delta and kappa receptors, but may require higher doses to antagonize the effects of delta and kappa ligands.

1 Naloxone

   a Often used to reverse the respiratory depression caused by opioid overdose, at doses of 1–5 µg/kg in aliquots of 0.04 mg.

   b Titration of intravenous naloxone is often used to reverse unwanted side-effects of pruritus, urinary retention, nausea, and vomiting without significantly affecting analgesia.

   c It is a short-acting medication (30–45 min); supplemental or intravenous infusion (5 µg/kg/h) may be needed in patients with long-acting opioid overdose.

   d Rapid intravenous injection may cause nausea and vomiting and cardiovascular stimulation (tachycardia, pulmonary edema, hypertension, dysrhythmia, ventricular fibrillation). This has been attributed to an increase in sympathetic nervous system activity.

2 Naltrexone

   a Acts mainly at the mu receptor, active after oral administration, and has a prolonged effect of up to 24 h.

CLINICAL APPLICATION OF OPIOID ANALGESICS

Despite the enormous amount of data available on the pharmacology of opioids, providing a patient with effective analgesia and a precise dosing schedule for a specific pain problem is often difficult and time-consuming. This is in part due to the subjectivity of pain and difficulties in measuring it, the individual variation in drug requirement, and the limited knowledge of the pharmacodynamic relationships of the analgesia and side-effects of these drugs. Therefore, several steps should be considered before prescribing analgesics for an individual patient:

1 Detailed history on effects of the opioids previously used, side-effects experienced, current opioid use, and tolerance.
2 Careful physical examination to determine the cause of the painful symptomatology.
3 After the diagnosis is established and the mechanism of pain determined, other factors should be considered prior to a therapeutic plan: patient's age, physical and nutritional status, renal and hepatic function, mental status, family support, and ability to follow instructions.

By taking into account all of the above factors, an effective analgesic regimen can be formulated. The basic idea is to use the most effective drug or combination of drugs for a specific pain state that will produce the least serious or distressful side-effects.

The clinical situations in which opioids might be used as an analgesic will only be considered in outline here. For more detailed information on specific situations, the reader should consult the relevant chapter.

Opioids in the management of acute pain

Following injury, pain generally disappears when the injuries are healed. Acute pain is often associated with objective physical signs of autonomic nervous system activity – tachycardia, hypertension, diaphoresis, mydriasis, and pallor. In cases where the causes are uncertain, establishing a diagnosis is a priority, but symptomatic treatment of pain should be given. In fact, a comfortable patient is better able to cooperate with history-taking and diagnostic procedures.

Opioid analgesia

- Opioid analgesics are the cornerstone in the management of moderate to severe acute pain. Effective use allows for postoperative activities such as deep breathing, coughing, ambulation, and physical therapy.
- When pain cannot be adequately controlled despite increasing the dose, other factors including residual surgical pathology or neuropathic pain should be considered.
- Tolerance and physiological dependence are unusual in short-term postoperative use. Similarly, psychological dependence and addiction are rare after the use of opioids for acute pain.[17,21,22]

Choice of agent

- Morphine is the standard agent for opioid therapy. If, because of sensitivity or allergy, morphine cannot be used, then another short-acting opioid such as hydromorphone or fentanyl can be substituted.
- Opioids with short half-lives are preferred for treatment of acute pain. Four to five half-lives are required before steady state is reached after dosing has begun or has been changed. The plasma concentration of a short half-life opioid would change rapidly and stabilize quickly after dose adjustment, and therefore is advantageous in an acute setting.
- Among the parenteral opioid formulations are methadone and levorphanol, which have half-lives long enough to compromise rapid dose adjustment and safety for uncontrolled severe pain. The use of these drugs for acute pain in routine clinical settings cannot be recommended.
- Meperidine should be reserved for very brief courses in patients who have demonstrated intolerance to other opioids. The active metabolite of meperidine, normeperidine, may accumulate with repetitive dosing and produce toxic effects. Accumulation is most likely to occur in patients with renal insufficiency, but normeperidine toxicity has been reported in patients with normal renal function after only a few days of repetitive dosing.
- Meperidine is contraindicated in patients who are receiving MAO inhibitors.
- The properties of agonist–antagonist opioids include a ceiling effect for respiratory depression and analgesia, the ability to reverse opioid effects in patients who are dependent on pure agonists, a lesser tendency for abuse, and a higher incidence of psychotomimetic effects. These inherent properties do not provide strong support for employing these drugs over the pure agonists in the management of acute pain, although patients with severe pulmonary disease may present a true indication for a drug with a ceiling effect for respiratory depression.

Dosage/schedule

- There is a large amount of patient intervariability in analgesic dose requirements and responses to opioids. The recommended dose may occasionally be inadequate. Subsequent dose titration is needed to maximize analgesia and minimize side-effects.

- Relative potency between opioids provides an approximation and a rational basis for selection of a starting dose, changing route of administration (e.g. intravenous to oral), or for switching opioids (Table 6.5).
- Patients who have been receiving opioid analgesics recently may require higher starting and maintenance doses.
- Analgesics should initially be administered on a regular time schedule during the acute stage. For example, if a patient is likely to have moderate to severe pain for 48 h, morphine may be ordered every 4 h around the clock for 36 h.
- Once the choice of opioid and duration of action is determined, the dosage frequency should be adjusted to maximize pain relief and prevent it from recurring.
- Later in the subacute stage, it may be acceptable to provide opioid analgesics on a p.r.n. basis or by changing to the oral route. This may provide pain relief while reducing the risk of adverse effects as the patient's analgesic requirement diminishes.
- Patients should be assessed at regular intervals to determine the efficacy of treatment, presence of side-effects, and the need for adjustment of dosage/interval or for supplemental doses for breakthrough pain.

Routes of administration

The intraspinal route is discussed in Chapters A12 and P32.

- *Intravenous*: this is the parenteral route of choice. It is suitable for bolus and continuous infusion and provides the most rapid onset of effect. Time to peak effect varies with drug lipid solubility, ranging from 1–5 min for fentanyl to 15–30 min for morphine.
- *Intramuscular*: causes pain and trauma and may deter patients from requesting pain medication. There are wide fluctuations in absorption from muscle and a 30–60 min lag to peak effect. Absorption may be more rapid after deltoid than after gluteal injection.
- *Rectal and sublingual*: these are alternatives to parenteral routes in patients unable to tolerate oral intake.
- *Oral*: most convenient and inexpensive. This route is appropriate if the oral route is tolerated, and is the mainstay of pain management in ambulatory patients.
- *Nasal*: transnasal administration offers an alternative and convenient route. Transnasal butorphanol appears to be safe and effective for the treatment of moderate to severe postoperative and migraine headache pain. Intranasal fentanyl has also been shown to be an effective alternative to its parenteral routes in postoperative patient.

Opioids in the management of cancer pain

Cancer pain may be acute, chronic, or intermittent, and often has a definable etiology, usually related to tumor recurrence or treatment. Long-term opioid treatment is the primary therapeutic approach to cancer pain. As many as 90% of patients benefit from optimal opioid therapy.[23] The predominant goals of cancer pain management focus on maintenance of function and comfort.

Drug choice

The World Health Organization (WHO) has developed a set of guidelines for the selection and administration of opioid drugs known as the "analgesic ladder" (Fig. 6.2).

- Pure opioid agonists are recommended for moderate or severe pain. The simplest approach for patients with moderate pain who have limited or no exposure to opioids involves a combination of opioids and either aspirin or acetaminophen. The opioid can be oxycodone, codeine, hydrocodone, or propoxyphene. The dose of these products can be increased until the maximal dose of coanalgesic is reached, e.g. limited by the maximum safe dose of acetaminophen (paracetamol) per day (4 g).
- For severe cancer pain, the selection of an opioid conventionally referred to as "strong" is empirically selected. Morphine is normally the preferred first-line drug based on extensive experience and availability of different formulations, including controlled release and sustained release forms with durations of 8–24 h.
- Other mu agonist opioids may be better tolerated in individual patients and may provide a better balance between analgesia and side-effects.
- Selection of an opioid is influenced by pharmacokinetic factors, the most essential of which is half-life. An opioid with a relatively short half-life is preferred for a quicker approach to steady state after dosing is initiated or changed. Long half-life opioids such as methadone and levorphanol are the most difficult to administer when rapid dose escalation is required during treatment of acute pain.
- Similarly, controlled release and sustained release formulations of opioid, including oral morphine and transdermal fentanyl, also require a long period to approach steady state. Steady state may not be reached for 1–2 days with morphine and 2–3 days for transdermal fentanyl.

Routes of administration

- The oral route is preferred in chronic cancer pain treatment owing to its safety, economy, and acceptability.
- The transdermal route of administration is available for highly lipophilic opioids such as fentanyl. It is

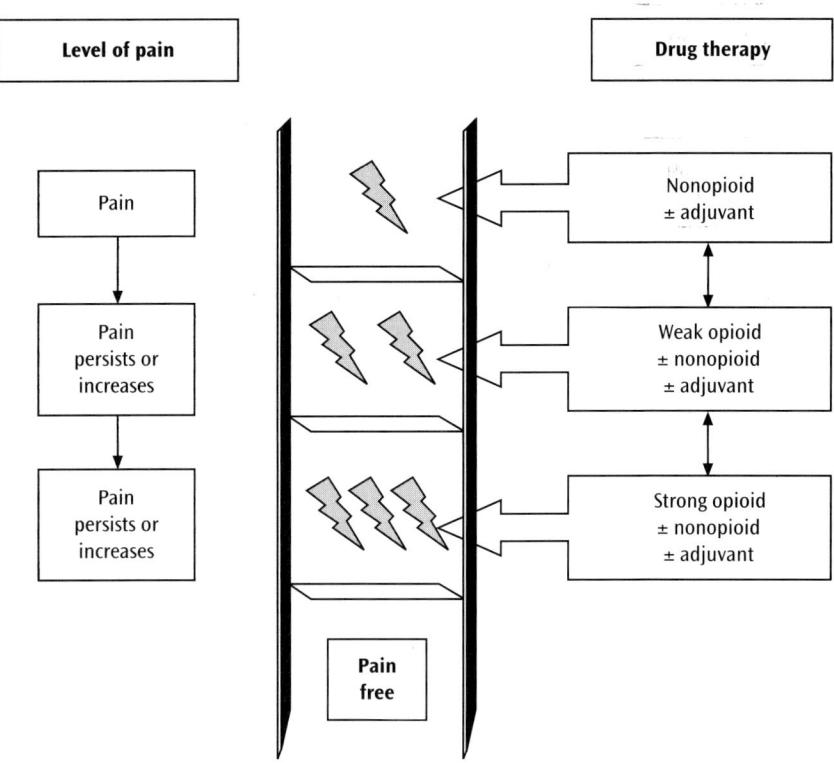

Figure 6.2 *WHO analgesic ladder.*

indicated for patients who cannot swallow or absorb an orally administered opioid, for those who are non-compliant with oral regimens or who would prefer an alternative, and for those in whom other opioid analgesics have failed to relieve their pains and who may thus benefit from a trial of fentanyl.

- The transnasal route is an alternative when patients are no longer able to tolerate the oral route. Butorphanol is the only commercially available opioid for transnasal application. However, because it is a mixed agonist–antagonist, this drug is not recommended for routine use in cancer pain treatment. Other agents currently being studied include fentanyl, sufentanil, and buprenorphine.
- Portable ambulatory infusion devices have also enhanced the clinical utility of infusion techniques. Patients who may require continuous opioid infusion, either intravenous or subcutaneous, can be managed in the ambulatory setting for long periods with this approach.
- Intraspinal opioid administration can provide potent analgesia at much lower doses than systemic administrations. This may reduce the adverse effects encountered with higher systemic dosing. The strongest indication for the intraspinal or epidural route is intolerable somnolence or confusion in the patient with adequate analgesia during systemic treatment. The preferred intraspinal opioids include morphine, hydromorphone, and fentanyl.

Administration guidelines

- Opioid dosing guidelines for cancer pain are highly effective and widely accepted. The usual starting dose in patients with limited opioid exposure is 5–10 mg of i.m. morphine every 4 h. For oral administration, an intramuscular to oral dose ratio of 1:3 should be used, thus 15–30 mg every 4 h or 45–90 mg of controlled release oral morphine every 12 h. An equianalgesic dose table should be consulted for selection of other opioids.
- In changing from one opioid to another, the new opioid's starting dose is also calculated using equi-analgesic conversion tables (Table 6.5). The dosing regimen based on the calculation should be reduced by at least 25–50% to account for interpatient variability and incomplete cross-tolerance between opioids. A larger reduction of up to 75% is prudent if the new drug is methadone or if the patient is sensitive to opioid side-effects, such as the elderly and those with major organ dysfunction.
- Whenever analgesia is not adequate, the dose of opioid should be increased until acceptable analgesia is produced or intolerable side-effects are encountered. A ceiling dose of pure opioid agonists has not been identified.
- Patients with constant pain can be managed with around-the-clock dosing and supplemented with "as needed" dosing for occasional breakthrough pain. The rescue dose is usually a short half-life drug

Table 6.5 *Opioid analgesics*

Class generic name: proprietary names	Route	Equianalgesic dose[a] (mg)	Peak[b] (h)	Duration[b] (h)	Half-life (h)	Pediatric dosing	Comments	Precautions
Agonists								
Naturally occurring opium derivatives								
Morphine	i.m.	10–15	0.5–1	3–5[d]	2–3.5	0.1 mg/kg q3–4 h	Standard of comparison for opioid-type analgesics; available in long-acting preparation	Impaired ventilation; bronchial asthma; increased intracranial pressure; liver failure; renal failure
	p.o.	30–60[c]	1.5–2	4		0.3 mg/kg q3–4 h		
Codeine	i.m.	120	0.5–1	4–6	3	Not suggested	Less potent than morphine; excellent oral availability	Like morphine
	p.o.	30–200		3–4		1 mg/kg q3–4 h		
Partially synthetic derivatives of morphine								
Hydromorphone	i.m.	1–2	0.5–1	3–4	2–3	0.015 mg/kg q3–4 h	Like diamorphine	Like morphine
	p.o.	7.5	1.5–2	4–6		0.06 mg/kg q3–4 h		
Oxymorphone	i.m.	1–1.5	0.5–1	3–5	NA	Not suggested	Like morphine	Like morphine
Diacetylmorphine	i.m.	4	4	3–4	2–3	Not suggested	Slightly shorter acting	Like morphine
Diamorphine	p.o.	4–8	4–8	3–4				
Oxycodone	p.o.	30	30	4–6	NA	0.2 mg/kg q3–4 h	Available alone, in combination with aspirin or acetaminophen and in a controlled-release preparation	Like morphine
Synthetic compounds								
Morphonans								
Levorphanol	i.m.	2	0.5–1	5–8	12–16	0.02 mg/kg q6–8 h	Like methadone	Like methadone
	p.o.	4	1.5–2			0.04 mg/kg q6–8 h		
Phenylheptylamines								
Methadone	i.m.	8–10	0.5–1	4–8	15–30	0.1 mg/kg q6–8 h	Good oral potency; long plasma half-life	Like morphine, accumulative with repeated doses
	p.o.	20	1.5–2	4–12		0.2 mg/kg q6–8 h		
Propoxyphene HCl	p.o.	130		4–6	3.5	Not suggested	"Weak" opioid, often used in combination with nonopioid analgesics	Accumulative with repeated doses, convulsions with overdose

Drug	Route	Dose				Maximal dose	Characteristics	Comments
Phenylpiperidines	i.m.	75–100	0.5–1	2–3		0.75 mg/kg q2–3 h	Shorter acting and about 10% as potent as morphine; has mild atropine-like antispasmodic effects	Normeperidine accumulates with repetitive dosing, causing CNS excitation; not for patients with impaired renal function or for those receiving monoamine oxidase inhibitors
Meperidine	p.o.	200–300	1–2	2–3		Not suggested		
Fentanyl	i.v.	50–100 µg		0.75–1		Not suggested	Short-acting potent opioid, mostly used in anesthesia or continuous infusion	More severe side-effects than morphine
Remifentanil	i.m.	0.5–1.0 µg	0.05	0.05–0.17	0.05	1.0 µg/kg q1 min	Very short acting, minutes vs. hours	Discontinuing dosage better than administering nalaxone
Agonist–antagonists								
Buprenorphine	i.m.	0.3–0.6	0.5–1	6–8	NA	0.004 mg/kg q6–8 h	Partial agonist of the morphine-type, less abuse liability than morphine	Can precipitate withdrawal in opioid-dependent patients
	s.l.	0.4–0.8	2–3	6–8		Not suggested	Not suggested	
Butorphanol	i.m.	2	0.5–1	4	2.5–3.5	Not suggested	Like nalbuphine	Like pentazocine
Pentazocine	i.m.	40–60	0.5–1	3–4	2–3	Not suggested	Mixed agonist–antagonist; less abuse liability than morphine; included in Schedule IV of Controlled Substances Act	Can cause psychotomimetic effects; might precipitate withdrawal in opioid-dependent patients, not for those with myocardial infarction
	p.o.	50–200	1.5–2	3–4		Not suggested		
Nalbuphine	i.m.	10–20	0.5–1	4–6	5	0.1 mg/kg q3–4 h	Like pentazocine but not scheduled	Incidence of psychotomimetic effects lower than with pentazocine

i.m., intramuscular; p.o., oral; s.l., sublingual; NA, not available; i.v., intravenous.
Acetaminophen (paracetamol); meperidine (pethidine); normeperidine (norpethidine).

a. These doses are recommended starting doses from which the optimal dose for each patient is determined by titration and the maximal dose is limited by adverse effects.
b. Peak time and duration of analgesia are based on mean values and refer to the stated equianalgesic doses.
c. For a single oral dose, the ratio of i.m./oral is 1:6; for repeated doses, the ratio is closer to 1:3.
d. Plasma half-life at least for morphine is age dependent; it increases with age.

offered "as needed" every 2–3 h at a dose equal to 5–15% of the total daily dose requirement.

Opioids in the management of chronic nonmalignant pain

The use of opioids to relieve chronic nonmalignant pain is subject to continuing debate because of concerns about addiction, tolerance, side-effects, and worsening disability. However, the published literature of clinical experience and critical evaluations of drug-related safety, efficacy, and addiction suggests that there is a subgroup of patients with chronic nonmalignant pain who can achieve sustained analgesia from opioid therapy – without occurrence of intolerable side-effects or development of aberrant drug-related behavior. If this perspective is agreeable, then the crucial role of the physician would involve patient selection and guidance in drug administration. The guidelines for opioid therapy in chronic nonmalignant pain highlight several patient issues.

- Once a full assessment in a multidisciplinary pain clinic has been completed, a therapeutic opioid trial may be initiated and either continued or discontinued depending on outcome. Side-effects, dose adjustments, and clinical endpoints, including pain relief, functional status, and development of aberrant drug-related behaviors, should be closely monitored.
- Patients are advised about the controversial nature of this therapy. Some physicians have adopted formal written consent and documentation in the medical record. The potential for physical dependence in babies born to women taking opioid therapy may need special emphasis.
- Basic knowledge of opioid pharmacology is mandatory. Some physicians believe that the selection of an opioid should avoid those with a rapid onset of action at mu receptors, the kinetics of which are linked to higher abuse potential.[24] There are some theoretical advantages for using agonist–antagonist opioids, but these appear to cause more practical problems during maintenance. Long-acting, slow onset, oral preparations such as methadone or sustained release morphine are preferable.
- An effective therapeutic trial requires individualization of the opioid dose. Unlike cancer pain where absolute dose is immaterial, for nonmalignant pain an intense dose titration may not be realistic and could distract attention from rehabilitative pursuits. If the opioid dose becomes unrealistic for the patient's clinical condition, the clinician should address it openly with the patient.
- Opioid therapy is not a substitute for a comprehensive pain management approach that focuses on psychological and rehabilitative therapies with the goal of functional restoration. For well-selected and highly motivated patients, opioid therapy could complement primary rehabilitative therapies.
- Finally, there should be continual observation for aberrant drug-related behaviors (Table 6.6). A "contract" between the patient and the physician is useful. There should be an agreement about discontinuation of medication following evidence of misuse. In such cases, highly structured instructions may be required to regain control over the therapy, such as more frequent visits, small prescriptions, and occasional urine drug screens.

Opioids in the management of pediatric pain

It has been clearly acknowledged that children of all ages do experience pain.[20,25,26] Pediatric patients deserve appropriate pain management of both surgical and other forms of pain. Except for neonates, the pharmacology of opioid analgesics appears to be similar in both children and adults. Like adults, children may develop tolerance during chronic opioid treatment, but tolerance is unusual in short-term postoperative use in opioid-naive patients. There is no evidence or known aspect of childhood development that may predispose children to higher risk for developing psychological dependence over the general population.

Points to consider when using opioid treatments for children:

- Choice of opioid agent is similar to other patient populations and types of pain, with morphine as the standard for therapy unless reaction or allergy necessitates changing to other opioids.
- Children vary in their response and dose requirements for opioids, therefore dose titration is prudent. The use of relative potency of opioids should help in determining the starting dose or an appropriate change from one opioid to another. Table 6.5 has recommended pediatric doses for the commonly used opioids.
- Children should receive analgesics at regular intervals to provide consistent pain relief and prevent breakthrough pain, which may provoke fear and anxiety and thus cause their pain to increase.
- Whenever possible, children should receive medications through routes that do not cause additional pain, such as intramuscular or subcutaneous injections. The simplest effective route is usually by mouth. If the oral route is not possible, drugs should be administered intravenously.

There are only a small number of dosing guidelines available for children. As a rough guideline, it is generally recommended that children 12 years and older receive full adult doses. Children between the ages of 7 and 12 years generally require 50% of the starting adult doses. Chil-

Table 6.6 *Aberrant drug-related behaviors that raise concern about the potential for addiction*

Behaviors more suggestive of an addiction disorder
Selling prescription drugs
Prescription forgery
Stealing or "borrowing" drugs from others
Injecting oral formulations
Obtaining prescription drugs from nonmedical sources
Concurrent abuse of alcohol or illicit drugs
Multiple dose escalations or other noncompliance with therapy despite warnings
Multiple episodes of prescription "loss"
Repeatedly seeking prescriptions from other clinicians or from emergency rooms without informing prescriber or after warnings to desist
Evidence of deterioration in the ability to function at work, in the family, or socially that appear to be related to drug use
Repeated resistance to changes in therapy despite clear evidence of adverse physical or psychologic effects from the drug

Behaviors less suggestive of an addiction disorder
Aggressive complaining about the need for more of drug
Drug hoarding during periods of reduced symptoms
Requesting specific drugs
Openly acquiring similar drugs from other medical sources
Unsanctioned dose escalation or other noncompliance with therapy on one or two occasions
Unapproved use of the drug to treat another symptom
Reporting psychic effects not intended by the clinician
Resistance to a change in therapy associated with "tolerable" adverse effects, with expressions of anxiety related to the return of severe symptoms

dren between 2 and 6 years require 20–25% of the starting adult dose. Neonates generally require lower doses of opioids according to body weight than older children.

CONCLUSION

As the understanding of the pharmacological aspects and clinical experience of opioids become more widespread in the medical communities, medical professionals have become more accepting of the use of opioids for the treatment of pain in both acute and chronic settings. The variety of opium derivatives, from naturally occurring to synthetic, allows medical personnel the flexibility to design a treatment regimen that takes into account the myriad of medical complexities, types of pain, and potential side-effects affecting their patients. Ongoing and future research and advances in the clinical use of opioid drugs, together with parallel growth in the understanding of opioid mechanisms, will hopefully counteract opiophobia and undertreatment of pain.

REFERENCES

1. Marks RM, Sachar EJ. Undertreatment of medical in-patients with narcotic analgesics. *Ann Intern Med* 1973; **78:** 173–81.

2. Evans CJ, Hammond DL, Frederickson RCA. The opioid peptides. In: Pasternak GW ed. *The Opiate Receptors.* Clifton Park, NJ: Humana Press, 1988: 23–71.

● 3. Benedetti C. Acute pain; a review of its effects and therapy with systemic opioids. In: Benedetti C, Chapman CR, Giron G eds. *Opioid Analgesia: Recent Advances in Systemic Administration, Advances in Pain Research and Therapy,* vol. 14. New York, NY: Raven, 1990: 367–424.

● 4. Stein C. Peripheral mechanisms of opioid analgesia. *Anesth Analg* 1993; **76:** 182–91.

5. Dalsgaard J, Flesby S, Juelsgaard P, *et al.* Low-dose intra-articular morphine analgesia in day-case knee arthroscopy: a randomized, double-blinded, prospective study. *Pain* 1994; **56:** 151–4.

6. Joshi GP, McCarroll SM, O'Brien TM, *et al.* Intrarticular analgesia following knee arthroscopy. *Anesth Analg* 1993; **76:** 333–6.

7. Jaffe JH, Martin WR. Opioid analgesics and antagonists. In: Gilman AG, Rall TW, Niesf AS, Taylor P eds. *The Pharmacological Basis of Therapeutics,* 8th edn. New York, NY: Pergamon Press, 1990: 485–521.

● 8. Pasternak GW. Pharmacological mechanisms of opioid analgesics. *Clin Neuropharmacol* 1993; **16:** 1–18.

● 9. Reisine T, Bell GI. Molecular biology of opioid receptors. *Trends Neurosci* 1993; **16:** 506–10.

◆ 10. Cousins MJ, Siddall PJ. Introduction to acute and chronic pain: implications for neural blockade. In: Cousins MJ, Bridenbaugh PO eds. *Neural Blockade in Clinical Anesthesia and Management of Pain.* Philadelphia, PA: Lippincott-Raven Publishers, 1998: 675–713.

◆ 11. Meunier JC, Mollereau C, Toll L, *et al*. Isolation and structure of the endogenous agonist of opioid receptor-like ORL1 receptor. *Nature* 1995; **377**: 532–5.

◆ 12. Reinscheid RK, Nothacker HP, Bourson A, *et al*. Orphanin FQ: a neuropeptide that activates an opioid like G protein-coupled receptor. *Science* 1995; **270**: 792–4.

● 13. Calo G, Bigoni R, Rizzi A, *et al*. Nociceptin/orphanin FQ receptor ligands. *Peptides* 2000; **21**: 935–47.

14. Carr DB, Jacox AK, Chapman CR, *et al*. *Acute Pain Management: Operative or Medical Procedures and Trauma*. Clinical Practice Guideline, AHCPR publication no. 92-0032. Rockville, MD: US Department of Health and Human Services, Public Health Service, Agency for Health Care Policy and Research, 1992.

● 15. Portenoy RK. Chronic opioid therapy in nonmalignant pain. *J Pain Symptom Manage* 1990; **5**: S46–62.

◆ 16. Yaksh TL. Tolerance: factors involved in changes in the dose–effect relationship with chronic drug exposure. In: Basbaum AI, Besson JM eds. *Towards a New Pharmacotherapy of Pain*. New York, NY: John Wiley & Sons, 1991: 157–80.

17. Ballantyne JC, Loach AB, Carr DB. Itching after epidural and spinal opiates. *Pain* 1988; **33**: 149–60.

18. Kaiko RF. Age and morphine analgesia in cancer patients with postoperative pain. *Clin Pharmacol Ther* 1980; **28**: 823–6.

19. Ventafridda V, Ripamonti C, DeConno F, *et al*. Antidepressants increase bioavailability of morphine in cancer patients. *Lancet* 1987; **1**: 1204.

20. Foley KM, Inturrisi CE. Pharmacokinetics of oral, intravenous, and continuous infusions of heroin. *Adv Pain Res Ther* 1986; **8**: 117–27.

21. Medina JL, Diamond S. Drug dependency in patients with chronic headache. *Headache* 1977; **17**: 12–14.

22. Porter J, Jick H. Addiction rare in patients treated with narcotics. *N Engl J Med* 1980; **302**: 123.

23. Ventafridda V, Tamburine M, Caraceni A, *et al*. A validation study of WHO method for cancer pain relief. *Cancer* 1987; **5**: 850.

24. Woods JH, Winger G. Opioids, receptors and abuse liability. In: Meltzer HY ed. *Neural Blockade in Clinical Anaesthesia and Management of Pain*, 2nd edn. Philadelphia, PA: Lippincott, 1988: 885–98.

25. Anand KJS, McGrath PJ eds. *Pain in Neonates*. New York, NY: Elsevier, 1993.

26. Anderson CTM, Zeltzer LK, Fanurik D. Procedural pain. In: Schechter NL, Berde CB, Yaster M eds. *Pain in Infants, Children and Adolescents*. Baltimore, MD: Williams & Wilkins, 1993: 435–57.

7

Treatment protocols for opioids in chronic nonmalignant pain

HARALD BREIVIK

Chronic nociceptive pain	77	Patient information and consent to opioid treatment	80
Chronic neuropathic pain	77	Drug-related behaviors that may raise concern	81
Indications for long-term treatment with a potent opioid analgesic in chronic non-neoplastic pain	78	Treatment of episodes of acute pain in patients on chronic opioid therapy for noncancer pain	81
Selection of patients, implementation, and follow-up of long-term potent opioid treatment	78	References	82
What is the evidence base for opioid treatment of chronic noncancer pain?	79		

This chapter will discuss the practical aspects of opioid therapy for chronic noncancer pain.

CHRONIC NOCICEPTIVE PAIN

There is increasing acceptance that potent opioids may be used with benefit in elderly patients with persistent or recurring nociceptive pain where causal therapy is unavailable or contraindicated. An example is an elderly lady with nightly pains and pain exacerbated by walking due to severe osteoarthritis in the knee joints. When such a patient cannot tolerate major surgery, a knee joint replacement is unavailable for socioeconomic reasons, or cyclo-oxygenase 1/2 (COX-1/2) inhibitors are ineffective, potent opioid analgesia can be an effective and humane way to help such a patient.

The following treatment protocols are appropriate:

1 Pain provoked by movement caused by necessary daily activities:
  a Immediate-release and controlled-release preparation, for example oxycodone q.s.,[1**] always in combination with acetaminophen (paracetamol) 500–1,000 mg.
  b General precautions and guidelines as described below for chronic noncancer pain.

2 Pain provoked by necessary/desirable activities in addition to daily activities (e.g. shopping, visiting family):
  a Add extra dose of immediate-release opioid for short-term activity.
  b Add extra dose of immediate-release plus controlled release preparation for activities lasting several hours.

3 Pain during the night, disturbing normal sleep:
  a Appropriate evening dose of slow-release opioid preparation.

CHRONIC NEUROPATHIC PAIN

Patients suffering from chronic noncancer pain often have neuropathic pain due to peripheral or central nervous system pathological mechanisms. This causes abnormal sensations provoked by innocuous stimuli and, together with an abnormal temporal profile, results in unpleasant, painful experiences.[2] A number of nonopioid drugs can modify these abnormal pain mechanisms and to some degree reduce suffering.[3***] Occasionally, it is appropriate to prescribe a potent opioid for patients suffering from chronic or persistently recurring non-nociceptive noncancer pain.[3***,4–10]

INDICATIONS FOR LONG-TERM TREATMENT WITH A POTENT OPIOID ANALGESIC IN CHRONIC NON-NEOPLASTIC PAIN

Long-term treatment in chronic non-neoplastic pain is justified if:

- other drugs and other methods with fewer side-effects have failed;
- pain relief from an opioid analgesic is sustained;
- the patient's quality of life is improved enough to tolerate side-effects and to accept the risk of long-term adverse effects of opioid therapy.

SELECTION OF PATIENTS, IMPLEMENTATION, AND FOLLOW-UP OF LONG-TERM POTENT OPIOID TREATMENT

This is not an easy task. It can be one of the most demanding treatment modalities that a pain clinician undertakes. There are several problems and practical challenges, initially as well as during long-term follow-up.

How to determine whether pain and quality of life improve with opioid treatment

Not all chronic pain patients respond to potent opioids.[11] Pain relief must be experienced as useful and sustained, with a dose and an administration form that make prolonged therapy feasible.

- A blinded intravenous test may give an indication of the responsiveness of the patient's pain to opioid treatment (see Chapter P4).
- However, only a trial period of 2–4 weeks with titrated oral administration can determine whether pain relief is sufficient to improve physical and social functioning.
- Since some degree of tolerance and withdrawal symptoms develop within a few days of starting opioid treatment, this trial period may lead directly to the following group of problems:
  - development of tolerance;
  - physical dependence;
  - withdrawal symptoms;
  - breakthrough pain;
  - pseudoaddiction.

The challenge of handling the complex problems of adjusting and controlling opioid intake is sometimes formidable: recognizing and correctly handling breakthrough pain to avoid unnecessary dose escalation; recognizing periods of "pseudoaddiction behavior" as such, rather than ruining the patient's trust in the doctor by handling a legitimate need for a higher dose as a symptom of addictive behavior.[12] Appropriate patient information

and a trustful collaboration with the patient is necessary to contain or avoid the physical withdrawal symptoms, the risk of psychological dependence, and the complex situation where a patient has become an iatrogenic, difficult-to-handle, opioid-using problem patient.[13]

Are some patients more prone to develop opioid treatment compliance problems than others?

The problems are potentially present in every patient, but they can be controlled better in those with pain that responds well to opioids and in those who have a stable psychosocial background and work situation.

An addictive disease process, such as alcoholism, affects 3–16% of the US population.[13] It is believed that this is due to a combination of factors, such as:

- biogenetic predisposition;
- psychological profile;
- sociocultural context;
- drug exposure and availability.

A previous personal or family history of alcoholism or other addictive disorders is the primary risk factor for developing difficult problems during opioid analgesic treatment for chronic pain.

These are relative contraindications[14] for starting a trial of opioid treatment for chronic noncancer pain.

Some opioid analgesics are safer than others

Unfortunately, problems with safety are present with all opioid analgesics: the very weak, such as tramadol; the weak, such as codeine/dihydrocodeine; the more potent, such as buprenorphine, oxycodone, and morphine; and the most potent opioids, such as fentanyl and sufentanil.

However, the problems develop more slowly with:

- weak opioids;
- opioid formulations and administration forms that have a slow onset and long, stable duration of effect.

Some administration modalities or routes are safer than others

Administration modalities that result in a slow onset and prolonged effect appear to be more easily controlled, such as:

- Oral administration of controlled-/sustained- release formulations.
- Possibly transdermal administrations of lipophilic opioids, e.g. fentanyl or buprenorphine. Time will show whether the present trend of increasing use of

transdermal fentanyl for chronic noncancer pain can be justified.[15]

Drugs with quick onset and short duration are more prone to control problems

- Parenteral injections of opioids for chronic pain is the administration form that is most difficult to handle and that eventually leads to escalation of dose and difficult compliance problems.

WHAT IS THE EVIDENCE BASE FOR OPIOID TREATMENT OF CHRONIC NONCANCER PAIN?

There are few double-blind, randomized, placebo-controlled clinical studies on the benefits and side-effects of opioid treatment for chronic non-neoplastic pain.[1,16] Long-term, double-blind, randomized clinical trials have not been performed and the many problems surrounding long-term opioid treatment of chronic pain are not going to be resolved by such trials. The numerous variables and confounding factors involved, the necessity of individually titrating doses, and the practical problems of maintaining blinding for several months make the challenges of such studies formidable. An ongoing, large, multicenter study of transdermal fentanyl for low back pain in which each patient will be treated for at least 12 months is not going to increase our knowledge on this issue since there is no control included in the study. Randomized, prospective, comparative studies without blinding may be the best we can hope for, but it is not very likely that we are going to see any of these soon. Not even major national or international agencies for medicines, who are responsible for the optimal use of drugs, are likely to take initiatives to clarify this important drug problem.

Suggested guidelines for treatment of chronic noncancer pain with opioids

Therefore, for the foreseeable future, guidelines will have to depend on the experience of long-term practitioners in pain medicine. National and international pain societies, together with others, have proposed guidelines for the rational use of opioid analgesics in the management of patients with chronic noncancer pain.[4-10]

The following outline of how one may approach this complex problem is expanded within several published guidelines in addition to the author's own experience over two decades of pain medicine practice.[13,17-19]

Assessment of the opioid response and justification for maintenance of opioid therapy

- Working diagnoses, differential diagnoses, diagnostic techniques, analyses of the pain condition with a con-

clusion as to the type of pain, and possible etiological and contributory pathogenic mechanisms.
- Specific statement of the medical indication for an attempt at assessment of opioid therapy:
  - Reasonable attempts (but unsuccessful) at treating the pain condition with available nonopioid medications and other interventions.
  - Markedly reduced quality of life.
- Potential contraindications to opioid treatment:
  - History of alcohol or substance abuse (relatively strong contraindication).
  - Unstable sociopsychological background (relative contraindication).
- Blinded opioid intravenous infusion test (morphine or alfentanil; see Chapter P4):
  - If there is a positive beneficial response after at least one opioid for pain intensity, and preferably some effect on sensory dysfunctional symptoms (allodynia), see next bullet point.
- Proceed with trial period of about 3 weeks of oral treatment with methadone or one of the controlled release opioid drugs, such as dihydrocodeine, oxycodone, morphine, or ketobemidone, with appropriate dose adjustments to provide:
  - Useful pain relief.
  - Improvement in function and quality of life.
  - Tolerable side-effects.
- If this treatment goal is not obtainable with any available long-term oral opioid [and the intravenous (i.v.) test was positive]:
  - Attempts at maintenance therapy with transdermal opioid may be considered.
  - The author strongly advises against parenteral opioid treatment. This is just too difficult to control for prolonged periods.

The objectives and treatment plan for maintenance opioid therapy

Objectives of treatment
- Reduction in pain.
- Improvement in social functioning.
- Ability to carry out daily activities.

The following must be measured, documented, and followed over time:

- Subjective pain assessment on a visual analog scale (or a 0–10 numeric rating scale) and a categorical verbal rating scale.
- Changes in physical and social functioning – are any changes due to opioid therapy?
- Daily activities – are any changes due to opioid therapy?

Treatment plan
- The treatment plan should aim at maintaining documented effects observed during the trial period.

- It should include the type of drug, administration form, and dosage.
- There should be a frequent review of medication use, effects, and overall benefits. Initially, this should be carried out twice weekly, then weekly, and, when stable, effects, side-effects, and dose required should be measured on at least a monthly basis.
- Included in patients' charts at every office/clinic visit, there should be:
  - Efficacy of treatment on pain rating scales.
  - Functional changes in ability to perform daily activities.
  - Changes in ability to function at home, at work, in the community, and with a social life.
  - Any adverse effects of opioid medication.
  - Assess compliance of drug use compared with agreed plan.
  - Review diagnosis and treatment plan.
- There should be unannounced urine or serum drug screens, when indicated.

Periodic reviews

At least every 6 months, there should be a review of the current status compared with previous documentation to determine whether continued opioid therapy is the best option for the patient.

PATIENT INFORMATION AND CONSENT TO OPIOID TREATMENT

Opioid treatment for chronic non-neoplastic pain can be safely managed, but this requires the patient to be well informed of the objectives, the effects, the short- and long-term adverse effects, and the very real risks of drug-related complications of addictive drugs:

- Verbal and written information should be given, including informed consent on starting treatment.
- The patient must be able to share responsibility for observing and reporting early symptoms of tolerance, physical dependence, and withdrawal.
- The patient is coresponsible for the dosing regime, compliance, adjusting dosage for breakthrough pain, and returning to baseline dosing.
- When appropriate, the patient should be made aware of the necessity of urine or serum medication level screening and checks for nonprescribed medications.

Both physician and patient awareness of the problems and responsibilities associated with opioid treatment should be documented in writing.

The patient must understand that complications associated with long-term opioid therapy include:

- *Confusion*, or other changes in mental state or cognitive and thinking abilities.
- *Coordination problems* and balance, which may make it unsafe to operate dangerous equipment or motor vehicles.

- *Increased sleepiness,* or drowsiness, especially when combined with other drugs or alcohol.
- *Constipation*, which requires prophylactic treatment from day one.
- *Respiratory depression,* breathing too slowly, especially when combined with night sedation and/or alcohol and if dose of opioid drug is rapidly increased.
- *Decreased appetite.*
- *Physical dependence*, the physiological adaptation to the opioid drug, characterized by the emergence of withdrawal syndrome during abstinence, which may be relieved by readministration of the opioid.
- *Physical dependence* is a predictable sequelae of regular, legitimate opioid use, and does NOT equate with addiction.
- *Withdrawal syndrome* is a specific constellation of signs and symptoms due to the abrupt cessation of, or reduction in, a regularly administered dose of opioid. It is characterized by three or more of the following symptoms that develop within hours to days after abrupt cessation of the opioid:
  - dysphoric mood;
  - anxiety;
  - nausea and vomiting;
  - muscle aches and abdominal cramps;
  - lacrimation or rhinorrhea (runny nose);
  - pupillary dilation;
  - piloerection ("goose flesh");
  - sweating;
  - diarrhea;
  - yawning;
  - fever;
  - insomnia.
- *Addiction*, which is a disease process involving use of opioid analgesic with:
  - loss of control of own behavior;
  - compulsive use;
  - continued use despite adverse social, physical, psychological, occupational, or economic consequences.
- *Tolerance* results from regular use of an opioid analgesic leading to a need for an increased dose of opioid to produce the desired effect. Tolerance is a predictable sequela of opioid use and does NOT imply addiction.
- *Breakthrough pain* and *pseudoaddiction* occur when pain for some reason increases transiently, requiring an extra opioid dose. If the patient is met with skepticism and breakthrough pain is not appropriately handled, the patient is liable to show behavior similar to truly addicted persons.
- *Pseudoaddiction behavior* may also occur when tolerance slowly develops and the opioid dose is not adjusted accordingly. This iatrogenic condition can be prevented/handled if there is a truly respectful and trusting relationship between patient and doctor.

- *Children born* to mothers on regular opioid medication are born physically dependent on the medication.
- *Logistic problems* relating to planned international travel must be anticipated and handled as required.

In addition to the above, there should be only one prescriber [with deputy prescriber(s) during absence for vacation, etc.] for all pain-related medication, and a single pharmacy should be used when possible.

There should be an agreed plan for monitoring compliance of treatment that includes:

- Number and frequency of all prescriptions.
- Urine or serum medication levels screening, including checks for nonprescribed medications. This should be carried out only when appropriate.

The reasons for discontinuing opioid therapy include violation of the written agreement, loss of demonstrable beneficial effects, and loss of control and trust.

DRUG-RELATED BEHAVIORS THAT MAY RAISE CONCERN

Drug-related behaviors that may raise concern about the potential for true addiction developing in medical patients who are prescribed opioids for chronic pain include:[18]

- Behaviors probably more predictive of true addiction:
  - Selling of prescription drugs.
  - Prescription forgery.
  - Stealing or "borrowing" drugs from others.
  - Injecting oral formulations.
  - Obtaining prescription drugs from nonmedical sources.
  - Concurrent abuse of alcohol or illicit drugs.
  - Multiple dose escalations or other noncompliance with therapy despite warnings.
  - Multiple episodes of prescription "loss."
  - Repeatedly seeking prescriptions from other clinicians or from emergency rooms without informing the physician responsible for medical treatment of the patient.
  - Evidence of deterioration in the ability to function at work, in the family, or socially that appears to be related to drug use.
  - Repeated resistance to changes in therapy despite clear evidence of adverse physical or psychological effects from the drug.
- Behaviors probably less predictive of addiction:
  - Aggressive complaining about the need for more drug.
  - Drug hoarding during periods of reduced symptoms.
  - Requesting specific drugs.
  - Openly acquiring similar drugs from other medical sources.
  - Unsanctioned dose escalation or other noncompliance with therapy on one or two occasions.
  - Reporting psychic effects not intended by the clinician.
  - Resistance to a change in therapy associated with "tolerable" adverse effects with expressions of anxiety related to the return of severe symptoms.

TREATMENT OF EPISODES OF ACUTE PAIN IN PATIENTS ON CHRONIC OPIOID THERAPY FOR NONCANCER PAIN

When these patients have surgery, suffer trauma, or need treatment in an intensive care unit, their need for analgesic therapy is often underestimated. Sometimes, even misguided attempts to wean them from opioid therapy are initiated. These patients do have opioid tolerance and need a tailored titration of potent shorter acting opioids. Trying to be restrictive with opioids in such a situation is not humane. Consider adding clonidine continuous intravenous infusion, starting with 1–2 µg/kg/h, which will suppress most of the autonomic and physical withdrawal symptoms, but withdrawal anxiety remains.

Whenever appropriate, a local or regional anesthetic technique, such as continuous femoral nerve or epidural block with a local anesthetic, an opioid, and adrenergic drug, should be used. In addition to a regional analgesic technique, opioid maintenance therapy is necessary to prevent tormenting the patient with withdrawal symptoms.

A case history illustrating problems facing the doctor and patient in long-term opioid treatment for noncancer pain

A middle-aged, former active student of political science and economics, now an unemployed single mother, suffered from psoriasis arthritis from the age of 12. Gradually, her joint pain increased, especially in the wrist joints, despite treatment with the customary regimens for arthritis. For analgesia, she took acetaminophen (until low-grade hepatitis C was diagnosed, caused, most likely, by a complication from a blood transfusion after the birth of her child) and codeine or dextropropoxyphene until the age of 31, when she underwent surgery to her right wrist joint with a synovectomy. Her right wrist pain increased, however, and she required surgical arthrodesis 6 months later. Her pain did not improve and she underwent surgery 4 years after the first operation, when one nerve entrapped in scar tissue was released, leading to a transient improvement of the pain. By now, the patient had acquired an iatrogenic complex regional pain syndrome in addition to her arthritis. For several years, she also had migraine and a gastrointestinal disorder with loose stools and abdominal cramps. This was aggravated by analgesic tablets, so she preferred the rectal administration of analgesics. Escalation of her opioid treatment started after the first operation, with occasional ketobemidone suppositories as rescue analgesia during periods of severe pain. From the age of 33, she was evaluated and treated at the pain clinic at a university hospital. She had little or no benefit from sympathetic blocks, amitriptyline, and clonazepam. She was maintained on pentazocine suppositories, which gave adequate pain relief for about 3 years. Gradually, the opioid was escalated to ketobemidone suppositories three to five times daily. From the age of 37, she was on an average dose of ketobemidone 5 mg four times daily, with two extra doses allowed every day for breakthrough pain. The patient moved to a smaller town in another part of the country. In this town, it was impossible for the patient to find a doctor who was willing to continue opioid prescription. The local health authorities accused her of being addicted to opioids and only offered her withdrawal treatment. An Enforcement Court rule made it possible for her to maintain contact with her former primary care physician, who continued to prescribe opioids. This was a difficult arrangement because of the distance. She was allowed to consult him four times a year. However, this arrangement became too difficult for everybody when the patient developed breakthrough pain and aggressive pseudoaddiction behavior. It was only after 2 years that a doctor in the local town was willing to assume opioid prescription responsibility for the patient. However, the patient had increasing difficulties with the child care authorities, who had received anonymous accusations of irresponsible care of her child due to opioid usage. The social circumstances in this town became impossible and she moved to the nearby community, where she had grown up as a child, and settled in the house in which her now ailing parents had lived until a few years ago. In this community, the district general practitioner had the knowledge and experience to take on the responsibility for managing her opioid treatment. He was able to establish a treatment regime based on a mutually trustful relationship which has been very successful for the patient. She has been able to decrease her drug usage, functions socially, and is able to care well for her child. She has confidence in her primary care physician and the previous, quite dramatic, episodes of breakthrough pain with aggressive pseudoaddiction behavior have now disappeared.

Comments

This patient illustrates that chronic noncancer pain can be treated with potent opioids for prolonged periods. The case also illustrates well how demanding this type of treatment is for the patient and the doctors involved. Pseudoaddiction can rapidly escalate into a major prob-

lem with a vicious circle of mistrust and accusations. This develops more easily when the doctor and patient do not know each other well, and the relationship can become very difficult when the patient is unwilling to accept the treating physician's diagnosis. Although the guidelines for chronic opioid treatment of noncancer pain are fairly straightforward, in practice they are quite demanding and many doctors and pain clinicians have been taken by surprise by the many unexpected difficulties that develop. Understanding and being prepared to tackle pseudoaddiction behavior makes this task easier. Clearly, multidisciplinary pain clinic expertise and resources are needed to help primary care physicians manage such challenging patients.

REFERENCES

1. Caldwell JR, Hale ME, Boyd RE, *et al*. Treatment of osteoarthritis pain with controlled release oxycodone or fixed combination oxycodone plus acetaminophen added to nonsteroidal antiinflammatory drugs: a double blind, randomized, multicenter, placebo controlled trial. *J Rheumatol* 1999; **26:** 862–9.

◆ 2. Woolf CJ, Mannion RJ. Neuropathic pain: aetiology, symptoms, mechanisms, and management. *Lancet* 1999; **353:** 1959–64

● 3. Sindrup SH, Jensen TS. Efficacy of pharmacological treatments of neuropathic pain: an update and effect related to mechanism of drug action. *Pain* 1999; **83:** 389–400.

● 4. Schug SA, Large RG. Opioids for chronic noncancer pain. In: *Pain: Clinical Updates*, vol. 3. Seattle, WA: International Association for the Study of Pain Press, 1995; **3:** 1–4.

5. Federation of State Medical Boards of the United States. Model Guidelines for the Use of Controlled Substances for the Treatment of Pain. Federation of State Medical Boards of the United States, Inc., 1998.

● 6. Portenoy RK. Opioid therapy for chronic nonmalignant pain: current status. In: Fields HL, Liebeskind JC eds. *Pharmacological Approaches to the Treatment of Chronic Pain: New Concepts and Critical Issues. Progress in Pain Research and Management*, vol. 1. Seattle, WA: IASP Press 1994: 247–87.

◆ 7. American Academy of Pain Medicine and the American Pain Society. The use of opioids for the treatment of chronic pain. A consensus statement from the American Academy of Pain Medicine and the American Pain Society. *Clin J Pain* 1997; **13:** 6–8.

◆ 8. Gramstad L, Haugtomt H, Breivik H. Use of opioids in chronic non-cancer pain – current status in Norway. In: Kalso E, Paakari P, Stenberg I eds. *Opioids in Chronic Non-cancer pain. Situation and Guidelines in the Nordic Countries*. Helsinki: National Agency for Medicines, 1999: 31–7.

9. McQuay H. Opioid use in chronic pain. *Acta Anaesthesiol Scand* 1997; **41:** 175–83.

◆ 10. Canadian Pain Society. Use of opioid analgesics for the treatment of chronic noncancer pain – a consensus statement and guidelines from the Canadian Pain Society. *Pain Res Manage* 1998; **3:** 197–208.

◆ 11. Arnér S, Meyerson BA. Lack of analgesic effect of opioids on neuropathic and idiopathic forms of pain. *Pain* 1988; **33:** 11–23.

◆ 12. Weissman DE, Haddox JD. Opioid pseudoaddiction – an iatrogenic syndrome. *Pain* 1989; **36:** 363–6.

◆ 13. Savage SR. Opioid therapy of chronic pain: assessment of consequences. *Acta Anaesthesiol Scand* 1999; **43:** 909–17.

14. Dunbar SA, Katz NP. Chronic opioid therapy for non-malignant pain in patients with a history of substance abuse: report of 20 cases. *J Pain Symptom Manage* 1996; **11:** 163–71.

15. Dellimijn P, van Duijn H, Vanneste J. Prolonged treatment with transdermal fentanyl in neuropathic pain. *J Pain Symptom Manage* 1998; **16:** 220–9.

◆ 16. Moulin DE, Iezzi A, Amireh R, *et al.* Randomised trial of oral morphine for chronic non-cancer pain. *Lancet* 1996; **347:** 143–7.

17. Breivik H. Strong opiate analgesics for chronic pain. *Tidsskr Nor Lægeforen* 1983; **103:** 1491–3.

◆ 18. Savage SR. Long-term opioid therapy: assessment of consequences and risks. *J Pain Symptom Manage* 1996; **11:** 274–86.

◆ 19. Kalso E, Paakari P, Stenberg I eds. *Opioids in Chronic Non-cancer pain. Situation and Guidelines in the Nordic Countries.* Helsinki: National Agency for Medicines, 1999: 31–7.

8

Subcutaneous drug infusions for the control of cancer pain

IVAN F TROTMAN AND FAEQA HAMI

Subcutaneous administration	85	Clinical studies	92
Indications for the use of subcutaneous infusions	86	Starting a subcutaneous infusion	95
Contraindications	86	Monitoring	95
Use of syringe drivers	86	Complications	96
Administration of drugs	88	Managerial issues	98
Choice of analgesic	88	Closing remarks	99
Drug combinations	92	References	99

Subcutaneous infusions for the control of cancer pain have become increasingly popular as a means of administering analgesic drugs (mostly opioids) since their use was first described in 1979. Subcutaneous infusions are usually delivered by means of a mechanical syringe driver. Drug infusions by this technique have also been found to be useful in alleviating a number of other symptoms, including agitation, vomiting, and intestinal obstruction, and to dry secretions in the terminal phase. Although some have argued that the syringe driver has been over-employed or inappropriately used as a medical "last rite" in dying patients, the benefits of the syringe driver in the overall management of cancer pain are unquestionable.[1]

Syringe drivers are portable battery- or clockwork-driven devices that are used to advance the plunger of a standard medical hypodermic syringe at a predetermined rate. Drugs previously mixed in the syringe can thus be administered to the patient via a catheter and an indwelling, usually subcutaneous, needle. Syringe drivers powered from the electrical mains can serve a similar purpose, but have the disadvantage of not being portable. Implantable pumps such as those used for chronic administration of intrathecal or epidural analgesia are beyond the scope of this chapter.

SUBCUTANEOUS ADMINISTRATION

The choice of the subcutaneous route for injection of drugs has evolved from common practice in UK hospices.[2,3] There are a number of advantages:

1 Ease of access. Drugs can be injected into a wide variety of sites over the body surface. The patient does not have to be moved or turned, therefore injections cause less disturbance and discomfort.
2 Safety. There are fewer complications than with intramuscular or intravenous injections. Nursing staff require few special skills or experience.
3 Avoidance of "bolus effect." Transient high peaks in plasma drug concentration are thought to be associated with an increased incidence of vomiting after morphine injection.
4 Possibly less painful for the patient, particularly if repeated injections are needed.

Subcutaneous infusions confer additional advantages, namely:

1 Portable devices allow the patient to remain ambulant and to be managed in the community, which is rarely possible using intravenous access.
2 The infusion can easily be resited if it becomes displaced without the need for specialist facilities or staff.
3 Savings in nursing time.
4 Reduced likelihood of the "last injection" phenomenon, in which a patient is perceived to die shortly after a drug is given with consequent distress among staff and blame from relatives.

5 The infusion pump (syringe driver) can be concealed beneath the bed covers or in a carrying pouch, causing less distraction and anxiety for the patient and family.

The use of subcutaneous infusions requires a number of assumptions:

1 That the physicochemical and pharmacological properties of drugs (either singly or in combination) are suitable for administration by this route.
2 That the drug remains stable in solution for the duration of the infusion.
3 That absorption from the subcutaneous tissues is reliable and constant.

Studies indicate that subcutaneous infusion of morphine achieves similar plasma concentrations to those found with intravenous infusion.[4] However, most of the data relating to the safety and efficacy of drugs given by subcutaneous infusion come from anecdotal evidence, case reports, or publications of small series. Moreover, in nearly all cases, the administration of drugs in this way is outside their indications, as licensed by the regulatory authorities. Their use in this manner therefore requires the exercise of clinical freedom and judgment.

INDICATIONS FOR THE USE OF SUBCUTANEOUS INFUSIONS

The principal indications for subcutaneous infusions by syringe driver are summarized in Table 8.1. Commonly, syringe drivers are used to manage the terminal phase of an illness because the patient is too weak to take oral medication or has become comatose. In patients who are dying, periods of wakefulness lessen, and oral medication can no longer be taken reliably. During this time, it is generally considered to be important that the patient continues to receive prescribed analgesia, and the only way to administer this is parenterally. The arguments against the routine use of syringe drivers in this situation are that not all patients require injectable analgesia, that adequate pain control can be maintained despite irregular dosing, and that possibly the requirement for strong (opioid) analgesics lessens during the dying process because of multiorgan failure.

For the patient who is vomiting and in pain, a syringe driver provides a tool for the dual management of symptoms with combinations of analgesic and antiemetic drugs.[5] Continuous administration of drugs by this route diminishes the need for, and discomfort of, intermittent injections. In uncontrolled pain, the use of a syringe driver is preferred to the use of "as required" injections for pain, not only for comfort but also to reduce the risk of tolerance and rapidly escalating opioid dose.[6]

Syringe drivers have an important role in the management of terminal delirium and intestinal obstruction. In

Table 8.1 *Indications for subcutaneous infusion*

Unconsciousness
Terminal care
Vomiting
Intestinal obstruction
Dysphagia
Pain control
Noncompliance
Use of specific drugs
Patient preference

these situations, sedatives or antisecretory agents are usually combined with appropriate doses of opioid analgesia.

CONTRAINDICATIONS

There are no absolute contraindications to the use of a subcutaneous infusion, and it is possible to administer very large volumes by this route. Severe clotting abnormalities, particularly a depressed platelet count, predispose to the risk of hemorrhage at the injection site. However, a clinician may consider the facility of a subcutaneous needle placement to outweigh the apparent risk of bleeding. The injection site should be inspected regularly. Occasionally, severe skin disease makes needle placement impossible, and subcutaneous needles should not be positioned into lymphedematous skin or into active tumor sites. Similarly, needles should not be inserted into skin that has been irradiated, and the insertion site should be away from joints.

Phobic anxiety states may preclude the effective use of a syringe driver, and patients with florid psychotic disturbance will often not tolerate their use until adequate sedation has been achieved or until the cause of the mental disturbance has been alleviated. The use of subcutaneous infusions by syringe driver requires appropriate consent from the patient.

USE OF SYRINGE DRIVERS

Syringe drivers are the most popular means of administering subcutaneous infusions. They are precision instruments that are calibrated to travel a fixed distance in a given time. The volume administered to a patient will vary according to the size of syringe fitted to the driver, and the dose of drug will depend upon its concentration within the syringe. There is potential for confusion in translating a prescription for a drug dose in milligrams to a driver speed in millimeters. The following need to be considered:

- choice of syringe driver;
- rate of administration;

- size and type of syringe;
- length and volume of the connection catheter.

Choice of syringe driver

There are several commercially available syringe drivers, and the choice of driver will often depend upon local availability and cost. Portable battery-driven units have gained widest acceptance for the management of pain in patients with cancer. In the UK, the most widely used syringe drivers are the Graseby models MS16(a) and MS26. A typical portable syringe driver is shown in Fig. 8.1. When drugs need to be administered in a large volume of diluent, a mains-operated device may be preferred because most portable syringe drivers will only accommodate a 30-ml syringe containing 20 ml of fluid (Fig. 8.2).

Portable syringe drivers enable the patient to be ambulant and to be easily transferred between hospital and community settings. The main disadvantages are that they are not fitted with malfunction alarms to warn if the device is inoperative, if the battery power is low, if the driver is overspeeding, or if there is inadvertent catheter disconnection. They do not allow significant bolus administration for breakthrough pain.

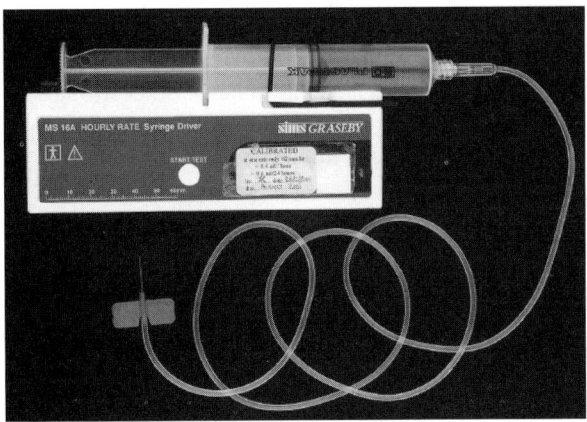

Figure 8.1 *Typical Graseby syringe driver with a "butterfly" subcutaneous needle connected.*

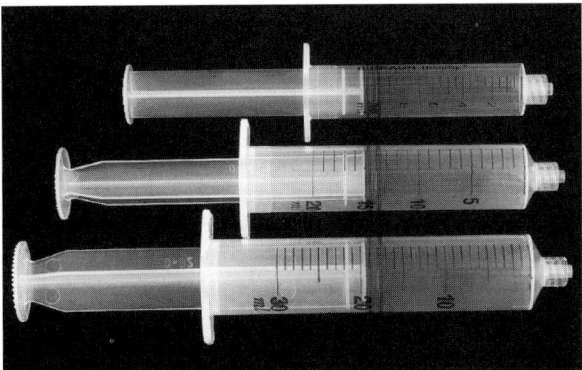

Figure 8.2 *Differing volume syringes (10, 20, and 30 ml) filled to 48 mm. Each would deliver its contents over 24 h when the syringe driver runs at 2 mm/h.*

Rate of administration

Most syringe drivers allow the rate of administration of the drug to be varied. However, it is recommended that only fixed rates of administration are used, and that, once set, the syringe driver speed is not altered. There are several reasons to prefer fixed rate drug administration to variable rate infusion:

1 Cancer pain is usually chronic and therefore requires stable doses of analgesia.
2 It is sometimes difficult to discriminate between breakthrough pain, escalation of pain, and incident pain (pain with movement or exertion). Breakthrough pain requires intermittent use of supplementary analgesia before pain returns to previous (controlled) levels; pain escalation requires an overall increase in analgesic dose; and incident pain calls for alternative strategies of pain management.
3 If opioid analgesia is used, poor background analgesia and perhaps inadequate supplementary dosing are likely to lead to early tolerance, with consequent apparent opioid unresponsiveness, high daily dosage, and emergence of unwanted effects.
4 When drugs are given subcutaneously, there is a delay between increasing the rate of administration and observing benefit.
5 The syringe driver is likely to run through prematurely and unpredictably, making it difficult to establish the true 24-h dose requirement once adequate pain control has been achieved.
6 It is common practice to mix two and sometimes more drugs in a syringe driver, and adjusting the rate of analgesic administration will also alter the dose of any co-therapy.
7 It is administratively safer to use fixed rate infusions. The patient may be cared for in a number of different health care environments, and uniformity of management of syringe drivers reduces the opportunity for prescribing error.

Devices that permit the patient to administer bolus doses of analgesia (patient controlled analgesia; PCA) have not gained wide acceptance in the control of cancer pain. Potentially, the use of PCA might allow rapid titration to stable doses in opioid-naive subjects or if changing from one opioid to another, when conversion factors are uncertain (e.g. morphine to fentanyl). However, the effective use of PCA requires intravenous access.

Caution is needed when changing from one syringe driver to another to ensure that the fixed rate of infusion is the same. Confusion can also occur when the infusion rate is specified in different units (millimeters per hour or millimeters per day).

Type of syringe

Most portable syringe drivers will accommodate 10-, 20-, or 30-ml syringes. However, the dimensions of the syringe may vary according to the manufacturer. The clinician needs to have confidence that syringes from the same manufacturer will conform to strict dimensional criteria. Because syringe drivers deliver the contents of a syringe in distance per unit time, fairly small variations in the internal diameter of the syringe will lead to significant changes in the volume delivered. When preparing drugs for administration, accurate dosing can only be assured by measuring the distance along the barrel of the syringe that is to be used (see Fig. 8.2).

Syringe quality should be such that the plunger moves easily within the barrel, is made of material sufficiently rigid to withstand distortion, and is intact, watertight, transparent, sterile and fitted with a Luer hub. Luer-locking syringes reduce the risk of inadvertent disconnection.

Connection tubing

It is customary to connect the syringe to a standard "butterfly"-type needle and administration set. Some manufacturers recommend and supply standard connection catheters and needles. Interpositioning lengths of manometer tubing (extension sets) can increase the length of catheter and thus allow the patient more mobility (Fig. 8.3). The length of the catheter and its volume have important implications when setting up or changing infusions, and this is considered in the section "Priming." For patients who experience reactions at the injection site, it is sometimes helpful to use plastic pediatric cannulas, such as those normally used for intravenous access.

ADMINISTRATION OF DRUGS

Many drugs have been given by subcutaneous infusion. Absorption of drugs by this route is reliable – the main limitation is irritation at the injection site. Decisions to give drugs by subcutaneous infusion have often been made on empirical grounds.

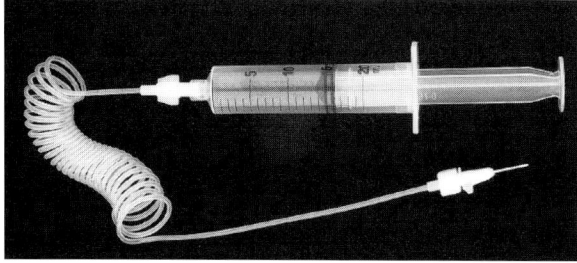

Figure 8.3 *Syringe with extendable connection tube and pediatric cannula.*

Drugs used in contemporary cancer care and the levels of evidence of their effect are listed in Tables 8.2–8.6. Most of the data for use of drugs in this way have been collected from experience in hospices and specialist palliative care units. As indicated previously, use of drugs by subcutaneous infusion is frequently outside of their licensed indications.

National policy, economic constraints, and local factors, including clinical preference and practice, will determine drug availability. Formulations may vary and not all drugs are available in all countries, e.g. although diamorphine is considered to be the opioid of first choice for use in subcutaneous infusions in the UK it is only available in a few other countries and is an illegal substance in the USA. Drug availability is important if a patient wishes to travel abroad or returns to die in their native country.

CHOICE OF ANALGESIC

Cancer pain is complex. It may arise directly from the tumor, from secondary deposits, or result from treatment. Pain in multiple sites is common and is often difficult to classify. Pain may have several different components (nociceptive or neuropathic), and these may vary with time. It has been estimated that 60% or more of patients will be prescribed morphine or other strong opioid during the course of their illness. Surveys of patients with advanced cancer receiving home care indicate a requirement for opioid analgesia in approximately 30%. It must be remembered that not all patients with cancer experience pain and that opioids may be used for other indications such as breathlessness or to relieve anxiety and distress. Cancer pain can rarely be managed by drug therapy alone. Even the most skillfully crafted prescription will be ineffective if no attention is paid to the other physical, emotional, and psychological aspects of a patient's care.

The choice of analgesic and dose for use by subcutaneous infusion is influenced by several factors:

- previous analgesic requirement and opioid use;
- availability of drug;
- type of pain.

In the management of cancer pain, most reports concern the use of opioid analgesia as they provide consistent and reliable pain relief.

Prescribing opioids

Most patients starting treatment by subcutaneous infusion will have had some exposure to opioids. If the previous opioid had been given by mouth, provided adequate pain relief, and is available for injection, equipotent analgesia can be obtained by using 50% of the oral dose. For

Table 8.2 *Use of opioids by subcutaneous infusion*

Opioid	Concentration	Potency ratio with morphine	Dose range	Evidence scoring
Morphine sulfate	10, 15, 20, 30 mg/ml	1	No upper limit	**
Morphine tartrate	120 mg/ml	1		
Diamorphine HCl	<250 mg/ml	2	No upper limit	**
Fentanyl	100 µg/2ml	100	25–50 µg/h	*
Alfentanil	1mg/2ml	4	0.5–1.0 mg/24 h No upper limit	0
Methadone HCl	10 mg/ml	1–10	No upper limit Use only if on oral methadone initially	*
Hydromorphone HCl	10, 20, 50 mg/ml	7.5	Range 1–35 mg/h No maximum dose	**
Oxycodone	Not available in UK	2		*
Dextromoramide	Parenteral form discontinued 1992	2		*
Meperidine	50 mg/ml	0.125	50 mg/h	*

Table 8.3 *Other analgesics*

Drug	Concentration	Dose range	Evidence scoring
Tramadol HCl	50 mg/ml	<400 mg/24 h	
Ketamine HCl	10, 50, 100 mg/ml	60–360 mg/24 h	*
Clonazepam	1 mg/ml	2–4 mg/24 h (for neuropathic pain)	
Ketorolac	10, 30 mg/ml	60–120 mg/24 h	*
Diclofenac	25 mg/ml	150 mg/24 h	

Table 8.4 *Sedatives*

Drug	Concentration	Dose range (per 24 h)
Midazolam HCl	5 mg/ml	5–60 mg
Haloperidol	5 mg/ml	5–30 mg
Methotrimeprazine HCl	25 mg/ml	12.5–200 mg
Phenobarbitone	30, 60, 200 mg/ml	50–200 mg (up to 1,200 mg)

Table 8.5 *Antiemetics*

Drug	Concentration	Dose range (per 24 h)
Metoclopramide HCl	5 mg/ml	30–60 mg
Haloperidol	5 mg/ml	5–20 mg
Methotrimeprazine HCl	25 mg/ml	6.25–50 mg
Cyclizine lactate	50 mg/ml	25–150 mg
Ondansetron	2 mg/ml	8–32 mg

opioids with relatively short half-lives (e.g. diamorphine, morphine, and hydromorphone), breakthrough pain is managed with bolus injections of the same opioid calculated as one-sixth of the total daily dose. If pain control is considered to be inadequate or there is a need for frequent breakthrough doses, the total dose in the infusion should be increased either by 25–30% (and sometimes more) or by summing the number of the supplementary (breakthrough) doses and adding this to the dose already in the infusion. In the latter situation, the amount added would depend upon the duration of the infusion. For example, if an infusion contains x mg of opioid and runs for 24 h and

Table 8.6 *Other drugs*

Drug	Concentration	Dose range (per 24 h)	Evidence scoring
Corticosteroids			
Dexamethasone	4 mg/ml	2–16 mg	*
Antisecretory agents			
Hyoscine hydrobromide	400 µg/ml	800–1,200 µg	*
Hyoscine butylbromide	20 mg/ml	60–120 mg	
Glycopyrronium bromide	200 µg/ml	800–1,200 µg	*
Octreotide acetate	50, 100, 200, 500 µg/ml	300–3,000 µg	*

Time not specified for dexamethasone dose range.

the patient requires y breakthrough injections of (usually) $x/6$ mg in a 24-h period, then the prescribed opioid dose for next 24 h would be $x + yx/6$ mg. An adjustment needs to be made for infusions of shorter duration.

Changing opioids

Sometimes, it is necessary to change from one opioid to another. This may occur if the opioid given by mouth is not available for injection or if a change in opioid might confer an advantage. Suggested equianalgesic doses of opioids are shown in Table 8.2, but caution is advised in their interpretation.[7,8] The concept of morphine equivalence is convenient for the design of clinical trials, where it is important to match groups of similar patients, but is of only limited value in treating patients. Most of the data from which equianalgesic doses of morphine are estimated derive from relatively low-dose studies and may not hold true at high doses or for chronic use. Particular caution is needed when changing from morphine to methadone, and large reductions in expected dose may be needed even though the two drugs have been traditionally regarded as equipotent.

Adequate and sustained pain control can usually be achieved by the use of just one opioid. However, there is a growing awareness that, for some patients, pain control becomes more difficult despite escalation in opioid dose and that severe unwanted events intervene. In this situation, a change from one opioid to another will often restore pain control with alleviation of adverse effects (usually hallucinations and confusion). Improvement in pain control following a change in opioid may be accompanied by a reduction in opioid requirement that can lead to the unanticipated emergence of narcosis. As a general rule, if a change in opioid is indicated, it is better to retitrate the dose or at least give less than that calculated from morphine equivalence data. Supplementary opioid analgesia can be given as required.

Opioid-naive subjects

Occasionally, a subcutaneous infusion will be started

in a patient who is in pain but who has not previously received opioid analgesia. The need for parenteral therapy may also indicate that the patient's clinical condition is deteriorating. Opioids should be started at very low doses, particularly in the elderly or in those with renal impairment. Subsequently, an assessment of the total daily requirement can be made from the need for supplementary injections. It is very difficult to estimate opioid requirements, and frequent clinical review is needed to ensure both absence of toxicity and achievement of pain relief. It may be possible to advance the dose of opioid very quickly in some patients. For those in very severe pain, it is occasionally necessary to administer supplementary doses on an hourly basis.

Opioid toxicity

Opioid toxicity can occur in a number of situations and can be considered in three distinct forms:

1 Narcosis. The classical form of opioid overdose with respiratory depression, hypotension, sedation, and small pupils. Apart from inadvertent overprescribing, it can occur in a number of special circumstances:
   a when changing from one opioid to another;
   b following a successful pain intervention (e.g. nerve block);
   c following introduction of cotherapy;
   d development of renal failure when using opioids eliminated by this route (e.g. morphine).
2 Unwanted effects. These are predictable and may improve as tolerance develops. Sometimes, they constitute an indication to stop or change the opioid. Such symptoms include:
   a nausea and vomiting;
   b sedation;
   c sweating;
   d bronchospasm;
   e blurred vision.
3 Adverse effects can arise unexpectedly and may be profoundly disabling. In many cases, the emergence of opioid toxicity of this type requires a major revision of the treatment plan. These symptoms can be

more distressing than those for which the opioid was prescribed. Adverse effects of this type are more common at very high opioid doses, where the dose has been increased very quickly, and where the pain is poorly opioid responsive. They are more common in the elderly. Examples of toxic adverse effects include:

a cognitive dysfunction;
b excessive sedation;
c hallucinations;
d myoclonus;
e allodynia.

The management of opioid toxicity requires mature decision-making and careful negotiation with the patient or, more usually, the family and carers. If a patient is dying, it is sometimes difficult to be certain that sedation or respiratory change is truly an opioid effect. Sedation, even to the point of unconsciousness, may be considered beneficial or an act of kindness. A balance has to be achieved between reducing the opioid dose and compromising symptom control. The use of specific opioid antagonists is rarely needed, but should be considered in the event of prescribing error, in the event of narcosis after opioids are first started in opioid-naive subjects, or when vital signs are severely impaired.

Narcosis can usually be managed by temporary discontinuation of the opioid infusion and restarting it after a few hours at a lower dose rate. Unwanted effects require explanation and often a coprescription (e.g. an antiemetic). In the event of a severe adverse event, a complete clinical reevaluation is mandatory. Other causes of symptoms should be sought, looking specifically for hypercalcemia, renal failure, diabetes, and infection. Mental changes raise the possibility of cerebral metastases, which can be excluded on clinical grounds or by scanning if appropriate. The treatment chart requires careful review, particularly of the number of supplementary doses of analgesic given or the use of concomitant therapy. Ultimately, the decision is whether to add treatments to counter the emergent problems, to change the opioid, or to explore alternative pain management techniques.

Opioid unresponsiveness

Pain that fails to respond to opioids is uncommon. When it is present, it is likely to have been recognized before the decision to use a subcutaneous infusion is made. Even those pain types generally regarded as opioid unresponsive (e.g. neuropathic pain) are rarely completely so. However, new pains frequently present themselves later in the course of an illness, and regular clinical review is essential. In the event of a pain apparently not responding to the prescribed opioid:

1 check that the patient is receiving the prescribed dose;
2 evaluate the new pain;

3 consider changing the opioid or adding another agent.

If a pain changes or a new pain emerges, consider the following factors:

1 Allodynia or cutaneous hypersensitivity may be induced by morphine: consider reducing the dose, changing the opioid, or exploring other agents for neuropathic pain. Sometimes, single bolus infusions of lidocaine (lignocaine) 100 mg intravenously may be effective.
2 Bed-bound, semiconscious patients may get pain from lying in the same position for prolonged periods. Regular turning, pressure-relieving mattresses, physiotherapy, or benzodiazepines may be helpful.
3 The appropriateness of adding another analgesic or using alternative pain management strategies. Weigh the patient's general condition and possible gain against the discomfort of other treatments, the lack of predictable benefit, and the risk of adverse events.
4 Fear and anxiety exert powerful influences on the cognitive perception of pain. The psychospiritual needs of the patient must be taken into account in any pain management plan.
5 Severe pain can arise from fractures, pressure sores, muscle spasms, cramps, constipation, and a distended bladder.

Nonopioid analgesics

Nonopioid analgesics have been used in subcutaneous infusions either alone or in combination with opioids. Nonsteroidal anti-inflammatory agents (NSAIDs) are promoted by the World Health Organization (WHO) as coanalgesics in the analgesic stepladder. Diclofenac, naproxen, and ketorolac have been given by subcutaneous infusion with benefit. Severe skin reactions may limit the use of diclofenac and naproxen.

Ketorolac has a marked morphine-sparing effect in some patients,[9] particularly those with predominately bone pain. The usual initial dose of ketorolac is 60 mg/day, with titration up to a maximum of 120 mg/day according to response. However, there are anecdotal reports of very high doses of ketorolac (240 mg in 24 h) being used without problems.

NSAIDs can precipitate renal failure and cause gastrointestinal hemorrhage. It is particularly important to recognize renal failure as this may lead to the development of toxicity from other drugs eliminated by renal excretion (see Opioid toxicity). If NSAIDs are thought to be indicated, the usual precautions to protect against gastrointestinal side-effects should be taken, particularly in the elderly. It may not be possible to provide adequate gastroprotection for patients who are unable to take drugs by mouth.

Ketamine is an antagonist of the *N*-methyl-D-aspartate receptor and has received increasing interest as an agent for neuropathic pain syndromes.[10] It can be given by subcutaneous infusion to good effect in patients with uncontrolled pain, or as a means to reduce the opioid dose in those experiencing severe adverse effects. Adverse events are common, particularly psychotomimetic effects with sedation, disorientation, hallucinations, and vivid dreams. Because of the high incidence of adverse effects, ketamine should be started at the lowest dose possible; some have recommended an initial test dose of 10 mg. Subcutaneous infusions starting at a dose of 1 mg/kg/day would seem appropriate, with subsequent upward titration according to response. Effective doses have been reported in the range 0.1–0.5 mg/kg/h. Adverse effects may necessitate stopping the drug, but can sometimes be managed with midazolam or haloperidol.

The use of both ketamine and ketorolac is sometimes associated with a dramatic improvement in pain relief. Therefore, it is prudent to reduce the opioid dose by 20–30% when either of these drugs is introduced for the first time. Both drugs are unsuitable for administration in water for injection. A list of drugs that must be prepared in normal saline is shown in Table 8.7.

Other agents

A number of other agents not generally regarded as analgesics may be helpful in the relief of pain. Drugs that can be given by subcutaneous infusion include:

1 Anxiolytics. Reducing fear and anxiety can alleviate pain. Midazolam (5–50 mg/day) can be added to the opioid infusion and supplementary doses may be equally as effective for breakthrough pain as bolus doses of opioid.
2 Sedatives such as methotrimeprazine (levomepromazine) (12.5–150 mg/day) have been considered to have some analgesic properties independent of sedation.
3 Antispasmodics such as hyoscine butylbromide (40–120 mg/day) may be effective in pain due to intestinal obstruction. Octreotide (300–3,000 μg/day), a synthetic analog of somatostatin, may also be effective by reducing intestinal secretion.
4 Corticosteroids (e.g. dexamethasone 4–16 mg/day) may be effective in reducing tumor swelling and are often useful in the management pain due to raised

Table 8.7 *Drugs to be mixed with normal saline*

Dexamethasone
Octreotide
Ondansetron
Ketamine
Ketorolac
Tramadol

intracranial pressure, intestinal obstruction, and neuropathic syndromes.

DRUG COMBINATIONS

Drug combinations have been used to anticipate or treat vomiting, to introduce coanalgesics, to provide sedation, and to reduce secretions.[2,5] It is common practice to use two drugs in combination from the time the infusion is first started. Some combinations of three or more drugs have been used and are summarized in Tables 8.8 and 8.9.

The potential for drugs to react with one another or with the delivery apparatus has been underinvestigated. Rigorous testing requires incubation of the drugs to be used for prolonged periods and at a range of concentrations. Visual inspection and high-power optical microscopy can assess chemical incompatibility, and high-pressure liquid chromatography can be used to determine the quantity of active drug that remains. Findings indicate that diamorphine is fully compatible with hyoscine.[11] Mixtures of diamorphine and haloperidol or cyclizine were only compatible at low concentrations. However, most of the data pertaining to drug combinations come from clinical observation and experience.[2,3,5,12–14]

CLINICAL STUDIES

There is a large collective experience of the use of opioids by subcutaneous infusion in the control of cancer pain. Apart from some special circumstances, there is no reason to believe that one opioid is superior to another. There may be minor differences in the incidence and severity of side-effects, but there have been very few controlled trials to prove this. One recent study indicated no difference between morphine and hydromorphone, but drew attention to the uncertain validity of using published conversion factors when changing from one opioid to another.[15]

Most of the published evidence for the value of opioids by continuous subcutaneous infusion outlines experiences gained in palliative care centers, where there has been little or no tradition of research. Most series describe the use of subcutaneous infusions in patients who are dying, and very few reports contain objective measurements of pain relief. Emphasis has been placed on demonstrating the safety and utility of opioid analgesics even at very high doses. Subcutaneous infusions have been continued successfully for prolonged periods (months in some cases), but mostly duration of infusion has been short (sometimes only a few hours).[2]

There are also a number of methodological problems in conducting clinical research in this area, namely but not exhaustively:

Table 8.8 *Two-drug combinations*

	Alfentanil	Clonazepam	Cyclizine	Dexamethasone	Diamorphine	Glycopyrrolate	Haloperidol	Hydromorphone	Hyoscine butylbromide	Hyoscine hydrobromide	Ketamine	Ketorolac	Methadone	Methotrimeprazine	Metoclopramide	Midazolam	Morphine sulfate	Octreotide	Ondansetron
Alfentanil		O	▽	O	O	O	O	O	O	O	O	O	O	O	O	O	O	O	O
Clonazepam	O				O		O			O							O		
Cyclizine	▽			▽	▽		▽		□			X			□		▽	X	
Dexamethasone	O		▽		O	X	O				O		O	X	O	O	O	O	O
Diamorphine	O	O	▽	O		O	O		O	O	O	O		O	O	O	O	O	O
Glycopyrrolate	O			X	O					O						O	O	O	
Haloperidol	O	O	▽	O	O					O		X	O	O	O	O	O	O	
Hydromorphone	O												O						
Hyoscine butylbromide	O		□		O						O				□	O	O	O	
Hyoscine hydrobromide	O	O			O	O	O									O	O		
Ketamine	O			O	O				O							O	O		
Ketorolac	O		X		O		X						O			X	O		
Methadone	O			O			O	O				O		O	O	O	O		
Methotrimeprazine	O			X	O		O						O		O	O	O		
Metoclopramide	O		□	O	O		O		□				O	O		O	O	O	
Midazolam	O			O	O	O	O		O	O	O	X	O	O	O		O	O	
Morphine sulfate	O	O	▽	O	O	O	O		O	O	O	O	O	O	O	O		O	
Octreotide	O		X	O	O	O	O		O						O	O	O		
Ondansetron	O			O	O														

Blank squares: no data; O, compatible; ▽, compatible at usual concentrations; □, occasionally incompatible; X, incompatible.

Table 8.9 *Three-drug combinations*

	Cyclizine	Dexamethasone	Glycopyrronium	Haloperidol	Hyoscine butylbromide	Hyoscine hydrobromide	Ketamine	Ketorolac	Methotrimeprazine	Metoclopramide	Midazolam	Octreotide	Diamorphine	Phenobarbitone
Diamorphine + cyclizine		▽	▽	▽	□	▽		X	▽	□	▽			
Diamorphine + dexamethasone	▽			○		○	○		X	○	○	○		
Diamorphine + glycopyrrolate	▽								○	○	○			
Diamorphine + haloperidol	▽	○			□	○	○	X	○	○	○	○		
Diamorphine + hyoscine butylbromide	□			□					○		○	○		
Diamorphine + hyoscine hydrobromide	▽	○		○					○	○	○			
Diamorphine + ketamine		○		○					○		○			
Diamorphine + ketorolac	X			X							X			
Diamorphine + methotrimeprazine	▽	X	○	○		○	○			○	○	○		
Diamorphine + metoclopramide	□	○	○	○		○			○		○			
Diamorphine + midazolam	▽	○	○	○	○		○	X	○	○		○		
Diamorphine + octreotide				○	○				○	○				
Diamorphine + ondansetron														
Dexamethasone + metoclopramide									○			○	○	
Dexamethasone + octreotide														○
Dexamethasone + ketamine											○			
Hyoscine butylbromide + haloperidol	X													
Hyoscine butylbromide + midazolam				○					○	○			○	
Haloperidol + midazolam	▽	○												

Blank squares: no data; ○, compatible; ▽, compatible at usual concentrations; □, occasionally incompatible; X, incompatible.

1 heterogeneity of patients;
2 multiple pain types and sites;
3 incidence of new pains;
4 deteriorating nature of the illness;
5 concomitant prescribing;
6 impact of radiotherapy, chemotherapy, and surgery;
7 cognitive loss or dysfunction;
8 changing priorities in care;
9 death.

This topic is dealt with in Chapter P37.

STARTING A SUBCUTANEOUS INFUSION

The procedure for starting a subcutaneous infusion can be considered under the headings:

- prescribing;
- preparing the infusion;
- priming;
- siting.

Prescribing

Prescriptions should be unambiguous and legible. They should also specify the drugs to be used, their doses, the diluent, and the duration over which they are to be infused. Standard prescription sheets may be used; however, for clarity and because the dose or combination of drugs may be changed, a purpose-designed prescription sheet might be preferred. The practitioner will need to comply with national legislation and local policies for prescription of controlled drugs.

Unless there are reasons to do otherwise, it is recommended that the doses be written in mg/24 h and that the infusion pump is set to run for this time.

Preparing the infusion

The following notes refer to the use of a syringe driver. If another type of infusion pump is used, reference should be made to the manufacturer's operating instructions. In all cases, drugs prescribed are reconstituted with diluent or drawn from ampoules and mixed together in a syringe.

1 Set the syringe driver to run at a fixed rate. A rate of 2 mm/h means that the driver will move the plunger of a syringe 48 mm in 24 h. Measure this distance on the barrel of the syringe to be used.
2 Check the volume that the syringe will hold when the plunger is pulled back 48 mm. Note that this volume may be slightly different from one syringe to the next, even though the distance is the same.
3 If this volume is less than that required to dissolve

and mix the drugs, a larger syringe will be needed; otherwise, add the drugs to the syringe using extra diluent to bring the plunger back 48 mm.
4 If the volume required to administer the drugs is greater than can be accommodated in a 30-ml syringe, the dose must be reduced and the rate of infusion increased (e.g. give 50% of the 24-h dose in 12 h). Alternatively, larger mains-driven pumps may be used.
5 Attach the syringe that is drawn up to 48 mm along its barrel to the syringe driver; ensure that the actuator mechanism engages with the flange on the end of the plunger and that the distal flange on the barrel locates tightly in the body of the driver.
6 Attach the connecting tubing by means of a Luer lock.
7 It is recommended that the syringe and its contents are protected from sunlight, usually by placing in a cloth sling bag.

Priming and siting

1 Prime the connection catheter and needle by allowing the syringe to empty some of its contents either by activating the motor or by manually depressing the plunger. Note that the volume required by some connection catheters may take up to 2 ml. This may reduce the time that the driver will run until the syringe is empty by several hours. When using large-volume connection catheters, it is better to use larger volume syringes and greater dilutions of drug.
2 Site the injection needle. Almost any part of the body can be used, but the most convenient sites include the upper chest (above the breasts), the outer upper arms or thighs, the abdomen, and sometimes over the shoulders. Cover the injection site with a transparent dressing.
3 Ensure that the battery is fitted and start the mechanism – a light will flash.
4 Keep and maintain records according to local policy, but particularly record the time that the infusion was started.

When the syringe has emptied, it should be replenished. The process of priming only needs to be repeated if the prescription is altered or a new needle and connecting tube is required.

MONITORING

Monitoring a subcutaneous infusion is essential. There are four main objectives:

1 to ensure that the infusion delivers the drugs as prescribed;
2 to monitor pain and symptom control;

3 to inspect the injection site;

4 to check for adverse events and toxicity.

Simple checklists can be used to ensure that an infusion is progressing in a satisfactory manner. These can be adapted to the clinical circumstances. The frequency of observations will depend on the availability of staff and the environment in which the patient receives care. In a specialist unit, observations every 4 h might be expected, whereas in the community these are inevitably less frequent. It is unnecessary and often inappropriate to perform a full profile of clinical measurements. Careful bedside observation is usually sufficient. Printed charts allow standardization of observation, act as a reminder, and are useful for audit. Important items to record include:

- the volume remaining before the syringe is empty – this not only provides a check that the infusion rate is as expected but also provides an estimate of when it will need to be replenished;
- that the infusion device is operating and that the connections are intact and not leaking;
- an inspection of the injection site.

Simultaneously, a brief clinical assessment of the patient will include their:

- level of consciousness/sedation;
- pulse and respiration;
- peripheral circulation, color, sweating;
- spontaneous movement or twitching;
- grimacing/moaning.

Monitoring pain control can be carried out using standard pain assessment tools. If the patient is awake and cooperative, simple visual analog scales or four-point verbal rating scores are most commonly used. If the patient is obtunded or unconscious, pain rating has to be performed by proxy, usually by the attending nurse and using visible nonverbal indicators of pain.

COMPLICATIONS

Complications during the use of subcutaneous infusions are uncommon. They can be considered under the following headings:

- equipment malfunction;
- reactions at injection site;
- drug reactions;
- prescribing errors.

Equipment malfunction

Modern infusion systems using syringe drivers are reliable and technical failure is unusual. Typical problems include:

- low power/battery failure;
- failure to recognize when the syringe is fully discharged;
- disconnection of delivery tubing;
- tube blockage;
- syringe displacement in the driver;
- cracked or leaking syringe;
- driver overspeed;
- backlash – delay in infusion because the plunger on the syringe is not closely opposed to the driver mechanism at start-up.

In each situation, the cause is usually obvious and can be remedied by appropriate action. Syringe drivers that malfunction should be inspected by an engineer and reapproved before further use. Many problems can be avoided by having local policies and procedures for the use of syringe drivers.

Reactions at the injection site

Minor reactions at the injection site are frequent and do not usually require intervention other than regular monitoring. On the other hand, reactions at the injection site are the commonest reason for having to resite the infusion. Reactions can vary from minor erythema to florid inflammatory lesions with abscess formation. With severe drug incompatibility, frank necrosis at the injection site may occur. The following should be considered when reactions are severe or frequent:

- Drug administered: some drugs are reported to cause more frequent reactions (cyclizine, diclofenac, ketamine, and methadone). Reactions to cyclizine may be related to its concentration. The risk of reactions is increased when drugs are mixed together in the same syringe.
- Is the correct diluent being used?
- Allergy/idiosyncrasy. There is some evidence that many of the minor reactions seen at injection sites are allergic in nature and will therefore happen in an unpredictable manner.[3] Allergic responses may occur to the metal needle as well as to the infused drugs.
- Infection.
- Host factors: severe clotting abnormalities, liver failure, renal failure, and immunosuppression may increase the likelihood of reactions.

Management of reactions will depend on severity. The infusion must be resited if the reaction is severe. Simple dressings are usually all that is required, but sometimes topical or systemic steroids, antibiotics, and surgical drainage or debridement are necessary. In all severe reactions, the cause should be sought.

Consideration must be given to:

- changing the drug or diluent;

- diluting the infusion, which may mean a larger syringe and changing the infusion rate;
- using single drug infusions and more than one syringe driver if several drugs are required;
- changing to a cannula made of plastic or Teflon rather than metal;
- adding low doses of corticosteroid to the infusion (dexamethasone, betamethasone, or prednisolone) is claimed to reduce the frequency that sites need to be changed; hyaluronidase has been thought to confer a similar advantage;
- using an alternative route of administration;
- ensuring an aseptic technique when preparing and dispensing an infusion.

Drug reactions

Drug reactions may occur in the infusion apparatus, the injection site, or in the body. Systemic drug reactions are no more or less common when the drug is given by subcutaneous infusion. However, there are some special circumstances that may lead to under- or overdosing. When opioids are infused there is a potential for narcosis, despite there being no apparent change in the prescribed amount of drug, in the following situations:

- The bioavailability of a drug may be altered when two or more are mixed together. If a change is made from one combination to another, or a decision is made to administer drugs singly, the opioid may become more (or less) active.
- Factors used to calculate the dose of opioid when converting from oral to subcutaneous infusion, or from one opioid to another, are only approximate and have large inter- and intrasubject variation. If a subcutaneous infusion is commenced because of vomiting or intestinal obstruction, inadvertent excess may be given because the patient had not been absorbing the prescribed opioid that was previously being given by mouth.
- At very high doses, it is unwise to apply the usual conversion factors when changing from one opioid to another as the second given opioid is likely to appear more effective. This observation has been used to advantage when opioid responsiveness is lost or adverse effects occur, and has led to the concept of "opioid rotation."
- Other concomitant pain interventions may reduce the opioid requirement. Large reductions in opioid.dose are sometimes needed if ketorolac or ketamine are added.
- The rate of absorption from the subcutaneous tissues may be enhanced if the patient is febrile, if topical heat is applied, or if the ambient temperature is high. Conversely, hypotensive patients with poor peripheral circulation may receive inadequate doses of analgesia.

Management of adverse events requires identification and withdrawal of the suspected drug. Regular inspection of the infusion will detect clouding or crystallization; new solutions should be prepared if this happens. The clinician needs to watch for the unexpected emergence of opioid toxicity and must be prepared to adjust the dose accordingly. In practice, serious opioid toxicity with subcutaneous infusions is uncommon. It is more likely to occur in opioid-naive subjects or in those for whom a concomitant pain intervention is successful and the opioid dose left unchanged.

Prescribing errors

Prescribing errors can put the patient at serious risk, are a cause of great anxiety to the clinical team, can destroy confidence, and may lead to subsequent litigation. They are nearly always avoidable. Errors can occur in writing and reading a prescription, in dispensing and preparing a drug, in identifying the recipient, and in monitoring drug administration. Although the use of subcutaneous infusion involves simple techniques, there are some important sources of error:

- Drugs need to be prepared and drawn up in solution in quantities that match a fixed distance along the barrel of a syringe. The volume to be used will only be the same if two syringes of identical type and size are used.
- The distance along the syringe that needs to be measured will depend upon the rate at which the driver unit is set to discharge the syringe contents.
- The rate at which the driver operates may be expressed in different units of distance and time from one driver to the next.
- The volume of the delivery catheter should be ignored when preparing the solution. It affects the time the syringe takes to empty when the infusion is started for the first time or after it has been resited, but does not affect the amount to be drawn up into the syringe.
- If the dose prescribed is altered, a completely new solution must be prepared with a new syringe. A new administration set may also be needed: large-volume extension sets will contain a dead-space that must be evacuated before the drug at the new concentration can be delivered.
- The size of the syringe is determined by the volume required to dissolve the prescribed amount of drug and is independent of the rate of infusion.
- It may not be possible to administer a full syringe because the jaws of the driver assembly will not open far enough. For example, in order to administer 20 ml, a 30-ml syringe may be needed (see Fig. 8.2).

Elimination of prescribing error is an important part of risk management for all clinicians and any organization engaged in patient care. The following are suggestions to help to achieve this:

- Clinicians should be fully conversant with a range of locally available drugs. Familiarity with a few drugs is better than a partial knowledge of many.
- Access to specialist services.
- Standardization of equipment across clinical areas.
- Published protocols and guidelines for the use of subcutaneous infusions.
- Documented procedures for setting up infusions and delivery systems.
- Record-keeping to ensure the standardization of prescription and monitoring of infusion.
- Regular servicing and calibration of equipment.
- Quality control and audit.
- Education and training.

MANAGERIAL ISSUES

The effective use of subcutaneous infusions in any health care environment requires the development of policies and procedures. These ensure uniformity of practice and are a safeguard for the patient, the practitioner, and the organization. They are an essential part of risk management. Protocols should be developed for the management of particular circumstances and guidelines published that are appropriate to the locality. Clear statements of objectives and desired outcomes of treatment are necessary; from these, standards can be evolved for subsequent audit.

Policies

Policies derive from statements of intent and outline a framework in which these can be achieved. They are prescriptive in nature and vary from broad generalizations such as "all patients with pain should have access to specialist pain services" to highly specific requirements such as those related to the use of controlled drugs. Policies outline the operational parameters that are expected of and supported by an organization. Policies for the use of subcutaneous infusions must consider:

- drug supply – what is available to the prescriber, storage, dispensing, mixing, record-keeping, etc;
- equipment – engineering specification, frequency of inspection, calibration, rate of administration, etc;
- circumstances of use – whether specialist units, hospitals, or community; the requirements for supervision, monitoring, informed consent, etc.;
- staffing – qualifications, training, experience, etc;
- education;
- quality control.

Procedures

Procedures often evolve from items of policy. They are instructions for specific circumstances and can be mandatory (e.g. reporting an accident) or advisory. Procedures may be needed for:

- handling, supply, preparation, and administration of drugs;
- setting up an infusion device;
- monitoring and record-keeping;
- reporting adverse events;
- disposal of consumables;
- cleaning, inspecting, and servicing instruments;
- lending equipment;
- handling complaints.

Protocols

Protocols are developed for particular situations, usually for use in just one locality (e.g. a cancer ward). They enable standardization of management and may relate to:

- specific clinical conditions;
- use of a particular item of equipment;
- drugs that require special precautions;
- mixing drugs;
- novel treatments.

Guidelines

Guidelines allow for information sharing among health care workers with similar client populations and problems. They enable uniformity of management and are particularly useful for patients with cancer, who frequently move from one health care environment to another. Guidelines are appropriate for:

- standardization and use of equipment;
- indications and use of specific drugs;
- drug combinations;
- managing adverse events.

Standards

Standards are measures that are applied to ascertain that desired objectives are achieved. They are essential to the conduct of an audit. They can be applied to assess both administrative and clinical issues. Standards have structure, process, and outcome. For example, a standard for the maintenance of infusion pumps might state "All pumps will be inspected and calibrated by a service engineer every 6 months." The structure is that there will be a procedure for servicing the pumps; the process that an engineer will do this; and an outcome that the engineer signs a label to this effect and attaches it to the pump. The standard can therefore be audited by inspecting the pumps and checking the labels. Standard-setting is particularly useful for:

- ensuring consistent and high levels of clinical care;
- identifying problems and highlighting areas for research;
- ensuring equipment remains functional;
- ensuring staff are adequately trained and updated;
- quality assurance.

CLOSING REMARKS

The introduction of the syringe driver was an important milestone in the evolution of symptom management for patients with cancer. This chapter outlines the use of subcutaneous infusions for the management of cancer pain. Much of the evidence for efficacy is anecdotal or from reports of experience gained in hospices and palliative care centers. There is an urgent need for good clinical trials, but there are a number of methodological difficulties. Nonetheless, the use of subcutaneous infusions has stood the test of time and remains an important tool in the armamentarium of the practicing physician, particularly those who care for patients who are dying.

REFERENCES

1. O'Neill WM. Subcutaneous infusions – a medical last rite. *Br Med J* 1994; **8:** 91–3.
● 2. David J. A survey of the use of syringe drivers in Marie Curie Centres. *Eur J Cancer Care* 1992; **4:** 23–8.
● 3. Oliver DJ. Syringe drivers in palliative care: a review. *Palliative Med* 1988; **2:** 21–6.
4. Dover SB. Syringe driver in terminal care. *Br Med J* 1987; **294:** 553–5.
◆ 5. Johnson I, Patterson S. Drugs used in combination in the syringe driver – a survey of hospice practice. *Palliative Med* 1992; **6:** 125–30.
6. Bruera E, Brenneis C, Michaud M, *et al*. Use of the subcutaneous route for the administration of narcotics in patients with cancer pain. *Cancer* 1988; **62:** 407–11.
◆ 7. Gordon GB, Stevenson KK, Griffie J, *et al*. Opioid equianalgesic calculations. *J Palliative Med* 1999; **2:** 209–18.
◆ 8. Twycross R, Wilcock A, Thorp S. *Palliative Care Formulary*. Oxford: Radcliffe Medical Press, 1998: 183–202.
9. Myers KG, Trotman IF. Use of ketorolac by continuous subcutaneous infusion for the control of cancer-related pain. *J Postgrad Med* 1994; **70:** 359–62.
10. Mercadente S, Lodi F, Spaio M, *et al*. Long-term ketamine subcutaneous continuous infusion in neuropathic cancer pain. *J Pain Symptom Manage* 1995; **10:** 310–14.
11. Regnard C, Pashley S, Westrope F. Anti-emetic/diamorphine mixture compatibility in infusion pumps. *Br J Pharm Pract* 1986; **8** (8): 218–220.
12. Bradley K. Swap data on drug compatibilities. *Pharm Pract* 1996; **6** (3): 69–72.
13. Grassby PF, Hutchings L. Drug combinations in syringe drivers: the compatibility and stability of diamorphine with cyclizine and haloperidol. *Palliative Med* 1997; **11:** 217–24.
● 14. O'Doherty CA, Hall EJ, Schofield L, Zeppetella J. Drugs and syringe drivers: a survey of adult specialist palliative care practice in the United Kingdom and Eire. *Palliative Med* 2001; **15:** 149–54.
15. Miller MG, McCarthy N, O'Boyle CA, Kearney M. Continuous subcutaneous infusion of morphine vs. hydromorphone: a controlled trial. *J Pain Symptom Manage* 1999; **18:** 9–16.

9

Antidepressants, antiepileptics, and antiarrhythmic drugs

SØREN H SINDRUP AND FLEMMING W BACH

Antidepressants	101	Antiarrhythmics	108
Antiepileptics	104	References	109

Some drugs within the antidepressant, anticonvulsant, and antiarrhythmic classes have become the preferred treatment of neuropathic pain for which conventional analgesics are apparently less efficacious. These drugs do not currently have a place in the treatment of nociceptive pain, although tricyclic antidepressants and sodium valproate have been successfully used in some headache conditions. The efficacy of antidepressants in neuropathic pain has been scientifically proven in a number of controlled clinical trials (see Chapter Ch18); however, the evidence for the effect of the other drug classes, with the exception of gabapentin, in neuropathic pain and headache is more scarce (see Chapter Ch19). The incomplete and often modest response seen with these drugs is accepted because, at present, there are no better alternatives.

ANTIDEPRESSANTS

Typical antidepressants used in pain treatment are:

1 Tricyclic antidepressants (TCAs)[1***,2***]
    a With balanced reuptake inhibition of norepinephrine (noradrenaline) and serotonin:
        Imipramine, amitriptyline, and clomipramine.
    b With relatively selective reuptake inhibition of norepinephrine:
        Desipramine, nortriptyline, and maprotiline.
2 Selective uptake inhibitors
    a Selective serotonin reuptake inhibitors (SSRIs):[2**]
        Paroxetine, citalopram, fluoxetine, and sertraline.
    b Serotonin and norepinephrine reuptake inhibitors (SNRIs):[2*,3*]
        Venlafaxine.

The conditions in which these drugs have been shown to have an effect are:

• painful polyneuropathy	TCAs, SSRIs, SNRIs
• postherpetic neuralgia	TCAs
• nerve injury pain	TCAs, SNRIs
• central poststroke pain	TCAs
• migraine prophylaxis	TCAs
• chronic tension type headache	TCAs

In neuropathic pain, the etiology is probably less important than the phenomenology and the mechanism of pain, which may be similar across the different conditions. There are no good data on this issue and it seems appropriate to consider the use of these drugs in neuropathic pain conditions independent of the etiology. Throughout the different neuropathic conditions, a clinically significant response with TCAs is seen in about 60% of patients; corrected for placebo response, two or three patients need to be treated in order to obtain one patient with > 50% pain relief. The response with SSRIs is equivocal, these drugs having only been tested in painful polyneuropathies. In this condition, about seven patients need to be treated in order to obtain one with > 50% pain relief. To date, there have been no publications of controlled studies on the SNRIs in pain treatment. In the UK, for example, regulatory approval has not been granted for any TCA for analgesic indications.

In migraine, two to five patients need to be treated with TCAs to obtain one patient with > 50% reduction in headache frequency, and in chronic tension-type headache three or four need to be treated. However, the data on both types of headache are equivocal. The SSRI citalopram has no effect in chronic tension-type headache and none of the SSRIs has been tested in migraine.

Contraindications

The majority of problems are with TCAs:

1 TCAs
   a recent myocardial infarction (< 6 months);
   b cardiac conduction disturbances, e.g. AV block;
   c uncontrolled congestive heart failure;
   d convulsive disorders;
   e untreated glaucoma;
   f treatment with monoamine oxidase inhibitors.
2 Selective uptake inhibitor (SSRIs and SNRIs)
   a treatment with monoamine oxidase inhibitors.

It is not clear whether SSRIs or SNRIs can be used in patients with convulsive disorders. Caution is also recommended when SSRIs and SNRIs are given to patients with other contraindications to TCAs.

The *serotonergic syndrome* characterized by hyperthermia and muscle spasms combined with changes in mental state, hyper- or hypotension, tachycardia, diarrhea, tremor, or problems with coordination may develop during treatment with all of these drugs. This syndrome may be seen with a single agent that potentiates serotonergic neurotransmission, but it is mainly seen as a drug–drug interaction when different drugs that potentiate serotonergic neurotransmission are combined and act either by the same or by different mechanisms.

Dosing and treatment schedule

TCAs, SSRIs, and SNRIs undergo hepatic metabolism before they are excreted in the urine. Hepatic metabolism for most of these drugs depends partially on a genetic polymorphic enzyme. This is the main cause for the pronounced pharmacokinetic variability which is seen in particular with TCAs (see Chapter Ch18). Together with the serum concentration–effect relationship, and the known toxicity for TCAs, this is the reason for recommending monitoring of serum drug concentration when TCAs are used. Monitoring is not necessary for SSRIs, which are less toxic and have no clear concentration–effect relationships. This situation for the SNRIs is as yet undetermined.

If there are no contraindications to TCA use, a treatment regimen as detailed in Fig. 9.1 can be tried for imipramine or amitriptyline. Clomipramine could also be prescribed using a similar regimen, the dose being increased to yield a maximum serum concentration of clomipramine plus desmethylclomipramine of around 400 nM. In patients suffering severe pain, the dose adjustment can be performed more rapidly in order to achieve an adequate effect sooner or to decide whether alternative treatments should be tried because the drugs are ineffective or cause side-effects. It should be noted that it is not necessary to titrate the dose for every patient treated

with imipramine to serum levels of about 400 nM nor every patient treated with amitriptyline to about 300 nM because some will have a satisfactory response at lower concentrations. The measurement of these serum drug concentrations are recommended, mainly to avoid toxicity. It is assumed that drug levels around 2,000 nM are toxic, i.e. only five times higher than the therapeutic concentration for imipramine. In the individual patient, it is impossible to know whether a poor response is due to inadequate dosing or whether the patient is a nonresponder. Thus, the reasons for employing therapeutic drug monitoring when TCAs are used are:

- Pronounced variability in pharmacokinetics: primarily due to genetic variability.
- Dosing according to effects and side-effects is not feasible: there are nonresponders, and side-effects may occur at subtherapeutic drug levels.
- Low therapeutic index: for example, for imipramine and amitriptyline there is a factor of 5–7 difference between therapeutic and toxic drug levels.
- Efficacy can be increased: for imipramine, it appears that the numbers needed to treat to obtain one patient with > 50% pain relief can be reduced from about 2 to 1.5 when dosing is guided by serum drug levels.

A summary of pretreatment safety measures and dosing schedules used for different antidepressants is given in Table 9.1. If the first-line tricyclic antidepressants are ineffective, it may be worth trying one of the other antidepressants as there is evidence that some patients respond better to the more selective compounds than those with a broader spectrum of actions. When contraindications to tricyclic antidepressants are present, the analgesic response is inadequate, or side-effects are intolerable, the treatment regimen detailed in Fig. 9.2 can be tried. The sequence in which the treatments, i.e. gabapentin, tramadol, selective serotonin reuptake inhibitors, etc., are tried is a matter of individual preference.

The SSRIs paroxetine, citalopram, and fluoxetine should be started at 10 or 20 mg daily and increased on a weekly basis to a maximum dose of 60 mg daily (Table 9.1). The place of the SNRIs in the treatment regimen still has to be established. Venlafaxine could be commenced at a starting dose of 37.5 mg twice daily, and if ineffective increased every second week by 75 mg until the maximum recommended dose for depression of 375 mg daily is reached (Table 9.1). Dose–effect and concentration–effect relations for TCAs in migraine and tension-type headache have not been studied in detail. In the studies performed, 10–150 mg/day of amitriptyline was used. If titration in this range is ineffective, it is suggested that a dosage regimen similar to that used in neuropathic pain is tried, but therapeutic drug monitoring is important for safety reasons – as in neuropathic pain.

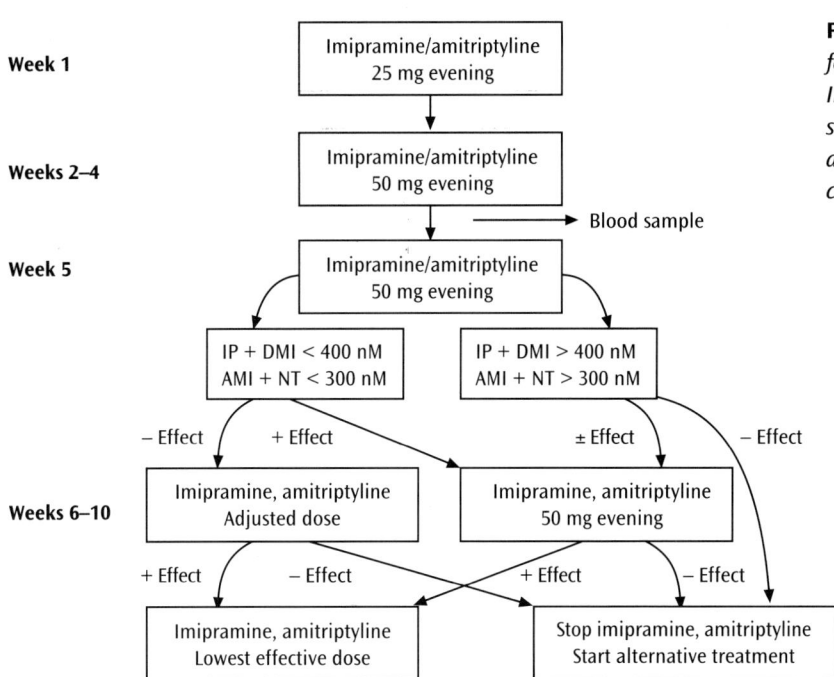

Figure 9.1 *Treatment schedule for imipramine and amitriptyline. IP + DMI, imipramine plus desipramine serum concentration; AMI + NT, amitriptyline plus nortriptyline serum concentration.*

Table 9.1 *Pretreatment safety measures and dosing of tricyclic antidepressants (TCAs), selective serotonin reuptake inhibitors (SSRIs), and serotonin norepinephrine reuptake inhibitors (SNRIs) in pain treatment*

	Drug group			
	TCAs	**SSRIs**		**SNRIs**
		Paroxetine Citalopram Fluoxetine	**Sertraline**	**Venlafaxine**
Caution	Liver disease Kidney disease Cardiac disease Orthostatic hypotension	Liver disease Kidney disease Hypertension	Liver disease Kidney disease	
Pretreatment tests	Liver function Kidney disease Blood pressure EKG	Liver function Kidney function	Liver function Kidney function Blood pressure	
Dosage interval (h)	12–24	24	24	12
Initial dose (mg/day)	25	10–20	50[a]	75
Dose increment	25 mg/week	10–20 mg/week	50 mg/week[a]	75 mg/2 weeks
Maximal dose	Individual[b]	60 mg/day	200 mg/day	375 mg/day
Monitoring of serum concentration	+	−	−	−

a. In elderly patients, 50 mg every second day and very slow dose titration.
b. Individually adjusted according to serum drug concentrations.
EKG, electrocardiograph.

Side-effects

It is well known that treatment with TCAs nearly always causes side-effects, and a substantial number of patients cannot accept chronic dosing with these drugs in a dose that is adequate to achieve pain relief. The SSRIs and SNRIs are better tolerated, probably because they are devoid of postsynaptic blocking effects, but these drugs are definitely not without side-effects.

1 TCAs
  a dry mouth, problems with accommodation;
  b constipation, urinary retention;

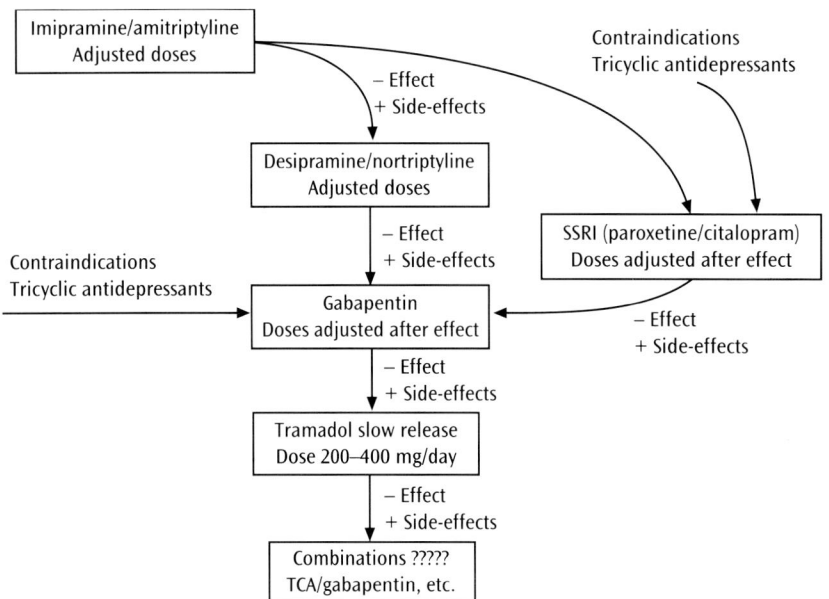

Figure 9.2 *Treatment schedule to be followed if imipramine/ amitriptyline is ineffective or causes intolerable side-effects, or if tricyclic antidepressants are contraindicated. TCA, tricyclic antidepressant; SSRI, selective serotonin reuptake inhibitors.*

   c sweating;
   d fatigue, sedation, mental change;
   e dizziness and orthostatic hypotension;
   f cardiac conduction disturbances (AV block, intraventricular blocks);
   g confusion (elderly).
2 Selective uptake inhibitors
   a SSRIs
     i nausea, vomiting;
     ii nervousness, anxiety, insomnia;
     iii sexual dysfunction (delayed ejaculation, impotence).
   b SNRIs
     i headache;
     ii nausea, vomiting;
     iii sweating;
     iv sedation, mental change;
     v hypertension.

The side-effects are most pronounced when treatment is started and as the dose increases. Patients should therefore be encouraged to stay on the treatment for at least a few weeks. The dry mouth which occurs with TCAs may be diminished by chewing gum, and it is probably wise to recommend a mild laxative initially in elderly patients. In particular, these patients should be warned about orthostatic phenomena, e.g. to be cautious when changing from a sitting or reclining position. The sedating properties of the TCAs can be used therapeutically by prescribing the drugs as single, evening doses because neuropathic pain is often aggravated at this time, causing sleep disturbance. However, patients should be advised against operating machinery or driving a motor vehicle until it is clear that the TCA is being administered at a stable dose which does not impair their ability to perform such tasks. Amitriptyline may be more sedating than the other TCAs with

balanced reuptake inhibition as it has potent antihistaminergic properties. However, the SSRIs should be dosed in the morning to avoid insomnia.

ANTIEPILEPTICS

Antiepileptics used in pain treatment comprise:

1 Nonspecific sodium channel blockers
   a phenytoin;[4]**
   b carbamazepine;[4]**
   c oxcarbazepine.[2]*
2 Specific sodium channel blockers
   a lamotrigine.[2]**,[5]**
3 Gabapentinoids
   a gabapentin.[2]***
4 Gabaergic drugs
   a sodium valproate.[6]**

The conditions in which antiepileptic drugs have been shown to have an effect are:

- Painful polyneuropathy (phenytoin, carbamazepine, gabapentin, lamotrigine).
- Postherpetic neuralgia (gabapentin).
- Central poststroke pain (carbamazepine, lamotrigine).
- Trigeminal neuralgia (carbamazepine, oxcarbazepine, lamotrigine).
- Migraine without aura (sodium valproate).

The etiology for neuropathic pain may be less important than the phenomenology and the mechanism of pain. There is no scientific evidence for the preferential use of antiepileptics in lancinating pains and antidepressants for steady burning-like pains. However, a superior outcome in the former type of pain is supported by the effectiveness of some of the antiepileptics in trigeminal neuralgia, in which there are no trials on antidepressants. In painful polyneuropathy, about two patients need to be treated with phenytoin (but combined data are equivocal), and about three patients with carbamazepine, to obtain one patient with > 50% pain relief. The figures are a little less favorable when carbamazepine is used for central pain and a little better when it is used in trigeminal neuralgia. When gabapentin is used, the numbers needed to treat are three or four patients for both painful polyneuropathy and postherpetic neuralgia. Phenytoin is used infrequently because it has too many side-effects in long-term treatment (see below). There is little evidence for the efficacy of oxcarbazepine in controlled trials, but it is frequently quoted that it has about the same potential to relieve neuropathic pain as carbamazepine, as in the case of the treatment of epilepsy. Lamotrigine has been adequately tested in trigeminal neuralgia, and more recently also in central pain and painful polyneuropathy. In the last condition, the number needed to treat for > 50% pain relief is 3.2.

Evidence for the benefit of sodium valproate has only been established in two trials in migraine without aura, but in this condition it was quite effective with only about two patients needing to be treated to obtain one patient with > 50% reduction in headache frequency. There are no trials on the use of sodium valproate for neuropathic pain.

At the time of writing, in the UK only, gabapentin is the only medication to have regulatory approval for the treatment of all neuropathic pain states (to a maximum dose of 1,800 mg/24 h). Carbamazepine and phenytoin have regulatory approval for the treatment of trigeminal neuralgia only, and phenytoin only as second-line therapy.

Contraindications

Several of these drugs can cause allergic skin eruptions, which is of course a contraindication to their use.

1 Phenytoin
   a AV block;
   b hepatic failure.
2 Carbamazepine
   a AV block;
   b treatment with monoamine oxidase inhibitors;
   c hepatic failure;
   d porphyria.
3 Oxcarbazepine
   a AV block;
   b treatment with monoamine oxidase inhibitors.
4 Lamotrigine
   a renal failure.
5 Gabapentin
   a none, but reduced doses in renal failure.
6 Sodium valproate
   a hepatic failure;
   b hepatic failure in relatives during treatment with sodium valproate;
   c Thrombocytopenia.

Dosing and treatment schedule

Phenytoin, carbamazepine, oxcarbazepine, and lamotrigine are metabolized and subsequently excreted, so these drugs should be used with caution in patients with liver disease. The active metabolite of oxcarbazepine (10-hydroxycarbazepine) is excreted via the kidneys, and gabapentin is excreted unchanged by the same route. Approximately 50% of an oral dose of sodium valproate is metabolized, and both the parent compound and the metabolites are excreted via the kidneys. Impaired renal function dictates that the dose of oxcarbazepine, gabapentin, and sodium valproate should be lowered. Plasma half-life, suggested dosage intervals, etc. for this class of drug are shown in Table 9.2.

The long-term efficacy of phenytoin may be predicted by an intravenous infusion test in which 15 mg phenytoin/kg body weight is infused over 30 min. In severe acute pain, for example with acute exacerbation of trigeminal neuralgia, intravenous loading with phenytoin may also be appropriate. Oral treatment is started with 50 mg twice daily and the dose can be increased weekly by 50 mg until a sufficient response or until the maximal recommended serum level is reached (Table 9.2). Dose increments should be monitored carefully at levels over 100 mg twice daily, since phenytoin exhibits saturation kinetics in which minor dose increments may cause major increases in serum drug concentrations at the higher dose levels.

When carbamazepine is used in the treatment of trigeminal neuralgia, an immediate effect is often desired. In this situation, the initial dose is 100 mg three times daily and it should be increased by 100 mg every second day until pain relief is achieved or intolerable side-effects are encountered. Later, the dose can be reduced cautiously to the lowest effective level. In less acute cases of trigeminal neuralgia or other pain states, the treatment should be initiated very slowly, i.e. with 100 mg in the evening and dose increments of 100 mg every 2–3 days up to a dose of 200 mg three times daily. Further increases in the dose are guided by effects, side-effects, and the upper recommended drug level (Table 9.2). Serum levels can be assessed every second week. In trigeminal neuralgia, it has been suggested that the effective drug level corresponds to the level recommended in the treatment of epilepsy.

If carbamazepine causes intolerable side-effects, a trial of oxcarbazepine is worthwhile. In this situation, the patient can be switched directly to oxcarbazepine in a corresponding or slightly higher dose. When the treat-

Table 9.2 *Pretreatment safety measures and dosing of antiepileptic drugs in pain treatment*

	Drug					
	Phenytoin	Carbamazepine	Oxcarbazepine	Lamotrigine	Gabapentin	Sodium valproate
Caution	Liver disease	Liver disease	Liver disease Kidney disease	Liver disease Kidney disease	Kidney disease	Liver disease Kidney disease Thrombocytopenia
Pretreatment tests	EKG Liver function	EKG Liver function Serum sodium White cell count	EKG Liver function Serum sodium White cell count	Liver function Kidney function	Kidney function	Liver function Kidney function Thrombocyte count White cell count
Half-life (h)	18–24[a]	10–20[b]	10–12[c]	25–30	5–7	6–15
Dosage interval (h)	12	8[d]	12	12	8	12
Maximum serum concentration[e] (μM)	80	40	120	–	–	700
Initial dose[f] (mg/day)	100	100	150	25	300	500
Maximal dose	Individual[g]	Individual[g]	Individual[g]	600 mg/day	4,800 mg/day	Individual[g]

a. Depends on the serum drug concentration owing to saturation kinetics.
b. After autoinduction with continuous treatment for weeks.
c. Refers to the active metabolite 10-hydroxycarbazepine.
d. With slow release formulation 12 h.
e. The suggested upper serum drug concentration in epilepsy treatment.
f. Low initial doses in order to minimize side-effects.
g. Individually adjusted according to serum drug concentrations.
EKG, electrocardiograph.

ment is started from scratch, the initial dose is 150 mg in the evening and increments of 150 mg daily are used until the dose is 450 mg twice daily. Further adjustments depend on the effect and side-effects, with a top dose level defined by the upper recommended serum drug concentration (Table 9.2).

From clinical practice, it has emerged that the initial low dosing of lamotrigine will reduce the risk of skin rashes. In the first 2 weeks, 25 mg is given in the morning, and over the next 2 weeks the dose is 25 mg twice daily. After this phase, the dose can be increased by 50 mg every second week until an acceptable response is achieved or a maximal total daily dose of 200–300 mg twice daily (Table 9.2). In trigeminal neuralgia, it has been suggested that the effect can be increased by using even higher doses in patients in which standard doses produce very low serum drug concentrations. In general, however, therapeutic drug monitoring with lamotrigine is not to be recommended because there is no clear concentration–effect relationship and no defined upper recommended serum drug level.

Gabapentin should also be started slowly to minimize side-effects. Over the first 2 days, 300 mg is given in the evening, then 300 mg twice daily for 2 days, and thereafter 300 mg three times daily (Table 9.2). If there is no effect, the dose can be increased by 300–600 mg every second week according to effects and side-effects, with an upper dose limit of 4,800 mg daily. Although gabapentin is claimed to be relatively well tolerated, clinical practice shows that daily doses ≥ 2,700 mg are often accompanied by intolerable sedation, and the maximum dose approved by the UK regulatory authorities is 1,800 mg daily.

In migraine, sodium valproate can be started at 500 mg/day, and the dose can be adjusted in steps of 500 mg every week to obtain the target serum drug concentration according to a serum drug level measured, for example, 3 weeks from the start of treatment (Table 9.2).

For all the drugs, it is well known that the response is often only partial and that side-effects may accompany any beneficial effect. Dosing according to effect may lead to unnecessary high drug consumption in the hope of further pain relief. It is therefore recommended that, after a positive response, the drug should be titrated to the lowest possible level for an individual optimal response.

Side-effects

The antiepileptic drugs will almost always cause some side-effects. The older drugs (phenytoin and carbamazepine) are more likely to do this, but the newer drugs can also cause side-effects.

1 Phenytoin
   a allergic manifestations (skin);
   b sedation;
   c problems with memory and attention;
   d nystagmus, double vision, ataxia, tremor;
   e nausea, constipation;
   f peripheral neuropathy (loss of deep tendon reflexes);
   g hirsutism;
   h gingival hypertrophy.
2 Carbamazepine
   a allergic manifestations (skin, mucosa, etc.);
   b sedation;
   c ataxia, dizziness, double vision;
   d problems with accommodation;
   e fluid retention, low sodium levels (clinical significance uncertain);
   f cardiac conduction disturbances (rare);
   g thrombocytopenia, agranulocytosis, aplastic anemia (rare);
   h confusion (elderly).
3 Oxcarbazepine
   a allergic manifestations (25% cross-reactivity with carbamazepine);
   b sedation;
   c headache;
   d ataxia, dizziness;
   e fluid retention, low sodium levels (clinical significance uncertain).
4 Lamotrigine
   a skin rash (see Dosing);
   b insomnia;
   c headache;
   d sedation, dizziness, nausea, double vision (high doses).
5 Gabapentin
   a sedation;
   b ataxia, dizziness;
   c headache, nausea, vomiting.
6 Sodium valproate
   a increased appetite and weight gain;
   b abdominal pain, nausea, and vomiting (rare, use enteric coated tablets);
   c sedation;
   d hand tremor;
   e alopecia (rare);
   f toxic hepatitis, pancreatitis (rare, mainly children).

Treatment with sodium valproate requires special attention because of the potentially serious side-effects. Before treatment is started, blood tests should be carried out to determine liver function and thrombocyte count. This should be repeated after 1 month and thereafter every 3 months during the first year of treatment. In addition, the patients should be aware of the symptoms of liver disease. Pretreatment safety measures for all the drugs are listed in Table 9.2.

In recent years, it has become clear that for many of the new antiepileptics the speed by which doses are increased is a major determinant of the degree of side-effects and therefore the tolerability of the drugs. This is probably also the case for the older antiepileptics and some of the other drug classes. *It is therefore recommended to "go low" and "go slow."*

ANTIARRHYTHMICS

Antiarrhythmics are used in the treatment of neuropathic pain. None of them has regulatory approval for this indication, although topical lidocaine (lignocaine) has been approved for use in postherpetic neuralgia in the USA.

1 Lidocaine: intravenous infusion; oral dosing is not possible because of the high first-pass metabolism.
2 Mexiletine: can be used orally; available as capsules.

Trials have also been performed with tocainide, procaine, and bupivacaine, but clinical utility is hampered by the high incidence of severe side-effects, fast elimination, and lack of effect respectively.

The conditions in which the effect of these drugs are documented[7]*** include:

- painful diabetic polyneuropathy;
- postherpetic neuralgia;
- nerve injury pain;
- central pain.

It has been argued that systemic local anesthetics are more likely to be effective in pain conditions arising from lesions in the peripheral nervous system, but several studies revealed benefit in conditions secondary to central nervous system lesions. Based on reports showing that systemic lidocaine is able to reduce secondary hyperalgesia and allodynia of several sensory modalities and is capable of reducing a spinally organized nociceptive reflex, it seems most likely that systemic anesthetics exert their effect mainly on the central nervous system. Systemic lidocaine has no impact on normal sensory thresholds.

The benefit of systemic lidocaine on spontaneous pain, pain paroxysms, dysesthesiae, and allodynia may vary between studies, but its effectiveness has been seen on all modalities in clinical trials. As sodium channel blockers may interact broadly in the currently accepted models for mechanisms of neuropathic pain, no recommendations can be given with respect to subtypes of neuropathic pain being more sensitive to antiarrhythmics than others. In the case of both systemic lidocaine and oral mexiletine, one should expect to treat more than 10 patients in order to see a patient with > 50% pain relief corrected for placebo.

Lidocaine infusions may be used to intervene in severe continuous painful conditions, often in the hope of a response of longer duration. Alternatively, it is used as a test to predict the effect of oral antiarrhythmics or other sodium channel blockers. However, firm evidence for such a predictive value is still lacking.

Contraindications

1 Systemic lidocaine
   a cardiac AV blocks II and III (if bifascicular, also type I);
   b supraventricular bradyarrythmias represent a relative contraindication;
   c allergy to this drug class.
2 Mexiletine
   a cardiac AV blocks II and III (if bifascicular, also type I);
   b hypotension;
   c allergy to this drug class.

Dosing and treatment schedule

Lidocaine (lidocaine hydrochloride) is infused *intravenously* as 5 mg/kg body weight over 30–45 min. Alternatively, a computer-controlled infusion paradigm can be used to obtain a serum lidocaine level of 3–4 μg/ml.[8] Doses should be reduced by 50% in heart failure or liver disease. Increases in blood pressure and heart rate are expected to occur during infusion (see Chapter P4).

1 Inform the patient about the procedure and side-effects and confirm that driving will not take place following the procedure.
2 Establish an intravenous line with 0.9% saline.
3 Measure blood pressure and start electrocardiograph (EKG) monitoring.
4 Begin controlled infusion of preservative-free lidocaine in 0.9% saline.
5 Observe the patient throughout the infusion and measure blood pressure every 15 min.
6 Continue observations as indicated above for 45 min following completion of the infusion.

Mexiletine is metabolized in the liver mainly by the isoenzyme CYP2D6. Because of the genetic polymorphism of this enzyme, variable pharmacokinetics and drug interactions need attention.

In order to increase compliance, initiate oral mexiletine treatment with a dose of 50 mg three times daily for 3 days, then 100 mg three times daily for 3 days, and thereafter 150–300 mg three times daily (approximately 10 mg/kg bodyweight). Preferably dosing should be in relation to meals.

A summary of pretreatment safety measures and dosing schedules used for different antiarrhythmics is given in Table 9.3.

Drug		
	Intravenous lidocaine	**Oral mexiletine**
Caution	Cardiac disease	Cardiac disease
	Liver disease	Liver disease
		Kidney disease
Pretreatment tests	EKG	EKG
	Blood pressure	Liver function
	Liver function	Kidney function
Half-life (h)	0.6–1.5	8–20
Dosage interval	–	8 h[a]
Maximum serum concentration (μmol/l)	15	16[b]
Initial dose	–	150 mg/day[c]
Maximal dose	450 mg	900 mg/day

Table 9.3 *Pretreatment safety measures and dosing of antiarrhythmics*

a. With slow-release formulation 12 h.
b. The suggested upper serum drug concentration in treatment of cardiac arrhythmias.
c. Low initial doses in order to minimize side-effects.
EKG, electrocardiograph.

Side-effects

Acute side-effects are common during intravenous lidocaine infusions at therapeutic doses:

- dizziness, sedation, confusion;
- perioral paresthesiae, slurred speech, blurred vision, euphoria, lightheadedness;
- nausea.

Side-effects disappear within minutes to hours following the end of infusion.

Oral mexiletine is often accompanied by side-effects:

- dizziness, lightheadedness, nausea, vomiting;
- fatigue, nervousness, tremor, unsteady gait, blurred vision;
- confusion, constipation or diarrhea, headache, paresthesiae, slurred speech;
- heartburn, chest pain.

The side-effects of oral mexiletine are often intolerable and it is possible that the apparent lower efficacy of this drug is because optimal doses cannot be used.

REFERENCES

● 1. McQuay HJ, Tramèr M, Nye BA, *et al.* A systematic review of antidepressants in neuropathic pain. *Pain* 1996; **68:** 217–27.

● 2. Sindrup SH, Jensen TS. Efficacy of pharmacological treatments of neuropathic pain. An update and effect related to mechanism of drug action. *Pain* 1999; **83:** 389–400.

3. Kunz NR, Goli V, Entsuah AR. Venlafaxine extended release in the treatment of pain associated with diabetic neuropathy. *Neurology* 2000; **54** (Suppl. 3): A441.

● 4. McQuay H, Carroll D, Jadad AR, *et al.* Anticonvulsant drugs for management of pain: a systematic review. *Br Med J* 1995; **311:** 1047–52.

5. Luria Y, Brecker C, Daoud D, *et al.* Lamotrigine in the treatment of painful diabetic neuropathy: a randomized, placebo-controlled study. In: Devor M, Rowbotham MC, Wiesenfeld-Hallin Z eds. *Progress in Pain Research and Management*, vol. 16. Seattle, WA: IASP Press, 2000: 857–62.

● 6. McQuay H, Moore A. *An Evidence-based Resource for Pain Relief*. Oxford: Oxford University Press, 1998: 221–48.

● 7. Chaplan SR, Bach FW, Yaksh TL. Systemic use of local anesthetics in pain states. In: Yaksh TL, Lynch C, Zapol WM *et al.* eds. *Anesthesia, Biologic Foundations*. Philadelphia, PA: Lippincott-Raven, 1997: 977–86.

● 8. Schnider TW, Gaeta R, Brose W, *et al.* Derivation and cross-validation of pharmacokinetic parameters for computer-controlled infusion of lidocaine in pain therapy. *Anesthesiology* 1996; **84:** 1043–50.

PART III

Psychological techniques

10

Self-regulation skills training for adults, including relaxation

DAVID SPIEGEL

Cortical modulation of pain	113	Hypnosis with children	116
Attention to pain	114	Mechanisms of hypnotic analgesia	116
Meaning of pain	114	Other forms of self-regulation for pain	116
Mood disorders and pain	114	Managing expectancy	117
Hypnosis	115	Conclusion	117
Self-hypnosis	116	References	117

Pain occurs in a psychophysiological context that can either exacerbate or diminish it. Pain usually occurs within the context of the subjective distress associated with a major medical illness or somatic trauma. The "pain experience" represents a combination of both tissue damage and the emotional reaction to it. There is ample evidence to suggest that psychological factors greatly influence the pain experience in either positive or negative ways. In fact, the intensity of pain is directly associated with its meaning. One critical factor that can amplify or diminish pain is the sense of helplessness that surrounds it. Helplessness is the key element underlying the intensity of reactions to trauma.[1,2,3]*** Pain is often intensified by the helplessness that accompanies it. Conversely, many pain patients report that they would find their pain tolerable if they could modulate it at least partially. The desire for control is a critical component of pain management.

Why, one might ask, would one contemplate utilizing a technique such as hypnosis, which is often thought to involve relinquishing control, in the treatment of a disorder that is better managed with enhanced control? Hypnosis is actually a normal state of highly focused attention, with a relative diminution in peripheral awareness.[4-6] Being hypnotized is akin to being so caught up in a good movie, play, or novel that one loses awareness of surroundings and enters the imagined world, a state termed "absorption."[7]* Indeed, people who have more such states spontaneously are more likely to be highly hypnotizable on formal testing.[8]* Although the suspension of disbelief involved in such absorption may make hypnotized people appear more suggestible, i.e. responsive to the instructions of the person inducing hypnosis, all hypnosis is in fact self-hypnosis, a means of altering one's inner state in the direction of an intensity of central focus. Thus, the very state that would appear to engender loss of control can be utilized quite effectively to enhance control, especially over unwanted sensations such as pain, which can be placed at the periphery of awareness, altered, or even eliminated.

CORTICAL MODULATION OF PAIN

Pain is the ultimate psychosomatic phenomenon. It is composed of both a somatic signal that something is wrong with the body and a message or interpretation of that signal involving attentional, cognitive, affective, and social factors. The limbic system and cortex provide a means of modulating pain signals,[9,10] by either amplifying them through excessive attention or affective dysregulation or by minimizing them through denial, inattention, relaxation, or attention-control techniques. It is well known that many athletes and soldiers sustain serious injuries in the heat of sport or combat and are unaware of the injury until someone points out bleeding or swelling. On the other hand, some individuals with comparatively minor physical disturbance report being totally immobilized and demoralized by pain. A single parent with a sarcoma complained of severe unremitting pain that was interlaced with tearful concern about her failure to discuss her terminal prognosis with her adolescent son. When an appropriate meeting was arranged to plan for his future and discuss her fate with him, the pain resolved.[11]

Pain perception is influenced by one's state of consciousness. For example, chronic pain tends to be worse during evenings and weekends when people are not distracted by routine activities. It is often reduced during sleep, but may in fact interfere with sleep; more severe kinds of pain can substantially reduce sleep efficiency. Many of the more potent drugs that treat pain reduce alertness and arousal, an often unwanted side-effect or one that can lead to abuse of analgesic medications.

ATTENTION TO PAIN

Like any other perceptual phenomenon, pain is modulated by attentional processes: you have to pay attention to pain for it to hurt. Novelty tends to enhance pain perception (as with an acute injury), although overwhelming and serious injury is sometimes accompanied by a surprising absence of pain perception until hours afterwards. This traumatic dissociation has been observed in victims of natural disaster, combat, and motor vehicle accidents.[12]

Somatic perception is modulated by the cortex, which enhances or diminishes awareness of incoming signals. Recent neuropsychological and brain-imaging research has demonstrated at least three attentional centers that modulate perception: a posterior parieto-occipital orienting system, a focusing system localized to the anterior cingulate gyrus, and an arousal–vigilance system in the right frontal lobe.[13,14***] These systems provide, among other things, for selective attention to incoming stimuli, allowing competing stimuli to be relegated to the periphery of awareness.

When Melzack and Wall[15] postulated the gate control theory of pain decades ago, they observed that higher cortical input could inhibit pain signals as well. They cited Pavlov's observation that repeated shocks to dogs eventually failed to elicit pain behavior, i.e. the dogs habituated to the painful signals, and this could only be explained as cortical inhibition of pain response. Thus, in their model, there is room for descending inhibition of pain via the substantia gelatinosa as well as competitive inhibition at the gate.[9] The important concept we gain from this theory is the interaction between central processing and perception of noxious stimuli at the periphery.

MEANING OF PAIN

It has been known for half a century that the meaning structure in which pain is embedded influences the intensity of pain. In his classic study, Beecher[16*]

noted with surprise that soldiers who were quite badly wounded on the Anzio beachhead seemed to require very little analgesic medication. He subsequently examined a matched group of civilian surgical patients at Massachusetts General Hospital with equal or less serious surgically induced wounds. They demanded far higher levels of analgesic medication than did the combat soldiers. Beecher concluded that this disparity was based on a difference in the meaning of the pain. To combat soldiers, the pain was almost welcome as an indication that they were likely to get out of combat alive, whereas to the surgical patients it represented an interference with life and a threat to survival. This means that patients who interpret pain signals as an ominous sign of the worsening of their disease are likely to experience a greater intensity of pain. This hypothesis has been confirmed, for example, among cancer patients. Those who believe the pain represents a worsening of their disease show more pain.[17*] Indeed, the meaning of the pain and associated anxiety and depression accounted for more variance in pain than did site of metastasis.

MOOD DISORDERS AND PAIN

Anxiety and depression are often associated with a profound sense of helplessness. They are noted as frequent concomitants of pain.[18,19*,20*] This early work implied that patients with psychopathology complained more about pain. Later work suggested that there is an interaction and that perhaps chronic pain amplifies or produces depression.[21*,22*] Indeed, the presence of significant pain among cancer patients is more strongly associated with major depressive symptoms than is a prior life history of depression.[23*]

Depression is the most frequently reported psychiatric diagnosis among chronic pain patients. Reports of depression among chronic pain populations range from 10% to 87%.[24*] Patients with two or more pain conditions have been found to be at elevated risk for major depression, whereas those patients with only one pain condition did not show such an elevated rate of mood disorder in a large sample of health maintenance organization (HMO) patients. The relative severity of the depression observed in chronic pain patients was illustrated by Katon and Sullivan,[25*] who showed that 32% of a sample of 37 pain patients met criteria for major depression and 43% had a past episode of major depression.

Anxiety is especially common among those with acute pain. Like depression, it may be an appropriate response to serious trauma through injury or illness. Pain may serve a signal function or be part of an anxious preoccupation, as in the case of the woman with the sarcoma cited above. Similarly, anxiety and pain may reinforce one another, producing a snowball effect of escalating and mutually reinforcing central and peripheral symptoms.

HYPNOSIS

Central psychological approaches to pain control can be highly effective analgesics and are underutilized.[26] It has been known since the middle of the 1800s that hypnosis is effective in controlling even severe surgical pain.[27] Hypnosis and similar techniques work through two primary mechanisms: muscle relaxation and a combination of perceptual alteration and cognitive distraction. Pain is not infrequently accompanied by reactive muscle tension. Patients frequently splint the part of their body that hurts. Yet, because muscle tension can by itself cause pain in normal tissue and because traction on a painful part of the body can produce more pain, techniques that induce greater physical relaxation can reduce pain in the periphery. Therefore, having patients enter a state of hypnosis so that they can concentrate on an image that connotes physical relaxation such as floating or lightness often produces physical relaxation and reduces pain.

The second major component of hypnotic analgesia is perceptual alteration. Patients can be taught to imagine that the affected body part is numb. This is especially useful for extremely hypnotizable individuals who can, for example, relive an experience of dental anesthesia and reproduce the drug-induced sensations of numbness in their cheek, which they can then transfer to the painful part of their body. They can also simply "switch off" perception of the pain with surprising effectiveness.[28,29] Temperature metaphors are often especially useful, which is not surprising given the fact that pain and temperature sensations are part of the same sensory system – the lateral spinothalamic tract. Thus, imagining that an affected body part is cooler or warmer using an image of dipping it in ice water or heating it in the sun can often help patients transform pain signals. Some patients prefer to imagine that the pain is a substance with dimensions that can be moved or can flow out of the body as if it were a viscous liquid. Others like to imagine that they can step outside their body to, for example, visit another room in the house. Less hypnotizable individuals often do better with distraction techniques that help them focus on competing sensations in another part of the body.

The specific technique employed may depend on the degree of hypnotic ability of the subject. For example, patients can be taught to develop a comfortable floating sensation on the affected body part. Highly hypnotizable individuals may simply imagine a shot of Novocain (procain hydrochloride) in the affected area, producing a sense of tingling numbness similar to that experienced in previous dental work. Other patients may prefer to move the pain to another part of their body, or to dissociate the affected part from the rest of the body. As an extreme form of hypnotically induced, controlled dissociation, some patients may imagine themselves floating above their own body, creating distance between themselves and the painful sensation or experience. To some more moderately hypnotizable patients, it may be easier to focus on a change in temperature, either warmth or coolness. A sensation of warmth could be elicited while imagining they are floating in a warm bath or applying a heating pad to a given area of the body. A cooling sensation can be elicited by imagining that the afflicted extremity is immersed in an ice-cold mountain stream or in a bucket of ice chips. Temperature metaphors are especially effective. This may be related to the fact that pain and temperature fibers run together in the lateral spinothalamic tract.

The images or metaphors used for pain control employ certain general principles. The first is that the hypnotically controlled image may serve to "filter the hurt out of the pain." They also learn to transform the pain experience. They acknowledge that it exists (the pain), but that there is a distinction between the signal itself and the discomfort the signal causes. The hypnotic experience, which they create and control, helps them transform the signal into one that is less uncomfortable. So patients expand their perceptual options by having them change from an experience in which either the pain is there or it is not to an experience in which they see a third option, in which the pain is there but transformed by the presence of such competing sensations as tingling, numbness, warmth, or coolness. Finally, patients are taught not to fight the pain. Fighting pain only enhances it by focusing attention on the pain, enhancing related anxiety and depression, and increasing physical tension that can literally put traction on painful parts of the body and increase the pain signals generated peripherally (Box 10.1).

For patients undergoing painful procedures, such as bone marrow aspirations, the main focus is on the hypnotic imagery *per se* rather than relaxation. This works especially well with children since they are so highly hypnotizable and easily absorbed in images.[30,31] Patients may be guided through the experience while the procedure is performed, or a given scenario can be suggested and later the patient can undergo the experience hypnotically while the procedure is under way. This enables them to restructure their experience of what is going on and

---

Box 10.1 *Components of pain treatment utilizing self-hypnosis*

- Explain hypnosis
- Measure hypnotizability
- Induce relaxation by concentrating on "floating"
- Hypnotic analgesia
  - Concentrate on a competing sensation:
  - Warmth, coolness, tingling, lightness, or heaviness
  - Filter the hurt out of the pain
- Anxiety control: screen technique
- Exit from self-hypnotic state
- Instructions in practicing self-hypnosis

dissociate themselves psychologically from pain and fear intrinsic to their immediate situation.

SELF-HYPNOSIS

Hypnotic techniques can easily be taught to patients for self-administration.[5,6] Pain patients can be taught to enter a state of self-hypnosis in a matter of seconds with some simple induction strategies, such as looking up while slowly closing their eyes, taking a deep breath and then letting the breath out, their eyes relax, their body floats, and one hand floats up in the air like a balloon. They are then instructed in the pain control exercise and taught to bring themselves out by reversing the induction procedure, again looking up, letting the eyes open, and letting the raised hand float back down. Patients can use this exercise every 1–2 h initially and any time they experience an attack of pain. They can evaluate their effectiveness in conducting the pain control exercise by rating on a scale from 0 to 10 the intensity of their pain before and after the self-hypnosis session. As with any pain treatment technique, hypnosis is more effective when employed early in the pain cycle, before the pain has become so overwhelming that it impairs concentration. Patients should be encouraged to use this technique early and often because it is simple and effective[32**] and has no side-effects.[33***] Indeed, it has been shown in a randomized trial in interventional radiology to produce better analgesia than that resulting from patient-controlled analgesia with midazolam and fentanyl, with less anxiety, fewer side-effects, and fewer procedural interruptions.[34**] This finding has been confirmed in a larger randomized trial involving 241 patients undergoing percutaneous vascular and renal radiological procedures. While pain increased linearly with procedure time in the routine care group, it did not in the group taught self-hypnosis, despite their use of half the analgesic medication through patient-controlled analgesia pumps. Most important, the hypnosis patients had fewer episodes of hemodynamic instability, and the average procedure time was 17 min (22%) shorter.[35**]

Although not all patients are sufficiently hypnotizable to benefit from these techniques, two out of three adults are at least somewhat hypnotizable,[4] and it has been estimated that hypnotic capacity is correlated at a 0.5 level with effectiveness in medical pain reduction.[36***] Furthermore, clinically effective hypnotic analgesia is not confined to those with high hypnotizability.[26]

HYPNOSIS WITH CHILDREN

Hypnosis is especially effective in comforting children who are in pain (see Chapter P13). Several good studies have shown greater efficacy than placebo attention control.[30**,31*,37] Hypnotic techniques, including going over favorite stories, are quite effective in removing the child from the immediacy of both pain and anxiety.[37] Hypnosis seems to have advantages over distraction, especially among young children undergoing medical procedures.[37] This is likely because children as a group are more hypnotizable than adults.[38*] Their imaginative capacities are so intense that separate relaxation exercises are not necessary. Children naturally relax when they mobilize their imagination during the sensory alteration component of hypnotic analgesia. Indeed, self-management utilizing hypnosis and related imagination exercises is becoming a first-line treatment for such problems as headaches among children.[39]

MECHANISMS OF HYPNOTIC ANALGESIA

Recent research indicates cortical effects of hypnotic analgesia exercises, including reduced ERP amplitude in response to somatosensory stimuli[40**] and increased frontal and parietal blood flow.[41*] A PET study indicated activation of the anterior cingulate gyrus during hypnotic analgesia.[42**] Thus, hypnotic alteration of nociception seems to involve cortical modulation of pain perception. A recent PET study of hypnotic alteration of color vision provides further evidence of changes in primary association cortex function.[43*] When highly hypnotizable subjects were instructed to perceive a gray-tone grid as filled with color, there was a significant increase in blood flow in the lingual gyrus, the primary brain site for color processing. Conversely, when a colored image was "drained" of color hypnotically, blood flow in that region decreased. Thus, with hypnosis, "believing is seeing," and hypnotic changes in sensation are accompanied by changes in brain function that indicate an actual change in perception, not merely in response to perception.

A number of studies have tested the idea that endogenous opiates are involved in hypnotic analgesia. But, with one partial exception,[44**] studies with both volunteers[45**] and patients in chronic pain[46**] have shown that hypnotic analgesia is not blocked and reversed by a substantial dose of naloxone given in double-blind, crossover fashion. Therefore, the cortical attention deployment mechanism is at the moment the most plausible explanation for hypnotic reduction of pain.

OTHER FORMS OF SELF-REGULATION FOR PAIN

Nearly every self-regulation technique that is used in the treatment of pain and related anxiety and depressive symptoms, including hypnosis, combines various forms of physical relaxation with cognitive restructuring. The principle of combining imagery with physical relaxation is associated with techniques such as systematic desensitization and progressive muscle relaxation. During these treatments, patients are instructed to maintain a physical sense of relaxation, while restructuring pain-related fears. A stimulus hierarchy is then developed from least to most stressful. Patients are taught to develop their own scenarios and to augment or reduce the intensity of the stimulus within seconds, as the therapist helps them to construct a graded hierarchy. These techniques are designed to disrupt the conditioned association between pain, anxiety about disease, and somatic tension which amplifies pain and focuses more attention on it.

Mindfulness-based stress reduction

One successful but somewhat different approach to self-regulation for pain has been mindfulness-based stress reduction. Based upon Eastern meditative traditions, the approach involves exercises aimed at altering the management of consciousness and the experience of perception in general, rather than influencing pain in particular.[47–50] In this practice, subjects are taught to spend about 30 min twice a day in a quiet state of meditation, focusing on present experience, inducing physical relaxation, and seeing anxieties as a focus on future possibilities that take away from enjoyment of the moment. Such techniques have proven quite effective with chronic pain, and have recently been shown to speed healing time for patients with psoriasis.[51**]

Biofeedback

A National Institutes of Health (NIH) Technology Assessment Panel reported that techniques such as hypnosis and biofeedback are effective in reducing chronic pain.[52***] Although hypnosis focuses on internally generated images, biofeedback utilizes external feedback from monitors that assess heart rate, skin conductance, skin temperature, blood pressure, muscle tension, and other physiological measures related to the functioning of the autonomic and peripheral nervous systems to facilitate anxiety and pain reduction.[53,54] Often, pain can be attenuated by altering peripheral skin temperature in the affected area. Similarly, skill in reducing muscle tension via muscle tension biofeedback may reduce secondary intensification of pain.[55] Thus, training in reducing physiological responses to pain such as muscle tension, sweating, and vasoconstriction can help to interrupt the feedback cycle of somatic distress and affective preoccupation that frequently intensifies pain.

MANAGING EXPECTANCY

Thus, it is particularly important to separate the expectation of efficacy from psychological self-management

treatments from a premise about etiology of the pain. Many patients (and doctors) assume that, if a psychological or placebo intervention reduces pain, the pain itself is "supratentorial." Nothing could be further from the truth. People can, as noted above, diminish or even ignore major injury and other forms of physical pain. The tissue injury is real, but they learn to dissociate themselves from it. To imply to a patient that such success means that the pain is not "real" undermines motivation and can be perceived by patients as insulting. Rather, it is best to utilize a "rehabilitation" model, teaching patients that they are learning to overcome a serious pain problem rather than proving that it was not so bad in the first place. In this way, patients can receive immediate emotional gratification from improvement, rather than feel ashamed of their ability to reduce pain.

CONCLUSION

The old dichotomy between peripheral and central pain is being replaced by a more complex and comprehensive analysis that evaluates central and peripheral components of pain and designs interventions that take advantage of therapeutic opportunities at all levels of pain perception processing. This point of view is important because it underscores the fact that successful psychosocial intervention for reducing pain may occur via understandable neurological mechanisms and does not prove that the pain is largely functional. In the same way, successful pharmacological intervention does not prove that the pain is completely peripheral in origin. Most pain syndromes are a combination of physical and neuropsychiatric distress and dysfunction and require a combination of biological and psychosocial intervention to be optimally effective. In particular, effective strategies such as hypnosis that provide a means for self-regulation of pain reduce the helplessness associated with pain, as well as inducing physical relaxation and altering perception. The strain in pain lies mainly in the brain.

REFERENCES

1. Koller P, Marmar CR, Kanas N. Psychodynamic group treatment of posttraumatic stress disorder in Vietnam veterans. *Int J Group Psychother* 1992; **42:** 225–46.
2. Spiegel D, Hypnosis in the treatment of victims of sexual abuse. *Psychiatr Clin North Am* 1989; **12:** 295–305.
● 3. Butler LD, *et al.* Hypnotizability and traumatic experience: a diathesis-stress model of dissociative symptomatology. *Am J Psychiatry* 1996; **153** (7): 42–63.
4. Spiegel H, Spiegel D. *Trance and Treatment: Clinical Uses of Hypnosis.* Washington, DC: American Psychiatric Press, 1987.
● 5. Spiegel D, Maldonado J. Hypnosis. In: Hales RE,

Yudofsky S, Talbott J eds. *American Psychiatric Press Textbook of Psychiatry*. Washington, DC: American Psychiatric Press, 1999.

6. Spiegel H, Greenleaf M, Spiegel D. Hypnosis. In: Sadock B, Sadock V eds. *Comprehensive Textbook of Psychiatry,* 7th edn. Philadelphia, PA: Lippincott Williams & Wilkins, 2000: 2128–46.

◆ 7. Tellegen A, Atkinson G. Openness to absorbing and self-altering experiences ("absorption"), a trait related to hypnotic susceptibility. *J Abnorm Psychol* 1974; **83:** 268–77.

8. Tellegen A. Practicing the two disciplines for relaxation and enlightenment: comment on "Role of the feedback signal in electromyograph biofeedback: the relevance of attention" by Qualls and Sheehan. *J Exp Psychol Gen* 1981; **110:** 217–31.

9. Melzack R. From the gate to the neuromatrix. *Pain* 1999; **6** (Suppl.): S121–6.

● 10. Brose WG, Spiegel D. Neuropsychiatric aspects of pain management. In: Yudofsky SC, Hales RE eds. *Synopsis of Neuropsychiatry*. Washington, DC: American Psychiatric Press, 1994.

11. Kuhn CC, Bradnan WA. Pain as a substitute for fear of death. *Psychosomatics* 1979; **20:** 494–5.

12. Spiegel D. Dissociation and hypnosis in post-traumatic stress disorder. *J Trauma Stress* 1988; **1:** 17–33.

13. Berger A, Posner MI. Pathologies of brain attentional networks. *Neurosci Biobehav Rev* 2000; **24:** 3–5.

◆ 14. Posner MI, Petersen SE. The attention system of the human brain. *Annu Rev Neurosci* 1990; **13:** 25–42.

◆ 15. Melzack R. Pain mechanisms: recent research. *Acupunct Electrother Res Int J* 1978; **3:** 109–12.

◆ 16. Beecher HK. Relationship of significance of wound to pain experiences. *JAMA* 1956; **161:** 1609–13.

17. Spiegel D, Bloom JR. Pain in metastatic breast cancer. *Cancer* 1983; **52:** 341–5.

18. Blumer D, *et al.* Biological markers for depression in chronic pain. *J Nerv Ment Dis* 1982; **170:** 425–8.

19. Bond MR. Personality studies in patients with pain secondary to organic disease. *J Psychosom Res* 1973; **17:** 257–63.

20. Woodforde JM, Fielding JR. Pain and cancer. *J Psychosom Res* 1970; **14:** 365–70.

21. Peteet J, *et al.* Pain characteristics and treatment in an outpatient cancer population. *Cancer* 1986; **57:** 1259–65.

22. Spiegel D, Sands SH. Pain management in the cancer patient. *J Psychosoc Oncol* 1988; **6:** 205–16.

◆ 23. Spiegel D, Sands S, Koopman C. Pain and depression in patients with cancer. *Cancer* 1994; **74:** 2570–8.

◆ 24. Dworkin SF, Von Korff M, LeResche L. Multiple pains and psychiatric disturbance. An epidemiologic investigation. *Arch Gen Psychiatry* 1990; **47:** 239–44.

25. Katon W, Sullivan M. Depression and chronic medical illness. *J Behav Med* 1990; **11:** 3–11.

◆ 26. Holroyd J. Hypnosis treatment of clinical pain: under-

standing why hypnosis is useful. *Int J Clin Exp Hypn* 1996; **44:** 33–51.

27. Esdaile J. *Hypnosis in Medicine and Surgery*. New York, NY: Julian Press, 1846 (reprinted 1957).

28. Miller ME, *et al.* Hypnotic analgesia: dissociated experience or dissociated control? *J Abnorm Psychol* 1993; **102:** 29–38.

29. Hargadon R, Bowers K, Woody E. Does counterpain imagery mediate hypnotic analgesia! *J Abnorm Psychol* 1995; **104:** 508–16.

◆ 30. Hilgard JR, LeBaron S. Relief of anxiety and pain in children and adolescents with cancer: quantitative measures and clinical observations. *Int J Clin Exp Hypn* 1982; **4:** 417–42.

◆ 31. Zeltzer L, LeBaron S. Hypnosis and nonhypnotic techniques for reduction of pain and anxiety during painful procedures in children and adolescents with cancer. *J Pediatr* 1982; **101:** 1032–5.

◆ 32. Spiegel D, Bloom JR. Group therapy and hypnosis reduce metastatic breast carcinoma pain. *Psychosom Med* 1983; **45:** 333–9.

● 33. Spiegel D. Oncological and pain syndromes. In: Hales R, Francis A eds. *American Psychiatric Association Annual Review,* vol. 5. Washington, DC: American Psychiatric Association Press, 1986.

34. Lang E, *et al.* Self-hypnotic relaxation during interventional radiological procedures: effects on pain perception and intravenous drug use. *Int J Clin Exp Hypn* 1996; **44:** 106–19.

◆ 35. Lang EV, *et al.* Adjunctive non-pharmacological analgesia for invasive medical procedures: a randomised trial. *Lancet* 2000; **355:** 1486–90.

● 36. Hilgard ER, Hilgard JR. *Hypnosis in the Relief of Pain*. Los Altos, CA: William Kauffman, 1975.

37. Kuttner L. Favorite stories: a hypnotic pain-reduction technique for children in acute pain. *Am J Clin Hypn* 1988; **30:** 289–95.

38. Morgan AH, Hilgard ER. Age differences in susceptibility to hypnosis. *Int J Clin Exp Hypn* 1972; **21:** 78–85.

● 39. Kuttner L. Managing pain in children. Changing treatment of headaches. *Can Fam Phys* 1993; **39:** 563–8.

◆ 40. Spiegel D, Bierre P, Rootenberg J. Hypnotic alteration of somatosensory perception. *Am J Psychiatry* 1989; **146:** 749–54.

41. Crawford HJ, *et al.* Effects of hypnosis on regional cerebral blood flow during ischemic pain with and without suggested hypnotic analgesia. *Int J Psychophysiol* 1993; **15:** 181–95.

◆ 42. Rainville P, *et al.* Pain affect encoded in human anterior cingulate but not somatosensory cortex. *Science* 1997; **277:** 968–71.

◆ 43. Kosslyn SM, *et al.* Hypnotic visual illusion alters color processing in the brain. *Am J Psychiatry* 2000; **157:** 1279–84.

44. Frid M, Singer G. Hypnotic analgesia in conditions of stress is partially reversed by naloxone. *Psychopharmacology* 1979; **63:** 211–15.

45. Goldstein A, Hilgard ER. Failure of the opiate antagonist naloxone to modify hypnotic analgesia. *Proc Natl Acad Sci USA* 1975; **72:** 2041–3.

46. Spiegel D, Albert L. Naloxone fails to reverse hypnotic alleviation of chronic pain. *Psychopharmacology* 1983; **81:** 140–3.

47. Kabat-Zinn J, *et al*. Meditation. In: Holland J ed. *Psychooncology*. New York, NY: Oxford University Press, 1998: 767–79.

48. Kabat-Zinn J. Mindfulness meditation: health benefits of an ancient Buddhist practice. In: Gurion GA ed. *Mind/Body Medicine*. New York, NY: Consumer Reports, 1993.

49. Kabat Zinn J. An outpatient program in behavioral medicine for chronic pain patients based on the practice of mindfulness meditation: theoretical considerations and preliminary results. *Revision* 1984; **7:** 71–2.

● 50. Kabat Zinn J, Lipworth L, Burney R. The clinical use of mindfulness meditation for the self-regulation of chronic pain. *J Behav Med* 1985; **8:** 163–90.

◆ 51. Kabat-Zinn J, *et al*. Influence of a mindfulness meditation-based stress reduction intervention on rates of skin clearing in patients with moderate to severe psoriasis undergoing phototherapy (UVB) and photochemotherapy (PUVA). *Psychosom Med* 1998; **60:** 625–32.

● 52. NIH Technology Assessment Panel on Integration of Behavioral and Relaxation Approaches into the Treatment of Chronic Pain and Insomnia, Integration of behavioral and relaxation approaches into the treatment of chronic pain and insomnia. *JAMA* 1996; **276:** 313–18.

53. Spiegel D. Facilitating emotional coping during treatment. *Cancer* 1990; **66** (Suppl. 6): 1422–6.

54. Titlebaum H. Relaxation. In: Zahourek RP ed. *Relaxation and Imagery: Tools for Therapeutic Communication and Intervention*. Philadelphia, PA: W. B. Saunders/Harcourt Brace Jovanovich, 1988: 28–52.

55. Wickramasekera I. How does biofeedback reduce clinical symptoms and do memories and beliefs have biological consequences? Toward a model of mind–body healing. *Appl Psychophysiol Biofeedback* 1999; **24:** 91–105.

11

Biofeedback

FRANK ANDRASIK AND HERTA FLOR

Approaches to biofeedback	121	Specific biofeedback approaches	130
Biofeedback as a general aid to relaxation	124	Evidence base	131
Select treatment considerations	125	References	132

Pain is a complex, multiply determined behavior that typically requires a multifaceted, multidimensional, and multidisciplinary approach. Biofeedback is often a component of treatment and, although this chapter focuses on biofeedback as an isolated technique, it is rarely if ever applied in isolation. At a minimum, it is combined with a host of allied relaxation-based treatments (see Chapters Ch5, P10, and P12). More typically, it is one of many options that patients and therapists consider.

Biofeedback has been defined as:[1]

> … a process in which a person learns to reliably influence physiological responses of two kinds: either responses which are not ordinarily under voluntary control or responses which ordinarily are easily regulated but for which regulation has broken down due to trauma or disease.

The process of biofeedback involves three operations. In the first operation, a biological response is detected and amplified by using certain measurement devices (or transducers) and electronic amplifiers. The bioelectrical potentials detected at this stage are in a form that is difficult to utilize in biofeedback. For example, raw or unprocessed muscle tension potentials resemble the static that one might hear between channels of a radio, and few individuals would be capable of detecting even gross changes in electrical activity. The second operation of biofeedback converts bioelectrical signals to a form that can be easily understood and easily processed by the patient. Averaging the electronic signal over a specified time period and filtering out unwanted aspects of the signals are examples of ways in which this is accomplished. The third operation involves the relatively immediate feedback of the signal to the patient. This feedback is most often presented in auditory and visual modalities and in either binary (signal on/signal off at a specified threshold value; commonly used when shaping is a goal) or continuous (as muscle tension decreases, the tone or click rate decreases) proportional fashion; on occasion, combinations of both are used. With all responses, care must be taken to ensure that areas of sensor placement are prepared adequately and that measurement devices are placed on the proper locations. These factors are especially crucial in electromyography (EMG) (and electroencephalography; EEG) because of the weak electrical signals that are detected. Here, electrode sites may need to be cleaned thoroughly with acetone or alcohol and lightly abraded (although advances in instrumentation are making this less necessary). With some recordings, a conductive gel or electrolyte is placed between the electrodes and the subject's skin to facilitate conductance and reduce measurement artifact. More detailed discussion of physiology, electrical theory, and bases of the primary responses utilized in biofeedback may be found in Peek[2] and various chapters within Cacioppo et al.[3] and Stern et al.[4] Various theories have been used to account for biofeedback, ranging from operant learning to cognitive and expectancy models.[5]

APPROACHES TO BIOFEEDBACK

Three different rationales or approaches have been offered for the use of biofeedback in pain management;[6,7] here, for simplicity, they will be termed general, specific, and indirect.

General approach

The "general" approach employs biofeedback as an aid to general or overall relaxation training. Two assumptions underlie this use. Assumption 1 is that a reduction in general arousal leads to a concurrent reduction in central processing of peripheral sensory inputs. Assumption 2 derives from the observed relationship between anxiety and pain – anxiety is associated with decreased pain tolerance and increased reports of pain. Therefore, achievement of a more relaxed state should lead to concomitant reductions in anxiety, which in turn enhance pain tolerance and decrease pain reports. One can make the case that most pain patients could benefit from relaxation and tension reduction, especially patients whose pain is associated with increased muscle tension. Thus, this approach is probably the most common. It also requires the least technical proficiency.

Specific approach

The "specific" biofeedback approach attempts to target and modify directly the physiological dysfunction or response system assumed to underlie the pain condition. This approach has its origins in the pain–spasm–pain cycle first described by Bonica.[8] In implementing this approach, therapists assess psychophysiological responding in the modalities assumed to be relevant to the condition under varied stimulus conditions. In the text to follow, comments will be restricted to peripheral measures, as these have garnered the greatest attention by researchers and clinicians. Most of the examples discussed here relate to muscle tension, as this is the response modality found most useful when working with pain patients. Readers seeking information about the much less studied central measures of pain are referred to Flor.[7]

Flor[7] has pointed out the functions, utility, and advantages of psychophysiological data collection in the "specific" approach to the treatment of chronic pain. These are:

- provide evidence for the role of psychological factors in maladaptive physiological functioning;
- satisfy, thus, a necessary prerequisite or justification for the use of biofeedback therapy;
- facilitate tailoring of treatments to patients;
- allow therapists and researchers to document efficacy, generalization, and transfer of treatment;
- identify predictors of treatment response;
- serve as a source of motivation (e.g. patients realize they are able to influence bodily processes by their own thoughts, emotions, and actions; feelings of helplessness decrease; openness to psychological approaches concurrently increases, etc.).

Key components of the psychophysiological assessment (or "psychophysiological stress profile," as some have labeled this approach) are summarized in Table 11.1 and are discussed more fully in Flor[7] and Arena and Schwartz,[9] among others. Brief comments about each component are in order.

Adaptation

The adaptation component is included for three main reasons:

- to allow patients to become familiar with the setting and recording procedure;
- to minimize presession effects (rushing to the appointment, temperature, and humidity differences between office and outdoors);
- to permit habituation of the orienting response and response stability to occur.

Although the need for a prebaseline period is widely acknowledged, scant research has been conducted to help identify key parameters of adaptation. Most, but not all, individuals will adapt within 5–20 min (some individuals, though, are not fully adapted even after a 60-min session). Practitioners are encouraged to extend this period until some stability is achieved for the key responses of interest. Patients are instructed merely to sit quietly during this period.

Baseline

Once adapted, the clinician will need to collect some type of baseline data. The baseline data serve as the basis of comparison for subsequent assessment phases and as the basis for gauging progress within and across future treatment sessions. Again, there are no definitive data to document the optimal approach – Should eyes be open or closed? Should the patient be fully reclined or sitting upright? Should conditions be neutral or designed to promote relaxation? – or the desired duration of baseline data collection. In clinical practice, the baseline period typically ranges from 1 to 5 min, during which time most responses will stabilize.

A second type of baseline may be helpful as well. This baseline is intended to assess preexisting abilities to regulate physiology. When the goal of biofeedback is generalized relaxation, it is useful to collect a second baseline during which the patient is instructed as follows: "I would now like to see what happens when you try to relax as deeply as you can. Use whatever means you believe will be helpful. Please let me know when you are as relaxed as possible."

It was once believed that elevated resting levels of muscle tension might be a unique characteristic of patients experiencing chronic pain. A review of 60 psychophysiological investigations conducted with headache, back, and temporomandibular pain and dysfunction (TMD) patients found minimal support for this notion.[10]*** Research on this topic is compounded by questions about measurement reliability and stability.[7,9]

Reactivity

The third component investigates psychophysiology in response to simulated stressors that are personally relevant or conditions that approximate real world

Table 11.1 *Components to a psychophysiological assessment for chronic pain*

Component	Brief description
Adaptation/habituation	Time to adjust to clinic/laboratory setting and to allow responses to stabilize
Baseline	
At rest	Serves as basis of comparison for subsequent data collection
Preexisting abilities	Assess current abilities to relax
Stress reactivity/real world Simulations	Simulate situations that occur in everyday life
Somatic	Body position and posture; dynamic movement, such as standing, sitting, bending, lifting, walking, etc.; work task, such as typing on a keyboard
Psychological	Stressful imagery, such as a negative encounter with a colleague or family member
Stress recovery	Time required to return to the baseline level
Muscle scanning	Brief sequential recordings from multiple bilateral sites under varied conditions
Muscle discrimination	Estimation of muscle tension levels

events that are associated with pain onset or exacerbation. Again, there is no standard, empirically validated approach. Some examples of commonly used stimulus conditions are:

- negative imagery, wherein a patient concentrates on a personally relevant unpleasant situation (the details of which have been obtained during the intake interview);
- cold exposure (e.g. Raynaud's disease) or cold pressor test (as a general physical stressor);
- movement, such as sitting, rising, bending, stooping, or walking;
- load bearing, such as lifting or carrying an object;
- operation of a keyboard.

Although baseline differences for EMG have not been found to reliably characterize pain disorders, symptom-specific responses to stimuli have been found for certain pain conditions on a more consistent basis (for a review, see Flor[7]).

Recovery

Another component involves recovery or return to baseline. If multiple stressful stimuli are presented to a patient, then a poststress recovery period is recommended after each stimulus presentation. This phase continues until the patient's physiology returns to a value close to that observed prior to stimulus presentation (often, responses do not fully return to their starting values).

The above components constitute the basic approach to psychophysiological assessment. The two remaining components listed in Table 11.1 are less common in practice, but may be useful as well.

Muscle scanning

Cram[11] has developed an approach that permits a therapist to quickly assess EMG activity from multiple sites, in a manner that does not require multiple recording channels (only two channels are needed). This approach is made possible by the use of two hand-held "post" electrodes, which are used to obtain brief (around 2 s/site)

sequential bilateral recordings while the patient is sitting and standing. Cram is developing a normative database designed to help the therapist determine whether any readings are abnormally high or low and whether any asymmetries (right side versus left side differences) exist, as these may be suggestive of bracing or favoring of a position or posture. The goal of biofeedback is to return aberrant readings to a more normal state. Although this type of approach seems straightforward at first, in actuality it is more complex. A number of factors can influence the readings obtained, including the angle and force by which the sensors are applied, the amount of adipose tissue present (fat acts as an insulator and dampens the signal), and the degree to which the sensors are placed in a similar location to that used for the norming sample (plus other variables that affect EMG in general).

Muscle discrimination

Some have speculated that an inability to perceive bodily states accurately may be a factor in maintaining chronic pain. Flor and colleagues found that patients with chronic pain were unable to perceive muscle tension levels accurately in both the affected and nonaffected muscles and that, when exposed to tasks requiring production of muscle tension, these patients overestimated physical symptoms, rated the task as more aversive, and reported greater pain.[12,13] These findings point to a heightened sensitivity.

Flor[7] has outlined a procedure that can be easily used to assess muscle discrimination abilities in a clinical setting:

- present the patient with a bar of varying height on a monitor;
- instruct the patient to tense a muscle to the level reflected in the height of the bar;
- vary the bar height from low to high;
- correlate the EMG readings obtained with the actual heights of the bars;
- define as "good" discrimination abilities correlation coefficients ≥ 0.80;

- define as "bad" or poor discrimination abilities correlation coefficients ≤ 0.50.

Summary

Finally, Flor[7] has summarized a number of recommendations for conducting psychophysiological assessment with pain patients. These are reproduced in Table 11.2.

Indirect approach

What is termed here as the "indirect" approach for employing biofeedback with pain patients is used more for clinical than for empirical reasons.[6] This model views biofeedback as a means of facilitating psychosomatic therapy. Take the case of the pain patient who steadfastly holds to a purely somatic view and refuses to accept the notion that other factors (emotional, behavioral, environmental) may be precipitating, perpetuating, or exacerbating pain and somatic symptoms. With such patients, a referral for biofeedback is likely to be less threatening (it is construed as a "physical" treatment for a "physical" problem) and to at least open the door for help. As "physiological insight" is acquired, such patients may begin to see the broader picture, i.e. the interplay of physical and psychological factors. In fact, it is not all that uncommon for a pain patient who denies psychological factors upon entry to therapy to make a request such as the following after just a few sessions of biofeedback: "Doc, how about turning off the biofeedback equipment today. I want to talk about a few things." From this point on, session time is divided between biofeedback and counseling. Nothing further will be said about this aspect.

BIOFEEDBACK AS A GENERAL AID TO RELAXATION

Any response modality indicative of heightened arousal theoretically can serve as a target for promoting relaxation. In practice, three have served most commonly as targets for overall relaxation – muscle tension, skin conductance (perhaps better known as sweat gland activity), and peripheral temperature. These modalities, termed the "workhorses" of the biofeedback general practitioner,[14] are easily collected, quantified, and interpreted and are discussed below. Other responses can be of value as well, including heart rate, respiration, and blood volume, but these will not be addressed further (for a discussion, see Flor[7]).

Electromyographic-assisted relaxation

The rationale for employing muscle tension (and skin conductance; see next section) feedback to facilitate relaxation is straightforward. The basis of the EMG signal is the small electrochemical changes that occur when a muscle contracts. By placing a series of electrodes along the muscle fibers, the muscle action potentials associated with the ion exchange across the membrane of the muscles can be detected and processed. (When single motor units are the focus of treatment, as in the case of muscle rehabilitation, fine wire electrodes that penetrate the skin surface are used.) EMG monitoring from surface sites is accomplished by the use of two active electrodes, separated by one ground electrode, to set up two separate circuits to detect electrical activity that leaks up to the skin surface. With this arrangement, the resultant signal is the difference between the two circuits (with the amount subtracted out considered to be noise). When EMG is used for generalized relaxation, sensors are typically placed on the forehead region (one active sensor about 2.5 cm above the pupil of each eye, with the ground or reference sensor placed above the bridge of the nose). This placement, which employs large-diameter sensors, is sensitive to muscle tension from adjacent areas, possibly down to the upper rib cage.[15] Originally, it was believed that reductions in forehead muscle tension would automatically generalize to most other untrained muscles (hence, promoting a state of "cultivated low arousal"). This does not automatically occur,[16]*** so clinicians may need to

---

Table 11.2 *Recommendations for psychophysiological assessment*

Use multiaxial classification of patients to identify specific somatic and psychosocial characteristics of the patients

If possible, use normative data from controls

Control for pain status (i.e. test in a pain-free and a painful state, if possible)

Control for medication (i.e. make sure patient has not taken analgesic or psychotropic medication for several days, if possible)

Use sites both proximal and distal to the painful site

Make sure that the measures selected are relevant for the specific type of pain being studied (e.g. temperature recordings for Raynaud syndrome, rather than EMG levels)

Use ecologically valid methods of stress induction (i.e. use self-selected stressors; test stressfulness by assessing subjective stress rating, heart rate, or skin conductance levels)

Use sufficiently long adaptation phases and baselines

Use a syndrome-specific and a general autonomic measure

Reproduced from Flor;[7] permission pending.

train patients from several sites in the course of general relaxation treatment (or combine biofeedback with other approaches).

Surface EMG has a power spectrum ranging from 20 to 10,000 Hz. Some of the commercially available biofeedback machines sample a very limited amount of this range. For example, some machines filter out EMG occurring below 100 Hz. This misses much of the EMG power spectrum and results in lower readings overall. Clinicians need to be aware of the "bandpass" of their equipment and to realize that readings obtained from one machine may not be comparable with those obtained on another machine where different settings may be employed. Some of the other factors affecting measurement quantity include sensor type and size, sensor placement on the muscle, and distance between sensors.

Skin conductance-assisted relaxation

Electrical activity of the skin, or sweating, has long been thought to be associated with arousal. In fact, in the late 1800s, Romain Virouroux included measures of skin resistance to facilitate understanding when working with cases of hysterical anesthesias.[2,17] Electrodermal activity became popular and thought of as a way to read the mind when used by Carl Jung in the early 1900s in word-association experiments. Two separate portions of the central nervous system are believed to responsible for control of the electrodermal activity.[18] Sensors are typically placed on body surface areas that are most densely populated with "eccrine" sweat glands (such as the palm of the hand or the fingers), as these respond primarily to psychological stimulation and are innervated by the sympathetic branch of the autonomic nervous system.[4] Conductance measures (the reciprocal of resistance; measured in micromhos or microsiemens), as opposed to resistance measures, are preferred in clinical application because the former measures have a linear relationship to the number of sweat glands that are activated. This permits a straightforward explanation to patients (as arousal increases, so does skin conductance; focusing on decreasing skin conductance helps to lower arousal and to achieve a state of relaxation).

Skin temperature-assisted relaxation

It is less obvious why skin temperature has been targeted for general relaxation. This is because the first clinical application resulted from a serendipitous finding by clinical researchers at the Menninger Clinic. During a standard laboratory evaluation, it was noticed that spontaneous termination of a migraine was accompanied by flushing in the hands and a rapid sizable rise in surface hand temperature.[19]* This led Sargent et al.[19] to pilot test as a treatment a procedure wherein migraineurs were given feedback to raise their hand temperatures as a way to regulate stress and headache activity. Treatment was augmented by components of autogenic training, leading to a procedure they termed "autogenic feedback." Noting that constriction of peripheral blood flow is under the control of the sympathetic branch of the nervous system, these researchers reasoned that decreases in sympathetic outflow led to increased vasodilation, blood flow, and a resultant rise in peripheral temperature (owing to the warmth of the blood). Thus, temperature feedback may best be thought of at the moment as yet another way to facilitate general relaxation. With migraine headache, other approaches, assumed to be tied more directly to the underlying physiology, have also been attempted. These include blood flow in various arteries and EEG. These approaches are either quite specialized and/or have not been the focus of extensive research, so they will not be discussed further.

SELECT TREATMENT CONSIDERATIONS

Individuals presenting for biofeedback treatment, either general or specific, may be confused about the nature of their disorder, anxious and depressed, discouraged, and uncertain about their chances for improvement. Brief instruction about factors underlying their condition, which points out those variables which potentially may be controlled by the patient, is often helpful in counteracting the patient's initial feelings of helplessness and in mobilizing his/her interest in treatment. This is followed by a description of biofeedback, what will be required during treatment (frequency and number of sessions, home practice, etc.), and any ancillary treatment that may be used. The explanation of biofeedback is best understood when accompanied by a live demonstration, which points out the steps involved in measurement and provision of feedback. Education remains an integral part of treatment, as patients continue to discover more about causes and new found ways to react (as it does in the other approaches described in Chapters Ch5 and P12).

When used for purposes of facilitating general relaxation, initial sessions are typically held in a quiet room, lights may be dimmed, and the patient semireclined in a comfortable chair that supports the entire body. Most clinicians adopt a "coaching" model. This involves:

- Sharing observations for discussion. "I noticed that a couple of minutes into the session, your EMG signal shot up. It seemed you might have been clenching your teeth then. How about dropping your lower jaw and moving it just a bit forward? I wonder if anything particular might have been on your mind then?"
- Determining when breaks and encouragement might be needed. Early attempts to lower EMG or skin conductance or to raise hand temperature often are met with the opposite effect, and this situation is para-

doxically worsened as patients try harder and harder; these occurrences can be of great therapeutic value as they help to demonstrate the relationship between thoughts and physiological functioning; explaining how and why this is happening helps to counteract frustration and to get the patient back on track.

- Helping patients to articulate and consolidate learning.
- Augmenting biofeedback with instruction in complementary relaxation approaches.

Biofeedback involves learning a skill that requires regular practice and eventually incorporating learned skills into day-to-day activities. Some patients become successful simply by concentrating on the feedback stimulus and becoming aware of corresponding sensations. Others engage in various mental games or attempt to empty their minds completely and think of nothing.[20] In the early sessions, patients are encouraged to experiment with various techniques, but to remain with a given technique long enough to give it an ample trial period. It may be most useful to view the therapist as a "coach" – someone who has special skills that the patient does not yet have but who can impart these skills by properly timed guidance. With experience, the therapist learns when the patient needs uninterrupted time to practice biofeedback and when support and assistance would be valuable. In fact, the only investigation of coaching during biofeedback found that learning was actually impeded when the therapist was overly active and intrusive.[21]

A typical treatment session involves the following components:

- Sensor attachment and time for adaptation.
- Initial progress review: discussion and review of data collection, attempts at applying skills, problems encountered, etc., while sensors are being attached and the patient is adapting.
- Resting baseline: to assess extent of change over time, as discussed previously.
- "Self-control" baseline: defined as the patient's ability to regulate the target response in the desired direction once training has begun but in the absence of feedback;[1] provides an index of the ability to perform the biofeedback skills outside of the treatment setting.
- Actual feedback for 20–40 min that is continuous or interrupted by breaks.
- Final resting or self-control baseline: to assess extent of learning within the session.
- Final progress review, homework assignment, etc.

Each session should end with a review of the strategies that were explored during the session and an appraisal of the effectiveness of each. Once the patient has shown some abilities to regulate target physiological levels in the clinic, practice outside of the office is encouraged. Initially, this practice is performed in a setting maximally conducive to achieving a relaxed state or concentrating on the task at hand. Subsequently, patients are instructed to practice during everyday, but low stress, activities (when driving, shopping, standing in line, during a coffee break, etc.). The final goal is to employ learned biofeedback skills to counteract the build-up of stress and physiological arousal. Skills have to be highly developed to be successful at this step.

Thus, the goals of biofeedback are for the patient to be able to discriminate when the target response is in need of control, effect the necessary change in the absence of feedback, apply the learned skills in the real world, and continue use of these skills over the long term. Therapists need, then, to be concerned with generalization and maintenance of learned skills. Lynn and Freedman[22] have identified a number of procedures for helping to make biofeedback training effects more durable. Among those which may be most easily implemented by the clinician are:

- overlearning the target response;
- incorporating booster treatments;
- fading or gradually removing feedback during treatment (increased use of self-control trials);
- training under stimulating or stressful conditions (during noise and distractions, while engaged in a physical or mental task, etc.);
- employing multiple therapists (possible in group practices);
- varying the physical setting;
- providing patients with portable biofeedback for use in real-life situations;
- augmenting biofeedback with other physiological interventions and with cognitive and behavioral procedures.

A number of procedures can be used to augment biofeedback treatments for pain, especially when biofeedback is used for general relaxation.

Imagery

The first and simplest is by imagining a pleasant or relaxing scene, such as lying on a blanket at the beach while listening to the waves roll in and back out or walking through a pleasant meadow on a warm, sunny day. It is best that patients avoid images that involve sexual content or vigorous physical activity (as these activities can increase rather than decrease arousal) and include as many sensory modalities (touch, sound, smell) and details as possible.[20] It is recommended that patients practice employing several different relaxing images, so that they can switch to another image if the selected one is not working at a given time. With practice, images can be recalled quickly and vividly and can be used effectively to provide mental escape when situations become seemingly overwhelming.

Diaphragmatic breathing

A second form involves relaxed or diaphragmatic breathing. Most patients find this to be a particularly useful procedure because breathing can be readily brought under voluntary control, and it is an activity that is vital to survival. The notion of relaxed breathing is deceptively simple, so most patients need detailed instructions for correct use. Improper application can lead to blood gas imbalance and hyper- or hypoventilation. Also, patients whose initial respiration rate is high (more than 30 breaths/min) may feel quite strange as their breathing rate approaches the relaxed range. Such patients are instructed to pay no particular attention to this and are informed that these peculiar feelings will pass with time. Gevirtz and Schwartz[23] provide an excellent discussion of the topic, which briefly reviews the physiology of breathing and provides instructions on how to teach patients to breathe slowly (to a target range of 5–8 breaths/min), deeply (to full lung capacity), and evenly (to facilitate the same rate for exhaling and for inhaling), while concentrating on the associated physiological sensations. Having the patient subvocalize a word associated with relaxation on each exhalation can help "cue" subsequent relaxation.

There are various ways to promote the desired breathing pattern. Patients can practice breathing:

- while holding their arms straight overhead (which minimizes chest movement);
- while lying on a firm surface, placing a medium weight book on the abdomen and raising and lowering the text with each cycle;
- while placing one hand on the chest and the other just below the rib cage, breathing in a manner that limits movement of the hand on the chest and maximizes movement of the hand on the abdomen.

Gevirtz and Schwartz[23] also discuss other approaches for promoting more relaxed breathing, including paced respiration, breath meditation, breath mindfulness, rebreathing, pursed-lip breathing, and instrument-based approaches. This very portable procedure can be easily combined with other relaxation techniques.

Autogenic training

A third form of relaxation borrows from the well-developed body of literature on autogenic training – a meditation-type relaxation. Autogenic training has an extensive history and involves having patients passively concentrate on key words and phrases selected for their ability to promote desired somatic responses.[24] When added to thermal biofeedback, clinicians typically utilize two of the total six components. Patients are instructed to focus on feelings/sensations of *warmth* and *heaviness* in the extremities, as this is believed to facilitate increased blood flow to the extremities, which accounts for peripheral warming and a reduction in sympathetic nervous arousal. It is recommended that patients develop their own phrasing and subvocalize these phrases numerous times (50–100) during practice in order to maximize effects.[20]

Progressive muscle relaxation training

The fourth and final technique, progressive muscle relaxation training, has the most extensive empirical basis (see the concluding section on the evidence base), but it is also the most complex. It involves having the patient engage in a systematic series of muscle-tensing and -releasing exercises, designed first to help the patient discriminate various levels of muscle tension, which makes it easier for the patient then to achieve an overall or generalized state of relaxation.

Andrasik[25] describes a typical relaxation training regimen, which is outlined in Table 11.3.

The following points are stressed when introducing this form of relaxation training:

- relaxation training consists of systematic tensing and relaxing of major muscle groups;
- tensing muscles even for a brief period results in them reflexively achieving a subsequent lower level of tension;
- experiencing a broad range of muscle tension levels enables clients to better discriminate when muscle tension is building;
- with improved discrimination abilities and once skills are acquired for rapidly relaxing muscles, this technique can be used to counteract tension build-up as it occurs throughout the day (termed applied relaxation);
- achieving a deep state of relaxation is a learned skill and requires regular practice;
- the procedure will first focus on all major muscle groups, but groups will subsequently be combined over time in order to permit rapid deployment.

The procedure the authors commonly employ begins by having the patient sequentially tense and relax 14 separate muscle groupings in the 18 steps indicated in Table 11.4. Prior to formal instruction, the patient is asked to complete a few practice tension–release cycles to ensure that the tension generated is proper (neither incomplete nor overly zealous) and is confined to the target group. Muscles that are very painful or that have been strained are omitted so as not to cause further problems. Target muscle groups are tensed for 5–7 s and then relaxed for 20–30 s, which constitutes a complete cycle. The patient is instructed to attend to the sensations associated with tension and relaxation during each cycle. If a patient prefers a different muscle sequence, it is acceptable to modify the sequence. However, once modified, it is important that the patient adheres to the same order. Patients may be periodically instructed to mentally scan select mus-

Table 11.3 *Outline of progressive muscle relaxation training program*

Week	Session	Introduction and treatment rationale	Number of muscle groups	Deepening exercises	Breathing exercises	Relaxing imagery	Muscle discrimination training	Relaxation by recall	Cue-controlled relaxation
1	1	X	14	X	X				
	2		14	X	X	X	X		
2	3		14	X	X	X	X		
	4		14	X	X	X	X		
3	5		8	X	X	X	X		
	6		8	X	X	X	X	X	
4	7		4	X	X	X	X	X	
5	8		4	X	X	X	X	X	X
6	9		4	X	X	X	X	X	X
7	None								
8	10		4	X	X	X	X	X	X

Based on Andrasik;[25] permission pending.

Table 11.4 *Fourteen initial muscle groups and procedures for tensing in 18 steps*

1 Right hand and lower arm (have client make fist, simultaneously tense lower arm)
2 Left hand and lower arm
3 Both hands and lower arms
4 Right upper arm (have client bring his/her hand to the shoulder and tense biceps)
5 Left upper arm
6 Both upper arms
7 Right lower leg and foot (have client point his/her toe while tensing the calf muscles)
8 Left lower leg and foot
9 Both lower legs and feet
10 Both thighs (have client press his/her knees and thighs tightly together)
11 Abdomen (have client draw abdominal muscles in tightly, as if bracing to receive a punch)
12 Chest (have client take a deep breath and hold it)
13 Shoulders and lower neck (have client "hunch" his/her shoulders or draw his/her shoulders up towards the ears)
14 Back of the neck (have the client press head backwards against headrest or chair)
15 Lips/mouth (have client press lips together tightly, but not so tight as to clench teeth; or have client place the tip of the tongue on the roof of the mouth behind upper front teeth)
16 Eyes (have client close the eyes tightly)
17 Lower forehead (have client frown and draw the eyebrows together)
18 Upper forehead (have client wrinkle the forehead area or raise the eyebrows)

Based on Andrasik[25] and Andrasik and Walch.[26]

cle groups that have been targeted previously in order to identify any residual tension. If detected, another tension–release cycle may be completed. Various procedures, all involving therapist suggestions, may also be used to promote a deepened sense of relaxation (such as having the therapist count out loud backwards from 5 to 1 and instructing the patient that a deeper level of relaxation will be experienced with each successive count). Relaxed breathing and imagery are added early on, in the manner discussed previously. Once the patient has made adequate progress at tensing and relaxing the 14 major muscle groups, the therapist begins to combine various muscle groups in order to abbreviate the procedure first to eight total muscle groupings and then to four groupings (see Table 11.5).

Muscle discrimination training can be added to facilitate abilities to detect even trace amounts of tension increases. To demonstrate this aspect, a patient is asked to engage in a complete tension–release cycle involving the hand and lower arm, then to tense these muscles by only half as much. This is followed by a tension cycle involving only one-quarter as much force. Once the concept of differential tension is understood, the patient is instructed to apply differential muscle tensing to the muscles most associated with pain. Final techniques concern relaxation by recall and cue-controlled relaxation. To implement relaxation by recall, the patient is instructed first to recall the sensations associated with relaxation and then to attempt to reproduce these sensations without the aid of tension and release cycles. Actual tension–release cycles are used only as needed to promote the desired somatic state. Practice outside of the office is necessary to maximize effects and patients are typically instructed to practice techniques taught them once or twice per day. Audiotapes, prepared commercially or by the therapist

during an actual session with the patient, can facilitate home practice.

The reader is referred to Andrasik,[25] Arena and Blanchard,[20] Lichstein,[27] or Smith[28] for further information about relaxation in general.

There are no firm criteria for deciding when to terminate biofeedback. In research investigations of biofeedback as a general relaxation technique, patients are typically provided a set number of treatments, typically ranging from 8 to 12. In practice, the number of sessions is determined according to clinical response, as gauged by the degree of symptom relief and/or adequacy of control of the target response. Skilled therapists come to sense when treatment has reached the point of diminishing returns or marginal utility (i.e. response reaches a plateau and further effort does not alter the situation). Some have argued for using a physiological training criterion as a

Table 11.5 *Abbreviated muscle groups*

Eight-muscle groups
1 Both hands and lower arms
2 Both legs and thighs
3 Abdomen
4 Chest
5 Shoulders
6 Back of neck
7 Eyes
8 Forehead

Four-muscle groups
1 Arms
2 Chest
3 Neck
4 Face (with a particular focus on the eyes and forehead)

Based on Andrasik and Walch.[26]

deciding factor, e.g. ability to reduce and keep EMG levels below a certain value for a specified time, ability to raise hand temperature above a certain value within a specified time period, etc. This intuitive notion has great clinical appeal, but we are not yet at a point where it is possible to advocate for a specific approach.

Few difficulties have been reported when using biofeedback as a general relaxation procedure. A small portion of clients may experience what has been termed "relaxation-induced anxiety," noted to be a sudden increase in anxiety during deep relaxation that can range from mild to moderate intensity and that can approach the level of a minor panic attack.[29] It is important for the therapist to remain calm, reassure the patient that the episode will pass, and, when possible, have the patient sit up for a few minutes or even walk about the office when this happens. With patients who are believed to be at risk for relaxation-induced anxiety, it may be helpful to instruct them to focus more on the somatic aspects as opposed to the cognitive aspects of training.[20] See Schwartz and Schwartz[30] for discussion of other problems and solutions.

SPECIFIC BIOFEEDBACK APPROACHES

Much of the research conducted to date has focused on the value of biofeedback as a general approach to decrease stress, tension, and pain. With certain pain conditions, more specific approaches are emerging as either alternative or preferred treatments for patients with certain characteristics. A few brief examples are given for purposes of illustration.

The studies used to support claims for efficacy of EMG biofeedback for recurrent headache have monitored muscle activity almost exclusively from the forehead area, despite patients reporting other sites as being central to their pain (such as occipital, temporal, neck, and shoulders). Support exists for feedback from the upper trapezius muscles[31]** and for an interesting and creative novel approach termed the frontal–posterior neck placement.

Nevins and Schwartz[32] noted over 15 years ago that the occipitalis area is a site of headache activity for certain tension-type patients. The difficulty for clinicians has been finding an easy way to monitor EMG activity from this site (without shaving the head). Nevins and Schwartz found that by placing one active electrode on the frontal area and the remaining active electrode on the posterior neck on the same side the summated electrical activity between these sites closely approximated that which occurred in the occipital area. Hudzynski and Lawrence[33] subjected this notion to a controlled experiment that compared a bifrontal forehead placement with bilateral frontal–posterior neck placements in tension headache subjects and headache-free controls. Bilateral EMG readings were also taken from the temple, mas-

seter, sternocleidomastoid, and cervical areas utilizing muscle scanning. Frontal–posterior neck readings best discriminated headache and nonheadache patients, and these readings could further distinguish headache from headache-free periods in headache patients. Hudzynski and Lawrence[34] have since published normative data to help clinicians gauge when EMG elevations, obtained when clients are both sitting and standing and when both narrow and wide filter settings are used, may be of clinical consequence. This approach warrants further investigation.

For TMD, in addition to frontal sites, biofeedback is provided from masseter and temporalis muscles.[35,36]

Work undertaken by Sherman[37] has helped to identify the most appropriate biofeedback treatment for patients experiencing phantom limb pain. Pain described as burning, throbbing, and tingling was associated with decreased temperature in the stump, whereas pain described as cramping was preceded by and associated with EMG changes. Targeting biofeedback accordingly leads to the greatest outcome.

Finally, some researchers have turned their attention to the psychophysiological model of Travell and Simons,[38] who postulated that a large percentage of chronic muscle pain resulted from trigger points. Hubbard and Berkoff[39] have expanded upon their view using the following line of reasoning:

- muscle tension and pain are sympathetically mediated hyperactivity of the muscle stretch receptors, or the muscle spindles;
- muscle spindles, which are scattered throughout the muscle belly (hundreds within the trapezius muscle), are encapsulated organs that contain their own muscle fibers;
- although traditionally viewed as a stretch sensor, the muscle spindle is recognized now to be a pain and pressure sensor and an organ that can be activated by sympathetic stimulation;
- thus, the pain associated with trigger points arises in the spindle capsule.

Support for this model comes from studies where careful needle electrode placements have detected high levels of EMG activity in the trigger point itself, but data collected from adjacent nontender sites just 1 cm away are relatively silent.[40] Further, when exposed to a stressful stimulus, EMG activity increases at the trigger point but not at the adjacent site.[41] This work provides further evidence of the link between behavioral and emotional factors and mechanisms of muscle pain. As a result of their basic research, Gevirtz et al.[42] have developed a comprehensive treatment program that uses EMG biofeedback to facilitate muscle tension awareness in sessions and in daily life activities, to identify stressors triggering increased EMG activity, and to assist patients in finding improved ways to cope with tension-producing situations.

EVIDENCE BASE

Multiple meta-analyses have been conducted for biofeedback, other active treatments (behavioral and pharmacological), and various control conditions for recurrent headache. The meta-analyses conducted to date are summarized in Table 11.6. Early meta-analyses excluded very few of the available studies; poorly designed studies were included along with expertly designed studies if sample sizes met a minimum criterion. More recent analyses have been much more selective about studies included for analysis. For example, the Agency for Health Care Policy and Research (AHCPR) meta-analysis[49]*** located 355 behavioral and physical treatment (acupuncture, transcutaneous electrical nerve stimulation, occlusal adjustment, cervical manipulation, and hyperbaric oxygen) articles. However, only 70 of the studies were *controlled trials* of behavioral treatments for migraine, and only 39 of these trials met criteria for inclusion in the analysis. Findings from the most recent meta-analyses may be best considered as providing lower bound estimates of effectiveness, under very tightly controlled conditions.

In addition to meta-analytic approaches, various groups have assembled panels to conduct evidence-based reviews, wherein rigorous methodological criteria are used to evaluate every study under consideration. Evidence-based analyses have been performed by the Division 12 Task Force of the American Psychological Association[50]*** and the US Headache Consortium (composed of the American Academy of Family Physicians, American Academy of Neurology, American Headache Society, American College of Emergency Physicians, American College of Physicians–American Society of Internal Medicine, American Osteopathic Association, and National Headache Foundation).[51]***

Consideration of the findings from the above evaluative sources leads to the following conclusions. (1) Biofeedback (and other relaxation or psychologically based approaches) led to significant reductions in headache activity, ranging from 30–60%. (2) Conversely, there is a sizeable number of patients who are nonresponders or partial responders (approximately 40–70%). Prediction of treatment response and careful treatment planning become particularly important when attempting to improve upon this outcome. (3) Improvements exceed those obtained for various control conditions. (4) Nonpharmacological treatments produce benefits similar to those obtained for pharmacological treatments. (5) Combining treatments can increment effectiveness, especially so for nonpharmacological combined with pharmacological. However, the net gain of adding a second treatment modality beyond a single treatment is sometimes relatively small, again stressing the importance of finding the "right" therapy fit for an individual patient. (6) Most studies of biofeedback and related approaches have included subjects that continued their consumption of any number of pharmacological agents while undergoing nonpharmacological interventions. Only a very few studies have systematically isolated pure treatments.

The US Headache Consortium concluded that behavioral treatments, such as biofeedback, may be particularly well suited for patients having one or more of the following characteristics:

- patient prefers such an approach;
- pharmacological treatment cannot be tolerated or is medically contraindicated;

Table 11.6 *Average improvement rates from separate meta-analyses*

Reference	EMG	REL	EMG + REL	BFCT	COG	PHARM	OTHER	PTCT	MDCT	WTLT
Tension-type headache										
43***	61	59	59					35	35	−5
44***	46	45	57	15						−4
45***	47	36	56		53	39	38	20		−5
46***	48	38	51		40	35[a]		17		3

Reference	ATFB	THBF	REL	VMBF	THBF + REL	EMG	COG	COG + BF	PTCT	MDCT	WTLT
Migraine headache											
43***	65	52	53							17	
47***		28	44	31	57						11
48***	49	27	48	43		29			26		13
49		37	32	33		40	49	35	9	5	

a Amitriptyline alone.
EMG, electromyographic biofeedback, generally provided from the frontal/forehead muscles; REL, relaxation therapy, generally of the muscle tensing and relaxing variety; BFCT, biofeedback control procedure, generally false or noncontingent biofeedback; COG, cognitive therapy, stress coping training, or problem-solving therapy; PHARM, various medications, ranging from aspirin and nonsteroidal inflammatory drugs to prophylactics to narcotics; OTHER, various approaches, other than BF, REL, or COG; PTCT, psychological or pseudotherapy control procedure; MDCT, medication control procedure; results taken from double-blind, placebo-controlled medication trials; WTLT, waiting list control procedure; no treatment; ATFB, thermal biofeedback augmented by components of autogenic training, as developed at the Menninger Clinic; THBF, thermal biofeedback by itself; VMBF, vasomotor biofeedback provided from the temporal artery. BF, EMG or thermal biofeedback.
Reproduced from Andrasik and Walch;[26] permission pending.

- response to pharmacological treatment is absent or minimal;
- patient is pregnant, has plans to become pregnant, or is nursing;
- patient has a long-standing history of frequent or excessive use of analgesic or acute medications that can aggravate headache;
- patient is faced with significant stressors or has deficient stress-coping skills.

A meta-analysis has recently been completed for biofeedback-based treatments for TMD. This analysis[52]*** revealed a mean improvement rate of 68.6% for active treatment compared with 34.7% for various control conditions. Effect size scores for pain measures were 1.04 and 0.47 and for examination results were 1.33 and 0.26 for biofeedback and controls respectively. Effects noted at the end of treatment were either maintained or improved during follow-up evaluations, some of which extended over 2 years.

In the research literature, biofeedback treatments for chronic pain other than headache and TMD are varied in their approach and fewer in number; limited direct replications have been attempted. Reviews by various panels[53]***,[54]*** and a meta-analysis[55]*** provide support for biofeedback as an effective treatment for chronic pain.

REFERENCES

1. Blanchard EB, Epstein LH. *A Biofeedback Primer*. Reading, MA: Addison-Wesley Publishing, 1978.
2. Peek, CJ. A primer of biofeedback instrumentation. In: Schwartz MS, Andrasik F eds. *Biofeedback: A Practitioner's Guide*, 3rd edn. New York, NY: Guilford Press, in press.
3. Cacioppo JT, Tassinary LG, Bernston GG eds. *Handbook of Psychophysiology*, 2nd edn. Cambridge: Cambridge University Press, 2000.
4. Stern RM, Ray WJ, Quigley KS. *Psychophysiological Recording*, 2nd edn. Oxford: Oxford University Press, 2001.
5. Schwartz NM, Schwartz, MS. Definitions. In: Schwartz MS, Andrasik F eds. *Biofeedback: A Practitioner's Guide*, 3rd edn. New York, NY: Guilford Press, in press.
◆ 6. Belar CD, Kibrick SA. Biofeedback in the treatment of chronic back pain. In: Holzman AD, Turk DC eds. *Pain Management: A Handbook of Psychological Treatment Approaches*. New York, NY: Pergamon Press, 1986: 131–50.
● 7. Flor H. Psychophysiological assessment of the patient
◆   with chronic pain. In: Turk DC, Melzack R eds. *Handbook of Pain Assessment*, 2nd edn. New York, NY: Guilford,2001: 76–96.
8. Bonica JJ. Management of myofascial pain syndromes in general practice. *JAMA* 1957; **164:** 732–8.
● 9. Arena JG, Schwartz MS. Psychophysiological assessment

◆   and biofeedback baselines for the front-line clinician: a primer. In: Schwartz MS, Andrasik F eds. *Biofeedback: A Practitioner's Guide*, 3rd edn. New York, NY: Guilford Press, in press.
10. Flor H, Turk DC. Psychophysiology of chronic pain: do chronic pain patients exhibit symptom-specific psychophysiological responses? *Psychol Bull* 1989; **105:** 219–59.
11. Cram JR. EMG muscle scanning and diagnostic manual for surface recordings. In: Cram JR *et al.* eds. *Clinical EMG for Surface Recordings*, vol. 2. Nevada City, CA: Clinical Resources, 1990: 1–141.
12. Flor H, Fürst M, Birbaumer N. Deficient discrimination of EMG levels and overestimation of perceived tension in chronic pain patients. *Appl Psychophysiol Biofeedback* 1999; **24:** 55–66.
13. Flor H, Schugens MM, Birbaumer N. Discrimination of muscle tension in chronic pain patients and healthy controls. *Biofeedback Selfregul* 1992; **17:** 165–77.
14. Andrasik F. Biofeedback. In: Mostofsky DI, Barlow DH eds. *The Management of Stress and Anxiety Disorders in Medical Disorders*. Boston, MA: Allyn & Bacon, 2000: 66–83.
15. Basmajian JV. Facts versus myths in EMG biofeedback. *Biofeedback Selfregul* 1976; **1:** 369–71.
16. Surwit RS, Keefe FJ. Frontalis EMG-feedback training: an electronic panacea? *Behav Ther* 1978; **9:** 779–72.
17. Neumann E, Blanton R. The early history of electrodermal research. *Psychophysiology*, 1970; **6:** 453–75.
18. Boucsein W. *Electrodermal Activity*. New York, NY: Plenum, 1992.
19. Sargent JD, Green EE, Walters ED. The use of autogenic training in a pilot study of migraine and tension headaches. *Headache* 1972; **12:** 120–4.
● 20. Arena JG, Blanchard EB. Biofeedback and relaxation therapy for chronic pain disorders. In: Gatchel RJ, Turk DC eds. *Psychological Approaches to Pain Management: A Practitioner's Handbook*. New York: Guilford Press, 1996: 179–230.
21. Borgeat F, Hade B, Larouche LM, Bedwani CN. Effect of therapist's active presence on EMG biofeedback training of headache patients. *Biofeedback Selfregul* 1980; **5:** 275–82.
22. Lynn SJ, Freedman RR. Transfer and evaluation of biofeedback treatment. In: Goldstein AP, Kanfer F eds. *Maximizing Treatment Gains: Transfer Enhancement in Psychotherapy*. New York, NY: Academic Press, 1979: 445–84.
23. Gevirtz RN, Schwartz MS. Breathing. In: Schwartz MS, Andrasik F eds. *Biofeedback: A Practitioner's Guide*, 3rd edn. New York, NY: Guilford Press, in press.
24. Schultz JH, Luthe W. *Autogenic Training*, vol. 1. New York, NY: Grune & Stratton, 1969.
25. Andrasik F. Relaxation and biofeedback for chronic headaches. In: Holzman AD, Turk DC eds. *Pain Management: A Handbook of Psychological Treatment Approaches*. New York, NY: Pergamon, 1986: 213–329.

● 26. Andrasik F, Walch SE. Biobehavioral assessment and
◆ treatment of recurrent headaches. In: Nezu AM, Nezu
CM, Geller PA eds. *Comprehensive Handbook of
Psychology*. Vol. 9. *Health Psychology*. New York, NY:
Wiley, in press.

◆ 27. Lichstein KL. *Clinical Relaxation Strategies*. New York,
NY: Wiley & Sons, 1988.

◆ 28. Smith JC. *Cognitive–Behavioral Relaxation Training: A
New System of Strategies for Treatment and Assessment*.
New York, NY: Springer Publishing Company, 1990.

29. Heide FJ, Borkovec TD. Relaxation-induced anxiety:
paradoxical anxiety enhancement due to relaxation
training. *J Consult Clin Psychol* 1983; **51:** 171–82.

30. Schwartz MS, Schwartz NM. Problems with relaxation
and biofeedback-assisted relaxation. In: Schwartz MS,
Andrasik F eds. *Biofeedback: A Practitioner's Guide*, 3rd
edn. New York, NY: Guilford Press, in press.

31. Arena JG, Bruno GM, Hannah SL, Meador KJ. A comparison of frontal electromyographic biofeedback training,
trapezius electromyographic biofeedback training, and
progressive muscle relaxation therapy in the treatment
of tension headache. *Headache* 1995; **35:** 411–19.

32. Nevins BG, Schwartz MS. An alternative placement
for EMG electrodes in the study and treatment of tension headaches. Paper presented at the 16th annual
meeting of the Biofeedback Society of America, New
Orleans, LA, 1985.

33. Hudzynski LG, Lawrence GS. Significance of EMG surface electrode placement models and headache findings. *Headache* 1988; **28:** 30–5.

34. Hudzynski LG, Lawrence GS. EMG surface electrode
normative data for muscle contraction headache and
biofeedback therapy. *Headache Q* 1990; **1:** 224–9.

35. Glass EG, Glaros AG, McGlynn FD. Myofascial pain dysfunction: treatments used by ADA members. *J Cranio-
mandibular Pract* 1993; **11:** 25–9.

◆ 36. Glaros AG, Lausten L. Temporomandibular disorders.
In: Schwartz MS, Andrasik F eds. *Biofeedback: A Practitioner's Guide*, 3rd edn. New York, NY: Guilford Press, in
press.

37. Sherman R. *Phantom Pain*. New York, NY: Plenum
Press, 1997.

38. Travell J, Simons D. *Myofascial Pain and Dysfunction:
The Trigger Point Manual*. New York, NY: Williams &
Wilkins, 1983.

39. Hubbard D. Chronic and recurrent muscle pain: pathophysiology and treatment, and review of pharmaco-
logic studies. *J Musculoskeletal Pain* 1996; **4:** 123–43.

40. Hubbard D, Berkoff G. Myofascial trigger points show
spontaneous EMG activity. *Spine* 1993; **18:** 1803–7.

41. McNulty E, Gevirtz R, Hubbard D, Berkoff G. Needle
electromyographic evaluation of trigger point response
to a psychological stressor. *Psychophysiology* 1994; **31:**
313–16.

◆ 42. Gevirtz RN, Hubbard DR, Harpin RE. Psychophysiologic
treatment of chronic lower back pain. *Professional Psychol Res Pract* 1996; **27:** 561–6.

43. Blanchard EB, Andrasik F, Ahles TA, *et al*. Migraine and
tension headache: a meta-analytic review. *Behav Ther*
1980; **14:** 613–31.

44. Holroyd KA, Penzien D. Client variables and the behavioral treatment of recurrent tension headache: a meta-
analytic review. *J Behav Med* 1986; **9:** 515–36.

45. Bogaards MC, ter Kuile MM. Treatment of recurrent
tension headache: a Meta-analytic review. *Clin J Pain*
1994; **10:** 174–90.

46. McCrory DC, Penzien DB, Hasselblad V, Gray RN. *Evidence Report: Behavioral and Physical Treatments for
Tension-type and Cervicogenic Headache*. Des Moines,
IA: Foundation for Chiropractic Education and Research
(product no. 2085), 2001.

47. Holroyd KA, Penzien DB, Holm JE, Hursey KG. Behavioral treatment of recurrent headache: what does the
literature say? Paper presented at the American Association for the Study of Headache, San Francisco. 1984,
June.

48. Blanchard EB, Andrasik F. Biofeedback treatment of
vascular headache. In: Hatch JP, Fisher JG, Rugh JD eds.
Biofeedback: Studies in Clinical Efficacy. New York, NY:
Plenum, 1987: 1–79.

49. Goslin RE, Gray RN, McCrory DC, *et al. Behavioral Physical Treatments for Migraine Headache. Technical Review
2.2*, February 1999 (prepared for the Agency for Health
Care Policy and Research under contract no. 290-94-
2025. Available from the National Technical Information Service; NTIS accession no. 127946), 1999.

50. Task Force on Promotion and Dissemination of Psychological Procedures. Training in and dissemination of
empirically-validated psychological treatments: report
and recommendations. *Clin Psychol* 1995; **48:** 3–23.

51. Campbell JK, Penzien DB, Wall EM. *Evidence-based
Guidelines for Migraine Headaches: Behavioral and
Physical Treatments*. Available on line at: http:
//www.aan.com/public/practiceguidelines/headache_
g1.htm, 2000.

52. Crider AB, Glaros AG. A meta-analysis of EMG biofeedback treatment of temporomandibular disorders. *J
Orofac Pain* 1999; **13:** 29–37.

53. Keefe FJ, Hoelscher TJ. Biofeedback in the management
of chronic pain syndromes. In: Hatch JP, Fisher JG, Rugh
JD eds. *Biofeedback: Studies in Clinical Efficacy*. New
York, NY: Plenum, 1987: 211–53.

54. NIH Technology Assessment Panel on Integration of
Behavioral and Relaxation Approaches into the Treatment of Chronic Pain and Insomnia. Integration of
behavioral and relaxation approaches into the treatment of chronic pain and insomnia. *JAMA* 1996; **276:**
313–18.

55. Morley S, Eccleston C, Williams A. Systematic review
and meta-analysis of randomized controlled trials of
cognitive behaviour therapy and behaviour therapy for
chronic pain in adults, excluding headache. *Pain* 1999;
80: 1–13.

12

Attentional regulation for adults with chronic pain

ELIZABETH ELLIOTT AND CHRIS ECCLESTON

Introducing the phases of treatment	136	Conclusion	146
Application of phases of treatment	137	References	146
A clinical case example	144		

Integral to current cognitive behavior treatments of chronic pain is the assumption that attention to pain exacerbates its detrimental effects and that distraction from the pain lessens these effects.[1,2] The importance of addressing attention to pain in chronic pain management programs has been highlighted in recent studies which have shown that the more one attends to pain and its potentially threatening consequences, the more likely one is to report higher pain intensity, emotional distress, psychological disability, and increased physician visits as a result of the pain.[3]

In this chapter, we present a clinical model of attention and pain focusing on the detail of treatment application. We stress the importance of attentional processes in the chronic pain experience and how learning to regulate attention can attenuate pain and reduce pain-associated disability. For the purposes of this chapter, we are labeling this model as "attention regulation" to incorporate both attention management strategies and the global process of change we believe accompanies attention management. Throughout this chapter, we emphasize the dynamic process of therapeutic engagement and therapeutic change. Our focus here is specifically on examples of the approach, using ideas of how to frame and word interventions. Our primary audience is clinical psychologists with experience of working in chronic pain management, so we assume some knowledge and shared language. Those untrained in cognitive methods and therapy process should not attempt the interventions outlined here. However, we hope that pain management teams and individual practitioners will find useful material here for reflection and discussion.

In order for pain to be processed, it must first capture attention that is already engaged with other thought and behavior.[4,5] Attending to pain, therefore, means that other attentional engagements are either lost or relegated in importance. This relationship between attention and pain has led to the hypothesis that other attentional engagements may displace pain from attention. Much of the work examining this hypothesis, however, has focused on time-limited or acute pain.[6,7] It is not a simple matter to transfer these methods to working with patients in chronic pain. Methods of distraction are not sensible strategies when faced with chronic and persistent pain. It can be insulting and counterintuitive to expect chronic pain patients to attend away from pain because sustained distraction from pain is effortful and generally ineffective. In addition, because the pain is chronic, one should remember that this persistent pain will capture attention: it is only a matter of time.[8]

The clinical pattern of chronic pain is one dominated by disability, fear, depression, and confusion. The result of repeated interruption by pain is the gradual loss of engagement in other activities and other interests. Patients often become interpersonally isolated and inhabit a pain-focused environment. The cognitive reality of this presentation is that patients present with habitual patterns of self-monitoring, attentional biases, and extensive and well-rehearsed patterns of destructive and denigrating self-talk. Focus on bodily sensation for contributory evidence of further pain and injury has its own detrimental consequences and is thought to maintain pain and disability.[3] In addition, worry that may follow repeated interruption by pain is also thought to be an important component to address in treatment.[9,10] We should remember that patients focus on their bodies and worry about a negative or catastrophic future for a reason: because they are *threatened* by persistent pain and disability. To engage in prolonged distraction from this fundamental threat is countercultural and makes no sense. For the chronic pain patient, attempts to avoid or distract from the pain may instead promote fear and promote unconscious patterns of avoidance. It is possible that repeated and failed attempts to distract from pain might become a problem rather than a solution. Avoidance of pain through attempting to distract oneself from it will prevent learning that exposure to pain may be less aversive than has been previously experienced or expected. Practitioners should, therefore, be aware that offering patients yet another strategy or treatment to relieve the pain could lead to further disappointment, reinforce a patient's mistrust of health care professionals, and make engagement in therapy more difficult.

An alternative to distraction as a means of controlling or lessening pain is for chronic pain patients to regulate their attention to pain by reengaging with aspects of themselves and their world that are changeable and that are controllable. Important in this approach is a focus on what is positive and controllable in an environment, not on what one is attending away from or avoiding. Rather than attempting to remove attention from something that constantly interrupts, attention regulation aims to reinterpret and provide new or lost meanings and behaviors to that which is being interrupted by pain (i.e. the rest of life). Clinical studies that have addressed cognitive coping techniques which teach purposeful focusing of attention to the here and now and the regulation of attention are in their infancy but are proving effective in a number of cognate areas.[11,12] The mechanism for attentional regulation is thought to be in interrupting and reducing threatening rumination about pain, disability, and its consequences.

In this chapter, we give an overview of the process for facilitating the regulation of attention in chronic pain. Our preferred model of treatment in pain management is of programmatic cognitive behavior therapy (CBT) delivered by an interdisciplinary team (see Chapter Ch24). Attention regulation is best delivered as a component of such a program. We exemplify the approach with extracts from our clinical experience, which has been largely with a residential program for adult chronic pain patients who were exposed to 14 CBT group sessions delivered for 1 h each day, Monday to Friday. For narrative purposes, we have chosen to organize the process within phases, which has some resonance with those outlined by Turk and his colleagues.[2] However, we recognize that the skilled clinician should be able to work within a session at different levels of engagement with the patient and across different phases of the therapy process.[13]

INTRODUCING THE PHASES OF TREATMENT

Phase 1: reconceptualizing the pain experience

Reconceptualizing the pain experience and developing a therapeutic alliance is important for the initiation and maintenance of CBT and therefore attention regulation. The patient's experience must be acknowledged in a nonblaming and accepting manner. This shared reconceptualization is essential for the development and maintenance of a therapeutic alliance throughout the process. This phase is delivered during the assessment of the patient and in the first treatment sessions.

Phase 2: developing awareness through objective observation

Developing an awareness of self, environment, and body through guided objective observation should facilitate the development of nonreactive observation. These methods increase both one's field of attention and reactivity to interruption. Methods in this phase aim to reengage the patient's attention to "able" rather than disabled aspects of themselves.[14] This phase in the process increases the patient's awareness of the interactions between thoughts, feelings, behaviors, and consequences of behaviors through self-monitoring observation.

Phase 3: the reengagement of attention to ability

Chronic pain patients are acutely aware of somatic changes and pain. Attempts to escape pain are unsuccessful and patients often become overly focused on activities that they perceive they are unable to do because of pain. The specific aims of phase 3 are to facilitate the refocusing of attention from "what cannot be done because of the pain" to "what can be done in spite of the pain."

Phase 4: the development of purposeful attention

Chronic pain patients are more likely to manage their pain by avoiding situations that can lead to increased pain or have in the past led to heightened pain. This includes unsuccessful attempts to not think about the pain. Purposeful attention is introduced to enable the patient to reconceptualize the experience and reduce the fear of pain. Attention is directed toward the pain, and using cognitive coping strategies the pain experience is perceived to be controllable and adapted. In the context of self-management, it also reintroduces patients to a more successful deployment of strategies that are normally used to disengage or distract attention from pain.

Phase 5: generalization and maintenance

Attention regulation is a lifestyle management regime within the context of CBT. Maintaining treatment gains requires continued practice of the skills and a return to using the strategies following a potential relapse. This crucial phase involves a reintroduction of hopefulness and planning for change by directing the focus of attention to realistic and achievable goals. The generalization of the use of attention regulation is encouraged as a part of daily living.

Facilitating attention regulation within the chronic pain setting is challenging and, we believe, requires the careful maneuvering between these five phases. We consider that phase 1 is essential for the delivery of all phases and therefore is a prerequisite for successful attention regulation. The delivery of the five phases can occur sequentially, e.g. before introducing phase 5 (generalization and maintenance strategies), phases 2, 3, and 4 should have been introduced. However, the phases are interdependent and one can order the intervention to suit each client or group. Also, it may be necessary to go back a phase if alliance is ruptured or the therapist needs to check that certain ideas are understood or skills practiced. We encourage the experienced psychologist to maneuver between phases (see the clinical case example at the end of this chapter).

The remainder of this chapter has been divided into five sections to accommodate the phase model of attention regulation. Each section aims to provide the reader with a rationale for implementing each phase. Phase 1 is described in more detail as it is considered essential for the success of all of the phases and occurs prior to engagement of the other phases. For phases 2–5, we have focused in each on:

- practical tips from our experience;
- describing useful clinical tools;
- stages in the delivery;
- complications that can arise.

We end with a clinical case example of phase 4 work that highlights the process of delivering attention regulation.

APPLICATION OF PHASES OF TREATMENT

Phase 1: reconceptualizing the pain experience

I believe you, your pain is real, and your worry is understandable.

Phase 1 of attention regulation encompasses assessment of the patient for a self-management approach and the first session of the group CBT program. Integral to facilitating the self-regulation of attention within pain management is a collaborative working relationship with the patient. This relationship aims to create a mutual understanding of the problem, contrast the patient's previous understanding of their pain with a cognitive formulation, and allow the patient the opportunity to choose the approach.

An established and trusted relationship with treating professionals who give consistent messages is essential in delivering a cognitive behavior therapeutic approach for pain management. A collaborative therapeutic relationship enables the patient to begin to reconceptualize and normalize their pain experience. Essential to achieving and maintaining this relationship is ongoing communication to the patient that you believe them and that their pain is real and not imaginary.

The first stage of engaging a patient in attention control methods is an increase in the patient's awareness of the effects of pain on their life and how they would like their life to be different. Assessment and session 1 aim to shift the person's perspective from pain as an isolated medical problem to one that encompasses their daily living routine, behaviors, thoughts and feelings, relationships, physical fitness, and future goals. Essential to the establishment of rapport are basic clinical and counseling skills in active listening, including paraphrasing, reflective questioning, and regular checks to determine whether clinician and patient continue to have a shared understanding of the problem.

Patients with chronic pain have an understandable hope that treatments, including self-regulatory techniques, will cure their pain. Repeated messages need to be given to allow patients to reconceptualize their pain experience. Particularly pertinent are the messages that:

- pain is not a reliable signal of injury or damage;
- there are currently no medical or surgical treatments that can be given to eliminate chronic pain;
- self-management techniques are designed to enable patients to begin doing more in spite of their pain.

The following aims of phase 1 are exemplified with typical examples of questions or frames that can be useful to establish a patient's understanding of their pain and also to begin to establish therapist–patient rapport. They can be used to start a more thorough interview of the effect of pain on the person's life.

Acknowledging pain

An important starting point for the building of a collaborative working relationship is to acknowledge the person's pain. Some examples for achieving this are:

Therapist: I have been reading your medical notes and also spoken with your doctor. It is clear that you have been experiencing a lot of distress and have undergone a number of treatments and investigations for your pain. Unfortunately, it seems that you have had no relief from your pain and the investigations have shed no light. This must be very worrying? I know that you have probably told many people now about the pain and they have all made notes, but I would like to start by hearing more directly, from you, about the pain. Will you tell me first about what led to your referral to this clinic, when your pain first began, and what has happened since then?

Developing an understanding of the patient's expectations and pain experience

Therapist: What do you understand by coming here today? What are you hoping for? What do you understand is causing your pain? What has been the best explanation that has been given to you to help you understand why you are still in pain? What is your greatest fear about what will happen in the future? What do you think the future holds for you with pain?

Giving difficult messages

Therapist: The reason that I am saying that we need to start thinking about another way of managing your pain is because chronic pain is pain that you can have that is no longer a signal of further injury or damage. This does not mean that your pain is imaginary or that it is all in your mind or head. Chronic pain is one of those unusual pain experiences. We do not fully understand what underlies it, but we do know that medical treatment has not been as helpful as we would have wished and that we must consider other ways of dealing with it because unfortunately when you have experienced pain for a long time it begins to affect more than your body. It affects how you feel about yourself, the way you relate to family and friends, what you do and do not do. It begins to take over your life. Other ways of dealing with your pain, then, are not about getting rid of your pain but enabling you to begin

doing things again in spite of your pain and to begin dealing with the effects of pain. Is this something that you have considered?

Establishing a rationale for self-management

Therapist: I have reviewed your medical records and it appears that you have been experiencing pain for quite a while. This must be very worrying for you. I understand that you have tried a number of treatments to help you with your pain but without success. This must be very frustrating and disappointing. I wonder what you think will be the next best step for you to take.

The aim of today is not to offer you another treatment or cure for your pain, but to consider another approach to dealing with it. We will be working with you to develop strategies to enable you to do things in another way so that pain does not take over, forcing everything else out so that it comes to dominate your life. This may not be an approach that you are ready to take right now but may be something that you would like to consider.

Reconceptualizing the pain experience

Therapist: From what you have been describing to me and from my experiences in speaking to others who have chronic pain, I would just like to show you my understanding of what may be happening for you and the reasons for considering another way of managing your pain. May I?

The therapist draws a diagram starting with the pain experience as the central point. The therapist begins by saying how they understand the pain to have affected the patient physically, including muscle tension, weakness, loss of flexibility, and postural changes. Next, the therapist should move on to how it has affected what the patient does (activity cycling, avoidance), their mood (down, worried), their specific thoughts (I can't cope, I may injure myself,), their relationships with others, and their financial situation. It is important to check back continually with the patient that each aspect of this diagram of pain-related disability is relevant. Ideally, the patient will generate the aspects and examples in each category. The more specific the better. Then show how each of these can affect each other, and how these can affect their pain. When the therapist has completed the model, they ask:

Therapist: Does this relate to your experience? A pain management approach to dealing with your pain aims to reduce the impact of the pain on your life. It focuses on helping in all of these areas that pain has affected. Is this approach something that you might like to consider?

Context

These messages need to be given in a context that enables rapport between the clinician and patient to be established. The clinician and patient should ideally be facing each other and the clinician should be fully attentive to the patient. The room should be one in which there will be no disturbance. Having a white board or flip chart is helpful to show the rationale and model for self-regulation and for acknowledging the patient's experience. It can be very affirming for the patient and their family members (if they attend the interview) to see what they have been describing. It can also be used to clarify differences in understandings and to guide the patient into considering an alternative explanation for their pain problem.

Complications

The person may have arrived with the following ways of understanding their predicament:

- that they have to live with pain; and/or
- that this assessment is the last hope;
- that it is all in their head;
- that they are not believed or taken seriously;
- that if this approach works then their pain must have been imaginary; or
- that they have to go through with this to satisfy other powerful agencies (e.g. legal, financial).

It is helpful to explore all of these expectations and to repeat the aims of pain management and to repeat that you believe the pain to be real but unhelpful, because it is no longer a sign of further injury or damage. Indeed, if the therapist realizes that they are seriously questioning the veracity of the patient's claims or the honesty of the patient, they should seek supervision. It is important to fully explore with the patient what they hope to achieve from the intervention. It is also useful to establish realistic expectations and achievable goals of therapy. Unrealistic expectations should be fully discussed with the patient (e.g. that pain management can rid one of pain). Sometimes what is an unrealistic expectation for the therapist will be unshakably realistic to or hoped for by the patient. In this case, the difference in opinion should be acknowledged. If patients view this approach as a final hope, the idea of what is meant by failure and its consequences should be explored.

Therapists should be mindful and respectful of the fact that some patients will understand that a different approach is being offered (that is rational and makes sense), but simply may not be ready or able to see its relevance to their own situation. The therapist should acknowledge that the patient may feel that other curative routes need (for them) to be pursued, but that the therapist thinks this approach is relevant for them and at any time they want to discuss it again they should feel free and unencumbered to do so.

Key points for phase 1

- Establish a collaborative relationship.
- Acknowledge pain.
- Give consistent messages.
- Guide the patient in considering an alternative approach to their pain by reviewing past treatments, investigations and diagnoses, and the consequences of these for their pain.

Phase 2: developing awareness through objective observation

What am I here in this treatment/program for? How has my life changed?

The second phase in the regulation of attention is the facilitation of the development of focused observation. This phase encompasses two to three sessions in the first week of a pain management program. These methods increase both the patient's field of attention and their ability to focus attention. The methods aim to reengage the patient's attention to "able" aspects of themselves. Common to these methods is the discouragement of the avoidance of unpleasant sensation, thought, and emotion and the prevention of illness attributions from normal symptoms arising from exercise, movement, or stress. This phase in the process enables patients to be purposefully aware of the interactions between their thoughts, feelings, behaviors, and the consequences of behaviors through self-observation strategies.

Successful purposeful observation is foundational to increasing the perception of self-regulation.

Practical tips for introducing concepts

- Patients should observe their tolerance or limit for physical activities such as sitting, lying, walking, and standing before setting their exercise and activity goals. In the early stages, goals for physical reactivity should also be set. Slowly introduce the idea of observing emotions and thoughts.
- Always emphasize that the thoughts, feelings, and behaviors are not causes of pain but effects of having pain for a long time.
- Patients will more likely maintain self-observation in between sessions if they own the reasons for why they are doing it.
- Often, a motivation for performing any of these strategies is the hope or expectation of pain relief. Patients may begin expressing their anger when the pain does not go away. Acknowledge the anger when it arises as understandable.
- To emphasize the importance of observation, it is important that the therapist asks about what the patient has been recording and to encourage patients to use their data in subsequent sessions.

Clinical tools for phase 2

See Table 12.1.

Stages in the delivery of phase 2

1 Observing behaviors, thoughts, moods, and physical reactions.
2 Noticing behavioral traps.
3 Noticing unhelpful or aversive patterns of thinking.

Complications for phase 2

- Self-monitoring can lead to an increase in symptom reporting or an increase in anxiety associated with pain. When this occurs, acknowledge the patient's worry and establish what their worry is and whether this symptom is different from their chronic pain.
- New symptoms can and do occur in treatment. If the symptom is a cause for concern, quick consultation with the pain program physician is necessary. The quick speed of this consultation is essential as unresolved new symptoms can halt the therapy process.
- If you are confident that a "new" symptom does not require medical intervention, it is helpful to delay or extinguish the urge for medical intervention by:
  - placing the control for the next step with the patient by asking them what they would usually do to manage this;
  - establishing what the patient predicts might happen if they do not act immediately;
  - what they plan to do in order to manage before reviewing the next step with you.

Key points for phase 2

- Encouraging patients to observe their behavior, physical reactions, thoughts and mood, and the consequences of these in relation to their goals to increase their awareness of what is and is not working for them in achieving their desired outcome.
- A therapeutic alliance is maintained through continual acknowledgement of what the patient expresses.

Phase 3: the reengagement of attention to ability

In spite of pain I am able to.

A common clinical experience is that chronic pain patients are more likely to focus their attention to what the pain is stopping them from doing. The aim of phase 3 is to facilitate the patient to refocus their attention from what they cannot do because of the pain to what they can do with the pain. The phase encompasses the next four sessions of the group CBT of an interdisciplinary pain management program. It is worth remembering that in this programmatic model of treatment delivery the components of CBT do not operate in isolation: their suc-

cess is interdependent with the success or failure of other treatment components such as physical therapy.

Practical tips

- As described in phase 2.
- Patients habitually focus on the absence of achievements and what cannot be attempted for fear of failure, self-rebuke, or social criticism. It is difficult for a pain patient who lives within a context of immediate negative consequences to think, first, about future consequences of behavior and, second, the possibility that these future consequences could be positive. It can be helpful to engage patients in the detailed analysis of how a new or renewed behavior (e.g. walking to a shop or telephoning a relative) will have consequences. The purpose will be to explore (1) the potential positive consequences and (2) how controllable the consequences can be.
- Making the tasks of focusing on abilities relevant and valid for patients is of crucial importance. Homework on observation of planning or nonplanning of behavior is essential to developing the skills of refocusing away from pain-related failure and the negative consequences of social withdrawal and disability.
- In addition to this reflective work, equally important is the successful adherence of patients to a program of therapy – an institutional routine that has demands and requirements of patients to participate fully despite pain.

Clinical tools for phase 3

See Table 12.2.

The process of delivery of phase 3

1 Noticing achievements.
2 Behavioral experiment.
3 Practice.
4 Introducing cognitive strategies.
5 Practice.

Complications for phase 3

- Patients may view cognitive coping statements as a trite instruction to think positively. This can lead patients to a further form of failure in attempting to think oneself out of unhappiness. If unaddressed, a "just think positively" trap can seriously challenge therapeutic alliance. If this happens, highlight the traps of positive thinking by taking the patient through possible problems, as discussed in phase 2.
- In this phase, a common observation is that patients' reports of abilities and insurmountable barriers to engaging in nonpain activities are at odds with (in contradiction to) their observed behavior. In other words, what they say that cannot do, you may see them do on a daily basis. This should be understood

Table 12.1 *Clinical tools for phase 2: developing awareness through objective observation*

Strategy	Description
1 Purposeful observation of behavioral traps: "What stops me from reengaging in an activity"?	Reflexive questioning heightens awareness of the behavioral traps that patients often find themselves in. The therapist, in a collaborative way, engages with the individual patient or group and through open-ended questioning leads them to discover cyclical traps often maintained by unhelpful thoughts or behavioral responses such as avoidance. A desire to be rid of pain in order to escape the vicious cycle can lead patients to become fixed in their efforts to problem-solve. At this stage, solutions are not offered by the clinician so that the patient can begin finding solutions other than getting rid of pain
2 Structured self-report diaries	There are many examples of structured self-report diaries used in CBT to enable patients to observe the triggers, responses, and consequences of their behaviors. These are helpful to give for homework at the end of sessions. The self-report diaries can offer data for future sessions. They can also be used to increase patient's ownership of all aspects of their pain management program through enabling them to observe and have a record of the changes that they are making. They are useful for self-governed exercise components of pain management as well as attention and cognitive components
3 Purposeful observation of the body	*Body scanning* aims to reestablish contact with the body through thorough and minute focusing on the body.[14] It involves developing concentration and flexibility of attention simultaneously. Self-managed exercise regimes introduce purposeful observation of somatic change and physical tolerances by engaging patients in observing their start points and tolerance levels for specific exercises and maintaining a record of these
4 Recognizing patterns of thinking and the consequences of these patterns	Focusing on thinking should enable one to recognize and reframe unhelpful patterns of thinking. A first step to achieving this is to begin observing thoughts as "just thoughts." There are ranges of different strategies described in CBT manuals to enable people to recognize patterns of thinking that can maintain and lead to difficulties with problem-solving. These are readily adaptable to the chronic pain situation, and experienced therapists should not be wary of adapting strategies to suit the special case of chronic pain

as only a sign that the patient is disengaged from their abilities, and focused upon pain as a barrier. Thought is not necessary for behavior.

- Observing well behavior can lead to patients being accused of dishonesty. If patients are threatened with accusations of dishonesty and/or overexaggeration, a typical reaction will be for a patient to recommunicate the extent of distress and disability suffered. If this occurs, the therapist should revisit aspects of phase 1.

Key points for phase three.

- There is a range of different strategies within all treatment components (physical, functional, and psychological) of an interdisciplinary pain management program that can be used to focus patients' attention from that which cannot be solved to that which can in spite of pain.
- Promote a well context, and preserve consistency and cohesiveness that maintains patients' attention to what they are doing and are able to do in spite of the pain.

Phase 4: the development of purposeful attention

You can play with your pain.

Chronic pain patients often report vivid imagery about their pain, and more often use strategies to avoid the images. The aims of phase 4 are first to reconceptualize the experience of pain, second to reduce or attenuate automatic catastrophic interpretations of the effects of pain, and third to increase controllability over pain. Attention strategies can facilitate the achievement of these aims first by teaching patients to focus their attention on the sensory components of pain and second by using imagery techniques to aid the patient in transforming their images of their pain. These techniques can be delivered over two to five sessions of an interdisciplinary pain management program.

Practical tips for phase 4

- Consider these as techniques to add to an overall management strategy and not the answer in themselves.

Table 12.2 *Clinical tools for phase 3: the reengagement of attention to ability*

Strategy	Description
1 The daily achievement diary	The daily achievement diary encourages patients to begin noticing and acknowledging the gains and changes that they are beginning to make no matter how small they are. It can be given to patients on the first day. These ideas are useful not only for attention training but also in maintaining and motivating change (phase 5)
2 Promoting consistency and cohesiveness across therapists	Integral to self-management are patients' attempts to regain control of critical aspects of their environment. One method of achieving this is for all therapists to maintain a consistent message that the pain is real but is not a sign of further damage. As a team, facilitating the patient and/or group to generate their own solutions provides a context in which the patient begins to repeatedly experience successful coping
3 Problem-solving strategies and self-evaluation	Generating a range of alternative solutions to a problem is a critical and often challenging first task in learning problem-solving skills and confidence. Patients should be encouraged to list as many solutions as possible regardless of their likelihood of success. Evaluation of the outcome of solutions to problems is an important component of effective problem-solving. Self-evaluation aims to shift attention to what has been achieved in spite of pain or in spite of what has not gone well. Problem-solving is a skill that requires practice
4 Coping self-statements	In addition to attentional strategies, self-statement analysis can lead to greater understanding of self-destructive and self-denigrating habitual thinking. Patients should be guided in providing evidence for their claims and providing counterevidence by attending to past achievements. Patients should also be encouraged to practice statementing during a painful stressor, rehearsing key statements to oneself such as "I can cope, I am coping with this," "I have coped with this before," and "This will not last"

Table 12.3 *Clinical tools for phase 4: the development of purposeful attention*

Strategy	Description
1 Sensation focusing	These strategies aim to reduce distress associated with pain through teaching purposeful attention to noxious sensations. Patients can become skilled in purposeful observation of painful sensations through distinguishing noxious sensations as isolated events. Patients are taught to first focus on their breathing and then extend their focus of attention to their body, their thoughts, sounds, and the environment surrounding them. Components of autogenic relaxation training can also be augmented with sensation focusing
2 Imagery	These strategies aim to transform the context in which the pain occurs or to transform the stimulus features of the pain. Strategies can be used with sensation-focusing techniques. They have been found to be effective in reducing acute pain. Other methods have been used in preparing people for an acute pain experience through advising them how long the pain will last and what the sensation will be like. Some examples of imagery are: <ul><li>Focusing on the pain and the sensations of the pain and imagining it as a color, e.g. patients may see their pain as the color red. The therapist can guide them to transform the color to one with less threatening associations</li><li>Imagining the sensations as a tight steel band and then loosening the bands</li><li>Focusing on the pain and then imagine moving the pain to another area of the body</li><li>Imagining a pleasant scene such as going to the beach or forest</li></ul>The most effective techniques are those produced by, and that are meaningful to, the patient. One can ask the patient to draw or enact an image of the pain to provide material for the task

Table 12.4 *Clinical tools for phase 5: generalization and maintenance*

Strategy	Description
1 The road of change: recognizing, preparing, and dealing with setbacks. "It can be more helpful to begin dealing with a setback before it becomes one"	To introduce the concept of a setback or a bad day can be challenging to patients as it triggers unhelpful thoughts, raises fears of going back, and can be received in a blaming way. We use a metaphor of the road of change that is rarely straightforward but that has ups and downs along the way. A bad day is defined as a blip in the journey; a setback as a deviation off track; and a total collapse is off the road completely. To aid discussion, it can be helpful to have patients draw their own road, beginning with the first day of the program to the point of discussion Therapists should feel free to develop their own extended metaphors or, ideally, to encourage the patient/group to develop their own metaphor
2 Goal setting: establishing areas for change and barriers to change	The likelihood of relapse is high in this population, so the therapist also aims to facilitate patients becoming aware of potential reasons for them not continuing with the strategies and potential resistance for using the strategies. Some examples of questions to elicit responses are: "What would I like to be doing at the end of the program?" "In 3 months' time?" "In 2 years' time?" "What might get in the way of me achieving this?" "What would be the advantages and disadvantages of changing?"
3 Developing a setback plan	A setback plan aims to enable patients to begin focusing their attention on the inevitability of continued pain in the future and their ability to manage. Developing a setback plan is conducted using aspects from all phases, for example: Phases 1 and 2: recognizing a setback Phase 3: identifying previous successful attempts, manage the setback, preparing for setbacks and evaluation of setback plan Phase 5: forward planning. The following questions may be helpful in facilitating patients' development of a setback plan: "What is the difference between a bad day, a setback, and a total collapse?" "What did you do or are you doing to manage a bad day?" "What would trigger a setback for me?" "What will enable me to get back on track?" "What did I do to deal with this setback?" "What worked and did not work?" "Why?" "What will I continue to do in the future?"

- If patients have been able to change their imagery, it is useful to emphasize the role of play. (You can play with something that you are in control of.)
- Not all of us have abilities to imagine creatively and not all patients are able to use imagery strategies; however, most patients can be guided to focus on sensations of pain.
- It is important to encourage patients to identify areas in which they have used distraction themselves and when it has been helpful and not helpful.
- It is important that the therapist or clinician does not put himself or herself in a position of being the magician. It is empowering for the patient to develop his or her own images and to practice at home.

Clinical tools for phase 4

See Table 12.3.

The process of delivery of phase 4

1 Awareness of the interaction of thoughts, feelings, somatic changes, behaviors, and pain.
2 Reframing unhelpful patterns of thinking.
3 Attention to achievements.
4 Purposeful attention to noxious sensations.
5 Disengagement of attention from noxious sensation.

Complications for phase 4

- For some patients, not being able to use imagery

reinforces a sense of hopelessness or failure. If this is expressed, highlight the past successful use of other forms of attention.

- For some patients, if imagery works in reducing the intensity or unpleasantness of pain, they may question the reality of their pain. This is why it is important to introduce these ideas after phases 1 and 2.

Key points for phase 4

- These strategies are not curative.
- Successful use of these strategies does not mean that pain is imaginary.
- These strategies are more effective when used with other strategies such as pacing.
- Attentional techniques are as effective with strong pain intensity as with mild pain intensity.

Phase 5: generalization and maintenance

How will I know I'm making gains?

Self-regulation of attention involves a change in behavior. To generalize and maintain the use of strategies, patients need to have opportunities to practice the ideas while in treatment and at home. As pain is complex and not likely to go away, pain "flare-ups," "setbacks," and bad days will occur and are not a sign of treatment failure. Patients are more likely to use the ideas again when they have experienced success and have owned their success. In relation to attention regulation, preparation and planning directs attention to what is predictable and controllable.

Practical tips for phase 5

- Normalizing setbacks as an everyday part of any progression can be useful. Here, creative use of allegory and metaphor are helpful. Any story of real progression will not demonstrate linear development. It will be more powerful if patients can draw upon their own interests or stories (in nonpain domains) that show how a path to success involves setbacks, wrong turns, obstacles, etc.
- The use of visual information such as road mapping techniques in which patients can visualize the idea that each gain is a small movement toward a goal, building on previous gains. In the same way, each loss or "setback" can be a small movement away from a goal or a distraction from the path to the goal, not a return to the beginning.
- Planning for strategy use during setbacks can be an effective tool. Throughout treatment, patients should be encouraged and coached to:
  - Attend to setbacks as they occur in treatment.

- Assess the antecedents of setbacks, attending away from immediate sensation to previous behavior.
- Develop a plan for dealing with setbacks. This can be a written or memorized plan. The success of such a plan is dependent upon its being tested and practiced in real situations.

Clinical tools for phase 5

See Table 12.4.

Process for the delivery of phase 5

1 Considering what can be different.
2 Considering barriers to change.
3 Recognizing bad days and setbacks.
4 Preparing for setbacks.
5 Planning for the future.

Complications for phase 5

- Patients can sometimes be reluctant to discuss bad days or setbacks because they fear that talking about them will invoke them.
- Patients also have hopes and expectations that if they try the strategies then they will be back to where they used to be before pain. Often, they set themselves unrealistic goals with no measures of achievement.
- Patients sometimes resist planning for the future because in the past their pain has thwarted their plans. To begin working with the resistance, it is often effective to focus on the benefits and costs of planning and when planning has been a useful strategy and when it has not.

Key points for phase 5

- Maintaining treatment gains in the context of persistent pain can be challenging. During periods of intense pain, negative emotional thoughts and images will be retrieved and will dominate consciousness.
- Methods are aimed at reducing the likelihood of behavioral traps being maintained by increasing perceived controllability through predicting when they will occur and developing and practicing management plans.

A CLINICAL CASE EXAMPLE

Below is an example of a clinical intervention delivered within the context of an interdisciplinary CBT chronic pain management program. The session is for 1 h and occurs in week 2 of a 3-week inpatient pain management program. The focus of the session is cognitive coping strategies. In relation to the phase model, this session would be phase 4 of attention regulation, but aspects of other phases are introduced as necessary by the therapist.

The development of purposeful attention

Establishing the patient's understanding of attention and developing a shared understanding of the problem

Therapist: In this session we are going to discuss the role of attention in pain. What do you understand by attention? [Highlight that attention is time-limited, selective, and easily interrupted.]

Therapist: Why do you think that we are introducing the ideas of attention in pain management?

Patient: It helps not to think about pain.

Therapist: Let's revisit the gate control theory of pain and how attention relates to our pain experience. As you can see, focused attention competes with the pain messages and for these reasons may help to turn down the volume of the pain.

Reengagement of attention on ability

Therapist: Can you give me some examples of what you do to take your mind off your pain?

Patient: I do the gardening or I read a book or I knit.

Therapist: Have you found these things to be helpful?

Patient: Sometimes when you are interested in something the pain is more bearable.

Developing awareness though objective observation

Therapist: Sometimes taking your mind off the pain can be so successful that you end up overdoing it. Lets look at an example, say gardening. What usually happens when you garden?

Patient: I get engrossed in it and want to finish what I am doing.

Therapist: And then what happens?

Patient: I tend to push myself.

Therapist: And then what happens?

Patient: I keep going because I know my pain will get worse when I stop.

Therapist: And then what happens?

Patient: My pain is excruciating.

Therapist: And what thoughts do you have afterwards?

Patient: I should have listened to my husband and not done the gardening. I am useless. I never seem to learn.

Therapist: And then what might you be feeling?

Patient: Pissed off with myself. Depressed.

Therapist: And then what happens when you feel this way?

Patient: I don't want to do gardening ever again. I will just stay inside the house.

Developing purposeful attention

Therapist: Often distraction is helpful in relieving your pain for a short time. However, as we have shown here, it can also be unhelpful, as you can become so involved in what you are doing that you overdo the activity and your pain afterwards is worse. An alternative to trying to escape from the pain may be to focus your attention on the pain. Some of you may find you can use imagery, others may find it is not at all helpful. This is okay as there is a range of different tools that you are already using. This is just one of the many. Let's experiment first.

Have the group or patient imagine a lemon using all their senses in the imagery, have them pick it up, feel its texture, smell it, cut it, and drink its juice. Most of the group will find they can taste the lemon, their faces will pucker and saliva will begin to form. Others will not have any response. This is okay. Point out that an image can affect the body, like dreaming, and that some people are more able to use imagery than others. Then introduce the following exercise:

Therapist: What I would like you to do is to begin by focusing your attention on your breathing, just noticing your breath as it moves past your nose. Notice the change in temperature as you breathe in and then out. Notice when your breath begins and ends. Just allow yourself to breathe.

Guide patients' attention to different areas of their body, for example eyelashes, tongue, fingers, toes, space between their body, the floor or chair, and space between sounds as they come and go. Remain attending to these for at least 60 s each.

Therapist: Now shift your attention to your pain. Notice the sensations of your pain as they come and go. Is there a beginning or an end to the sensations? Is each sensation the same or do they vary? Just allow yourself to be fully present with your pain.

Therapist: Now transform your pain into a color. It can be any color you would like it to be. Now change the color into one that is warm, healing, and calm. Now breathe into the pain and allow it to completely fill your body. Now expand it further to completely fill the room. Just be with this for a moment. Return your attention back to your breath and when you are ready move your body and open your eyes.

Reengagement of attention to ability (self-evaluation)

Therapist: What was that like for you?

Patient: I found it really hard to focus on my pain. It was scary but I found after a while it was okay.

Therapist: Tell me what happened?

Patient: I was able to give my pain a color, it was red, and then I changed it to pink.
Therapist: Did this surprise you that you were able to do this with your pain?
Patient: Yes! Is this like hypnotherapy or something?
Therapist: Sort of. Did it surprise you that you could do it?
Patient: Yes!
Therapist: Were you able to expand your pain? What was that like?
Patient: That was really scary, but after a while I found it really relaxing.

Acknowledging the pain as real

Therapist: Were you surprised that you were able to do this?
Patient: Yes! But does this mean my pain is imaginary?
Therapist: No. It is possible that you can begin to play with real pain, changing it, controlling it.

Generalization and maintenance

Therapist: What would stop you from using this strategy?
Patient: If it did not work?
Therapist: How would you know it did not work?
Patient: I just could not relax and the pain was still there.
Therapist: What would get in the way of you relaxing?
Patient: The pain.
Therapist: Is it possible to find other ways to relax with the pain?
Patient: I don't know, I guess I could say to myself to stay calm or have a bath or do something I enjoy.

CONCLUSION

The evidence is excellent for the effectiveness of CBT in producing meaningful clinical change in various domains of pain experience, including reduced pain-related distress and disability (see Chapter Ch24).[15]*** However, only now are the components of this successful therapy being subjected to scrutiny. Clinical and experimental research is placing increasingly more emphasis on the role of attention, acceptance, and the avoidance of pain-related fear as critical factors that maintain pain-associated disability.[16,17] Now, attempts are being made to examine interventions or components of interventions. See, for example, Chapter P14. Although CBT for chronic pain in adults is now well established, there are very few source texts for clinicians on the framework and instantiation of interventions. More work is needed on the development of worked examples and comprehensive manuals. This chapter provides one worked example of therapy that can be used for instruction or training within multidisciplinary teams delivering programmatic group or individual treatments.

REFERENCES

1. Melzack R, Wall PD. *The Challenge of Pain*. New York, NY: Penguin, 1982.
● 2. Turk DC, Meichenbaum D, Genest M. *Pain and Behavioural Medicine: A Cognitive Behavioural Perspective*. New York, NY: Guildford Press, 1983.
3. McCracken LM. Attention to pain in persons with chronic pain: a behavioural approach. *Behav Ther* 1997; **28**: 271–84.
4. Melzack R. Pain: past, present, and future. *Can J Exp Psychol* 1993; **47**: 615–29.
5. Price DD. *Psychological and Neural Mechanisms of Pain*. New York, NY: Raven Press, 1988.
◆ 6. McCaul KD, Malott JM. Distraction and coping with pain. *Psychol Bull* 1984; **95**: 516–33.
◆ 7. Eccleston C. The attentional control of pain: methodological and theoretical concerns. *Pain* 1995; **63**: 3–10.
● 8. Eccleston C, Crombez G. Pain demands attention: a cognitive–affective model of the interruptive function of pain. *Psychol Bull* 1999; **125**: 356–66.
● 9. Aldrich S, Eccleston C, Crombez, G. Worrying about chronic pain: vigilance to threat and misdirected problem solving. *Behav Res Ther* 2000; **38**: 425–536.
10. Keefe FJ, Van Horn V. Cognitive–behavioural treatment of rheumatoid arthritis pain: maintaining treatment gains. *Arthritis Care Res* 1993; **6**: 213–22.
◆ 11. Kabat-Zinn J, Lipworth L, Burney R. The clinical use of mindfulness meditation for the self-regulation of chronic pain. *J Behav Med* 1985; **8**: 163–90.
12. Teasdale JD, Segal Z, Williams JMG. How does cognitive therapy prevent depressive relapse and why should attentional control (mindfulness) training help? *Behav Res Ther* 1995; **33**: 25–39.
13. Roth A, Fonagy P. *What Works for Whom? A Critical Review of Psychotherapy Research*. New York, NY: Guildford Press, 1996.
14. Kabat-Zinn J. An outpatient programme in behavioural medicine for chronic pain patients based on the practice of mindfulness meditation: theoretical consideration and preliminary results. *Gen Hosp Psychiatry* 1992; **4**: 33–47.
15. Morley S, Eccleston C, Williams ACdeC. Systematic review and meta-analysis of randomized controlled trials of cognitive behaviour therapy for chronic pain in adults, excluding headache. *Pain* 1999; **80**: 1–13.
16. McCracken LM. Behavioural constituents of chronic pain acceptance: results from factor analysis of the Chronic Pain Acceptance Questionnaire. *J Back Musculoskeletal Rehabil* 1999; **13**: 93–100.
17. Van den Hout JHC, Vlaeyen JWS, Houben RMA, *et al*. The effects of failure feedback and pain-related fear on pain report, pain tolerance, and pain avoidance in chronic low back pain patients. *Pain* 2001; **92**: 247–57.

13

Hypnosis, biofeedback, and self-regulation skills for children in pain

LEORA KUTTNER AND TIMOTHY CULBERT

Developmental issues	147	Integrated approaches	157
Benefits for children and adolescents	148	Theoretical rationale: mechanisms of change	160
Anxiety, fear, and pain	149	Common features of self-regulatory methods	161
Diaphragmatic breathing	149	Training in hypnosis and training and professional	
Bubble blowing	150	certification in biofeedback	161
Relaxation	150	Conclusion	161
Hypnosis with children in pain	150	References	162
Biofeedback	155		

The pain experience is inherently psychophysiologic in nature. It always includes both a biologic, objective component – the actual tissue damage or insult – and an affective, cognitive subjective component – the experience of discomfort, suffering, and the attribution of the sensation as painful and unpleasant. Self-regulation techniques, such as hypnosis and biofeedback, represent integrative approaches that directly address this essential mind–body unity.

Hypnosis, biofeedback, and related self-regulation approaches have come to the forefront as evidence-based, practical, and potent therapeutic strategies[1-3] for children and adolescents with a variety of acute, recurrent, and chronic pain problems (Tables 13.1 and 13.2). In addition, because these strategies tap into children's innate developmental drives for mastery, fantasy, and curiosity, they serve as ideal vehicles for teaching children to actively help themselves through pain and associated anxiety symptoms.

Self-regulation skills are defined as psychophysiological strategies that use focused attention and practice to train a person to identify and control unwanted symptoms and modify undesirable physiologic responses, so that the desired level of health and wellness is achieved. Applied psychophysiology is the area of study that examines links between behavioral/emotional/cognitive phenomena and physiologic response patterns. A number of self-regulation methods fall into this area (Table 13.3).

This chapter covers some key pediatric concerns in the pain research literature, describes the techniques of diaphragmatic breathing and relaxation therapy, and then provides in-depth clinical applications with illustrative case examples of hypnosis and biofeedback as the prototype self-management strategies for children and adolescents to manage acute, recurrent, and chronic pain. The chapter closes with the theoretical rationale and communality of these self-regulatory techniques in therapeutic practice and the limitations for their use.

DEVELOPMENTAL ISSUES

Traditionally, young children have been regarded as too young to understand their physiological processes and too immature to cooperate and learn how to modify them. The concept that young children can regulate their pain sensation and perception may seem radical, but it is well within a preschooler's ability.[3-5] Adapted to each stage of development from age 3 to the teenage years, self-regulation methods such as bubble blowing, regulated breathing, relaxation techniques, imagery, hypnosis, and biofeedback methods, using updated interesting

Table 13.1 *Pain-related conditions for which self-regulation approaches are helpful*

Chronic/recurrent pain	Neuromuscular disorders
Headache: migraine, tension type, mixed	Orthopedic conditions/procedures
Recurrent abdominal pain	Sickle cell anemia
Somatization/somatoform disorders	Cancer
Gastrointestinal problems (severe constipation, anismus)	HIV/AIDS
Irritable bowel syndrome	Burns
Raynaud syndrome	Fibromyalgia
Reflex sympathetic dystrophy	Juvenile rheumatoid arthritis
Pain related to chronic medical conditions	

HIV, human immunodeficiency virus; AIDS, acquired immune deficiency syndrome.

Table 13.2 *Pain-related procedures for which self-regulation approaches are helpful*

Acute pain	Trauma
Procedural pain	Surgical procedures
Venipuncture	Dressing changes
Bone marrow aspiration	Preoperative
Intravenous placement/infusion	Perioperative
Sutures	Throat culture
Gynecological examination	

Table 13.3 *Self-regulation techniques*

Self-hypnosis (mental imagery)
Biofeedback
Breath control training
Progressive muscle relaxation
Mind–body education
Self-monitoring

computer tracking programs, can be taught to children in pain or who are anticipating pain and distress.

It is essential to correctly gauge each child's emotional and cognitive age so that information is accurately understood, age-appropriate language is used, and the therapeutic partnership is productive and not confusing or boring. Chronological age is not always an accurate measure, as anxiety and pain tend to make a child regress. Consequently, the clinician must be creative and sensitive, and must observe the child closely during the introduction to select the best-suited self-regulation method and adjust the direction and coaching to the changes in the child. This becomes more challenging when the techniques are used to modify pain perception during medical procedures. Under these conditions, the clinician must coordinate with the team and pace the child to maximize self-coping during the more painful part of the procedure.

With developmentally appropriate language, adequate support, and trust, children of all ages can learn coping and self-regulation skills to reduce pain and anxiety for surgery, invasive medical procedures, chronic diseases, and recurring painful conditions.[1-4] Whatever the child's age, when successfully integrated by the child as a

way of dealing with pain and discomfort, these methods have long-term benefits[6] and can be used throughout the person's life for other incidental or accidental pain, well beyond the original reason for the pain management referral. When well established in the child's repertoire, developed skills can also play a crucial part in easing the approach to death, as part of the palliative therapeutic regimen.

BENEFITS FOR CHILDREN AND ADOLESCENTS

There are substantial advantages for children and adolescents who do learn and practice these methods of self-regulation. Their active participation in the therapeutic process leads to greater maturity and independence in managing their pain symptoms, enhanced self-confidence, reduced disabling effects of recurring or long-term pain, and increased ability to participate in normal daily activities. There is consistent clinical evidence that children learn these methods more rapidly than do adults, and generally children are more adept than adults in using hypnotherapy for control of pain. Children are also more proficient at physiologic control, as demonstrated by Attansio *et al.*[7] and confirmed by others. Thus, children are excellent candidates for self-regulatory training.

More has been written about the use of self-regulatory methods with adults than with children and adolescents. However, over the last 10 years, there has been a notable increase in the demand for training in the clinical application of pediatric self-regulatory methods within children's hospitals in North America and Europe by pediatric health care professionals, including nurses, psychologists, pediatricians, anesthesiologists, and child life specialists. (In the last 10 years, the number of attendees and requests for training workshops by the Society for Developmental & Behavioral Pediatrics, the American Clinical Hypnosis Society, Professional Pediatric Pain Seminars, and the Association for Applied Psychophysiology and Biofeedback has notably increased.) The practical benefits and ease of implementation of self-regulatory methods within pediatric settings is making them acceptable and more commonly practiced in North America and some parts of Europe. Parents are increasingly interested in mind–body, nonmedication approaches for their children.

ANXIETY, FEAR, AND PAIN

Even in the best of situations, because of the intrinsically disturbing aspects of experiencing pain, children become sensitized and develop specific fears and generalized anxiety about medical procedures and interventions perceived to cause pain.[8,9] Successful pain management almost always includes interventions for the anticipatory anxiety component of pain. This includes a thorough pain history, previous pain experiences, and family and cultural pain attitudes. Self-regulation therapies tend to address both the anxiety and the pain experience simultaneously as illustrated below.

Case example

Abbi, a 12-year-old, was referred for self-regulation training to control severe needle phobia. She needed immunizations within a few weeks to go on a family overseas trip, and the referring pediatrician had been unsuccessful in gaining Abbi's cooperation for these vaccinations. She screamed and cried uncontrollably and her parents and professional staff were at a loss to know how to help her.

Abbi recalled only one other experience, a few years back, when she had venipuncture, which required many attempts to get the sample. She recalls feeling out of control as people held her down. Since that time, she has had a strong fear of needles. Despite those fears, she expressed the desire to help herself.

During the first session, we began with basic electromyography (EMG) and breathing training, emphasizing control and mastery themes. Abbi enjoyed this and did well. During the next session, she was trained in electrodermal activity (EDA) as an easy way for her to track her own nervous system's anxiety responses to needles. Over that and the two subsequent sessions, Abbi focused on controlling her sympathetic nervous system (SNS) response with graduated exposure to elements of the vaccination experience. She learned to control her breathing, heart rate, and SNS activity, as reflected in her maintenance of low EDA readings. She particularly liked a biofeedback screen called "kaleidoscope," in which she erased a complex design of colorful lines and shapes as she decreased her EDA to the desired threshold level.

A vaccination visit plan was then discussed and role-played using actual equipment, but stopped short of giving the injection. She practiced by playing the nurse and giving a play vaccination to her favorite stuffed animal. Mental imagery was added to her practice regimen, including the idea of imagining herself getting the vaccination, maintaining good control, and noticing how proud she felt. The following week in the biofeedback room, with her EDA sensor attached and running, Abbi demonstrated her self-regulation skills by keeping her EDA at desired levels, staying in control, and receiving her vaccination with minimal distress. She was very proud of her accomplishment.

Comment

Needle phobia is a common problem in a variety of settings for children of all ages. Many children report afterwards that the anticipatory anxiety and emotional distress is often worse than the actual "shot" itself. Direct desensitization with the monitoring of a relevant physiologic modality such as EDA, breathing, or heart rate offers an excellent opportunity to reinforce the desired behavioral change. The engaging nature of visual feedback and the ability to set concrete "goals" are helpful for many young children to reinforce their sense of control. Finally, the use of these techniques can heighten curiosity, thus enhancing the focus on something other than the injection pain.

DIAPHRAGMATIC BREATHING

Regulated and rhythmic diaphragmatic breathing is an easy first step to teach the beginnings of self-regulation[10] and yields immediate results in "being boss of your own body." Little preparation is required, and as such it is useful in first encounters with a fearful child in an acute or procedural pain situation. To start, the child is instructed to "exhale" rather than the conventional request to "inhale." Releasing breath allows a frightened child to "let go" tension and then breathe in more deeply. Emphasizing "Blow out!" interrupts mounting anxiety and enables the child or teenager to gain a modicum of self-control.

Physiologically, acute pain and acute anxiety are manifested as a shift into sympathetic arousal, and are seen behaviorally in the child's shallow rapid breathing, sometimes hyperventilation, increased muscular tension, attentional vigilance, and often whimpering or tears. The instruction to "Breathe out the pain – blow it far away!" interrupts the mounting fight or flight response. Maintained over three to five exhalations, with encouragement to slow these exhalations down, physiological markers change. The child's breathing shifts from the quicker and more shallow chest breathing to the deeper diaphragmatic breathing, which is more relaxing. Children then report feeling more in control and less overwhelmed by the pain, anxiety, or panic. This physiological shift can be achieved and stable within 5 min and hence is ideal for blood draws and intravenous (i.v.) injections. In a survey of children who participated in a biofeedback program for a variety of psychophysiological disorders, 80% identified "breathing stuff" as the component of the training that they used the most and retained the longest.[10]

In acute pain, many children hyperventilate, which intensifies feelings of discomfort and lack of control. Coaching them to slow down and be "in charge" of their breathing is a positive first step, providing a focus apart from the pain itself. In addition, there is some evidence that with panic- or anxiety-induced hyperventilation, the resulting drop in CO_2 levels and subsequent alkalosis leads to decreased cerebral blood flow.[11] This distorts cognitive processing so that understanding, making decisions, judgments, and coping are impaired. Development of a controlled diaphragmatic pattern, with return to normal exhaled CO_2 levels, often induces muscle relaxation and decreased SNS arousal, both of which further promotes pain modulation and a sense of well-being.

BUBBLE BLOWING

With children 10 years and under, blowing bubbles is a more child-centered way of placing the child in charge of the process, maintaining the breathing, and diverting attention away from the pain onto the task of creating, tracking, and counting the bubbles. This technique has surprised us with its usefulness, particularly for immunizations and other minor painful pediatric procedures.[4,5] Furthermore, bubble blowing and regulated deep breathing establishes the concept of self-regulation and the awareness of how to modify body responses. It has been effective with toddlers and preschoolers in acute pain, for anticipatory anxiety prior to a procedure, or during invasive medical procedures.

RELAXATION

Relaxation is a pleasant experience for children aged 6 years and older as a second step in the self-regulation training of physiologic pain processes. With younger children, relaxation generally happens automatically. As a general rule, they do not yet have the degree of kinesthetic awareness to control and release specific muscle groups without an active biofeedback signal. Of course, there are individual differences, and if physical tension is a concern for a child younger than 6 the "Raggedy Ann" doll game is developmentally appropriate to teach relaxation without the child having to lie down and close their eyes.

Raggedy Ann

Demonstrating with a floppy doll how each of her limbs flops and her body bends and hangs down comfortably, the preschool child is encouraged to imitate the doll with floppy arms and legs and finally to hang loosely over the arm of the clinician "like a floppy, happy Raggedy Ann." Parents and the child are then instructed to practice being a floppy Raggedy Ann before the feared procedure, or when the child gets pain, so that it does not hurt as much and the pain can drain away.

Relaxation with older children

Muscle relaxation

Muscle tightness and muscle group asymmetries can cause and/or contribute to a variety of pain conditions. Muscle relaxation helps children to become more aware of their bodies in helpful ways, and to refocus and relax. Alternating sequentially through the body between tightening and relaxing different muscles groups, children are taught discrimination and control of areas of muscle tension. After completion of several rounds of squeezing and letting go, many older children and teenagers are able to discharge excessive nervous and muscle tension, improving their level of comfort.

Progressive relaxation

An alternative and less demanding relaxation technique is to cover the older child with a blanket and invite him or her to "Close your eyes and let the relaxation begin to seep into your body." Starting at the child's toes, move slowly up the body and describe each part of the body becoming heavier, warmer, and more relaxed. Over a 5- to 7-min period, slowly guide the child's attention to the growing comfort and release that is occurring in their body, particularly in and around the areas of pain or ache. Making an audio-taped recording of this enables the child to regularly practice relaxation, increasing the ability to release muscle tension, pain, and discomfort. This method is particularly helpful for bed-ridden children who are compromised by disease, surgery, treatments, such as during bone marrow transplantation, or who are in end-of-life care.

HYPNOSIS WITH CHILDREN IN PAIN

Hypnosis is essentially an altered state of consciousness that changes a child's perception and experience of pain without complete conscious effort. It is an internal imaginative process that differs from other techniques such as distraction, which focuses the child's attention on external objects. Hypnosis uses the child's imagination as the agent of change.[1] The clinician enters the child's world, using the child's frame of reference and language to create an alternate experience, then addresses the pain through suggestions for altering sensations and increasing comfort. As such, the therapeutic process of hypnosis is in step with the apparent involuntary nature and manifestation of pain.

The therapeutic use of hypnosis for pain is clinically

highly valued. It has been said that there is no other psychological tool so efficacious in creating comfort out of discomfort yet with none of the adverse side-effects associated with medical treatments of similar efficacy.

The goal of using hypnosis during pain is to:

- Shift the child from being fearful of the pain and dependent on others to a personal understanding of the pain signals.
- Reduce the intensity of the pain and/or create distance from the pain, altering its distressing impact.
- Use the child's innate cognitive abilities to retrain his/her nervous system in order that the frequency and intensity of recurring or ongoing pain lessens and the child is willing to actively cope, so that the pain does not control the child's life and activities.

A hypnotic trance state is an altered state of consciousness in which perception, memory, emotions, and sensation can be therapeutically changed.

To ease a child's pain, a trance is created during which the following occur:

- The child's attention is intensified and narrowed during hypnotic inductions and imaginative involvements to create an alternate or competitive experience.
- Suggestions for positive change that are immediate or posthypnotic are provided.
- The pain sensations are positively reframed as having signal value to which strategies that diminish nociception can be used.
- Time distortion for long-term benefit and for a reduction of energy fatigue is provided.

Hypnoanalgesia

- Much of the evidence for the effectiveness of the use of hypnoanalgesia has been derived from studies in the emergency room[1,8*,9] and on treatments for procedural pain in oncology treatments, addressing the pain and distress associated with lumbar punctures and bone marrow aspirations for children with leukemias. As a therapy, hypnosis is ideally suited to acute and chronic pain.
- Goldie,[9*] in one of the earliest controlled studies with hypnosis, used hypnoanesthesia in the emergency room during surgery for patients aged 3–57 years. When hypnosis was used, Goldie noted a significant reduction in the percentage of patients needing pharmacotherapeutic analgesia or anesthesia for suturing and the reduction of fractures.
- Over the intervening years, there have been a number of studies on the use of hypnosis as an adjunct to pediatric anesthesia in order to decrease the use of preoperative medication, to enable greater ease during anesthetic induction, to reduce the amount of

anesthesia and requirements for analgesics postoperatively, and to increase postoperative comfort.[1]

- In a prospective, controlled, randomized trial comparing hypnoanalgesia with propranolol and placebo, Olness et al.[12**] found that the use of hypnosis was significantly more effective in reducing the frequency of headaches than either propranolol or placebo, which did not differ from each other.

Hypnoanalgesia promotes dissociation from the pain, such as the "pain switch" technique or the "magic glove" (for video demonstrations, see references 4 and 5).

In the *pain switch technique*, the child is told how the brain receives and interprets nerve signals from all parts of the body:

> Right now the nerves in your body are sending a lot of pain information about your e.g. broken wrist. Your brain instantly understands these nerve signals, and sends messages back to the body, that keeps you aware of the pain. Now, I'm going to teach you how to focus your attention on the switches in your brain that control those incoming pain signals so that you can turn them down. As you do that your body will receive weaker pain messages and therefore feel less pain. The more you practice this the better you'll get at turning the pain switches down more quickly. And you'll feel less pain and be in more control.

During hypnotic induction, the child moves into a trance and is instructed to focus on the switch inside their brain that goes to the painful body part. This is the deepening process of the hypnotic trance (Fig. 13.1). With each deep exhalation during diaphragmatic deep breathing, the child is guided to turn down the pain switch as much as possible until comfort is experienced, or until a satisfactory plateau in the pain perception is achieved. The child is encouraged through posthypnotic suggestion to maintain that decreased pain level, and with each subsequent practice to achieve greater levels of comfort and pain relief. The child is then brought out of the trance state.

The criterion for success is that the child feels a significant difference between the pain levels before and after the hypnotic trance. It is important to emphasize that the goal of the "pain switch" is not to remove all pain, which is often an unrealistic goal, but to decrease the perceived pain and to increase the child's mastery over this pain. Obviously, this method has particular value for children with recurring or chronic pain conditions.

Case example

Jonathan, a 14-year-old, traumatically amputated the top joints of two fingers on his right hand during a woodworking class. After plastic surgery to reshape tips for these fingers, he was discharged with acetaminophen (paracetamol) with codeine to control his pain. He was referred for hypnosis by his family physician. Jonathan

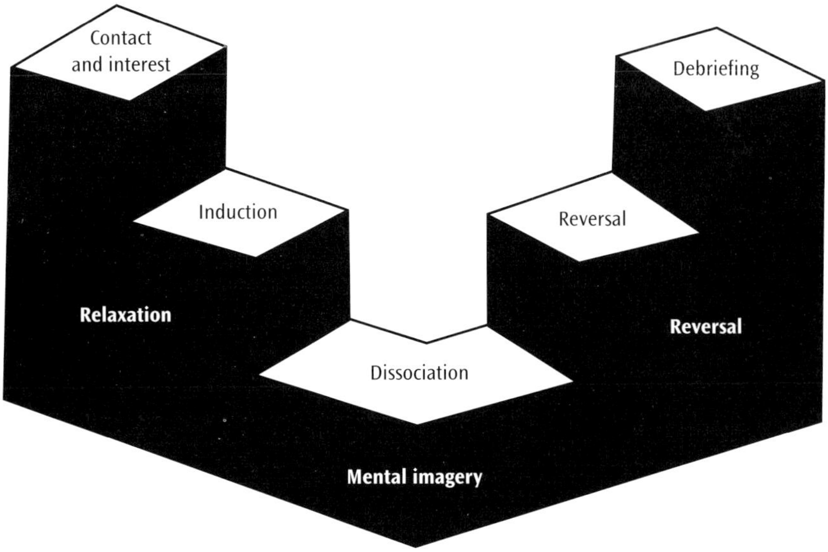

Figure 13.1 *The process of hypnosis. (Reproduced with kind permission of Dr Richard Solomon, NCI Pediatric Pain Management: A Professional Course. East Lansing, MI: Michigan State University, 1995.)*

was in shock that his hand was forever altered and experienced throbbing pain in the top of his digits, which he rated 6 out of 10. In the first session, he was trained to use the pain switch and was able to reduce the pain to 3 out of 10. He was also given posthypnotic suggestions for seeing his hand as normal and being able to use it naturally with comfort and growing ease.

An audio tape was made of the hypnotic process so that he could practice it as often as he needed during the subsequent days. His progress was rapid, and on the second session 5 days later he reported pain levels of 3 and the ability to get the pain down to 1 using the hypnotic tape. His hand was continuing to heal well and he was feeling less self-conscious about displaying it. The third session was a follow-up 2 weeks later – Jonathan reported that "the nightmare was over." His new finger tips were somewhat sensitive, but no longer painful, and he was getting accustomed to using them again. He planned to return to his passion of drumming.

Comment

With the traumatic nature of this injury, the therapeutic concern was that Jonathan could develop phantom digit pain. Since the trauma, shock, and pain were addressed simultaneously, he did not develop this distressing phenomenon. In acute situations, only a few hypnotic interventions are needed as part of the pain therapy to improve the course of recovery.

Hypnosis in emergency

In an emergency – a startling environment for most – children often spontaneously move into a hypnotic trance with narrowed absorption and attention to the pain. In this situation, relaxation is not required; rather, a spontaneous active–alert trance often occurs. The child in this altered state of awareness is highly suggestible. The

clinician's task is to recognize and use this spontaneously altered state of consciousness to diminish pain perception and distress, and to promote rapid healing.[8]*

A simple and highly effective hypnotic intervention for trauma pain is to talk calmly and directly, defining with the child precisely *where the pain is* and *where the pain is not*. Defining where it is not is as important as knowing the areas of pain. It draws the child's attention to the limits of the pain. This enables the clinician to provide suggestions for reducing the area affected by the pain and for increasing the spread of comfort from the nonaffected areas. This intervention works synergistically with any needed analgesics, increasing the efficacy of both.

The therapeutic work is to sustain the child's absorption so that they no longer feel overwhelmed. Panic and anxiety are reduced by providing limits to the pain sensation, which was feared to be endless.

Hypnosis with the preschool child

Since hypnosis with preschool age children is so different from that with the school-age child and adolescent, it is not strictly accurate to refer to the experience as true hypnosis. A better term for the preschoolers trance is protohypnosis or imaginative involvement.[1]

The different manifestations with the younger child are that:

- Closing eyes is invariably associated with going to sleep – something that no alert or anxious preschoolers will willingly do, particularly when in pain in an unfamiliar environment.
- Their grasp of their world shifts fluidly between the world of fantasy and reality. This is the age of imaginary playmates and the spontaneous playing out of fears or concerns.
- Younger children do not easily settle and become still. They are usually unfamiliar with the concept of relax-

ing and so instructions "to relax" may be meaningless.

- Their active imagination is often physically expressed through movement. Their hypnotic trance thus occurs with eyes open, and sometimes wriggling and moving.

Children under 6 years old consequently require an informal, activity-based method during which they are free to move around. Props such as puppets, teddy-bears, bubbles, music, or a favorite story can also be helpful in promoting and maintaining the child's trance. It is important to be highly flexible, engaging, and informal, and to speak in a manner that absorbs attention and not the quiet soothing tone used with adults.

Despite these differences, children as young as 3 years have been found capable of significantly altering their sensations and relieving pain during painful medical procedures.[5] These effects occur rapidly, and young children can create partial anesthesia or sensation alteration within a few minutes.[5,8*,9*] Sometimes during hypnosis, the child's gaze often becomes more fixed – a sign of greater absorption.

Inviting a very young child to enter a hypnotic trance to cope with pain requires a creative fit between the type of pain and the child's frame of reference.

Case example

Taylor, 28 months old, was diagnosed with juvenile diabetes type 1 that required two insulin injections – one at breakfast and the other at evening meal. Because of the fragile nature of her diabetes, she needed finger sticks a few times during the day to check her blood sugar levels. Initially, she put up a worthy fight, exhausting her parents, who were overwhelmed by the diagnosis and were feeling guilty about the frequent pain they induced. A dissociative imaginative involvement method was developed incorporating blowing out, ice, and her passion for her Dolly. Taylor was invited to imagine herself as Dolly, who got her insulin "pokes" easily:

> Dolly has diabetes. Let's sit her close on Mom's lap and to cuddle Mommy. Dolly now has to have her shot, but we can help her to feel okay. … Right. … Let's rub her leg with the ice-cube so that it can go cold and it won't bother her … now remind Dolly that she can blow out "blow out." Now that's it, Dolly. Now it's all done!
>
> Now Taylor, let's pretend you are Dolly. Nice happy Dolly. Come Dolly, sit on Mom's lap and cuddle her. That's it. Let's rub Dolly-Taylor's leg with ice, so that it's nice and cold so that nothing bothers her. Remember now "Blow out, blow out" and Dolly-Taylor's poke is over – just like Dolly. Clever girl!

Comment

The parent's confusion, guilt, and discomfort with the procedure had escalated the drama of Taylor's proce-

dures. Once a feasible ritual was established, the focus was more on the play with Dolly rather than the needle. The parents became a more effective team, so Taylor accepted and cooperated with their routine. At the follow-up visit, she mentioned that now all of her toys had diabetes!

Position for intramuscular injections

We have found that the positioning of preschoolers for intramuscular injections is very important. Place the child's thigh between the parent's legs and have the parent wrap their arms firmly around the child, containing the child's arms. The other adult does the preparation and gives the injection. With practice, this ritual becomes simplified over time, and two adults may not always be needed.

Hypnosis with school-age children and adolescents

Fit the trance to the nature of the child's pain, their interests, and their beliefs. Gather this information from the child or adolescent, parent, or nurse and incorporate it within the trance experience to increase absorption and improve outcome.

Useful questions to ask are:

- Where would you rather be than here?
- What helped you best when you were in pain before?
- What did you do or think that best helped the pain to go away?
- Where are your favorite places/what are your favorite things to do?

Use this information to weave a relevant and absorbing trance for the child:

- The peak of children's hypnotizability is from 8 to 12 years.[1]
- Most children 6 years or older are able to sit or lie still, attend, respond to verbal direction, and easily move into a hypnotic trance. They can close their eyes and follow the process of relaxing and releasing muscle tension around the painful site.
- Adolescents' trances more closely resemble those of adults: they will often need longer trances for therapeutic benefit; they take longer to relax and shift away from present reality and longer to return back.
- After their hypnotic trances, children often report their own spontaneous elaborations that reveal the degree to which the child made the trance his own relevant experience. These can be included in future hypnotic sessions.

Case example

Michael, a somewhat obsessive 10-year-old, suffered for 3 years with frequent tension migraine headaches. When asked the questions above, he answered that he would rather be snorkeling in Hawaii. He felt best when he was away from his sister (significantly, he misheard the second question) and he did not have anything that helped the pain go away, which is a common reply from children with a long history of chronic or recurring pain.

Using an ideomotor finger induction,[1,5] Mathew moved rapidly into trance and confirmed that he was snorkeling in Hawaii. He was able to identify the fish that swam by, the underwater sea life forms he encountered, and continued to provide minute details of this inner experience as it unfolded. He was encouraged to let the sea water wash his headache pain out of his forehead and temples, and to note that the further he went into the coral reef the better and better his head felt. Four minutes into the experience, he reported no headache remaining. With a posthypnotic suggestion that with each practice the pain would drain away faster and he would remain headache free for longer and longer periods, he was invited to return to the room.

Comment

The need for control in this intense, somewhat obsessive, boy made it appropriate that he take the lead in developing his trance experience. The more he invested himself in this experience, the more effective it would be. His lead would also ensure a quicker relief from pain. Michael required only one session as follow-up. He remained in charge of his now infrequent headaches and at follow-up proudly confirmed that they were "not a hassle" anymore.

Self-regulatory techniques as an aid in diagnosis

The process of training children and adolescents in the use of self-regulation methods can serve as a diagnostic aid to understanding more about puzzling, complex, ongoing pain problems in which one form of therapy has not been effective in controlling the pain. The child's and parents' responses to self-regulation training often reveal beliefs and attitudes to pain and the degree of the child's motivation to get well again.

Through the standard procedure of training, we note how ready the child or adolescent is to engage with the preliminary exercises, what degree of response there is, the accompanying affect, and the parental reaction in the early stages. Children and adolescents are asked to keep a log of pain episodes, noting important features, prior activity and mood, "helpers" the child used, and the pain rating out of 10. This enables the clinician to "finetune" the therapy, to ascertain the pain triggers, practice efficacy, and rate and efficacy of response, and to determine whether there are any other issues hampering the patient's ability to competently manage the pain.

Case example

Twelve-year-old Cathy was referred with idiopathic diffuse pain syndrome by a rheumatology department because her pain was not being managed. She complained of widespread pain that had started in her legs and soles of her feet a year earlier, when she was intensely involved in swimming. The pain had since spread throughout her body and was particularly painful in her shoulders, arms, and back. She had stopped going to school and was quickly moving toward increased disability by isolating herself from friends and remaining indoors because of the pain. She cried her way through physiotherapy, finding gentle pressure and the exercises exquisitely painful, and ceased going. Her mother, a lawyer, was exasperated with her daughter, expressing that "she was no good at being a nurse!" Her parents were divorced and Cathy was distant from her father, who had a passion for athletics.

Cathy was invited to learn the "pain switch," as are many children with recurrent and chronic pain. She agreed and cooperated in the induction. However, in the deepening of the hypnotic process, she began frowning and said "my pain is getting worse." Relaxation is the key component of hypnosis: however much pain the patient is in, the process of letting go tends to provide some easing of the pain. It is rare that the pain worsens. Her response indicated some reluctance, perhaps distrust of the process, fear of letting go, or perhaps disbelief that she could ever feel better.

Her response during the pain switch has remained characteristic of her response to therapy to date. Whenever something is offered to her, she refutes its capacity to help her pain or demonstrates that it is useless. With anger and depression more prominent, she was given paroxetine 20 mg for both its pain and antidepressant properties. Over the last 3 months, she has made very gradual progress, demonstrating little insight into her emotional distress and complaining "Can you give me something more to stop the pain?" When invited to combine the "pain switch" with her medication "to help both become more effective," she refuses, saying "both don't help." She comes promptly to her sessions, displays anger and distress, discusses perceived misunderstandings, and rejects any suggestion that some of these personal pains may be expressed in physical pain as well. Her mother has become a key part of her recovery, as she is a critical part of her problems.

Comment

Our experience with self-regulatory methods is that children who are psychologically healthy are usually eager to help themselves get well, so that their pain is less of a presence in their lives. For children such as Cathy, pain is performing a purpose, however dysfunctional it may appear. Within the family, it has successfully thwarted her parents. It prevented her father from putting her under greater pressure to succeed at swimming, and it has drawn her mother in closer in order to take better care of her and be the "nurse" she never wanted to be but that her daughter wants her to be. This "arrangement" is not without its therapeutic challenges. After 3 months of treatments, including individual therapy with her divorced parents, Cathy is not as depressed, but reports little progress in relief from pain and has not yet reengaged in her life. This clinical picture of chronic pain and depression, complicated by family dysfunction, often requires long-term treatment for approximately 18–24 months.

BIOFEEDBACK

Biofeedback refers to the use of electronic or electromechanical equipment to measure and then feedback information about physiologic functions. The child or adolescent uses this physiologic information to improve body awareness and gain control of the selected physiologic response in the desired direction. Feedback is provided in a variety of auditory, visual, and even multimedia "game" formats that the patient finds most appealing and understandable.

Biofeedback is an ideal self-regulation skill for many children and adolescents because of its immediacy.[2] Patients quickly and convincingly see the evidence of physiologic control and also dramatically see the evidence for mind–body connections. We have found that children delight in seeing profound, rapid changes in heart rate, breathing, muscle tension, and other physiologic parameters achieved simply by imagining different situations (active versus passive activities) or by thinking of different emotional states (fear versus happiness). With improved somatic awareness and mastery in physiologic control, children can truly see that "a change in thinking causes a change in your body's response." Armed with this confidence, children can take charge of pain-related symptoms in a variety of ways.

Biofeedback adds precision to the self-regulation skills training experience for both the child in pain and the clinician. For example:

- Biofeedback therapy is designed to enhance each child's sense of mastery and control, promoting a shift from a more external to a more internal "locus of control."
- In certain pain-related conditions, such as headache and Raynaud syndrome, mastering physiologic change in specific ways to specific thresholds, for example increasing peripheral temperature to greater than 92°F, is very helpful in eliminating pain.
- For chronic and recurring pain, physiological control training via biofeedback builds confidence and often allows the tapering of pain medication. The child develops more trust in the internal healing ability and pain coping strategies, and becomes less reliant on the external help of medication.

- It is highly beneficial in teaching children to control excessive sympathetic nervous system activity and dysfunctional breathing patterns, commonly associated with the anxiety component of the pain experience.
- Because of its game-like quality, biofeedback is a user-friendly strategy that is culturally syntonic with today's high-technology youth. It provides immediate, concrete reinforcement with rapid attainment of skill.

Studies have shown that children are excellent at physiologic control of a variety of physiologic functions and are usually better than adults. Biofeedback is currently being used in inpatient and outpatient medical settings and in school-based and community mental health centers. Biofeedback modalities that are most commonly utilized are described in Table 13.4.

Components of biofeedback training

The schedule

- Most children can be taught and coached in biofeedback techniques within six to eight 40-min biofeedback sessions, spaced 1–2 weeks apart.
- In the first biofeedback session, the coached children develop an increase in body awareness and physiological control, which is immediately and strongly reinforcing.
- The first three or four sessions are scheduled about 1 week apart and subsequent sessions are spaced at 2-week intervals.

The practice

- The practicing of these self-regulation and relaxation skills at home, at school, and in other relevant settings is underscored as being of prime importance.
- Some patients do best with scheduling daily practice sessions at home in an organized routine, e.g. a minimum of two 5-min practice sessions at home per day. Other patients do best with situation-specific practice, e.g. prior to your math test, breath deeply and relax your muscles.
- Brief (30 s to 1 min) and frequent relaxation mini-breaks are also helpful for children with persistent pain complaints.
- Children are asked to keep a daily log or "symptom

Table 13.4 *Biofeedback modalities and abbreviations*

Peripheral temperature (thermography)	TMP
Breathing (pneumography)	PNG
Exhaled carbon dioxide level (capnography)	CAP
Heart rate (photoplethmysography)	PPG
Muscle tension (electromyography)	EMG
Sweat gland activity (electrodermal activity)	EDA
Electrical brain activity (electroencephalography)	EEG

diary" that details practice progress and describes symptoms using a visual analog scale (VAS) rating system for symptom severity.

- Eventually, a number of cues can be developed with the patient that serve as helpful reminders to use their chosen pain control technique.

Parental involvement

In the first one or two sessions, parents are invited to observe in order to get a general sense of the process, what the practice expectations are, and their role in coaching their child at home. After that, children are usually invited to participate alone with the clinician, so that they give their full attention. This emphasizes their responsibility, choice, and sense of partnership in participating in the therapeutic process.

Physiologic modality

A variety of physiologic modalities may be explored to determine what would be the most responsive to ameliorate the pain symptom. For certain patients, the modality to be trained, for example temperature, muscle tension, or breathing, is determined by their particular pain symptom. For others, the physiologic modality that is most "hotly" reactive is identified and then trained. There is some debate within the biofeedback field about whether training the specific modality is more important or whether the general process issues are more important.

For certain problems where specific etiologic mechanisms can be identified, training to that parameter is indicated:

- Migraine headaches have a vascular reactivity component. Training peripheral finger temperature to increase to levels above 92–95°F on a regular basis seems to decrease the migraine's frequency and severity. The mechanism includes autonomic nervous system balance changes that may then affect vascular reactivity patterns.
- Chronic tension headaches display tight and/or asymmetric muscle groups on electromyography (EMG) evaluation in the neck, face, and shoulders. Training in muscle relaxation and symmetry can decrease symptoms.
- Reflex sympathetic dystrophy shows sympathetic nervous system (SNS) dysfunction in the affected limb. Electrodermal activity (EDA) training to decrease excess SNS can be helpful.
- Raynaud's disorder involves decreased blood flow to the hands and feet, causing pain particularly in cold weather. Peripheral temperature biofeedback training restores normal blood flow ability and ameliorates these symptoms.
- Fibromyalgia is thought to display parasympathetic imbalance. Using respiratory sinus arrhythmia (RSA) and/or EDA may be helpful in this condition.

Electroencephalography (EEG) protocols for pain conditions that include depression are being developed to identify brain wave patterns (neurosignatures) that can be altered to modify pain.

Beyond its value in providing information to the pediatric patient about their body, biofeedback equipment provides physiologic data that are helpful for therapy. Some clinicians routinely monitor physiologic changes during sessions, but do not initially disclose the information. Watching SNS activity and changes when talking about sensitive or uncomfortable topics gives helpful data in determining which themes, topics, and life experiences affect the patient and which are particularly distressing or stimulating. This is particularly helpful with complex pain or somatization disorders in which the physiologic monitoring helps to identify possible emotional and other triggers that, at a minimum, may be exacerbating the child's pain.

Physiologic monitoring can also evaluate progress with other self-regulatory strategies, such as relaxation training or response to certain types of thematic material or mental imagery. These data can be reviewed at a later time in order to facilitate understanding certain response patterns to pain or to reinforce progress or the possibilities for change.

The technique

In each biofeedback training session, thought is given to select the visual screen displays and auditory feedback options that optimally engage and appropriately challenge each child. Additional therapeutic techniques are used within any one session and across subsequent sessions:

- Mental imagery is commonly employed to provide the opportunity for imaginary or "*in vivo*" rehearsal, to enhance physiologic change, and to deepen the relaxation experience.
- Reframing the problem in manageable terms and with an emphasis on daily function, rather than the limitations created by the symptom.
- A positive self-talk repertoire is developed to form part of the therapeutic repertoire. As with hypnosis, adjustments to language should reflect each child's developmental level, individual interests, and perspectives.

Discern–control–generalize

In clinical biofeedback training, it is best to follow a hierarchical structure of tasks from the discerning phase to the developing control phase and then to generalize this learning to the child's everyday life.

In the *discern* phase of training, children are taught about mind–body links and physiologic control and are assisted in learning to discriminate differences between states of relaxation (low SNS arousal) and tension or anxiety (high SNS arousal), negative and positive sensations, and notice-associated sensations. They are also coached to carefully and completely tune into inner bodily events and sensations. For example, for the child with muscle tension as part of their pain symptom complex, early recognition of tension in specific muscle groups (such as trapezia or neck muscles) is important in the discern phase. "How does your muscle feel; how fast is your heart beating? Notice your breathing – is it fast or slow? Are you breathing in your chest or shoulders or down in your belly?" Part of the process is to then to ask what these symptoms and body sensations mean to the child. Being optimally aware of the range of internal messages associated with the pain prepares the child to respond more readily toward therapeutic change.

An efficient and enjoyable way to train an initial sense of body awareness is by discrimination training with surface EMG. Children can quickly learn to identify even low levels of tension and/or muscle asymmetry with biofeedback and then correct this problem. Eventually, they can do this without the presence of immediate visual or auditory feedback. They develop acute awareness of the target symptom or sensation and then can act preemptively to control it. One of the distinct benefits of biofeedback training is the enhanced capacity for "somatic awareness."

It is important to note that, for children, baseline values for individual physiologic modalities may vary somewhat. Baseline values across sessions can also vary, particularly for EDA and peripheral temperature.

In the *control* phase of training, patients are coached to master specific skills and to achieve certain trends or threshold goals in training a specific physiologic function. For example:

- The child might be helped to consistently maintain a bifrontal EMG reading below $3\,\mu V$, an EDA below $5\,\mu V$ with directed relaxation, or a finger temperature of 93–95°F. All of these would be common goals and would reflect a desirable level of lowered SNS activity.
- With diaphragmatic breathing, children master the ability to relax chest and thoracic musculature, achieve good abdominal movement, breathe at a slow pace, and maintain an inhalation time of 3–4 s with an exhalation time of 6–10 s.

We begin with a home practice recommendation of 5 min twice a day to foster comfort, confidence, and experience with these techniques. Note that for children it is not necessary to achieve rigidly defined predetermined goals for any given modality. General trends in certain modalities are indicative of the desired trend in or magnitude of physiologic change. In this training phase, many children find that specific mental imagery enhances the rapidity with which they can regulate their level of change for a given modality. For example, imagining warmth- and relaxation-related experiences to facilitate their own peripheral temperature change.

The *generalize* phase is often the most challenging part of biofeedback training as the patient begins to apply the learned skills successfully in the appropriate real-life situation or environment without the machine or the clinician. Most children enjoy quick success in the *discern* and *control* sessions, and within three to five sessions most are achieving the desired physiologic control goals in the biweekly office-based sessions.

For transfer of skills to take place:

- Triggers and cues are identified with the patient that will alert them to apply their self-management skills. Early pain signals that were previously ignored now cue the child to engage in the selected helpful strategies.
- Parents and teachers are encouraged to help cue in ways that are agreed upon with the child.
- Role playing specific situations with the patient to elicit emotional arousal and/or imaginal rehearsal techniques can prepare them for the real-life stimulus.
- Usually, one or two long-term follow-up sessions or refresher sessions are set up 2–4 months from the initial sessions to check on long-term progress and to offer any support and adjustments needed to the plan.

Psychophysiologic profile

Early in the biofeedback experience, it is useful to complete a psychophysiologic stress profile on each child. This identifies the unique pattern of ANS reactivity (an individual's ANS "fingerprint") to different types of stressful stimuli and their ability to recover from such stress. During this procedure, the child is attached to various sensors [temperature, EMG, EDA, photoplethmysography (PPG), and breathing] and a 2- to 4-min baseline is recorded of one relaxation condition with eyes open followed by one with eyes closed. The child is then led through a set of different standardized stressors (such as: cognitive stressor, doing a rapid series of age-appropriate math calculations; physical stressor, painful stimulus such as placing an extremity in an ice-water bath).

The profile can be reviewed with the child as a dramatic example of mind–body connections and as evidence for their ability to recover from stressors. Information about preferred response modality helps to determine which modality to train in subsequent sessions. For example, some children will be sensitive temperature responders with rapid and large changes across each condition in the profile, whereas for others the heart rate or EDA responds more dramatically.

INTEGRATED APPROACHES

Biofeedback can be used to facilitate the therapeutic relationship:[13]*

- It is a comfortable, nonthreatening, and quite playful way to begin the pain management process, build rapport, and elicit a sense of curiosity.
- Relaxation enhances emotional comfort and willingness to communicate.
- Biofeedback is similar to that of induction techniques used in hypnosis and hypnotherapy. Watching the visual feedback and listening to a monotonous auditory-guiding feedback tone tends to narrow attention and increase awareness of internal body events and sensations, which open the door to further discussion of these phenomena.
- These states of deep relaxation enhance access to unconscious material and facilitate fantasy and imagery. With the development of an alternative state of awareness during biofeedback training, the child may be more open to therapeutic suggestion for pain and distress reduction.
- Self-hypnosis can be very useful in the later stages of self-regulation training. Adding "age progression," in which the child sees himself in the future as healthy, functional, and pain free, brings that possibility closer and sets a positive expectation for symptom control in a finite time span.

Case example

Fifteen-year-old Jenni was referred for chronic daily headaches, which began 8 months earlier when school started. Previously, she had experienced only occasional minor headaches. The headaches she reported had continued, unabated, every day since the beginning of the school year. Rated on a visual analog scale to be a "7," Jenni described them as bitemporal and somewhat diffuse and as occurring each day from the time she awoke until midday. In addition, approximately once every 2 weeks, she would have a more severe, pounding headache associated with nausea which she would have to "sleep off." These were likely migraine. She was missing school more often and her mother was concerned. Ibuprofen and propranolol had not been helpful, and Jenni did not want to try other medications. Jenni liked school, was a good student, and had a close group of friends. She thought stress played some role in the exacerbation of her headaches, which had become a topic of frequent discussion at home.

At the first session, a psychophysiologic stress profile was completed and Jenni saw with interest that even with a mild cognitive stressor (she was asked to do some challenging math problems) her SNS reacted briskly with a decrease in peripheral temperature, increases in heart rate and EDA, and changes in breathing. She recovered to baseline quickly after stress, and this was pointed out as a healthy sign. She learned a basic progressive muscle relaxation and mental imagery exercise and how to track her headaches in a symptom diary.

One week later, at the second session, she brought her calendar and her ratings had not changed much. Diaphragmatic breathing and self-hypnosis on themes of control, healthy functioning, and decreased pain were explored and developed. Jenni was encouraged to reframe her thoughts about headaches and the control they were exerting over her life and, instead, focus on the things she enjoyed doing and could do.

At the third session, Jenni noted she had begun to experience a drop in her daily pain ratings from an unchanging "7" on her VAS to an occasional "4–6 range" rating on some days. She reported that she forgot about headaches altogether while doing her self-hypnosis practice. She had had one probable migraine event that week and had missed one day of school. Her mother also commented that Jenni seemed to be talking less about her headaches at home. At this session, the link between peripheral (finger) temperature and headaches was explored with Jenni. Her baseline finger temperature (nondominant hand, index finger) was 78°F. With direct visual feedback using a colorful pyramid display, Jenni was able to increase finger temp to 90°F after 8 min of relaxation. Specific images about warmth and blood flow were explored as another way to facilitate the finger-warming phenomena. Jenni was given temperature bands for home training and instructed in their use, so she could see the same benefits and success with her home practice.

By the fourth session, Jenni was doing much better and had experienced several headache-free days and no migraine episodes. With home training combining breathing, self-hypnosis, and muscle relaxation, she was consistently achieving finger temperatures of 90–92°F. At long-term follow-up a few months later, she had only rare headaches and was utilizing her self-management skills in both preventative and abortive modes for headache control. She felt confident about her pain control skill, and no longer felt the need to use medication.

Comment

The literature supporting biofeedback and relaxation skills training as effective for relieving juvenile migraine and tension-type headaches is quite robust. Randomized, controlled trials and meta-analyses have described the long- and short-term benefits of self-regulation training as being superior to pharmacotherapy.[12]** Bifrontal EMG and peripheral temperature training are particularly successful, although the mechanisms by which they effect therapeutic change are not completely understood.

Children and adolescents with chronic, mixed headaches, such as in Jenni's case, can be the most refractory to any treatments. Self-regulation training coupled with effective education about mind–body links and stress management are key ingredients for success. In our experience, the majority of children who suffer from migraine can taper or eliminate medication use, whether it be abortive or preventative medication, after self-regulation training. Decreased reliance on medication and increased self-efficacy are the keys to a successful outcome for this complex pain problem.

Limitations for biofeedback and hypnosis

Biofeedback and hypnosis are not panaceas, and care must be taken to understand their indications, contraindications, and limitations:[1]

- Biofeedback training and hypnosis are usually not suitable for children who are psychotic or severely depressed, and should be undertaken with extreme caution in children with post-traumatic stress disorder (PTSD) and other severe emotional problems.
- In certain cases, the scientific literature supports the use of a specific biofeedback modality for a specific disorder. Seek supervision and case consultation when in doubt.
- Only use biofeedback training with children who present with pain complaints/diagnoses that are well within one's scope of training and expertise.
- Be honest with parents and with patients about the expected length of therapy and reasonable expectations for hypnosis and the biofeedback training process.

In a 1987 study, Olness and Libbey[14] found that 20% of children referred for self-regulation training (primarily hypnosis) had a previously undiagnosed biologic etiology for their condition. This study underscores that all children presenting with psychophysiologic symptoms require thorough medical and neurologic evaluation to rule out organic conditions that may contribute to the presenting symptom. For example, children with headaches and abdominal pain need specific medical and neurologic evaluation to rule out tumor, infectious, and metabolic problems that can cause recurrent pain.

Concurrent use of psychotropic medication is not a contraindication to biofeedback and/or relaxation training, but needs to be carefully reviewed on a case-by-case basis. Certain psychotropic agents will change ANS responsivity and so may affect baseline measurements and the child's ability to modulate certain modalities, such as peripheral temperature, heart rate, and skin conductance. Some children can reduce or even eliminate the need for certain medications when biofeedback training is successful (e.g. analgesic use in juvenile migraine). This must be carefully coordinated with the prescribing physician.

Case example

Mitchell, a 10-year-old athletic-looking boy, was referred by a local pediatric neurologist for biofeedback training for lower back and other muscle pain. Mitchell described experiencing severe, debilitating muscle cramping and pain several months earlier, with no specific history of trauma or other initiating event. The muscle spasms, cramping, and associated pain had waxed and waned for months with no predictable pattern. Several specialty consults and full laboratory evaluation, including neurologic, rheumatologic, and other tests, had not identified any clear etiology. Mitchell was very active, participating in downhill skiing and snowboarding at the time the symptoms developed. Occasionally, on the day after he skied, he would experience a flare-up of the pain, but this was not always consistent. Bed rest, warm baths, and anti-inflammatory agents were all tried without good benefit.

By the time he was referred for biofeedback training, the pain was mostly centered around his mid- to lower back, in the paraspinal area. Mitchell had begun missing school with increasing frequency because of his pain episodes. He liked school and had good friends and was a good student. Mitchell's mother was very distressed by his severe episodes. On a visual analog scale of 0–10, Mitchell described these episodes as an "11!" The working diagnosis at the time of referral was muscular back pain/strain with a possible "functional" component.

At the first biofeedback session, a back, shoulder, and neck muscle scan was completed in both sitting and standing positions. At the time of the scan, Mitchell was not experiencing any pain. Scan results identified pockets of muscle asymmetry and elevated tension primarily in the paraspinal area of the midback and also in the cervical area. These findings were explained to Mitchell. Mitchell was then taught a basic progressive muscle relaxation (PMR) exercise involving the alternate tightening then relaxing of a variety of muscle groups. During PMR training, Mitchell was taught to tighten and then relax a variety of specific muscle groups and to begin focusing his attention on the discrimination of levels of muscle tension in different body areas. At first, direct visual and auditory EMG feedback was provided; later on, Mitchell could describe a level of muscle tension for a given muscle or group very accurately with no external feedback. He enjoyed playing EMG-controlled biofeedback games with sports themes. In Bioball, the goal is to relax the target muscle group while waiting for a pitch; if your muscles are relaxed to a preset threshold, you are successful and hit a home run.

His initial home assignment was to practice PMR two or three times each day and track his own VAS pain ratings on a calendar each day. At the second session, 1 week later, Mitchell reported practicing regularly and a few better days. Bilateral EMG on midback paraspinals showed better symmetry and decreased muscle tension levels (bilaterally to below $5\,\mu V$). We then moved into teaching Mitchell slow, rhythmic, diaphragmatic breathing as another deep relaxation method. He added breathing to his home practice regimen.

One week before his next session, Mitchell again had a few very severe episodes of pain with muscle spasm and rippling. He experienced hyperphagia and feeling "hot" at the beginning of these episodes and somnolent afterwards. In reviewing the situation, the presenting picture did not sound like typical muscular back strain, nor did it fit the picture of a somatization disorder. Referral was made to a neuromuscular specialist and, after extensive testing, a diagnosis of a rare mitochondrial myopathy was made.

Although medications, dietary changes, and physical therapy were prescribed, Mitchell's pain still occurs episodically with little relief. He did find, however, that his self-regulation techniques were helpful and continued to practice. At his next session, we agreed that, beyond relaxation-related techniques, we would develop other direct pain management strategies. We started self-hypnosis training. Mitchell really enjoyed this and with practice experienced benefit. He found imagery involving favorite places and activities helpful for distraction. He also utilized specific suggestions about changing the character of the pain, decreasing the perceived intensity and developing feelings of "coolness" when he felt overheated. Although Mitchell continues to have episodes of spasm and associated pain, he has maintained a positive, confident attitude about his ability to actively use self-directed pain management strategies. He is attending school much more regularly and continues to ski and snowboard.

Comment

This case highlights how the clinician needs to stay alert to the diagnostic picture indicated by the pain, and that self-regulatory methods are helpful for a broad range of pain problems. Here, an integrated approach was taught using self-awareness and simple muscle relaxation and then more complex hypnotherapeutic pain control techniques were added. Because medications had largely been ineffective, the feeling of active control and multiple nonpharmacological choices for pain management that Mitchell developed with self-regulation were invaluable in keeping him from greater functional impairment, despite his disease and ongoing pain.

THEORETICAL RATIONALE: MECHANISMS OF CHANGE

Thoughts and emotions directly influence physiologic response systems and processes, such as blood flow, muscle tension, release of hormones, neuropeptides, and inflammatory mediators, and immune system changes, all of which play a role in the production of pain. In addition to spinal control mechanisms of nociceptive transmission, descending pathways that originate in the cortex and thalamus can play a significant role in modulating each person's pain perception and experience. The gate control theory of pain suggests that thoughts, beliefs, and emotions may affect how much pain you feel from any given physical sensation. The ability to plan and actively modulate pain perception via connecting pathways from

the central nervous system (CNS) gives rise to consideration of a number of therapeutic interventions that may work centrally to "close the gates" via these descending CNS influences.

Melzack[15] postulates an essential interplay between central and peripheral nervous systems with regard to the pain experience and pain experience pathways that are partly innate and partly learned. Calling this neural network "the neuromatrix," the likely basis for one's physical wiring, he proposes that it plays a role in pain and somatic awareness. Being somewhat malleable, it acquires its individual reaction patterns or "neurosignature" through repeated activation. Perhaps self-regulatory strategies modify these pain reaction pathways both consciously and unconsciously to reconfigure an individual's response tendency.

Hypnosis

We do not fully understand the hypnotic process, but it is agreed that, as a state of altered consciousness, hypnosis is different both from the normal waking state and from the different stages of sleep. Hypnosis resembles various meditative states, with its narrowly focused attention, primary process thinking, and ego-receptivity.[1,12]** Some have postulated that hypnosis decreases anxiety rather than affecting the pain sensation itself. Hypnosis does decrease anxiety and thereby increases pain tolerance, but this is certainly not the predominant mechanism of action for hypnoanalgesia and hypnoanesthesia.

With the discovery of endorphins, there was speculation that the key to the mechanism of action of hypnoanalgesia had been found. The hypothesis that hypnosis is the natural way of releasing endorphins has not yet been supported by research. Hypnotic analgesia for experimental pain was not reversed by the administration of naloxone hydrochloride. Furthermore, in contrast to the elevated endorphin levels in patients experiencing acupuncture, patients experiencing hypnotic analgesia showed no increase in endorphin levels. Current findings in this intriguing area of inquiry may have methodological pitfalls, particularly problems in measurement. Melzack and Wall's gate control theory of pain provides one rationale for the effectiveness of hypnosis in the control of pain. The theory is far from a full explanation of hypnotic action.

Research suggests that successful self-regulation strategies operate on multiple levels with multifactorial mechanisms of therapeutic change.[12]** A variety of potential mediators in pain control, both specific and nonspecific, may play a role.

Potential specific mechanisms of pain control with biofeedback and hypnosis

• Decreased sympathetic nervous system activity: there

is evidence that SNS activity upmodulates pain conduction.[16]

- Specific physiologic changes that are condition specific: such as muscle relaxation and symmetry training in tension headache; reduction in excessive SNS activity in irritable bowel syndrome; reduction in inflammatory mediators secondary to specific therapeutic suggestion for burns.
- Downregulation of the descending pathway.
- Release of endogenous pain neuropeptides.
- Unidentified neuroelectrical/neurochemical/neurometabolic/somatic changes.

Potential nonspecific mechanisms of pain control

- The shift from an external to a more internal locus of control enhances self-efficacy in the self-control of pain.
- Positive expectancy, also called placebo factor, "faith factor," and hopefulness.
- The active partnership and rapport with the clinician.
- Cognitive reframing of the pain, which occurs particularly in the biofeedback and hypnosis process, does not necessarily change pain intensity but shifts its relevance, quality, attention, secondary gain factors, coping strategies, and level of functional impairment.

COMMON FEATURES OF SELF-REGULATORY METHODS

- It may be that the hypnotic induction experience and biofeedback training are two pathways to the same endpoint – a state of heightened suggestibility where patients can make choices about pain perception, control, and change.[12★★]
- Diaphragmatic breathing, relaxation methods, biofeedback, and hypnosis are commonly integrated in the therapeutic process of relieving a child's pain. In fact, for most pediatric patients, biofeedback training leads to an altered state of awareness with narrowed, highly focused attention, facilitation of a state of comfort and relaxation, and facilitation of a sense of control – just like that described in hypnosis.
- Some children and adolescents enjoy the added visual and sensory feedback elements and find that they accelerate their somatic awareness and subsequent pain modulation ability. Others move quickly beyond the need for external feedback cues and cultivate the "internal" imagery experience in mastering their pain symptoms.
- Simply training a child to change a physiologic modality such as heart rate or breathing does not necessarily result in immediate pain reduction. However, by integrating this body control training with somatic

awareness, therapeutic suggestions, and new ways of self-control, many children experience benefits.

- Children and adolescents are highly active participants in therapy and are offered several approaches or options depending on their interests, developmental level, and coping style. Our role is as a "coach." The ultimate responsibility for success rests with the patient. Nevertheless, skilled guidance, rapport, honesty, and a true sense of partnership are key ingredients in this undertaking to control pain.

TRAINING IN HYPNOSIS AND TRAINING AND PROFESSIONAL CERTIFICATION IN BIOFEEDBACK

Formal training is recommended for those interested in applying this powerful group of techniques. Training in hypnosis occurs through the Society for Developmental & Behavioral Pediatrics Workshops (9 Station Lane, Philadelphia, PA 19118-2939, USA) and The American Society for Clinical Hypnosis (Suite 402, Chicago, IL 60610, USA). Training in biofeedback is available by contacting the Association for Applied Psychophysiology and Biofeedback (10200 W 44th Ave., Wheat Ridge, CO 80033, USA). Professional certification is available through the Biofeedback Certification Institute of America. Training includes both course work and clinical supervision as well as written and practical exams.

CONCLUSION

One aspect of our "humanness" is the capacity to examine, appreciate, and regulate our inner experience and reactions to pain. Self-regulation strategies, such as hypnosis and biofeedback, uniquely and directly cultivate these internal abilities to modulate and reduce pain phenomena. Within the last decade, self-regulation strategies have moved to the front lines as evidence-based, practical approaches for clinical pediatric pain management. These uniquely valuable tools for managing pain in children and adolescents are (1) biofeedback, with its "hi-tech" appeal, (2) hypnosis, which uses innate imaginative abilities, (3) diaphragmatic breathing, a fundamental physiological index of distress and pain, and (4) relaxation, a training to counteract the tension and preoccupation of pain.

Pain drains a child's energy and their ability to cope. The experience of pain is demonstrated to have long-lasting effects on children and adolescents. Supporting the practice of self-regulatory techniques seems to mitigate much of the negative impact of pain on children and their functioning. Since these methods facilitate competency and a sense of mastery over nociception, anxiety, and distress, they enable children to take a more active part in and responsibility for their treatment and recovery.

Individuals that are actively engaged in some form of self-regulation appear to have an improved quality of life. Children who master self-regulation skills acquire special "life skills" to serve them in future pain encounters. Early training in self-regulation skills, self-hypnosis, or biofeedback may also be an important disease-prevention tool in pediatrics. There is growing evidence that when a child or adolescent is in pain and knows how to mediate and regulate both the pain and the concomitant anxiety or fear the long-term prognosis is improved.

The most commonly raised objection from medical and nursing staff to the use of self-regulatory strategies is "I don't have time." This assumes that self-regulation training is lengthy and removed from medical treatment. It need not be. Over the last 15 years, we have learned a great deal about how rapidly patients in pain respond to hypnosis, and how shock and anxiety increase a person's receptivity to suggestion. In addition, teaching children about mind–body connections does not necessarily require expensive computerized biofeedback equipment. A thermometer in the clinic room, a pulse oximeter in the emergency room, and a scale in the triage room can all be used as "biofeedback" devices to help patients to understand their bodies and begin to develop self-control, confidence, and relief from pain. What is required by the practitioner is the ability to engage with children, creativity, flexibility, commitment, and a sense of humor. It remains a puzzle then why self-regulation is not even more widely utilized in pediatric training and practice.

REFERENCES

◆ 1. Olness K, Kohen DP. *Hypnosis and Hypnotherapy with Children*, 3rd edn. New York, NY: Guilford Press, 1996.

● 2. Culbert, T. Biofeedback with children and adolescents. In: Schaefer C ed. *Innovative Psychotherapy Techniques in Child and Adolescent Therapy*, 2nd edn. New York, NY: John Wiley & Sons, 1999.

3. Kuttner L. *A Child in Pain, How to Help, What to Do*. Vancouver: Hartley & Marks, 1996.

4. Sugarman L. *Imaginative Medicine: Hypnosis is Pediatric Practice*. Video documentary (70 min), 1997. Available from 2233 Clinton Ave, S. Rochester, NY 14618-2632 USA.

5. Kuttner L. *No Fears, No Tears, Children with Cancer Coping with Pain*. Video documentary (27 min), 1985. Available from Canadian Cancer Society, 855 W.10th Ave, Vancouver BC V5Z 4J4 Canada.

6. Kuttner L. *No Fears, No Tears –13 Years Later*. Video documentary on the long-term impact of children's pain control, 1998. Available from 203–1089 W. Broadway, V6H 1E5 Canada.

● 7. Attansio V, Andrasik F, Burke E, *et al*. Clinical issues in utilizing biofeedback with children. *Clin Biofeedback Health* 1985; **8:** 134–41.

8. Kohen D. Application of relaxation mental imagery in pediatric emergencies. *Int J Clin Exp Hypn* 1986; **34:** 283–94.

9. Goldie C. Hypnosis in the casualty department. *Br Med J* 1956; **2:** 1340–2.

10. Kajander R, Peper E. Teaching diaphragmatic breathing to children. *Biofeedback* 1998; **26:** 14–17.

11. Mars D Biofeedback assisted psychotherapy using multimodal biofeedback including capnography. *Biofeedback* 1998; **26:** 4–7.

12. Olness K, MacDonald J, Uden D. Prospective study comparing propranolol, placebo and hypnosis in management of juvenile migraine. *Pediatrics* 1987; **79:** 593–7.

13. Culbert T, Rearney J, Kohen D. Cyberphysiologic strategies for children: the clinical hypnosis, biofeedback interface. *Int J Clin Exp Hypn* 1994; **442:** 97–117.

14. Olness K, Libbey P. Unrecognized biologic basis for behavioral symptoms in children referred for hypnotherapy. *Am J Clin Hypn* 1987; **30:** 1–8.

15. Melzack R. Phantom limb pains and the concept of the neuromatrix. *Trends Neurosci* 1990; **13:** 88–92.

16. Baron, R. Levine JD, Fields HL. Causalgia and reflex sympathetic dystrophy: does the sympathetic nervous system contribute to the generation of pain? *Muscle Nerve* 1999; **22:** 678–95.

14

Graded exposure *in vivo* for pain-related fear

JOHAN W S VLAEYEN, JEROEN DE JONG, PETER H T G HEUTS, AND GEERT CROMBEZ

Characteristics of pain-related fear	163	Education	169
Pain-related fear and attention	164	Exposure *in vivo*	169
Disconfirmations of harm beliefs	164	Effectiveness	173
Graded *in vivo* exposure versus graded activity	165	Summary	174
Cognitive–behavioral assessment	165	References	174

In an attempt to explain how and why some individuals with musculoskeletal pain develop a chronic pain syndrome, biopsychosocial models have been developed, including the "fear-avoidance model of exaggerated pain perception,"[1] and, more recently, a cognitive–behavioral model of fear of movement/(re)injury.[2,3] The central concept of these models is "fear of pain," or the more specific "fear that physical activity will cause (re)injury." Two opposing behavioral responses to pain are postulated: "confrontation" and "avoidance." In the absence of any serious somatic pathology, confrontation is conceptualized as an adaptive response that eventually may lead to the reduction of fear and the promotion of recovery of pain or function. In contrast, avoidance leads to the maintenance or exacerbation of fear, possibly resulting in a condition similar to a phobia. The avoidance results in the reduction of both social and physical activities, which in turn leads to a number of physical and psychological consequences augmenting the disability.[4] Prospective studies in acute low back pain patients[5] and healthy people[6] have provided support for the idea that pain-related fear may be an important precursor of pain disability.

What are the clinical consequences of these findings? In this chapter, we will first highlight the typical characteristics of pain-related fear, and the association between pain-related fear and attentional, cognitive, and behavioral processes. From a clinician's point of view, we will address cognitive–behavioral assessment methods in patients who report excessive pain-related fears. We will then describe a novel treatment approach for patients with musculoskeletal pain which is based on the treatment methods developed for people with anxiety disorders. An adapted form of exposure *in vivo* with behavioral experiments is described which aims to provide personal evidence that the anticipated catastrophic consequences of physical performance do not occur. We critically appraise the currently available data on the effectiveness of this novel approach and address some of the complicating factors. Finally, we will provide some directions for future research and development.

CHARACTERISTICS OF PAIN-RELATED FEAR

In 1990, Kori *et al.*[7] introduced the term "kinesiophobia" (kinesis = movement) for the condition in which a patient has "an excessive, irrational, and debilitating fear of physical movement and activity resulting from a feeling of vulnerability to painful injury or reinjury." Recent evidence revealed that, during confrontation with feared movements, chronic low back pain patients who are fearful of movement/(re)injury typically show cognitive (worry), psychophysiological (muscle reactivity), and behavioral (escape and avoidance) responses, rendering support for the idea that chronic pain and chronic fear share important characteristics.[4,8,9]

There is evidence that pain-related fear is associated with specific worries, often referred to as pain catastrophizing. Pain catastrophizing is considered an exaggerated negative orientation toward noxious stimuli, and has been shown to mediate distress reactions to painful stimulation.[10] Crombez *et al.*[11] found that pain-free volunteers with a high frequency of catastrophic thinking about pain became more fearful when threatened with the possibility of occurrence of intense pain than students with a low frequency of catastrophic thinking. In line with these findings, a strong association has been found between pain-related fear and pain catastrophizing in chronic pain patients, and it has been suggested that pain catastrophizing is likely to be a precursor of pain-related fear.[2,12]

The reactivity of lumbar musculature in fearful chronic low back pain (CLBP) patients was studied in an experiment in which the subjects watched a neutral nature documentary, followed by a fear-eliciting video displaying a person vigorously performing physical activity.[13] Although self-reported tension increased from the nature documentary to the activity exposure in the fearful CLBP patients, there was a general decrease in muscular reactivity in both subgroups, probably due to initial contextual fear. This decrease, however, was less in fearful patients, who remained at about the same reactivity level.

It has repeatedly been shown that pain-related fear is associated with escape/avoidance behaviors. In a study in which chronic pain sufferers volunteered to undergo cold pressor pain, it was shown that expected danger significantly predicted avoidance of another cold pressor immersion.[14] Chronic pain patients who associate pain with damage tend to avoid activities that produce pain. Other studies that used physical performance tests reported that poor behavioral performance appeared to be more strongly associated with pain-related fear than with pain severity[15] and biomedical findings.[3]

The effects of pain-related fear on behavioral performance also appear to generalize to restrictions in daily life situations. Waddell *et al.*[16] demonstrated that fear-avoidance beliefs about work are strongly related to disability of daily living and work lost in the past year, and more so than pain variables such as anatomical pattern of pain, time pattern, and pain severity, and concluded that "Fear of pain and what we do about it may be more disabling than pain itself."

PAIN-RELATED FEAR AND ATTENTION

The cognitive theory of anxiety put forward by Eysenck[17] makes the assumption that the most important function of anxiety is to facilitate the early detection of potentially threatening situations. In other words, highly anxious individuals demonstrate hypervigilance, both generally and specifically. General hypervigilance (or distractibility) refers to the propensity to attend to any irrelevant stimuli being presented. Specific hypervigilance involves the inclination to attend selectively to threat-related rather than to neutral stimuli. So far, there has been little research that directly examined hypervigilance in pain patients who report pain-related fear. Based on their study investigating the construct validity of the McGill

Pain Questionnaire, Pearce and Morley[18] suggested that patients with chronic pain be characterized by a selective attention toward cues that are thematically related to pain and its consequences. A more recent replication with the dot-probe paradigm found that individuals with chronic pain with low anxiety sensitivity were able to shift their attention away from stimuli related to pain, in contrast to the subjects with high pain sensitivity.[19] In other words, they found evidence for a specific form of hypervigilance. These findings are in line with the observation that chronic back pain patients who avoid back-straining activities report not only high fear of pain and fear of (re)injury but also high attention to back sensations.[20,21] Using a body-scanning reaction time paradigm, Peters *et al.*[22] found that in a group of fibromyalgia patients detection latency for innocuous electrical stimuli in the arm was predicted by scores on the Pain Anxiety Symptoms Scale, and was most consistent with the cognitive anxiety subscale. Indirect evidence on association between pain-related fear and body hypervigilance is found using a primary task paradigm in which chronic pain patients are requested to direct their attentional focus toward an attentionally demanding task. Degradation in task performance on the cognitive task can be taken as an index of attentional interference due to hypervigilance. A number of studies have demonstrated that disruption of performance to an attentionally demanding task was most pronounced in chronic pain patients who reported high negative affect, somatic awareness, and high pain intensity[23] and fear of (re)injury.[24]

DISCONFIRMATIONS OF HARM BELIEFS

What are the clinical implications of the above-mentioned findings? Philips[4] was one of the first to argue for the systematic application of graded exposure in order to produce disconfirmations between expectations of pain and harm, the actual pain, and the other consequences of the activity. She further suggested that "These disconfirmations can be made more obvious to the sufferer by helping to clarify the expectations he/she is working with, and by delineating the conditions or stimuli which he feels are likely to fulfill his expectations. Repeated, graded, and controlled exposures to such situations under optimal conditions are likely to produce the largest and most powerful disconfirmations."[4] Experimental support for this idea is provided by the match/mismatch model of pain,[25] which states that people initially tend to overpredict how much pain they will experience, but after some exposures these predictions tend to be corrected to match with the actual experience. A similar pattern was found by Crombez *et al.*[26] in a sample of CLBP patients who were requested to perform four exercise bouts (two with each leg) at maximal force. During each exercise bout, the baseline pain, the expected pain, and the experienced pain were recorded. As predicted, the CLBP patients initially overpredicted pain, but after repetition of the exercise bout the overprediction was readily corrected. The expectancy did not seem to generalize to the exercise bout with the other leg as a small increase in pain expectancy reemerged. Also here, expectancies were immediately corrected after another performance. In sum, it is quite plausible that, in analogy with the treatment of phobias, graded exposure to back-stressing movements may indeed be a successful treatment approach for back pain patients reporting substantial fear of movement/ (re)injury.

GRADED *IN VIVO* EXPOSURE VERSUS GRADED ACTIVITY

From a distance, graded *in vivo* exposure may appear to be quite similar to the usual graded activity programs[27*,28**] in that it gradually increases activity levels despite pain. However, both conceptually and practically, exposure *in vivo* is quite different from graded activity. First, graded activity is based on instrumental learning principles, and selected health behaviors are shaped through positively reinforcing predefined quota of activities. Exposure *in vivo*, originally based on extinction of pavlovian conditioning,[29] is currently viewed as a cognitive process during which fear is activated and catastrophic expectations are being challenged and disconfirmed, resulting in reductions in the threat value of the originally fearful stimuli. Second, during graded activity, special attention goes to the identification of positive reinforcers that can be provided when the individual quotas are met, whereas graded exposure pays special attention to the establishment of an individual hierarchy of the pain-related fear stimuli. Third, usual graded activity programs include individual exercises according to functional capacity and observed individual physical work demands, while graded exposure includes activities that are selected based on the fear hierarchy and the idiosyncratic aspects of the fear stimuli. For example, if the patient fears the repetitive spinal compression produced by riding a bicycle on a bumpy road, then the graded exposure should include an activity that mimics that specific activity and not just a stationary bicycle.

According to the suggestions made by Butler[30] for the cognitive–behavioral treatment of phobic disorders, and Turner[31] for the application of behavioral interventions of back pain in primary care, we suggest that the intervention generally be designed in three steps: cognitive–behavioral assessment, education, and exposure with behavioral experiments.

COGNITIVE–BEHAVIORAL ASSESSMENT

In this section, we will deal with specific questionnaires, the interview, the establishment of graded hierarchies, and the behavioral tests that can be applied in order to gain sufficient information about the idiosyncratic aspects of pain-related fear responses in patients with chronic musculoskeletal pain.

Specific questionnaires

A basic question that may be asked is what the patient is afraid of or, in other words, what is the nature of the perceived threat? An answer to this question is not as simple as it seems. Patients may not view their problem as involving fear at all and may simply see difficulty in performing certain movements or activities. In addition, the specific nature of pain-related fear varies considerably, making an idiosyncratic approach almost indispensable. Some patients fear pain. Other patients may fear not so much current pain but pain that will be experienced at a later time, e.g. the day after a physical exercise. Finally, patients may not fear pain itself, but the impending (re)injury that it is supposed to indicate, or they fear becoming permanently handicapped. The literature reflects this variety of fear stimuli by discussing measures for the assessment of fear of pain, fear of work and physical activity, and fear of (re)injury as a result of movement.

Fear of pain

- An early attempt to assess fear of pain is the Pain and Impairment Relationship Scale (PAIRS), which was developed to study chronic pain patients' attitudes concerning activity and pain.[32] The scale has 15 items which are rated on seven-point Likert scales, and it has been found to have good psychometric characteristics. The original study demonstrated that beliefs that activity would increase pain were related to physical impairment.
- The Fear of Pain Questionnaire (FPQ[33]) consists of 30 items concerning fear of minor pains (biting on one's tongue during eating), severe pains (breaking an arm), and medical pain (such as pain caused by a syringe). The scale has shown good reliability. Criterion validity is supported by high correlations with pain catastrophizing and pain ratings during a cold pressor test.
- In 1992, the Pain Anxiety Symptoms Scale (PASS[34]) was developed to measure cognitive anxiety symptoms, escape and avoidance responses, fearful appraisals of pain, and physiologic anxiety symptoms related to pain. It is a 40-item questionnaire with internally consistent subscales. The validity of the PASS has been supported by positive correlations with measures of anxiety, cognitive errors, depression, and disability. A more recent exploratory factor analysis revealed five factors which could be labeled as catastrophic: thoughts, physiological anxiety symptoms, escape/avoidance behaviors, cognitive interference, and coping strategies.[35]

Fear of work-related activities

- The *Fear-Avoidance Beliefs Questionnaire* (FABQ[16]) focuses on the patient's beliefs about how work and physical activity affect his/her low back pain. The FABQ consists of two scales: fear-avoidance beliefs of physical activity and fear-avoidance beliefs of work, the latter being consistently the stronger. The authors found that fear-avoidance beliefs about work are strongly related to disability of daily living and work lost in the past year; this was not the case for biomedical variables such as anatomical pattern of pain, time pattern, and severity of pain. On the other hand, the FABQ physical subscale is much stronger in predicting behavioral performance tests.[15]

Fear of movement/(re)injury

- The *Survey of Pain Attitudes* (SOPA[36]) was developed to assess patients' attitudes towards five dimensions of the chronic pain experience: pain control, pain-related disability, medical cures for pain, solicitude of others, and medication for pain. Because of the authors' clinical observation of an association between chronic patients' hesitancy to exercise and the expressed fear of possible injury, a new scale (Harm) was added to the original instrument. As well as the Disability Scale and the Control Scale, the Harm Scale appeared to independently predict levels of dysfunction.
- The *Tampa Scale for Kinesiophobia* (TSK[37]) is a 17-item questionnaire that is aimed at the assessment of fear of (re)injury due to movement. Each item is provided with a Likert scale, with scoring alternatives ranging from "strongly agree" to "strongly disagree." Most psychometric research has been carried out with the Dutch version of the TSK, which appears to be sufficiently reliable ($\alpha = 0.77$) and valid.[2] Modest but significant correlations were found with measures of pain intensity, catastrophizing, impact of pain on daily life activities, and generalized fear. Regression analyses revealed that levels of disability were best predicted by pain-related fear, and that this was best predicted by catastrophizing. Pain intensity levels and biomedical findings were significantly less predictive of both pain-related fear and disability levels.[3] Moreover, the TSK discriminated well between avoiders and confronters during a behavioral performance task.[2,15] A factor analysis revealed four nonorthogonal factors, to which the following labels were assigned: harm, fear of (re)injury, importance of exercise, avoidance of activity.[3] Because of the relatively high intercorrelations among the subscales and the more favorable internal consistency and construct validity of the TSK total score, the TSK total score is preferable to the subscales.

In sum, questionnaires for the assessment of pain-related fear are now available, although the validity of some of them need to be further explored. For clinical purposes, these questionnaires seem to be appropriate as a first screening to identify patients who suffer excessive pain-related fear. However, the questionnaires do not tell us what the individual is exactly fearful of.

Interview

General issues

For elevated scores, the above-mentioned fear questionnaires are only indicative of the presence of pain-related fear. The assessment should be continued to further validate the hypothesis that the patient's disability is mainly determined by these fears. The semistructured interview is an additional and important tool to obtain information about the behavioral, psychophysiological, and cognitive aspects of the symptoms and to better estimate the role of pain-related fear in the maintenance of the pain problem (see Box 14.1). It also includes information about the antecedents (situational or internal) of the pain-related fear, and about the direct and indirect consequences. This screening might also include other areas of life stresses, as they might increase arousal levels and indirectly fuel pain-related fear. The etiologic model (Fig. 14.1) is shown to be a useful model that the clinician can keep in mind during the interview. Factors that often seem to be associated with the development of the fear are the characteristics of pain onset and the ambiguity around the presence or absence of positive findings on medicodiagnostics. For example, a person involved in a traffic accident may develop a fear of driving as a result of the traumatic experience. Likewise, a back pain patient may develop a fear of lifting after experiencing pain while lifting or after receiving information from a medical doctor that lifting can damage nerves in the spinal cord. Of interest is that CLBP patients who retrospectively reported a sudden traumatic

---

Box 14.1 *Items addressed during the interview*

1. What does your pain feel like?
2. When did the pain start?
3. What were the circumstances of the pain onset?
4. If there was a sudden pain onset, what did you do, feel, and think at that moment?
5. What are you not doing because of the pain problem?
6. What do you think is causing your pain?
7. What do you think will happen in the near future if the pain remains untreated?
8. What is the influence of deep relaxation on your pain?

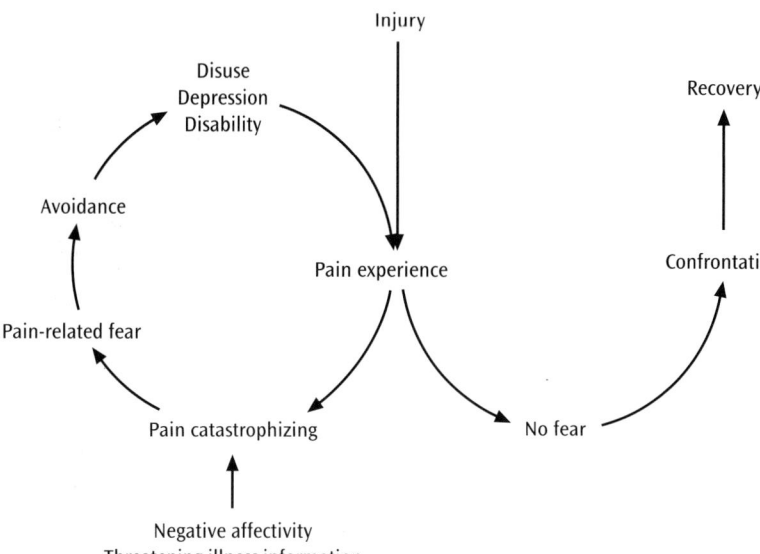

Figure 14.1 *The cognitive–behavioral model of pain-related fear (based on Vlaeyen and Linton,[9] with permission).*

pain onset scored higher on the TSK than patients who had reported that the pain complaints started gradually. Most chronic back pain patients who present with pain-related fear appear to base their conviction about vulnerability to (re)injury on the results of diagnostics tests such as radiographs and magnetic resonance imaging (MRI). The combination of (threatening) information conveyed by the medical specialist and the experience of pain and discomfort seem to strengthen that conviction. The visual confrontation with the radiographs and just hearing the diagnosis can be quite upsetting to some patients, as this information may be interpreted as being more threatening than intended by the specialist.

Although reports about misconceptions and misinterpretations of information can be used during the educational part of the intervention, it is more useful to identify the current level of severity and the maintaining factors of the pain problem and associated pain-related fear. The severity can often be estimated by inquiring about the extent to which the pain problem interferes with daily life, including the ability to carry on paid work, leisure activities, and normal relationships. Maintaining factors usually are negative thoughts about the danger of the physical activities, the avoidance of these activities, and hypervigilance to signals of threat. Negative thoughts can be elicited by inquiring about the client's personal theory about his pain and associated functional incapacity. Expectations about the future are also worth inquiring about: "What do you think will happen if the pain is left untreated?" For example, the back and pelvic pain complaints of a female patient started during her first pregnancy and increased after the delivery. She started worrying about the future because a relative who had received the same diagnosis finally became wheelchair bound. Her main belief was that during certain movements the tissue and nerves around the ridged symphysis pubis could be damaged or ruptured, possibly resulting in

paralysis of the lower limbs. In most cases, these thoughts make people alert to bodily sensations that may signal impending danger. Situations that provoke these sensations are fearfully avoided. To gain insight into avoidance behaviors, the therapist may ask questions such as "What does the pain prevent you from doing?" and "If you no longer had this pain problem, what differences would it make to your daily life?" One can also ask directly about the situations that may worsen the pain problem. Finally, the assessment should also clarify whether other problems such as major depression, marital conflicts, or disability claims warrant specific attention before or after treatment. If more complicated problems are expected to arise as the pain problem diminishes, it may be better to leave the pain problem untreated.

Determining treatment goals

There are several reasons why it is wise to spend some time on the determination of treatment goals.[38] First, cognitive–behavioral treatments for pain, including exposure *in vivo*, never aim at the reduction of pain but at the restoration of functional abilities despite pain. It helps to make this general goal explicit, and both patient and therapist should agree on one or more realistic and specific goals that are formulated in positive terms. Typical examples are being able to go shopping to the supermarket alone or go swimming twice a week for half an hour. In cases where the goal is to return to work, it may be wise to consult with the occupational physician or vocational counselor. Often, the exposure treatment can be synchronized with a graded resumption of work activities. Second, setting goals also helps to structure the treatment and to design the hierarchy of stimuli that will be introduced during the actual exposure *in vivo*. For example, if a patient wishes to resume his sports activities, the therapist will make sure that aspects of these will be included in the graded exposure activities. Third, setting functional goals also redirects the focus of attention from pain and physical symptoms toward daily life activities with the emphasis on the possibility of change away from the disability status. Finally, as the patient is invited to formulate his or her own goals, goal setting inadvertently reinforces the notion that active participation is an essential part of the treatment.

Graded hierarchies

Once it has become clear that pain-related fear is pivotal in the maintenance of a person's pain disability, it is useful to inquire about the essential stimuli: What is the patient actually afraid of? So far, there is a lack of standardized tools for identifying these stimuli. In our experience, it is quite difficult for pain patients to verbally estimate the threat value of different situations. One of the problems is that the avoidance behaviors are not really acknowledged to be the consequences of fear but to be a direct consequence of the pain and the experienced vulnerability for (re)injury. In addition to checklists of daily activities, the presentation of visual materials such as pictures of back-stressing activities and movements might be worthwhile. They can be quite helpful in the development of graded hierarchies, reflecting the full range of situations avoided by the patient, beginning with those that provoke only mild discomfort and ending with activities or situations that are beyond the patient's present abilities. The Photograph Series of Daily Activities (PHODA[39]) is a standardized method that appears to be appropriate to design graded hierarchies. PHODA uses 98 photographs representing various physical daily life activities, including lifting, bending, walking, bicycling, etc., that are presented to the patients, who are requested to place each photograph along a fear thermometer. (A CD-rom version of PHODA, including 98 pictures and a brief manual, is available and can be requested from phoda@hszuyd.nl) This scale consists of a vertical line with 11 anchor points (ranging from 0 to 100) printed on a piece of cardboard that measures 60 cm × 40 cm (Fig. 14.2). The fear thermometer is placed on a table in front of the patient with the following instruction: "Please look at each photograph carefully, and try to imagine yourself performing the same movement. Place the photograph on the thermometer according to the extent to which you feel that this movement is harmful to your back." In our experience, abrupt changes in movement (e.g. suddenly being hit) or activities consisting of repetitive spinal compressions (riding a bicycle on a bumpy road) are frequently mentioned stimuli in chronic back pain patients who score high for pain-related fear measures. These situations are feared because of beliefs about the causes of pain, such as ruptured or severely damaged nerves: "If I lift heavy weights, the nerves in my back might be damaged." For examples of a graded hierarchy, see Tables 14.1 and 14.3. Also of interest

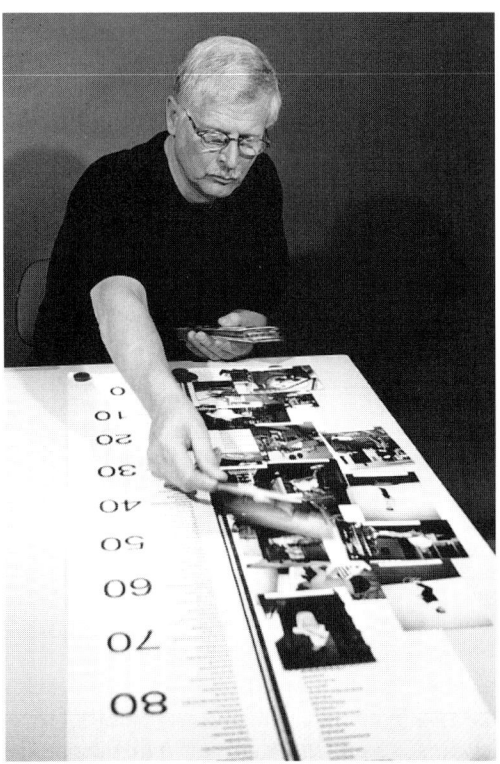

Figure 14.2 *The use of PHODA[39] in establishing fear hierarchy.*

is that the same activity can be rated differently depending on the context in which the activity is performed. For example, the activity "running" receives an 80 when performed in a wood, and 50 when performed on an even terrain. It is therefore a good idea to expose patients to physical activities in a variety of contexts.

Behavioral tests

Sometimes, patients find it hard to estimate the harmfulness of an activity when it has been avoided extensively. In such cases, behavioral tests can be introduced. They consist of performing an activity that has been avoided previously while performance indices (such as time, distance, or number of repetitions) are measured. Target behaviors can be derived from the PHODA items, and in most cases the behavioral tests can be considered as a variant of the exercise tolerance test described by Fordyce.[40] To assess the extent to which avoidance occurs, patients are asked to perform the activity "… until pain, weakness, fatigue or any other reason causes you to wish to stop" (reference 40, p. 170). Behavioral tests have the advantage that anticipatory anxiety and the anxiety during exposure can be measured separately.[30] In addition, they provide a more objective measure of avoidance behavior.

EDUCATION

The first session of graded exposure *in vivo* always consists of unambiguously educating the patient in a way that the patient views their pain as a common condition that can be self-managed, rather than as a serious disease or a condition that needs careful protection. The aim is to correct the misinterpretations and misconceptions that have occurred early on during the development of the pain-related fear. Each patient is given a careful explanation of the fear-avoidance model, using the patient's individual symptoms, beliefs, and behaviors to illustrate how vicious circles (pain → catastrophic thought → fear → avoidance → disability → pain) maintain the pain problem. In cases where the pain-related fear appears to be fuelled by having a ("positive") diagnostic test, it may be useful to review these tests together with a physician. It can be explained to patients that they probably have overestimated the value of these tests, and that in symptom-free people similar abnormalities can also be found. One of the effects of this education is that it increases the patient's willingness to finally engage in activities that they have been avoiding for a long time. Additionally, the provision of a more fluid, less localized understanding of pain could provide a greater sense of legitimacy for the pain in the absence of positive test results.[41]

EXPOSURE *IN VIVO*

Exposure

Current treatments of excessive fears and anxiety are based on the experimental psychological work of Wolpe,[42] who reported on systematic desensitization. In this keystone treatment method, individuals progress through increasingly more anxiety-provoking encounters with phobic stimuli while utilizing relaxation as a reciprocal inhibitor of rising anxiety. Because relaxation was intended to compete with the anxiety response, a graded format was chosen to keep anxiety levels as weak as possible. Later studies revealed that exposure to the feared stimuli appeared to be the most essential component of the systematic desensitization, and when applied without relaxation produced similar effects.[43] For a fearful patient, experiencing first-hand the results of changes in their behavior is far more convincing than rational argument; therefore, the most essential step consists of graded exposure to the situations that the patient has identified as "dangerous" or "threatening." Subsequently, individually tailored practice tasks are developed based on the graded hierarchy of fear-eliciting situations, thereby following the general principles for exposure. The patient agrees to perform certain activities or movements that they used to avoid. Patients are also encouraged to engage in these fearful activities as much as possible until anxiety levels have decreased. Each activity or movement is first modeled by the therapist, who demonstrates how the activity can be performed in the most ergonomically efficient manner. The presence of the therapist, who may initially encourage further exposures, is gradually withdrawn to facilitate independence and to create contexts that mimic those of the home situation.

Behavioral experiments

Following on from cognitive theory, which assumes that cognitive "errors" can be corrected through conscious reasoning, behavioral experiments have been developed for which the basis is a collaborative empiricism. The essence of a behavioral experiment is that the patient performs an activity to challenge the validity of his catastrophic expectations and misinterpretations. These interpretations take the form of "if … then …" statements, and are empirically tested during a behavioral experiment. Three steps can be distinguished. First, the patient formulates a hypothesis, e.g. a back pain patient may expect that jumping down from a stair will inevitably cause nerve damage in the spine and excruciating pain. Second, an experiment is designed, e.g. if the patient is convinced that jumping down is harmful then the therapist can further inquire about the minimal height that is needed to cause nerve injury. Finally, the experiment is carried out and evaluated. The therapist invites the patient to jump down from the stair and the consequences are assessed (see Box 14.2). In practice, behavioral experiments are difficult to separate from mere exposure, and they can best be used simultaneously.

Case illustrations

Although many patients with chronic musculoskeletal pain have similar fears (fear of physical activities that produce pain or that are assumed to cause reinjury), the origin of their fears may be different. Rachman suggested three pathways for the acquisition of excessive fears: direct trauma (classical conditioning), vicarious observation (social learning), and informational transmission. Each of these can be recognized in the pain histories of fearful patients who seek treatment at our center. We will describe two patients, one of whom developed fear as a result of direct trauma and one as a result of informational transmission.

Ms X was a 40-year-old married woman who worked for a cleaning service. Her pain started 5 years before referral to the rehabilitation center while lifting a trash bag and throwing it into a big container. During this movement, she heard a "crack" in her lower back, immediately followed by a "shooting" pain. She was very frightened that she might have injured herself seriously because she had never felt anything similar and did not understand what was going on. The smallest movement was very painful. From then on, she experienced about four to six of these "cracks" a day, which she interpreted as signs of tissue or nerve damage. She could almost predict which movements provoked these frightening cracks, and tried to avoid them as much as possible. She had been told by different specialists and therapists that these cracks were not normal and she was afraid of becoming paralyzed. For 3 years, she took part in numerous sessions of physical therapy, but without much success. Finally, she was referred to the rehabilitation center for a comprehensive assessment and treatment program.

The exposure part of the program consisted of nine sessions, each lasting about 60–90 min, spread over 3 weeks. During the educational part, it was made clear to the patient that "cracks" may occur without causing damage, and the vicious circle was explained with the message that she was suffering from excessive avoidance behavior because of her misbelief that "cracks" are dangerous. Table 14.1 gives an overview of the graded hierarchy based on PHODA. One of the essential stimuli was bending forward, and we chose to start the exposure with simply bending at the knees and coming up again by putting small objects on the floor and picking them up. Before each trial, the patient's expectations of pain and harm were noted, and after the actual performance the experienced pain and harm were evaluated (Table 14.2). Gradually, the activities became physically more intense.

During the last sessions, Ms X was bicycling over rough terrain, jumping from a 75-cm-high stool, playing badminton, and performing all of the daily household chores. Because Ms X was included in a controlled outcome study, the exposure treatment was followed by a period of graded activity of equal length.

Ms Y was a 35-year-old married woman whose back and pelvic pain complaints started during her first pregnancy, 6 years ago, and increased after the delivery. After a second and third pregnancy, her pain complaints increased, and she remained unable to carry out a number of daily activities. An orthopedic assessment was performed and radiographs of the pelvis showed a ridged symphysis pubis and a pelvic instability. The visual confrontation with the radiographs was upsetting to her, and she became quite worried after hearing the diagnosis. She started worrying about the future because a relative who had received the same diagnosis finally became wheelchair bound. Her main belief was that during certain movements the tissue and nerves around the ridged symphysis pubis could be damaged or ruptured, possibly resulting in paralysis of the lower limbs.

During the educational part of the program, the rehabilitation physician explained to her that the so-called abnormal findings on the radiographs were, in fact, not unusual and were often seen in asymptomatic people. When the physician reviewed the radiographs with her, Ms Y preferred not to look at them, and revealed that she found these and other images of body parts very repulsive. Using a three-dimensional model of the spine, the

Table 14.1 *Graded hierarchy of pain-related fear stimuli for Ms X*

Pretreatment hierarchy	(PHODA) item	Post-treatment PHODA score
100	Throwing a trash bag	0
90	Lifting a child from squat	20
80	–	–
70	Making up the bed	0
60	Mopping the floor	10
50	Carrying a shopping bag on both arms	0
40	–	–
30	Rolling over in bed	0
20	Walking up and down stairs	0
10	Hanging out something on the clothes line	0

Table 14.2 *Graded hierarchy of pain-related fear stimuli for Ms Y*

Pretreatment hierarchy	(PHODA) item	Post-treatment PHODA score
100	Carrying a small child on the shoulders	10
90	Raking leaves into a heap	20
80	Lifting a laundry basket	0
70	Riding off a curbstone with a bicycle	0
60	Lacing one's shoes while bending forward	10
50	Washing the dishes	0
40	–	–
30	Making up the bed	20
20	Emptying a dishwasher	0
10	Hanging something on a coat hook	0

physician explained to her that her strongest fear, i.e. becoming paralyzed by a ruptured symphysis or displacement of disks because of movement, could never happen in daily life. Although Ms Y seemed reassured, she was not totally convinced. The therapist subsequently proposed to test the activity–harm assumption by exposing her to the activities that she had fearfully avoided. Box 14.2 displays the graded hierarchy based on PHODA. Because Ms Y was included in a controlled outcome study, the exposure treatment was preceded by a period of graded activity of equal length. The treatment course was quite similar to that of Ms X, with a steep decrease in levels of fear and catastrophizing.

Complicating factors

Pain increases

Although patients have agreed that the treatment is not primarily aimed at reducing pain levels, it is very frightening to experience a sudden pain attack during the exposure treatment. This is what happened to Ms Z, a 46-year-old woman with chronic low back pain, who was given a regular rehabilitation program of mainly exercise therapy without success. Half-way through the treatment, Ms Z was discharged because "she appeared not to be motivated." One year later, she was again referred to the hospital, and because of her elevated score on the TSK she

---

Box 14.2 *Dialogue between Ms X and therapist during a behavioral experiment*

Therapist:	OK, today we'll start with the next activity. Why don't we try lifting this empty crate. What do you think?
Patient:	[sighs] I don't think I can manage that.
Therapist:	What do you think might happen?
Patient:	I'm sure I'll get more pain. The disks in my back can't take such pressure. It may further damage the nerves there.
Therapist:	How would you notice this?
Patient:	My back will collapse, I won't be able to stand, and I may become paralyzed.
Therapist:	How likely is it that this will happen when lifting this crate, on a scale 0 (not likely) to 100 (very likely)?
Patient:	I am not sure, around 70.
Therapist:	OK, well why don't we try and see what happens. I'll do it first, and then it's your turn. [At this point the therapist models the lifting task, and invites the patient to do the same, and while the patient is holding the case the therapist goes on inquiring about what happens.]
Therapist:	Good. You're doing very well. How did it go?
Patient:	OK, I guess. It did hurt somewhat, but my back could hold it quite well. It did not collapse.
Therapist:	Right, despite the pain, you managed to lift this crate, right? Suppose we do this again, how would you rate the chances of your becoming paralyzed?
Patient:	Well, I would say a 40, but there was no crack.
Therapist:	Would the situation be different if you had felt a crack?
Patient:	Oh yes, definitely.
Therapist:	How could we induce such a crack.
Patient:	When I was still working, I usually carried heavier weights than the one I just lifted.
Therapist:	Shall we make this one a bit heavier?
Patient:	[Laughs nervously] OK then.
Therapist:	OK, go ahead and add more bottles. [The patient fills the whole case with bottles. After that, the therapist models the activity before the patient attempts it herself.]
Therapist:	Did you feel a crack?
Patient:	Not really, but, you know, suppose I should turn to this side [left] while lifting – that would make the situation much more dangerous.
Therapist:	OK, is that worrying you more than lifting objects?
Patient:	I think so, yes.

By doing this behavioral experiment, a new stimulus is introduced: rotating while lifting. At this point, the therapist invites the patient to show what she means by rotating. Thereafter, a new behavioral experiment is carried out incorporating this new stimulus, and the process of challenging expectations is repeated over again.

was then offered an *in vivo* exposure treatment, which she accepted. A graded hierarchy was planned, she agreed to keep daily measurements of her levels of fear, catastrophizing, and pain intensity, and the various physical activities were successfully approached. Of interest was that her current pain level decreased almost synonymously with her fear ratings (Fig. 14.3). Before starting the fifth session, she complained of a severe, sharp pain that struck her in the morning while getting out of bed. She described this event as being very similar to the beginning of her pain problem. She was quite worried that this again was a sign of something being seriously wrong in her back. Her major concern was that too much movement would only worsen the situation, and she suggested that she should not take part in the program that day. The therapist briefly explored the circumstances of the pain attack and concluded with the patient that there was no reason for further medical examination. Ms Z did not think that this attack was caused by her increased activity level, and both she and the therapist decided to continue with the treatment and chose badminton for the activity as Ms Z liked it very much. As Ms Z experienced no increase in her pain during this activity, she gradually became more confident, and the session was completed almost as planned. It is clear from Fig. 14.3, which shows the patient's daily ratings of pain and fear, that after 4 days the ratings were back down again.

Maintenance of change

Expanding contexts

What is actually learned during exposure? Although some researchers assume that exposure leads to a disconfirmation of overpredictions of the aversive characteristics of fear stimuli, there is growing evidence that exposure cannot simply be equated with unlearning. Studies have demonstrated that a competition occurs between the original threatening (excitatory) meaning of the stimuli and a new (inhibitory) meaning. In other words, during successful exposure, exceptions to the rule are learned rather

than a fundamental change of that rule.[29] Crombez *et al.*[44] showed that, in chronic low back pain patients, exposure to one movement (bending forward) did not generalize toward another dissimilar movement (straight leg raising). This pattern of results was only characteristic for high pain catastrophizers. The treatment implications of these findings are lengthy exposures to the full variety of contexts and natural settings in which fear has been experienced. PHODA might be a useful tool in eliciting information about these contexts in chronic pain patients.

Other forms of exposure

The form of graded *in vivo* exposure described above is specifically developed for patients with chronic musculoskeletal pain, particularly back pain, who are moderately to severely disabled and who report substantial pain-related fear. Nevertheless, one has to bear in mind that the literature on the cognitive–behavioral treatment of phobias describes several variations in the way exposure can be conducted, of which most have not been systematically evaluated. One could, for example, consider imaginal exposure or exposure using virtual reality instead of *in vivo*. Patients with an ability to create vivid images may be asked to imagine themselves performing the "harmful" physical activities they tend to avoid. Instead of the massed version we described above (once every day for several weeks), a spaced version (one every week for several months) may also be an option. Rather than approaching the fearful stimuli in a graded fashion, an interesting question is to what extent the process of change would be accelerated by directly exposing patients to the most intensely feared stimuli. Finally, the treatment would be made more accessible to a larger group of patients if self-exposure, with a manual, were as effective as the therapist-guided exposure we describe here. The reason we have chosen graded exposure with the aid of a therapist is that, based on our experience, it would provide the most credible, safe, and effective treatment approach.

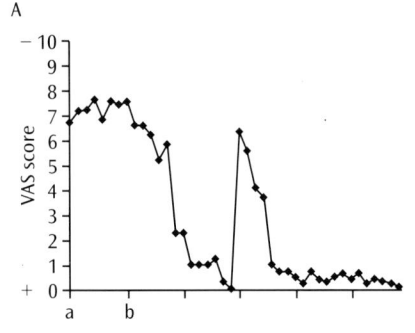
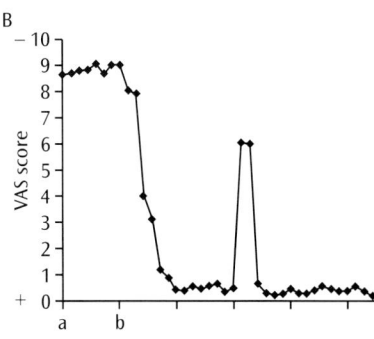

Figure 14.3 *Daily measures of fear of pain severity (A; visual analog scale) and movement/(re)injury (B) for subject Z across baseline and exposure* in vivo. *a, start baseline; b, start exposure* in vivo.

EFFECTIVENESS

Despite the fact that the importance of pain-related fear continued to be highlighted by behavioral theorists, empirical investigations including clinical outcome studies lagged behind theoretical thinking. We recently conducted two empirical studies to examine the effectiveness of a graded *in vivo* exposure treatment with behavioral experiments compared with the usual graded activity in reducing pain-related fears, catastrophizing, and pain disability in CLBP patients reporting substantial fear of movement/(re)injury.[45,*46*] A replicated single-case crossover design was applied, one with four and one with six consecutive CLBP patients. Only patients who reported substantial fear of movement/(re)injury (TSK score > 40), and who were referred for outpatient behavioral rehabilitation, were included. After a no-treatment baseline measurement period, the patients were randomly assigned to one of two interventions. In intervention A, patients received the exposure first, followed by graded activity. In intervention B, the sequence of treatment modules was reversed. Daily measures of pain-related cognitions and fears were recorded using visual analog scales. Before and after the treatment, the following measures were taken: pain-related fear, pain catastrophizing, pain control, and pain disability.

Figure 14.4 displays the daily measures for fear of movement/(re)injury, fear of pain, and pain catastro-

phizing. Although the supplemental value of this "background" treatment program cannot be ruled out in this study, the remarkable improvements that are observed whenever the graded exposure was initiated suggests that the therapeutic power of the graded exposure is much stronger. The crossover design gave us the opportunity to examine the differential effects of graded exposure and graded activity and also the additional treatment effect of the second treatment module. As the order of treatment modules did not make any difference to the final outcome, no such effect was found in this study. On the other hand, carryover effects were clearly observed when graded exposure was followed by graded activity. What can be said about the possible mediators of treatment effects? The treatment duration was much too short to produce significant increases in muscle strength. The abrupt change in the daily measures is suggestive of cognitive changes. Although the exposure lasted for a period of 3 weeks, the reduction in catastrophizing and fear was achieved within 7 days, or three exposure sessions. Rachman and Whittal[47] proposed that such abrupt changes are more characteristic of insight learning, rather than the usual gradual progression of trial and error learning. In our study, the presentation of the rationale at the start of the exposure might have contributed to this insight. Many patients reported that, for the first time, they received a credible rationale for their current level of disability.

Although these first results are quite promising, there

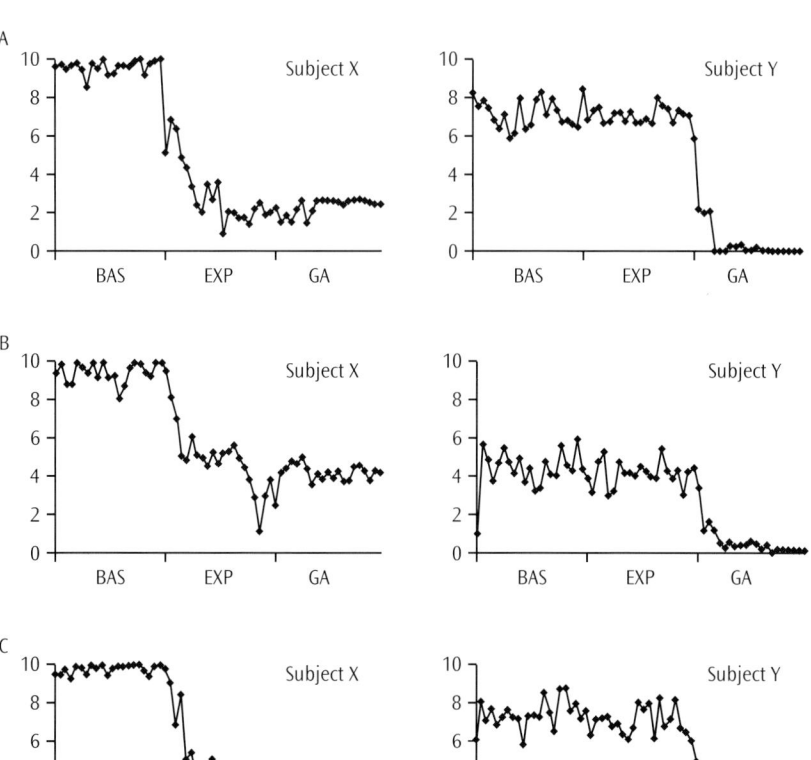

Figure 14.4 *Daily measures of fear of movement/(re)injury for subjects X and Y across baseline (days 0–21) and both treatment modes (days 22–42 and days 43–63). A, fear of movement/(re)injury; B, fear of pain; C, pain catastrophizing. BAS, baseline; EXP, exposure in vivo; GA, graded activity (based on Vlaeyen et al.,[45] with permission from Elsevier, BV).*

are a number of caveats to be considered. First, the preliminary evidence reported here is limited in that it included a small number of patients. On the other hand, a single-case experimental design was chosen with appropriate time series statistical analyses. In the crossover design, all patients received both interventions; therefore, long-term differential effects could not be established. Replication studies in the form of randomized controlled trials using larger samples and long-term follow-up measurements are warranted.

SUMMARY

"Fear of pain and what we do about it may be more disabling than pain itself" (reference 16, p. 164). According to this statement, the intuitively appealing idea that the lowered ability to accomplish tasks of daily living in chronic pain patients is merely the consequence of pain severity is refuted. The recent literature supports the early conjecture that chronic pain and phobia share important characteristics. Indeed, studies have shown that, during confrontation with feared movements, CLBP patients who are fearful of movement/(re)injury typically show psychophysiological (muscle reactivity), behavioral (escape and avoidance), and cognitive (worry) responses. It was not until recently that this line of thought was extended to the behavioral assessment and management of chronic pain. Specific pain-related fear measures, by which pain patients whose level of disability is likely to be controlled by pain-related fears, have been developed. As a result, a screening questionnaire that is aimed at the identification of acute back pain patients at risk has been developed for use in primary care and includes several items about fear and avoidance.[48,49] In addition, the cognitive-behavioral assessment also includes the semistructured interview, the development of graded hierarchies, and the application of behavioral tests. This chapter describes an *in vivo* exposure treatment for the reduction of pain-related fear in CLBP patients. Preliminary outcome data show that an exposure *in vivo* consists of individually tailored practice tasks based on a graded hierarchy of fear-eliciting situations, and not just a physical training program or usual graded activity that does not take into account these essential and idiosyncratic fear stimuli. These data also show that exposure *in vivo* may help the patient to confront rather than avoid physical movement, and that a reduction in self-reported disability levels follows. Although cognitive–behavioral treatments for chronic pain are quite favorable,[50**] there is an urgent need for further refinement of our treatments, including a better match between treatment modalities and patient characteristics. The approach described in this chapter may contribute to the process of customization of cognitive–behavioral treatments in the care of chronic pain patients.

Acknowledgments The authors wish to thank Mario Geilen, Herman Mulder, Noel Dortu, and the staff at the Department of Pain Rehabilitation of the Hoensbroeck Rehabilitation Center for their contribution in making the application of the exposure treatment possible. This contribution is supported by grant 904–65–090 from the Council for Medical and Health Research of the Netherlands (NWO-MW) to the first author.

REFERENCES

◆ 1. Lethem J, Slade PD, Troup JD, Bentley G. Outline of a fear-avoidance model of exaggerated pain perception. I. *Behav Res Ther* 1983; **21:** 401–8.

◆ 2. Vlaeyen JW, Kole-Snijders AM, Boeren RG, van Eek H. Fear of movement/(re)injury in chronic low back pain and its relation to behavioral performance. *Pain* 1995; **62:** 363–72.

3. Vlaeyen JWS, Kole Snijders AMJ, Rotteveel AM, *et al*. The role of fear of movement/(re)injury in pain disability. *J Occup Rehabil* 1995; **5:** 235–52.

◆ 4. Philips HC. Avoidance behaviour and its role in sustaining chronic pain. *Behav Res Ther* 1987; **25:** 273–9.

5. Klenerman L, Slade PD, Stanley IM, *et al*. The prediction of chronicity in patients with an acute attack of low back pain in a general practice setting. *Spine* 1995; **20:** 478–84.

6. Linton SJ, Buer N, Vlaeyen JWS, Hellsing A-L. Are fear-avoidance beliefs related to the inception of an episode of back pain? A prospective study. *Psychol Health* 2000; **14:** 1051–9.

◆ 7. Kori SH, Miller RP, Todd DD. Kinesiophobia: a new view of chronic pain behavior. *Pain Manage* 1990; **Jan/Feb:** 35–43.

◆ 8. Asmundson GJ, Norton PJ, Norton GR. Beyond pain: the role of fear and avoidance in chronicity. *Clin Psychol Rev* 1999; **19:** 97–119.

◆ 9. Vlaeyen JW, Linton SJ. Fear-avoidance and its consequences in chronic musculoskeletal pain: a state of the art. *Pain* 2000; **85:** 317–32.

10. Sullivan MJL, Bishop SR, Pivik J. The pain catastrophizing scale: development and validation. *Psychol Assess* 1995; **7:** 524–32.

11. Crombez G, Eccleston C, Baeyens F, Eelen P. When somatic information threatens, catastrophic thinking enhances attentional interference. *Pain* 1998; **75:** 187–98.

12. McCracken LM, Gross RT. Does anxiety affect coping with chronic pain? *Clin J Pain* 1993; **9:** 253–9.

13. Vlaeyen JW, Seelen HA, Peters M, *et al*. Fear of movement/(re)injury and muscular reactivity in chronic low back pain patients: an experimental investigation. *Pain* 1999; **82:** 297–304.

14. Cipher DJ, Fernandez E. Expectancy variables predicting tolerance and avoidance of pain in chronic pain patients. *Behav Res Ther* 1997; **35:** 437–44.

◆ 15. Crombez G, Vlaeyen JW, Heuts PH, Lysens R. Pain-related fear is more disabling than pain itself: evidence on the role of pain-related fear in chronic back pain disability. *Pain* 1999; **80:** 329–39.

◆ 16. Waddell G, Newton M, Henderson I, *et al.* A Fear-Avoidance Beliefs Questionnaire (FABQ) and the role of fear-avoidance beliefs in chronic low back pain and disability. *Pain* 1993; **52:** 157–68.

17. Eysenck MW. *Anxiety and Cognition. A Unified Theory.* Hove: Psychology Press, 1997.

18. Pearce J, Morley S. An experimental investigation of the construct validity of the McGill Pain Questionnaire. *Pain* 1989; **39:** 115–21.

19. Asmundson GJ, Kuperos JL, Norton GR. Do patients with chronic pain selectively attend to pain-related information?: preliminary evidence for the mediating role of fear. *Pain* 1997; **72:** 27–32.

20. Crombez G, Vervaet L, Lysens R, *et al.* Avoidance and confrontation of painful, back-straining movements in chronic back pain patients. *Behav Modif* 1998; **22:** 62–77.

◆ 21. McCracken LM. "Attention" to pain in persons with chronic pain: a behavioral approach. *Behav Ther* 1997; **28:** 271–81.

22. Peters ML, Vlaeyen JW, van Drunen C. Do fibromyalgia patients display hypervigilance for innocuous somatosensory stimuli? Application of a body scanning reaction time paradigm. *Pain* 2000; **86:** 283–92.

23. Eccleston C, Crombez G, Aldrich S, Stannard C. Attention and somatic awareness in chronic pain. *Pain* 1997; **72:** 209–15.

24. Crombez G, Eccleston C, Baeyens F, *et al.* Attention to chronic pain is dependent upon pain-related fear. *J Psychosom Res* 1999; **47:** 403–10.

25. Rachman S. The overprediction of fear: a review. *Behav Res Ther* 1994; **32:** 683–90.

26. Crombez G, Vervaet L, Baeyens F, *et al.* Do pain expectancies cause pain in chronic low back patients? A clinical investigation. *Behav Res Ther* 1996; **34:** 919–25.

27. Fordyce WE, Brockway JA, Bergman JA, Spengler D. Acute back pain: a control-group comparison of behavioral vs traditional management methods. *J Behav Med* 1986; **9:** 127–40.

28. Lindstrom I, Ohlund C, Eek C, *et al.* The effect of graded activity on patients with subacute low back pain: a randomized prospective clinical study with an operant-conditioning behavioral approach. *Phys Ther* 1992; **72:** 279–90; Discussion 291–3.

29. Bouton ME. Context and ambiguity in the extinction of emotional learning: implications for exposure therapy. *Behav Res Ther* 1988; **26:** 137–49.

30. Butler G. Phobic disorders. In: Hawton K, Salkovskis PM, Kirk J, Clark DM eds. *Cognitive Behaviour Therapy for Psychiatric Problems. A Practical Guide.* Oxford: Oxford University Press, 1989: 97–128.

31. Turner JA. Educational and behavioral interventions for back pain in primary care. *Spine* 1996; **21:** 2851–7; discussion 2858–9.

32. Riley JF, Ahern DK, Follick MJ. Chronic pain and functional impairment: assessing beliefs about their relationship. *Arch Phys Med Rehabil* 1988; **69:** 579–82.

33. McNeil DW, Rainwater AJ. Development of the Fear of Pain Questionnaire-III. *J Behav Med* 1998; **21:** 389–410.

34. McCracken LM, Zayfert C, Gross RT. The Pain Anxiety Symptoms Scale: development and validation of a scale to measure fear of pain. *Pain* 1992; **50:** 67–73.

35. Larsen DK, Taylor S, Asmundson GJ. Exploratory factor analysis of the Pain Anxiety Symptoms Scale in patients with chronic pain complaints. *Pain* 1997; **69:** 27–34.

36. Jensen MP, Karoly P. Pain-specific beliefs, perceived symptom severity, and adjustment to chronic pain. *Clin J Pain* 1992; **8:** 123–30.

37. Miller RP, Kori SH, Todd DD. The Tampa Scale for Kinisophobia. Unpublished report. 1991.

38. Kirk J. Cognitive–behavioural assessment. In: Hawton K, Salkovskis PM, Kirk J, Clark DM eds. *Cognitive Behaviour Therapy for Psychiatric Problems. A Practical Guide.* Oxford: Oxford University Press, 1989: 13–51.

39. Kugler K, Wijn J, Geilen M, *et al.* The Photograph series of Daily Activities (PHODA). CD-rom version 1.0. Heerlen: Institute for Rehabilitation Research and School for Physiotherapy, The Netherlands, 1999.

40. Fordyce WE. *Behavioral Methods for Chronic Pain and Illness.* St Louis, MO: Mosby, 1976.

41. Rhodes LA, McPhillips-Tangum CA, Markham C, Klenk R. The power of the visible: the meaning of diagnostic tests in chronic back pain. *Soc Sci Med* 1999; **48:** 1189–203.

42. Wolpe J. *Psychotherapy by Reciprocal Inhibition.* Stanford, CA: Stanford University Press, 1958.

43. Craske MG, Rowe MK. A comparison of behavioral and cognitive treatments of phobias. In: Davey GCL, ed. *Phobias. A Handbook of Theory, Research and Treatment.* Chichester: Wiley & Sons, 1997: 247–80.

44. Crombez G, Eccleston C, Vansteenwegen D, Vlaeyen JWS, *et al.* Exposure to movement in low back pain patients: restricted effects of generalisation. *Health Psychol* (in press).

◆ 45. Vlaeyen JW, de Jong J, Geilen M, *et al.* Graded exposure *in vivo* in the treatment of pain-related fear: a replicated single-case experimental design in four patients with chronic low back pain. *Behav Res Ther* 2001; **39:** 151–66.

46. Vlaeyen JWS, de Jong J, Geilen M, *et al.* The treatment of fear of movement/(re)injury in chronic low back pain: further evidence for the effectiveness of exposure *in vivo. Clin J Pain* (in press).

47. Rachman S, Whittal M. Fast, slow and sudden reductions in fear. *Behav Res Ther* 1989; **27:** 613–20.

48. Kendall NAS, Linton SJ, Main CJ. *Guide to Assessing Psychosocial Yellow Flags in Acute Low Back Pain: Risk Fac-*

tors for Long-term Disability and Work Loss. Wellington: Accident Compensation Corporation, 1997.

49. Linton SJ, Hallden K. Can we screen for problematic back pain? A screening questionnaire for predicting outcome in acute and subacute back pain. *Clin J Pain* 1998; **14:** 209–15.

50. Morley S, Eccleston C, Williams A. Systematic review and meta-analysis of randomized controlled trials of cognitive behaviour therapy and behaviour therapy for chronic pain in adults, excluding headache. *Pain* 1999; **80:** 1–13.

PART IV

Physical therapy and rehabilitation protocols

Physiotherapy

ANNE ELISABETH LJUNGGREN AND JAN MAGNUS BJORDAL

Pain and the physiotherapy process   179
Examination   180
Treatment   181
Inter-disciplinary cooperation   186
References   186

Within the discipline of physiotherapy, medical knowledge is combined with psychological insight and social comprehension of the patient's situation. The human body and movements are core fields, with the central goal being to achieve optimal physical function. At the same time, psychological and social factors are considered. Physiotherapy concerns health problems on all functional levels, dealing with impairments, daily activities, and social participation – and always considering contextual factors. In most countries, patients are referred to physiotherapists by physicians.

The treatment process comprises several approaches. The physical situation is intertwined with attitudes of interrelationships, and all kinds of resources should be considered. Treatment of patients in pain is based upon attentive, systematic, and conscientious examination, with every procedure presupposing mutual trust. The explicit expression of goals to be reached is of utmost importance. For the patient as well as the therapist, goals should be realistic. Mostly, it is necessary to define intermediary goals to reach the main goal, and even to rank the goals. Sometimes, the goal is very modest, and could even be to prevent a deterioration (Fig. 15.1).

In physiotherapy, the ultimate goals are to help patients perform daily activities optimally and to enable them to return to work or their premorbid functional status. This means that, in applying interventions, the relationship between the patient's own resources and the demands placed on them have to be considered. Patients should realize the association between problem-provoking factors and pain and other symptoms. Patients should be encouraged to make use of activities that will facilitate a natural cure. The best goal always comprises elements of prevention.

PAIN AND THE PHYSIOTHERAPY PROCESS

Nobody can live their whole life without pain and discomfort. The human being is subject to a broad and manifold spectrum of suffering involving both affective and cognitive mechanism, which are difficult to evaluate. By its very nature, pain is a subjective phenomenon, and pain perception is modified by many factors. The perception encompasses physical dysfunction as well as psychological problems, often in combination. Nociceptive pain resulting from tissue damage is modulated by a variety of neurophysiologic and emotional systems and psychosocial interactions. In therapy, physiotherapists utilize pain-inhibiting mechanisms.

There is a hierarchy of pain varieties. It is usual to distinguish among nociceptive, neurogenic, and psychogenic pain, and even existential pain, but in clinical practice it can be difficult to differentiate among these. It is common to assume that psychopathology and psychosocial problems are the results of pain, and not the causes. Each individual pain experience can be influenced by a number of factors, such as anxiety, low self-esteem, dissatisfaction with work, insufficient social network, or poor coping strategies.

Physiotherapy is the main gateway to the human body; however, during the physiotherapy process, treatment is not restricted to organ dysfunction. Patients often communicate feelings that profoundly influence their lives, such as uncertainty and anxiety associated with pain. Accordingly, physiotherapy cannot be limited to an understanding of the human body alone.

Because of the complex physiotherapy process (Fig. 15.1), patient and therapist meet over a long period of time. This represents a special situation that makes com-

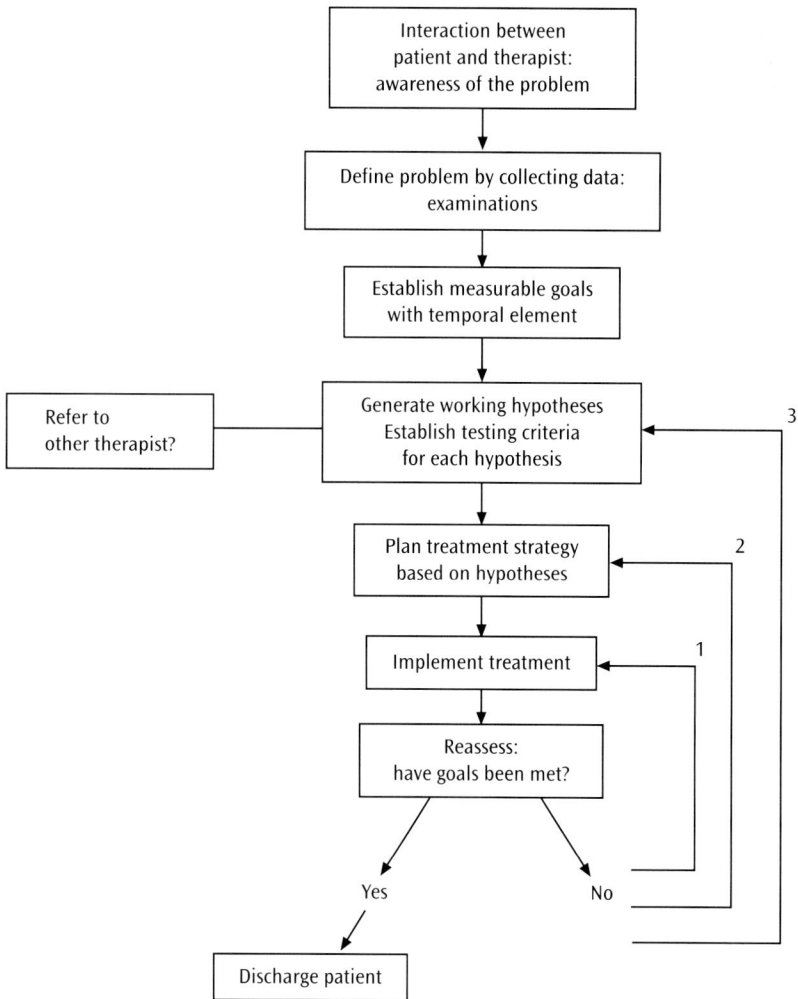

Interaction between
patient and therapist:
awareness of the problem

Define problem by collecting data:
examinations

Establish measurable goals
with temporal element

Refer to
other therapist?

Generate working hypotheses
Establish testing criteria
for each hypothesis

3

Plan treatment strategy
based on hypotheses

2

Implement treatment

1

Reassess:
have goals been met?

Yes   No

Discharge patient

Figure 15.1 *The physiotherapy process represents a hypothesis-oriented algorithm, in which part goals are continuously assessed. Precise goal setting provides the opportunity to tailor outcomes to the individual patient. When goals are not met, questions such as (1) "Was the implementation correct?", (2) "Was the strategy correct?", or (3) "Was the hypothesis viable?" may be asked.*

munication possible on several levels. Communication opens up many possibilities for changing a patient's misinterpretations, attitudes, and pain behavior. The therapy situation could be likened to the relationship between an athlete and his/her coach. Just like the coach, the physiotherapist seeks to make the patient use his/her resources in a way in which optimizing and improving physical performance is the goal. In order to achieve this, the physiotherapist can use a number of tools and techniques. These include creating a climate of trust and confidence, which is vital for successful physiotherapy.

It is fundamental to distinguish between acute and so-called chronic pain. Acute pain, which is a warning and protection signal, rarely represents any big problem in physiotherapy. Similarly, in subacute conditions, it is possible to give causal treatment. In pain linked to a delayed onset of recovery, the challenge for the physiotherapist is to find the factors that are predisposing the patient to pain and that are maintaining it. However, when pain persists for 3–6 months or longer, the whole pain experience is different. Pain expresses itself as functional suffering at different levels, and patients with persistent pain often present with combinations of organic, psychological, and socioeconomic problems. The subjective pain experience

may even be associated with a motive of secondary gain. Physiotherapists can combine professional care with insight and knowledge about the relationship between suffering and the pattern of living in work and leisure. The expression "chronic" has, however, connotations to something which is incurable, and should be replaced by, for instance, "long-lasting."

EXAMINATION

Decision-making is ... something which concerns all of us, both as makers of the choice and as sufferers of the consequences.

Lindley (English clinician)[1]

In physiotherapy, diagnosis is not a goal in itself, but represents a valuable basis for prognostic considerations and therapeutic decisions. Clinical decision-making includes the gathering of data that describe the clinical picture, the patient expressing subjective phenomena, and the physiotherapist mapping symptoms and more objective signs by performing a physical examination.[2] The examination should include the whole body and should list both problems and resources. When it comes to clinical decision-making, a physiotherapy treatment program is based just as much upon the patient's physical resources as the organic dysfunction itself.

The clinical history is fundamental to understanding the interplay among the patient, the disease, and the pain, and to evaluate the potential for change. The patient's verbal expressions and body language make it possible to determine the patient's understanding of the situation. The clinical history should include information about such factors as previous diseases, time off work, treatment experience, work, economy, family relationships, and social network. The pain itself should be mapped with regard to localization, duration, variation, and quality. It is also essential to determine the factors that affect, provoke, and maintain the pain, as well as factors relieving the pain.

For a physiotherapist, the specific clinical findings are important because interventions often aim to improve functional impairments and activities. Depending on the nature of the disease, the physical examination should cover a range of functions, e.g. body posture and habitual positions, active and passive motions, movement patterns and motor skills, respiration and certain sounds, appearance and consistency of the structures of the soft tissues, pain behavior, and motivation for treatment.[2] By combining a verbal clinical history with the physical information gathered from clinical signs, physiotherapists have the opportunity to evaluate a patient's knowledge and understanding of their situation and the potential for successful treatment.

Regularly, physicians refer patients for physiotherapy because of a medical diagnosis that is based on the International Classification of Diseases (ICD) or other classification system. However, most functional problems do not fit into these diagnostic systems. Physiotherapists make functional diagnoses that give information about the consequences of diseases and that cover the whole hierarchy of functions. In contrast to medical diagnoses, functional diagnoses are changeable, and are often immediately influenced by therapy. The recently revised International Classification of Functioning Disabilty and Health (ICIDH-2)[3] considers the consequences of disease at various functional levels and within different fields. Physiotherapists use a battery of instruments to measure and evaluate function in patients with different types of pain, considering discriminative, predictive, and evaluative types of measurements.

TREATMENT

Primum non nocere.

Hippocrates, *c.* 400 BC

No single intervention represents a panacea. Within physiotherapy, the choice of treatment is based on the principle of parsimony. The treatment choice presupposes sufficient knowledge of the natural course of the disease. In performing treatment procedures, physiotherapists formulate hypotheses about the causes of signs and symptoms, and test the hypotheses through the results obtained after performing the treatment (Fig. 15.1). It may be important to distinguish between causal and symptomatic treatment, although there is no clear distinction between these two main types. Therapy used to alleviate symptoms can address their cause, and vice versa. It is essential that the therapist, and preferably also the patient, is fully aware of the aims of treatment. Physiotherapy consists of several empirically developed treatment modalities that have been frequently criticized for a lack of scientific evidence on effects. However, many of the reviews on physiotherapy treatment modalities have not searched the physiotherapy literature outside Medline, or have used poor reviewing methods.[4***] It is also important to emphasize that modern physiotherapy normally consists of a combination of treatment modalities. Controlled trials on a single modality may overlook beneficial interactions between modalities or important cognitive effects of the physiotherapy process. Physiotherapy has the advantage of possessing a large battery of interventions that can address aspects of pain on a physical, psychological, and social level.

Causal treatment

Mens sana in corpore sana.

Juvenalis, *c.* AD 100

Causal treatment modalities aim to improve or normalize the tissue and organ functions influencing the cause of suffering. In the presence of psychopathology, mechanisms of action are complex and may be long-lasting.

In western societies, more money is probably spent on musculoskeletal diseases than on any other type of disease. Musculoskeletal diseases are mostly the result of the long adaptation time of soft tissue. The nutrition of collagen tissue is poor compared with muscular tissue: it takes about a whole year to heal a ligament after massive injury compared with about 1 month for a muscle. Accordingly, skeletal muscles may violate their own tendons and cause local overloading. In the intervertebral disk, turn-over time amounts to 2 years. Thus, tissue vulnerability during the healing phase may be manifest. Both immobilization and overloading give degenerative changes, and both correlate with pain and other symptoms (Fig. 15.2). Accordingly, progressive, dynamic training are important key tasks for all of us, whether we are in pain or not, and should be a life-long activity.

Cognitive interventions

Physiotherapy interventions often take place over a long period of time when subacute or chronic pain syndromes

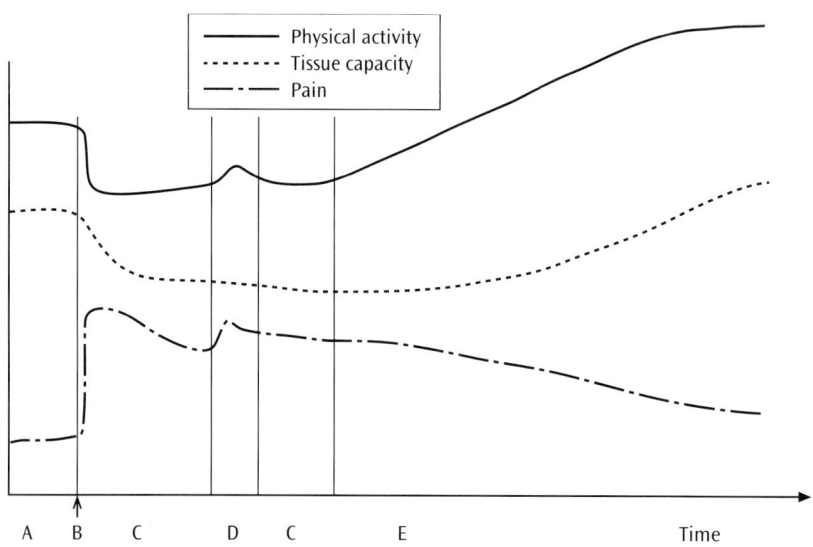

Figure 15.2 *Hypothetical collocation showing the relationship between physical activity, pain, and tissue properties with time. A, healthy period; B, injury; C, inactivity; D, attempts to increase activity; E, rehabilitation by progressive exercises.*

are treated. The long contact between the patient and therapist makes it possible to both give and receive information, which may influence insight into disease and suffering.

In the physiotherapy process (Fig. 15.1), several tools can be used. They all aim at initiating a cognitive change in the patient's understanding of symptoms and how movement patterns and physical activity affect the sensation of pain. Patients often misinterpret the somatic symptoms, which leads to physical inactivity. It is a challenge for the physiotherapist to understand the patient's misinterpretations and to reduce the fear and anxiety that are connected to movement and physical activity. Strategies of information, reassurance, encouragement, relaxation techniques, alternative ways of coping with stress, and changing of focus away from pain are all useful alternatives employed by the physiotherapist. These tools are the key elements in cognitive–behavior therapy that have been proved to be effective in the treatment of long-lasting pain.[5]***

Ergonomic advice

Treating patients in pain includes preventive interventions – just changing the work environment is not sufficient. In both primary and secondary prevention, the goal is to impart knowledge and to help patients to help themselves.

A range of pain schools and low back, neck, and shoulder schools exists, some of which are cross-diciplinary.[6]*** Most of these work with classes of patients, practicing principles of pain-deprogramming activities. Ergonomic knowledge is used in its broadest meaning, and advice and interventions are based upon biomechanical considerations and psychological insight. To make such teaching arrangements successful, the information has to be consistent, and factors such as patient's knowledge, attitudes, and behavior should be supervised and followed up over time. Patients with long-lasting

pain often take part in pain schools. Job satisfaction combined with exercise can be the best painkiller. A recent Cochrane review concluded that little is known about the cost-effectiveness of back schools, which may be effective in patients with recurrent and long-lasting low back pain in occupational settings.

Physical training

Physiotherapists are teachers of motor skills. Active exercise therapy is considered to be the most important of all the physiotherapy treatments, not least in pain conditions.[7] By practicing the application of movement pattern variability, with pauses in the movement, pain can be prevented. Both ligaments and joint capsules represent important proprioceptive organs for the awareness and understanding of movements and positions, as well as for dispersing muscular tension. Condition and endurance training dynamically activate large muscle groups and improve tissue nutrition, which is of importance in both prevention and therapy. In back pain, there has been no evidence that one particular training program is better than another. It seems that pain is efficiently reduced by long-term exercise (more than 1 h), which increases β-endorphin levels. Exercise should be both motivational and simple to carry out. Outdoor training in the fresh air might be preferred. Walking, jogging, cross-country skiing, swimming, and dancing, all at a sensible pace, are excellent activities. Such exercises also improve coordination, which is often impaired in long-lasting pain conditions. They may also have a positive effect upon trunk rotation, which is one of the first movements to be impaired with inactivity. But to increase the range of motion is scarcely an aim in itself. Stretching after activity has been recommended, however too much stretching may result in impairment of the viscoelastic properties of connective tissue.

Worldwide, there are combined activity programs,

comprising high-intensity exercises, that may be undertaken individually or in groups, both with and without equipment. While practicing progressive training, one has to consider behavior patterns, work demands, and social network. Patients should be motivated to take responsibility for their exercise. In itself attractive and varied, physical manual work represents a valuable intervention in pain prevention and therapy. The treatment program should result in the patients themselves experiencing success, perhaps reflecting the demands placed on them by society.

The McKenzie approach

The McKenzie approach is a concept of diagnosis and therapy for the whole spine, which is also applicable to the peripheral joints and their surrounding tissues. Symptoms in mechanical low back pain are categorized into postural, dysfunctional, and derangement syndromes, which should be treated as separate entities. In derangement syndrome, repeated movements in the direction that is claimed to decrease the accumulation of nuclear material will give a reduction and centralization of pain, whereas stretching of shortened structures through repeated movements seems to be adequate in dysfunctional syndrome. The patients are taught to practice self-mobilization and self-manipulation of their own spine.[8]**

Medical exercise therapy

Medical exercise therapy (MET) was developed in Norway and is now used worldwide.[9] The aim of the exercises is to normalize function, using specific exercises for mobilizing hypomobile areas and designing stabilizing exercises for other parts. Thus, stability, muscular control, and coordination are learned, as well as mobility and endurance. Treatment implies a conscientiously dosed regimen, even with negative loading. Progression is made possible by the use of specially designed exercise equipment (Fig. 15.3). Under continuous supervision by the physiotherapist, MET is given for 1 h to groups of a maximum of five patients. Each patient has an individually designed exercise program, related to symptoms, clinical diagnosis, needs, and expectations.[10]**

Manual therapy

The extensive field of manual medicine, or manual therapy (MT),[11] consists of an eclectic set of diagnostic and therapeutic procedures, from *manipulation* and *mobilization* to *classical medical massage (soft-tissue handling)* and *manual traction*. Within this field, pioneers have combined the best elements from orthopedics, osteopathy, chiropractic, and folk medicine, as well as physical activity and fitness. MT aims at normalizing physical function, mostly at the impairment level. The risk of damage associated with manipulation implies that such maneuvers should be avoided in patients with suspected disk herniation. Internationally, MT is used by physicians, chiropractors, osteopaths, and physiotherapists.

A

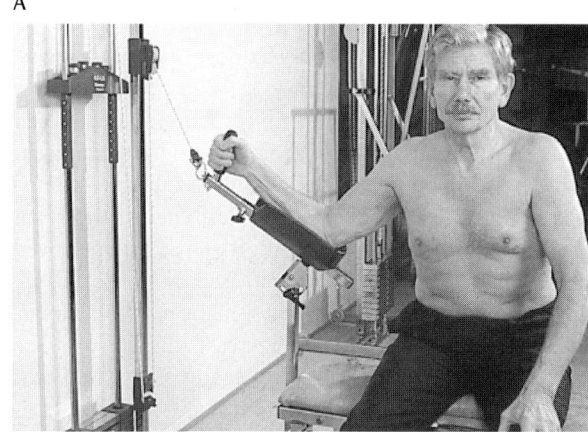

B

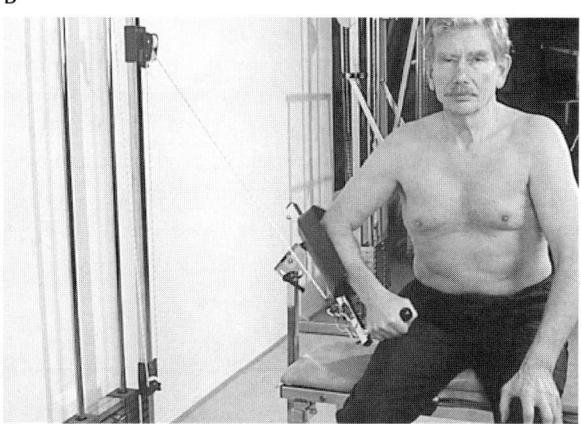

Figure 15.3 *One example among 7–9 exercises in the treatment of shoulder pain using the medical exercise therapy system, showing a patient with long-lasting subacromial pain syndrome using the shoulder rotator device attached to the multipurpose bench and the pulley apparatus. (A) starting position. (B) End position. The shoulder rotation exercise is performed with 45° of abduction in the shoulder doing three sets of 30 repetitions internally and three sets of 30 repetitions externally, alternating between internal and external rotation (in total six sets of 30 repetitions). The attachment of the rope from the pulley is easily changed from internal to external rotation and vice versa. (From: Torstensen TA. Medical Exercise Therapy. Exercise Manual for Shoulder, Elbow and Wrist Pain. Dysfunction of the Upper Extremity. Holten Institute (www.holteninstitute.com), Stockholm, 1998, pp. 1–104, with permission from the author and the patient.) Extensive description of a treatment process is to be found in Torstensen TA, Meen HDM, Stiris M. The effect of medical exercise therapy on a patient with chronic supraspinatus tendinitis. Diagnostic ultrasound-tissue regeneration: A case study. J Orthop Sports Phys Ther 1994; 20 (6):19–327.*

Psychomotor physiotherapy

Psychomotor physiotherapy was developed in Norway, and is based upon the knowledge that posture, movements, muscular tension, and respiration affect each other mutually, and that psychological and physical reactions have to be considered simultaneously.[12] Its aims are to produce a process of physical change based on the resources of patients, giving the patient improved coping patterns through an increased awareness of the connection between mental and somatic reactions. Treatment effects may include an increased ability to relax, decreased pain, and emotional changes. Psychomotor physiotherapy is different from local and symptom-oriented therapy and is often indicated for long-lasting pain conditions, which usually spread and give additional problems. Closely linked to psychomotor physiotherapy are psychodynamic body therapy and psychiatric physiotherapy. Psychomotor physiotherapy is only performed by specially trained physiotherapists.

Other methods within the field of psychiatric and psychosomatic physiotherapy include classical and modern variants focusing on body consciousness, such as Jacobson's progressive training and autogenic training.[13]

Symptomatic treatment

> Natura curat, non medica.
>
> Hippocrates, c. 400 BC

In aiming to reduce pain and discomfort, some symptomatic treatment types can, at the same time, have a causal effect. It is often relevant to apply symptomatic treatment in the introductory phase, preparing the body for more active treatment types. This is relevant during a single treatment session as well as during a series of treatments. Whenever possible, passive treatment types should not be used, and symptomatic treatment types should be reduced. However, in order to prevent central sensitization and development of long-lasting pain, it is of the utmost importance to stop peripheral pain signals as soon as possible. To achieve this aim, it can be appropriate to apply symptomatic treatment types.

Unloading

Empirical evidence has shown that rest, immobilization, and deloading all reduce acute pain. However, such methods have to be applied with care. In long-lasting pain, bed rest is not recommended because the deloading effect will be counteracted by a series of complications. Most patients with acute lumbago without nerve root symptoms are recommended not to stay in bed for more than 2 days. With serious nerve root affliction, the period of bed rest could have a duration of up to 2 weeks. Most patients are able to modify their activities and can manage to perform light physical work.

The use of a belt, corset, or walking aid is a compromise between bed rest and upright activities (Fig. 15.4). Corsets and other orthoses can influence mobility and muscular and mechanoreceptor activity, and can often increase temperature locally and give a positive placebo effect.

Traction is directed toward mechanically separate joint surfaces. The treatment can be applied intermittently or continuously, manually or with apparatus, and may be administered to all joints in the body. The patients can also generate the traction force themselves. Depending on symptoms and reaction to treatment, the period of traction can vary from seconds to minutes. Randomized controlled trials on traction treatment in the lumbar and cervical regions have shown results that vary from none to good pain-relieving effect.[14***] A positive effect may be explained by the unloading of tender structures and stretching of soft tissue, thus increasing circulation.

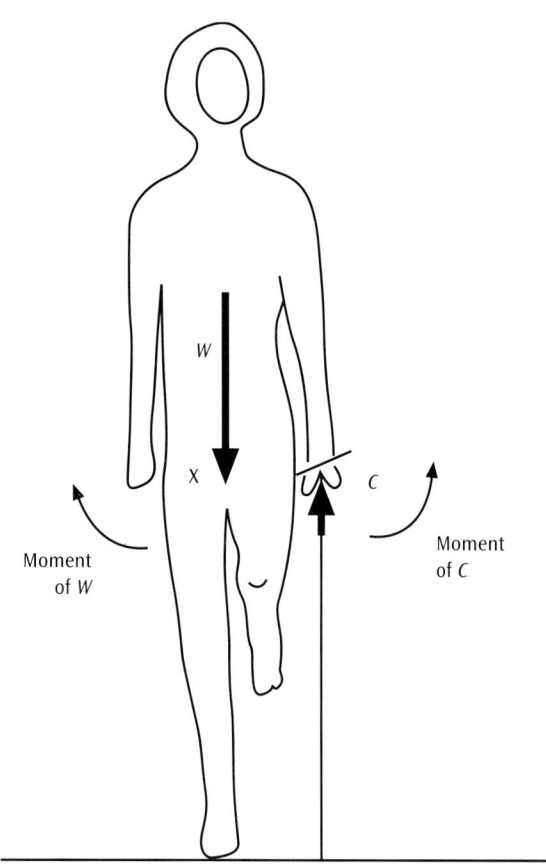

Figure 15.4 *Principle for the unloading effect upon the hip joint (X) by using a crutch in the opposite hand. Vector W denotes the force produced by the body weight, and vector C the force from the crutch. When W = 600 N and C = 150 N, the hip joint reaction force is approximately 2,000 N when standing on one leg without support. The unloading effect from the crutch is estimated to be about seven times the force from the crutch, i.e. halving the joint reaction force.*

Massage

Classical medical massage comprises the passive handling of soft tissues such as skin, muscles, fascias, and tendons. A variety of grips are used, such as effleurage, pétrissage, and frictions.

Massage is among the oldest treatment varieties within physiotherapy. Over the last decade, massage has been looked upon with growing skepticism. This view is based upon the increasing amount of scientific evidence that shows patients with long-lasting pain benefit from treatment which involves active participation, such as exercise and behavioral therapy. However, more recently, skepticism on the effect of massage has to some degree been refuted. Scientific evidence in favor of massage is still weak, but the number of randomized controlled trials is slowly increasing. Short-term clinical effects have even been reported in those trials where massage was administered as monotherapy. In addition to pain reduction, these effects include reduced stiffness and muscular and mental relaxation.[15**,16**] In modern physiotherapy, massage is usually combined with advice, mobilization, traction, or active exercises. Recent randomized controlled trials have proved that a combination of these modalities provides good results compared with other established therapies.[10**,17**]

Physical agents

The use of physical agents by physiotherapists has a long tradition in the treatment of pain. The modalities include thermal agents, electrotherapeutic techniques, and pneumatic compression, and they have been used and developed from empirical knowledge ever since physiotherapy became an independent profession in the nineteenth century. Today, they normally serve as adjuncts, aiming at reducing pain prior to other treatments such as massage, joint mobilization, therapeutic exercises, or training for improvement of motor control.

Heat
Heat can be applied on the skin by hot packs, paraffin wax, parafango (mud bath), or heated water, which transmit the heat energy to the body through conduction or convection. The effect on pain seems to be induced primarily through a central gating mechanism. Some experimental evidence also suggests that an increase in local sensory threshold of peripheral nerves plays a role in the pain-relieving effect from heat therapy. Heat therapy produces immediate, but transient, pain relief in long-lasting conditions such as arthritis, vertebrogenic low back pain, and myofascial pain.

In heat therapy, the temperature is increased mostly in the subcutaneous layers, but a clinically relevant increase can be measured down to 1.5–2 cm after application of heat on the skin surface. Heat therapy should be avoided in the acute stages of soft-tissue injuries, as heat then will increase the formation of edema. Deeper tissues can be heated by radiation from ultrasound, shortwave, or microwave diathermy. However, there is a paucity of controlled trials elucidating whether high doses of radiation from ultrasound, shortwave, or microwave diathermy are clinically effective. Recent research findings[18] suggest that nonthermal effects of ultrasound and shortwave therapy are clinically more important than was previously thought (for references, see Electrotherapeutic techniques).

Cold
Pain after acute injury is associated with increased sensitivity of afferent pain receptors and pressure-induced pain from edema in the injured soft tissue. Cryotherapy is often used to reduce acute pain and the formation of local edema. Decreased temperature reduces blood flow and hematoma and lessens the increase in interstitial fluid pressure following acute soft-tissue injuries. Mild cryotherapy applied for 20 min every second hour for the first 2 days after injury may reduce both pain and swelling.[19***] Application times shorter than 10 minutes have led to reactive hyperemia and subsequently an increase in tissue temperature. The use of cryotherapy seems to be less popular than heat therapy for patients with arthritis, which may be due to the side-effect of reduced elasticity in connective tissue that is induced by cold.

Electrotherapeutic techniques
Such techniques can roughly be divided into two categories:

1 *Electrical stimulation* that acts through the induction of action potentials in peripheral sensor/motor nerves which leads to muscle contraction and/or activation of central gating mechanisms that modulate pain perception.

Electrical stimulation can be used for symptomatic pain control or to increase local blood flow or metabolism through electrically induced muscle contractions. The most frequently used modality for pain control is probably transcutaneous electrical nerve stimulation (TENS), which can be delivered by small pocket-size stimulators. Electrodes are placed in the painful area or over superficially situated nerve trunks that innervate the painful area. The best effect is achieved when the intensity of the electrical current is set at a strong, but subnoxious, sensation by the patient. Pulsewidths of 100–300 μs and pulse frequencies with ranges of 1–5 Hz (acupuncture-like TENS) or 60–110 Hz seem to produce the best clinical response. Stimulation times should be 15–30 min, and the majority of patients will then report 50% pain relief or more during stimulation and for up to 0.5–2 h after stimulation.

In clinical use, TENS is effective in the treatment of acute pain, yielding pain reduction in about 80% of patients.[20**] In some patients with long-lasting conditions, the effect of TENS seems more short lived. For these patients, the response to TENS is high during the first sessions, but the effect on pain diminishes over time.[21]* Patients that still experience pain reduction after 4 weeks of daily use are likely to have a lasting effect that can reduce the need for other analgesics or therapy for years. Besides adequate pain relief, an increase in physical and social activity are the most common effects of TENS in patients with long-lasting pain.[22]* TENS is also a useful adjunct before exercise therapy, and may increase muscle activation and reduce the time for rehabilitation after surgery.

Other forms of electrical stimulation, such as interferential current therapy and diadynamic currents, probably act through the same mechanism as TENS. Electrical muscle stimulation (EMS) promotes local circulation and metabolism and reduces hypotrophy of inactive muscles. This method differs from TENS by using stimulating intermittent muscle contraction for 2–5 s. The combination of TENS and EMS has proven effective in the treatment of low back pain.[23]**

A recently developed form of electrotherapy – cutaneous field stimulation – seems to reduce itch effectively and may have a potential in the treatment of pain. Electric shocks are delivered at low frequency through little sharp needles, which penetrate slightly into the epidermis. The needles are mounted on a flexible plate, which covers the cutaneous field to be stimulated.

2   *Electromagnetic fields*, *laser*, or *ultrasound* can induce beneficial effects on the biochemical environment and metabolism of soft tissue. Shortwave therapy (ST) penetrates deep into the tissues and can reduce inflammatory response and pain after acute soft-tissue injuries.[19]*** Low-level laser therapy (LLLT) has limited penetration ability, but has been shown to improve healing in superficially situated subacute and chronic tendinitis.[24]** Both ST and LLLT speed up the healing process in the proliferative and remodeling phases after soft-tissue injuries. Pain originating from long-lasting joint disorders may be symptomatically reduced after treatment with ST or LLLT. Myofascial pain has also been successfully reduced by LLLT.[24]*

Ultrasound (US) therapy can be used for the same indications as ST and LLLT. Although US is the most common form of electrotherapy in many countries, the clinical effect has been more uncertain than for LLLT and ST.[25]*** However, recent clinical trials have found clinical effects on tendon disorders.[25] In investigating chronic carpal tunnel syndrome under rigorous conditions, US was found to be clearly more effective than placebo US.[26]***

INTER-DISCIPLINARY COOPERATION

A physician can prescribe or just suggest a treatment. In most countries, a physiotherapist can implement the treatment that the physician considers to be the most appropriate. However, if the physiotherapist considers that a different treatment would be more appropriate, the physician should be consulted and approve the change. The aim of physiotherapy should be pointed out by the physician, who should also give adequate medical and laboratory findings as supplements to the medical diagnosis. The referral system presupposes good collaboration between the physician and the therapist, who have a responsibility to give feedback to each other on the patient's progress. It is a presupposition of that collaboration that the physiotherapist is able to take responsibility for the patient's care and to make decisions. In some parts of the world, physiotherapists have become the first, and responsible, contact in primary health care for patients with pain conditions of musculoskeletal origin.

It is essential to make demands on patients. If patients do not cooperate, or treatment shows no result after four to six treatment sessions, then that particular treatment should be considered to have ended. It is a challenge to find new approaches and to find new resources. Sometimes, we must look for other, underlying, causes, for example environmental conditions, occupational situations, social elements, and psychological factors. These, rather than elements emanating from the patient, may be responsible for the condition. It can be necessary to send the patient to another physiotherapist, for both personal and professional reasons. As always in therapy, the challenge is to find the right therapy for a given patient as well as to find the right patient for a given therapy. In most cases, patients with long-lasting pain need inter-disciplinary evaluation and treatment. It is essential to carry out follow-up examinations.

REFERENCES

1. Lindley DV. *Making Decisions*. London: Wiley Interscience, 1971.
2. Gross J, Fetto J, Rosen E. *Musculoskeletal Examination*. Cambridge: Blackwell Science, 1996.
3. International Classification of Functioning, Disability and Health (ICIDH 2) Final draft. Full version. *Classification, Assessment, Surveys and Terminology Team*. Geneva: World health organization, 2001.
● 4. Bjordal JM, Greve G. What may alter the conclusions of reviews? *Phys Ther Rev* 1998; **3:** 121–32.
● 5. Morley S, Eccleston C, Williams A. Systematic review and meta-analysis of randomized controlled trials of cognitive behaviour therapy for chronic pain in adults, excluding headache. *Pain* 1999; **80:** 1–14.
● 6. Klingenstierna U. Back schools: a review. *Clin Rev Phys Rehabil Med* 1991; **3:** 155–71.
● 7. Nordin M, Campello M. Physical therapy. Exercises and the modalities: when, what and why? *Neurol Clin North Am* 1999; **17:** 75–89.

8. Stankovic R, Johnell O. Conservative treatment of acute low back pain. A 5 year follow-up study of two methods of treatment. *Spine* 1995; **20:** 469–72.

9. Torstensen TA. The physical therapy approach. In: Frymoyer JW, Ducker TB, Hadler NM, *et al.* eds. *The Adult Spine: Principles and Practice*, 2nd edn. Philadelphia, PA: Lippincott-Raven, 1997: 1797–805.

◆ 10. Torstensen TA, Ljunggren AE, Meen HD, *et al.* Efficiency and costs of medical exercise therapy, conventional physiotherapy, and self-exercise in patients with chronic low back pain. A pragmatic, randomized, single-blinded, controlled trial with 1-year follow-up. *Spine* 1998; **23:** 2616–24.

◆ 11. Harris JD, McPartland JM. Historical perspectives of manual medicine. In: Stanton DF, Mein EA eds. *Physical Medicine and Rehabilitation. Manual Medicine.* Philadelphia, PA: W. B. Saunders, 1996: 679–93.

12. Thornquist E, Bunkan BH. *What is Psychomotor Therapy?* Oslo: Norwegian University Press, 1991.

● 13. Linton SJ. Chronic back pain: integrating psychological and physical therapy – an overview. *Behav Med* 1994; **20:** 101–4.

● 14. van der Heijden GF, Beurskens AJ, Koes BW, *et al.* The efficacy of traction for back and neck pain: a systematic, blinded review of randomized clinical trial methods. *Phys Ther* 1995; **75:** 93–104.

15. Sunshine W, Field TM, Quintino O, *et al.* Fibromyalgia benefits from massage therapy and transcutaneous electrical stimulation. *J Clin Rheumatol* 1996; **2:** 18–22.

16. Field T, Hernandez-Reif M, Seligman S, *et al.* Juvenile rheumatoid arthritis: benefits from massage therapy. *J Ped Psychol* 1997; **22:** 607–17.

17. Preyde M. Effectiveness of massage therapy for sub-acute low-back pain. A randomized controlled trial. *Can Med Assoc J* 2000; **162:** 1815–20.

18. Nussbaum E. To heat or not to heat – that is the question. *Phys Ther Reviews* 1997; **2:** 59–72.

● 19. Ogilvie-Harris DJ, Gilbart M. Treatment modalities for soft tissue injuries of the ankle: a critical review. *Clin J Sports Med* 1995; **5:** 175–86.

◆ 20. Benedetti F, Amanzio M, Casadio C, *et al.* Control of postoperative pain by transcutaneous electrical nerve stimulation after thoracic operations. *Ann Thorac Surg* 1997; **63:** 773–6.

21. Woolf CJ, Thompson JW. Stimulation-induced analgesia: transcutaneous electrical nerve stimulation (TENS) and vibration. In: Wall PD, Melzack R eds. *Textbook of Pain.* Edinburgh: Churchill Livingstone, 1994: 1191–208.

22. Chabal C, Fishbain DA, Weaver M, Heine LW. Long-term TENS use: impact on medication utilization and physical therapy costs. *Clin J Pain* 1998; **14:** 66–73.

23. Moore SR, Shurman J. Combined neuromuscular electrical stimulation and transcutaneous electrical nerve stimulation for treatment of chronic back pain: a double-blind, repeated measures comparison. *Arch Phys Med Rehabil* 1997; **78:** 55–60.

24. Lögdberg-Andersson M, Mutzell S, Hazel Å. Low level laser therapy of tendinitis and myofascial pain. A randomised double-blind controlled study. *Laser Ther* 1997; **9:** 79–86.

25. Ebenbichler GR, Resch KL, Nicolakis P, *et al.* Ultrasound treatment for treating the carpal tunnel syndrome: a randomized "sham" controlled trial. *Br Med J* 1998; **316:** 731–5.

● 26. van der Windt DAWM, van der Heijden GJMG, van den Berg SGM, *et al.* Ultrasound therapy for musculoskeletal disorders: a systematic review. *Pain* 1999; **81:** 257–71.

16

Manual medicine

SOMAYAJI RAMAMURTHY AND PHILIP E GREENMAN

Structural diagnosis	189	Results	192
Imaging studies	191	Complications	192
Management	191	References	193

Manual medicine, which includes treatments such as mobilization or manipulation, has been utilized in the health care system since before the time of Hippocrates.[1] The art of manual medicine is not a part of the curriculum of Western medical schools (allopathy), but members of the general public are happy to seek the services of manual medicine practitioners such as osteopathic physicians and chiropractors. Although many physicians believe that manual medicine has little to offer in the management of pain, over the past 10 years the authors have had the opportunity, in the University Health System Pain Management Center, to observe, practice, and evaluate manual medical approaches in the management of acute and chronic pain. The results of this noninvasive therapy are very impressive, and there has been a reduction in the number of injections used for the treatment of many common pain problems that in the past were treated with invasive modalities.

The efficacy of manipulative therapy in the treatment of acute and chronic low back pain has been the subject of numerous well-controlled studies. However, the fact that 80–90% of patients with low back pain report improvement whether or not they have received therapeutic intervention presents a confounding problem in the planning of controlled studies. Some studies have found no difference in outcome with manual medicine.[2**,3] Other well-controlled studies document objective improvement in the range of motion, pain level, speed of recovery, and use of analgesic medication and muscle relaxants.[4–8*] In patients with acute back pain of less than 1 months' duration, manipulation seems to provide benefit compared with standard therapy. However, chronic back pain does not seem to respond as well as acute pain, and thus manipulation provides no advantage over standard therapy.[9**,10**] Anderson et al.,[11*] in a recent well-controlled study, concluded that manual medicine and standard medical care produce similar clinical results in patients with back pain of 3 weeks' to 6 months' duration; however, the use of medication is greater in patients receiving standard care. Vicenzino et al.[12] reported statistically significant improvement in objective measures and decreased pain following cervical spine manipulative physiotherapy in the treatment of patients with lateral epicondyle dysfunction. We believe that manual medicine is an important and effective tool in the armamentarium of the pain medicine physician.

STRUCTURAL DIAGNOSIS

Structural diagnosis[1,13,14] is part of the physical examination of a patient in our pain clinic. It consists in various maneuvers involving the loading of the joints, for example the facet joints or sacroiliac joint, and assessing the range of motion in various body positions. This examination enables the levels at which there is significant dysfunction to be determined. Lack of mobility of a particular rib with inspiration and expiration or of a facet joint in the cervical or lumbar area or of the sacroiliac joint can also be identified. Thus, the range of motion can be assessed and joint asymmetry and tissue texture abnormality can be determined. Frequently, the area of dysfunction is also a specific area of tenderness. For example, if there is rib dysfunction, tenderness is typically present all along the rib: anteriorly, laterally, and posteriorly.

Common pain syndromes diagnosed by manual medicine

Facet joint dysfunction at different levels in the spine is probably the single most common syndrome that is amenable to manual medical therapy.

Cervical facet dysfunction

All the joints of the neck, beginning at the atlanto-occipital joint and including all the facet joints, can be dysfunctional and produce pain. Common causes include sudden movement, so-called whiplash injury,[15] and sleeping in an abnormal position, although it also sometimes occurs in the absence of any identifiable cause. Examination reveals a decreased range of motion in the affected segment. This restriction can be clearly identified by appropriate movements that isolate the range of motion for that particular segment. We have found that palpation over the facet invariably corroborates the structural diagnosis. Commonly, cervical pain is accompanied by referred pain over the head, neck, and shoulder, and sometimes also pain referred to the arm, depending on the level. In the case of dysfunction of the upper joints, including the atlanto-occipital and the upper facet joints, pain is referred to the upper part of the neck and back of the head. Pain from the middle and the lower joints is referred to the neck and the upper extremity. The zones of reference of the individual facet joints have been mapped by the injection of hypertonic saline into these joints.

There may be accompanying myofascial pain,[16] which can be identified with careful palpation of the sternocleidomastoid, trapezius, splenius capitis, levator scapulae, and scalene muscles. Many patients with joint restriction and myofascial pain develop headache, which is often misdiagnosed as a migraine.

Thoracic facet and rib dysfunction

The thoracic facet joints and ribs are a functional unit. Dysfunction usually involves rotational injury and is commonly seen in golfers. In many instances, pain is precipitated by rotational movement of the thorax and is accompanied by muscular pain of the paraspinals and referred pain from the back, sometimes radiating to the front of the chest, and frequently mistaken for angina or pulmonary problems. We have come across patients whose gallbladder has been removed because they suffered from right-sided mid-thoracic pain but in whom pain continued after surgery and was relieved by mobilization of the T7–8 ribs, followed by appropriate stretching exercises. Such patients are likely to have tenderness over the facet paraspinally, and the pain can be reproduced by careful palpation of the rib all along posterior, lateral, and anterior aspects. This particular feature differentiates it from myofascial pain originating from the rhomboids and serratus anterior muscles.

First rib dysfunction commonly produces pain along the medial aspect of the arm and the forearm, including the little finger. Some affected patients are mistakenly diagnosed as having thoracic outlet syndrome or many have undergone ulnar nerve transposition. We have been able to relieve these patients' pain by mobilization of the first rib. Dysfunction of the third and fourth ribs is extremely common and is associated with thoracic pain worsened by deep breathing. These ribs can easily be mobilized to relieve the pain.

Lumbar facet dysfunction

Lumbar facet dysfunction commonly causes low back pain. Usually, the restriction is identified by flexion and extension and can be isolated to a particular segment, such as L4–5 or L5–S1. By loading the facets, for example by quadrant loading, in which the upper body is rotated to one side at the same time as extending the spine, the patient is usually able to pinpoint the level at which the pain originates. This can also be accomplished by extending the hip with the patient in the prone position. Patients are able to localize the pain exactly to the level of facet involved. This maneuver usually loads the lower facets, most commonly L4–5 and L5–S1. In our experience, this maneuver does not load the sacroiliac joint.

Sacroiliac joint dysfunction

The sacroiliac joints[13,14] normally have one or two degrees of motion. Even this tiny range of motion, if impaired, can produce a very significant impairment of function and pain. Most commonly, this pain is worse when the patient is seated. The pain is commonly referred to the buttock and the posterior thigh, and occasionally to the groin and to the symphysis pubis. Usually, one side of the hemipelvis is immobile and dysfunctional. This dysfunction can be identified by various maneuvers directed at assessing the movement of the S1 joint. One of the simplest such maneuvers is to ask the patient to lie in the prone position with knees together bent at 90° and let the ankles fall out into hip internal rotation. Internal rotation will usually be noticeably decreased on the side affected by sacroiliac joint restriction. The relative motion of the S1 joints can also be assessed by springing, but this seems to be a very subjective test.

In the Gillette test,[14] the patient lifts the knee very high while in the standing position with support. Motion of the sacroiliac joint is assessed by placing one thumb under the posterior superior iliac spine on the side of hip flexion with the other thumb in the midline roughly at the S2 level. To begin with the thumbs are at the same level, one at the midline and one just below the posterior superior iliac spine. Normally, the thumb under the posterior superior iliac spine drops inferiorly and laterally with hip flexion. Restriction is indicated by decreased motion compared with the normal side. The levels of the anterior and posterior superior iliac spines are likely to be different in the supine and prone positions depending upon the rotational deformity and restriction. Anterior rotation causes the posterior superior spine to be higher and the anterior superior spine lower on the affected side. The side of restriction with motion testing determines whether the involved side is "high" or "low."

Very commonly, sacroiliac joint dysfunction results in a clear leg length difference, although usually of not more than 1/2 to 1 inch. A particular type of dysfunction called a superior shear commonly occurs after an event that directs force upward through the leg or buttock. This results in superior displacement of the hemipelvis on the affected side in such a manner that when the levels of the ischial tuberosities and iliac crests are compared the affected side is clearly elevated. This is often accompanied by significant shortening of the lower extremity on the affected side, but the shortening is above the knee level. Shortening of the lower extremity with superior shear is best identified in the unload, i.e. supine or prone, positions and not while standing.

There continues to be confusion about the role of shear dysfunction in the true short leg/pelvic tilt syndrome. This can be assessed when the knees are flexed in the prone position. The distance from the knee to the heel will be the same on both sides. Tenderness and tension over the sacroiliac ligament[1] is a common finding in patients with sacroiliac joint dysfunction. Often, patients with sacroiliac joint dysfunction also have tenderness over the symphysis pubis. Because of the dysfunction of the sacroiliac joint, the muscles attached to the hemipelvis are also dysfunctional. Whenever examination reveals tightness of the piriformis, adductor, hamstring, quadratus, or psoas muscles, sacroiliac joint dysfunction should be suspected. This shortening of the muscles and tightness of the muscle is significantly relieved soon after mobilizing the sacroiliac joint.

IMAGING STUDIES

Unfortunately, imaging techniques[17**,18] such as radiography, magnetic resonance imaging (MRI), and computed tomography (CT) do not provide any information regarding dysfunction of these joints.

Even clinical evaluation has its pitfalls. In a study carried out at our institution, we[19**] found that 20% of asymptomatic individuals have clinically restricted sacroiliac joint motion on one side. This makes it difficult to diagnose sacroiliac joint dysfunction in a patient with back pain. In addition, studies that attempt to correlate clinical examination and the sacroiliac joint and facet joint involvement have not been able to predict accurately the result of local anesthetic injection into these joints. Poor inter-rater reliability has been found in studies of clinical evaluation of sacroiliac joint dysfunction.

MANAGEMENT

Various types of maneuvers can be used to relieve pain resulting from joint dysfunction:

- soft-tissue techniques;
- muscle energy technique;
- mobilization without impulse;
- high-velocity, low-amplitude thrust (mobilization with thrust);
- myofascial release;
- functional release by position;
- cranial sacrum.

Soft-tissue techniques

Soft-tissue techniques include massage, traction, and stretching of the muscles. They are usually used in preparation for the utilization of other techniques.

Muscle energy technique

We commonly utilize this technique prior to the use of articular techniques. It involves using what is essentially a contract–relax technique to restore normal motion in a joint. For example, in a patient who is suspected of having a posterior position of the pelvis, the clinician will manually rotate the pelvis anteriorly, or into the motion barrier; this is followed by a 3–7 s submaximal effort by the patient against the practitioner. The patient relaxes, then the procedure is repeated 3–5 times and the restriction reassessed. This technique is most commonly used in patients who are elderly and have severe osteoporosis, sometimes secondary to the use of corticosteroids.

Articular procedures

Mobilization without impulse is the articular procedure most often practiced in our clinic. We prefer to define manipulation as skilful and dexterous treatment by hand. In the chiropractic literature and some of the German literature the term "manipulation" is used to mean mobilization with thrust (high-velocity thrust technique). When an area appears to be restricted, a series of repetitions of operator oscillation of the joint is performed. This procedure appears to influence the mechanical behavior of the articulation and the articular tissues, restoring the normal joint mechanics.

High-velocity, low-amplitude thrust

This technique is most commonly used by chiropractors and is referred to as mobilization with impulse or high-velocity, low-amplitude thrust. These procedures are directed primarily toward an articulation and related periarticular structures. During a high-velocity thrust, operative forces are directed into the joint in the direction of restriction and are frequently associated with a popping sound.

Myofascial release

This technique is utilized by some practitioners. We do not use this technique in our clinic. Nor do we employ the craniosacral system of manual medicine, which involves mobilizing the sutures of the cranium.

RESULTS

There are few well-controlled studies documenting the effectiveness of manual medicine. Most of the information is anecdotal. In our clinic, we use a physical therapist to provide manual treatment of joint restriction before considering any invasive procedures. Approximately 45% of our patients with dysfunction of various joints significantly improve following manual medicine modalities.

We also find that mobilization and manipulation is ideally followed by a stretching exercise program. Patients are instructed in the exercises to follow and should adhere strictly to the program. Stretching exercises restore the muscles and ligaments to their normal length, maintain joint mobility, and prevent the resumption of the dysfunctional pattern. When the manual medicine techniques produce partial or no benefit, we proceed to diagnostic injections of these joints.

Varying degrees of relief are achieved by manipulative therapy. Approximately 45% of patients show remarkable improvement and are discharged from the clinic with the recommendation to continue the exercises. Some patients achieve only temporary pain relief and the mechanical dysfunction returns despite frequent mobilization. In these patients, we use orthotic devices such as the sacroiliac belt. In some patients, pain and joint tenderness persist despite correction of mechanical dysfunction and restoration of the normal range of motion.

In patients who do not experience complete benefit with manipulative therapy, we proceed to diagnostic injections. Usually, if the diagnosis is correct, patients achieve complete relief of the pain with a local anesthetic injection. The duration of relief coincides with the duration of action of the short-acting or long-acting local anesthetic. Some patients achieve prolonged pain relief with the use of intra-articular steroids. When intra-articular steroids do not provide long-term relief, we use the radiofrequency lesioning of the medial branches of the cervical, thoracic, or lumbar facet joints.

Manipulation of joints with anesthesia (MUJA)[20*]

Manipulation under anesthesia is employed if the patient finds mobilization uncomfortable. In these instances we mobilize the joint after providing analgesia.

We have been able to mobilize joints easily following local anesthetic block of the sacroiliac joint and facet joints. The force necessary to mobilize the joint is significantly reduced. Injection of local anesthetic into the facet and sacroiliac joints provides excellent analgesia for subsequent manual medicine modalities. Local anesthetic medial branch blocks provide excellent analgesia for the mobilization of cervical, thoracic, and lumbar facet joints. Sacroiliac joint mobilization can be facilitated by analgesia provided by local anesthetic injection along the lateral margin of the sacrum at the joint level.

Manipulation under general anesthesia is employed by some practitioners. We do not find general anesthesia necessary for this purpose. Regional anesthesia is an effective, safe alternative.

COMPLICATIONS

Serious complications from manual medicine are very rare. Dvorak and von Orelli[21] report an incidence of 1 in 400,000 for symptom exacerbation and 1 in 400,000 for true complications.

1 Temporarily increased discomfort in the mobilized joint commonly lasts 2–3 days. It normally responds to ice, heat, and nonsteroidal anti-inflammatory drugs.
2 Elderly patients or patients with significant osteoporosis on corticosteroids may sustain fractures following mobilization. These usually are hairline nondisplaced fractures and respond to standard immobilization and analgesics.
3 Fractures in the cervical vertebra have resulted in injury to the vertebral[22***] arteries, resulting in hemiplegia and even death. Prolonged extension and rotation of the cervical spine increases the risk of injury to the vertebral artery.
4 Patients with rheumatoid arthritic or patients with significant degenerative changes in upper cervical vertebrae need to be carefully assessed with imaging studies before attempting mobilization. Clinical assessments of vertebral arterial function are not reliable.

In conclusion, mechanical dysfunction of various joints is a common cause of pain in a significant number of patients. Usually, Western medical practitioners do not take this into consideration, and patients are misdiagnosed. The majority of patients can be treated very effectively with noninvasive methods. When patients are treated in a setting in which there is a multidisciplinary approach, the correct diagnosis can be made. Unfortunately, these modalities are typically available only in unimodality clinics. Incorporating manual medicine in Western medical practice will help a large number of patients using noninvasive techniques.

REFERENCES

● 1. Greenman PE. Syndromes of the lumbar spine, pelvis and sacrum. *Phys Med Rehabil Clin N Am* 1996; **7**: 773–85.

◆ 2. Godfrey CM, Morgan PP, Schatzker J. A randomized trial of manipulation for low-back pain in a medical setting. *Spine* 1984; **9**: 301–2.

◆ 3. Doran DML, Newell DJ. Manipulation in treatment of low back pain: a multicentre study. *Br Med J* 1975; **2**: 161–4.

◆ 4. Cibulka MT, Delitto A, Koldenhoff RM. Changes in innominate tilt after manipulation of the sacroiliac joint in patients with low back pain. *Phys Ther* 1988; **68**: 1359–63.

● 5. Twomey L, Taylor J. Exercise and spinal manipulation in the treatment of low back pain. *Spine* 1994; **20**: 615–19.

● 6. Shekelle PG, Adams AH, Chassin MR, *et al*. Spinal manipulation for low-back pain. *Ann Intern Med* 1992; **117**: 590–8.

7. Cibulka MT. The treatment of the sacroiliac joint component to low back pain: a case report. *Phys Ther* 1992; **72**: 917–92.

8. Nwuga VCB. Relative therapeutic efficacy of vertebral manipulation and conventional treatment in back pain management. *Am J Phys Med* 1982; **61**: 273–8.

9. Sims-Williams H, Jayson MIV, Young SMS, *et al*. Controlled trial of mobilization and manipulation for low back pain: hospital patients. *Br Med J* 1979; **2**: 1318–20.

10. Sims-Williams H, Jayson MIV, Young SMS, *et al*. Controlled trial of mobilization and manipulation for patients with low back pain in general practice. *Br Med J* 1978; **2**: 1338–40.

11. Anderson GBJ, Lucente T, Davis AM, *et al*. A comparison of osteopathic spinal manipulation with standard care for patients with low back pain. *N Engl J Med* 1999; **341**: 1426–31.

12. Vicenzio B, Collins D, Wright A. The initial effects of a cervical spine manipulative physiotherapy treatment on the pain and dysfunction of lateral epicondylalgia. *Pain* 1996; **68**: 69–74.

● 13. Greenman PE. The osteopathic approach to rehabilitation. In: Kirkaldy-Willia W, Bernard TN eds. *Managing Low Back Pain,* 4th edn. New York, NY: Churchill Livingstone, 1997: 341–50.

● 14. Greenman PE. The osteopathic view of acute spinal disorders. In: Mayer TG, Mooney V, Gatchel R eds. *Contemporary Care of Painful Spinal Disorders*: Philadelphia, PA: Lea & Febriger 1991: 181–90.

● 15. Greenman PE. Manual and manipulative therapy in whiplash injuries. *Spine: State of the Art Reviews* 1993; **7**: 517–30.

● 16. Travell JG, Simmons DG. Myofascial pain and dysfunction. In: Travel JG, Simmons DG eds. *The Trigger Point Manual.* Baltimore, MD: Williams & Wilkins, 1983.

17. Jensen MC, Brant-Zawadzki MN, Obuchowski N, *et al*. Magnetic resonance imaging of the lumbar spine in people without back pain. *N Engl J Med* 1994; **331**: 69–73.

18. Powell MC, Wilson M, Szypryt P, *et al*. Prevalence of lumbar disc degeneration observed by magnetic resonance in symptomless women. *Lancet* 1986; **2**: 1366–7.

19. Dreyfuss P, Dryer S, Griffin J, *et al*. Positive sacroiliac screening tests in asymptomatic adults. *Spine* 1994; **19**: 1138–43.

20. Dreyfuss P, Michaelsen M, Horne M. MUJA: manipulation under joint anesthesia/analgesia: a treatment approach for recalcitrant low back pain of synovial joint origin. *J Manipulative Physiol Ther* 1995; **8**: 537–46.

21. Dvorak J, von Orelli F. The frequency of complications after manipulation of the cervical spine (case report and epidemiology). *Schweiz Rundschau Med Praxis* 1982; **71**: 64–9.

22. Haldeman S, Kohlbeck FJ, McGregor M. Risk factors and precipitating neck movements causing vertebrobasilar artery dissection after cervical trauma and spinal manipulation. *Spine* 1999; **24**: 785–94.

PART V

Interventions

17

Peripheral nerve blocks: practical aspects

DAVID HILL

Agents and techniques for peripheral nerve blocks	197	Nerve blocks of the lower limb	219
Nerve blocks of the head and neck	200	Nerve blocks of the pelvis	230
Nerve blocks of the upper limb	204	References	232
Nerve blocks of the thorax and abdomen	215		

The ability to perform peripheral nerve blocks is an essential skill in the comprehensive management of acute, chronic, and cancer pain. The main prerequisite for successful peripheral nerve blocks is a full understanding of the relevant topographical landmarks, the structures between the skin and the relevant nerve, and the course and immediate relations of the nerve. Accurate location of the target nerve often requires competence in the use of a peripheral nerve stimulator; however, this is not a substitute for adequate anatomical knowledge.

The Holy Grail of peripheral nerve blockade is a long-lasting local anesthetic that is completely reversible. However, in the absence of such an agent, pain management still occasionally necessitates the use of chemical, thermal, or cryogenic destructive techniques, especially near the end of life.

AGENTS AND TECHNIQUES FOR PERIPHERAL NERVE BLOCKS

Local anesthetics

Local anesthetics are sodium channel-blocking drugs that are unique in their ability to block nerve impulses conducted proximally (pain relief) and impulses conducted distally (motor blockade) in any peripheral nerve. Unlike neurolytic agents, local anesthetics produce a conduction block that is painless and completely reversible. Nerve fiber types vary in their sensitivity to local anesthetics, so that injection of differing concentrations selectively blocks different types of fiber. Differential blockade is a useful diagnostic tool and has several practical uses in pain management:

- Attributing pain to a single nerve.
- Differential block to identify the neural pathway that subserves the pain.
- Permits precise targeting prior to a destructive procedure.
- Allows the patient to experience temporary before permanent blockade.
- Repeated at intervals, temporary blockade may have a long-lasting effect (e.g. scar neuromas or muscle trigger point injections).

Local anesthetic blocks are both diagnostic and therapeutic and may obviate the need for permanent neurolysis.

Individual agents[1]

Lidocaine (lignocaine)

- Rapid onset and short duration (hours).
- Maximum recommended dose in adult is 200 mg (data sheet), although doses of 4–7 mg/kg have been advocated.
- Lidocaine causes vasodilatation at the site of injection.
- Addition of 1:200,000 epinephrine (adrenaline) may slow systemic absorption and prolong duration of the block.
- Large doses (35 mg/kg) combined with 1:1,000,000 epinephrine by subcutaneous infiltration have been used for liposuction.
- Available preparations may contain the preservatives sodium metabisulfite and methylparahydroxybenzoate, both of which may cause nerve injury.

Prilocaine

- Rapid onset and duration.

- Similar potency to lidocaine.
- Readily hydrolyzed, reducing risk of systemic toxicity.
- Aminophenol metabolites oxidize hemoglobin to methemoglobin.
- Maximum dose 10 mg/kg (total maximum adult dose 600 mg).
- Has no vasoactivity.
- Multidose vials contain methylparahydroxybenzoate as preservative.

Bupivacaine (racemic)

- Slow onset and long duration (lasts two to three times longer than lidocaine).
- Maximum recommended dose in adults 150 mg, dosage should not exceed 2 mg/kg.
- Epinephrine does not seem to reduce systemic absorption or prolong duration of block.
- Main disadvantage is low threshold for cardiotoxicity. Experimentally, epinephrine enhances cardiotoxicity.
- Epinephrine-containing preparations contain sodium metabisulfite.
- Opioid–bupivacaine mixtures provide analgesia in a synergistic manner.

Levobupivacaine

- This S-enantiomer of bupivacaine is less cardiotoxic.
- Equipotent to racemic bupivacaine by the epidural route.
- Still to be fully evaluated clinically in peripheral nerve blockade.

Ropivacaine

- Claims a greater degree of separation between sensory and motor nerve block (differential block).
- Claims of less toxicity may be secondary to its potency being lower than bupivacaine.
- Ropivacaine causes vasoconstriction and prolongation of nerve blockade compared with bupivacaine.
- The addition of epinephrine probably confers no additional benefit.
- Maximum recommended dose 2 mg/kg.

Neurolytic agents and techniques for peripheral nerve blockade[2]**

Neurolysis of peripheral nerves by chemical, thermal, or cryogenic means is indicated for patients with limited life expectancy. Peripheral neurolysis has several disadvantages:

- The analgesia is not permanent.
- It is associated with neuritis and deafferentation pain.
- It can produce unwanted motor blockade.
- It can damage surrounding tissues.

Therefore, it is usually performed under the following circumstances:

- The pain is severe and other methods have failed.
- The pain is in the distribution of an identifiable peripheral nerve.
- A trial block of local anesthetic has been successful.
- The effects of the local anesthetic block are acceptable to the patient.

The most undesirable complication of peripheral neurolysis is the onset of neuropathic pain. This has been reported following treatment in up to 28% of cases. Comparisons of different volumes and concentrations of neurolytic agents have not been reported. It would seem logical to use a small amount of agent to minimize damage to nontarget tissue; however, incomplete lesions may make neuropathic pain more likely. Repeat injections are often necessary to achieve success.

Neurolytic agents

Alcohol and phenol are the most commonly used agents. The incidence of neuropathic pain is believed to be greater following peripheral neurolysis with alcohol.

Alcohol

- Generally used undiluted for peripheral nerve blockade.
- Injection is immediately followed by burning pain along the distribution of the nerve, followed by warm numbness.
- Pain relief increases over a few days and is maximal by a week.

Phenol

- Various concentrations are available as an aqueous preparation or in glycerin. A maximum of 6.7% can be dissolved in water at room temperature.
- Aqueous phenol can be injected down smaller gauge needles.
- Following injection, an initial local anesthetic effect subsides to neurolysis, which may take 3–7 days to become apparent.
- The density and duration of the block is felt to be less than that of alcohol; 5% phenol is equivalent to 40% alcohol in neurolytic potency.

Neurolytic techniques

Cryoanalgesia
The basic principle is as follows:

- Freezing of a nerve segment to –60°C with a 2-mm probe.
- Achieved by rapid expansion of carbon dioxide or nitrous oxide gas.
- The probe is left in contact with the nerve for 1–2 min and allowed to thaw before removal.
- An acute injury produces analgesia for 2–20 weeks.
- The basal lamina of the nerve is left intact, allowing eventual regeneration.

Although cryoanalgesia has its proponents, results can be disappointing. The technique requires accurate placement of a bulky probe, which is difficult to achieve when inserted percutaneously. Placement under direct vision is not usually a realistic option in pain management clinics. The main advantage of cryoanalgesia is the low risk of neuritis.

Pulsed radiofrequency

- A pulsed radiofrequency (RF) lesion is achieved by applying energy with a pulsed time cycle of $2 \times 20\,ms/s$ at temperatures not exceeding 42°C.
- The mechanism of neuromodulation is unclear, but the electromagnetic field energy may interrupt nerve transmission.
- Pulsed RF has been used with benefit for blockade of most peripheral nerves and ganglia.
- A typical lesion is 42°C for 120 s repeated three times.

Nerve location by peripheral nerve stimulation[3]

A peripheral nerve stimulator (PNS) is not a substitute for anatomical knowledge and should not be used to hunt blindly for nerves. Its main use is to place a needle close to the target nerve, especially when a nerve or plexus has a characteristic pattern of muscle movement in response to stimulation. The distinct endpoint is pulse-synchronous muscle movement or paresthesiae attributable to the target nerve.

Principles of nerve location

- Use a PNS that has a variable current output up to 5 mA.
- Set for short duration of impulse (less than 100 µs) at a frequency of 1–2 Hz so that motor nerves are stimulated preferentially.
- Connect anode (+ve) to a large ground electrode well away from the site of the nerve block to ensure current flows through the target nerve.
- Initially set delivered current at 3 mA.
- Connect cathode (–ve) to block the needle.
- Using a standard approach to the nerve, advance needle until within the expected vicinity of nerve.
- When using a current of around 3 mA or less, the nerve will not be stimulated unless the needle tip is within 1 cm.
- Painful levels of stimulation will be needed if the nerve is more than 2 cm away.
- Look for pulse-synchronous muscle movement to indicate that the needle tip is close to the nerve.
- Carefully adjust the needle tip position so that "just discernible" muscle movement is seen with a current of 0.1–0.5 mA.
- Sudden pain or exaggerated muscle movement may

indicate direct contact with the nerve.
- The exact current depends on the target nerve. Small nerves such as the median nerve require 0.1–0.3 mA whereas the sciatic nerve may require 2 mA.
- Elderly patients or the presence of neuropathy require greater current.
- Following injection of local anesthetic, muscle movement will increase because of increased current conduction and then fade as the nerve is displaced by the volume of the injection.

Insulated or noninsulated needles

- Insulated needles prevent current loss in surrounding tissue.
- Insulated needles require half the current of noninsulated needles.
- There is a greater variety and availability of noninsulated needles.
- For most uses, noninsulated needles are satisfactory.
- There is no evidence that one needle over another is more successful or minimizes the risk of neural damage.

General principles of practice

This chapter is essentially a "how to do it" guide, and detailed discussions of the indications and efficacy of the blocks for various pain conditions are not discussed. This information can be found in the relevant chapters elsewhere or in the reference included with each block.

Resuscitation equipment

- Infrequently, systemic toxicity from the administration of local anesthetic and neurolytic agents can occur.
- These techniques should not be performed without immediate availability of, and skill in using, airway and cardiovascular resuscitation facilities.

Aseptic technique

- All equipment should be sterile and preferably disposable.
- Cleaning fluids should be disposed of prior to drawing up local anesthetic solutions to avoid error.
- Both gloves and a mask should be worn.

Needles

- Preliminary skin infiltration and wheals are performed with 23-gauge or 25-gauge hypodermic needles.
- There is no consensus on which design of needle to use for peripheral nerve block, both long and short beveled needles have been shown to produce nerve trauma.

- Short, beveled needles (angle approximately 45°) offer more feedback to the operator.
- Pencil-point needles (side port) are designed to prevent intraneural injection and may yet prove to be beneficial.

NERVE BLOCKS OF THE HEAD AND NECK

Occipital nerve block[4]**

Indications

- Diagnosis and treatment of occipital neuralgia.
- Scalp anesthesia for surgical procedures.

As defined by the International Headache Society, occipital neuralgia is diagnosed by successful local anesthetic block of that nerve. Chronic occipital neuralgia can be treated by repeated injections of local anesthetic and depot steroid.

Relevant anatomy

- The greater occipital nerves originate from the posterior rami of C2, often with a branch from C3.
- Interneuronal connections within the upper spinal cord may allow occipital pain to be referred to the trigeminal distribution.
- The nerve becomes subcutaneous inferior to the superior nuchal line, 3 cm lateral to the occipital protuberance, and lies immediately medial to the occipital artery.
- The lesser occipital nerve originates from the anterior rami of C2 and C3.
- The nerve runs upwards along the posterior border of the sternomastoid muscle to supply the lateral and posterior scalp.
- The lesser occipital nerve lies superficial to, and becomes lateral to, the occipital artery.

Landmarks

- Greater occipital protuberance.
- Mastoid process.
- Occipital artery.

Practical steps (Fig. 17.1)

- Best position is sitting with the head flexed.
- Selection of nerve for block is based on reproduction of pain with nerve palpation.
- Identify the line between the occipital protuberance and the mastoid process.
- Insert a 25-gauge needle subcutaneously 2 cm lateral to the occipital protuberance, and medial to the pulsation of the occipital artery.

- Inject 4–5 ml of solution to block the greater occipital nerve.
- Redirect the needle along the line between the bony landmarks toward the mastoid process and inject a further 3–4 ml subcutaneously to block the lesser occipital nerve.

Complications

- The superficial nature of the block should make complications rare.

Peripheral branches of the trigeminal nerve[5]

Blockade of the more peripheral branches (mental nerve, infraorbital nerve, supraorbital nerve, and supratrochlear nerve) has the advantage of a lower incidence of unwanted motor blockade and sensory disturbances than blockade of the Gasserian ganglion.

Indications

See Table 17.1.

Relevant anatomy (Fig. 17.2)

- The three foramina for the mental nerve, the infraorbital nerve, and the supraorbital nerve all lie in the same plane, which passes through the pupil in its resting position.
- The supratrochlear nerve lies medial to the supraorbital nerve.

Mental nerve block

The mental nerve can be blocked by an intraoral or an extraoral route. The extraoral route will be described.

Landmarks

- Mental foramen.

Practical steps

- Palpation to identify the mental foramen.
- Clean skin.
- A 25-gauge needle is inserted toward the foramen.
- The needle should not be placed in the canal, to avoid nerve damage.
- Aspirate for blood.
- Inject 2–3 ml of local anesthetic.
- Neurolysis can be achieved with incremental injections of 0.1 ml of glycerol or phenol in glycerin after trail block with local anesthetic. Cryoanalgesia can also be performed, but a small scar may occur.

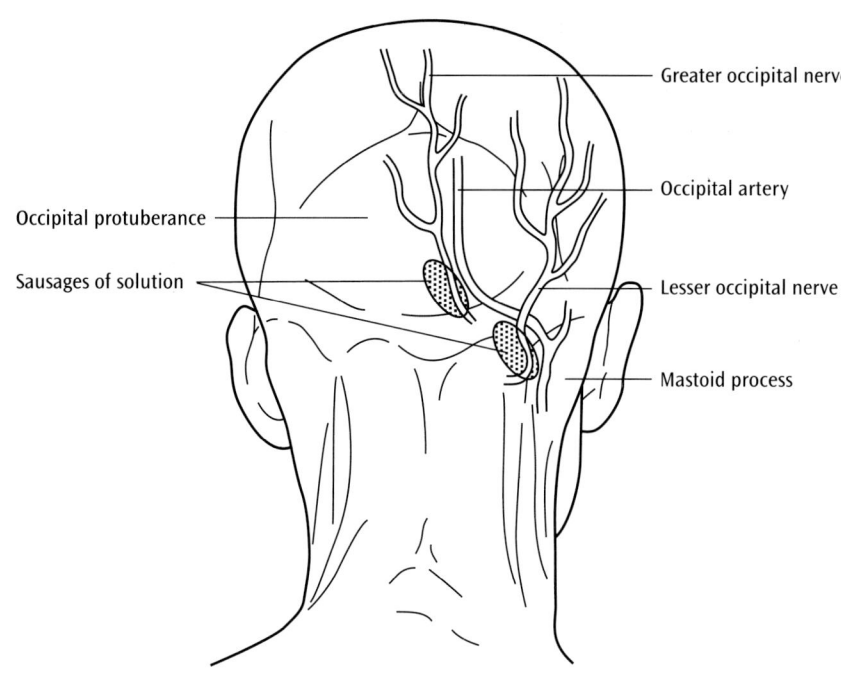

Figure 17.1 *Occipital nerve block. Landmarks for blockade of the greater and lesser occipital nerves.*

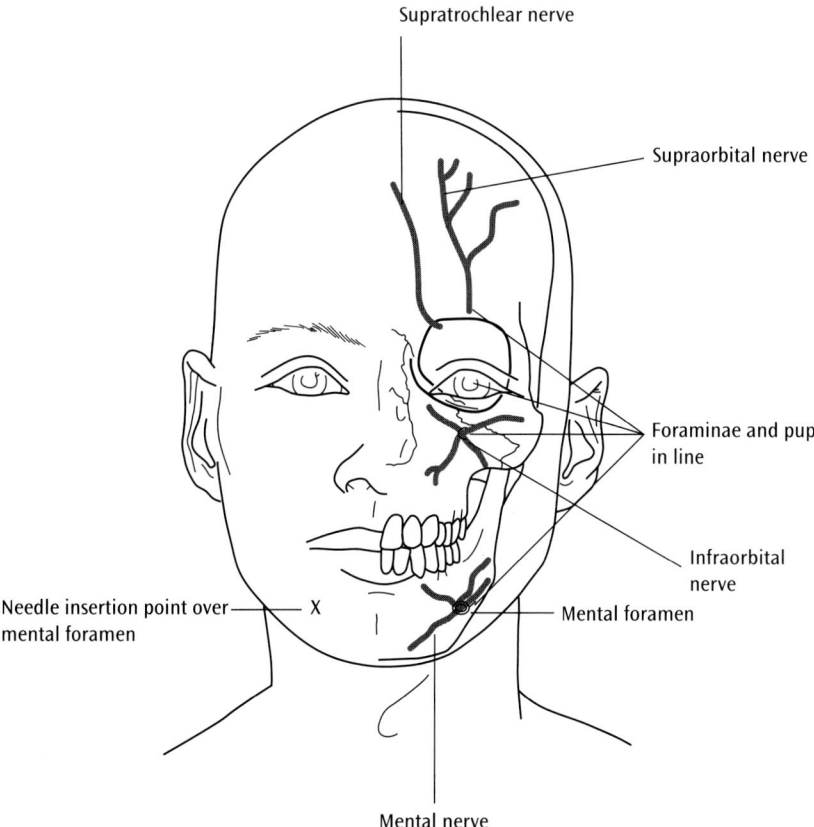

Figure 17.2 *Peripheral branches of the trigeminal nerve. Landmarks for blockade of supraorbital, infraorbital, and mental nerves.*

Infraorbital nerve block

Landmarks
- Infraorbital foramen.

Practical steps
- Palpate infraorbital foramen (1 cm lateral to external nares and 1 cm below the lower border of the orbit).
- Insert a 25-gauge needle subcutaneously towards the foramen.
- Avoid entering the canal with the needle.
- Aspirate for blood.
- Inject 2–3 ml of local anesthetic.
- Neurolysis as above.

Table 17.1 *Indications for blockade of the peripheral branches of the trigeminal nerve*

Local anesthetic block	Local anesthetic and steroid block	Neurolytic block
Surgical anesthesia	Adjunct to pharmacological treatment of trigeminal neuralgia	Cancer pain
Differential neural block	Atypical facial pain	Trigeminal neuralgia
Trial block prior to neurolysis	Cluster headaches	Cluster headache
Palliation in acute emergencies	Facial trauma	
Palliation of acute shingles		

Supraorbital and supratrochlear nerve blocks

Landmarks

- Supraorbital notch.
- Bridge of nose.

Practical steps

- Palpate supraorbital notch.
- Clean skin, avoiding the eye.
- Move 25-gauge needle subcutaneously toward notch.
- Avoid entering foramen.
- Aspirate for blood.
- Inject 3–4 ml of local anesthetic.
- Redirect needle medially toward the bridge of the nose.
- Aspirate for blood.
- Inject a further 3–4 ml of local anesthetic.
- For bilateral block, insert the needle in the midpoint of the bridge of the nose.
- Neurolysis as above; avoid damaging hair follicles in the eyebrow with cryoanalgesia.

Complications

- Trauma to nerves (compression).
- Facial hematoma.
- Infection.
- Activation of herpes zoster.
- Postneurolytic dysesthesia.

Spinal accessory nerve block[6]

Primarily, this block was advocated for the treatment of cervical dystonias. However, the efficacy and safety of botulinum toxin injections has largely made this block redundant.

Indications

- Diagnosis and treatment of spasm of sternomastoid or trapezius muscles (multiple sclerosis, posterior fossa tumors, collagen diseases, or myopathies).
- Neurodestruction of the nerve has been carried out by chemical, cryogenic, radiofrequency, or surgical lesions.

Relevant anatomy

- Origin – nucleus ambiguus.
- Exits the skull through the jugular foramen.

- The nerve traverses the posterior border of the sternomastoid muscle in the upper third of the muscle.
- Along with the cervical plexus, the nerve innervates the trapezius muscle.

Landmarks

- Posterior border of the sternomastoid.

Practical steps (Fig. 17.3)

- Patient lies supine looking away from the side of the block.
- Patient lifts the head against resistance to outline the posterior border of the sternomastoid muscle.
- Insert a 25-gauge needle at the junction of the upper one-third with the lower two-thirds of the posterior border of the muscle.
- Direct the needle slightly anteriorly to a depth of approximately 2 cm.
- Aspirate for blood.
- Inject 10 ml of local anesthetic, which may be combined with steroid (up to 80 mg depot methyl-prednisolone).

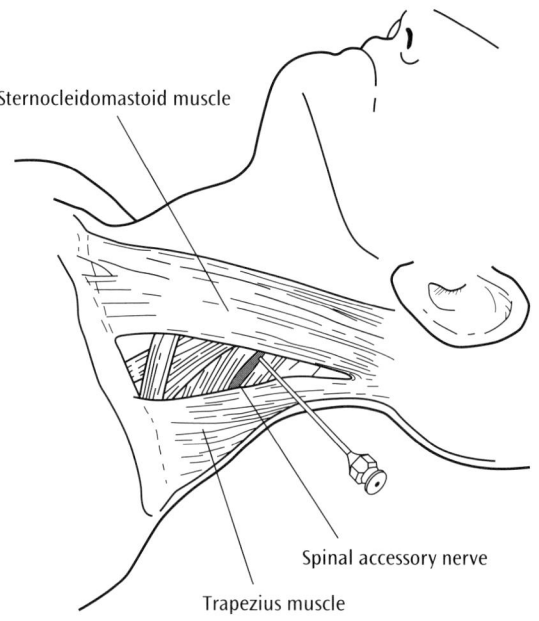

Sternocleidomastoid muscle

Spinal accessory nerve

Trapezius muscle

Figure 17.3 *Spinal accessory nerve block. Landmarks for blockade of the spinal accessory nerve.*

Complications

- Inadvertent intravascular injection (jugular vessels).
- Hematoma (reduced by applying pressure or ice packs).
- Inadvertent block of phrenic, recurrent laryngeal, vagus, or glossopharyngeal nerves.
- Inadvertent central neural block.

Cervical plexus block[7]

Cervical plexus block can be deep or superficial; the deep block also provides muscle relaxation (motor block).

Indications

- Surgery of the neck (usually carotid endarterectomy).
- Pharyngeal cancer pain.
- Occipital and posterior auricular neuralgia.

Superficial cervical plexus block

Relevant anatomy (Fig. 17.4A)

- The superficial branches of the plexus (C2–4) are cutaneous and emerge from behind the posterior border of the sternomastoid muscle at its midpoint.
- They penetrate the cervical fascia and radiate out subcutaneously.
- Innervates the skin of the scalp and ear (lesser occipital and great auricular nerve).
- Innervates the skin of the submandibular area, the neck, top of the shoulders, and anterior chest wall (anterior cutaneous nerve and supraclavicular nerves).

Landmarks

- Posterior border of the sternomastoid.
- Cricoid cartilage.

Practical steps

- Position patient supine with head turned away from side of block.
- Single injection technique (Fig. 17.4B)
  - A line drawn laterally from the cricoid cartilage usually crosses the middle of the posterior border of the sternomastoid muscle where the nerves emerge.
  - Insert a 22-gauge needle immediately behind the muscle at the midpoint and at right angles to the skin until it "pops" through the cervical fascia.
  - Inject 10 ml of local anesthetic solution, which if correctly placed will be seen flowing up and down the posterior border of the muscle.
- Superficial injection technique (Fig. 17.4C)
  - Insert a 22-gauge needle subcutaneously and infiltrate along the middle one-third of the posterior border of the sternomastoid.
  - Inject 5–10 ml of local anesthetic.

Deep cervical plexus block (Labat method)

Relevant anatomy

- The cervical roots emerge from the intervertebral foraminae.
- They lie in the sulcus of the transverse processes before combining to form the plexus.
- A deep plexus block is in effect a cervical paravertebral block of C2–4.

Landmarks (Fig. 17.5)

- Mastoid process.
- Chassaignac's tubercle (C6).
- Cricoid cartilage.

Practical steps (Fig. 17.5)

- The patient lies supine with the head turned away from the side of the block.
- A line is drawn from the mastoid process to the anterior tubercle of C6 at the level of the cricoid cartilage.
- This line indicates the position of the cervical transverse processes.
- On this line, the transverse processes of C2–4 are palpated (approximately 1.5-cm intervals below the mastoid process).
- C3 lies at the level of the hyoid bone.
- C4 lies at the level of the upper border of the thyroid cartilage.
- The skin is infiltrated overlying the transverse processes of C2, 3, and 4.
- A 22-gauge, 3.5-cm needle is inserted medially and downwards onto the transverse processes at these three points (usually less than 2 cm deep, they become more superficial as they descend).
- The needle is then walked laterally off the transverse process.
- Aspirate for blood and cerebrospinal fluid (CSF).
- Inject 3–5 ml of local anesthetic.

The needle must locate the transverse process as far laterally as possible to avoid the vertebral artery. The downward direction of the needle avoids insertion into the intervertebral foramen, and risk of epidural or subarachnoid injection.

Complications

- Inadequate block for surgery.
- Intravascular injection of local anesthetic (vertebral artery, jugular veins).
- Hematoma (tear of vein).
- Compression of carotid sheath (large volumes of local anesthetic).
- Central neural blockade.
- Recurrent laryngeal nerve block (2%).
- Phrenic nerve block (50%).
- Hypoglossal nerve block.
- Injury of spinal cord.

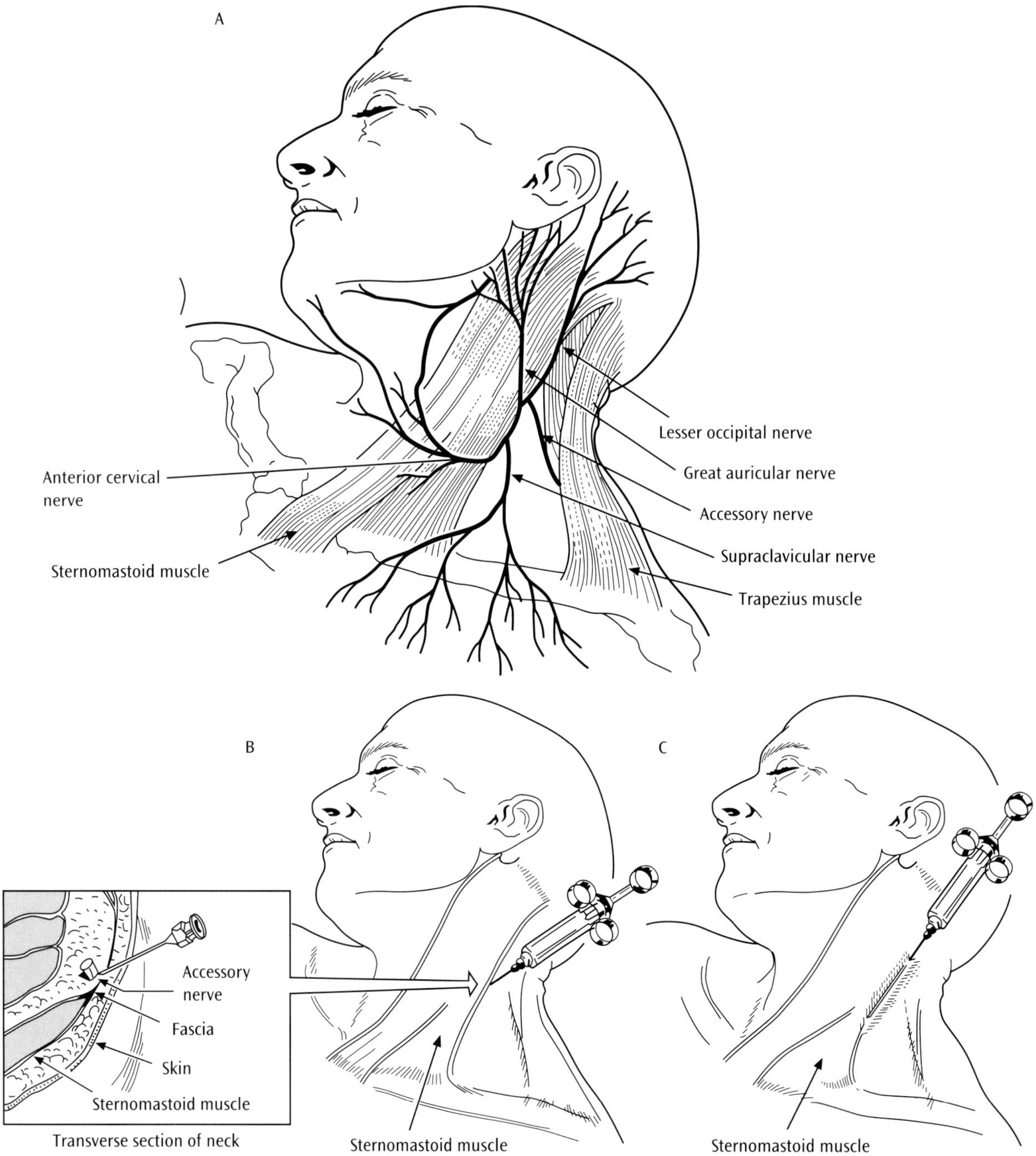

A

Lesser occipital nerve

Great auricular nerve

Accessory nerve

Supraclavicular nerve

Trapezius muscle

Anterior cervical nerve

Sternomastoid muscle

B

Accessory nerve

Fascia

Skin

Sternomastoid muscle

Transverse section of neck

Sternomastoid muscle

C

Sternomastoid muscle

Figure 17.4 *(A) Cervical plexus. (B) Superficial cervical plexus block; landmarks for the single-injection technique. (C) Superficial cervical plexus block; landmarks for the superficial injection technique.*

NERVE BLOCKS OF THE UPPER LIMB

Brachial plexus block[8]

The literature describes over 40 different techniques, which fall into four approaches: interscalene, supraclavicular, infraclavicular, and axillary.

- No one technique is clearly better than another.
- The axillary approach is the easiest to learn with the fewest complications.

- The infraclavicular approach is the least popular as it requires a peripheral nerve stimulator connected to an 8-cm needle, which can be uncomfortable for the conscious patient.
- The use of 40 ml of solution (in a healthy male patient) combined with digital pressure should produce a satisfactory block, whatever approach is used.
- The "immobile needle" technique is important. Using a 10- to 20-cm extension tube, the needle can be isolated from the movements of the syringe (aspiration, injection, and changing of syringes).

- A short, beveled needle may give better sensation when the brachial plexus sheath is breached.
- A peripheral nerve stimulator is often used to confirm the needle position, and pulse synchronous muscle movements are easily detected in the arm.
- Onset of block may take up to 40 min with bupivacaine.

Indications

- Surgical anesthesia of the shoulder, arm, or hand.
- Postsurgical analgesia employing continuous infusion.

- Chronic pain management employing intermittent bolus or continuous infusion.
  - Differential block.
  - Complex regional pain syndrome (to facilitate physical therapy).
  - Brachial plexus invasion by tumor.

Relevant anatomy (Fig. 17.6)

(The ramifications and various junctions of the roots on their way to becoming peripheral nerves is not clini-

Figure 17.5 *Deep cervical plexus block. Landmarks and needle insertion points for deep cervical plexus block.*

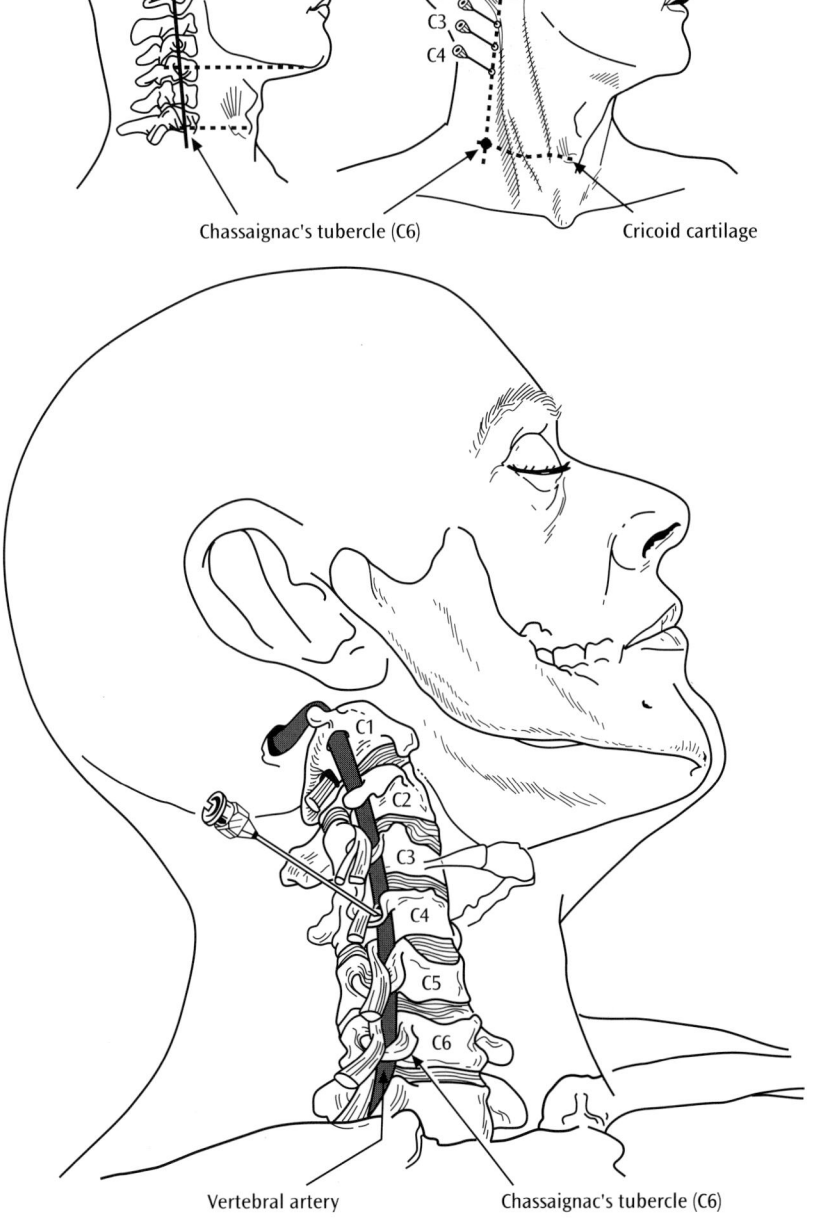

cally relevant, only the anatomy of practical use will be described.)

- Roots arise from C4–T1.
- The radial nerve supplies all dorsal muscles in the upper arm below the shoulder.
- The musculocutaneous nerve supplies the muscles in the arm and skin sensation in the forearm.
- The median and ulnar nerves are nerves of passage in the arm, but result in motor function in the forearm and hand together with sensation in the hand.
- The median nerve is mainly responsible for forearm innervation, whereas the hand is more heavily innervated by the ulnar nerve.
- The four main peripheral nerves can be checked using the "four Ps" (Table 17.2).
- The vertebral arteries leave the brachiocephalic or subclavian arteries and travel upwards to enter a bony canal in the transverse process of C6. It is important to be aware of needle tip position in this area.
- The phrenic nerve passes through the neck to the thorax on the ventral surface of the anterior scalene muscle. It is always blocked with the interscalene approach.

Interscalene block

- Best for shoulder analgesia.
- Often the ulnar nerve is spared.
- Can be performed with arm in any position.

Landmarks

- Cricoid cartilage.
- Posterior border of the sternomastoid muscle.
- Interscalene groove.

Practical steps (Fig. 17.7)

- Position the patient supine with the head on a pillow, and turned away from the side of the block.
- Push patient's shoulder to lower the clavicle.
- A line drawn laterally from the cricoid cartilage crosses the midpoint of the sternomastoid.
- Locate the interscalene groove behind the midpoint of the posterior border of sternomastoid (roll fingers).
- The interscalene groove is at an oblique angle to the sternomastoid (it is not parallel to the sternomastoid).
- Asking the patient to sniff or inspire vigorously will relax the scalene muscles enough to feel the transverse process of C6.
- At this point, insert a 22-gauge, 3.5-cm needle aiming slightly caudad, posterior, and medially (an extension of the needle would exit the neck through the spinous process of T1).
- The plexus sheath will usually be breached at 1–2.5 cm deep; remember this should be a very superficial block.
- Advance the needle carefully until paresthesiae are elicited or there is a motor response with a nerve stimulator.

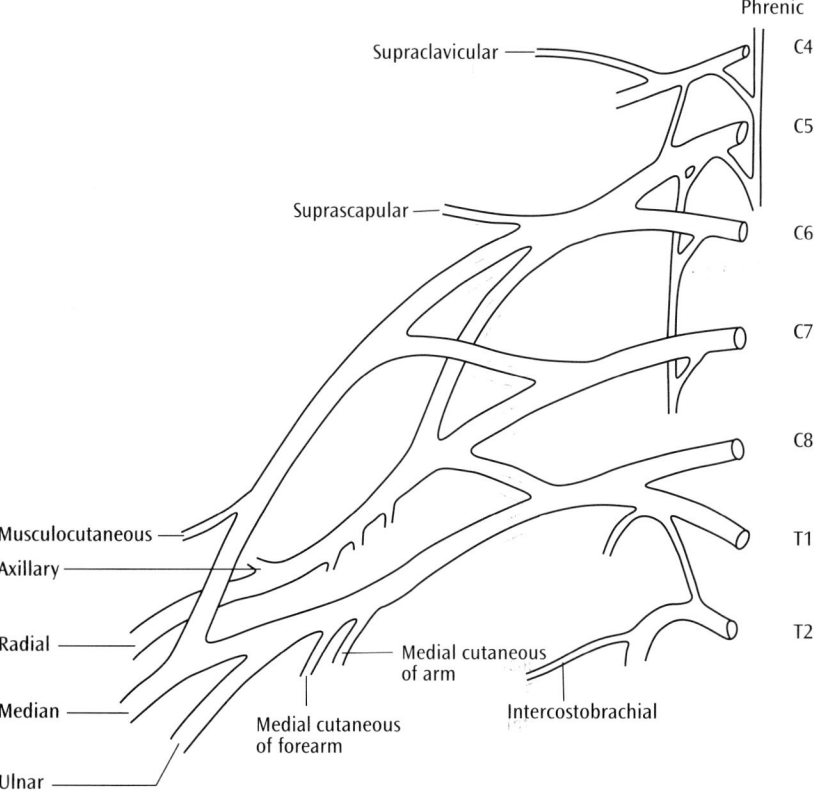

Figure 17.6 *Brachial plexus. Basic anatomy of the brachial plexus.*

Table 17.2 *Testing of four main peripheral nerves of the brachial plexus*

"Four Ps"	Action	Nerve checked
Push	Extend arm with triceps	Radial
Pull	Flex arm with biceps	Musculocutaneous
Pinch	Fifth digit	Ulnar
Pinch	Index finger	Median

- Aspirate for blood or CSF.
- Inject slowly and incrementally.

Supraclavicular block (subclavian perivascular technique)

- Best chance of blocking the entire arm.
- Delayed onset of pneumothorax may preclude use as an outpatient procedure.
- Block carried out at the "division" level of the plexus.

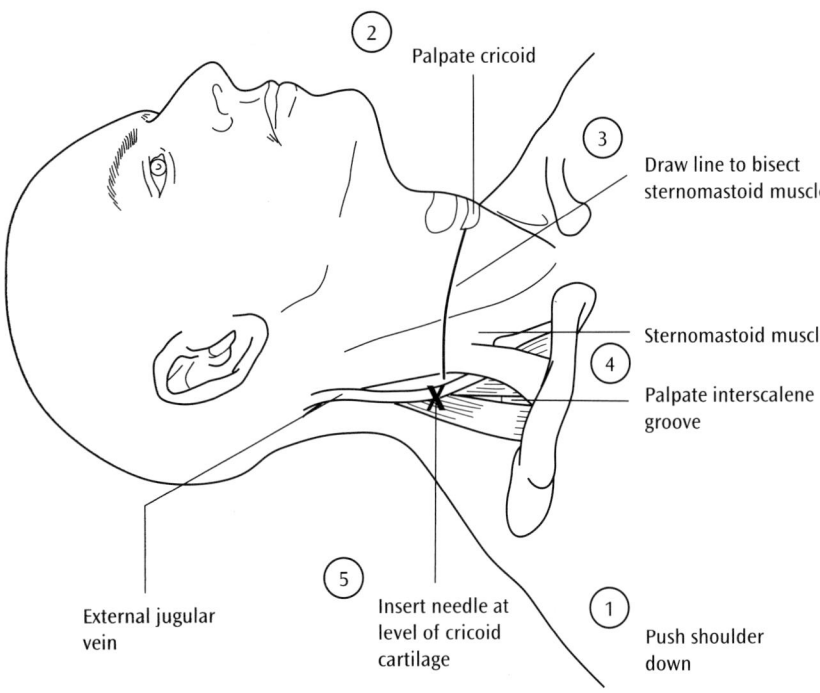

Figure 17.7 *Interscalene block. Landmarks and steps for performing interscalene brachial plexus block.*

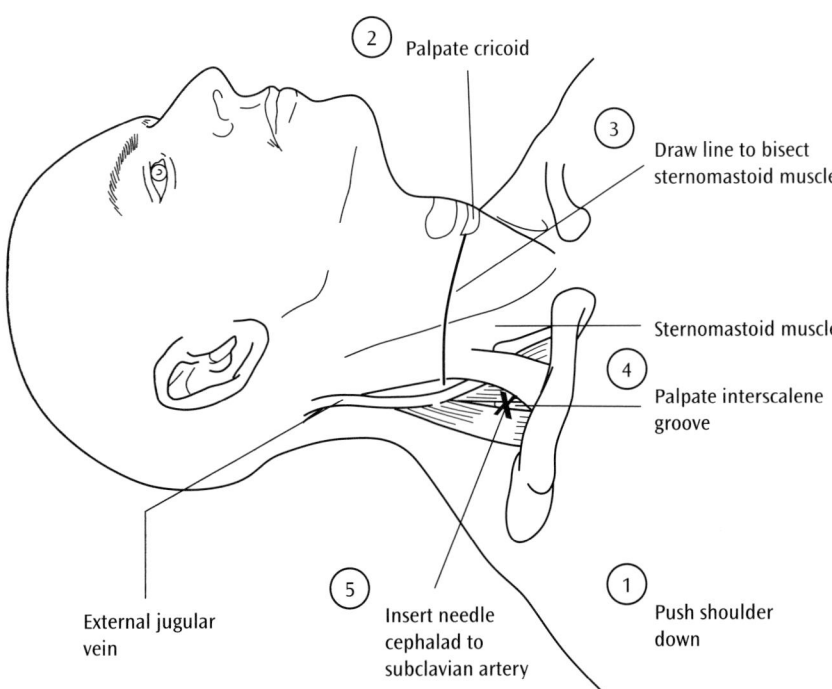

Figure 17.8 *Supraclavicular block. Landmarks and steps for performing supraclavicular brachial plexus block.*

Landmarks

- Cricoid cartilage.
- Posterior border of the sternomastoid.
- Clavicle.
- Pulsation of subclavian artery.

Practical steps (Fig. 17.8)

- Patient lies supine with a small pillow, head turned away from the side of the block.
- Locate the interscalene groove as above.
- Follow the interscalene groove distally until it meets the clavicle.
- The pulsation of the subclavian artery can be felt in the interscalene groove 1 cm superior to the clavicle at its midpoint.
- The ideal position for needle insertion is just above the pulsation of the subclavian artery.
- Insert a 22-gauge, 3.5-cm needle caudally in the horizontal plane, parallel to the neck.
- The needle should pierce the plexus sheath 1–2 cm deep to the skin.
- Paresthesiae may occur immediately, and usually occur in the distribution of the superior trunk.
- A peripheral nerve stimulator may be used to confirm the needle position.
- Hold the needle in a steady position and aspirate for blood.
- Inject local anesthetic solution using digital pressure to encourage proximal or distal spread of local anesthetic as desired.
- Sheath should be seen distending.
- Subcutaneous swelling indicates an extrasheath injection.

Infraclavicular block (method of Raj)

- Often used for continuous plexus analgesia.
- Needle crosses the pectoral muscle and is more painful than other approaches.
- Sedation may be required.

Landmarks

- Chassaignac's tubercle (C6).
- Brachial artery.
- Midclavicular point.

Practical steps (Fig. 17.9)

- Patient lies supine with arm abducted.
- A line is drawn between the transverse process of C6 and the brachial artery through the midpoint of the clavicle.
- The site of needle insertion is a point 2.5 cm caudad to the midclavicle.
- A 22-gauge, 10-cm needle or cannula is inserted in a direction from the insertion site toward the imagined brachial artery in the proximal axilla (i.e. directed laterally).

- A peripheral nerve stimulator is useful as it allows the patient to be sedated (needle insertion can be painful).
- Aspirate for blood (axillary artery or vein).
- Inject local anesthetic solution incrementally.

Axillary block

- Most effective for analgesia distal to the elbow.
- Risk of complications is low.
- Block can be single shot or continuous.
- Since the axillary artery lies at the center of a four-quadrant neurovascular bundle, some favor multiple injections to improve the quality of block.
- The block does not have to be performed high in the axilla, needle insertion in the mid to lower portion of the axillary hair patch may be easier and equally effective.
- The musculocutaneous nerve may be spared and require separate block.
- The intercostobrachial nerve is not part of the plexus and is blocked separately by subcutaneous infiltration in the medial axilla (prevents tourniquet pain).

Landmarks

- Axillary artery pulsation.
- Lateral border of pectoralis major.

Practical steps (Fig. 17.10)

Position patient supine with arm abducted to 90° at the shoulder and the elbow flexed to 90° (overabduction may compress the axillary artery).

- Single injection or insertion of the cannula
  - Palpate the pulsation of the axillary artery at the level of the lateral border of the pectoralis major.
  - Fix the artery with the palpating finger.
  - Insert a 22-gauge, 3.5-cm needle or cannula just superior to the artery and parallel to it as if going to cannulate the artery.
  - As the plexus sheath is pierced, a change of resistance should be felt.
  - Paresthesiae indicate correct needle placement.
  - A peripheral nerve stimulator can confirm the needle position.
  - Aspirate for blood.
  - Inject local anesthetic solution using digital pressure to encourage proximal spread of solution.
  - If the axillary artery is inadvertently entered, the needle can either be withdrawn or it can be advanced beyond the artery and the injection made deep to the artery (transarterial technique).
  - Successful injection is indicated by a "sausage-shaped" distension of the plexus sheath, whereas subcutaneous injection is indicated by a "hamburger-shaped" distension in the axilla.
- Multiple injections (Fig. 17.11)
  - Palpate and fix the axillary artery.

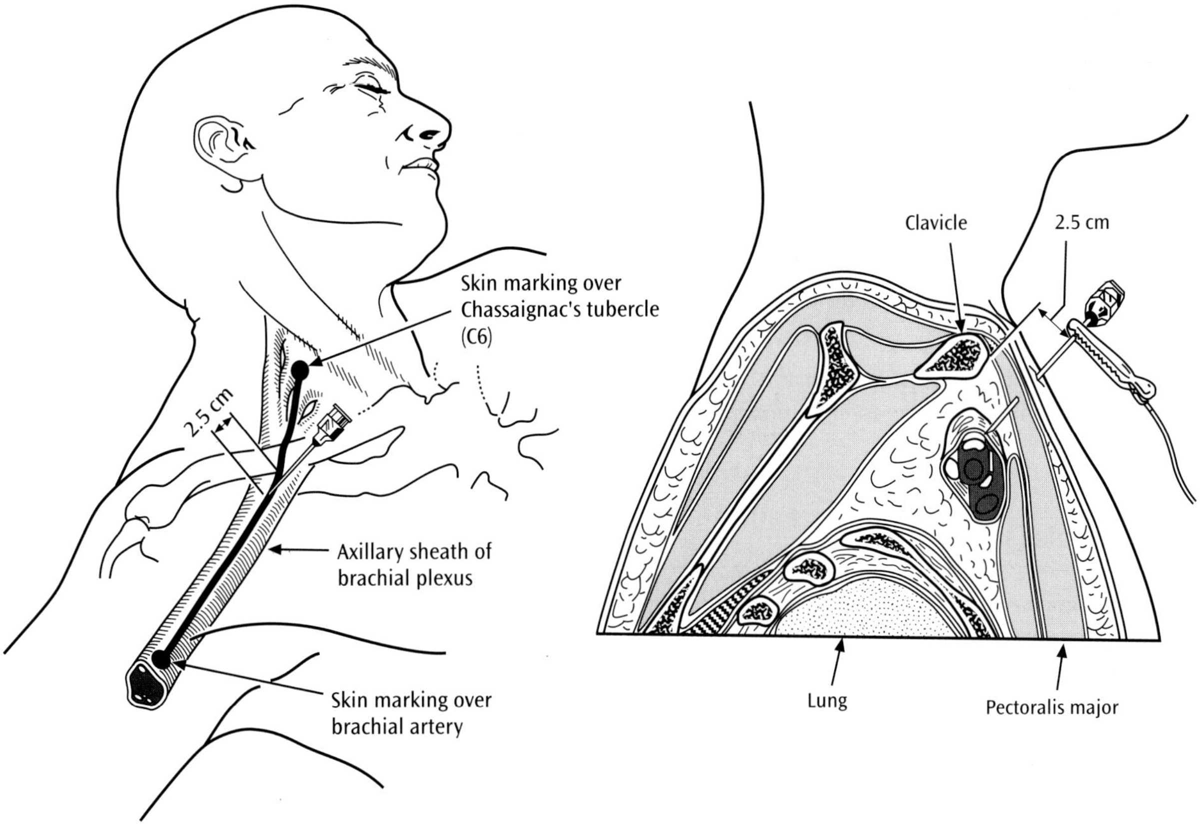

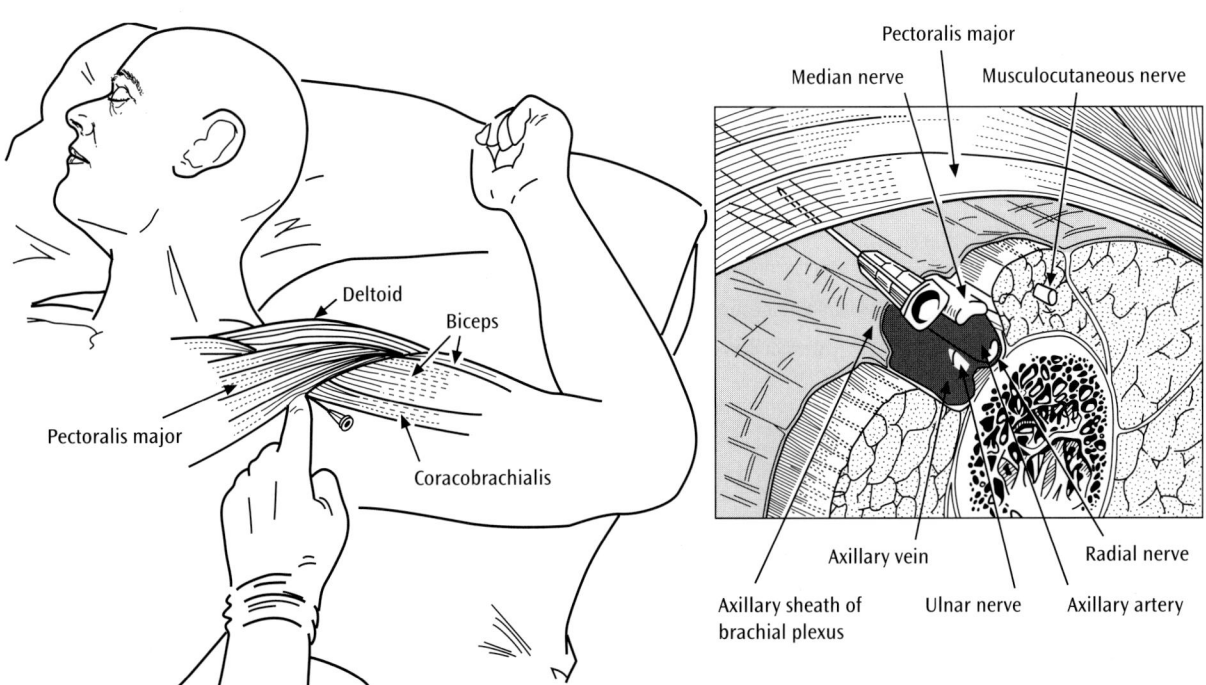

Figure 17.9 *Infraclavicular block. Landmarks for infraclavicular block.*

Figure 17.10 *Axillary block. Landmarks for axillary brachial plexus block.*

- Inject around the axillary artery in a "fan-like" manner.
- Divide the local anesthetic dose into four quadrant injections.
- The median nerve is found in the 12-to-3 quadrant (as on a clock).
- The ulnar nerve in the 3-to-6 quadrant.
- The radial nerve in the 6-to-9 quadrant.
- The musculocutaneous nerve in the 9-to-12 quadrant within the substance of the coracobrachialis muscle.

Complications of brachial plexus block

For a description of possible complications, see Table 17.3.

Suprascapular nerve block[9]

The suprascapular nerve can be blocked by the anterior, posterior, or superior approach. Only the posterior approach will be described

Indications

Local anesthetic block

- Postsurgical pain relief.
- Assessment of shoulder pain (differential block).
- Trial block prior to neurolysis.

Local anesthetic and depot steroid block

- To facilitate physical therapy of the shoulder joint (capsulitis, bursitis, tendinitis).
- Shoulder stiffness and pain secondary to complex regional pain syndrome.

Neurolytic block

- Cancer pain.

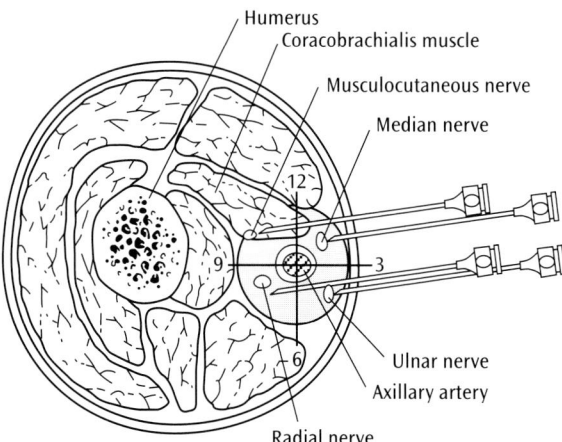

Figure 17.11 *Axillary block: multiple injection technique. Needle insertion points for performing axillary brachial plexus block by multiple injection technique.*

Relevant anatomy

- The suprascapular nerve is a branch of the brachial plexus (C4–6).
- The nerve passes under the coracoclavicular ligament through the suprascapular notch.
- The artery and vein accompany the nerve through the notch.
- The nerve supplies sensation of the shoulder joint.
- The nerve innervates infraspinatus and supraspinatus muscles.

Landmarks

- Spine of scapula.

Practical steps (Fig. 17.12)

- The posterior approach is only suitable for conscious patients because the patient is sitting.
- Palpate the spine of the scapula and identify its midpoint.
- The suprascapular notch lies about 1 cm above.
- Insert a 22-gauge, short, beveled needle at right angles to the skin until bony contact is made (usually 2–3 cm).
- "Walk" the needle upwards to the edge of the suprascapular notch.
- Paresthesiae may occur.
- Avoid entering the notch too deeply and causing nerve damage or pneumothorax.
- Avoid angling the needle superiorly and passing over the top of the scapula.
- Aspirate for blood.
- Inject 10 ml of local anesthetic (± steroid).

Complications

- Intravascular injection.
- Pneumothorax.

Nerve blocks at the elbow[10]

- The ulnar, median, and radial nerves may be blocked at the elbow.
- This provides sensory loss to the hand and motor loss to forearm and hand muscles.
- Sensory loss to the forearm requires block of the lateral, medial, and posterior cutaneous nerves of the forearm.

Indications

- Minor surgery or postsurgery analgesia distal to the elbow.
- Supplementation of brachial plexus block.
- Localization of pain to a single nerve.

Table 17.3 *Complications of brachial plexus blocks*

	Axillary	Infraclavicular	Supraclavicular	Interscalene	
Vertebral artery injection	–	–	+/–	++	Rare but can be lethal
Subarachnoid/epidural injection	–	–	+	++	Rare but dangerous
Phrenic nerve palsy asymptomatic	+/–	+/–	++	+++	36–90% usually
Recurrent laryngeal nerve palsy	–	–	+	+	1.5–6% incidence
Stellate ganglion block	+	+	++	+++	50–90% incidence
Pneumothorax	+/–	+/–	+++	+	0.6–25% usually asymptomatic

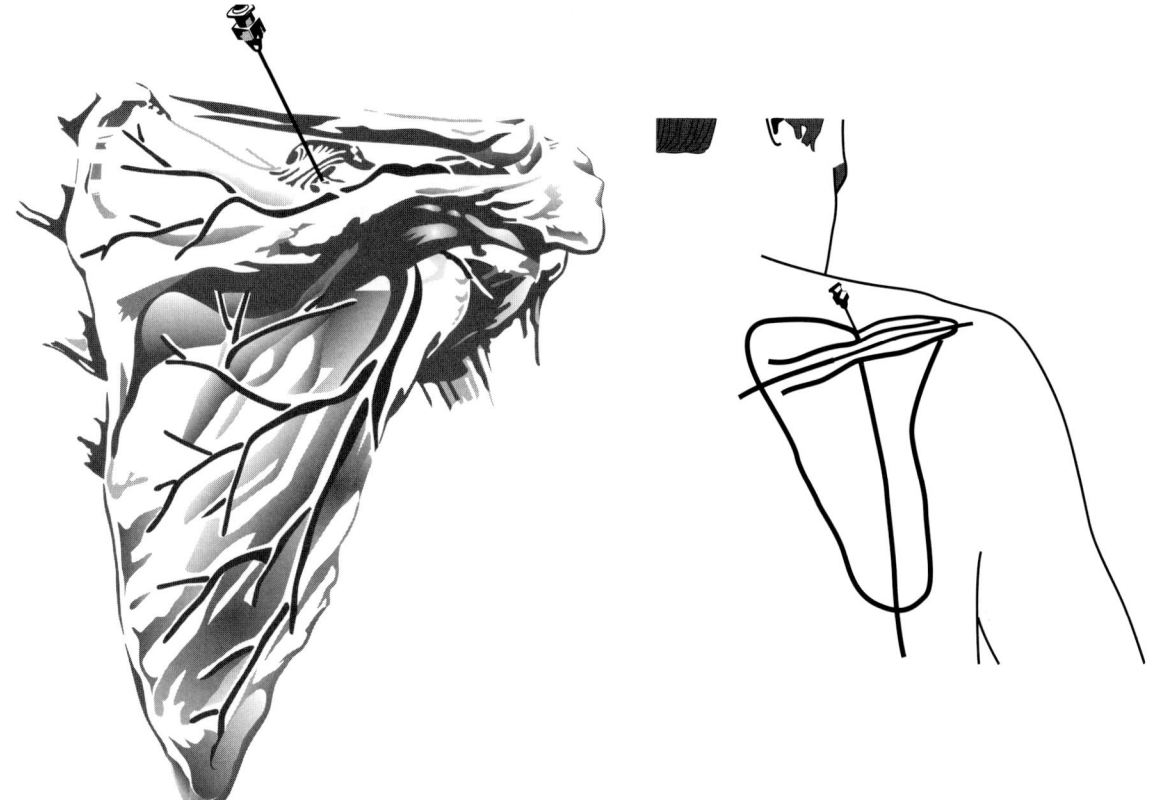

Figure 17.12 *Suprascapular nerve block. Landmarks and needle insertion point for suprascapular nerve block (posterior approach).*

Relevant anatomy

- The ulnar nerve enters the forearm by passing behind the medial epicondyle of the humerus before passing down the ulnar side of the forearm.
- The median nerve lies immediately medial to the brachial artery just proximal to the flexor skin crease of the elbow. It lies just deep to the bicipital aponeurosis.
- The medial cutaneous nerve of the forearm lies subcutaneously above the bicipital aponeurosis.
- The radial nerve is the largest branch of the plexus. It crosses in front of the lateral epicondyle of the humerus, in a groove deep to the brachioradialis muscle and lateral to the biceps tendon to enter the forearm.
- The lateral cutaneous nerve of the forearm is the con-tinuation of the musculocutaneous nerve and lies just below the deep fascia, lateral to the biceps tendon.
- The posterior cutaneous nerve of the forearm is a proximal branch of the radial nerve and lies subcutaneously over the lateral epicondyle of the humerus.

Ulnar nerve block

Landmarks
- Medial epicondyle of humerus.
- Ulnar sulcus.

Practical steps (Fig. 17.13)
- Place the hand behind the head under a pillow.
- At the elbow, palpate the medial epicondyle.
- Needle insertion site is 1 cm proximal to the epicondyle, where it may be possible to palpate the nerve.

- Insert a 25-gauge, 3.5-cm needle horizontally, 1–2 cm deep to the skin, until paresthesiae are elicited.
- If bone is contacted, reposition the needle.
- Nerve is superficial.
- Take care not to inject into nerve.
- Inject 5 ml of local anesthetic solution.
- Avoid the ulnar nerve sulcus within the epicondyle as the nerve is fixed and easily damaged by a needle or compression by local anesthetic.

Median nerve and medial cutaneous nerve of the forearm blocks

Landmarks

- Antecubital fossa.
- Pulse of brachial artery.
- Medial border of biceps tendon.
- Head of pronator teres.

Practical steps (Fig. 17.14)

- With the arm abducted to 45°, palpate the intermuscular groove between the biceps tendon and pronator teres.
- Locate the brachial pulse within this groove.
- At this point, insert a 25-gauge, 3.5-cm needle just medial to the artery and just proximal to the elbow crease, angled at 45° to the skin.
- Piercing of the biceps aponeurosis may be felt.
- Once paresthesiae are elicited, inject 5 ml of local anesthetic solution slowly.
- On completion of the median nerve block, withdraw the needle until subcutaneous.

- Redirect proximally along intermuscular groove, injecting a "sausage" of local anesthetic (5–7 ml of solution).

Radial nerve and lateral cutaneous nerve of the forearm blocks

Landmarks

- Antecubital fossa.
- Lateral epicondyle of humerus.
- Lateral border of biceps tendon.
- Medial border of brachioradialis muscle.

Practical steps (Fig. 17.14)

- Palpate the intermuscular groove between the biceps and brachioradialis muscles just proximal to the flexor skin crease of the antecubital fossa.
- The nerve runs deep to the brachioradialis at this point.
- A nerve stimulator is useful as nerve location can be difficult.
- Insert a 25-gauge, 3.5-cm needle directed proximally to reach the anterior aspect of the lateral epicondyle.
- After contact with bone, inject 5 ml of local anesthetic solution.
- While withdrawing the needle, inject a further 5 ml of solution to block the lateral cutaneous nerve, which lies just deep to the fascia lateral to the biceps tendon.

Posterior cutaneous nerve of forearm block

- Flex arm across the chest of the patient.

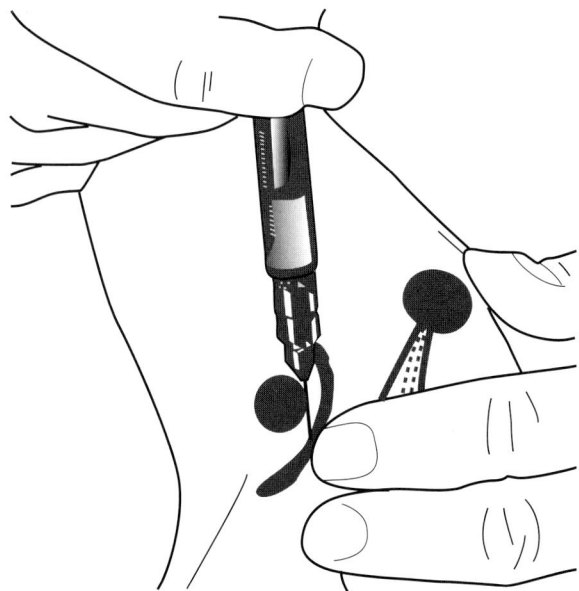

Figure 17.13 *Ulnar nerve block. Landmarks and needle insertion point for ulnar nerve block.*

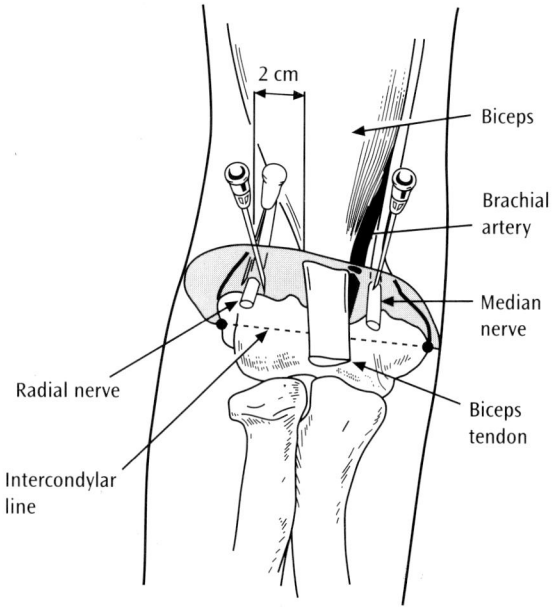

Figure 17.14 *Median and radial nerve blocks. Landmarks and needle insertion point for median and radial nerve blocks at the elbow.*

- Inject a subcutaneous "sausage" over the lateral epicondyle toward the olecranon process.
- Inject 5 ml of local anesthetic solution.

Complications

- Risk of nerve damage with intraneural injection.
- Compression of nerve with a large volume of local anesthetic.
- Hematoma.

Nerve blocks at the wrist[11]

This produces sensory block of the hand and motor block of the intrinsic hand muscles. The flexor and extensor muscle of the forearm are left intact.

Indications

- Minor surgery of all or part of the hand.
- Complex hand surgery where ability to use forearm muscles is required.
- Postsurgical analgesia (after brachial plexus block, to regain control of arm).
- Localization of pain in the territory of a single nerve.

Relevant anatomy

- The median nerve lies superficially at the level of the proximal skin crease, between the tendon of palmaris longus and the tendon of flexor carpi radialis.
- The ulnar nerve is lateral and deep to the flexor carpi ulnaris tendon, medial to the artery.
- The radial nerve emerges deep to the brachioradialis tendon and winds round the radius onto the dorsum of the wrist.

Ulnar nerve block (medial approach)

- The ulnar nerve divides into a dorsal and a palmar branch, both branches need to be blocked.
- The nerve can be blocked by a ventral or a medial approach. The medial approach allows both nerve branches to be blocked from the same needle insertion site. The medial approach is less likely to damage the artery.

Landmarks

- Flexor carpi ulnaris tendon.
- Ulnar artery pulse.
- Pisiform bone.

Practical steps (Fig. 17.15)

- Position arm supine and abducted.
- At 1 cm proximal to the pisiform bone at the wrist, insert a 25-gauge needle at 90° to the skin immediately deep to the flexor carpi ulnaris.
- Advance the needle to a depth of 1–2 cm and aspirate for blood.
- Inject 4 ml of local anesthetic solution.
- Withdraw the needle until subcutaneous and redirect both dorsally and ventrally to block the dorsal and palmar branches with 2 ml of solution.

Median nerve block

Landmarks

- Flexor carpi radialis tendon.
- Palmaris longus tendon (if present).

Practical steps (Fig. 17.16)

- Ask the patient to flex their wrist against resistance to outline the tendon of palmaris longus.
- If present, insert a 25-gauge needle just lateral to the tendon.
- If not present, insert needle 1 cm medial to the ulnar border of the flexor carpi radialis tendon.
- The flexor retinaculum should be encountered at a depth of less than 1 cm.
- Advance the needle a further 2–3 mm as the nerve lies immediately deep to the retinaculum.
- Move needle fanwise to elicit paresthesiae.
- Immobilize needle and inject 3 ml of local anesthetic solution.
- Resistance to injection should not occur (withdraw to prevent intraneural injection).
- Withdraw needle until subcutaneous, and inject a further 2 ml to block the palmar cutaneous branch.

Radial nerve block

Landmarks

- "Anatomical snuff box."
- Radial styloid.
- Ulnar styloid.

Practical steps (Fig. 17.17)

- At the level of the "anatomical snuff box," the radial nerve is superficial.
- Insert a 25-gauge needle and raise a subcutaneous "sausage" of local anesthetic solution in a ring from across the base of the anatomical snuff box toward the ulnar border of the wrist in a line joining both styloid processes together.
- Inject 7–10 ml of local anesthetic solution.
- This technique more resembles a "field block."

Complications

- Nerve blocks at the wrist are superficial and complications are few.
- Risk of nerve damage if intraneural injection occurs.
- Hematoma.

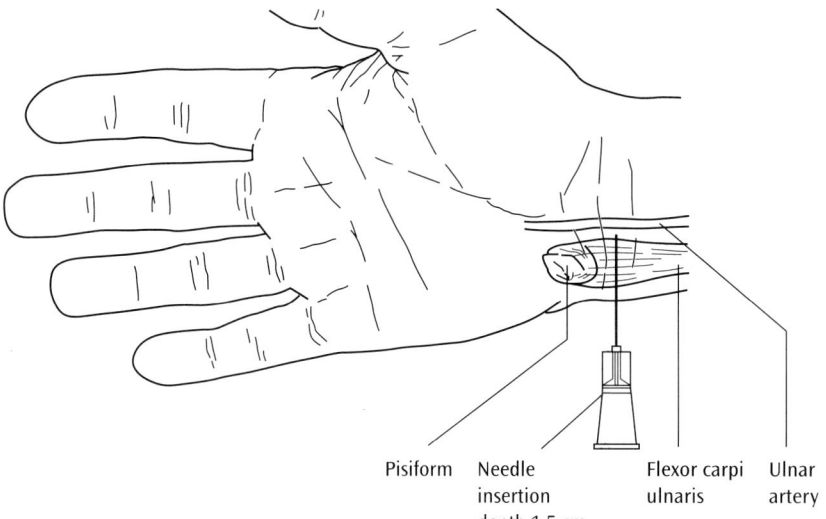

Figure 17.15 *Ulnar nerve block. Landmarks and needle insertion point for ulnar nerve block at the wrist.*

Pisiform   Needle insertion depth 1.5 cm   Flexor carpi ulnaris   Ulnar artery

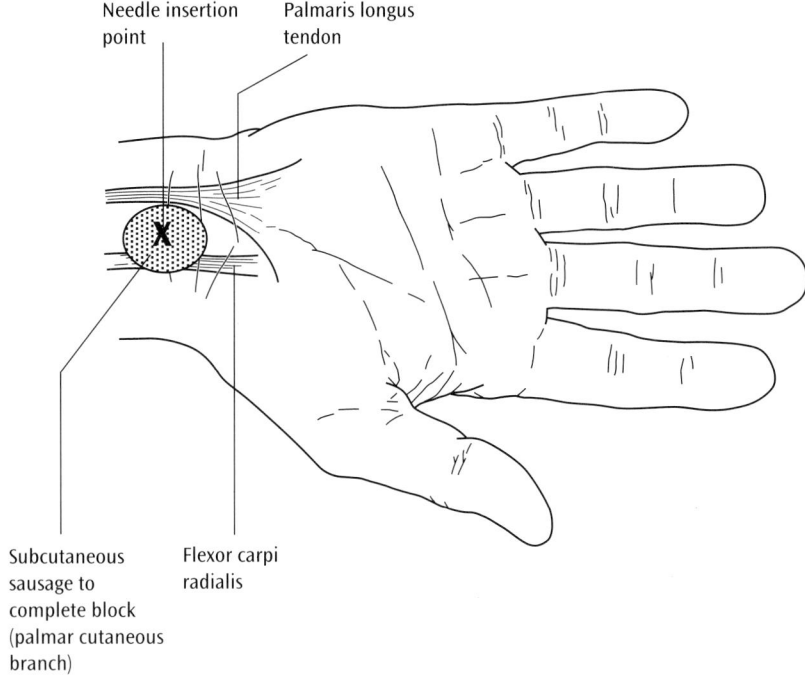

Needle insertion point   Palmaris longus tendon

Figure 17.16 *Median nerve block. Landmarks and needle insertion point for median nerve block at the wrist.*

Subcutaneous sausage to complete block (palmar cutaneous branch)   Flexor carpi radialis

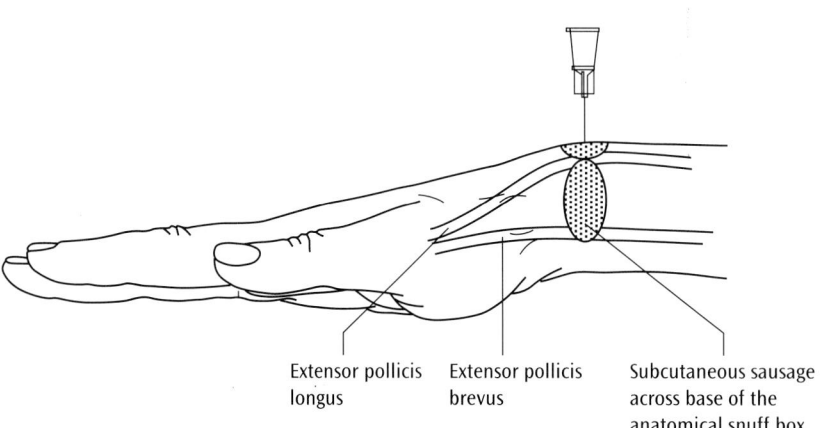

Figure 17.17 *Radial nerve block. Landmarks and needle insertion point for radial nerve block at the wrist:*

Extensor pollicis longus   Extensor pollicis brevus   Subcutaneous sausage across base of the anatomical snuff box

NERVE BLOCKS OF THE THORAX AND ABDOMEN

Thoracic paravertebral block[12]

Indications

Local anesthetic block

- Analgesia following thoracotomy or nephrectomy.
- Fractured ribs.
- Thoracic vertebral collapse or compression fracture.
- Acute herpes zoster.
- Differential block for evaluation of chest wall, upper abdominal, and thoracic spinal pain.
- Prognostic block prior to neurolysis.

Local anesthetic and steroid block

- Post-thoracotomy pain.
- Postherpetic neuralgia.
- Rib fractures.

Neurolytic block (phenol, cryoneurolysis, or radiofrequency)

- Cancer of thoracic spine, ribs, chest wall, and abdominal wall.

Relevant anatomy

- The spinal cord gives rise to 12 pairs of thoracic nerves (T1–12).
- The thoracic paravertebral nerves pass below the transverse process of the vertebra after leaving their intervertebral foramina.
- A branch loops back through the intervertebral foramina to supply the spinal ligaments, meninges, and vertebra.
- Within the paravertebral space, the thoracic nerve communicates with the sympathetic nervous system and then divides into a posterior and anterior primary division.
- The posterior division supplies the interfacetal joints, muscles, and skin of the back.
- The anterior division passes into the subcostal groove beneath the rib to become the intercostal nerve.
- The 12th thoracic nerve lies beneath the 12th rib and becomes the subcostal nerve.
- The intercostal and subcostal nerves supply skin, muscles, ribs, parietal pleura, and parietal peritoneum.

Landmarks

- Thoracic vertebral spinous processes.

Practical steps (Fig. 17.18)

- Patient may be positioned prone or lateral.
- Identify the spinous process of the vertebra above the nerve to be blocked.
- Mark a point 3 cm lateral to the upper (cephalad) border of the spinous process.
- At this point, insert a 22-gauge, 8-cm spinal needle perpendicular to the skin and advance the needle aiming for the transverse process (usual depth 3–4 cm).
- Withdraw the needle slightly and redirect upwards (cephalad) so that the needle tip "walks off" the upper border of the transverse process.
- Once bony contact is lost, advance the needle a further 2–3 cm.
- Avoid directing the needle too medial as an epidural or intrathecal injection may occur.
- Avoid directing the needle too lateral as an intercostal or interpleural injection may occur.
- As the needle is advanced beyond the transverse process, a loss of resistance may be felt as the costo-transverse ligament is crossed.
- Loss of resistance to saline can be used to confirm the needle position.
- Occasionally, paresthesiae may occur.
- A nerve stimulator can be used, when pulse synchronous movement of the rectus muscle will be seen.
- Aspirate for CSF or blood.
- Inject 5 ml of local anesthetic solution to block three or four dermatomes.
- If continuous analgesia is planned, the procedure can be performed using an peridural kit, leaving behind a catheter in the paravertebral space.

Complications

- Pneumothorax (up to 20% incidence).
- Epidural, subdural, or intrathecal injection.
- Trauma to nerve roots.
- Hematoma.
- Infection (immunocompromised patients).

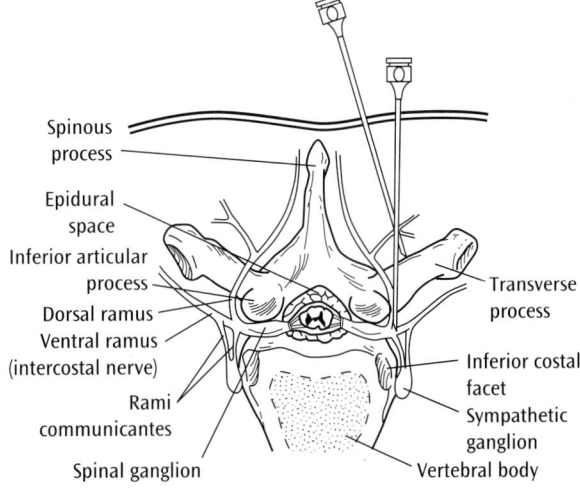

Figure 17.18 *Thoracic paravertebral block. Landmarks and needle insertion point for thoracic paravertebral block.*

Intercostal nerve block[13]*

Indications

Local anesthetic block

- Rib fractures.
- Chest wall contusion.
- Pleurisy.
- Fractured sternum.
- Insertion of chest drain.
- Analgesia after thoracic or abdominal surgery.
- Diagnostic block in visceral versus somatic pain.

Local anesthetic and steroid

- Acute herpes zoster.
- Postherpetic neuralgia.
- Post-thoracotomy pain.

Neurolytic block

- Rib or chest wall invasion by tumor.

Relevant anatomy

- Intercostal nerves are the continuation of the anterior primary division of thoracic nerves. T1 contributes to the brachial plexus; T2–3 forms a cutaneous branch to the arm (intercostobrachial nerve); T12 forms the subcostal nerve, which descends in the abdominal wall and communicates with L1.
- The classic vein, artery, and nerve pattern below each rib only occurs in 17% of people. The nerve varies from midcostal (73%) to supracostal (10%). Intercostal nerves may split into two distinctive bundles, which may later rejoin.
- Each intercostal nerve usually gives off four branches (Table 17.4).

Landmarks

- Angle of rib.
- Midaxillary line.

Practical steps (Fig. 17.19)

Posterior approach

The block is performed posteriorly at the angle of the rib, just lateral to the sacrospinous muscles (usually 8 cm lateral to the spinous process).

- Count ribs upwards from 12th rib and identify angle of required rib.
- Retract skin and subcutaneous tissues upwards.
- Insert a 25-gauge, 3.5-cm needle onto the rib.
- Withdraw the needle and redirect to "walk off" the lower border of the rib.
- Aspirate for blood.
- Inject 3–4 ml of local anesthetic solution.
- Multiple blocks are often carried out together and can be painful.

Table 17.4 *Branches of the intercostal nerves*

Branch	Innervation
Gray rami communicantes	Sympathetic ganglion
Posterior cutaneous branch	Paravertebral muscles and skin
Lateral cutaneous division	Anterior and lateral skin sensation
Anterior cutaneous branch	Midline chest and abdominal skin

Midaxillary approach

- This block is performed in the midaxillary line. The lateral cutaneous branch may be missed, but this can be blocked by infiltrating subcutaneously on withdrawal of the needle.
- Suitable for supine patients that cannot be turned.
- Upper intercostal nerves can be blocked by raising the patient's arm to access the axilla.

Anterior approach

- The intercostal nerves can be blocked anterior to the midaxillary line.
- Parasternal blocks may used after sternotomy or rectus sheath blocks for abdominal wall analgesia.

Complications

- Pneumothorax (related to the experience of the operator and failure to control the depth of the needle).
- Systemic toxicity.
- Hypotension (central spread of local anesthetic).
- Respiratory depression (effective nerve block after systemic opioids).

Interpleural block[14]

The exact mechanism of action is not understood, but it has been shown that sensory and autonomic fibers are blocked, and often a unilateral block has bilateral effects.

Interpleural block should not be attempted bilaterally as the risk of pneumothorax is too great.

Indications

Postsurgical analgesia

- Unilateral subcostal analgesia after surgery.
- Breast surgery.
- Renal surgery.
- Multiple rib fractures.
- Cardiac surgery.

Chronic pain

- Chronic pancreatitis.
- Postherpetic neuralgia.
- Complex regional pain syndrome.

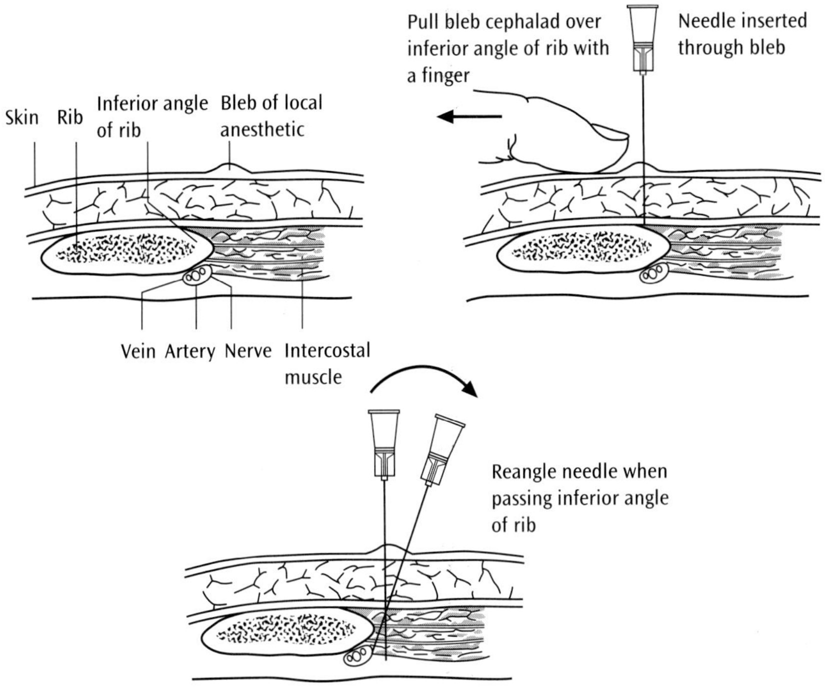

Figure 17.19 *Intercostal nerve block. Landmarks and needle insertion point for intercostal nerve block.*

Cancer pain
- Pancreatic cancer.
- Upper abdominal cancer.
- Breast cancer.
- Chest wall cancer.

Relative contraindications

- Significant respiratory disease (pneumothorax would be disastrous).
- Bronchopleural fistula.
- Prior pleurodesis.

Relevant anatomy

- The pleural space is 10–20 μm wide and 2,000 cm^2 in area (in an adult male).
- The interpleural space lies between the visceral pleura lining the heart and lungs and the parietal pleura covering the thoracic cage.
- Interpleural pressure varies from –12 cmH$_2$O at the lung apices to –5 cmH$_2$O at the lung bases.

Landmarks

- Angle of sixth or seventh rib.

Practical steps (Fig. 17.20)

The patient's position is determined by the requirement of the block.

- Sensory block of intercostal nerves: position the patient with affected side down with head down tilt (20°) to block T1–9.

- Sympathetic block: affected side up with head down tilt for cervical sympathetic chain.
- Combined sensory and sympathetic block: initially, affected side up, then turn patient supine.
  - With the patient in the lateral position, identify the angle of the sixth or seventh rib.
  - Insert an 18-gauge Tuohy needle attached to a "loss-of-resistance" device (either a syringe of saline or a 500-ml bag of saline).
  - Aim the needle at 45° toward the upper edge of the rib.
  - Once contact has been made with the rib, walk the needle off the upper border of the rib and advance into the pleural space.
  - At this point, the saline will run easily or can be injected easily.
  - Hold needle immobile with one hand and either insert a catheter or slowly inject 20 ml of local anesthetic solution.
  - The technique can be refined using one of several commercially available devices. Special "closed system" kits are available with "one-way valves" to prevent the entrainment of air.
  - The needle is best inserted at the end of expiration to minimize risk of lung damage.
  - A postblock chest radiograph is advised, particularly after catheter insertion.

Complications

- Pneumothorax (5%).
- Pleural effusion (0.4%).
- Systemic toxicity of local anesthetic.

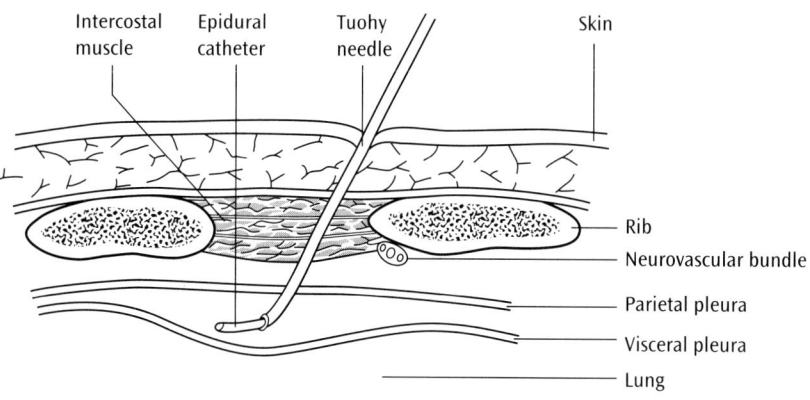

Figure 17.20 *Interpleural block. Landmarks and needle insertion point for interpleural block.*

- Malposition of catheter.
- Infection.
- Bronchopleural fistula.

Ilioinguinal, iliohypogastric, and genitofemoral nerve blocks[15]

Indications

- Inguinal hernia surgery.
- Postsurgical analgesia.
- Ilioinguinal–iliohypogastric neuralgia.
- Genitofemoral neuralgia.
- Chronic testicular pain.
- Neuroma.

Relevant anatomy

- The iliohypogastric nerve (L1) runs between transversus abdominus and internal oblique muscles reaching the lower abdomen 4 cm medial to the anterior superior iliac spine to supply the skin above the inguinal ligament.
- The ilioinguinal nerve (L1) runs parallel to, but deep to, the iliohypogastric nerve. The nerve passes through the external inguinal ring and gives branches to the scrotum (labia majora).
- The genitofemoral nerve (L1 and L2) splits into two on the psoas muscle just above the inguinal ligament to give the genital and femoral branches. The genital branch follows the spermatic cord and supplies the cremasteric muscle and skin of the scrotum (labia majora), while the femoral branch supplies the skin overlying the femoral triangle.

Landmarks

- Anterior superior iliac spins (ASIS).
- Pubic tubercle.
- External inguinal ring.

Practical steps (Fig. 17.21)

Iliohypogastric and ilioinguinal nerve blocks

- Position the patient supine.
- Identify the ASIS.
- Mark a point 2 cm medial and inferior to the ASIS.
- Insert a 22-gauge, 3.5-cm needle at this point, advancing until the resistance of the aponeurosis of the external oblique muscle is felt.
- The needle is advanced slowly until the aponeurosis is pierced, the iliohypogastric nerve lies just deep to the aponeurosis.
- Aspirate for blood, and inject 5 ml of local anesthetic solution.
- Advance the needle further through the internal oblique muscle (1–2 cm) and inject a further 5 ml of solution to block the ilioinguinal nerve.

Genitofemoral nerve block

- Invaginate the skin of the scrotum through the external ring to exclude hernia contents in the canal.
- Palpate the line between the ASIS and the pubic tubercle; 1 cm above its midpoint, the deep inguinal ring can be felt – place a finger at this point.
- Insert a 22-gauge, 3.5-cm needle parallel to the canal, 1 cm distal to the finger overlying the deep ring.
- Often a loss of resistance is felt as the needle pierces the external oblique aponeurosis to enter the inguinal canal.
- Aspirate for blood and inject 5 ml of local anesthetic solution.
- The femoral vessels and nerve lie immediately deep to the canal; therefore, the needle depth should be controlled.

Complications

- Hematoma.
- Damage to the spermatic cord.
- Damage to the bowel.
- Inadvertent femoral nerve block.

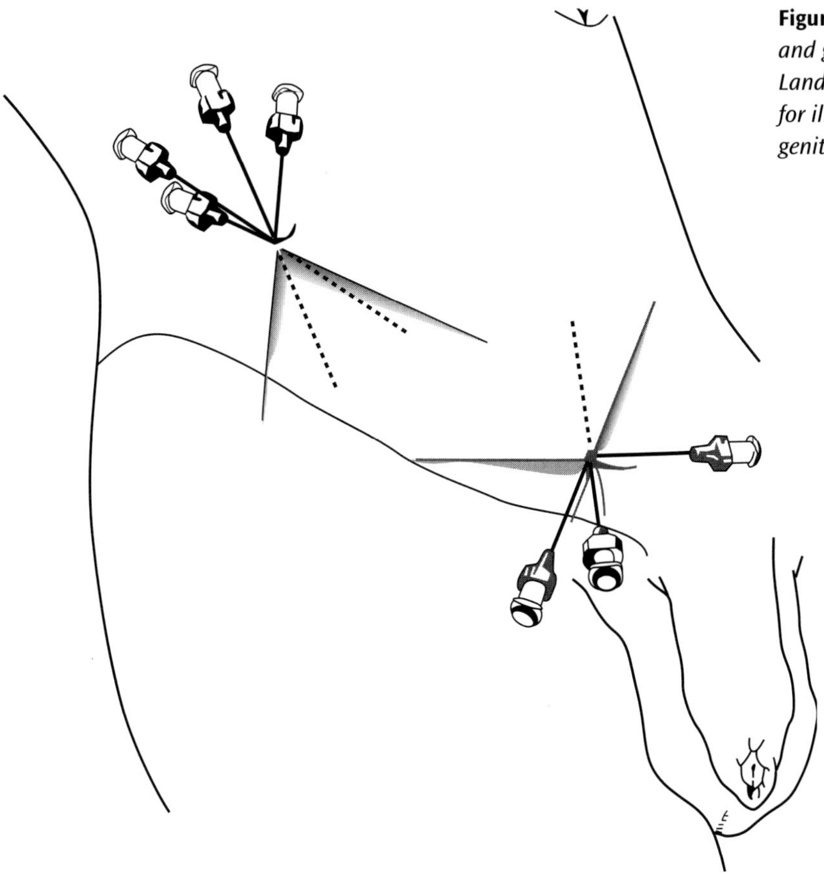

Figure 17.21 *Ilioinguinal, iliohypogastric, and genitofemoral nerve blocks. Landmarks and needle insertion positions for ilioinguinal, iliohypogastric, and genitofemoral nerve blocks.*

NERVE BLOCKS OF THE LOWER LIMB[16]

Nerve blocks of the lower limb are not popular owing to the more easily accomplished central nerve blockade. However, in those patients in which central nerve blockade is contraindicated or patients who cannot tolerate the cardiovascular effects, peripheral nerve blocks still have a place. Discrete nerve blockade always has a place in diagnosis and treatment of chronic pain syndromes.

The nerve supply to the lower limb comprises two plexus and five major terminal branches.

Lumbar plexus block[17]

The lumbar plexus can be blocked by two proximal techniques: a paravertebral technique which blocks the nerve roots and the lumbar plexus block or psoas compartment block which blocks the loops of the plexus. A distal technique has also been advocated, referred to as either the "Winnie three-in-one block" or the "inguinal paravascular block."

Indications

- Surgery of hip, thigh, or upper leg.
- Postsurgical analgesia.
- Cancer of hip or upper femur.

Blockade of the lower limb is not achieved without also blocking the sacral plexus.

Relevant anatomy

- The lumbar plexus is formed by the anterior divisions of L1–4; T12 is included in 50% and occasionally L5.
- The plexus is formed in front of the lumbar transverse processes and then lies as deep loops within a "compartment" deep in the psoas muscle at the medial border of quadratum lumborum.
- The individual nerves then course to their site of innervation.
- The lumbar sympathetic chain is closely related: it lies on the anterolateral surface of the lumbar and sacral bodies medial to the anterior foramina.
- There are connections between the lumbar plexus and the sympathetic chain, despite being separated anatomically.
- Lumbar spinous processes are nearly horizontal and are usually 3–4 cm deep.
- Lumbar transverse processes are short (3 cm). The average depth of a transverse process to skin is 5 cm.

Landmarks

- Spinous process of lumbar vertebrae.

Practical steps (Fig. 17.22)

The classical technique describes multiple paravertebral injections; however, single injection techniques between L2 and L5 have been advocated (psoas compartment block).

- Position the patient with the side of the block uppermost or, alternatively, prone with a pillow under the abdomen.
- Identify spinous process of L3 and mark a point 3 cm lateral.
- At this point, insert a 22-gauge, 8-cm spinal needle, at right angles to the skin until the tip contacts the transverse process (usually 5 cm deep).
- Withdraw needle slightly and redirect.

Paravertebral technique

Redirect the needle cephalad and medially so that the tip just passes above and 2–3 cm deep to the transverse process. Paresthesiae may occur. Aspirate for blood or CSF and inject local anesthetic solution: either 5-ml boluses at multiple levels or a single injection of 15–20 ml.

Lumbar plexus (psoas compartment) technique

Redirect needle cephalad only. Advance the needle until parallel to the midline about 2 cm deep to the transverse process. Entry into the psoas compartment will be indicated by a loss of resistance, which can be confirmed with a syringe of saline. Aspirate for blood and inject local anesthetic solution (15–20 ml).

Distal technique (Winnie three-in-one, or inguinal paravascular block)

- Position patient supine.
- Mark a point just lateral to the femoral artery and just below the inguinal ligament.

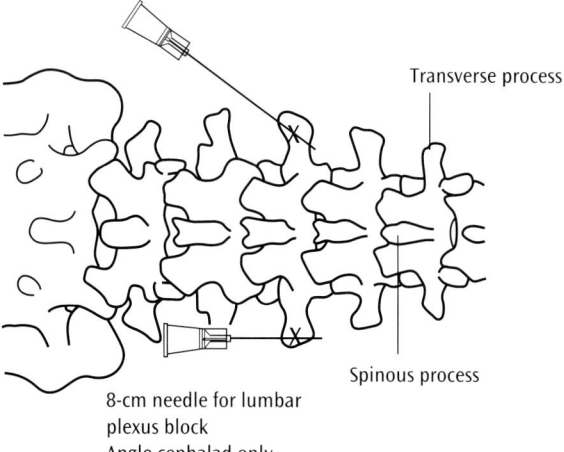

8-cm needle for paravertebral block
Angle medially and cephalad

Transverse process

Spinous process

8-cm needle for lumbar plexus block
Angle cephalad only

Figure 17.22 *Lumbar plexus block. Landmarks and needle insertion points for the "paravertebral" and "psoas compartment" techniques.*

- At this point, insert a 22-gauge, 8-cm needle or a 20-gauge cannula at an angle of 20° to the skin. Direct the needle cephalad and parallel to the artery – a distinct give will be felt as the needle penetrates the fascia lata and then the iliopectineal fascia around the nerve.
- Needle position can be confirmed by a syringe of saline demonstrating a "loss of resistance" or a nerve stimulator causing pulse-synchronous movement of the sartorius muscle.
- Aspirate for blood.
- Inject 20–30 ml of local anesthetic solution, which should block the femoral, obturator, and lateral cutaneous nerve of the thigh.

This distal approach to the lumbar plexus is not always reliable. The lateral cutaneous nerve of the thigh is frequently missed. The block may also spill over to involve the sacral plexus and the sciatic nerve may be blocked.

Complications

- Inadvertent epidural or intrathecal injection (proximal techniques).
- Inadvertent puncture of major vessels (needle too deep).
- Nerve trauma.
- Infection.

Sacral plexus block

This is a paravertebral block which, when combined with the lumbar plexus block, anesthetizes the lower limb; S1–3 contributes to the sciatic nerve.

Indications

- Temporary relief of sciatica.
- Cancer pain in the distribution of sacral nerve roots.
- In combination with lumbar plexus block for surgery of leg, thigh, or hip.

Relevant anatomy

- The sacral plexus comprises L4–5 and S1–3 nerves and part of S4.
- It lies on the anterior surface of the sacrum on top of the piriformis muscle.
- It is covered by pelvic fascia and anterior to the plexus and fascia lie the ureter, bowel, and iliac vessels.
- The plexus divides into two branches.
- The collateral branches supply the pudendal plexus, the hip joint, and gluteal, adductor, and hamstring muscles.
- The terminal branches supply the greater and lesser sciatic nerves.
- The sacrum has two rows of openings on its posterior surface (posterior sacral foramina).

- These rows of foramina are not parallel to the edges of the sacrum – they angle less steeply to the midline as they descend.
- The transacral canal is narrow, being 2.5 cm deep at S1 and 0.5 cm deep at S4.

Landmarks

- Posterior superior iliac spine.
- Sacral cornu.

Practical steps (Fig. 17.23)

- Position patient prone with a pillow under the pelvis.
- Draw a line from a point 1 cm medial and 1 cm below the posterior superior iliac spine to a point 1 cm lateral and 1 cm above the sacral cornu. A third point is marked at the midpoint of this line. This identifies the foramina of S2–4.
- Soft tissues overlying the foramina are greatest over the upper foramina, but the S2 foramina is often easiest to identify.
- A 22-gauge, 8-cm needle is inserted toward the posterior surface of the sacrum until it contacts bone.
- The needle is withdrawn slightly and adjusted medially until it enters the foramina.
- Advance the needle 2 cm into the upper foramina and less than 0.5 cm for the lowest foramina.
- A peripheral nerve stimulator can be helpful for confirming the needle position.
- Aspirate for blood and CSF.
- Inject 5 ml of local anesthetic solution.
- Repeat at several foramina if blocking the entire plexus.

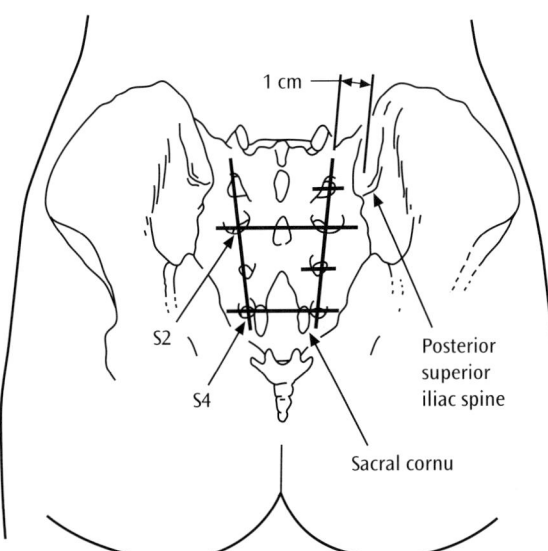

Figure 17.23 *Sacral plexus block. Landmarks and needle insertion points for sacral nerve blocks.*

Complications

- Loss of parasympathetic function to bladder and bowel.
- Inadvertent intrathecal injection.
- Inadvertent vascular injection.
- Inadvertent puncture of bowel.

Peripheral branches of the lumbosacral plexus[18]

The lumbar and sacral plexuses have five peripheral branches: femoral, obturator, lateral cutaneous, sciatic, and posterior cutaneous nerves.

The femoral, obturator, and lateral cutaneous nerves can be blocked simultaneously by the "three-in-one block" and is described above under blocks of the lumbar plexus. In this section, blocks of the individual nerves will be described.

femoral nerve block

Indications
- Analgesia after femoral fracture.
- Surgery or postsurgical analgesia of the knee (along with sciatic, obturator, and lateral cutaneous nerve block).

Relevant anatomy
- The femoral nerve is the largest branch of the plexus.
- It enters the leg below the inguinal ligament lateral to the femoral vessels.
- It is covered in its own fascial sheath (iliopectineal fascia) and lies deep to the fascia lata.
- It has an anterior and posterior division.
- The anterior division is motor to sartorius and sensory to the anterior and medial skin of the thigh, including the knee.
- The posterior division is motor to quadriceps femoris, sensory to the knee, and ends as the saphenous nerve.

Landmarks
- Inguinal ligament.
- Femoral artery.

Practical steps (Fig. 17.24)
- Identify and mark a point 1 cm lateral to the femoral artery 1 cm below the inguinal ligament.
- Insert a 22-gauge, 3.5-cm needle to a depth of 3 cm (deeper than the artery).
- A peripheral nerve stimulator, showing pulse-synchronous movement of the sartorius muscle, can confirm needle placement.
- Aspirate for blood.
- Inject 10 ml of local anesthetic solution.
- Withdraw the needle, redirect it 3 cm lateral to the

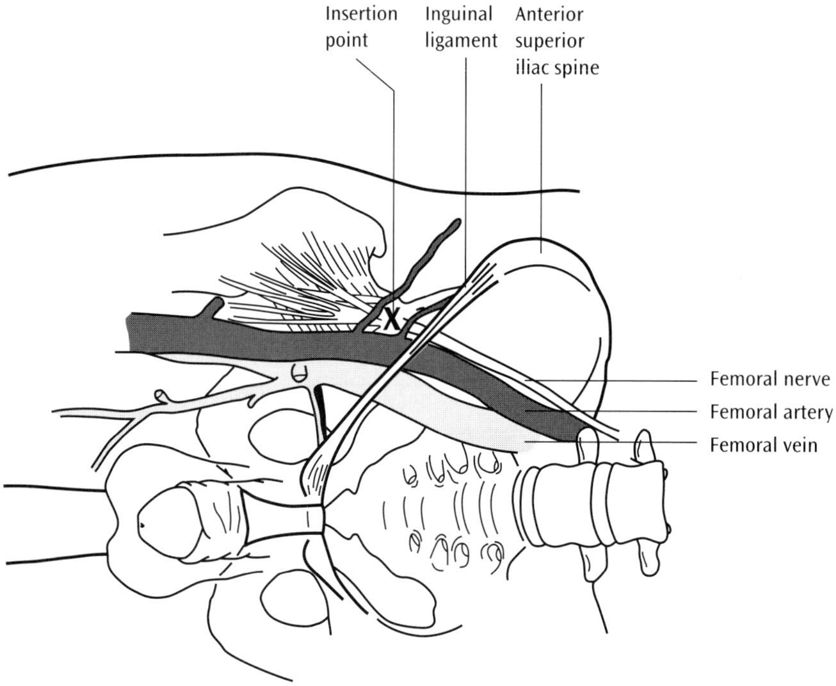

Figure 17.24 *Femoral nerve block. Landmarks and needle insertion point for femoral nerve block.*

artery, and inject a further 5 ml of solution as often the nerve has already divided into two.

- If the artery is punctured, pressure should be applied for at least 5 min to minimize the hematoma.

Complications

- Hematoma.
- Nerve trauma.
- Pain at site of injection.
- Infection.

Obturator nerve block

The obturator nerve can be blocked by either a direct or an indirect approach (Winnie three-in-one block). The Winnie three-in-one block may not reliably block the obturator nerve, and has been described above.

Indications

- Surgery or postsurgical analgesia of the knee (in conjunction with sciatic, femoral, and lateral cutaneous block).
- To abolish stimulation by diathermy during bladder surgery.
- Diagnosis of obturator nerve entrapment.
- Neurolytic block in adductor muscle spasticity (phenol or radiofrequency).

Relevant anatomy

- The obturator nerve enters the leg through the obturator foramen.
- It divides into two branches, the anterior and posterior branch, which are separated by the adductor brevis muscle.
- The anterior branch is sensory to the hip and medial aspect of the thigh and is motor to the anterior adductor muscles.
- The posterior branch is sensory to the capsule of the knee and is motor to the deep adductor muscles.

Landmarks

- Pubic tubercle.

Practical steps (Fig. 17.25)

- The direct approach blocks the nerve as it passes through the obturator foramen below the superior ramus of the pubic bone.
- Position the patient supine with the leg to be blocked abducted.
- Protect the genitalia from cleaning solutions.
- Mark a point 1–2 cm below and 1–2 cm lateral to the pubic tubercle.
- At this point, insert a 22-gauge, 8-cm needle vertically downwards onto the pubis bone. Redirect the needle laterally and superiorly to enter the obturator foramen below the superior ramus.
- The needle should only be advanced 2–3 cm into the obturator foramen to avoid bladder damage.
- A peripheral nerve stimulator is helpful and pulse-synchronous movement of the adductor muscles confirms needle placement.
- Aspirate for blood.
- Inject 10 ml of local anesthetic solution.

Complications

- Hematoma.
- Nerve trauma.
- Bladder damage.
- Infection.
- Pain at site of injection.

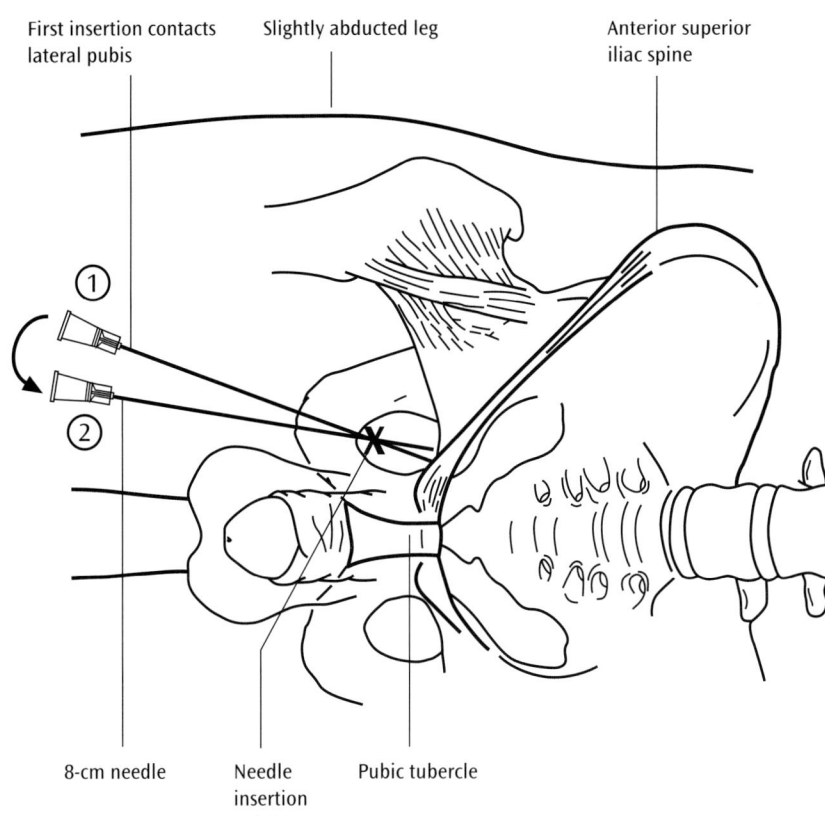

First insertion contacts lateral pubis

Slightly abducted leg

Anterior superior iliac spine

① ②

8-cm needle

Needle insertion point

Pubic tubercle

Figure 17.25 *Obturator nerve block. Landmarks and needle insertion point for obturator nerve block.*

Lateral cutaneous nerve of the thigh

Indications

- Diagnosis and treatment of meralgia paresthetica.
- Postsurgical analgesia after hip surgery.
- Anesthesia for skin graft harvesting or muscle biopsy.

Relevant anatomy

- The nerve emerges at the lateral border of the psoas muscle below, passing obliquely under the iliac fascia to enter the thigh either deep to or through the inguinal ligament 2 cm medial to the anterior superior iliac spine.
- The course of the nerve varies as it crosses the inguinal ligament.
- Beyond the inguinal ligament, the nerve divides into anterior and posterior branches.
- The anterior branch becomes superficial about 10 cm distal to the anterior superior iliac spine and supplies the anterior and lateral thigh down to the knee.
- The posterior branch becomes superficial before the anterior branch and supplies the lateral thigh from the greater trochanter to mid-thigh.

Landmarks

- Anterior superior iliac spine (ASIS).
- Inguinal ligament.

Practical steps (Fig. 17.26)

- Position patient supine.

- Mark a point 2–3 cm medial and 2–3 cm inferior to the ASIS.
- At this point, insert a 22-gauge, 3.5-cm needle at right angles to the skin.
- Direct the needle downwards until it lies deep to the fascia lata. A "give" should be felt in the needle.
- Fan-wise injection of 10 ml of local anesthetic is deposited above and below the fascia lata by moving the needle "in and out."
- If this block is supplementing a sciatic and femoral block, the total dose of local anesthetic must be controlled.
- A nerve stimulator may be used to confirm paresthesiae in the skin of the thigh, but patients with nerve entrapment may not be able to distinguish this.

Complications

- Nerve trauma.
- Local anesthetic toxicity (see above).
- Inadvertent femoral nerve block (needle too medial and deep).
- Hematoma.
- Infection.

Sciatic nerve block

As the nerve is deep, a peripheral nerve stimulator makes success more likely and avoids multiple needle redirections in a conscious patient. Because the nerve is large, high concentrations of local anesthetic are used (e.g.

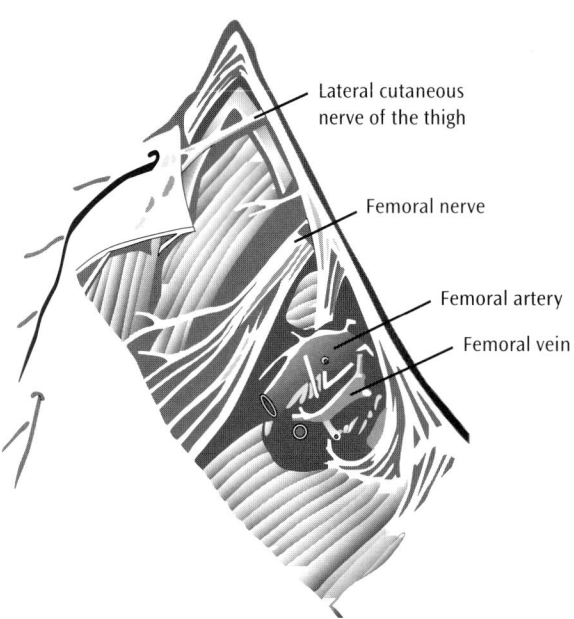

Figure 17.26 *Lateral cutaneous nerve of the thigh block. Landmarks for the lateral cutaneous nerve of thigh and its relationship to the femoral nerve.*

0.75% bupivacaine) and the block may take 45–60 min to develop completely.

Four approaches have been advocated for this block:

- The posterior (classical) approach is the most proximal and is the most likely to produce a complete block of all the branches of the sciatic nerve. It also is the best route for a sciatic nerve catheter.
- The lithotomy approach is the easiest to learn as the nerve is at its most superficial, and the landmarks are identifiable in an obese limb. Assistance is needed to support the leg, and this position may be difficult if the patient has painful joints.
- The anterior and lateral approaches do not require the patient to be moved. Some find the lateral approach difficult to locate the nerve.

Indications

- Postsurgical analgesia of the knee (in combination with femoral, obturator, and lateral cutaneous blocks).
- Analgesia for fractures below the knee.
- Complex regional pain syndromes of leg.
- Ischemic pain of leg.

Relevant anatomy

- Sciatic nerve supplied by L4–S3.
- Largest nerve in body (2 cm wide as exits pelvis).
- Divides into peroneal and tibial branches anywhere from the sciatic foramen to the lower thigh.
- The sciatic nerve supplies the hip joint and hamstring muscles.
- The tibial nerve supplies the knee and ankle joint, the muscles of the calf, and plantar muscles of the foot. Cutaneous innervation is via the sural nerve, which supplies the posterolateral skin of the lower leg.
- The peroneal nerve supplies the knee and skin of

the proximal and lateral part of the lower leg and the dorsum of the foot.

Sciatic nerve block: posterior approach

Landmarks

- Posterior superior iliac spine (PSIS).
- Sacrococcygeal joint.
- Greater trochanter.

Practical steps (Fig. 17.27)

- Position the patient in the lateral position, with the side to be blocked uppermost.
- Flex the top leg to 90° to stabilize the patient ("recovery position").
- Draw a line from the greater trochanter to the PSIS.
- Draw a second line from the greater trochanter to the sacrococcygeal joint (1–2 cm below the sacral cornu).
- Draw a third line at 90° from the midpoint of the first line.
- Where this line bisects the second line represents a point overlying the sciatic nerve as it leaves the sciatic foramen.
- At this point, insert a 22-gauge, 8-cm needle perpendicular to the skin and advance through the gluteal muscles.
- If bone is contacted (5–6 cm deep), redirect the needle until it passes through the sciatic foramen.
- At this stage, connect the peripheral nerve stimulator and advance the needle until pulse-synchronous dorsiflexion and eversion of foot are produced (usually at a depth of 6–8 cm).
- In obese patients, a 10-cm needle may be necessary.
- Aspirate for blood and inject 10–15 ml of local anesthetic solution.

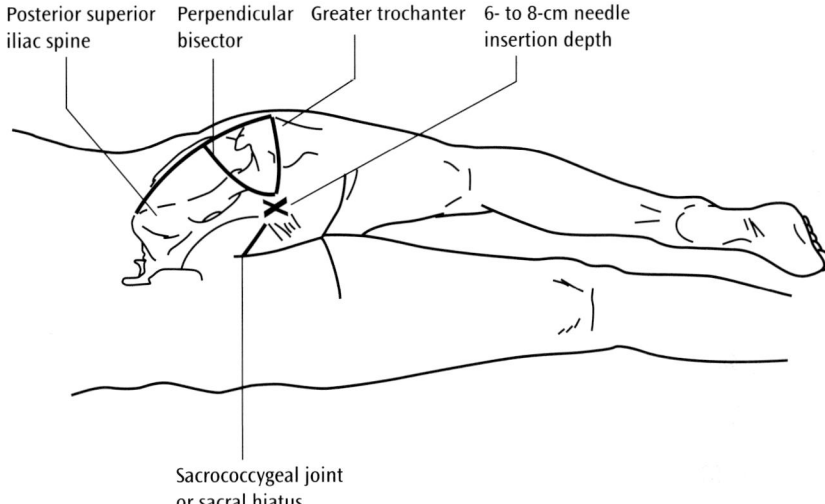

Figure 17.27 *Sciatic nerve block: posterior approach. Landmarks and needle insertion point for a posterior approach to the sciatic nerve block.*

Sciatic nerve block: lithotomy approach

Landmarks
- Greater trochanter.
- Ischial tuberosity.

Practical steps (Fig. 17.28)
- Position the patient supine with the leg to be blocked in the lithotomy position (knee and hip at 90°).
- Draw a line between the greater trochanter and the ischial tuberosity.
- Mark a point 1 cm above the midpoint of this line.
- At this point, insert a 22-gauge, 8-cm needle perpendicular to the skin.
- Advance the needle through the intermuscular septum between biceps femoris and semitendinosus muscles.

- The nerve lies 5–7 cm deep to the skin.
- If bony contact is made, redirect the needle medially to miss the greater trochanter.
- A nerve stimulator will produce pulse-synchronous muscle movement of either the tibial (plantar flexion and inversion of foot) or peroneal (dorsiflexion and eversion of foot) nerve.
- Painful stiff joints may prevent this approach.

Sciatic nerve block: anterior approach

Landmarks
- Greater trochanter.
- Inguinal ligament.

Practical steps (Fig. 17.29)
- Position the patient supine (leg slightly abducted).

Figure 17.28 *Sciatic nerve block: lithotomy approach. Landmarks and needle insertion point for a lithotomy approach to the sciatic nerve block.*

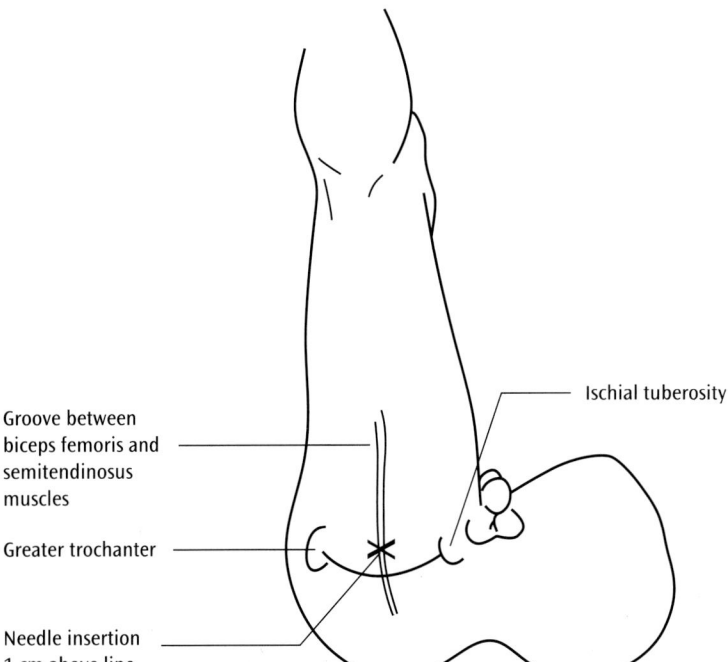

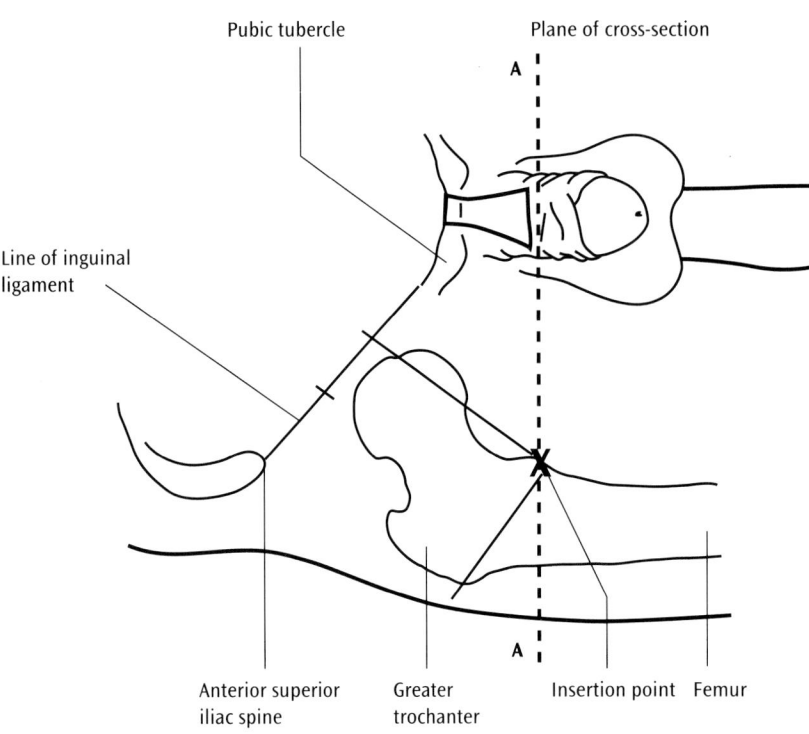

Pubic tubercle
Plane of cross-section
A
Line of inguinal ligament
A
Anterior superior iliac spine
Greater trochanter
Insertion point
Femur

Figure 17.29 *Sciatic nerve block: anterior approach. Landmarks and needle insertion point for an anterior approach to the sciatic nerve block.*

- Draw a line the length of the inguinal ligament and divide it into three equal parts.
- Mark the junction between the middle and medial third.
- Draw a second line, parallel to the inguinal ligament from the greater trochanter across the anterior thigh.
- Draw a third line perpendicular to both lines. Starting from the junction, mark on the first line to a point where it bisects the second parallel line.
- At this point, insert a 22-gauge, 10-cm needle vertically downwards through the skin to pass medial to the femur.
- Bony contact is frequently made (femur) – correct by redirecting the needle more medial.
- The nerve lies just deep to the lesser trochanter behind the adductor magnus.
- A "give" may be felt as the needle enters this space (usually 8–10 cm deep).
- A nerve stimulator may confirm the needle position by demonstrating pulse-synchronous muscle movement (see above).
- Aspirate for blood.
- Inject 10–15 ml of local anesthetic solution.

Sciatic nerve block: lateral approach

Landmarks
- Lateral prominence of the greater trochanter.
- Inferior border of femur.

Practical steps (Fig. 17.30)
- Position the patient supine.

- Mark a point on the inferior border of the femur 3 cm from the lateral tuberosity of the greater trochanter.
- Insert a 22-gauge, 15-cm needle perpendicular to the skin until it contacts the femoral shaft.
- Withdraw the needle and redirect to pass beneath the femur.
- Connect the needle to a peripheral nerve stimulator and advance to a depth of 8–12 cm, when pulse-synchronous muscle movements should occur (see above).
- Aspirate for blood and inject 15 ml of local anesthetic solution.

Complications of sciatic nerve block

- Procedure may be painful in the conscious patient.
- Nerve trauma.
- Vasoconstriction in contralateral leg.
- Hematoma.
- Infection.

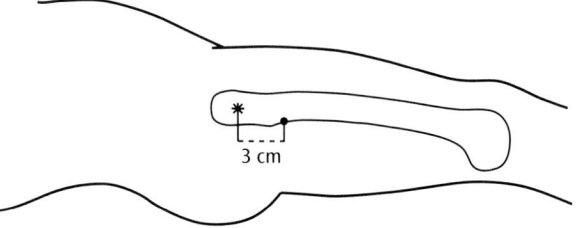

3 cm

Figure 17.30 *Sciatic nerve block: lateral approach. Landmarks and needle insertion point for a lateral approach to the sciatic nerve block.*

Posterior cutaneous nerve of the thigh

- The posterior cutaneous nerve (S1–3) innervates the posterior aspect of the thigh and upper part of calf.
- The nerve exits the greater sciatic foramen alongside the sciatic nerve and is inevitably blocked with the sciatic nerve.

Nerve blocks around the knee

Four nerve blocks are commonly performed at the knee: saphenous nerve block, tibial and peroneal nerve blocks (popliteal fossa block), and intra-articular block within the knee itself.

Indications

- Postsurgical analgesia for knee surgery (intra-articular block) or surgery on the foot (saphenous, tibial, and peroneal block).
- Chronic pain syndromes of the knee (intra-articular block).

Relevant anatomy

- The saphenous nerve is the continuation of the femoral nerve and supplies the medial half of the lower leg from above the knee to the ball of the great toe. The nerve become subcutaneous at the medial side of the knee, immediately below the sartorius muscle.
- The peroneal and tibial nerves are the continuation of the sciatic nerve.
- The tibial nerve arises at the upper border of the popliteal fossa and is the larger branch.
- The peroneal nerve enters the popliteal fossa at its upper border and exits by winding round the head of the fibula (prone to damage).

Nerve blocks around the knee: saphenous nerve block

Landmarks

- Medial tibial condyle.
- Tibial tuberosity.

Practical steps (Fig. 17.31)

- Position the patient supine.
- Identify the medial border of the medial tibial condyle where the nerve lies subcutaneously.
- At a point 2 cm posteromedial to the medial condyle, insert a 22-gauge, 3.5-cm needle and, keeping the needle subcutaneous, inject a ring of local anesthetic solution (10 ml) inferiorly toward the posterior border of the condyle.

Complications

- Nerve trauma.

- Intravenous injection (beware varicose veins).
- Hematoma.
- Infection.

Nerve blocks around the knee: popliteal fossa block

Both the tibial and peroneal nerves can be blocked by a single injection in the upper triangle within the "diamond-shaped" popliteal fossa.

Landmarks

- Diamond-shaped popliteal fossa.
- Femoral condyles.
- Popliteal artery pulse.

Practical steps (Fig. 17.32)

- Position the patient prone.
- Draw a line between the femoral condyles (posterior skin crease).
- Identify the popliteal artery pulse along this line.
- Mark a point just lateral to the pulse and 2–3 cm above the intercondyle line.
- At this point, insert a 22-gauge, 3.5-cm needle.
- Advance the needle 2–3 cm deep to locate the nerve by paresthesiae in the foot or pulse-synchronous movement of the foot (peripheral nerve stimulator).
- Aspirate for blood.
- Inject 10–15 ml of local anesthetic solution which should flow easily.

Complications

- Nerve trauma.
- Painful procedure.
- Intravenous injection.
- Hematoma.
- Infection.

Nerve blocks around the knee: intra-articular block

This block has become popular for providing postsurgical analgesia following arthroscopy and depends on peripheral opioid receptors within the knee joint.

Indications

- Postsurgical analgesia.
- Chronic pain syndromes of the knee (LA and steroid).

Landmarks

- Medial border of the patella.
- Groove between the patella and femur.

Practical steps (Fig. 17.33)

- With the patient's leg extended, identify the groove between the medial border of the patella and the femur.

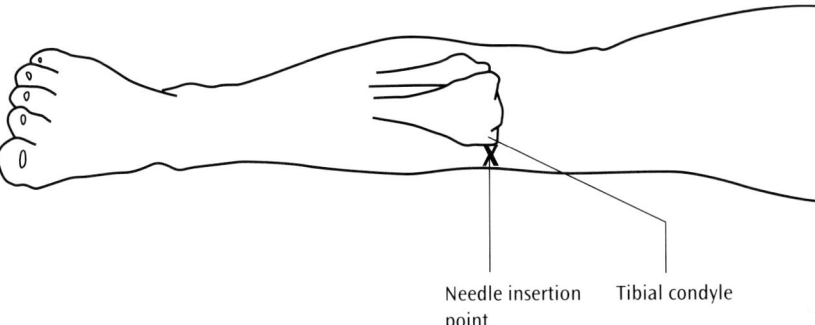

Figure 17.31 *Saphenous nerve block. Landmarks and needle insertion point for a saphenous nerve block.*

Needle insertion point   Tibial condyle

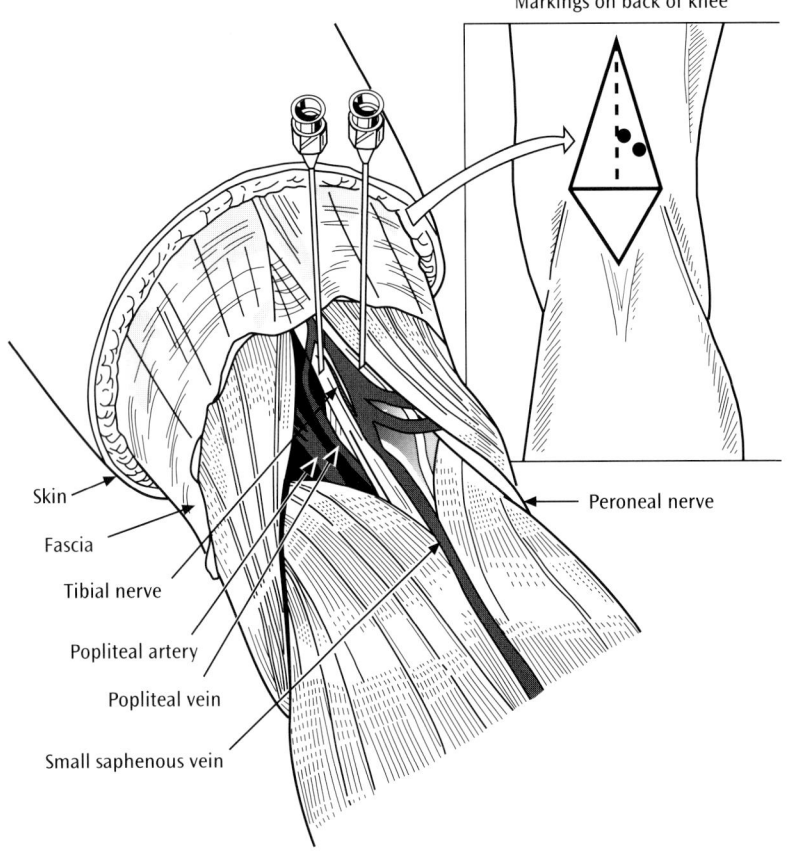

Markings on back of knee

Skin
Fascia
Tibial nerve
Popliteal artery
Popliteal vein
Small saphenous vein

Peroneal nerve

Figure 17.32 *Tibial and peroneal nerve blocks. Landmarks and needle insertion points for the tibial and peroneal nerve blocks.*

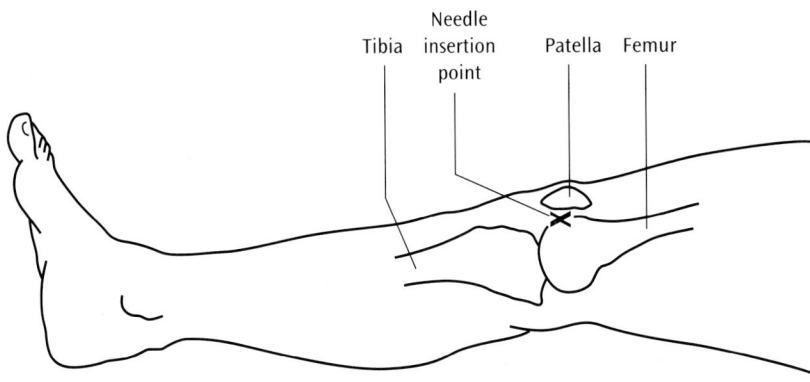

Tibia   Needle insertion point   Patella   Femur

Figure 17.33 *Intra-articular block of the knee. Landmarks and needle insertion point for an intra-articular block of the knee.*

- Insert a 25-gauge, 3.5-cm needle into the knee joint along this groove.
- Avoid impaling the needle tip into the articular cartilage.
- Inject local anesthetic solution into the knee, up to 30 ml [with epinephrine (adrenaline)] may be injected.
- The injection should meet little resistance.
- Methylprednisolone may be injected for chronic pain syndromes or morphine 1–2 mg for postsurgical analgesia.
- This block does not cause any sensory or motor effects that would prevent ambulation.
- Careful asepsis must be followed to avoid an infected joint.

Complications
- Painful procedure.
- Damage to articular cartilage.
- Infection.
- Local anesthetic toxicity.

Nerve blocks at the ankle

The nerve supply to the foot is provided by five terminal nerves: superficial and deep peroneal, saphenous, sural, and tibial (Fig. 17.34).

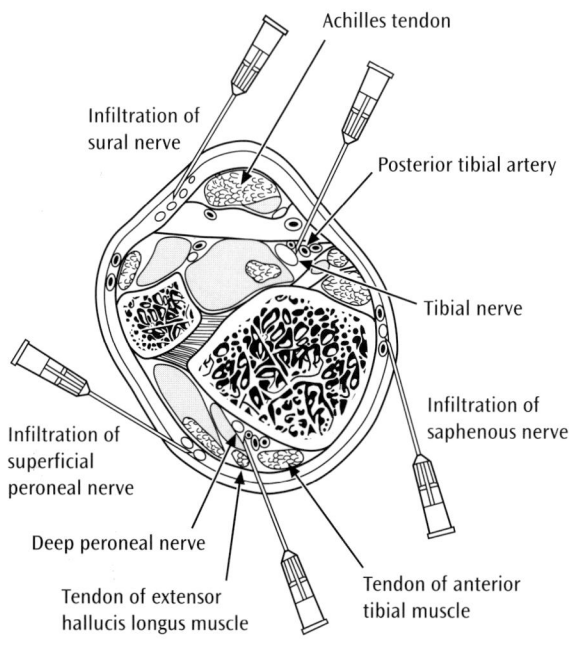

Figure 17.34 *Nerve blocks at the ankle. Landmarks and needle insertion points for nerve blocks at the ankle.*

Indications
- Anesthesia for surgery of the foot.

Relevant anatomy
- The skin of the dorsum of the foot is supplied by the superficial and deep peroneal nerves.
- The lateral border of the fifth toe is supplied by the sural nerve.
- The superficial and deep nerves are blocked in combination because of their overlapping skin innervation.
- The saphenous nerve supplies the medial surface of the foot. It divides into two branches at the medial malleolus.
- The sole of the foot is supplied by four branches of the tibial nerve: medial calcaneal, medial plantar, lateral plantar, and sural nerves.
- The sural nerve branches off the tibial nerve in the popliteal fossa and passes between the lateral malleolus and calcaneum to supply the lateral border of the foot.

Sural nerve block (Fig. 17.34)

Landmarks
- Achilles tendon.
- Lateral malleolus.

Practical steps
- Traditionally, the patient is positioned prone, alternatively the patient can lie supine with the foot inverted.
- Insert a 25-gauge, 3.5-cm needle immediately posterior to the lateral malleolus, and direct the needle tip toward the lateral border of the Achilles tendon.
- Inject a subcutaneous sausage of local anesthetic solution (5–7 ml) between the lateral malleolus and the Achilles tendon.

Saphenous nerve block (Fig. 17.34)

Landmarks
- Medial malleolus.
- Long saphenous vein.

Practical steps
- Position the patient supine and externally rotate the foot.
- Identify a point 1 cm proximal and 1 cm anterior to the medial malleolus.
- Identify the long saphenous vein, which lies in close proximity to the nerve.
- At this point, insert a 25-gauge, 3.5-cm needle and inject 5 ml of local anesthetic solution around the long saphenous vein.
- Avoid intravenous injection.

Tibial nerve block (Fig. 17.34)

Landmarks

- Posterior tibial artery.
- Medial malleolus.

Practical steps

- Traditionally, the patient is positioned prone, alternatively the patient can remain supine.
- Identify the posterior tibial artery.
- Insert a 25-gauge, 3.5-cm needle immediately inferior to this point at 45° to the skin parallel to the long axis of the tibia and advance toward the bone.
- Paresthesiae may be elicited before contacting bone.
- Inject 5 ml of local anesthetic solution.

Superficial and deep peroneal nerve block (Fig. 17.34)

Landmarks

- Dorsalis pedis artery.

Practical steps

- Position patient supine, with the foot supported in extension.
- Palpate the dorsalis pedis pulse.
- Insert a 25-gauge, 3.5-cm needle immediately medial to the artery.
- Advance the needle 1 cm cephalad and deep.
- If the needle contacts bone or tendon, withdraw tip slightly.
- Aspirate for blood.
- Inject 5 ml of local anesthetic solution.
- Withdraw the needle to the subcutaneous plane and deposit a sausage of local anesthetic solution laterally toward the lateral malleolus (blocks superficial branch).

Complications of ankle blocks

- Nerve trauma.
- Hematoma.
- Vascular occlusion if local anesthetic volume too great.
- Infection.

NERVE BLOCKS OF THE PELVIS[19,20]

Pudendal nerve block

This block provides analgesia of the lower vagina and perineum, and can be carried out via a transvaginal or a transperineal approach. The transvaginal approach is preferred as it is more reliable. Many would consider a caudal block more straightforward, with better effect.

Indications

- Analgesia for childbirth (second stage).
- Analgesia for episiotomy.
- Analgesia for suturing perineum.

Relevant anatomy

- The pudendal nerve is a branch of the sacral plexus.
- It runs lateral and posterior to the ischial spin and sacrospinous ligament.
- It has two branches: the dorsal nerve and the perineal nerve.
- The dorsal branch passes under the symphysis pubis to supply the clitoris/penis.
- The perineal branch supplies the inferoposterior aspect of the scrotum or the labia majora.
- The pudendal nerve is blocked as it passes the ischial spine.

Landmarks

- Ischial spine.
- Sacrospinous ligament.

Practical steps (transvaginal approach) (Fig. 17.35)

- Position patient supine in the lithotomy position.
- Palpate the ischial spine and sacrospinous ligament transvaginally with the index and middle finger of one hand.
- Guide a 20-gauge, 14-cm needle attached to a 10-ml syringe to the ligament just below the ischial spine.
- Advance the needle tip just through the ligament.
- Aspirate for blood (pudendal vessels run near the nerve).

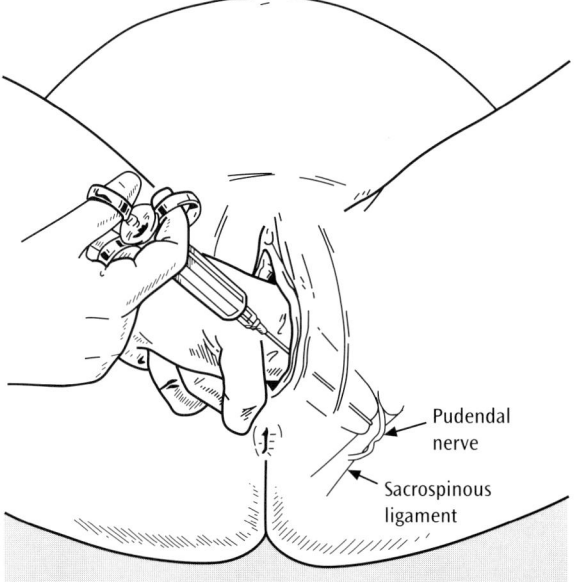

Figure 17.35 *Pudendal nerve block. Landmarks and needle insertion point for a pudendal nerve block.*

- Inject 10 ml of local anesthetic solution.
- The procedure is repeated for the opposite nerve.
- Special needle guides (Kobak needle) have been advocated to limit the penetration of the needle.

Complications

- Inadvertent intravenous injection of local anesthetic.
- Hematoma.
- Nerve trauma.
- Infection.

Paracervical block

Epidural analgesia for labor has made this block almost obsolete.

Indications

- Short lived analgesia for the first stage of labor (40–90 min).

- Analgesia for delivery, in combination with pudendal blocks.

Relevant anatomy

- Pain of uterine contractions, and cervical dilatation, is mediated via sympathetic fibers.
- The sympathetic fibers from the pelvic sympathetic plexus communicates via the lumbar and lower thoracic sympathetic chain to the rami communicantes of T11 and T12.
- The paracervical block acts on the sympathetic fibers in the loose parametrial tissue around the cervix.

Landmarks

- Lateral fornices of the vagina.

Practical steps (Fig. 17.36)

- The patient is positioned supine in the lithotomy position.

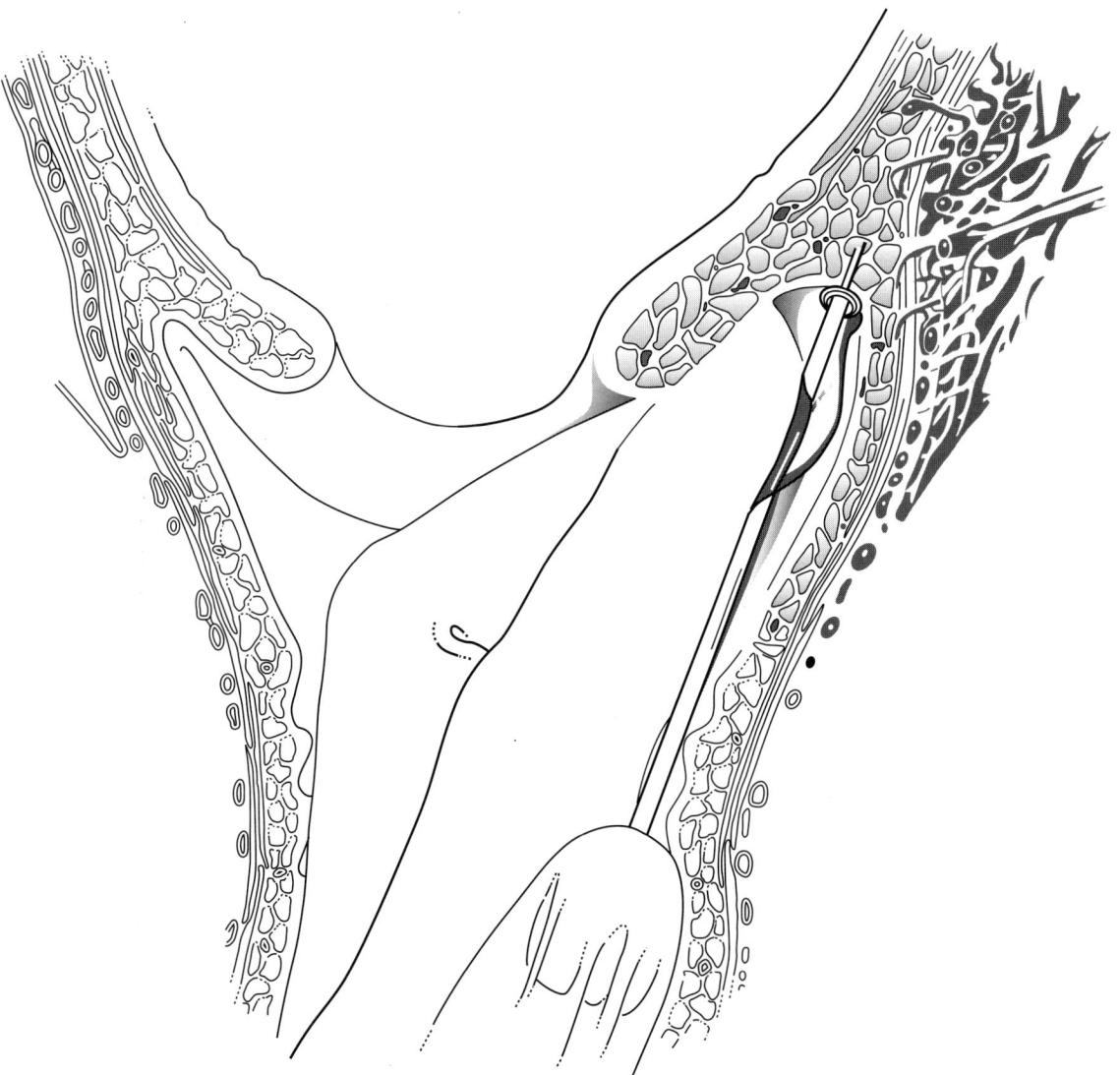

Figure 17.36 *Paracervical nerve block. Landmarks and needle insertion point for a paracervical nerve block.*

- A 20-gauge, 14-cm needle is directed into the lateral fornices at 3–4 o'clock and at 8–9 o'clock.
- A needle depth-limiting device (Kobak needle guide) is useful to limit needle tip penetration to 5–7 mm.
- Advance the needle tip until it pierces the mucosa.
- Aspirate for blood.
- Inject 10 ml of local anesthetic solution.

Complications

- Intravenous injection/absorption of local anesthetic.
- Fetal heart rate abnormalities.
- Unexpected fetal death.

REFERENCES

● 1. de Jong RH. Local anesthetics in clinical practice. In: Waldman SD ed. *Interventional Pain Management*. Philadelphia, PA: WB Saunders, 2001: 201–19.

2. Ramamurthy S, Walsh NE, Schoenfeld LS, Hoffman J. Evaluation of neurolytic blocks using phenol and cryogenic block in the management of chronic pain. *J Pain Symptom Manage* 1989; **4**: 72.

● 3. Pither CE, Raj PP, Ford DJ. The use of peripheral nerve stimulators for regional anesthesia. A review of experimental characteristics, technique, and clinical applications. *Reg Anesth* 1985; **10**: 49–58.

4. Bovim G, Sand T. Cervicogenic headache, migraine without aura and tension-type headache: diagnostic blockade of greater occipital and supra-orbital nerves. *Pain* 1992; **51**: 41–8.

◆ 5. Waldman SD. Trigeminal nerve block. In: Weiner RS ed. *Innovations in Pain Management*, vol. I. Orlando, FL: PMD Press, 1990: 10–15.

6. Katz J. Vagus nerve block. In: Katz J ed. *Atlas of Regional Anesthesia*. Norwalk, CT: Appleton-Century-Crofts, 1995: 52–3.

● 7. Pappas JL, Warfield CA. Cervical plexus blockade. In: Waldman SD ed. *Interventional Pain Management*. Philadelphia: WB Saunders, 2001: 342–61.

◆ 8. Brown DL. Brachial plexus block: an update. *ASA Refresher Lectures* 2000; **153**: 1–7.

9. Bonica JJ. Musculoskeletal disorders of the upper limb. In: Bonica JJ ed. *The Management of Pain*, 2nd edn. Philadelphia, PA: Lea & Febiger, 1990: 891–3.

10. Pinnock CA, Fischer HBJ, Jones RP. Nerve blocks at the elbow. In: Pinnock CA, Fischer HBJ, Jones RP eds. *Peripheral Nerve Blockade*. London: Churchill Livingstone, 1996: 118–25.

11. Lofstrom B. Nerve block at the wrist. In: Eriksson E ed. *Illustrated Handbook in Local Anaesthesia*. London: Lloyd-Luke, 1979: 90–2.

● 12. Richardson J, Lonqvist PA. Thoracic paravertebral block. *Br J Anaesth* 1998; **81**: 230–8.

13. Moore D, Bush W, Scurlock J. Intercostal nerve block: a roentgenographic anatomic study of technique and absorption in humans. *Anesth Analg* 1980; **59**: 815.

● 14. Murphy DF. Interpleural analgesia. *Br J Anaesth* 1993; **71**: 426–34.

15. Racz GB, Hagstrom D. Iliohypogastric and ilioinguinal nerve entrapment: diagnosis and treatment. *Pain Digest* 1992; **2**: 43–8.

16. Bridenbaugh PO. The lower extremity: somatic blockade. In: Cousins MJ, Bridenbaugh PO eds. *Neural Blockade in Clinical Anesthesia and Management of Pain*. Philadelphia, PA: JB Lippincott, 1988: 417–36.

◆ 17. ChayenD, Nathan H, Chayen M. The psoas compartment block. *Anesthesiology* 1976; **45**: 95–9.

● 18. Tagariello V. Sciatic nerve blocks: approaches, techniques, local anaesthetics and manipulations. *Anaesthesia* 1998; **53**: 15–17.

19. Englesson S. Pudendal nerve block. In: Eriksson E ed. *Illustrated Handbook in Local Anaesthesia*. London: Lloyd-Luke, 1979: 98–100.

20. Englesson S. Paracervical block. In: Eriksson E ed. *Illustrated Handbook in Local Anaesthesia*. London: Lloyd-Luke, 1979: 96–7.

18

Sympathetic blocks

HARALD BREIVIK

Anatomy of the sympathetic nervous system	233	Thoracic sympathetic block	240
Indications for sympathetic neural blockade	235	Lumbar sympathetic block	241
Testing for completeness of sympathetic blockade	236	Intravenous regional sympathetic block	243
Tests of sympathetic function, blood flow, and pain	236	References	245
Stellate ganglion block	237		

The sympathetic nervous system maintains a constrictor tone in blood vessels of the skin. The classic indication for sympathetic neural blockade and surgical sympathectomy has been to help in the healing of ischemic cutaneous ulcers and to relieve foot pain at rest.[1] Although vascular surgery helps many such patients, rest pain due to ischemic conditions of the lower extremity is still an appropriate indication for lumbar sympathetic neural blockade.*[1]

Sympathetically maintained pain is indicated by pain relief in complex regional pain syndromes subsequent to either systemic alpha blockade (i.v. phentolamine test;[2] see Chapter P4) or regional sympathetic block. This can be with repeated local anesthetic blocks, neurolytic sympathetic blocks, or radiofrequency (Chapter P26) or surgical neurolysis. The most common indication for sympathectomies nowadays seems to be hyperhidrosis. However, this is now recognized as a significant cause of persistent pain because as many as 10% of patients develop postsympathectomy neuropathic pain after open or endoscopic sympathectomy for hyperhidrosis.***[3]

Sympathetic afferent and efferent pain impulses are stopped by brachial plexus, spinal, or epidural local anesthetic blocks. These effects are exploited with continuous brachial plexus blocks, obstetric epidurals, and postoperative epidurals using local anesthetic for the relief of visceral pain. Visceral sympathetic inhibition increases gastrointestinal motility after surgery (see Chapter A12). It is, however, the more specific sympathetic blocks, made possible by the separation in peripheral anatomy of sympathetic and somatic nervous structures, that will be described in this chapter.

Specific sympathetic blockade is possible at the cervi-cothoracic and lumbar areas as well as at the celiac and hypogastric sympathetic plexa. Specific interruption of sympathetic afferent or efferent nerves at these three vertebral areas is possible because the sympathetic ganglia and plexa are sufficiently anatomically separated from somatic nerves that it is possible to achieve sympathetic blockade without blocking sensory or motor functions (Fig. 18.1).

Lumbar sympathetic block for rest pain of the legs and celiac plexus block for abdominal visceral pain from cancer are two of the most beneficial neural blockade techniques available.*[1]

Celiac plexus blockade, superior hypogastric plexus block, and ganglion impar block are described in Chapter P19.

ANATOMY OF THE SYMPATHETIC NERVOUS SYSTEM

The peripheral sympathetic nervous system originates in efferent neurons in the intermediolateral column of the spinal cord, passing preganglionic fibers to the ventral roots from T1 to L2 out of the spinal canal as the white rami communicantes to the sympathetic chain (Fig. 18.2). The sympathetic chain lies at the anterolateral aspect of the vertebral bodies in the cervical region. In the thorax, it is adjacent to the neck of the ribs, relatively close to the somatic nerve roots, whereas in the lumbar region the sympathetic chain again lies anterolateral to the bodies of the vertebrae and is separated from the somatic nerve roots by the psoas muscle and psoas fascia. The pregan-

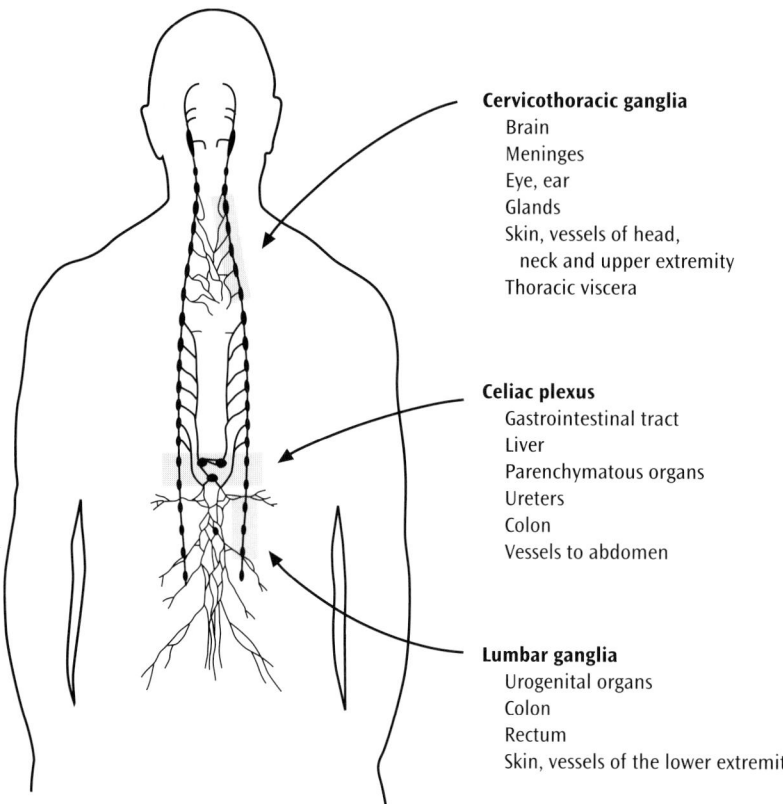

Figure 18.1 *Sympathetic nervous system outlined. (Reproduced with permission of Lippincott Williams & Wilkins© from Breivik et al.[1])*

Cervicothoracic ganglia
Brain
Meninges
Eye, ear
Glands
Skin, vessels of head,
    neck and upper extremity
Thoracic viscera

Celiac plexus
Gastrointestinal tract
Liver
Parenchymatous organs
Ureters
Colon
Vessels to abdomen

Lumbar ganglia
Urogenital organs
Colon
Rectum
Skin, vessels of the lower extremity

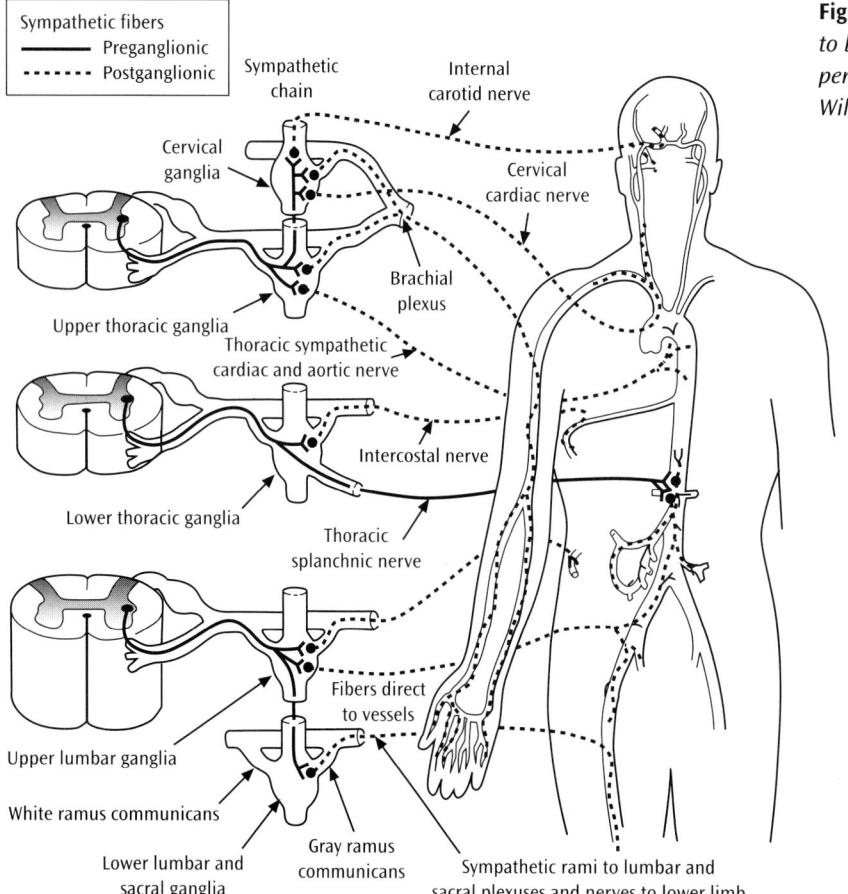

Figure 18.2 *Sympathetic nerve supply to blood vessels. (Reproduced with permission of Lippincott Williams & Wilkins© from Breivik et al.[1])*

Sympathetic fibers
—— Preganglionic
····· Postganglionic

Sympathetic chain
Internal carotid nerve
Cervical ganglia
Cervical cardiac nerve
Upper thoracic ganglia
Brachial plexus
Thoracic sympathetic cardiac and aortic nerve
Intercostal nerve
Lower thoracic ganglia
Thoracic splanchnic nerve
Fibers direct to vessels
Upper lumbar ganglia
White ramus communicans
Lower lumbar and sacral ganglia
Gray ramus communicans
Sympathetic rami to lumbar and sacral plexuses and nerves to lower limb

glionic fibers run a variable distance within the sympathetic chain to ganglia in the chain up or down from the segment of the spinal cord where they originate, or they may pass to peripherally located ganglia in the gastrointestinal or urogenital tracts (Fig. 18.2).

This variable level of relay between the preganglionic and the postganglionic neurons within the sympathetic chain is one reason for variable results from an apparently technically successful block, and also for regeneration of sympathetic function after a successful sympathetic block and recurrence of the symptoms that indicated the sympathetic blockade.

There are three or four cervical sympathetic ganglia, 12 thoracic, four or five lumbar, and four sacral sympathetic ganglia. There is one coccygeal sympathetic ganglion – the ganglion impar.

The fibers from the sympathetic ganglion cells are widely distributed to join peripheral nerves via the gray rami communicantes and also to join blood vessels to various organs.

The sympathetic chain receives efferent preganglionic fibers from the spinal cord as well as afferent visceral fibers carrying pain impulses from the extremities, the head and neck, and the abdominal and pelvic viscera, including the urogenital system. The carotid arteries, aorta, and vena cava receive direct postganglionic nerves from nearby sympathetic ganglia and plexuses (Fig. 18.2). Sympathetic nerve fibers may arrive at the vessel wall from adjacent ganglia, via postganglionic fibers passing in somatic nerves to the vessels and postganglionic fibers that pass up or down the sympathetic chain, or fibers synapsing in the prevertebral plexuses before they pass to the vessels. All these sympathetic vascular nerves and filaments meet in extensive perivascular and adventitial sympathetic networks. Local anesthetic blockade using perivascular brachial plexus approaches will inhibit sympathetic nervous functions very effectively in the upper extremity, a fact exploited well by continuous brachial plexus block after reimplantation surgery of the extremity.

The functions and role of the sympathetic nervous system in chronic pain are described in Chapter Ch29 and are reviewed by Breivik et al.[1] and Jänig and Stanton-Hicks.[4]

INDICATIONS FOR SYMPATHETIC NEURAL BLOCKADE*[1,3–5]

The following clinical conditions may benefit from interruption of sympathetic efferent and afferent nerves.

Acute pain

- Acute pancreatitis.

- Renal colic.
- Cardiac pain.
- Visceral pain from uterine contractions.
- Acute ischemic pain from accidental intra-arterial injections of irritating drugs such as thiopentone.
- Frostbite.
- Vascular surgery and reimplantation surgery (to reduce postoperative pain and improve postoperative blood flow).
- Acute exacerbation of Raynaud's disease.

Chronic pain

- Obliterative arterial disease causing rest pain in the lower extremities (when vascular surgery is not indicated).
- Complex regional pain syndromes (CRPS types I and II).[4]
- Phantom limb pain.
- Central pain.
- Chronic pancreatitis.
- Cancer pain from upper abdominal viscera.
- Cancer pain from pelvic viscera.

There is considerable disagreement on whether complex regional pain syndromes are indications for sympathetic blockade.[4] This was formerly called reflex sympathetic dystrophy (RSD), but the diagnosis was often made without ascertaining whether sympathetic block relieved the pain.[4] Clearly, patients with a picture of what clinically was called "reflex sympathetic dystrophy" did not always have pain relief after sympathetic blocks. It is now realized that sympathetically maintained pain is present in only about one-third of patients with a clinical presentation of complex regional pain syndrome (CRPS type I or type II).[1,4]

Only intravenous phentolamine tests (see Chapter P4) or diagnostic sympathetic blocks will indicate whether the patient has a component of sympathetically maintained pain in their complex regional pain syndrome. Only one in three or one in four CRPS patients have sympathetically maintained pain.[4]

Studies on the pain-relieving effects of sympathetic neural blockade, in which patients with the clinical presentation of "RSD" or "CRPS" were included without documenting that they had sympathetically maintained pain, obviously must have had a very low sensitivity: any beneficial effects on the few patients with sympathetically maintained pain would have disappeared into the majority of nonresponding patients included simply because they did not have sympathetically maintained pain. Such studies will have a very high risk of false-negative results. Unfortunately, there are many publications of poorly designed "randomized controlled" trials with such obvious flaws that invalidate their conclusions.

Unfortunately, long-standing complex regional pain

syndromes with a component of sympathetically maintained pain do not often have long-lasting pain relief after sympathethic blockade. Some patients who initially had good pain relief with sympathetic blockade gradually, after several years, lost their component of sympathetically maintained pain.[*6]

Even more worrisome is the fact that sympathectomy by radiofrequency destruction – surgical removal of parts of the sympathetic chain – or (less frequently) neurolytic chemical sympathectomy can produce new neuropathic pain problems in some unfortunate patients with chronic complex regional pain syndromes.[*3,5] This does not happen after sympathetic blockade performed with traditional local anesthetic drugs, nor after regional intravenous guanethidine sympathetic blockade (Fig. 18.3).

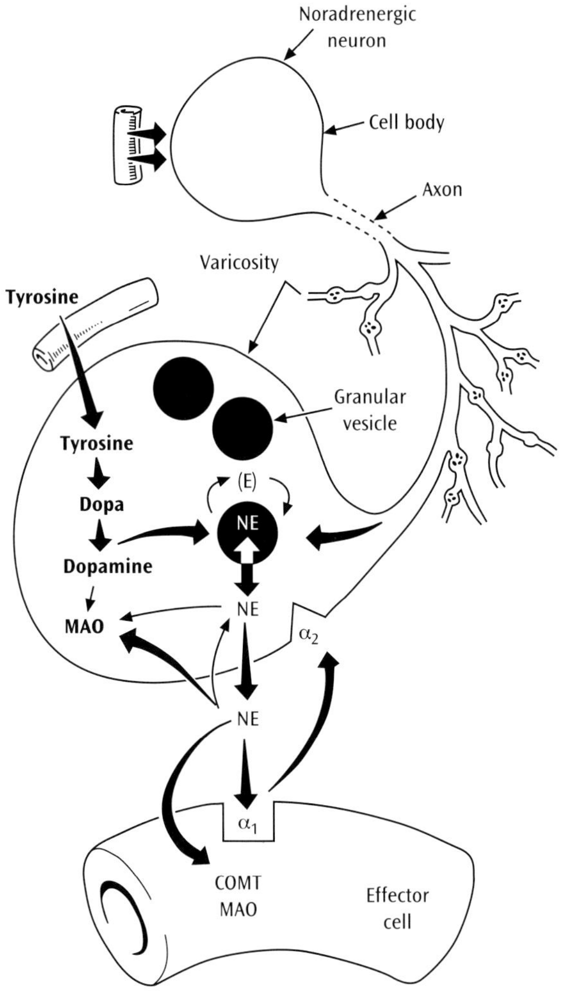

TESTING FOR COMPLETENESS OF SYMPATHETIC BLOCKADE

In patients with a reasonably healthy vascular system, a clear-cut, objective, easily documented peripheral vasodilatation occurs after a sympathetic block. An increase in skin temperature of several centigrade can be felt and measured.

TESTS OF SYMPATHETIC FUNCTION, BLOOD FLOW, AND PAIN[1]

Sympathetic function

- Skin conductance response.
- Sweat test.
- Skin plethysmography and ice response.

Blood flow

- Plethysmography.
- Laser Doppler flowmeter.
- Pulse wave changes.
- Temperature.

Pain

- Subjective pain intensity score (visual analog scale, verbal categorical scale, numeric rating scale).
- Subjective pain relief score.
- Analgesic drug consumption.

Function

Improved functions that were inhibited by pain (e.g. claudication distance).

Skin temperature measurements

These can be carried out quite simply and reliably in clinical practice by measuring skin temperature with a thermocouple probe and a telethermometer. Reliable results are obtained by measuring the distal part of the extremity at 10 different points (below each toe, in the middle of the sole, on the dorsum pedis; or similar points on the upper extremity) on each side.

Figure 18.3 *Sympathetic nerve endings and receptors. Norepinephrine (NE; noradrenaline) is released as the transmitter substance on depolarization of the presynaptic neuron. This is inhibited by local anesthetic blocking drugs. Reuptake of NE back into the presynaptic nerve terminals is blocked for several days by guanethidine. MAO, monoamine oxidase (Reproduced with permission of Lippincott Williams & Wilkins© from Breivik et al.[1])*

At an appropriate time after the block has been performed (at least 30 min), expose both extremities to cold air. This will cause the temperature to drop on the unblocked side and remain unchanged or increase up to several degrees, depending on the state of the vessels of the patient, on the blocked side.

Skin conductance response and skin potential response

These two tests are reasonably reliable, they require some special equipment, and the results depend on the degree of arousal of the central nervous system. Sedation, drugs that alter sympathetic activity, anticholinergic drugs, and steroids all interfere with these tests.[1]

Pain assessment

Whenever the indication for sympathetic block is acute or chronic pain, a visual analog scale or numerical rating scale of present pain intensity should be used before and after the block, as well as a categorical scale of pain relief.

Duration of any pain relief, and its effects on functions that have been inhibited by the pain, must be documented in a pain diary.

Contraindications

Patients with an increased bleeding tendency and those who are anticoagulated cannot have any of the major sympathetic blocks performed. The risk of deep-sited bleeding, which cannot be stopped by compression, is significant. For these patients, intravenous regional sympathetic block with guanethidine, where available, may be an alternative to sympathetic blocks of the sympathetic chain or prevertebral sympathetic plexuses.

Bilateral sympathetic blocks should *not* be performed on the same day because the risk of orthostatic hypotension increases. Bilateral lumbar sympathetic block may cause loss of ejaculation and may be contraindicated in some patients. Clearly, this must be discussed thoroughly with the patient.

Sympathetic blockade with local anesthetic drugs

For diagnostic and prognostic sympathetic blocks, lidocaine (lignocaine), mepivacaine, bupivacaine, or ropivacaine can all be used. Carrying out a double-blind block with either a short-acting or a long-acting local anesthetic may help to evaluate the placebo effect in the response to the block.

Mepivacaine and lidocaine should have a sympathetic block duration of 1.5–3 h; bupivacaine and ropivacaine 3–10 h.[1]

A double-blind, true placebo-controlled block is usually not feasible. However, Tenicela and coworkers managed to perform a truly placebo-controlled trial of stellate ganglion block for herpes zoster of the trigeminal nerve, providing evidence for a prophylactic effect on postherpetic neuralgia.***[7]

Image intensifier and contrast enhancement for verification of location of blocking solution

For those who have radiographic image intensifier facilities to visualize the procedure, the local anesthetic should be mixed with a small amount of iohexol (Omnipaque) or Conray 420.[1]

For neurolytic blocks

- Phenol 6% (60 mg/ml) in water or dissolved in Omnipaque.
- Ethanol 50–100% may be used for celiac plexus block.

Major complications due to neurolytic sympathetic blocks

- For the sympathetic ganglion chain (cervical or lumbar), ethanol carries a significant risk of inducing new neuropathic (neuralgic) pain.[1,5] Phenol is probably a little safer in this respect.
- One can never eliminate the risk of injecting into the wall or lumen of a radicular artery supplying the spinal cord, or injection into a peripheral epidural sleeve. The risk is lower in the cervical and lumbar segments than in the thoracic segments, but it is never zero. These accidents result in permanent, major neurological sequelae.

STELLATE GANGLION BLOCK

The cervicothoracic sympathetic chain is located in the space between the fascia overlying the prevertebral muscles and the carotid sheath (Fig. 18.4).

The sympathetic preganglionic fibers supplying the head, neck, and the upper extremities emerge from the spinal cord segments T1–T6. They converge and pass to the cervicothoracic sympathetic chain of ganglia, the upper thoracic and lower cervical ganglion in front of the neck of the first rib forming the *stellate ganglion*. Immediately below the stellate ganglion lies the *cupula of the pleura*, and directly posterior to the stellate ganglion lies

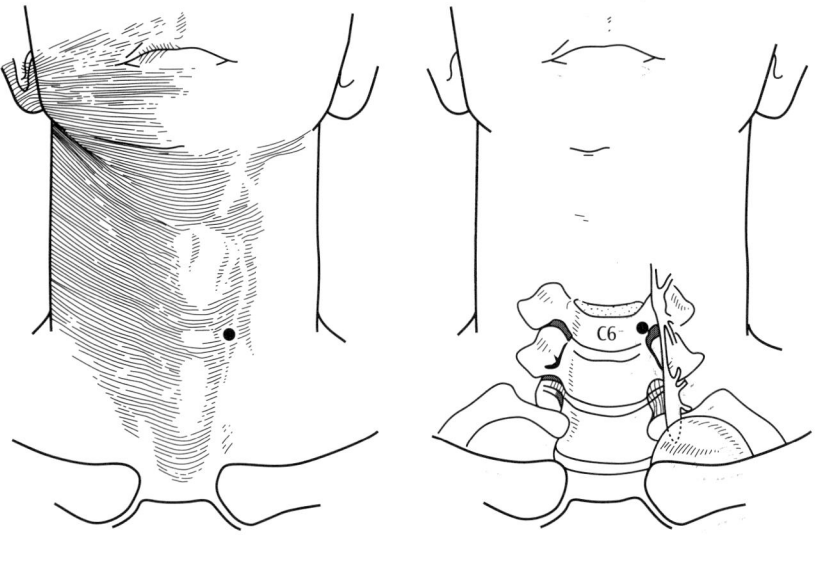

Figure 18.4 *Cervicothoracic sympathetic ganglion chain. Prevertebral muscles (1). The middle cervical ganglion (2). The ganglion stellatum (3) is located on the neck of the first rib (6–8), extending up to the transverse process of C7. At this level, the vertebral artery is lateral and anterior to the ganglion; at the C7 level, the artery has dived posteriorly, safely into the foramen intertransversarium. The top of the pleura (9) is also well below the transverse process of C6 (Chassaignac's tubercle). Anterior (4) and middle (5) scalene muscles (see text). (Reproduced with permission of Lippincott Williams & Wilkins© from Breivik et al.[1])*

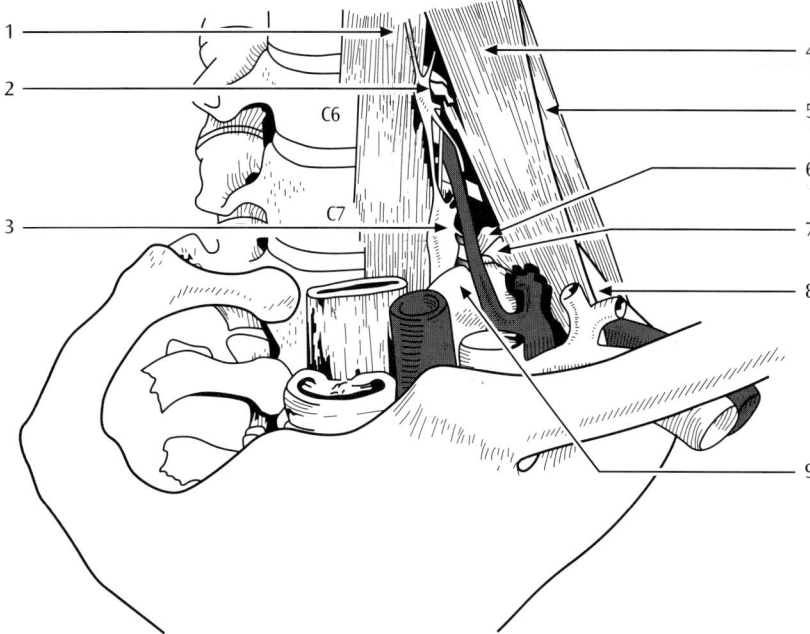

the *vertebral artery*. The intermediate cervical ganglion lies in front of the medial part of the transverse process of C7, the middle cervical ganglion on the medial part of the transverse process of C5. The superior cervical ganglion is at the level of C2–C3.

The safe approach to the cervicothoracic sympathetic chain of ganglia is to aim for the transverse process of C6 (Chassaignac's tubercle) and inject a sufficient volume of the local anesthetic solution, with radio-opaque contrast medium added if a radiographic record of the spread is desired. Aiming directly toward the stellate ganglion risks causing pneumothorax or even injuring the vertebral artery. Injection into the vertebral artery results in major *grand mal* seizures as an immediate consequence.

Technique of cervicothoracic sympathetic ganglion (stellate ganglion) block

With the patient supine, head resting on a thin pillow:

- The neck should be slightly extended at the atlanto-occipital joint. This stretches the esophagus and moves it away from the needle path.
- Slightly opening the mouth relaxes some neck muscles.
- The carotid pulse is palpated lateral to the trachea at the level of the cricoid cartilage. The artery and sternocleidomastoideus muscle are gently moved laterally and the resistance of the prominent transverse pro-

cess of C6 (Chassaignac's tubercle) is felt and placed between the index and the ring finger on the left hand.

- A fine needle (25 gauge) on a 20-ml syringe filled with the chosen local anesthetic solution (plus radiographic contrast medium if desired) is gently advanced toward the Chassaignac's tubercle.
- When bone is met, the needle is retracted slightly (about 2 mm); the needle and syringe are fixed with the left hand.
- Aspiration is performed and a small test dose of 0.3–0.5 ml is injected while the patient's face is continuously monitored by the anesthesiologist performing the block, preferably maintaining eye contact with the patient.
- Another 0.5-ml test dose is injected slowly, and may be repeated three times at about 10-s intervals.
- When no reaction occurs, slightly larger injections are performed repeatedly, until the desired volume (up to 20 ml) has been injected.
- The patient is then helped into a sitting position so that the injected local anesthetic solution may gravitate downwards toward the stellate ganglion.
- The patient will usually feel a "lump in the throat" and should be warned in advance that the voice may become hoarse.

An alternative technique is a two-operator technique, with one operator concentrating on placing the needle correctly in front of the Chassaignac's tubercle while the other aspirates and injects the solution via an extension tube. The author would recommend a one-operator technique as the safest, but it requires more manual dexterity.

Signs of cervicothoracic sympathetic ganglion block

Within seconds to a couple of minutes, the patient feels the eyelid drooping and:

- Ptosis can be observed.
- Miosis (a shrinking pupil) develops.
- Sinking of the eyeball (enophthalmos) develops.
- These signs and dry, warm, pinkish skin on the blocked side of the face are the signs of Horner's syndrome.
- The patient experiences a feeling of a blocked nose because of swelling of the nasal mucosa from vasodilatation, and the conjunctiva becomes reddish from vasodilatation.

The temperature of the hand and fingers of the upper extremities should be measured, with preferably cold exposure to accentuate the skin temperature differences between the blocked and unblocked side (see above).

Horner syndrome alone does not confirm a sympathetic block of the upper extremity. Temperature or the clear feeling of warm and dry skin of the palm on the blocked side are indications that the sympathetic fibers to the upper extremity are also blocked.

Complications

Life-threatening complications

A stellate ganglion block is a very simple block to learn and to perform (unless the patient has a short and obese neck); however:

- intra-arterial (vertebral artery or carotid artery) and
- intrathecal injections are easily done and are dangerous.

The practitioner must therefore be prepared to treat such complications immediately if they occur. No one should attempt a stellate ganglion blockade without studying the anatomy closely, and this block should never be performed by anyone who is not very well experienced in resuscitation techniques. Injection of even a 0.5- to 1-ml volume directly into the vertebral artery will cause immediate *grand mal* seizures, leading to a situation which is dramatic and difficult to treat. The seizures may last for many minutes.

Obviously, stellate ganglion blockade should not be performed without having an intravenous catheter in place, together with drugs and resuscitation equipment available for the treatment of such complications.

An intrathecal injection into a dural sleeve will cause more gradual onset of a high spinal anesthetic, with respiratory muscle paralysis and hypotension. Again, expert anesthesiologic resuscitation skills, drugs, and equipment must be at hand.

Less dramatic adverse effects

- Local anesthetic block of the *recurrent laryngeal nerve* causes temporary hoarseness and a feeling of a lump in the throat. This can be unpleasant but is not dangerous (bilateral stellate ganglion block should not be performed for this reason).
- Some patients experience Horner syndrome as unpleasant. Eye drops with phenylephrine will reduce the pupillary changes as well as the enophthalmos and the red eye.
- A cervical hematoma may occur, but is usually not dramatic or dangerous unless the patient is anticoagulated or has another reason for increased bleeding (which are contraindications for this block).
- Some patients have a feeling of paresthesiae along the chest wall and on the inside of the upper arm. This is transient.
- The *brachial plexus* may be blocked, in which case the patient does not have an isolated sympathetic block and the diagnostic value of the block is unreliable.

- *Phrenic nerve block* may occur; this is another reason why bilateral blocks should not be performed and care should be taken in patients with chronic obstructive lung disease.
- *Pneumothorax* may occur; still another reason why bilateral stellate ganglion block should never be performed.

Neurolytic stellate ganglion block

Phenol 6% (60 mg/ml) in water or X-ray contrast medium, in a volume of 2 ml in front of the transverse process of C6 will cause incomplete cervicothoracic sympathetic block. This block may cause a persistent Horner's syndrome, and if sympathetic blockade of the upper extremity is intended, the results are not reliable.

THORACIC SYMPATHETIC BLOCK

The chain of sympathetic ganglia in the thoracic region is located close to the neck of the ribs and quite close to the somatic nerve roots and their epidural sleeves (Fig.

18.5). This is different from the cervical region, where the sympathetic ganglia are separated from the somatic roots by the longus colli and the anterior scalene muscles, and is also different from the lumbar region, where the psoas major muscle separates the sympathetic ganglia from the somatic nerve roots. The close proximity to the pleura is a concern.

Indications

In order to obtain complete interruption of the sympathetic outflow to the *upper extremity*, the upper thoracic ganglia (down to T6) must be blocked. Because of the high risk of damaging somatic nerve roots and intrathecal injections, blind (or even image intensifier) techniques using neurolytic agents have now generally been replaced by thoracoscopic techniques.[1]

Pain from *coronary insufficiency* can be treated with continuous stellate ganglion and upper thoracic sympathetic ganglion blocks. Even for these indications thoracic sympathetic block has been replaced by alternative techniques, such as epidural spinal cord stimulation and epidural or intrathecal opioid and local anesthetic drug infusions.

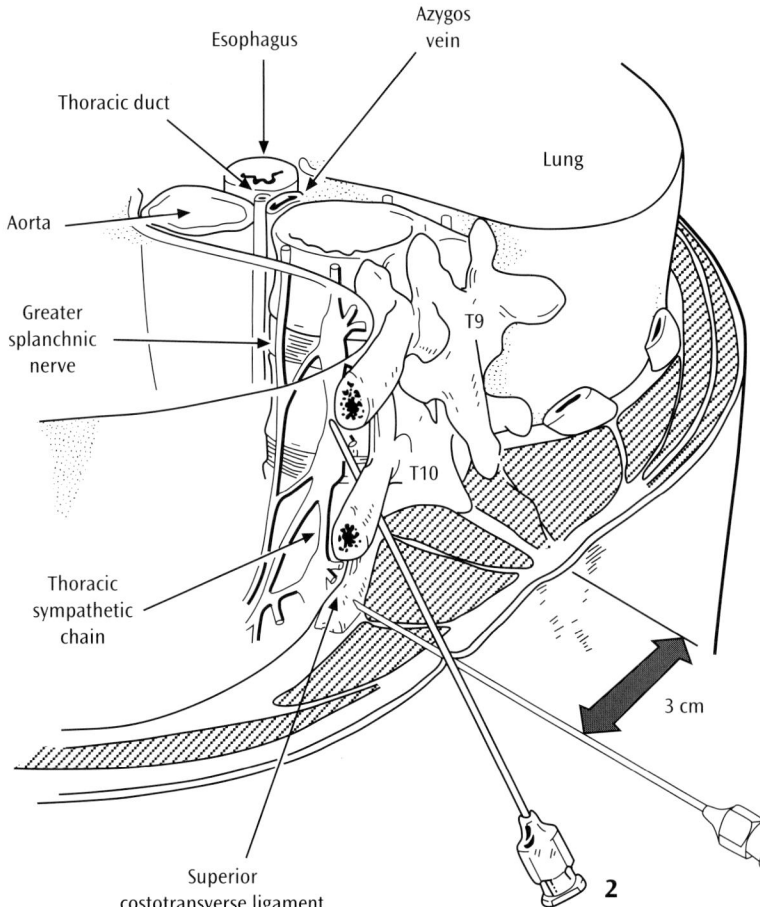

Figure 18.5 *Thoracic sympathetic ganglia are lying close to spinal nerve roots and their dural sleeves. The pleura is very close anteriorly. The needle is positioned correctly for a thoracic sympathetic ganglion block, but proximity to these structures means that this block has a high risk of complications (see text). (Reproduced with permission of Lippincott Williams & Wilkins© from Breivik et al.[1])*

Technique

A needle enters the skin about 3 cm from the midline of the upper thoracic spinous processes and is advanced medially toward the vertebral body. A superficial contact with bone means that the rib has been hit, and the needle will have to be placed a little higher or lower to enter the intercostal space and advanced toward the body of the vertebra in the paravertebral space. At this point, 2 ml of a local anesthetic is deposited about 1 cm behind the crest of the vertebral body. A warm, dry hand indicates correct siting of the injection. Formerly, 6% (60 mg/ml) aqueous phenol (2 ml) or a similar amount of phenol dissolved in Omnipaque or Conray 420 was occasionally employed for neurolytic blocks, but the risks of neurological complications are considerable (see above for alternative techniques).

Complications

Somatic nerve root injury and spinal cord damage from intrathecal (or intra-arterial) injections of neurolytic solutions, as well as pneumothorax, are high-risk complications of this specific thoracic sympathetic chain blockade.

LUMBAR SYMPATHETIC BLOCK

The ganglia of the sympathetic chain lie close to the anterior part of the lateral side of the lumbar vertebral bodies, being separated from the somatic nerves by the psoas fascia and the psoas muscle (Fig. 18.6). One injection of about 20 ml of local anesthetic solution at the level of L2 or L3 in the correct fascial plane will spread upwards and downwards and achieve an adequate longitudinal spread for a complete sympathetic block of the lower extremity. For diagnostic and prognostic blocks, this may be a sufficiently precise technique; however, if neurolytic agents, such as phenol, are used, separate needles at levels L2, L3, and L4 are required.

Technique of lumbar sympathetic block

The spinous processes of L1 and L4 should be marked as reference points: L1 is at the level where the 12th ribs meet the lateral sides of the erector spina muscles. The L4 spinous process is at the level of the posterior superior iliac crests (Fig. 18.7).

- A 12-cm-long, 20- to 22-gauge needle is introduced 8–10 cm lateral to the middle of the spinous process of L4 and another one at L2.
- A marker (piece of rubber or plastic) should be placed on the needle before entering the skin. The needle is then advanced medially towards the body of the vertebrae (of L2 or L4).
- If bone is met after about 4–5 cm from the skin, this will be the transverse process. The transverse process is about half the distance from the skin to the depth of the sympathetic chain on the anterolateral part of the vertebral body.
- If the transverse process is used as a marker of depth, the rubber marker should be placed (after withdrawing the needle to the subcutaneous tissue) about twice the distance from the tip of the needle (about 10 cm from the tip of the needle).
- The needle should be redirected in a cranial or caudad direction to avoid the transverse process, and advanced until contact with bone is made again.
- The needle should be withdrawn to the subcutaneous tissue (to avoid bending the needle) before changing direction to advance it to the depth of the rubber

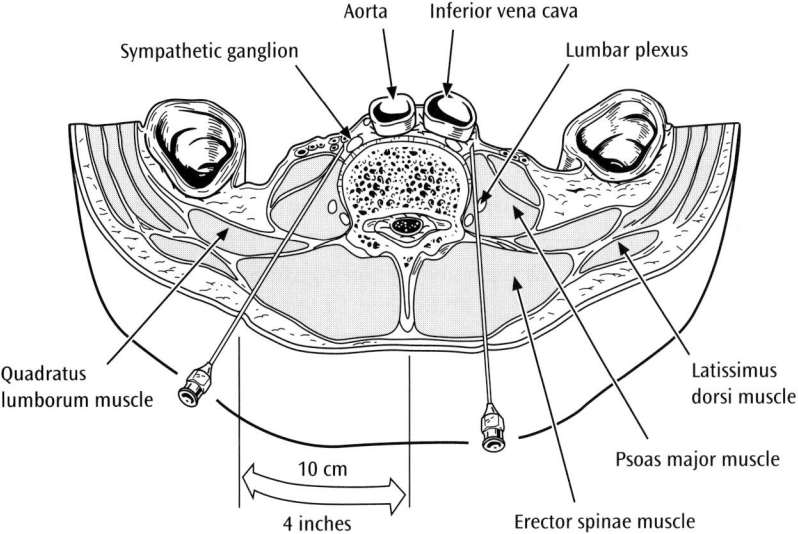

Figure 18.6 *Lumbar sympathetic block of ganglia at L2, L3, and L4, which are lying on the anterolateral aspect of the vertebral bodies well separated from other nervous tissues and blood vessels (see text). (Reproduced with permission of Lippincott Williams & Wilkins© from Breivik et al.[1])*

Aorta

Inferior vena cava

Sympathetic ganglion

Lumbar plexus

Quadratus lumborum muscle

Latissimus dorsi muscle

Psoas major muscle

Erector spinae muscle

10 cm

4 inches

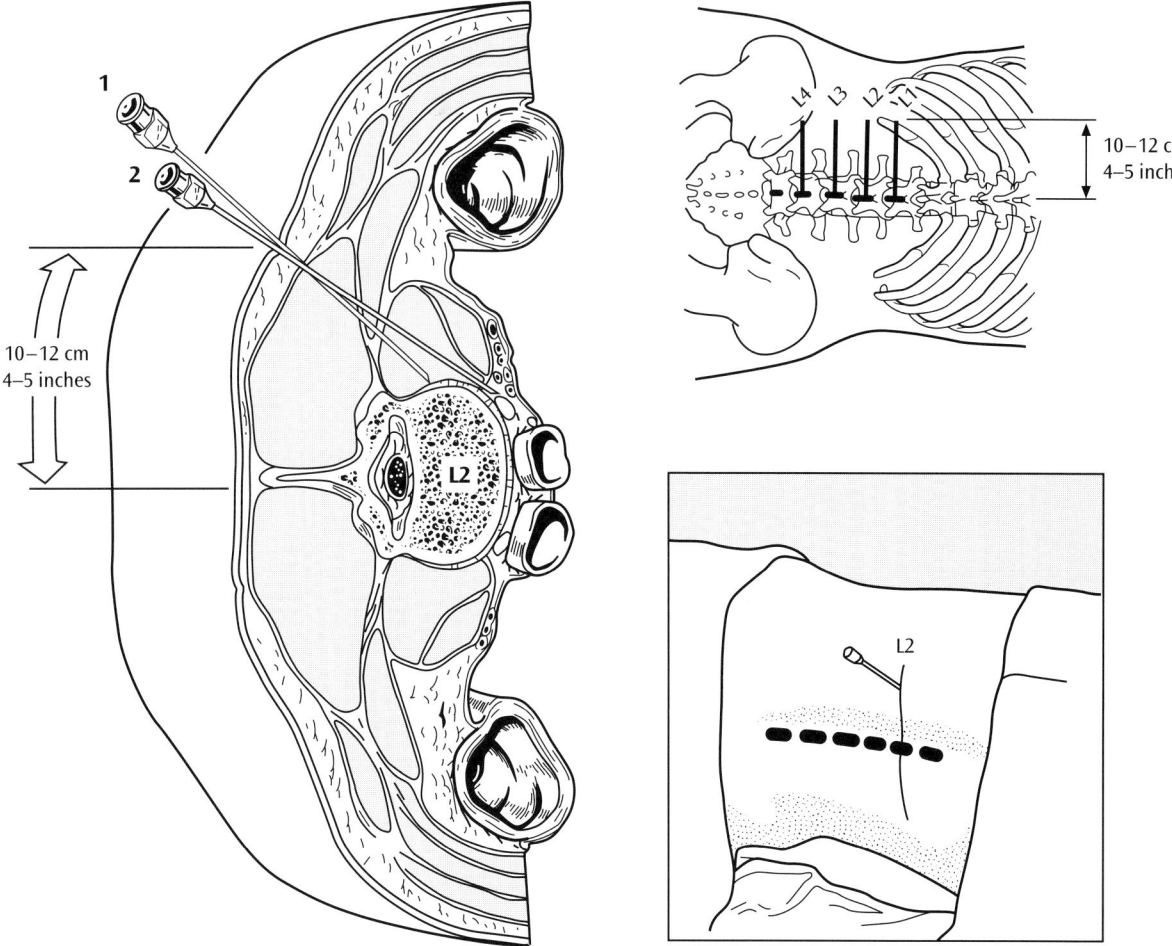

Figure 18.7 *Lumbar sympathetic ganglion block (see text). (Reproduced with permission of Lippincott Williams & Wilkins© from Breivik et al.[1])*

marker, or until the needle tip slides off the anterolateral phase of the vertebral body.

- In thin patients with less back muscle tissue, the distance is less than 10 cm; in bigger patients with more back muscle tissue, the distance is more than 10 cm from the skin.
- The correct position of the needle tip can be verified by use of a loss-of-resistance technique as the needle penetrates the psoas fascia.
- If the needle at L2 is placed first, the second needle at L4 will usually have to be introduced slightly deeper.
- Careful aspiration for blood and cerebrospinal fluid (CSF) is carried out before a test dose injection, which should not meet resistance.
- Resistance to injection means that the needle is in the wrong place, such as the wall of the aorta or vena cava, an abdominal viscus, or inside an intervertebral disk.
- Radiographic confirmation with a local anesthetic mixed with a contrast medium allows verification of the correct needle tip position.[8]

Dose of local anesthetic

If the indication for the block is to relieve visceral pain, 20–30 ml of bupivacaine 2.5 mg/ml (0.25%) at L2 will eradicate pain from, for instance, renal colic. If the indication for the block is to evaluate or prognosticate the effect of a possible neurolytic block, then 5 ml of a local anesthetic mixed with contrast medium is injected at L2 and at L4.

Continuous lumbar sympathetic blockade

This is possible by placing an 18-gauge long epidural needle at L2 and one at L4, positioning a catheter through each needle and injecting bupivacaine 2.5 mg/ml 5 ml in each catheter every 6 h for up to several days. However, the catheters tend to shift with vertebral body movement. Verification of the position of the catheters is needed (with radiographic contrast) if the block becomes less effective.

Single needle injection technique[9]

The tip of the 12th rib indicates the lower border of L2. A needle is placed 2–3 cm below and medial to the tip of the 12th rib and directed medially until the vertebral body of L3 is encountered at a depth of about 10 cm. Sufficient solution (15–25 ml) with radiographic contrast medium is added, and image intensifier control will indicate whether the most important ganglia of L2, L3, and L4 are covered by the solution.[9]

Neurolytic blocks of the lumbar sympathetic ganglia

When vascular surgeons refer patients who cannot be helped by vascular surgery for neurolytic lumber sympathectomy, the indications are usually severe ischemic rest pain, an ulcer that does not heal, or the desire to obtain a demarcation between viable and nonviable tissue before leg amputation. These patients are usually quite ill, have a high incidence of ischemic heart disease, and often have chronic pulmonary disease, diabetes mellitus with complications, and other ailments of old age. There is less risk with a neurolytic sympathectomy than even radiofrequency neurolysis, and surgical sympathectomy may not be tolerated by these patients.[1]

Agents for lumbar sympathetic blocks

Phenol 6% (60 mg/ml) in water is preferred, although up to 10% phenol in iohexol (Omnipaque) or Conray-420 has the advantage of being visible under image intensifier.

Technique

- With the image intensifier[1] or biplanar image intensifier, lateral and anteroposterior views are obtained, tilting the patient ventrally and dorsally to thoroughly check the position of the needle.
- A 1-ml test dose of local anesthetic followed by 0.5-ml boluses (up to 3–4 ml of the phenol-containing contrast medium) with image intensifier verification of correct positioning is injected.
- The injected neurolytic solution with radiographic contrast should cover each level (L2, L3, and L4) in the correct anterolateral position.[1]
- Before withdrawing the needles, 0.5 ml of a local anesthetic is injected through the needle to avoid leaving neurolytic solution on somatic nerve roots or spinal nerves during the removal of the needle.
- Patients should remain on their side for about 5 min to prevent the solution from spreading laterally.

- Patients are kept supine for 30–60 min while the skin temperature of the lower extremities, blood pressure, and heart rate are monitored.
- After about 1 h, patients are mobilized slowly and their blood pressure is checked for orthostatic hypotension.
- Most patients are able to leave the clinic after a few hours. Unstable elderly patients should be monitored as inpatients for at least 24 h after the block.
- The block can be repeated on the other side after a day, depending on the reaction to the first block.

Complications

Provided needle placement is executed carefully and verified by a local anesthetic test dose and/or radiographic contrast with image intensifier, complications are infrequent. However, injection of local anesthetic or neurolytic drugs into the cerebrospinal fluid, adjacent to spinal nerve roots or spinal nerves, and intravascularly is always possible.

- *Transient postsympathectomy neuropathic pain* occurs in up to 50% of patients in the anterolateral proximal part of the lower extremity.
- Neurolytic agents may reach the genitofemoral nerve (Fig. 18.8). Genitofemoral neuralgia is infrequent when phenol is employed (5–10%), and in most cases it is transient. However, when alcohol is used, more severe and protracted pain in the groin from genitofemoral ethanol neuritis occurs.
- The ureter may be damaged by phenol or alcohol.
- If bilateral upper level lumbar sympathectomy is performed, ejaculatory failure may follow.
- Postsympathectomy hyperesthesia (allodynia), most frequently occurring in the L1 dermatomal area, may be due to genitofemoral nerve damage from a neurolytic agent, but it may also result from a postsympathectomy denervation hyperesthesia. This occurs more frequently in younger patients having surgical sympathectomy for hyperhidrosis than with phenol sympathetic blocks. This neuropathic-type pain persists after cervicodorsal and lumbar surgical sympathectomy (also radiofrequency ablation) in 10–15% of patients.[3] Hyperesthetic burning discomfort in the groin and anterolateral part of the thigh may also persist for 2–5 weeks after phenol sympathetic blocks.[10]

INTRAVENOUS REGIONAL SYMPATHETIC BLOCK

A technique that provides a simple and efficient means of producing long-term sympathetic blockade was described by Hannington-Kiff using guanethidine (Ismeline) in an

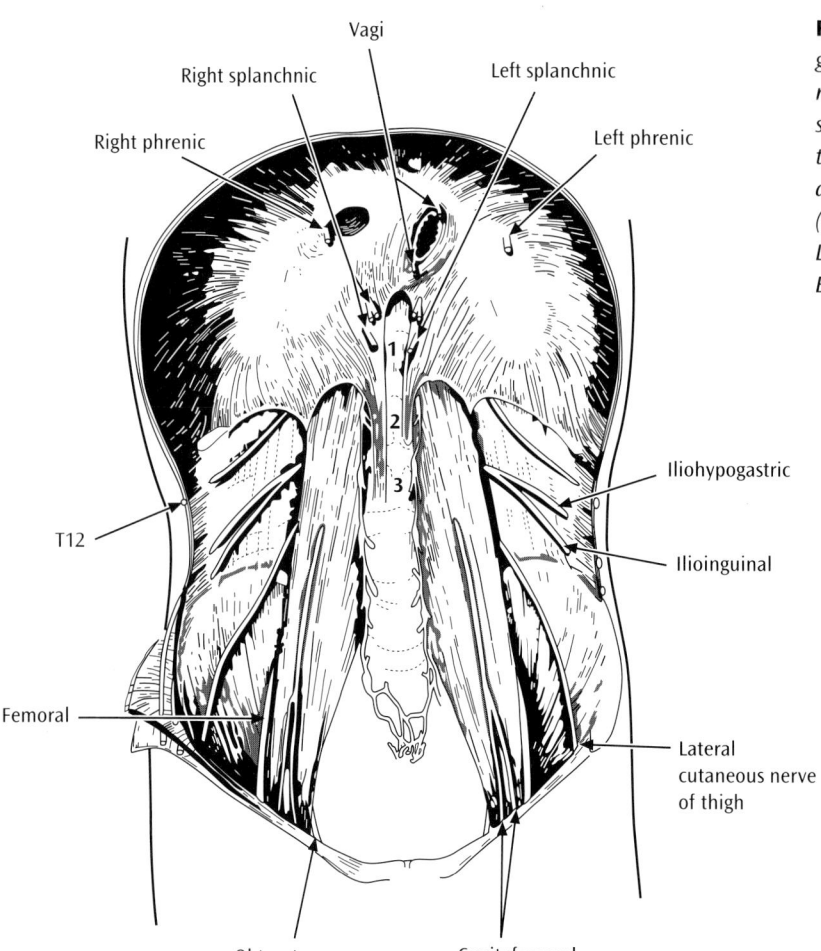

Vagi
Right splanchnic
Left splanchnic
Right phrenic
Left phrenic
Iliohypogastric
T12
Ilioinguinal
Femoral
Lateral
cutaneous nerve
of thigh
Obturator
Genitofemoral

Figure 18.8 *Illustration of position of genitofemoral nerve making spread of neurolytic solutions from a posterior sympathetic ganglion blockade to this nerve possible, causing neuritis and neuropathic pain (see text). (Reproduced with permission of Lippincott Williams & Wilkins© from Breivik et al.[1])*

intravenous regional sympathetic functional block.[11] Its value has been reconfirmed by several pain clinicians and clinical neurophysiologists.***[1,2,6,12–16]

Unfortunately, a "randomized controlled trial" with three major flaws has been influential in weakening the reputation and widespread use of this valuable technique.[17] That study included a group of patients with "reflex sympathetic dystrophy" without documented sympathetically maintained pain. In such a group of pain patients, any positive effect of sympathetic blockade will disappear among confounding factors.

The second flaw in such studies has been diluting the guanethidine with a local anesthetic solution. The local anesthetic inhibits the release of norepinephrine (noradrenaline) from the sympathetic nerve endings. The sympathetic functional blocking effect of guanethidine occurs as a result of inhibition of reuptake of released norepinephrine back into the sympathetic nerve endings (Fig. 18.3). The presence of a local anesthetic will therefore prevent the effect of guanethidine from occurring.

Even a third flaw is possible in studies dissolving the guanethidine in a local anesthetic solution. The systemic effects of lidocaine (and other sodium channel-blocking local anesthetic drugs) on neuropathic pain are well documented. When guanethidine dissolved in a lido-

caine solution was compared with a "placebo" (i.e. lidocaine solution i.v.), this placebo-controlled treatment was shown to be an active and effective therapy for neuropathic pain in about one-third of patients. No wonder there has been no demonstrable difference between guanethidine in lidocaine and lidocaine alone.

Unfortunately, such flawed publications seem to have led to the unavailability of guanethidine for sympathetic blocks in some countries. Fortunately, it is still available in western Europe. Alternatives to guanethidine for i.v. regional sympathetic blocks (e.g. bretyllium, phentolamine) do not result in prolonged functional sympathetic blockades.

Duration of guanethidine sympathetic functional block

Compared with stellate ganglion block with lidocaine, which results in vasodilatation lasting for about 1h, a regional intravenous sympathetic block with guanethidine increases the temperature of the cold extremity for as long as 3 days after block.[14]

Arnér showed that intravenous phentolamine predicts the long-term effect of regional intravenous sympathetic block with guanethidine.*[2] Olsson *et al.* documented the excellent, often curative, clinical effect on complex regional pain syndrome in adolescents.*[15]

Regional intravenous sympathetic block with guanethidine

This is less stressful than the alternative techniques, which are more invasive and carry more risks. There is no contraindication to this technique in the presence of anticoagulation or bleeding disorders.

The technique should therefore still be available as it remains a valuable alternative in pain clinics treating patients with complex regional pain syndromes, where sympathetically maintained pain is a significant component of many patients' suffering.[16]

Technique of regional intravenous block

- Normal saline should be used to dilute 10 mg of guanethidine (10 mg for the first block, up to 30 mg for repeat blocks).
- About 25 ml of normal saline is used for the upper limb and about 40 ml for the lower limb.
- An intravenous cannula is placed in the affected limb, as close to the painful area as possible.
- A second cannula is placed in a vein on a nonaffected limb for analgesia and sedation if needed during the procedure.
- It is important not to use a local anesthetic to dilute the guanethidine (see above).
- A wide cuff of appropriate size is placed around the upper arm or thigh, the extremity lifted to drain as much venous and capillary blood as possible.
- The cuff is then inflated to about 50 mm above systolic blood pressure.
- The diluted guanethidine is injected intravenously in the affected limb and the cuff is maintained inflated for a minimum of 20 min.
- It is often necessary to give the patient intravenous opioid with rapid onset (e.g. alfentanil), in titrated doses to make the patient comfortable during the procedure.
- When the blood pressure cuff is released and circulation reestablished in the treated extremity, norepinephrine released from sympathetic nerve endings by guanethidine will flood into the systemic circulation.
  - This creates a transient increase in blood pressure and heart rate.
  - During the block procedure, soon after injection of the guanethidine solution, the patient's sympathetically maintained painful sensation will often increase because of the same mechanism of norepinephrine release.

- This should be treated with intravenous rapidly acting opioid rather than injecting a local anesthetic with the guanethidine, which will prevent the beneficial effect of the guanethidine (see above).

Adverse effects

- Some patients will have a stuffy nose due to the systemic distribution of guanethidine after release of the cuff.
- Occasionally, some orthostatic hypotension occurs during the first 1–2 days after an intravenous regional sympathetic guanethidine block. Patients should be warned to take proper precautions.
- Patients with paroxysmal cardiac arrhythmias may occasionally have an attack of cardiac arrhythmia precipitated by the guanethidine.

REFERENCES

1. Breivik H, Cousins MJ, Löfström JB. Sympathetic neural blockade of upper and lower extremity. In: Cousins MJ, Bridenbaugh PO eds. *Neural Blockade in Clinical Anesthesia and Management of Pain*, 3rd edn. Philadelphia, PA: Lippincott-Raven Publishers, 1998: 411–45.
2. Arnér S. Intravenous phentolamine test: diagnostic and prognostic use in reflex sympathetic dystrophy. *Pain* 1991; **46:** 17–22.
3. Furlan AD, Mailis A, Papagapiou M. Are we paying a high price for surgical sympathectomy? A systematic literature review of late complications. *J Pain* 2000; **1:** 245–57.
4. Jänig W, Stanton-Hicks M eds. *Reflex Sympathetic Dystrophy: A Reappraisal. Progress in Pain Research and Management.* Seattle, WA: IASP Press, 1996: 1–249.
5. Cousins MJ, Walker S. Chronic pain: management strategies that work. *Anesth Analg* 2001; **92** (Suppl.): 15–25.
6. Wahren LK, Gordh T, Torebjörk E. Effects of regional intravenous guanethidine in patients with neuralgia in the hand; a follow-up study over a decade. *Pain* 1995; **62:** 379–85.
7. Tenicela R, Lovasik D, Eaglstein W. Treatment of herpes zoster with sympathetic blocks. *Clin J Pain* 1985; **1:** 63–7.
8. Walker SM, Cousins MJ. Complex regional pain syndromes: including "reflex sympathetic dystrophy" and "causalgia." *Anaesth Intensive Care* 1997; **25:** 113–16.
9. Hatangdi VS, Boas RV. Lumbar sympathectomy: a single needle technique. *Br J Anaesth* 1985; **57:** 285–90.
10. Cousins MJ, Reeve TS, Glynn CH, *et al.* Neurolytic lumbar sympathetic blockade: duration of denervation and relief of rest pain. *Anaesth Intensive Care* 1979; **7:** 121–5.

◆ 11. Hannington-Kiff JG. *Pain Relief*. London: Heinemann Press, 1974: 68.

◆ 12. Holland AJC, Davies KH, Wallace DH. Sympathetic blockade of isolated limbs by intravenous guanethedine. *Can Anaesth Soc J* 1977; **24:** 597–602.

◆ 13. McKain CW, Bruno JU, Goldner JL. The effects of intravenous regional guanethedine and reserpine. *J Bone Joint Surg* 1983; **6:** 808–15.

◆ 14. Bonelli S, Conoscente F, Movilia PG, *et al*. Regional intravenous guanethedine vs. stellate ganglion block in reflex sympathetic dystrophies: a randomized trial. *Pain* 1983; **16:** 297–305.

◆ 15. Olsson GL, Arnér S, Hirsch G. Reflex sympathetic dystrophy in children. In: Tyler DC, Krane EL eds. *Advances in Pain Research and Therapy*. New York, NY: Raven Press, 1990: 323–31.

● 16. Breivik H. Chronic pain and the sympathetic nervous system. *Acta Anaesthesiol Scand* 1997; **41:** 131–4.

17. Kaplan R, Claudio M, Kepes E, Gu XF. Intravenous guanethidine in patients with reflex sympathetic dystrophy. *Acta Anaesthesiol Scand* 1996; **40:** 1216–22.

19

Neurolytic blocks

ÉTIENNE DE MÉDICIS AND OSCAR A DE LEON-CASASOLA

Interpleural phenol blocks	247	Ganglion impar block	252
Celiac plexus block	248	Conclusions	253
Superior hypogastric plexus block	251	References	253

Pain associated with cancer may be somatic, visceral, and neuropathic in origin, and about 50% of all cancer patients have a combination of pain types at the time of diagnosis. When visceral structures are stretched, compressed, invaded, or distended, a poorly localized noxious pain is reported. Patients experiencing visceral pain often describe the pain as vague, deep, squeezing, crampy, or colicky in nature. Other signs and symptoms include referred pain, such as shoulder pain that appears when the diaphragm is invaded with tumor, and nausea/vomiting.

Visceral pain associated with cancer may be relieved with oral pharmacological therapy that includes combinations of nonsteroidal anti-inflammatory agents, opioids, and coadjuvant therapy. Neurolytic blocks of the sympathetic axis are also extremely effective in controlling visceral cancer pain. Thus, neurolysis of the sympathetic axis should be judged as an important adjunct to pharmacological therapy for the relief of severe pain experienced by cancer patients. As such, these blocks can rarely eliminate cancer pain because patients frequently experience coexisting somatic and neuropathic pain as well. Thus, oral pharmacological therapy must be continued, albeit at lower doses. The goal of performing a neurolytic block of the sympathetic axis is to (1) maximize the analgesic effect of opioid or nonopioid analgesics and (2) reduce the dosage of these agents to alleviate untoward side-effects.

Neurolysis techniques have a narrow risk–benefit ratio. Thus, sound clinical judgment and complete patient understanding are essential to minimize undesirable effects. The detailed description of the techniques for these blocks is beyond the scope of this chapter. Thus, the reader is directed to other publications for this purpose.[1]

INTERPLEURAL PHENOL BLOCKS

The role of interpleural analgesia (IPA) in both acute and chronic pain management is still undergoing clinical scrutiny. Original work with this technique showed that IPA could provide analgesia in patients with subcostal incisions and fractured ribs.[2,3]

The technique for insertion of an interpleural catheter is relatively easy, and an epidural tray can be utilized. Local anesthetics [0.5% bupivacaine or 2% lidocaine (lignocaine)] have been traditionally utilized via intermittent bolus or a continuous infusion. Recently, interpleural phenol[4] has been described as an alternative for the treatment of visceral pain associated with esophageal cancer. Unpublished data suggest that this is an effective technique to treat visceral pain associated with cancer of the esophagus, liver, biliary tree, stomach, and pancreas. A multicenter study is under way to determine the efficacy of this block in the treatment of pain associated with the above-mentioned malignancies (H Silva, R Plancarte, and OA de Leon-Casasola, personal communication).

Drugs and dosing

For neurolytic blocks, the utilization of increasing concentrations of phenol is recommended. Since patients with cancer of the esophagus or the chest wall frequently exhibit pleural effusions, several injections through a catheter are indicated. Initially, 10 ml of 6% phenol is recommended, and a progressive increase up to 10% according to the results is encouraged because the pleural effusion acts as a diluting agent. However, experience with patients with pleural effusions suggests that administration of 5–10 ml of 6% phenol will render adequate results (H Silva, R Plancarte, and OA de Leon-Casasola, personal communication).

For analgesia associated with cancer, a continuous infusion of 0.25–0.375% bupivacaine (8–10 ml/h) or intermittent bolus doses of 0.5% bupivacaine (10–15 ml every 8 h) also provide adequate analgesia. However, if the higher concentration of bupivacaine is chosen, the risk of toxicity is greater. Thus, the use of 0.375–0.5% ropivacaine as a continuous infusion, or 0.5% ropivacaine 10–15 ml every 8 h, would be a better choice in these patients.

Technique

The key to a successful analgesic response is proper positioning of the patient. For all blocks except multiple intercostal rib blocks sparing the thoracic sympathetic chain, the patient should be positioned with the affected side upward. Since the block works by mass action, delivery of the agent is by gravity to thoracic spinal nerves emanating from the paravertebral area. The patient is turned to an oblique position, with the side to be blocked uppermost. The operator stands to face the patient's back. The head may be placed up or down 20° depending on the area to be blocked in order to facilitate the spread of the injectate by gravity. For upper abdominal visceral pain, and sympathetic block for pain originating from the upper abdomen, the patient can be placed in a sitting position and the block performed on the left side for pancreas, stomach, and spleen pain and on the right side for liver pain.

Once the patient is positioned properly and supported by a pillow, a skin wheal is raised immediately superiorly to the eighth rib in the seventh intercostal space, approximately 10 cm lateral to the midline. If a continuous technique is selected, a needle allowing passage of a catheter (often epidural) is selected. If a single injection technique is used, then a short, beveled needle of sufficient length is used. Before inserting the needle, a syringe containing approximately 2 ml of saline is inserted immediately superiorly to the eighth rib, using a passive loss-of-resistance technique. When the needle tip is in the pleural space, injection will be easy. If a catheter is used, it should be threaded approximately 10 cm into the pleural space, taking care to reduce air trapped in the needle.

Complications

Complications from this procedure can be divided into two categories: traumatic injuries produced by either the needle or the catheter and those produced if the neurolytic agent is injected into the interpleural space. Thus, pneumothorax may occur in 2% of patients,[5] and lung injury when a rigid catheter is utilized has been reported.[5] Phrenic nerve palsy resulting in respiratory failure may also occur following this block. Thus, bilateral blocks should be avoided.

Systemic effects from drug absorption may also occur since the pleural membranes are highly vascularized. Thus, the doses of phenol should be limited to 10 ml of a 10% solution.

Efficacy

There is no outcome information to determine the efficacy of this block for the treatment of visceral pain. The published literature on this block is limited to a case report; the effects in a large population have not been reported.

CELIAC PLEXUS BLOCK

The celiac plexus is situated retroperitoneally in the upper abdomen. It is at the level of the T12 and L1 vertebrae, anterior to the crura of the diaphragm. It surrounds the abdominal aorta and the celiac and superior mesenteric arteries.

The plexus is composed of a network of nerve fibers, from both the sympathetic and parasympathetic systems. It contains two large ganglia, which receive sympathetic fibers from the three splanchnic nerves (greater, lesser, and least). The plexus also receives parasympathetic fibers from the vagus nerve.

Autonomic supply to the liver, pancreas, gallbladder, stomach, spleen, kidneys, intestines, and adrenal glands, as well as to the blood vessels, arises in the celiac plexus.

Indications

Neurolytic blocks of the celiac plexus have been used for malignant and chronic nonmalignant pain. In patients with acute or chronic pancreatitis, they have been used with significant success.[6] Likewise, patients with cancer in the upper abdomen who have a significant visceral pain component have responded well to this block.[7]**

Technique

There are three approaches to block nociceptive impulses from the viscera of the upper abdomen. These approaches are the retrocrural or classic approach, the anterocrural approach, and neurolysis of the splanchnic nerves. With all these approaches, the needles are inserted at the level of the first lumbar vertebra, 5–7 cm from the midline. Then, the tip of the needle is directed toward the body of L1 for the retrocrural and anterocrural approaches and to the body of T12 for neurolysis of the splanchnic nerves.

Figures 19.1–19.3 illustrate the final position of the needles and the expected spread of contrast medium after successful placement. More recently, computed tomography and ultrasound techniques have allowed pain specialists to perform neurolysis of the celiac plexus via a transabdominal approach. This approach is frequently used when patients are not able to tolerate either the prone or lateral decubitus position, or when the liver is so enlarged that a posterior approach is not feasible.

Drugs and dosing

For neurolytic blocks, 50–100% alcohol, 20 ml per side, is utilized. Injected by itself, alcohol can produce severe pain. Thus, it is recommended to first inject 5–10 ml of 0.25% bupivacaine 5 min before injection of alcohol, or to dilute 100% alcohol by 50% with local anesthetic (0.25% bupivacaine). Phenol in a 10% final concentration may also be used and has the advantage of being painless on injection. Both agents appear to have the same efficacy.

Complications

Complications associated with celiac plexus blocks appear to be related to the technique used – retrocrural, transcrural,[8,9] or transaortic.[10] In a prospective, randomized study of 61 patients with cancer of the pancreas, Ischia et al.[7]** compared the efficacy and the incidence of complications associated with three different approaches with celiac plexus neurolysis. Orthostatic hypotension was more frequent in patients who had a retrocrural (50%) or splanchnic nerve block technique (52%) than those who underwent an anterocrural approach (10%).

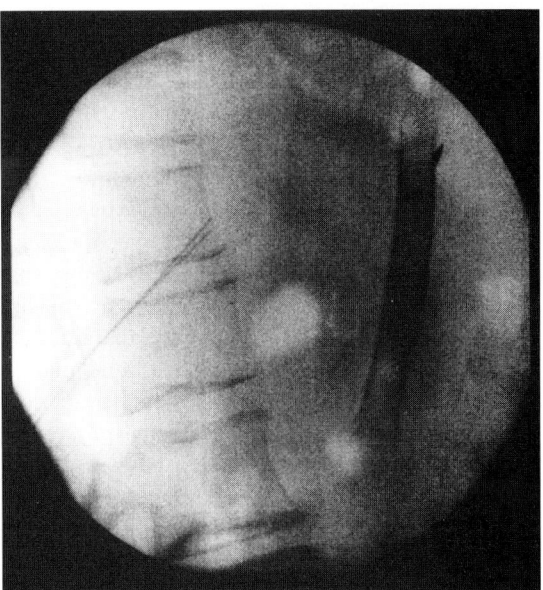

Figure 19.2 *Lateral view demonstrating correct needle positioning for splanchnic nerve blocks.*

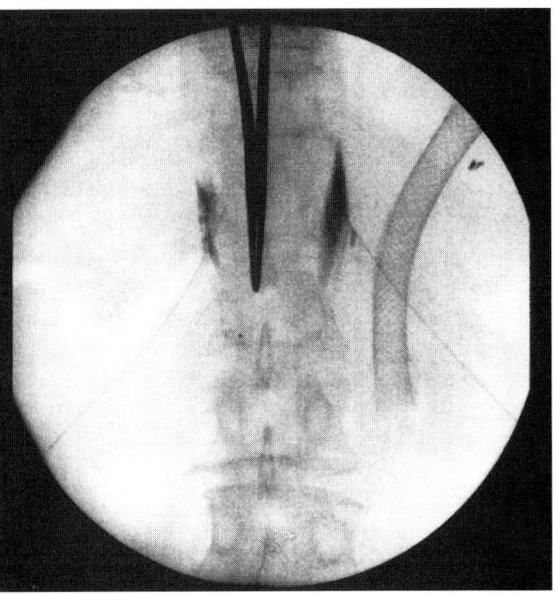

Figure 19.3 *AP view demonstrating correct needle positioning and contrast medium spread for splanchnic nerve blocks.*

In contrast, transient diarrhea was more frequent in patients who had an anterocrural approach (65%) than in those having a splanchnic nerve block technique (5%), but not the retrocrural approach (25%). The incidence of dysesthesiae, interscapular back pain, reactive pleurisy, hiccupping, or hematuria was not statistically different among the three groups.

The incidence of complications from neurolytic celiac plexus blocks was recently determined by Davis[11] in 2,730 patients having blocks performed from 1986 to 1990. The overall incidence of major complications, such as paraplegia and bladder and bowel dysfunction, was 1 in 683

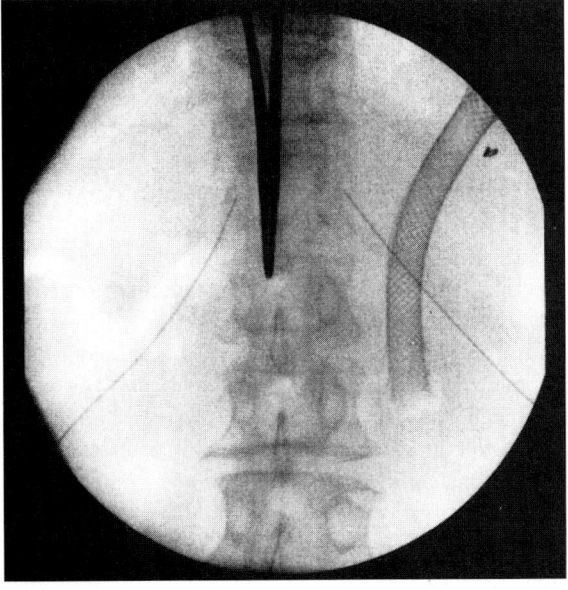

Figure 19.1 *AP view demonstrating correct needle positioning for splanchnic nerve blocks.*

procedures. However, the report does not describe which approach or approaches were utilized for the performance of the blocks.

Important aspects in the diagnosis and management of specific complications include:

1 Malposition of the needle should always be ruled out with radiologic imaging prior to the injection of a neurolytic agent, as the needle's tip may be intravascular, in the peritoneal cavity, or in a viscus. Imaging techniques currently used include biplanar fluoroscopy, computed tomography, or ultrasound guidance. However, no study has evaluated the superiority of one technique over the others. Wong and Brown[12] suggested that the use of radiologic imaging does not alter the quality of the block or the incidence of complications, based on a retrospective study of 136 patients with pancreatic cancer pain treated with a celiac plexus block with or without radiological control of the position of the needle's tip. However, it is not clear how many of those patients had radiologic imaging. Assuming that half of the patients did not, the upper 95% confidence limit for complications is 5%.[13]

2 Orthostatic hypotension may occur after the block in 1–3% of the patients for up to 5 days. Treatment includes bed rest, avoidance of sudden changes in position, and fluid replacement. Once compensatory vascular reflexes are fully activated, this side-effect disappears. Wrapping of the lower extremities from the toe to the upper thighs with elastic bandages has been used with success in patients who developed orthostatic hypotension and needed to ambulate during the first week after the block.

3 Backache may result from:
   a local trauma during the needle placement resulting in a retroperitoneal hematoma;
   b alcohol irritation of the retroperitoneal structures;
   c injury to the lumbar plexus.

   Patients with a backache should have at least two hematocrit measurements at 1-h intervals. If there is a decrease in the hematocrit, radiologic imaging is indicated to rule out a retroperitoneal hematoma. A urine analysis positive for red blood cells suggests renal injury.

4 Retroperitoneal hemorrhage is rare, but has also been reported. Thus, in patients who present with orthostatic hypotension, one must rule out hemorrhage before assuming that it is a physiologic response to the block. Patients who present with backache and orthostatic hypotension after a celiac plexus block should be admitted to the hospital for serial hematocrit monitoring. If a low or a decreasing hematocrit is demonstrated, patients should undergo radiological evaluation to rule out injury to the kidneys, the aorta, or other vascular structures. A surgical consult should be obtained as soon as feasible.

5 Diarrhea may occur as a result of the sympathetic block of the bowel. Treatment includes hydration and antidiarrheal agents. Oral loperamide is a good choice, although any anticholinergic may be used. Matson et al.[14] reported near-fatal dehydration from diarrhea after this block. Thus, in debilitated patients, it must be treated aggressively.

6 Abdominal aortic dissection has also been reported.[15,16] The mechanisms of aortic injury are direct damage with the needle during the performance of the block. As expected, the anterocrural approach is more frequently associated with this complication. Thus, if there is evidence of atherosclerotic disease of the abdominal aorta, it would seem appropriate to avoid this approach.

7 Paraplegia and transient motor paralysis has occurred after celiac plexus block.[17–22] Current thinking is that these neurologic complications may occur because of a spasm of the lumbar segmental arteries that perfuse the spinal cord.[23] In fact, canine lumbar arteries undergo contraction when exposed to low concentrations of alcohol.[24**] Thus, it is empirically suggested that if there is evidence of significant atherosclerotic disease of the aorta, suggesting that the circulation to the spinal cord may also be impaired, alcohol should not be used. However, there is also a report of paraplegia after phenol use,[25] suggesting that other factors such as direct vascular or neurologic injury, or retrograde spread to the spinal cord, may come into play. These complications further support the use of radiologic imaging during the performance of the block.

Efficacy

There are only two randomized controlled trials[7**,26] and one prospective study[27] evaluating the efficacy of celiac plexus neurolysis in pain due to cancer of the upper abdomen. One of the studies evaluated the efficacy of three different approaches to celiac plexus neurolysis in pancreatic cancer in a prospective, randomized fashion.[8] In this study, 48% (29/61 patients) experienced *complete* pain relief after the neurolytic block. The remaining patients [32 (52%)] required further therapy for residual visceral pain owing to technical failure in 15 patients (20%) or neuropathic/somatic pains in 17 patients (28%). The other study[26] compared the procedure with oral pharmacological therapy in 20 patients. The author concluded that celiac plexus neurolysis resulted in the same reduction in visual analog pain scores as therapy with a nonsteroidal anti-inflammatory drug (NSAID)–opioid combination. However, opioid consumption was significantly lower in the group of patients who underwent neurolysis than in the group receiving oral pharmacological therapy during the 7 weeks of the study. Moreover, the incidence of side-effects was greater in the group of patients receiving oral pharmacological therapy than in those in the block group.

In the other prospective, nonrandomized study,[27] 41 patients treated according to the World Health Organization (WHO) guidelines for cancer pain relief were compared with 21 patients treated with a neurolytic celiac plexus block. The authors concluded that this technique can play an important role in the management of pancreatic cancer pain.

Since one of the two studies that used a randomized controlled design compared different approaches to the celiac plexus and had no control group,[7**] and the other compared the procedure with an analgesic drug,[26] it is not possible to estimate the success rate of this technique. In contrast, the results of a meta-analysis that evaluated the results of 21 *retrospective* studies in 1,145 patients concluded that adequate to excellent pain relief was achieved in 89% of the patients during the first 2 weeks after the block.[28***] Partial to complete pain relief continued in approximately 90% of the patients that were alive at the 3-month follow-up, and in 70–90% of the patients during the time period between the 3-month follow-up to death. Moreover, the efficacy was similar in patients with pancreatic cancer to those with other intra-abdominal malignancies of the upper abdomen. However, it is important to recognize that these results are based on *retrospective* evaluations, which may not yield reliable information or may be subject to publication bias. In addition, statistical techniques used for the analysis must account for the heterogeneity produced by the patient's selection criteria, technical differences in the performance of the blocks, choice of neurolytic agents and doses, diversity in the tools for the evaluation of pain, goals of therapy, etc. Thus, the meta-analysis must be interpreted with caution as the results may be overly enthusiastic.

New perspectives

As previously discussed, oral pharmacological therapy with opioids, nonsteroidal anti-inflammatory agents, and coadjuvants is frequently used for the treatment of cancer pain. However, there is evidence to suggest that chronic use of high doses of opioids may have a negative effect on immunity.[29] Thus, analgesic techniques that lower opioid consumption should have positive effects on patient outcomes. Lillimoe *et al.*[30] showed in a prospective, randomized trial that patients with nonresectable cancer of the pancreas receiving a splanchnic neurolysis had a longer survival than patients who did not. These findings may be the result of lower opioid use in the group of patients randomized to neurolysis, resulting in (1) a better preserved immune function and (2) a reduced incidence of side-effects such as nausea and vomiting, which allows patients to eat better. This hypothesis is currently being tested in a prospective, randomized trial.

SUPERIOR HYPOGASTRIC PLEXUS BLOCK

Cancer patients with tumor extension into the pelvis may experience severe pain unresponsive to oral or parenteral opioids. Moreover, some patients may complain of excessive sedation or other side-effects which limit the acceptability and usefulness of oral opioid therapy. Thus, a more invasive approach may be needed to control pain and improve their quality of life.

Pelvic pain associated with cancer and chronic nonmalignant conditions may be alleviated by blocking the superior hypogastric plexus.[31-34] Analgesia to the organs in the pelvis is possible because the afferent fibers innervating these structures travel with the sympathetic nerves, trunks, ganglia, and rami and are accessible for neurolytic blocks. Thus, a sympathectomy for visceral pain is analogous to a peripheral neurectomy or dorsal rhizotomy for somatic pain. A recent study has suggested that, even in advanced stages, visceral pain is an important component of the cancer pain syndrome experienced by patients with cancer of the pelvis.[32**] Thus, it appears that percutaneous neurolytic blocks of the superior hypogastric plexus should be offered more frequently to patients with advanced stages of pelvic cancer.

The superior hypogastric plexus is situated in the retroperitoneum, bilaterally extending from the lower third of the fifth lumbar vertebral body to the upper third of the first sacral vertebral body. The technique for the blockade has been described elsewhere.[31,32**,33**]

Technique

Patients are placed in the prone position with a pillow under the pelvis to flatten the lumbar lordosis. Plancarte *et al.*[31] preceded some of their blocks with a "single-shot" L4–5 epidural injection of 8–10 ml of 1% lidocaine to enhance patient cooperation, reduce reflex muscle spasm, and ameliorate discomfort. Alternatively, local infiltration of the intervening muscle planes can be performed. Needle insertion sites are 5–7 cm lateral to the midline, depending on patient's height and girth, at the level of the L4-L5 interspace. Two 17.5- to 22.5-cm (7–9 inch), 22-gauge, short, beveled needles (Chiba type) are inserted with the bevel directed medially 45° mesiad and 30° caudad so that the tips lay anterolateral to the L5–S1 intervertebral space. Aspiration is important to avoid injection into the iliac vessels. If blood is aspirated, a transvascular approach can be used.

Biplanar fluoroscopy is used to verify accurate needle placement. Anterior–posterior (AP) views should reveal the tip of the needle at the level of the junction of the L5 and S1 vertebral bodies. Lateral views will confirm placement of the needle tip just beyond the vertebral body's anterolateral margin. The injection of 2–3 ml of water-soluble contrast medium is used to verify accurate needle placement and to rule out intravascular injection. In the AP view, the spread of contrast should be confined to the midline region. In the lateral view, a smooth posterior contour corresponding to the anterior psoas fascia indicates that the needle is at the appropriate depth. Figures 19.4 and 19.5 show adequate needle placement and contrast medium spread prior to neurolysis of the superior hypogastric plexus.

For a prognostic hypogastric plexus blockade, a volume of 6–8 ml of 0.25% bupivacaine through each needle is recommended. For therapeutic purposes, a total of 6–8 ml of 10% aqueous phenol through each needle can be injected.

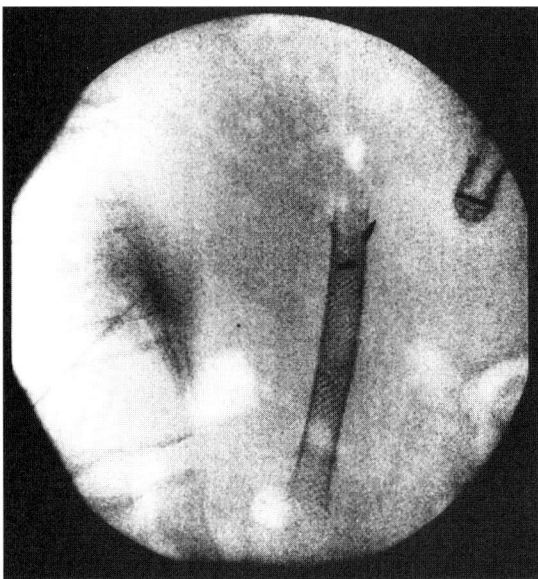

Figure 19.4 *Lateral view demonstrating correct needle positioning and contrast medium spread for splanchnic nerve blocks.*

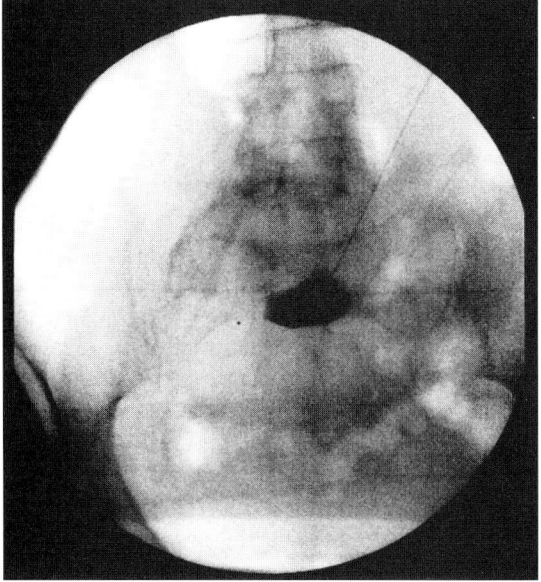

Figure 19.5 *AP view demonstrating correct needle positioning and contrast medium spread for superior hypogastric plexus block.*

Complications

A combined experience of more than 200 cases from the Mexican Institute of Cancer, Roswell Park Cancer Institute, and M.D. Anderson Cancer Center has failed to detect neurologic complications associated with this block.[33]**

Efficacy

The effectiveness of the block was originally demonstrated by documenting a significant decrease in pain scores via a visual analog pain scale (VAS).[31] In this study, Plancarte *et al.* showed that this block was effective in reducing VAS scores in 70% of the patients with pelvic pain associated with cancer.[31] The great majority of the patients enrolled had a diagnosis of cervical cancer. In a subsequent study, 69% of the patients experienced a decrease in VAS scores. Moreover, a mean daily opioid morphine reduction of 67% was seen in the success group (736 ± 633 to 251 ± 191 mg/day), and 45% in the failure group (1,443 ± 703 to 800 ± 345 mg/day).[32] In a more recent multicentric study, 159 patients with pelvic pain associated with cancer were evaluated. Overall, 115 patients (72%) had satisfactory pain relief after one or two neurolytic procedures. Mean opioid use decreased by 40% from 58 ± 43 to 35 ± 18 equianalgesic mg/day of morphine, 3 weeks after treatment, in all the studied patients. This decrease in opioid consumption was significant for both the success group (56 ± 32 to 32 ± 16 mg/day) and the failure group (65 ± 28 to 48 ± 21 mg/day).[33] Success was defined in these two studies as the ability to reduce opioid consumption by at least 50% in the 3 weeks following the block and a decrease in the pain scores below 4/10 on the visual analog pain scale.[32,33]

In a recent case report, Rosenberg *et al.*[34] reported on the efficacy of this block in a patient with severe chronic nonmalignant penile pain after transurethral resection of the prostate. Although the patient did not receive a neurolytic agent, a diagnostic block performed with 0.25% bupivacaine and 20 mg of methylprednisolone acetate was effective in relieving the pain for more than 6 months. The usefulness of this block in chronic benign pain conditions has not been adequately documented.

GANGLION IMPAR BLOCK

The ganglion impar is a solitary retroperitoneal structure located at the level of the sacrococcygeal junction. This ganglion marks the end of the two sympathetic chains.

Visceral pain in the perineal area associated with malignancies may be effectively treated with neurolysis of the ganglion impar (Walther's).[35,36] Patients who will benefit from this blockade will frequently present with vague and poorly localized pain which is burning in character and frequently accompanied by sensations of burning and urgency. However, the clinical value of this block is not clear as the published experienced is limited (three case series).

Technique

This block may be performed with the patient in the left lateral decubitus position with the knees flexed, the lithotomy position, or in the prone position. The easiest approach is with the patient in the prone position, where a 20-G, 3.8-cm (1.5 inch) needle is inserted through the sacrococcygeal ligament in the midline. The needle is then advanced until the tip is placed posterior to the rectum. Figure 19.6 illustrates adequate needle placement and contrast medium spread.

Complications

No complications have been reported with this block.

CONCLUSIONS

Neurolysis of the sympathetic axis is a safe and cost-effective way to treat visceral pain associated with cancer. The benefits are improved analgesia and a decrease in opioid consumption. These factors may have not only economic implications but also important clinical effects owing to the effects of high doses of chronic opioid therapy in the immune and gastrointestinal systems. Current knowledge and techniques to perform these blocks allow patients to undergo these procedures in a safe and expeditious manner. Thus, pain practitioners should consider

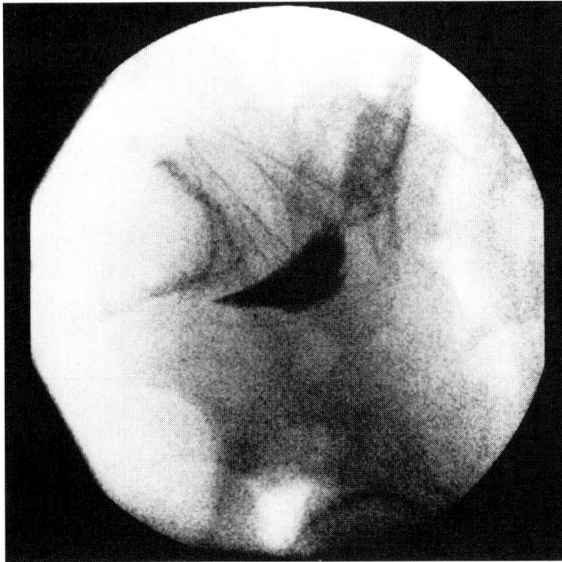

Figure 19.6 *Lateral view demonstrating correct needle positioning and contrast medium spread for superior hypogastric plexus block.*

them as adjuvant therapy for the successful treatment of cancer pain.

REFERENCES

1. Regional anesthetic techniques for the management of cancer pain. In: *Techniques in Regional Anesthesia and Pain Management*, vol. 1. Urmey WF ed. Philadelphia, PA: W. B. Saunders, 1997.
2. Reiestad FL, Stromskag KE. Interpleural catheter in the management of postoperative pain. A preliminary report. *Reg Anesth* 1986; **11:** 89.
3. Rocco A, Reiestand F, Gudman J, *et al.* Intrapleural administration of local anesthetics for pain relief in patients with multiple rib fractures. Preliminary report. *Reg Anesth* 1987; **12:** 10–14.
4. Lema MJ, Myers DP, de Leon-Casasola OA. Interpleural phenol therapy for the treatment of chronic esophageal cancer pain. *Reg Anesth* 1992; **17:** 166–70.
5. Stromskag KE, Reiestad F, Holmquist EVO, *et al.* Intrapleural administration of 0.25%, 0.375%, and 0.5% bupivacaine with epinephrine after cholecystectomy. *Anesth Analg* 1988; **67:** 430–44.
6. Rykowski JJ, Hilgier M. Continuous celiac plexus block in acute pancreatitis. *Reg Anesth* 1995; **20:** 528–32.
7. Ischia S, Ischia A, Polati E, Finco G. Three posterior percutaneous celiac plexus block techniques: a prospective randomized study in 61 patients with pancreatic cancer pain. *Anesthesiology* 1992; **76:** 534–40.
8. Singer RC. An improved technique for alcohol neurolysis of the celiac plexus block. *Anesthesiology* 1982; **56:** 137–41.
9. Hilgier M, Rykowski JJ. One needle transcrural celiac plexus block: single shot, or continuous technique, or both. *Reg Anesth* 1994; **19:** 277–83.
10. Ischia S, Luzzani A, Ischia A, Faggion S. A new approach to the neurolytic block for coeliac plexus: the transaortic technique. *Pain* 1983; **16:** 333–41.
11. Davis DD. Incidence of major complications of neurolytic coeliac plexus block. *J R Soc Med* 1993; **86:** 264–6.
12. Womg GY, Brown Dl. Celiac plexus block for cancer pain. *Techniques Reg Anesth Pain Manage* 1997; **1:** 18–26.
13. Hanley JA, Lippman-Hand A. If nothing goes wrong, is everything all right. *JAMA* 1983; **249:** 1743–5.
14. Matson JA, Ghia JN, Levy JH. A case report of a potentially fatal complications associated with Ischia's transaortic method of celiac plexus block. *Reg Anesth* 1985; **10:** 193–6.
15. Sett SS, Taylor DC. Aortic pseudoaneurysm secondary to celiac plexus block. *Ann Vasc Surg* 1991; **5:** 88–91.
16. Kaplan R, Schiff-Keren B, Alt E. Aortic dissection as a complication of celiac plexus block. *Anesthesiology* 1995; **83:** 632–5.

17. Galizia EJ, Lahiri SK. Paraplegia following coeliac plexus block with phenol. *Br J Anaesth* 1974; **46:** 539–40.

18. Lo JN, Buckley JJ. Spinal cord ischemia a complication of celiac plexus block. *Reg Anesth* 1982; **7:** 66–8.

19. Cherry DA, Lamberty J. Paraplegia following coeliac plexus block. *Anaesth Intensive Care* 1984; **12:** 59–72.

20. Woodham MJ, Hanna MH. Paraplegia after coeliac plexus block. *Anaesthesia* 1989; **44:** 487–9.

21. Van Dongen RTM, Crul BJP. Paraplegia following coeliac plexus block. *Anaesthesia* 1991; **46:** 862–3.

22. Jabbal SS, Hunton J. Reversible paraplegia following coeliac plexus block. *Anaesthesia* 1992; **47:** 857–8.

23. Wong GY, Brown DL. Transient paraplegia following alcohol celiac plexus block. *Reg Anesth* 1995; **20:** 352–5.

24. Brown DL, Rorie DK. Altered reactivity of isolated segmental lumbar arteries of dogs following exposure to ethanol and phenol. *Pain* 1994; **56:** 139–43.

25. Galizia EJ, Lahiri SK. Paraplegia following coeliac plexus block with phenol. *Br J Anaesth* 1974; **46:** 539–40.

◆ 26. Mercadante S. Celiac plexus block versus analgesics in pancreatic cancer pain. *Pain* 1993; **52:** 187–92.

◆ 27. Ventafridda GV, Caraceni AT, Sbanotto AM, *et al.* Pain treatment in cancer of the pancreas. *Eur J Surg Oncol* 1990; **16:** 1–6.

◆ 28. Eisenberg E, Carr DB, Chalmers TC. Neurolytic celiac plexus block for the treatment of cancer pain: a meta-analysis. *Anesth Analg* 1995; **80:** 290–5.

29. Yeager MP. Morphine inhibits spontaneous and cyto-kine-enhanced natural killer cell cytotoxicity in volunteers. *Anesthesiology* 1995; **83:** 500–8.

30. Lillimoe KD, Cameron JL, Kaufman HS, *et al.* Chemical splanchnicectomy in patients with unresectable pancreatic cancer. *Ann Surg* 1993; **217:** 447–57.

◆ 31. Plancarte R, Amescua C, Patt RB, Aldrete JA. Superior hypogastric plexus block for pelvic cancer pain. *Anesthesiology* 1990; **73:** 236–9.

◆ 32. de Leon-Casasola OA, Kent E, Lema MJ. Neurolytic superior hypogastric plexus block for chronic pelvic pain associated with cancer. *Pain* 1993; **54:** 145–51.

◆ 33. Plancarte R, de Leon-Casasola OA, El-Helealy M, *et al.* Neurolytic superior hypogastric plexus block for chronic pelvic pain associated with cancer. *Reg Anesth* 1997; **22:** 562–8.

34. Rosenberg SK, Tewari R, Boswell MV, *et al.* Superior hypogastric plexus block successfully treats severe penile pain after transurethral resection of the prostate. *Reg Anesth Pain Med* 1998; **23:** 618–20.

◆ 35. Plancarte R, Amescua C, Patt RB. Presacral blockade of the ganglion of Walther (ganglion impar). *Anesthesiology* 1990; **73:** A751.

36. Swofford JB, Ratzman DM. A transarticular approach to blockade of the ganglion impar (ganglion of Walther). *Reg Anesth* 1998; **23** (3S): 203.

20

Intra-articular injections

JOHN ETHERINGTON AND SIMON PAUL

Evidence for effectiveness of joint injection	255	Complications	259
General principles	256	Equipment	259
General technique	257	Drugs	259
Indications	258	Joint injection methods	260
Contraindications	258	References	267

Corticosteroids were first introduced for the treatment of rheumatoid arthritis in 1948. Since that time, they have been widely used in the treatment of inflammatory polyarthropathies, although their optimal systemic use has still to be determined.[1] In an attempt to maximize the therapeutic benefits and minimize the side-effects, Hollander introduced and developed the intra-articular injection of hydrocortisone into the knee joint.[2] Subsequently, his colleague McCarty improved on the technique by using the synthetic triamcinolone hexacetonide in other joints, including the small joints of the hand.

This therapy is now widely used by rheumatologists, orthopedic surgeons, family physicians, and general practitioners. The procedures are inexpensive and appear to be highly effective in the treatment of inflammatory arthropathies and in certain musculoskeletal conditions. However, evidence for their efficacy from randomized control trials and subsequent systematic reviews is limited.

In part, this paucity of evidence is the result of the treatment being established long before the concept of evidence-based medicine. In addition, there are many different techniques used for a heterogeneous group of diseases. Outcome measures in musculoskeletal disease are weak, and arthropathies are prone to spontaneous remission, all of which complicates the assessment of treatment response. The evidence that is available will be discussed.

EVIDENCE FOR EFFECTIVENESS OF JOINT INJECTION

There are very few systematic reviews of the effectiveness of corticosteroid injection – they have been mainly confined to the shoulder, elbow, and knee and they are disappointing in their conclusions.

Two systematic reviews of intra-articular injection of the glenohumeral joint have found no evidence of effect.[3***,4] These reviews identified two randomized, controlled trials (RCTs) that showed no benefit in either pain or range of movement when compared with placebo.[5**,6] One RCT in adhesive capsulitis that compared dosages of triamcinolone (20 mg versus 40 mg) found the higher dose more effective at relieving pain, restriction of movement, and functional impairment. One small RCT in adhesive capsulitis showed a benefit combining steroid injection with hydrodistension of the joint [using 19 ml of 0.5% lidocaine (lignocaine)] when compared with injection alone.[7**] There were only 20 patients in the study, so the results should be interpreted with caution. However, at 12 weeks, there were improvements in the range of motion and in the physician's global assessment, although not in pain. Hydrodistension is not a routine procedure, although it has been used beneficially in other studies.[8*]

Subacromial injection has been subjected to a systematic review[3***] that identified two placebo-controlled RCTs of corticosteroid injection for rotator cuff tendinitis. The first, which had 50 cases, was a study of subacromial injection alone;[9**] the second was a study of subacromial and intra-articular injection (40 cases).[10**] The review concluded that there was evidence of an improved range of abduction of the shoulder at 4 weeks but not of improvement in the pain. An additional RCT with 55 cases, which compared methylprednisolone and lidocaine with lidocaine alone, found no difference in either pain or abduction at 12 weeks.[11**] All these studies are limited by their small size, and the systematic reviews emphasized the lack of uniformity of the studies, poor study methods, and the heterogeneity of study populations and outcome measures.

A systematic review of injection therapy in lateral epicondyle elbow pain identified 12 RCTs, but these were of overall poor to moderate quality.[12]*** There did appear to be a short-term benefit from steroid injection, and the studies of better methodological quality indicated more favorable results. No conclusions could be drawn about the optimal form or dose of corticosteroid, and there were similar findings in an RCT of medial epicondylitis.[13]**

Corticosteroid injection is frequently used in the knee, particularly in rheumatoid arthritis but also in osteoarthritis (OA) where the indications for use are less clear.[14] A systematic review in OA identified 10 RCTs, but found little benefit in terms of pain relief over placebo.[15]*** A subsequent RCT demonstrated only short-term benefit in pain for the corticosteroid injection group.[16]** However, the American College of Rheumatology advocates the "judicious" use of corticosteroid injections, as mono- or combination therapy, in OA of the knee in patients with symptomatic effusions.[17] Although a further RCT showed a positive effect on pain from intra-articular methylprednisolone acetate at 3 weeks compared with both baseline and placebo, no clinical predictors of response could be identified.[18]** This supports the clinical impression that therapy may be effective in certain patients with OA, but identifying the patient group beforehand is often difficult.

Intra-articular injection is predominantly used in the treatment of adult joint disease, but there is evidence of successful use in children.[19,20] Full remission of joint inflammation lasting >6 months following injection was achieved in 82% of injections in children, but in 18% of the injected joints the inflammation recurred within 6 months of injection. Despite concerns for the possible side-effects of growth retardation, there appears to have been a reduction in leg-length discrepancy in those children who received steroid injection for juvenile chronic arthritis.[21]* However, the study was retrospective and involved small numbers. On balance, children should not be excluded from this treatment simply because of their age.[22]

Conclusion

Although clinically the effects of intra-articular injection can appear dramatic, there is a very poor-quality evidence base for its use. Nevertheless, it remains a mainstay of treatment in the inflammatory arthropathies and in many other musculoskeletal conditions. The absence of evidence for its effectiveness is at least balanced by good evidence of its safety, which improves the risk–benefit assessment when contemplating the therapy in an individual patient.

GENERAL PRINCIPLES

This chapter will deal principally with intra-articular injections, but will include some elements of local soft-tissue injection that may be of relevance to the pain specialist.

The aim of therapy is to deliver an anti-inflammatory agent – a corticosteroid – into an area of active inflammation. This is frequently combined with a local anesthetic agent that acts to provide immediate pain relief, confirm accurate placement of the corticosteroid agent, and possibly contribute a secondary pain blockade which may be longer lasting than would be expected from the pharmacological effect of the agent.

The corticosteroid may act in a number of ways to derive a therapeutic response: as a local anti-inflammatory;[23] by suppression of the hypothalamic–pituitary–adrenal axis; by alteration of monocyte and lymphocyte trafficking; and by suppression of the release of tumor necrosis factor α by stimulated peripheral blood monocytes.[24] Clinical response to intra-articular steroid therapy is accompanied by a decreased expression of the genes that play a role in the articular destruction of rheumatoid arthritis, such as those for collagenase, the tissue inhibitor of metalloproteinases, and HLA-DR.[25] There also appear to be effects on surface-active phospholipid in the joint that may contribute to improved joint lubrication[26] and improvements in measures of muscle strength, probably because of a decrease in the reflex muscular inhibition associated with synovitis of a joint.[27]

Effective therapy requires an understanding of:

- Diagnostic techniques.
- Musculoskeletal anatomy.
- The essential need for an aseptic technique.
- The accurate placement of an injection, which may include the use of imaging techniques.
- The contraindications and complications of treatment.
- The need for adequate counseling of the patient.

Injection therapy should usually be part of a program of rehabilitation that might combine education, physiotherapy, occupational therapy, and other pharmacological interventions.

Aseptic technique is essential for the injection, but the procedure does not need to be carried out in an operating room with staff gloved and gowned. There is considerable evidence for the safety of the procedure when carried out in an outpatient department or clinical office.[2*,28–31] The operator needs to clean the skin, use single-use disposable vials, and a no-touch technique. Domestically clean, dry hands are satisfactory; sterile gloves are not required, although it is reasonable to use gloves to protect against spillage of body fluids onto the operator. The incidence of postinjection septic arthritis is extremely small.

Counseling the patient involves explanation of:

- the diagnosis;
- aims of treatment;
- limitations of treatment;
- risks and type of complications;
- advice on postinjection management.

An understanding of the diagnosis on the part of the patient will help to frame patient expectations and modify the rate of return to activity. It may allow identification and avoidance of precipitating factors in the case of overuse injuries. The aims of treatment should be explained in order to avoid raising expectations beyond what can be delivered. A full outline of potential complications should be given, and these are outlined in the key points on complications. They may be delivered to the patient as an information sheet.

Patients should be advised to rest as much as possible postinjection, as long-term efficacy is improved.[32]** In the case of injection adjacent to weight-bearing tendon structures, strenuous physical activity should be avoided for 10–14 days after injection.

GENERAL TECHNIQUE

Each anatomical area has specific techniques for successful injection. These will be covered in sequence, but there are a number of technical principles that can be generalized for all joints.

The general technique is summarized in the key points below.

Key points 1: preparation

- Accurate diagnosis.
- Patient explanation of procedure, including verbal consent.
- Ensure both the patient and the doctor are in a comfortable position before administration of the injection.
- Confirm local anatomy.
- Mark injection spot.
- Clean skin.
- The skin should be cleaned at this stage with alcohol wipes or other appropriate antibacterial agent. Iodine solutions should be avoided because of staining and possible allergic reactions.
- Cleaning the skin at this point allows for the alcohol to evaporate and have its bactericidal effect before the injection.
- Draw up drugs.

Key points 2: carrying out the procedure

- Anesthetize with:
  - ethyl chloride;
  - local anesthetic.

- Insert needle.
- Aspirate.
- Inject:
  - there should be minimal resistance during injection into an intra-articular space.
- Aspirate on withdrawing needle:
  - negative pressure within the syringe draws residual steroid from the needle to avoid contamination of subcutaneous tissues, which reduces the risk of subcutaneous fat atrophy or depigmentation.
- Apply pressure.
- Apply dressing.
- Patient to rest.
- Final advice.

Steroid and local anesthetic may be delivered in a number of combinations, as outlined in Table 20.1.

The authors prefer the first option, corticosteroid and local anesthetic mixed together in the syringe. The use of ethyl chloride spray will successfully anesthetize the skin, there will be immediate confirmation of the successful location of the injection, and there will be only one intracapsular injection, thereby minimizing the risk of infection. A firm and smooth injection technique with good prior ascertainment of surface landmarks will ensure minimal discomfort during this procedure.

Correct placement of the injection is critical to success. In a study by Eustace et al.[33]* of injections into the shoulder of steroid combined with radiographic contrast material, only 37% were judged to be accurately placed: 29% of attempted subacromial injections and 42% of the attempted glenohumeral injections. There were significant differences in relation to outcome between the accurately placed and the inaccurately placed groups. Other techniques used include ultrasound[34] and fluoroscopy.[35] Most injections are still carried out without imaging, probably because of the logistic difficulties of doing otherwise. Methods of determining correct placement are outlined in Table 20.2.

There is limited evidence on the optimum frequency of injection. The key points outlining the advice on administration (Key points 3) contain some general principles that constitute best practice in the area. The interval between injections is set as 4–6 weeks. This is based on the concept that most long-acting steroids will have a similar duration of effect and that reinjection prior to this is unlikely to improve the effectiveness of the treatment. Three injections per joint per year is a compromise between the need to repeatedly inject in some conditions and the possibility of joint damage, although evidence for the latter is limited. As a rule, if a condition does not improve after three injections there should be a review of the diagnosis and management. For example, a joint affected by rheumatoid arthritis that has not responded to injection on three separate occasions would indicate the need to review the patient's systemic antirheumatic therapy or consider surgical intervention such as arthroscopic washout or joint replacement.

Table 20.1 *Methods of delivering corticosteroid into an area of inflammation*

Mode of delivery	Advantages	Disadvantages
Corticosteroid and local anesthetic mixed in same syringe	Single injection Immediate effect May be some amelioration of postinjection flare	No local anesthetic delivered to skin Consider use of ethyl chloride anesthetic spray
Local anesthetic to skin and capsule of joint	Pain-free injection of corticosteroid	Requires two injections
Local anesthetic into joint *Then* corticosteroid	Pain-free injection of cortico-steroid Confirmation of correct injection site – pain-free movement of joint	Two intra-articular injections – doubles risk of infection

Table 20.2 *Confirmation of correct placement of injection*

Method	Confirmation
Use of intralesional/intra-articular LA	Repetition of painful movement immediately post injection, e.g. subacromial injection for supraspinatus tendinitis resulting in immediate loss of painful arc and loss of pain on the resisted action of the muscle
Simultaneous arthrography	Contrast seen within joint, e.g. in injection of hip joint
Ultrasound guidance	Particularly around tendon sheaths
Clinical response	Review of outcome 2–6 weeks later

LA, local anesthetic.

Recently, there has been a tendency to perform multiple joint injections in the early presentations of acute inflammatory joint disease, with the aim of rapid and early control of disease activity. The number of joints injected will depend on disease activity and the ability of the patient to tolerate the procedures. Large doses of corticosteroids will inevitably have systemic effects,[24]* which may contribute to this regimen's effectiveness.

Key points 3: general advice on administration

- There should be 4–6 weeks between injections.
- Three injections per joint per year.
- Any number of joints can be injected at any one time, provided the patient can tolerate it.

INDICATIONS

Local injection therapy usually carried out in one of two contexts, i.e. injection into or adjacent to:

- Synovial space
  - the joint space;
  - around a tendon sheath;
  - in a bursa.
- Painful soft-tissue structure
  - an enthesis;
  - adjacent to nerve entrapment.

The general indications for treatment are listed below (Key points 4). For the purposes of this chapter, we will concentrate on injections into the synovial space, with some reference to injection around an enthesis.

Key points 4: indications for treatment

- Inflammatory arthritis.
- Bursitis.
- Paratendinitis.
- Soft-tissue inflammatory lesions
  - inflamed cysts;
  - entheseopathies.
- Nerve compressions.

CONTRAINDICATIONS

There are few contraindications to injection therapy. The major concerns are listed below (Key points 5). The only absolute contraindication is concurrent peri- or intra-articular sepsis. However, the consequences of injecting into an infected joint might not be as dire as suspected. In rabbits injected with intra-articular *Staphylococcus epidermidis* and then treated with intra-articular antibiotics, the addition of local corticosteroids appeared harmless and seemed to improve the joint histological–histochemical parameters of the infection.[36] The remaining contraindications are relative and, in some circumstances, weighing the benefits of injection against the risks and having obtained fully informed consent the procedure may be appropriate.

The authors do not inject hip joints as they are inaccessible except with radiographs or ultrasound imaging and there are few indications for the approach, although some groups have found it beneficial in rheumatoid and osteoarthritis.[37]* Osteoarthritis demonstrates an unpredictable response to steroid injection. If joint damage is limited, pain can be improved by weight loss, walking aids, and the appropriate exercises. If severe, this may be an indication for joint arthroplasty. The first response in treating inflammatory arthropathies should be systemic control of the disease.

Key points 5: contraindications

- Absolute
  - current peri/intra-articular sepsis.
- Relative
  - uncertain diagnosis;
  - bleeding diathesis;
  - joint prosthesis;
  - acute articular/cartilaginous damage;
  - history of tuberculosis;
  - intra-articular fracture;
  - bacteremia;
  - absence of an inflammatory process.

COMPLICATIONS

Complications in the use of intra-articular injection are uncommon and usually mild. The commonest complication is postinjection flare, which has an estimated prevalence of between 2% and 3%. This takes the form of an exacerbation of joint pain which is usually of short duration (24–48 h) and which may be accompanied by superficial erythema. The patient should be warned before the injection of this potential complication and reassured of its transient and inconsequential nature. They can be advised to use a nonsteroidal anti-inflammatory drug (NSAID) and ice compresses to reduce the pain and swelling if it occurs. This probably occurs as the result of a crystal synovitis, and neutrophil phagocytosis of steroid crystals has been described.

Intra-articular infection is uncommon using the techniques described, with a quoted incidence of between 1: 10,000 and 1:50,000 injections.[2*,28,31] There may be a further reduction in the incidence of this complication if a corticosteroid prepackaged within a sterile syringe is used.[29*]

Exacerbation of an arthropathy or deterioration of articular cartilage following repeated intra-articular injection is debatable. Studies of steroid-induced arthropathy have largely been based on subprimates.[38] Although there appears to be a deleterious effect on cartilage in some studies,[39] this impression is confused by other studies which suggest that steroids may protect the dog anterior cruciate ligament (ACL)-deficient knee from the development of OA.[40] The effects on primates have been less clear, and limiting dosage and number of injections will probably prevent any deleterious effects. Studies in humans have usually been in joints with established arthropathy, confounding a true assessment of the causal effect of steroids on deteriorating arthropathy. In a retrospective study of rheumatoid patients, injection therapy was not associated with a higher risk of arthroplasty.[41*]

The incidence of tendon rupture is similarly difficult to assess. Advice is frequently given to avoid intratendinous injection, although the pressures required to inject into a normal tendon are probably prohibitive. The studies of tendon rupture after adjacent injection are confounded by the presence of underlying tendinopathies,[42*] and the risk next to normal tendons is likely to be minimal. The biggest concern is the Achilles tendon. Nevertheless, given the possible changes in tendon reported in animals,[43] it is recommended to advise a reduction in weight-bearing activity for 10–14 days after injection adjacent to a tendon.[44***]

There have been a number of other complications described including anaphylaxis, which is rare, but resuscitation facilities should be available.[45] Suppression of the hypothalamic–pituitary axis is a recognized complication, but is of questionable clinical significance.[46,47]

Key points 6: complications

- Postinjection flare: steroid crystal-induced synovitis.
- Introduction of articular infection: 1:10,000–50,000 injections.
- Enhanced joint damage: debatable.
- Aseptic necrosis.
- Tendon rupture.
- Soft-tissue atrophy and hypopigmentation.
- Hypothalamic–pituitary–adrenal axis suppression.
- Anaphylaxis.

EQUIPMENT

The equipment (outlined in key points 7) required for joint injection is minimal and inexpensive.

Key points 7: equipment

- Syringes: 2, 5, 10 ml.
- Needles: 21 gauge, 23 gauge, 25 gauge.
- Gloves: nonsterile.
- Alcohol swabs.
- Ethyl chloride: anesthetic spray.
- Sticking plaster.

DRUGS

The medications outlined below are sufficient for most circumstances. They should be used from once-only vials to prevent the possibility of cross-infection. Short-acting steroids should be used adjacent to weight-bearing tendons and for superficial injections where tracking of steroid into the subcutaneous tissues could lead to fat and skin atrophy. They should also be used in the context of a diagnostic trial. Longer acting steroids are more useful for deeper injections, particularly where there is a need to provide sustained anti-inflammatory relief, e.g. in an inflammatory arthropathy. Recently, triamcinolone hexacetonide has been withdrawn from the market and methylprednisolone acetate is therefore used as an example of a long-acting steroid.

Key points 8: medication

- Corticosteroids
  - short acting: hydrocortisone acetate (5–25 mg).
  - prolonged acting: methylprednisolone acetate (40–80 mg).
- Local anesthetic
  - lidocaine (1% or 2%): *without epinephrine*.

JOINT INJECTION METHODS

Techniques for injecting the knee joint

The knee joint is one of the commonest and easiest joints to inject. This can be done via the following two approaches:

1 Medial or lateral. The techniques for these approaches are similar, but require placement of the needle on either side of the patella. The choice of side depends on the ease of access and the site at which there is maximal palpable effusion. These approaches are better for knees with large effusions
2 Anterior. This approach is better for injecting knees where there is no palpable effusion, as there are fewer prospects of traumatizing the subarticular cartilage of the patella and inducing pain.

The principal indication for these techniques is inflammatory joint disease, e.g. rheumatoid and seronegative arthropathy and inflammatory features of osteoarthritis.

Medial and lateral approach

Patent positioning
The patient is supine with the knee fully extended.

Siting the injection
Palpate the lateral/medial border of the patella and place the site of injection at the junction of its middle and upper thirds. Mark the site of puncture with a cross using a ballpoint pen.

The needle should be inserted posterior to the under surface of the patella and pointing slightly superiorly (Fig. 20.1).

Equipment

- Corticosteroid
  - methylprednisolone acetate (40–80 mg)
  - mixed with 1% lidocaine hydrochloride (10 mg/ml, 5 ml).
- Nonpermanent ballpoint pen.
- Ethyl chloride anesthetic spray.
- Alcohol-based swabs.
- Two 21-gauge sterile, prepacked needles: one for drawing up, the other for joint injection.
- One 10-ml sterile, repacked syringe.
- Sterile gauze swab.
- Small elastic adhesive plaster.

Procedure

1 Describe the procedure to the patient and obtain consent.
2 Mark site.
3 Swab away center of the ballpoint pen cross with an alcohol swab so as to leave the arms of the cross pointing to the exact site of puncture.
4 Draw up steroid and local anesthetic into the 10-ml syringe and mix thoroughly.
5 Change the drawing up needle to a sterile, sheathed 21-gauge needle.
6 Use ethyl chloride spray to anesthetize skin until skin turns white.
7 Insert needle through the skin and direct slightly posterosuperiorly underneath the patella.
8 Aspirate fluid from the joint, if present, using a separate syringe.
9 Inject steroid/anesthetic solution, taking care not to displace the needle from the joint. Minimal pressure on the syringe should be required.
10 Withdraw needle, aspirating simultaneously to avoid tracking of steroid along the puncture wound.
11 Apply pressure with a gauze swab if necessary and cover with a small adhesive plaster if not allergic.
12 Dispose of all needles and syringes safely to avoid needle-stick injury.
13 Advise the patient to rest the knee over the next 24–48 h. Strenuous activity is to be avoided. Bed rest if possible.

Anterior approach

Patent positioning
The patient lies supine with the knee flexed and the foot resting on the couch.

Siting the injection
Palpate either side of the patellar tendon. There is a natural gutter formed between the tendon, femoral condyles, and the tibial plateau. Mark the site of the puncture with a cross using a ballpoint pen.

The needle should be inserted perpendicularly

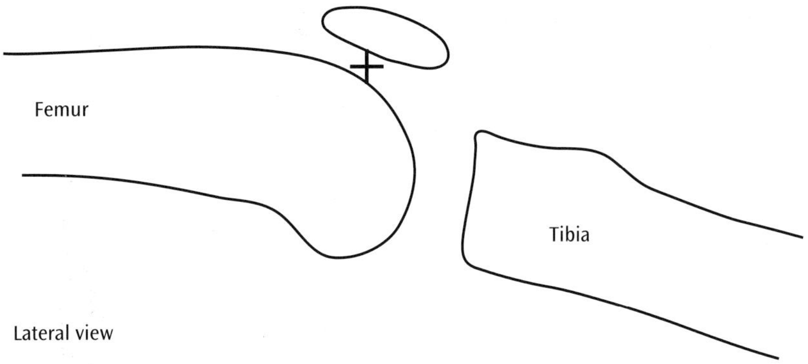

Femur

Tibia

Lateral view

Figure 20.1 *Medial/lateral approach to injection of the knee joint. The needle should be inserted into the joint at the point of the cross from the viewpoint of the reader.*

through the skin posteriorly into the joint. It will need to be inserted approximately 3 cm to avoid the fat pad. The equipment and procedure is otherwise the same as the medial and lateral approach (Fig. 20.2).

Technique for injecting the ankle (talocrural) joint

The ankle joint is best approached anteriorly.

Patient positioning
The patient can sit up or be supine on the treatment couch. The hip and knees should be flexed with the sole of the foot resting flat on the surface of the couch.

Siting the injection
Ask the patient to dorsiflex the ankle against resistance to demonstrate the tibialis anterior tendon. Palpate the dorsalis pedis artery to ascertain that the injection will not be in line with its path. The injection will go just laterally to this tendon and inferiorly to the distal end of tibia. Mark the site of puncture (Fig. 20.3).

Principal indications
The principal indications are inflammatory joint disease, for example rheumatoid or seronegative arthropathy and inflammatory features in osteoarthritis, and post-traumatic chronic synovitis.

Equipment

- Corticosteroid
  - methylprednisolone acetate (40 mg);
  - mixed with 1% lidocaine hydrochloride (10 mg/ ml, 5 ml).
- The remaining equipment is as described for injecting the knee joint.

Procedure

1 Preparation is as for injecting into the knee joint.
2 Insert the 21-gauge needle perpendicularly to the skin, and slightly superiorly, up to a depth of about 2–3.5 cm. Aspirate on the syringe to ensure that the needle is in ankle joint.

Technique for injecting around the foot

Metatarsophalangeal joint of the hallux

The metatarsophalangeal (MTP) of the hallux is best approached medially.

Patient positioning
The patient should lie on their side on the treatment couch with the affected foot down-most, allowing easy access to the medial joint line.

Siting the injection
The joint line is usually easy to feel and the medial puncture site is just below the extensor tendon of the hallux. Mark the site of puncture with a cross using a ballpoint pen.

Principal indications
The principal indications are inflammatory arthritis, for

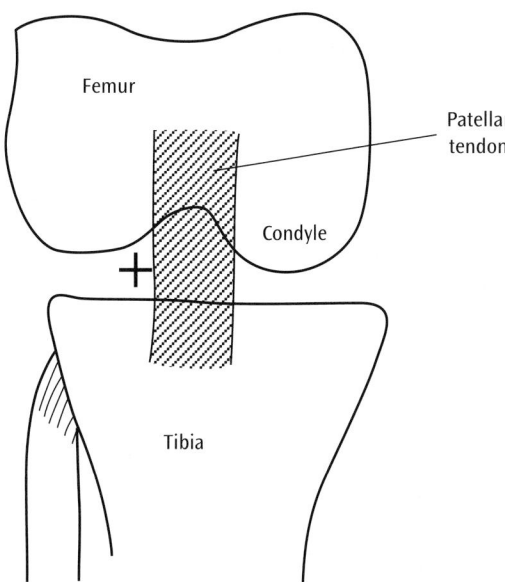

Figure 20.2 *Anterior approach to injection of the knee joint. The needle should be inserted into the joint at the point of the cross from the viewpoint of the reader.*

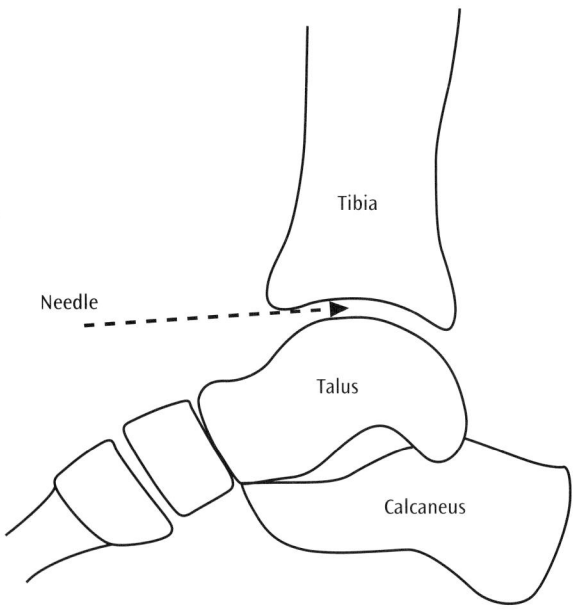

Figure 20.3 *Anterior injection of the talocrural joint.*

example rheumatoid arthritis, refractory crystal synovitis, for example gout, and osteoarthritis.

Equipment
- Corticosteroid
  - either hydrocortisone acetate (25 mg/ml, 0.5–1 ml) or methylprednisolone acetate (40 mg/ml, 0.5–1 ml);
  - mixed with 1% lidocaine hydrochloride (10 mg/ml, 1–2 ml).
- One 21-gauge sterile, prepacked needle for drawing up; a 25-gauge needle for the joint injection.
- One 2-ml sterile, prepacked syringe.
- The remaining equipment is as described for injecting into the knee.

Procedure

1 Preparation is as for injecting into the knee joint.
2 Change the drawing up needle to a sterile sheathed 25-gauge needle.
3 Insert the needle perpendicularly to the skin and direct laterally to a depth of about 0.5–1 cm. Aspirate with the syringe to ensure that there has been no accidental cannulation of vessels.
4 Aspirate fluid from the joint if present.
5 Inject steroid/anesthetic solution with firm pressure, taking care not to displace needle from the joint. It will usually accept 0.5–1 ml of fluid. Resistance to injection usually indicates that the needle has been inserted too far. Withdraw a couple of millimeters and attempt to inject again.

Technique for injecting the shoulder

Subacromial bursa

Patient positioning
The patient lies resting against the backrest of the couch, which should be set at around 45°. The forearm on the affected side is allowed to rest in a relaxed position in the lap of the patient.

Siting the injection
Palpate the lateral border of the acromion process by tracing the clavicle from the sternoclavicular joint. You will feel a gap between the tip of the acromion process and the head of the humerus. Gentle distraction of the upper arm downward will accentuate this space. Mark the spot with a cross (Fig. 20. 4).

Principal indications

- Supraspinatus lesions: tears, tendinopathy, calcific tendinitis.
- Subacromial bursitis.
- Subacromial impingement: injection will help to resolve mild cases of this and will temporarily alleviate symptoms in most cases. However, recurrence of symptoms after one or two injections combined with positive signs of impingement would indicate the need for a surgical opinion for decompression.
- Inflammatory joint disease, e.g. rheumatoid arthritis.

In most cases where this injection is indicated, there will be a painful arc on abduction of the shoulder. This pain will frequently disappear when repeating the movement immediately after an accurately placed injection. The patient should be informed that the pain may return after the local anesthetic effect has worn off, but should improve again when the steroid starts to take effect.

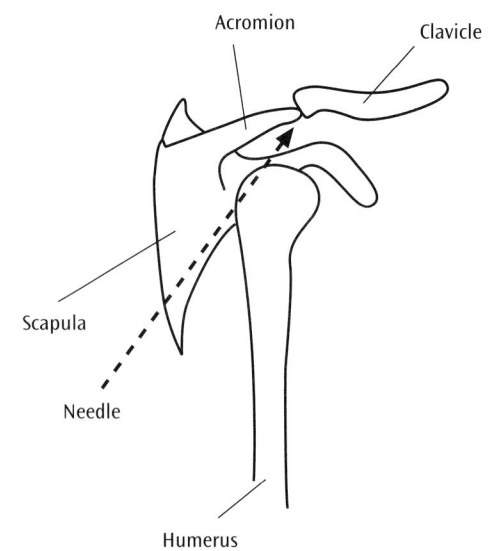

Figure 20.4 *Injection of the subacromial space.*

Equipment

- Corticosteroid
  - methylprednisolone acetate (40 mg);
  - mixed with 1% lidocaine hydrochloride (10 mg/ml, 5 ml).
- The remaining equipment is as described for injecting into the knee.

Procedure

1 Preparation is as for injecting into the knee joint.
2 Insert the needle perpendicularly to the skin into the gap between the inferior margin of the acromion and the superior aspect of the humerus slightly posteriorly by about 2.5 cm. Aspirate with the syringe to ensure that there has been no accidental cannulation of vessels.
3 Aspirate fluid from the joint, if present.
4 Inject steroid/anesthetic solution, taking care not to displace the needle from the joint. Minimal pressure on the syringe should be required. Resistance to injection usually indicates that the needle has been inserted too far. Withdraw a couple of millimeters before aspirating and attempting to inject again.

Glenohumeral joint

Access to the glenohumeral joint (GHJ) can be achieved using the posterior or anterior route. The approach taken depends largely on personal preference.

Glenohumeral joint: posterior approach

Patient positioning
The patient sits relaxed on the couch with their arm by their side.

Siting the injection
- Standing behind the patient, palpate the coracoid process on the anterior aspect of the affected shoulder at the deltopectoral triangle.
- Identify the GHJ line by rotating the arm. Mark the posterior joint line.
- The needle should be inserted from the posterior joint line toward the lateral side of the coracoid process (Fig. 20.5).

Equipment

- Corticosteroid
  - methylprednisolone acetate (40 mg)
  - mixed with 1% lidocaine hydrochloride (10 mg/ml, 5 ml).
- The remaining equipment is as described for injecting into the knee.

Procedure

1 Preparation is as described for injecting into the knee.

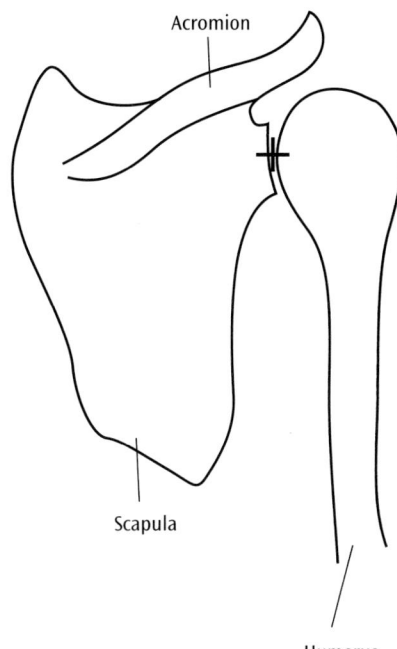

Figure 20.5 *Posterior injection of the glenohumeral joint. The needle should be inserted into the joint at the point of the cross from the viewpoint of the reader.*

2 Insert needle perpendicularly to the skin, and direct toward the lateral side of the coracoid process.
3 Aspirate on the syringe to ensure that the needle is in the GHJ.
4 Inject steroid/anesthetic solution with firm pressure, taking care not to displace needle. There should be little resistance.

Glenohumeral joint: anterior approach

This approach is suited to aspiration of large GHJ effusions.

Patient positioning
The patient sits up against the backrest of the treatment couch. The doctor rotates the arm to locate the coracoid process and joint line anteriorly and the acromion posteriorly. The arm is rested across the patient's abdomen to aid internal rotation.

Siting the injection
The injection is made just lateral to the tip of the coracoid with the needle directed to the tip of the acromion. Confirmation of correct placement can be made by gentle passive external rotation of the shoulder, movement will be felt from the needle tip (Fig. 20.6).

Procedure
The volume and technique is the same as for posterior injection.

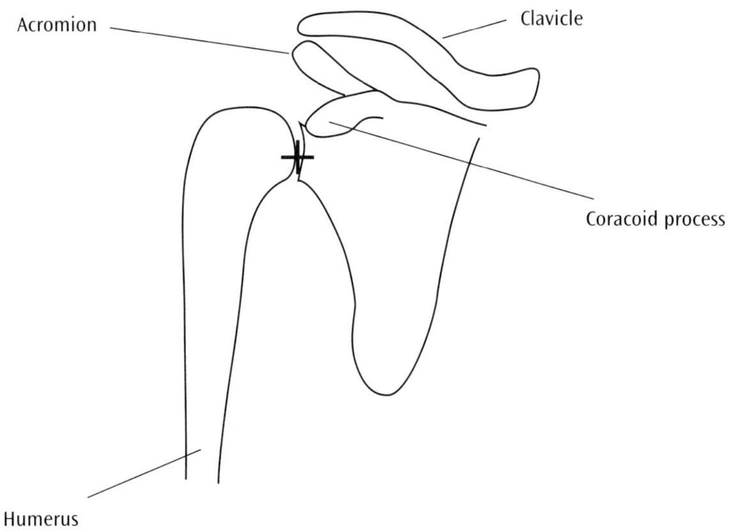

Figure 20.6 *Anterior injection of the glenohumeral joint. The needle should be inserted into the joint at the point of the cross from the viewpoint of the reader.*

Technique for injecting around the elbow joint

Posterior approach into the elbow joint

The posterior approach to the elbow joint is the easiest.

Patient positioning
The patient is seated on a chair with the affected elbow relaxed in a flexed position on a cushioned table.

Siting the injection
Feel for the depression in the midline at the back of the flexed elbow between the two halves of the triceps that is created by the olecranon fossa of the humerus. The needle will be passed perpendicularly to the skin just above the olecranon process. Mark the site of the puncture with a cross using a ballpoint pen (Fig. 20.7).

Principle indication
The principal indication is inflammatory joint disease, e.g. rheumatoid arthritis.

Equipment

- Corticosteroid
  - methylprednisolone acetate (40 mg);
  - mixed with 1% lidocaine hydrochloride (10 mg/ml, 2–3 ml).
- The remaining equipment is as described for injecting into the knee.

Procedure

1 Preparation is as described for injecting into the knee.
2 Insert the needle perpendicularly to the skin to a depth of about 2 cm. Aspirate with the syringe to ensure that there has been no accidental cannulation of vessels.
3 Aspirate fluid from the joint if present.
4 Inject steroid/anesthetic solution with firm pressure, taking care not to displace the needle from the joint. Resistance to injection usually indicates that the nee-

dle has been inserted too far. Withdraw a couple of millimeters and attempt to inject again.

Lateral epicondyle

The injection is made into the enthesis between the common extensor tendon and lateral epicondyle (Fig. 20.8).

Patient positioning
The patient is seated with the elbow supported in a flexed and supinated position on a cushioned surface.

Siting the injection
The injection site is found by locating the point of maximal tenderness around the lateral epicondyle. Mark the site of puncture with a cross using a ballpoint pen.

Equipment

- Corticosteroid
  - either hydrocortisone acetate (25 mg/ml, 0.5–1 ml) or methylprednisolone acetate (40 mg/ml, 0.5–1 ml);
  - mixed with 1% lidocaine hydrochloride (10 mg/ml, 1–2 ml).
- One 21-gauge sterile, prepacked needle for drawing up; a 25-gauge or a 23-gauge needle for the joint injection.
- One 2-ml sterile, prepacked syringe.
- The remaining equipment is as described for injecting into the knee.

Procedure

1 Preparation is as described for injecting into the knee.
2 Change the drawing up needle to a sterile sheathed 25-gauge or 23-gauge needle.
3 Inject steroid/anesthetic solution with firm pressure, taking care not to displace the needle from the site of maximal tenderness. More pressure is needed on the syringe plunger when injecting into the soft tissues than when injecting into a joint. However, exces-

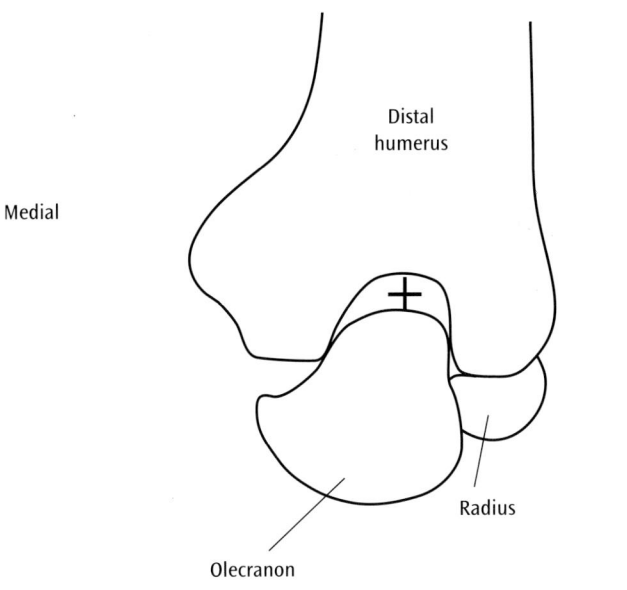

Figure 20.7 *Posterior approach into the elbow joint. The needle should be inserted into the joint at the point of the cross from the viewpoint of the reader. The needle should travel parallel to the line of the ulna.*

Medial

Lateral

Distal humerus

Radius

Olecranon

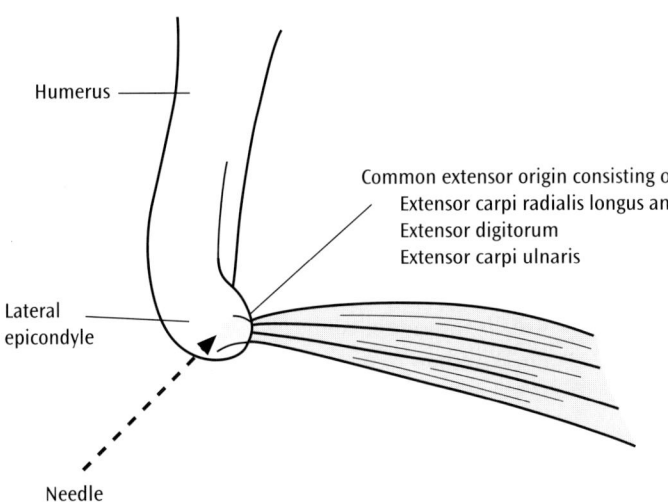

Figure 20.8 *Injection into common extensor tendon origin at the lateral epicondyle.*

Humerus

Common extensor origin consisting of the origins of:
Extensor carpi radialis longus and brevis
Extensor digitorum
Extensor carpi ulnaris

Lateral epicondyle

Needle

sive resistance to injection usually indicates that the needle has been inserted too far. Withdraw a couple of millimeters and attempt to inject again. An attempt must be made to inject around the enthesis and into the periosteum. This can be painful and the patient needs to be warned of this.

4 Fanning out the injection over the painful area by partial needle withdrawal and reinsertion will distribute the mixture more effectively.

Medial epicondyle

The injection is made into the enthesis of the common flexor tendon and medial humeral epicondyle. The medial approach is taken and patient positioning, equipment, and volumes used are identical to those used in lateral epicondylitis.

The difference is in siting the injection. Once again, the point of maximal tenderness at the enthesis of the flexor tendon and epicondyle is located by palpation.

The ulnar nerve rests in the groove behind the medial epicondyle, and its close proximity to the site of injection merits particular care.

Technique for injecting the wrist

The radiocarpal joint

Patient positioning
The patient is sitting comfortably with the affected hand relaxed in a pronated position on a cushioned table, allowing easy access to the joint line.

Siting the injection
The joint is felt as a gap between the distal radius and the proximal carpal bones. Mark the site of puncture with a cross using a ballpoint pen (Fig. 20.9).

Principal indication
The principal indication is inflammatory arthritis, e.g. rheumatoid arthritis.

Equipment

- Corticosteroid
  - either hydrocortisone acetate (25 mg/ml, 0.5–1 ml) or methylprednisolone acetate (40 mg/ml, 0.5–1 ml);

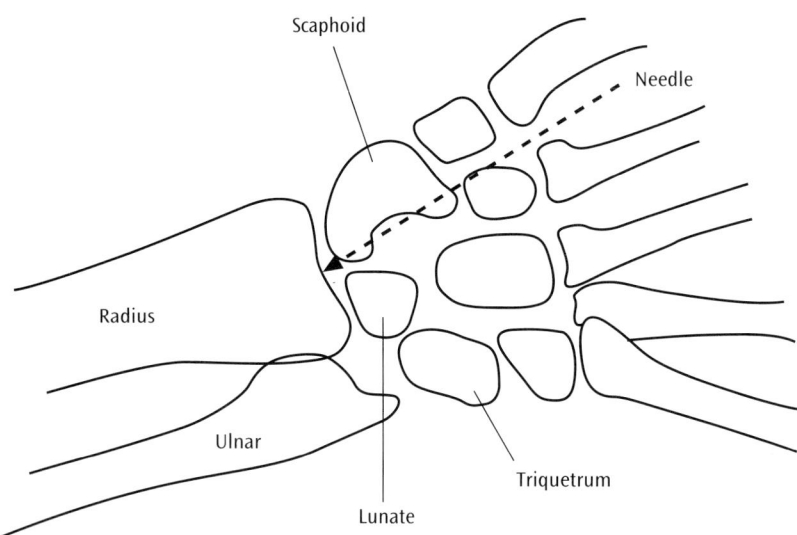

Figure 20.9 *Injection of the radiocarpal joint of the wrist.*

– mixed with 1% lidocaine hydrochloride (10 mg/ml, 1–2 ml).
- One 21-gauge sterile, prepacked needle for drawing up; a 25-gauge needle for the joint injection.
- One 2-ml sterile, prepacked syringe.
- The remaining equipment is as described for injecting into the knee.

Procedure

1 Preparation is as described for injecting into the knee. Change the drawing up needle to a sterile sheathed 25-gauge needle.
2 Insert the needle at 45° to the skin and direct slightly proximally to a depth of about 1 cm. Aspirate with the syringe to ensure that there has been no accidental cannulation of vessels.
3 Aspirate fluid from the joint if present.
4 Inject steroid/anesthetic solution with firm pressure, taking care not to displace the needle from the joint. It will usually accept 1–2 ml of fluid. Resistance to injection usually indicates that the needle has been inserted too far. Withdraw a couple of millimeters and attempt to inject again.

The distal radioulnar joint

Patient positioning
The patient is sitting comfortably with the affected hand relaxed in a pronated position on a cushioned table allowing easy access to the joint line.

Siting the injection
The joint line is felt as a gap at the distal radius and ulnar when pronating and supinating the patient's forearm.

Principal indication
This is inflammatory arthritis, e.g. rheumatoid arthritis.

Equipment
As for injecting the radiocarpal joint.

Procedure

1 The procedure is similar to that for injecting the radiocarpal joint, but in this case the needle is inserted tangentially under the dorsal ligaments of the wrist to a depth of about 1 cm into the radioulnar joint space. Aspirate with the syringe to ensure that there has been no accidental cannulation of vessels.
2 Aspirate fluid from the joint if present.
3 Inject steroid/anesthetic solution. The joint will usually accept 1–2 ml of fluid. Resistance to injection usually indicates that the needle has been inserted too far. Withdraw a couple of millimeters and attempt to inject again.

Technique for injecting the joints of the hand

Metacarpophalangeal joint

The metacarpophalangeal (MCP) joint of the hand concerned is best approached via the medial or lateral approaches.

Patient positioning
The patient is sitting comfortably with the affected hand relaxed in a pronated position on a cushioned table or couch, allowing easy access to the joint line.

Siting the injection
The joint line is usually easier to feel after distraction with the finger slightly flexed. The MCP joint does not always lie under the knuckle (Fig. 20.10). Mark the site of puncture with a cross using a ballpoint pen.

Principal indications
These are inflammatory arthritis, for example rheumatoid arthritis, or osteoarthritis.

Equipment

- Corticosteroid

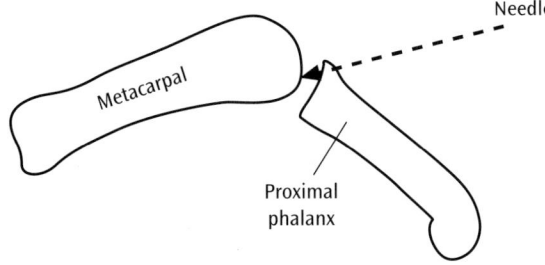

Figure 20.10 *Injection of the metacarpophalangeal joint of the index finger.*

- either hydrocortisone acetate (25 mg/ml, 0.5 ml) or methylprednisolone acetate (40 mg/ml, 0.5 ml);
- mixed with 1% lidocaine hydrochloride (10 mg/ml, 0.5–1 ml).
- One 21-gauge sterile, prepacked needle for drawing up; a 25-gauge needle for the joint injection.
- One 2-ml sterile, prepacked syringe.
- The remaining equipment is as described for injecting into the knee.

Procedure

1 Preparation is as described for injecting into the knee.
2 Change the drawing up needle to a sterile sheathed 25-gauge needle.
3 Insert the needle perpendicularly to the skin lateral or medial to the extensor tendon, and then direct tangentially under it to a depth of about 0.5 cm. Aspirate with the syringe to ensure that there has been no accidental cannulation of vessels.
4 Aspirate fluid from the joint if present.
5 Inject steroid/anesthetic solution with firm pressure, taking care not to displace the needle from the joint. It will usually accept 0.5 ml of fluid. Resistance to injection usually indicates that the needle has been inserted too far. Withdraw a couple of millimeters and attempt to inject again.

Proximal interphalangeal joint

The equipment and procedure for injecting the proximal interphalangeal joint (PIP) joint are exactly as described for the MCP joint. However, because of the small size of the joint, accessibility may be more difficult and the volumes of fluid which can be injected may be correspondingly less.

The main indications will be rheumatoid and osteoarthritis.

REFERENCES

1. Kirwan JR, Russell AS. Systemic glucocorticoid treatment in rheumatoid arthritis – a debate. *Scand J Rheumatol* 1998; **27:** 247–51.
2. Hollander JL. The use of intra-articular hydrocortisone, its analogues and its higher esters in arthritis. *Md Med J* 1970; **61:** 511.
3. Green S, Buchbinder R., Glazier R, Forbes A. Systematic review of randomised controlled trials of interventions for painful shoulder: selection criteria, outcome assessment and efficacy. *Br Med J* 1998; **316:** 354–60.
4. Van der Windt DAWM, Van der Heijden GJMG, Scholten RJPM, *et al.* The efficacy of non-steroidal anti-inflammatory drugs for shoulder complaints. A systematic review. *J Clin Epidemiol* 1995; **48:** 691–704.
5. Berry H, Fernandes L, Bloom B, *et al.* Clinical study comparing acupuncture, physiotherapy, injection and oral anti-inflammatory therapy in the shoulder. *Curr Med Res Opin* 1980; **7:** 121–6.
6. Rizk T, Pinals R, Talaiver A. Corticosteroid injections in adhesive capsulitis: investigation of their value and site. *Arch Phys Med* 1991; **72:** 20–2.
7. Gam AN, Schydlowsky P, Rossel I, *et al.* Treatment of "frozen shoulder" with distension and glucorticoid compared with glucorticoid alone. A randomised controlled trial. *Scand J Rheumatol* 1998; **27:** 425–30.
8. Laroche M, Ighilahriz O, Moulinier L, *et al.* Adhesive capsulitis of the shoulder: an open study of 40 cases treated by joint distention during arthrography followed by an intra-articular corticosteroid injection and immediate physical therapy. *Rev Rhum* [English edition] 1998; **65:** 313–19.
9. Adebajo AO, Nash P, Hazleman BL. A prospective double blind dummy placebo controlled study comparing triamcinolone hexacetonide injection with oral diclofenac 50 mg TDS in patients with rotator cuff tendinitis. *J Rheumatol* 1990; **17:** 1207–10.
10. Petri M, Dobrow R, Neiman R, *et al.* Randomized, double-blind, placebo-controlled study of the treatment of the painful shoulder. *Arthritis Rheum* 1987; **30:** 1040–5.
11. Vecchio PC, Hazleman BL, King RH. A double-blind trial comparing subacromial methylprednisolone and lignocaine in acute rotator cuff tendinitis. *Br J Rheumatol* 1993; **32:** 743–5.
12. Assendelft WJ, Hay EM, Adshead R, Bouter LM. Corticosteroid injections for lateral epicondylitis: a systematic overview. *Br J Gen Pract* 1996; **46:** 209–16.
13. Stahl S, Kaufman T. The efficacy of an injection of steroids for medial epicondylitis. A prospective study of sixty elbows. *J Bone Joint Surg* [American edition] 1997; **79:** 1648–52.
14. Creamer P. Intra-articular corticosteroid injections in osteoarthritis: do they work and if so, how? *Ann Rheum Dis* 1997; **56:** 634–6.
15. Kirwan JR, Rankin E. Intra-articular therapy in osteoarthritis. *Baillieres Clin Rheumatol* 1997; **11:** 769–94.
16. Ravaud P, Moulinier L, Giraudeau B, *et al.* Effects of joint lavage and steroid injection in patients with osteoarthritis of the knee: results of a multicenter, randomized, controlled trial. *Arthritis Rheum* 1999; **42:** 475–82.
17. Hochberg MC, Altman RD, Brandt KD, *et al.* Guidelines for the medical management of osteoarthritis. Part II.

Osteoarthritis of the knee. American College of Rheumatology. *Arthritis Rheum* 1995; **38:** 1541–6.

◆ 18. Sheeran TP, Roobottom CA, Wanklyn PD, *et al*. The effect of bed rest and intra-articular steroids on the acute phase response in rheumatoid arthritis. Intra-articular corticosteroids are effective in osteoarthritis but there are no clinical predictors of response. *Clin Exp Rheumatol* 1993; **11:** 49–52.

19. Padeh S, Passwell JH. Intraarticular corticosteroid injection in the management of children with chronic arthritis. *Arthritis Rheum* 1998; **41:** 1210–14.

● 20. See Y. Intra-synovial corticosteroid injections in juvenile chronic arthritis – a review. *Ann Acad Med Singapore* 1998; **27:** 105–11.

21. Sherry DD, Stein LD, Reed AM, *et al*. Prevention of leg length discrepancy in young children with pauciarticular juvenile rheumatoid arthritis by treatment with intraarticular steroids. *Arthritis Rheum* 1999; **42:** 2330–4.

22. Dent PB, Walker N. Intra-articular corticosteroids in the treatment of juvenile rheumatoid arthritis. *Curr Opin Rheumatol* 1998; **10:** 475–80.

23. Buris LF, Bodor N, Buris L. Loteprednol etabonate, a new soft steroid is effective in a rabbit acute experimental model for arthritis. *Pharmazie* 1999; **54:** 58–61.

24. Steer JH, Ma DT, Dusci L, *et al*. Altered leucocyte trafficking and suppressed tumour necrosis factor alpha release from peripheral blood monocytes after intra-articular glucocorticoid treatment. *Ann Rheum Dis* 1998; **57:** 732–7.

25. Firestein GS, Paine MM, Littman BH. Gene expression (collagenase, tissue inhibitor of metalloproteinases, complement, and HLA-DR) in rheumatoid arthritis and osteoarthritis synovium. Quantitative analysis and effect of intraarticular corticosteroids. *Arthritis Rheum* 1991; **34:** 1094–105.

26. Hills BA, Ethell MT, Hodgson DR. Release of lubricating synovial surfactant by intra-articular steroid. *Br J Rheumatol* 1998; **37:** 649–52.

27. Geborek P, Mansson B, Wollheim FA, Moritz U. Intraarticular corticosteroid injection into rheumatoid arthritis knees improves extensor muscles strength. *Rheumatol Int* 1990; **9** (6): 265–70.

28. Gray RG, Gottlieb NL. Intra-articular corticosteroids. An updated assessment. *Clin Orthop* 1983; **177:** 235–63.

◆ 29. Seror P, Pluvinage P, d'Andre FL, *et al*. Frequency of sepsis after local corticosteroid injection (an inquiry on 1160000 injections in rheumatological private practice in France). *Rheumatology* 1999; **38:** 1272–4.

● 30. Rozental TD, Sculco TP. Intra-articular corticosteroids: an updated overview. *Am J Orthop* 2000; **29:** 18–23.

31. Hunter JA, Blyth TH. A risk–benefit assessment of intra-articular corticosteroids in rheumatic disorders. *Drug Safety* 1999; **21:** 353–65.

◆ 32. Chakravarty K, Pharoah PD, Scott DG. A randomized controlled study of post-injection rest following intra-articular steroid therapy for knee synovitis. *Br J Rheumatol* 1994; **33:** 464–8.

◆ 33. Eustace JA, Brophy DP, Gibney RP, *et al*. Comparison of the accuracy of steroid placement with clinical outcome in patients with shoulder symptoms. *Ann Rheum Dis* 1997; **56:** 59–63.

34. Grassi W, Lamanna G, Farina A, Cervini C. Synovitis of small joints: sonographic guided diagnostic and therapeutic approach. *Ann Rheum Dis* 1999; **58:** 595–7.

35. Lucas PE, Hurwitz SR, Kaplan PA, *et al*. Fluoroscopically guided injections into the foot and ankle: localization of the source of pain as a guide to treatment – prospective study. *Radiology* 1997; **204:** 411–15.

36. Wysenbeek AJ, Volchek J, Amit M, *et al*. Treatment of staphylococcal septic arthritis in rabbits by systemic antibiotics and intra-articular corticosteroids. *Ann Rheum Dis* 1998; **57:** 687–90.

37. Plant MJ, Borg AA, Dziedzic K, *et al*. Radiographic patterns and response to corticosteroid hip injection. *Ann Rheum Dis* 1997; **56:** 476–80.

38. Papacrhistou G, Anagnostou S, Katsorhis T. The effect of intraarticular hydrocortisone injection on the articular cartilage of rabbits. *Acta Orthop Scand* 1997; **275** (Suppl.): 132–4.

39. Murray RC, DeBowes RM, Gaughan EM, *et al*. The effects of intra-articular methylprednisolone and exercise on the mechanical properties of articular cartilage in the horse. *Osteoarthritis Cartilage* 1998; **6:** 106–14.

40. Pelletier JP, Martel-Pelletier J. *In vivo* protective effects of prophylactic treatment with tiaprofenic acid or intraarticular corticosteroids on osteoarthritic lesions in the experimental dog model. *J Rheumatol* 1991; **27:** 127–30.

41. Roberts WN, Babcock EA, Breitbach SA, *et al*. Corticosteroid injection in rheumatoid arthritis does not increase rate of total joint arthroplasty. *J Rheumatol* 1996; **23:** 1001–4.

42. Read MT, Motto SG. Tendo Achilles pain: steroids and outcome. *Br J Sports Med* 1992; **26:** 15–21.

43. Martin DF, Carlson CS, Berry J, *et al*. Effect of injected versus iontophoretic corticosteroid on the rabbit tendon. *South Med J* 1999; **92:** 600–8.

44. Shrier I, Matheson GO, Kohl HW. Achilles tendonitis: are corticosteroid injections useful or harmful? *Clin J Sport Med* 1996; **6:** 245–50.

45. Mace S, Vadas P, Pruzanski W. Anaphylactic shock induced by intraarticular injection of methylprednisolone acetate. *J Rheumatol* 1997; **24:** 1191–4.

46. Huppertz HI, Pfuller H. Transient suppression of endogenous cortisol production after intraarticular steroid therapy for chronic arthritis in children. *J Rheumatol* 1997; **24:** 1833–7.

47. Lazarevic MB, Skosey JL, Djordjevic-Denic G, *et al*. Reduction of cortisol levels after single intra-articular and intramuscular steroid injection. *Am J Med* 1995; **99:** 370–3.

21

Facet (zygapophyseal) joint injections and medial branch blocks

RON COOPER

Applied anatomy	269	Complications of zygapophyseal blocks	274
Indications	270	Evidence for the use of zygapophyseal joint blocks	274
Contraindications	271	Conclusion	275
Limitations of treatment	271	References	275
Preparation for zygapophyseal blocks	271		

Chronic spinal pain, especially that involving the lumbar and cervical regions, is commonly encountered in pain clinic practice. It has been estimated that it will be experienced by 60–70% of the adult population at some time in their lives.[1]

The exact diagnosis of low back pain can be difficult. At the turn of the twentieth century, mechanical disorders of the sacroiliac joint, such as distraction or dislocation, were considered common causes for low back pain. Goldthwait, in 1911,[2] suggested that zygapophyseal or facet joint disturbances were mainly responsible for low back pain and instability. Contemporary surgical practice focused on intervertebral disk herniation as a cause for low back pain and sciatica.[3] As laminectomy and nerve root decompression did not always relieve symptoms, interest was directed toward other causes for spinal pain.

In over 85% of patients with lumbar and cervical pain no specific spinal pathology can be identified as the cause.[4***] Both lumbar and cervical zygapophyseal joints have been considered a significant source of chronic low back and neck pain.

The term *facet joint syndrome* (lumbar spine) was first attributed to Ghormley in 1933,[5] when he described this pain syndrome as usually occurring after a sudden twisting injury to the lumbar spine, producing low back pain, usually without sciatica.

Mooney and Robertson, in 1976,[6*] demonstrated that the pain patterns resulting from lumbar zygapophyseal joint injections of hypertonic saline could be relieved by subsequent intra-articular injections of local anesthetic. More recently, it has been recognized that a similar pain syndrome can occur in the cervical spine. Aprill and colleagues, in 1990, described the pain patterns associated with cervical disease, conducting studies in healthy volunteers and patients with chronic neck pain.[7*,8*]

APPLIED ANATOMY

The reader is referred to the extensive work of Bogduk for a detailed description of the anatomy of the zygapophyseal joints, and only a brief outline will be given here.[9,10] Any two consecutive vertebrae articulate to form three joints: the large joint between the two vertebral bodies and the two paired (right and left) zygapophyseal joints, which are formed between the superior articular process of one vertebra and the inferior articular process of the vertebra above. The term "facet joint" is used in clinical practice to describe these paired synovial joints, which are also referred to as the posterior intervertebral joints.

Posterolaterally, a firm fibrous capsule covers the joint, while anteriorly the softer ligament flavum contacts the synovium. The fatty tissue around the exiting spinal nerve is continuous with that in the superior recess of the joint. This provides a direct route to the epidural space. This point has a practical significance, as the joint volume in the lumbar spine is in the order of 1–2 ml. Injected volumes larger than this can distend the joint capsule and spread directly into the epidural space, confounding any observed results from diagnostic blocks. Drugs injected on one side can spread to the opposite side at the same level, or to an adjacent level on the same side.[11] The zygapophyseal joints help to resist the associated shearing movements with forward flexion and the compressive forces with rotational spinal movements.

The nerve supply of the zygapophyseal joints is derived from the posterior primary ramus of the nerve root. The spinal nerve divides into anterior (ventral) and posterior (dorsal) rami as it emerges through the intervertebral foramen (Fig. 21.1).

The medial branch of the posterior primary ramus is responsible for joint sensation. Innervation from the medial branch divides to supply the lower pole at its own level, and also the upper pole of the joint below. Terminal branches of the medial branch nerve supply the ligaments and periosteum of the vertebral arches posterior cervical muscles, as well as the multifidus and interspinalis muscles. Successive medial branches from above and below supply each joint. This dual-segment innervation has important implications for zygapophyseal nerve block and denervation procedures, as both branches need to be blocked to completely denervate a single joint.

The course of the medial branch of the posterior ramus is fixed anatomically at two points: at its origin near the superior aspect of the base of the transverse process and distally where it emerges from the canal formed by the mammilloaccessory ligament.

In the cervical spine, nerves supplying the zygapophyseal joints are more specific and make only a small contribution to cervical posterior muscle sensation.[12]

INDICATIONS

The zygapophyseal facet joints are regarded as a common source of spinal pain, particularly in the lumbar and cervical regions.[9,10,12–14] The clinical diagnosis of zygapophyseal joint pain is poorly defined and nonspecific. Features of zygapophyseal joint pain include:

- deep, dull, aching pain;
- uni- or bilateral;
- paravertebral tenderness;
- associated muscle spasm;
- lateral bending or rotational movements increase pain intensity;
- extension rather than flexion movements increase pain intensity;
- Valsalva maneuver and straight-leg raising (SLR) do not affect pain intensity;
- segmental referral pattern in relation to the joint origin.

Cervical zygapophyseal joint pain occurs in the following regions:

- occiput and behind ear C1/2;
- vertex and upper neck C2/3;
- posterolateral neck C3/4;
- supraclavicular fossa C4/5;
- deltoid C5/6;
- posterior scapular C6/7.

Lumbar zygapophyseal joint pain occurs in the following regions:

- groin T12/L1;
- hips L1/2;
- buttocks L2/3;
- thighs L3/4;
- usually above the knee.

Clinical history and examination, including radiologic investigations such as computed tomography (CT) scans, are not particularly useful in its accurate diagnosis.[15,16]

Relief of pain rather than provocation of pain is con-

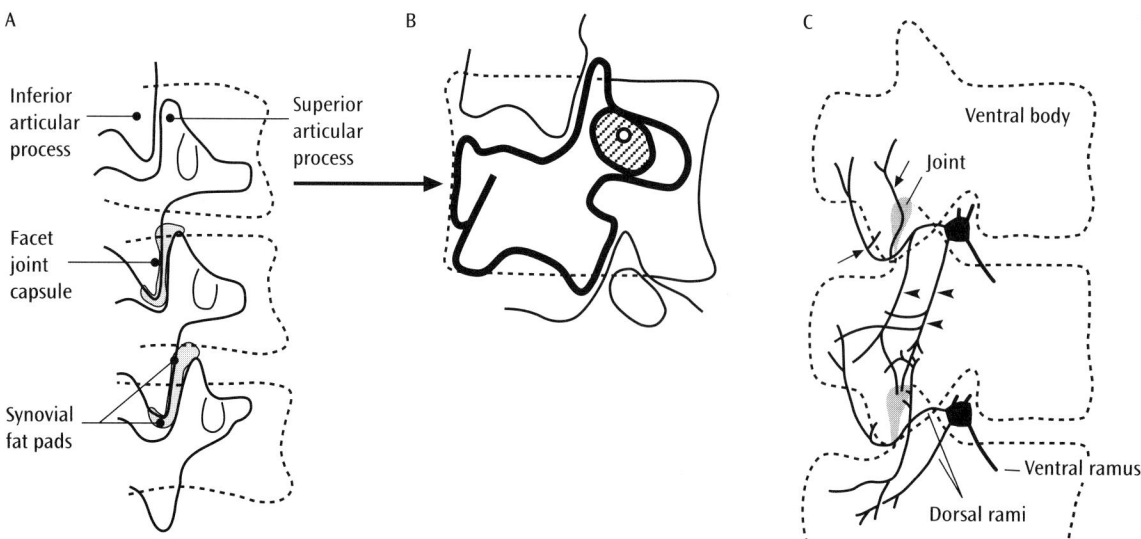

Figure 21.1 *Zygapophyseal joint anatomy.*

sidered the more reliable test.[17] Either intra-articular injections at the suspected painful level, using 1–2 ml of local anesthetic, or medial branch nerve blocks using 0.5–1 ml of local anesthetic, are used to achieve this. Care should be taken to avoid false-positive results, which can confound the interpretation of the procedure, particularly if neurolysis is planned after diagnostic blocks. Excessive doses of local anesthetic can result in spread to other structures, such as the epidural space, producing a false-positive result. Vascular uptake of local anesthetic from the site of injection, by reducing the effective drug dose, can result in a false-negative result. Psychological factors associated with the block can instill in patients a false sense of expectation that their pain will be relieved. Some individuals are therefore likely to have false-positive results. False-positive rates in patients undergoing diagnostic blocks have been reported to be between 25% and 50%.[18, 19**,20**]

Repeat blocks using different local anesthetics with different duration of action, or placebo blocks with saline, are sometimes used to try and overcome these hurdles. This is particularly important in patients with suspected secondary gain phenomena. However, such methods are not without ethical problems and should be undertaken only after careful consideration and discussion with patients and their advisors.

Zygapophyseal joint blocks performed in a meticulous standardized manner avoid the subjectivity associated with clinical assessment, which has been shown to be very unreliable, and allow an objective assessment to be made for the individual patient.

CONTRAINDICATIONS

The same contraindications apply to zygapophyseal blocks as for any other block used in pain management. These include:

- coagulopathies;
- infection either systemically or at the injection site;
- pregnancy (X-rays);
- allergy to contrast media or local anesthetics.

LIMITATIONS OF TREATMENT

Informed consent for the procedure should be obtained and the patient advised that the procedure is primarily diagnostic rather than therapeutic. It is important not to build up expectations or introduce bias before carrying out the procedure, which is ideally done using a placebo control. Patients should be advised to record the duration of any pain relief obtained.

The aim of any zygapophyseal joint block is either to anesthetize the target joint by intra-articular injection

of small dose of local anesthetic or to block the medial branch that innervates the joint. The practical preparation of the patient is similar for both lumbar and cervical spines, but differences in technique due to the anatomy of each region will be described.

PREPARATION FOR ZYGAPOPHYSEAL BLOCKS

The following should be available:

- resuscitation facilities;
- operating room/radiology suite with C-arm fluoroscopy;
- needles, sterile basic pack;
- skin preparation solutions;
- local anesthetics;
- radiographic contrast media;
- staff to position patient/C-arm, carry out observations, and allay patient anxiety.

Patients should understand what to expect during and after the procedure. In particular, they should be aware that the procedures are carried out while conscious, with anxiolysis if required. Cooperation is needed to determine provocation of pain and analgesia during and after the procedure. Skin infiltration with local anesthetics will reduce pain associated with needle passage during localization of the target joints. The usefulness and safety of the procedure are reduced if patients are excessively sedated and unable to respond verbally or to cooperate with the operator.

Radiographic screening of needle insertions is mandatory for all of these procedures. The use of a fluoroscopic C-arm allows the beam to be directed at variable angles to the target. Any changes in either depth or direction of the needle is immediately checked by screening. The use of a water-soluble contrast medium can assist this. A printed image showing positioning of the needle in two planes, with or without contrast, is desirable, particularly when a neurolytic procedure is being undertaken.

The procedure is carried out aseptically after adequate skin preparation using an iodine-based solution (e.g. Povidone-Iodine), chlorhexidine, or alcohol-based antiseptic (e.g. chlorhexidine 0.5% in 70% alcohol). Sterile drapes are used both on the patient and over the C-arm, and strict aseptic techniques, using gowns, gloves, and minimal-touch technique, should be adhered to.

A skilled radiographic assistant with knowledge of the particular screening projections needed for this procedure is desirable. All personnel should be careful to protect themselves and others against unnecessary exposure to the hazards of radiation. Special thin radioabsorbent sterile gloves and protective eyewear can be worn by the operator to reduce absorption of radiation in these areas during the procedure.

A 22- to 25-gauge spinal needle is used for intra-articular injections, whereas medial branch blocks and radio-frequency procedures are generally carried out using a 22-gauge needle. Long needles (100 mm) are generally required for lumbar procedures, whereas needles of half this length are sufficient for cervical procedures. However, longer needles may be required if the patient is particularly obese. Luer-lock needles are useful but not essential.

Intravenous access is obtained, and if needed an anxiolytic such as midazolam may be administered. Verbal contact must be maintained with the patient throughout the procedure, particularly when medial branch blocks or neurolysis are being performed.

Trained staff familiar with the procedure should be present to assist the operator. Routine noninvasive monitoring of the patient should include electrocardiography, blood pressure, and heart rate during the procedure. This is particularly important during cervical procedures, during which sudden untoward cardiovascular changes or transient loss of consciousness could occur during injection of local anesthetics. In order to maximize the usefulness of diagnostic procedures there is no place for carrying out these without radiological screening. Precision is required and screening with the C-arm should be carried out to check every change of needle position. Following medial branch denervation patients in our clinic are allowed to leave with an adult escort half an hour after lumbar procedures (2 h for cervical procedures), provided observations are satisfactory.

Lumbar zygapophyseal blocks

For lumbar procedures the patient is initially placed prone with a pillow under the upper abdomen and the legs slightly abducted.

Intra-articular blocks

Patients must be positioned so that an oblique view of the lumbar spine is obtained (Fig. 21.2). The patient has to lie in a semiprone position on the X-ray-translucent table with a pillow under the abdomen. Alternatively, the C-arm may be rotated to direct the beam obliquely through the target area. This view is necessary to visualize the joint cavity, which must be seen clearly at the target level and can require up to a 45° oblique projection from the sagittal plane. This angle decreases as one ascends the spine.

The joint to be blocked should be identified and marked. Following skin preparation, local anesthetic is infiltrated into the skin and deeper tissues over the joint. The needle is inserted in the line of sight along the direction of the X-ray beam, with its target being the midpoint of the joint. Contact with bone should be achieved to allow a depth assessment of the target joint. The needle is then guided to the joint cavity, when some "give" is initially felt on entry, followed by a firmer gripping sensation on the needle tip. A small amount of radiocontrast (not

more than 0.3 ml) is injected to produce an arthrogram. This is seen as either a slit or dumb-bell shape in outline, and confirms intra-articular location of the needle. At this point the C-arm can be rotated in the sagittal plane to confirm that the needle is indeed located in an intra-articular position. Up to 1.5 ml of local anesthetic or a mixture of local anesthetic with steroid is injected.

Medial branch blocks

Initially an anteroposterior view is used and the C-arm is rotated obliquely through 15° in order to visualize the target point of the medial branch nerves. The "Scottie dog" image is seen with the target point lying high on the "eye" of the "dog" (Fig. 21.1B).

The spinal needle or radiofrequency electrode is introduced in the line of sight along the direction of the X-ray beam. The skin entry point is at the junction between the upper edge of the transverse process and the lateral edge of the superior articular process. Contact is made with bone at this target junction, then the needle is redirected more cephalad and laterally until loss of bone contact occurs in this groove (Fig. 21.3). Lateral radiographic views are taken to check the depth of the needle or electrode, which should lie level with a line joining the posterior intervertebral part of the intervertebral foramina. If it lies anterior to this line it should be withdrawn and rechecked on screening.

The preferred technique is to use a radiofrequency electrode or pole needle to permit sensory threshold testing. Stimulation at 100 Hz to detect proximity to the medial branch nerve should be elicited below 1.5 V, and this is repeated at 2 Hz to exclude proximity to the emerging segmental spinal nerve. No motor stimulation should be detected at up to 2 V. When both sensory threshold testing and radiographic screening in oblique and lateral views indicate satisfactory electrode positioning, a small volume of contrast medium (0.2 ml) can be injected to exclude any vascular uptake. If this is satisfactory, 0.5–1.0 ml of local anesthetic is then injected to produce a diagnostic block. If neurolysis is desired, then a radiofrequency lesion can be made for 60 s at 80°C using a temperature-controlled electrode. Both medial branch nerves which supply the target joint are blocked separately.

Cervical zygapophyseal blocks

For cervical procedures, the patient is placed in the supine position with the head and neck slightly extended.

Intra-articular blocks

The neck is screened using a lateral view. This permits visualization of the outline of both the right and left articular pillars superimposed. It is then necessary to rotate the C-arm slightly to separate the images. This is confirmed when the intervertebral foramina and asso-

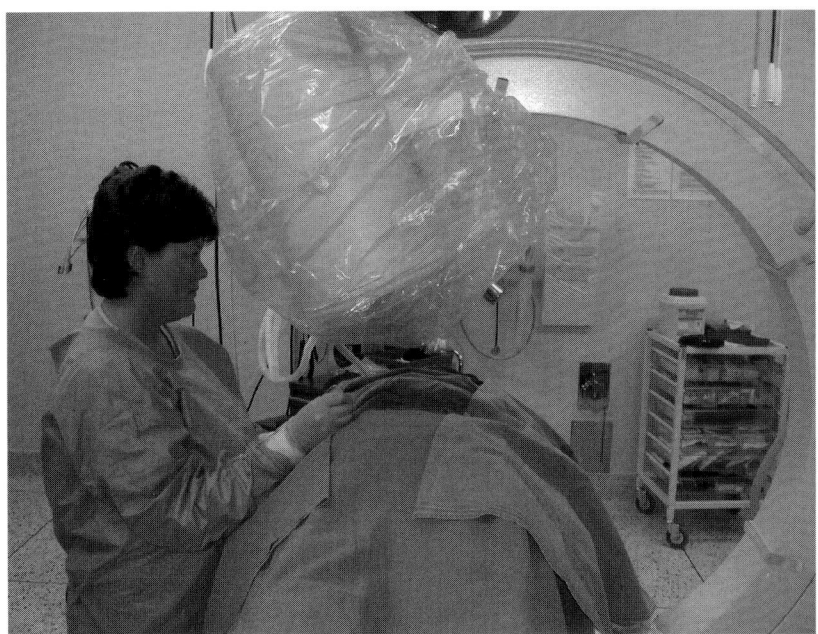

Figure 21.2 *Positioning of C-arm for "line of vision" introduction of needle toward target in lumbar spine.*

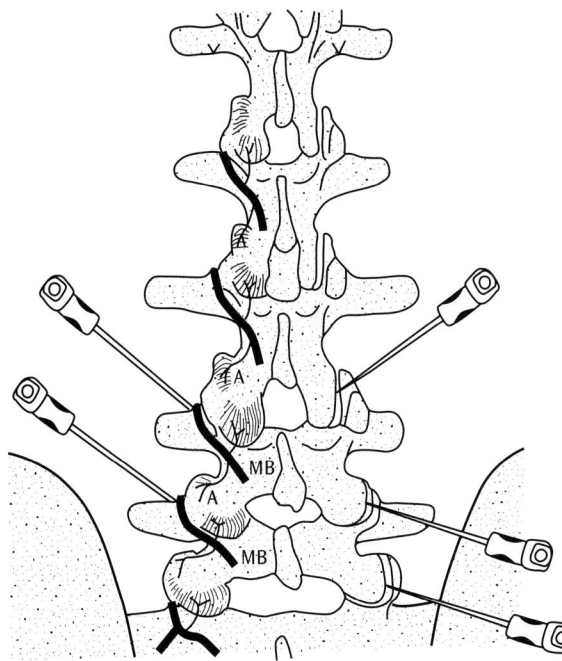

Figure 21.3 *Needle positioning for lumbar intra-articular zygapophyseal and medial branch blocks. Medial branches (MB) of the dorsal rami, and articular branches (A) are shown on the left, with needles placed L3–4, L4–5, and L5 S1 on the right. Reproduced with permission from Bogduk N. Back pain: zygapophyseal blocks and epidural Steroids. In: Cousins MJ, Bridenbaugh PO eds.* Neural Blockade in Clinical Anesthesia and Management of Pain, *2nd edn. Philadelphia, PA: JB Lippincott 1998: 935–46.*

ciated zygapophyseal joints are easily seen. Preparation and draping can be carried out once the C-arm has been set up in the appropriate position. After infiltration of the skin with local anesthetic at the entry site, just behind the posterior edge of the sternomastoid muscle, a 25-gauge

50-mm spinal needle is directed toward the target joint, already identified by radiographic screening.

This is achieved by carefully observing the image during tilting of the beam from the lateral to oblique position while the needle is in contact with bone. The joint image will appear to move in the same direction as the needle, confirming the correct target image. The degree of C-arm tilt that gives the clearest image, with the widest joint cavity view, should be used before attempting to enter the joint. If the true lateral view is not confirmed there is a risk of passing the needle through the spinal canal toward the opposite side.

To assure safety during the procedure, the needle should be in contact with bone on either the superior or inferior articular process of the target joint, and then toward the joint edge and into the joint cavity, when it is felt to "give." An arthrogram using not more than 0.3 ml of contrast confirms positioning when a sigmoid shape can be seen. Up to 1.5 ml of local anesthetic or anesthetic and steroid is then injected into the joint.

For C2–3 joints the lateral view will not show the target joint cavity particularly well, and it is necessary to turn the patient's head from the neutral position into the table to give a better view of the joint cavity, which slopes downwards and medially.

Medial branch blocks

The C-arm is initially positioned in the anterior–posterior projection and then rotated obliquely to approximately 20° and 10° caudocranially. This is to direct the X-ray beam parallel to the axis of the intervertebral foramen, and the emerging segmental nerves will also be parallel to the X-ray beam.

As the posterior primary ramus traverses the base of the superior articular process, which is easily viewed in this projection, it allows the operator to judge safely the depth between the segmental nerve and the needle tip. The entry site is behind the posterior border of the facet column and slightly below the target joint. The needle or electrode is advanced anteriorly and cranially to make bone contact with the posterior facetal column; the C-arm is then rotated to obtain an anteroposterior view. The tip of the needle should lie at the "waist" of the articular pillars on the target joint (Figs 21.4 and 21.5).

Electrical sensory threshold testing is then carried out as for the lumbar spine. Stimulation at 100 Hz should elicit sensation in the neck at below 1 V, and at 2 Hz there should be absence of motor stimulation at up to 2 V. A diagnostic block using 0.5–1.0 ml of local anesthetic is performed, following which a radiofrequency thermal lesion at 80°C for 60 s can be made if desired.

COMPLICATIONS OF ZYGAPOPHYSEAL BLOCKS

Most patients will experience significant muscular pain for several days after the procedure, but the following problems have been reported:

- motor block from spinal anesthesia;
- meningitis due to chemical irritation;
- hematoma, particularly in cervical spine procedures;
- transient ataxia and disturbed gait after upper cervical blocks;
- postdenervation pain and dysesthesia;
- local anesthetic reactions;
- superficial skin infections;
- skin burns from faulty electrodes.

Complications from radiofrequency lumbar facet denervation are uncommon if the procedure is performed carefully and with precision. Postprocedure neuritis, which manifests as a sunburn-like feeling in the area of the lesion, can occur after radiofrequency neurolysis and is often distressing to patients.. The condition usually resolves spontaneously within 6–8 weeks, and the majority of patients require only reassurance. The etiology is unknown but may be related to the denervation of the lateral branch as well as the medial branch fibers. If it is particularly distressing, a short (2-month) trial of a membrane-stabilizing drug such as carbamazepine or gabapentin can be helpful. Regeneration of the medial branch nerve may be responsible for the return of pain in patients who initially achieved good pain relief after denervation.

Relying on these interventional procedures alone is not usually sufficient to achieve prolonged relief of pain. They are considered to be best carried out in conjunction with ongoing physiotherapy and pain management treatments in order to maintain any symptomatic improvements achieved from a reduction in spinal nociceptive input.

EVIDENCE FOR THE USE OF ZYGAPOPHYSEAL JOINT BLOCKS

The reported results from zygapophyseal joint blocks vary considerably. The results of cervical spine procedures tend to be more favorable than the results of procedures in the lumbar area (16–69% vs. 69–86% effectiveness[21]). Similar outcomes have been reported whether intra-articular or medial branch blocks have been carried out.[22**,23**] In a population of patients with chronic low

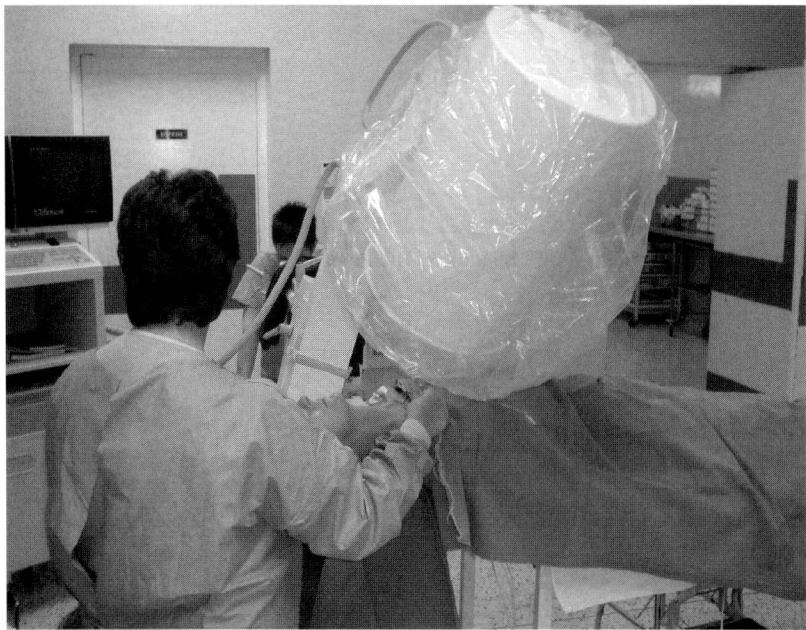

Figure 21.4 *Positioning of C-arm for "line of vision" introduction of needle toward target in cervical spine.*

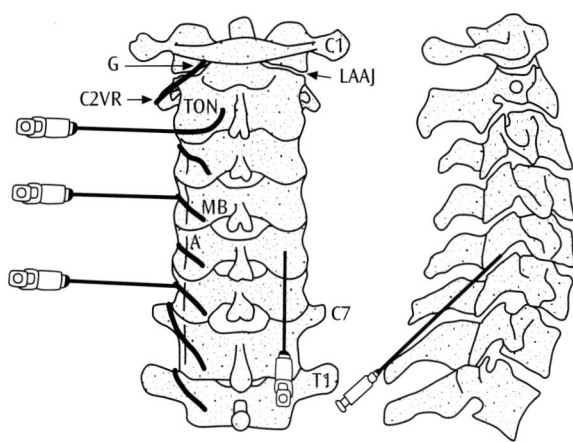

Figure 21.5 *Needle placement for cervical medial branch and intra-articular zygapophyseal blocks. Posterior view showing C2 ganglion (G) location behind the lateral atlantoaxial joint (LAAJ), C2 anterior ramus C2 UR, courses of the medial branches of the cervical dorsal rami (MB) and articular branches (A), 3rd occipital nerve (TON). Needles show position for blocking. C4 and C6 medial branches and 3rd occipital nerve. Lateral view showing needle directed into C5–6 zygapophyseal joint.Reproduced with permission from Bogduk N. Back pain: zygapophyseal blocks and epidural Steroids. In: Cousins MJ, Bridenbaugh PO eds. Neural Blockade in Clinical Anesthesia and Management of Pain, 2nd edn. Philadelphia, PA: JB Lippincott 1998: 935–46.*

back pain who received intra-articular blocks with local anesthetics, Mooney and Robertson demonstrated 60% initial relief, with 20% continuing to have complete relief at 6 months.[6*] In 1990 Silvers[24] was unable to demonstrate any benefit from using blocks with dilute phenol compared with local anesthetic and steroid. In a randomized-controlled trial Carette et al.[25**] demonstrated that zygapophyseal joint injections were of no value in patients with low back pain. In a randomized controlled study to assess the efficacy of radiofrequency denervation in patients with chronic low back pain Gallagher et al.[19**] reported a significant improvement in pain scores after denervation compared with placebo.

Sluijter and Koetsveld-Baart[26] carried out an investigation on the radiofrequency lesioning of cervical zygapophyseal joints and/or the dorsal root ganglion in patients with chronic neck pain and cervicobrachalgia. An improvement of more than 40% pain relief in 60% of the patients treated was reported. Lord et al., in 1995,[27] observed that 70% of patients achieved effective pain relief following lower cervical denervations, compared with 44% who had upper cervical denervations. This was an open prospective study and selection was based on relief of pain after diagnostic medial branch nerve blocks. In 1996, Lord et al.[28**] reported a randomized, controlled, double-blind trial of radiofrequency lesions in the lower cervical spine. In patients with chronic neck pain following whiplash injury duration of pain relief was greater when radiofrequency medial branch denervation was carried out compared with local anesthetic nerve blocks alone.

CONCLUSION

There is evidence that facet joint or medial branch blocks can alleviate chronic spinal pain of facet joint origin. These confirm the diagnosis, and longer pain relief can be achieved by denervation, usually with radiofrequency lesioning. Although these procedures are not overly difficult to perform, a standardized, meticulous technique, based on applied anatomy and supported by radiological imaging, should be used. Procedures should be carried out in an environment with immediately available resuscitation facilities.

REFERENCES

1. *Epidemiological Evidence on Back Pain*. Report of a CSAG Committee on Back Pain. London: HMSO Publications Centre, 1994: 9–21.
2. Goldthwait JR. The lumbosacral articulation: an explanation of many cases of lumbago, sciatica and paraplegia. *Boston Med Surg J* 1911; **164:** 365.
3. Mixter WJ, Barr JS. Rupture of the intervertebral disc with involvement of the spinal canal. *N Engl J Med* 1934; **211:** 210–15.
4. Bardense GAM, Weber W, van Kleef M. Treatment of spinal pain by means of radiofrequency procedures – Part I: The lumbar area. *Pain Rev* 1999; **6:** 143–54.
5. Ghormley RK. Low back pain with special reference to the articular facet, with presentation of an operative procedure. *J Am Med Assoc* 1933; **101:** 1773–7.
6. Mooney V, Robertson J. The facet syndrome. *Clin Orthop* 1976; **115:** 149–56.
7. Dwyer A, Aprill C, Bogduk N. Cervical zygapophyseal joint pain patterns. I. A study in normal volunteers. *Spine* 1990; **15:** 453–7.
8. Aprill C, Dwyer A, Bogduk N. Cervical zygapophysial joint pain patterns. II. A clinical evaluation. *Spine* 1990; **15:** 458–61.
9. Bogduk N. The lumbar vertebrae. In: *Clinical Anatomy of the Lumbar Spine and Sacrum*, 3rd edn. London: Churchill Livingstone, 1997: 1–11.
10. Bogduk N. The clinical anatomy of the cervical dorsal rami. *Spine* 1982; **7:** 319–30.
11. McCormick CC, Taylor JR, Twang LT: Facet joint arthrography in lumbar spondylosis: anatomic basis for spread of contrast medium. *Radiology* 1989; **171:** 193–6.
12. Bogduk N, Long DM. The anatomy of the so-called "articular nerves" and their relationship to facet denervation in the treatment of low back pain. *J Neurosurg* 1979; **51:** 172–7.

13. Raymond J, Dumas J. Intra-articular facet block: diagnostic test or therapeutic procedure? *Radiology* 1984; **151:** 333–6.

14. Bogduk N, Marsland A. The cervical zygapophysial joints as a source of neck pain. *Spine* 1988; **13:** 610–617.

15. Schwarzer AC, Aprill CN, Derby R, *et al*. Clinical features of patients with pain stemming from the lumbar zygapophysial joints. Is the lumbar facet syndrome a clinical entity? *Spine* 1994; **19:** 1132–7.

16. Schwarzer AC, Wang S, O'Driscoll D, Harrington T, Bogduk N, Laurent R. The ability of computed tomography to identify a painful zygapophysial joint in patients with chronic low back pain. *Spine* 1995; **20:** 907–912.

17. Schwarzer AC, Derby R, Aprill CN, *et al*. The value of the provocation response in lumbar zygapophysial joint injections. *Clin J Pain* 1994; **10:** 309–13.

18. Barnsley L, Lord S, Wallis B, Bogduk N. False positive rates of cervical zygapophysial joint blocks. *Clin J Pain* 1993; **9:** 12–30.

◆ 19. Gallagher J, Vadi PLPD, Wedley JR, *et al*. Radiofrequency facet joint denervation in the treatment of low back pain: a prospective controlled double-blind study to assess its efficacy. *Pain Clin* 1994; **7:** 193–8.

◆ 20. North RB, Kidd DH, Zahurak M, Pantiadosi S. Specificity of diagnostic nerve blocks: a prospective, randomized study of sciatica due to lumbosacral spine disease. *Pain* 1996; **65:** 77–85.

21. Pawl RP. Headache, cervical spondylosis, and anterior cervical fusion. *Surgical Annual* 1971; **9:** 391.

◆ 22. Marks RC, Houston T, Thulbourne T. Facet joint injection and facet nerve block. A randomised comparison in 86 patients with chronic low back pain. *Pain* 1992; **49:** 325 – 328.

◆ 23. Barnsley L, Lord S, Wallis B, Bogduk N. Lack of effect of intraarticular corticosteroids for chronic pain in the cervical zygapophyseal joints. *N Engl J Med* 1994; **330:** 1047–50.

24 Silvers RH. Lumbar percutaneous facet rhizotomy. *Spine* 1990; **15:** 36–40.

◆ 25. Carette S, Marcoux S, Truchon R. A controlled trial of corticosteroid injections into facet joints for chronic low back pain. *N Engl J Med* 1991; **325:** 1002–7.

26. Sluijter M, Koetsveld-Baart C. Interruption of pain pathways in the treatment of the cervical syndrome. *Anaesthesia* 1980; **35:** 302–7.

27. Lord SM, Barnsley L, Bogduk N. Percutaneous radiofrequency neurotomy in the treatment of cervical zygapophyseal joint pain: a caution. *Neurosurgery* 1995; **36:** 732–9.

◆ 28. Lord SM, Barnsley L, Wallis BJ, *et al*. Percutaneous radiofrequency neurotomy for chronic cervical zygapophyseal joint pain. *N Engl J Med* 1996; **335:** 1721–6.

22

Botulinum toxin injections

LAUREN C SEEBERGER AND CHRISTOPHER F O'BRIEN

History	277	Dose selection	280
Mechanism of action	277	Duration of benefit/additional treatments/outcomes	280
Preparation of the toxin	278	Suboptimal response or treatment failure	280
Equipment and patient considerations	278	Summary	282
Injection techniques	279	References	282

Botulinum toxin (BTX), one of the most potent neurotoxins known to man, has been harnessed for use in a variety of conditions. The attenuation and purification of the compound has led to practical everyday use without danger of causing botulism at therapeutic dosages. Although initially developed for use in conditions of eye muscle overactivity, BTX injections are used routinely for non-Food and Drug Administration-approved indications, including dystonia, spasticity, temporomandibular joint dysfunction, gastrointestinal disorders, headache, hyperhydrosis, and cosmetic muscle relaxation.[1]

HISTORY

While investigating an outbreak of food poisoning in a village in Belgium at the end of the nineteenth century, Professor van Ermengem first identified the anerobic bacillus *Clostridium botulinum*, which produces the toxin that causes botulism.[2] Subsequent isolation and purification was undertaken, with much of the research being driven by the United States National Academy of Sciences during World War II. Two important events – the crystallization of the toxin and the discovery that the toxin acts peripherally on neuromuscular junctions – led to greater understanding and the subsequent use of the toxin for experimental purposes.

In the early 1970s, Dr Alan Scott explored the medical use of BTX in monkeys with strabismus and, in 1980, results of the first clinical trial of using the type A serotype (BTX-A) were published.[3] BTX-A, Botox (Allergan), was subsequently approved in 1989 by the US Food and Drug Administration (FDA) for blepharospasm, strabis-

mus, and hemifacial spasm. Nearly a decade later, it was approved for the treatment of cervical dystonia. Dysport (Ipsen) is a different formulation of BTX-A and is currently available in Europe. The BTX type B (BTX-B), registered under the trade name Myobloc in the US and Neurobloc in Europe (Elan Pharmaceuticals), was FDA approved in December 2000. The product was shown to be beneficial in BTX-A-responsive as well as BTX-A-resistant patients.[4,5]

MECHANISM OF ACTION

There are seven structurally similar but antigenically distinct serotypes of BTX, designated A–G. The primary amino acid sequences of the neurotoxins are known for A–F. All have a similar region where activation takes place. However, the different toxin serotypes have different binding sites as well as individualized intracellular activity. The toxins primarily restrict their activity to motor nerve terminals by inhibiting acetylcholine release from pre- and postganglionic nerve endings of the autonomic nervous system. At therapeutic doses, intramuscular injection of BTX effects a dose-dependent reversible paralysis, alleviating excessive muscle contractions.[6]

For all BTX serotypes, the neurotoxin protein itself is synthesized as a single polypeptide chain with a molecular weight of about 150 kDa.[7] In this state, the neurotoxin is relatively nontoxic. However, proteolytic cleavage or "nicking" within a specific region activates the toxin, forming a di-chain compound, consisting of a heavy chain and a light chain linked by a disulfide bond. This cleavage usually occurs before the release of the toxin by the bacterium. Each chain has a specific role. The heavy chain confers extreme specificity to the molecule because of its avid binding to acceptors on the neuronal cell membrane. The heavy chain also contains the region that contributes to the unique antigenicity of each serotype. Thus, neutralizing antibodies developed against one serotype do not neutralize the effects of another.[8] The light chain is responsible for intracellular toxicity. The disulfide bond serves only to hold the chains together.

BTX proceeds through three steps to inhibit neuromuscular conduction (Fig. 22.1):[9]

1 Binding of the heavy chain to the serotype-specific acceptor on the nerve terminal. Importantly, each serotype has its own unique acceptor binding sites.
2 Internalization of the molecule. The toxin crosses the plasma membrane, and the light chain is released into the cytosol by a pH-dependent mechanism.
3 Enzymatic cleavage of one of the synaptic proteins required for docking and fusion of acetylcholine-containing vesicles. BTX-A cleaves synaptosome-associated protein (SNAP-25), whereas BTX-B cleaves synaptobrevin.

Ultimately, new nerve terminals sprout and establish temporary connections with the muscle. Evidence suggests that the new nerve terminals will fade as the original neuromuscular junction is revived and starts releasing quanta of acetylcholine.[10] Thus, BTX may act to prevent release of acetylcholine by blocking exocytosis from the nerve cell but does not interfere with storage or synthesis of acetylcholine. The action is not permanent as the neuromuscular junction will be reestablished and there are no long-term muscle fiber changes known.

PREPARATION OF THE TOXIN

The two available BTX-A products, Botox and Dysport, are lyophilized powder preparations that must be reconstituted before use. For most purposes, Botox is diluted using 1–2 ml of diluent per 100-unit vial; Dysport is diluted using 1–2 ml of diluent per 500-unit vial. The steps for reconstituting BTX-A are outlined in Table 22.1. Unlike the BTX-A products, Myobloc is produced as a liquid formulation and therefore does not require reconstitution before use. Myobloc is stable for at least 36 months in the refrigerator,[11] whereas Botox and Dysport are stored in the freezer.

Importantly, the units of toxin required for intramuscular injection differ among the available toxin preparations, a point that must be kept in mind when selecting dosages for patients. A universal system using the mouse LD_{50} bioassay has been developed to determine potency, but is not standardized. Using this system, BTX is defined in units. One unit is equivalent to the dose that is lethal in 50% of mice following an intraperitoneal injection (LD_{50}).[12] Toxicity in mice, however, does not translate to effects seen in humans. It is known that animal species are differentially sensitive to the different BTX serotypes. In nonhuman primates, the LD_{50} of BTX-A is about 24 U/kg,[13] whereas for BTX-B this dose is 1,920 U/kg.[14] In both cases, extrapolation to humans would indicate a relatively large margin for safety when used at therapeutic doses.

Clinical trials have shown that the type A preparations Dysport and Botox are not equivalent.[15] The potency ratio is 3–5 units of Dysport to 1 unit of Botox. The reason for this unit-for-unit discrepancy is not known but may reflect differing binding capabilities, diffusion, or assay techniques.[16–18] No dose conversion ratios are available comparing different BTX serotypes.

EQUIPMENT AND PATIENT CONSIDERATIONS

The patient should be placed in a comfortable position, and muscles to be injected should be fully accessible. Equipment needs are listed in Table 22.2. Beyond the initial needle penetration, BTX injections are generally not uncomfortable, and topical or subcutaneous anesthetics are usually not necessary. However, for sensitive patients or areas, topical anesthetic creams may improve tolerability of injections. Such agents should be applied 30–60 min

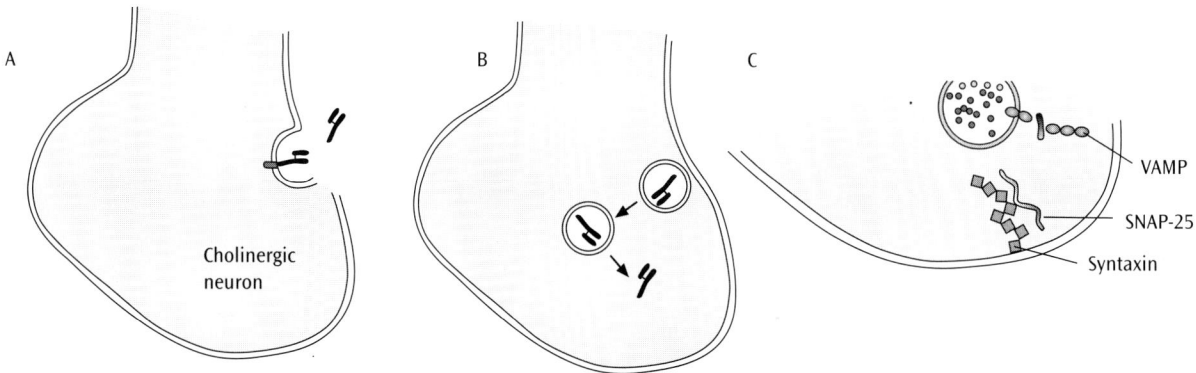

Figure 22.1 *Mechanism of action of botulinum toxin. (A) Binding. (B) Internalization. (C) Toxic action. SNAP-25, synaptosome-associated protein; VAMP, vesicle-associated membrane protein.*

Table 22.1 *Preparation of BTX-A and BTX-B*

BTX-A	BTX-B
Keep frozen at −5°C until ready to use	Keep refrigerated (≤ 36 months) or at room temperature (≤ 9 months)
Use a buffered, nonpyrogenic solution of 0.9% NaCl	
Draw up NaCl using a 25-gauge or larger needle	May dilute with 0.9% NaCl
Slowly introduce NaCl into vial, avoiding agitation and bubbling	Draw up NaCl using a 25-gauge or larger needle
	Use toxin within 4 h (for sterility)
Gently swirl mixture then withdraw using 25-gauge or larger needle	Dispose vial containing residual toxin in proper biohazardous waste container
Use toxin within 4 h (for sterility)	
Dispose of vial containing residual toxin in proper biohazardous waste container	

Table 22.2 *Equipment requirements for electromyographic (EMG)-guided injections*

Teflon-coated, hollow-bore EMG needle
Reference lead with surface electrode
Standard or portable EMG machine
Syringe with 25-gauge needle or larger for mixing
Gauze and alcohol wipes
Preservative-free, nonpyrogenic 0.9% NaCl
BTX product
Freezer storage for BTX-A; BTX-B can be refrigerated

Table 22.3 *Potential adverse effects of BTX*

Weakness of injected and adjacent muscles
Hematoma/bruising
Infection at injection site
Transient swelling
Focal atrophy
Influenza-like symptoms
Increased pain
Brachial plexopathy (rare)
Allergic reaction (rare)

Table 22.4 *BTX contraindications*

Pregnant or lactating women
Patients with myasthenia gravis or Eaton–Lambert syndrome
Patients with motor neuron disease (ALS)
Aminoglycoside antibiotics
Infection at injection site

ALS, amyotrophic lateral sclerosis.

prior to injections for maximal effect. Dilution of either BTX-A or BTX-B with preserved saline may reduce local pain on injection.[19]

A full explanation of the potential risks and benefits of BTX injection should be provided to the patient. The most common adverse effect is weakness in the injected and adjacent muscles. Patients can be assured, however, that the weakness will be temporary. Special consideration is given to areas where excessive weakness can have profound implications, such as dysphagia following laryngeal injections. In these situations, appropriate supportive care is required (e.g. alteration of diet or placement of nasogastric tube to prevent aspiration). Influenza-like symptoms occurring the day after injections have been reported; however, this effect is self-limited and not associated with fever or vomiting. Patients may experience increased pain as the injections become effective because of shifts in muscle use patterns. Potential risks of BTX injections are listed in Table 22.3. Contraindications are listed in Table 22.4.

Care must be used in patients with muscular diseases and/or already present weakness (e.g. multiple sclerosis). Patients on anticoagulation therapy may be injected safely as long as adequate measures are taken to avoid hematoma formation. It is not contraindicated to give patients injections if they are on antibiotics, with the exception of aminoglycosides. Patients can drive afterwards, do not need to be accompanied, and may resume usual activities and medications after BTX injections.

INJECTION TECHNIQUES

There remains controversy about the best method of injecting BTX. Some advocate injection near motor endplates whereas others report no difference in effectiveness of the toxin using this tedious approach. Likewise, reports of increased benefit associated with electromyographic (EMG) guidance balance those suggesting no additional benefit from the technique.[20,21]

EMG guidance may help to assist in precise localization of the needle tip in target muscles.[20] Target muscles are first selected based upon observed biomechanics (e.g. excessive forearm pronation, cervical rotation). Then, target muscles are localized by clinical assessment using palpation of muscle belly and tendon accompanied by passive and active range of motion of the affected joint. Motor unit potentials are recorded from the tip of the EMG needle and localization can be confirmed by repeating active and passive maneuvers of the selected muscle. Crisp-sounding, well-formed motor unit potentials indicate close proximity to a contracting muscle fascicle. The needle should be repositioned if poorly formed or "distant-sounding" units are encountered.

Adjacent nontarget muscles should also be tested to avoid inadvertent injection and unwanted weakness. EMG studies in nonhuman primates show that BTX-B exhibits significantly less denervation to distant noninjected muscles than BTX-A, which may have implications in terms of dosing.[11] Confirmation of correct needle placement in the intended muscle is outlined in Table 22.5. Once placement has been properly confirmed, injections can be initiated. It is suggested that multiple small (volume) dose injections be used. More than 0.5 ml of fluid may disrupt muscle fibers. A full discussion of EMG setup, technique, and interpretation is beyond the scope of this chapter.

DOSE SELECTION

There are no set BTX dosages for any particular muscle, but guidelines have been established for the most commonly injected muscles. The doses used for treatment of spasticity are provided in Table 22.6. Dosing guidelines for other conditions (e.g. cervical dystonia) and other muscles may be accessed online at www.wemove.org. One of the most difficult tasks is to determine appropriate dosages when many muscles are involved without exceeding dose limitations. In this case, one must select target muscles for specific functional goals and choose the optimal dose possible to achieve the desired clinical effect. When selecting dose, many factors must be considered: muscle size, severity of muscle spasm, preexisting weakness, and the desired weakness from the procedure. For patients who have already undergone injections, assessment of their clinical response is critical in determining future placement and doses of BTX. When becoming familiar with BTX, it is valuable to see patients several weeks after injection for a better understanding of intervention and outcome.

Table 22.5 *Steps to ensure correct electromyographic (EMG) needle placement*

Insert EMG needle into selected muscle

Encourage the patient to relax if muscle activity immediately present (muscles in spasm may have constant activation)

Move selected muscle/tendon unit through passive range of motion and monitor EMG activity (should be active and crisp sounding)

Move nontarget muscle/tendon unit through passive range of motion and monitor EMG activity (should be minimal or absent in nontargeted area)

Have patient attempt active range of motion of selected muscle/tendon unit while monitoring EMG activity

Have patient attempt active range of motion of nonselected muscle/tendon unit while monitoring EMG activity

DURATION OF BENEFIT/ADDITIONAL TREATMENTS/OUTCOMES

Onset of effect with BTX is usually 2–14 days. The average duration of clinical benefit is 12–16 weeks. Duration of subclinical electrophysiologic effect may last up to 12 months. Patients with severe spasticity may have shorter duration of clinical benefit, whereas patients with dystonia of small facial muscles may have a longer duration of benefit. The degree of benefit is greater than the weakness caused by the toxin, a fact that suggests selective blocking of the most active nerve terminals, as is seen in experimental animal models. Hallett and colleagues[22] contend that encouraging frequent muscle contraction during BTX binding could improve outcome. Stimulation of the injected muscles after BTX may improve clinical effect, possibly allowing the use of lower doses.[23,24]

If the purpose of the injections is to improve mobility and joint range of motion, then early physical or occupational therapy is warranted. Physical and occupational therapists are extremely helpful in determining goals for the patient as well as assessing improvement following the procedure. Stretching is an important part of the posttreatment plan, as is strengthening of opposing muscles. Patients should not try to strengthen target muscles as the injections are meant to cause graded muscle weakness and relaxation. Clinical scales assessing the primary goal of treatment should be performed at baseline, at 2 weeks, and at 12 weeks postinjection.

The following are allowed after BTX injections:

- acupuncture;
- massage;
- transcutaneous electrical nerve stimulation (TENS);
- physical therapy, adaptive equipment as needed;
- occupational therapy, adaptive equipment as needed;
- stretching;
- serial casting;
- oral agents for spasticity or pain;
- intrathecal agents for spasticity or pain.

SUBOPTIMAL RESPONSE OR TREATMENT FAILURE

The most common causes of poor response to BTX are incorrect dosage, incorrect muscle choice, or inappropriate selection of treatment goal. Examination of the injected muscles should show weakness or atrophy in muscle groups injected, and EMG testing should confirm denervation changes. Over time, some patients exposed to BTX may form neutralizing antibodies that lead to clinical nonresponsiveness with subsequent injections. Neutralizing antibodies have been reported in up to 10–17% of patients treated with BTX-A.[25–27] Data addressing the occurrence of antibody formation with BTX-B are

Table 22.6 *Dosing guidelines for BTX-A (Botox) and BTX-B (Myobloc) in the treatment of spasticity*

Clinical pattern	Potential muscles involved	Botox Dose range (units)	Botox Number of injection sites	Myobloc Dose range (units)	Myobloc Number of injection sites
Upper limbs					
Adducted/internally rotated shoulder	Pectoralis complex	75–150	2–4	2,500–5,000	2–6
	Latissimus dorsi	50–150	3 or 4	2,500–5,000	2–6
	Teres major	25–100	1 or 2	1,000–3,000	1–4
	Subscapularis	50–100	1 or 2	1,000–3,000	1 or 2
Flexed elbow	Brachioradialis	25–100	1–3	1,000–3,000	2–4
	Biceps	75–200	2–4	2,500–5,000	2–4
	Brachialis	40–100	2	1,000–3,000	2
Pronated forearm	Pronator quadratus	10–50	1	1,000–2,500	1 or 2
	Pronator teres	25–75	1 or 2	1,000–2,500	1 or 2
Flexed wrist	Flexor carpi radialis	25–100	2	1,000–3,000	1 or 2
	Flexor carpi ulnaris	20–70	2	1,000–3,000	1 or 2
Thumb-in-palm	Flexor pollicis longus	10–30	1	1,000–2,500	1 or 2
	Adductor pollicis	5–25	1	500–2,500	1
	Opponens	5–25	1	500–1,500	1
Clenched fist/fingers	Flexor digitorum superficialis	20–40	1	1,000–3,000	1 or 2
	Flexor digitorum profundus	20–40	1	1,000–3,000	1 or 2
Intrinsic hand	Lumbricales/interossei (per hand)	5–10	1	1,500–4,500	3
Lower limbs					
Flexed hip	Iliacus/iliopsoas	50–200	2	3,000–7,500	2 or 3
	Psoas	50–200	2	3,000–7,500	1 or 2
	Rectus femoris	75–200	3	2,500–5,000	1–3
Flexed knee	Medial hamstrings	50–200	3	2,500–7,500	2–4
	Gastrocnemius (as knee flexor)	50–150	4	3,000–7,500	2–4
	Lateral hamstrings	100–200	3	2,500–7,500	2–4
Adducted thighs	Adductor brevis/longus/magnus	75–300	6	5,000–10,000	2–6
Stiff (extended) knee	Quadriceps	50–200	6	5,000–7,500	2–6
Equinovarus foot	Gastrocnemius	50–250	4	3,000–7,500	2–4
	Soleus	50–200	2	2,500–5,000	1–3
	Tibialis posterior	50–150	2	3,000–7,500	1–3
	Tibialis anterior	50–150	2 or 3	2,500–5,000	1 or 2
	Flexor digitorum longus	50–100	3	2,500–5,000	1 or 2
	Flexor digitorum brevis	20–40	1	2,500–5,000	1 or 2
	Flexor hallucis longus	25–75	2	1,500–3,500	1 or 2
Striatal toe	Extensor hallucis longus	20–100	2	2,000–4,000	1 or 2
Neck					
	Sternocleidomastoid	25–100	3	1,000–3,000	1–4
	Scalenus complex	15–50	3	1,000–3,000	2–4
	Splenius capitis	50–150	3	1,000–5,000	2–4
	Semispinalis capitis	50–150	3	1,000–5,000	2–4
	Longissimus capitis	50–150	3	1,000–5,000	2–4
	Trapezius	50–150	3	1,000–5,000	2–6
	Levator scapulae	25–100	3	1,000–4,000	2–4

Information obtained from WeMove website (www.wemove.org).

currently not available, although estimates of prevalence in cervical dystonia patients of 18% are listed in the prescribing information for BTX-B. Again, neutralizing antibodies to one serotype have not been reported to affect the activity of another. Therefore, if treatment resistance against one serotype is confirmed in a patient, benefits can still be attained with an alternate serotype.

The primary factors in developing antibodies appear to be younger age at onset of illness, higher mean dose of BTX per visit, and overall high cumulative dose.[28] Additionally, giving booster doses within 1 month after injections increases the likelihood of developing immunity.[25] To decrease the risk of resistance, patients initiated on BTX therapy should be injected as infrequently as possible (no more than once every 3 months), the lowest effective doses should be used, and booster injections should be avoided (Table 22.7).

If uncertainty as to resistance persists, a test dose of BTX may be administered in the frontalis muscle unilaterally and the patient reevaluated after 2 weeks (Fig. 22.2). If the patient is able to move the injected muscle at this time, then he/she is considered to be resistant to that toxin. For Botox, the test dose is 15 units, divided into two 7.5-unit doses. For Myobloc, preliminary studies indicate that 750–1,000 units is appropriate.

Serological tests can be used to determine the presence of BTX antibodies in sera. The mouse LD_{50} bioassay is most commonly used for this purpose. This assay has been found to be highly specific but is rather low in sensitivity.[29] Recently, Hanna and colleagues[30] compared the immunoprecipitation assay (IPA)[31] with the mouse bioassay. They evaluated clinical response in 83 patients previously treated with Botox, and found that the IPA was more sensitive and nearly as specific as the mouse bioassay in detecting neutralizing antibodies. Advantages of IPA are its quantitative nature permitting serial measurements of antibody titers and lack of need for live animal testing. Neither IPA nor mouse bioassay are commercially available yet. Importantly, tests of nonresponsiveness using unilateral brow or frontalis injections correlate well with patient clinical status, lending more weight to the use of this simple tool to determine resistance to BTX. The overall clinical significance of antibody testing remains unknown.

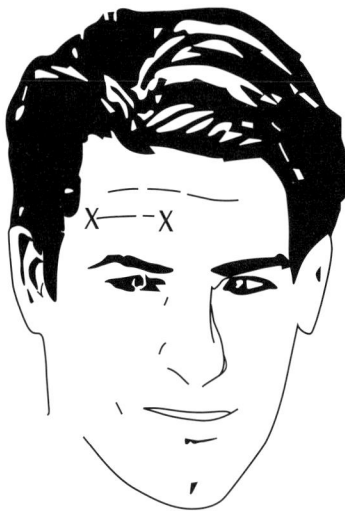

Figure 22.2 *Injection sites for test doses. The frontalis injection sites are indicated by an X (= 7.5 units Botox or 500 units Myobloc).*

SUMMARY

BTX has become a valuable treatment tool for a variety of clinical conditions that involve muscle overactivity. Two BTX-A preparations, Botox and Dysport, and a new liquid preparation of BTX-B, Myobloc, are currently available (Dysport available in Europe only). The toxins have similar structural, pharmacological, and clinical properties. However, in terms of binding sites, target protein, formulation (i.e. lyophilized powder versus liquid), spread effects, and units for dosing, they are uniquely distinct, such that each should be considered its own chemical entity. Clinical studies to establish the use of these agents in numerous therapeutic areas are already under way and should show promising results.

REFERENCES

● 1. Bell MS, Vermeulen LC, Sperling KB. Pharmacotherapy with botulinum toxin: harnessing nature's most potent neurotoxin. *Pharmacotherapy* 2000; **20:** 1079–91.

2. van Ermengen E. Ueber einem neuen anaeroben Bacillus und seine eziehungen zum Botulismus. *Z Hyg Infektionskrankh* 1887; **26:** 1–56 (in English: *Rev Infect Dis* 1979; **1:** 701–19).

3. Scott AB. Botulinum toxin injection into extraocular muscles as an alternative to strabismus surgery. *Ophthalmology* 1980; **87:** 1044–9.

◆ 4. Brashear A, Lew MF, Dykstra DD, *et al.* Safety and efficacy of Neurobloc (botulinum toxin type B) in type-A responsive cervical dystonia. *Neurology* 1999; **53:** 1439–46.

◆ 5. Brin MF, Lew MF, Adler CH, *et al.* Safety and efficacy of

Table 22.7 *Guidelines for reducing the risk of resistance to BTX[a]*

Inject at 12 weeks or longer interval
Use lowest effective dose
Avoid booster injections, even if benefit is less than desired

a. Consider "test" injections in the eyebrow or frontalis muscle to confirm whether patient is nonresponsive.

NeuroBloc (botulinum toxin type B) in type-A resistant cervical dystonia. *Neurology* 1999; **53:** 1431–8.

6. Hambleton P. Clostridium botulinum toxins: a general review of involvement in disease, structure, mode of action and preparation for clinical use. *J Neurol* 1992; **239:** 16–20.

● 7. Montecucco C, Schiavo G. Structure and function of tetanus and botulinum neurotoxins. *Q Rev Biophys* 1995;28:423–72.

8. Halpern JL, Smith LA, Seamon KB, *et al.* Sequence homology between tetanus and botulinum toxins detected by an antipeptide antibody. *Infect Immun* 1989; **57:** 18–22.

9. Oguma K, Fujinaga Y, Inouek. Structure and function of Clostridium botulinum toxins. *Microbiol Immunol* 1995; **39:** 161–8.

10. De Paiva A, Meunier FA, Molgo J, *et al.* Functional repair of motor endplates after botulinum neurotoxin type A poisoning: biphasic switch of synaptic activity between nerve sprouts and their parent terminals. *Proc Natl Acad Sci USA* 1999; **96:** 3200–5.

● 11. Callaway J, Arezzo JC, Grethlein AJ. Botulinum toxin type B: an overview of its biochemistry and preclinical pharmacology. *Semin Cutan Med Surg* 2001; **20:** 127–36.

12. Schantz EJ, Kautter DA. Standardization assay for Clostridium botulinum toxins. *J Assoc Off Anal Chem* 1978; **61:** 96–9.

13. Botox® Product Monograph. Botox® botulinum toxin type A purified neurotoxin complex. Allergan, Inc., Irvine, CA, 1998.

14. Meyer KE, Caputo FA, Gasper C, Shopp GM. Botulinum toxin type B, NeuroBloc: comparable systemic toxicities in adult and juvenile cynomolgus monkeys. *Mov Disord* 2000; **15** (Suppl. 3): 158–9.

15. Brin MF, Blitzer A. Botulinum toxin: dangerous terminology errors. *J R Soc Med* 1993; **86:** 493–4.

◆ 16. Odergren T, Hjaltason H, Kaakkola S, *et al.* A double-blind, randomized, parallel group study to investigate the dose equivalence of Dysport and Botox in the treatment of cervical dystonia. *J Neurol Neurosurg Psychiatry* 1998; **64:** 6–12.

17. Van den Bergh P, Lison DF. Dose standardization of botulinum toxin in dystonia. In: Fahn S, Marsden CD, DeLong M eds. *Advances in Neurology*. Philadelphia, PA: Lippincott-Raven Publishers, 1998; 231–5.

18. Whurr R, Brookes G, Barnes C. Comparison of dosage effects between the American and the British botuli-num toxin A product in the treatment of spasmodic dysphonia. *Mov Disord* 1995; **10:** 56.

19. Alam M, Dover JS, Arndt KA. Pain associated with injection of botulinum A exotoxin reconstituted using isotonic sodium chloride with and without preservative: a double-blind, randomized controlled trial. Archives Dermatol 2002; **138** (4): 510–4.

● 20. Barbano RL. Needle EMG guidance for injection of botulinum toxin: needle EMG guidance is useful. *Muscle Nerve* 2001; **24:** 567–8.

21. Jankovic J. Needle EMG guidance for injection of botulinum toxin: needle EMG guidance is rarely required. *Muscle Nerve* 2001; **24:** 568–70.

22. Hallett M, Glocker FX, Deuschl G. Mechanism of action of botulinum toxin. *Ann Neurol* 1994; **36:** 449.

23. Hesse S, Reiter F, Konrad M, Jahnke MT. Botulinum toxin type A and short-term electrical stimulation in the treatment of upper limb flexor spasticity after stroke: a randomized, double-blind, placebo-controlled trial. *Clin Rehabil* 1998; **12:** 381–8.

24. Hesse S, Jahnke MT, Luecke D, Mauritz KH. Short-term electrical stimulation enhances the effectiveness of botulinum toxin in the treatment of lower limb spasticity in hemiparetic patients. *Neurosci Lett* 1995; **201:** 37–40.

25. Greene P, Fahn S, Diamond B. Development of resistance to botulinum toxin type A in patients with torticollis. *Mov Disord* 1994; **9:** 213–17.

26. Jankovic J, Schwartz KS. Clinical correlates of response to botulinum toxin injections. *Arch Neurol* 1991; **48:** 1253–6.

27. Zuber M, Sebald M, Bathien N, *et al.* Botulinum antibodies in dystonic patients treated with type A botulinum toxin: frequency and significance. *Neurology* 1993; **43:** 1715–18.

28. Jankovic J, Schwartz K. Response and immunoresistance to botulinum toxin injections. *Neurology* 1995; **45:** 1743–6.

◆ 29. Hanna PA, Jankovic J. Mouse bioassay versus western blot assay for botulinum toxin antibodies: correlation with clinical response. *Neurology* 1998; **50:** 1624–9.

30. Hanna PA, Jankovic J, Vincent A. Comparison of mouse bioassay and immunoprecipitation assay for botulinum toxin antibodies. *J Neurol Neurosurg Psychiatry* 1999; **66:** 612–16.

31. Palace J, Nairne A, Hyman N, *et al.* A radioimmunoprecipitation assay for antibodies to botulinum A. *Neurology* 1998; **50:** 1463–6.

23

Long-term intrathecal and intracisternal treatment of malignant- and nonmalignant-related pain using external pumps

PETRE V NITESCU, LENNART K APPELGREN (DECEASED), AND IOAN D CURELARU

History	285	Side-effects and complications of intrathecal pain treatment and their management	300
Applied anatomy and physiology	286		
Indications	286	Side-effects and complications of high cervical intrathecal–intracisternal pain treatment and their management	302
Limitations	288		
Technique of intrathecal catheterization	288		
Technique of high cervical (intrathecal) and intracisternal catheterization	295	Advantages of the intrathecal/intracisternal pain treatment	303
Insertion complications	295	Advantages of externalized intrathecal catheters and pumps over implanted intrathecal catheters and pumps	303
Solutions (drugs, concentrations, mixtures, proportions)	295		
Guidelines for adjustment of the intrathecal pain treatment	297	Disadvantages of the intrathecal pain treatment	304
Clinical results	298	Efficiency of the intrathecal pain treatment	304
Care of the patient and of the infusion system	298	References	305

The data presented in this chapter are based on the results obtained from 548 patients – 406 with malignant and 142 with nonmalignant "refractory" pain conditions – treated with intrathecal administration of bupivacaine with or without opioids (morphine or buprenorphine, $n = 519$), or with intracisternal infusions of bupivacaine alone ($n = 29$, 15 with malignant and 14 with nonmalignant pain), between 16 December 1985 and 1 March 1999.

HISTORY

Intrathecal catheterization

In 1985, Arnér and Arnér[1]* reported on the inefficacy of epidural morphine alone to relieve some types of pain, such as:

- neurogenic/neuropathic pain;
- intermittent nociceptive pain of both somatic and visceral origin;
- severe, refractory pain from mucocutaneous ulcers.

In 1986, Hjortsjø et al.[2]* reported on the potentiation of spinal morphine antinociception by spinal bupivacaine. The following year, Kroin et al.[3] reported on the effects of chronic subarachnoid bupivacaine infusion in dogs.

In 1990, in a clinical crossover study with administration of bupivacaine/morphine infusions by the epidural–intrathecal route, Nitescu et al.[4]** demonstrated the superiority of the latter. The following year, Nitescu et al.[5] described a technique for long-term intrathecal catheterization for the treatment of chronic pain and Sjöberg et al.[6]* reported on the first series of 52 patients with refractory cancer pain treated with long-term intrathecal administration of morphine and bupivacaine.

High intrathecal–intracisternal catheterization

Crul *et al.*[7] reported in 1994 on the long-term continuous intrathecal administration of morphine and bupivacaine into the anterior subarachnoid space at the upper cervical level accessed by a lateral C1–C2 puncture.

In 1996, Appelgren *et al.*[8]* reported on the continuous intracisternal administration of bupivacaine infusions for long-term treatment of refractory malignant and nonmalignant pain.

APPLIED ANATOMY AND PHYSIOLOGY

The spinal intrathecal space

This space is confined between the inside of the dura mater (theca) and the outside of the spinal cord and is divided into two compartments:

1 The spinal subdural space is located between the inside of the dura mater and the outside of the arachnoid. This space is usually virtual, having a sagittal diameter of 0.05–0.25 mm.
2 The spinal subarachnoid space is situated between the inside of the arachnoid and the outside of the spinal cord covered by the pia mater. The subarachnoid space is divided into two compartments (anterior and posterior) that are separated by the denticulate ligaments.

In adult patients, the dorsal subarachnoid space has sagittal diameters ranging from 4.75 to 5.75 mm. This is sufficiently wide to accommodate the bevel of a 17-gauge Tuohy needle (~ 3 mm) or of an intrathecal catheter with an outer diameter of 1.1 mm (Fig. 23.1).

The subarachnoid space is filled with cerebrospinal fluid (CSF), which is produced by the arterial choroid plexus by secretion and ultrafiltration. The daily production of the CSF is as large as its total volume, i.e. approximately 150 ml, of which 25–30 ml is located in the spinal subarachnoid space. After a small loss of CSF, its production may increase from ~ 150 to 432 ml/day, and after a larger loss to about 800 ml/day. At 37°C, the CSF specific weight ranges between 1.003 and 1.009, and its physiological pH between 7.4 and 7.6. A small CSF loss of 20 ml results in headache, which is promptly relieved (within 2–4 min) by a subarachnoid injection of 20 ml isotonic saline.[9] A loss of ~ 245 ml CSF per day after a dural puncture with a 23-gauge needle has been reported.[10] The daily CSF loss after a puncture with a 17-gauge Tuohy needle is unknown.

We have found that the distance from the skin to the subarachnoid space punctured at the L2–L3 interspace, measured in 30 adult patients, ranged from 3.5 to 8.0 cm (median = 5.5 cm).

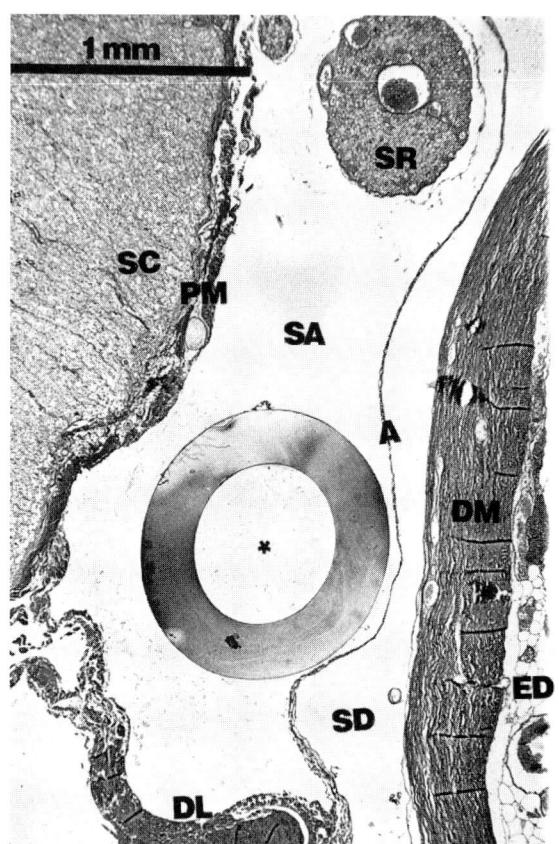

Figure 23.1 *Neurohistopathologic image showing catheterization of the subarachnoid space. SC, spinal cord; PM, pia mater; SR, spinal root in the subarachnoid space (SA); asterisk, intrathecal catheter lumen; A, arachnoid; SD, subdural space; DM, dura mater; ED, epidural space filled with loose connective tissue; DL, denticulate ligament. There is no sign of reaction on the catheter surface and the adjacent nerve roots. Staining method: van Gieson.*

The intracisternal space

The cerebellomedullary cistern or cisterna magna is an expansion of the subarachnoid space lying between the cerebellum and the medulla oblongata (Fig. 23.2). The cerebellomedullary cistern has a length of 5–6 cm and a depth (distance between the arachnoid and the posterior surfaces of the spinal cord and medulla oblongata) of 1.5 cm.[11] A needle inserted from the back of the neck, just above the spine of axis, having its tip directed towards the nose root *(glabella)*, would reach the medullary part of the cisterna magna after 3–5 cm.

INDICATIONS

Intrathecal administration of opioids and bupivacaine

The intrathecal administration of opioids and bupivacaine is indicated for:

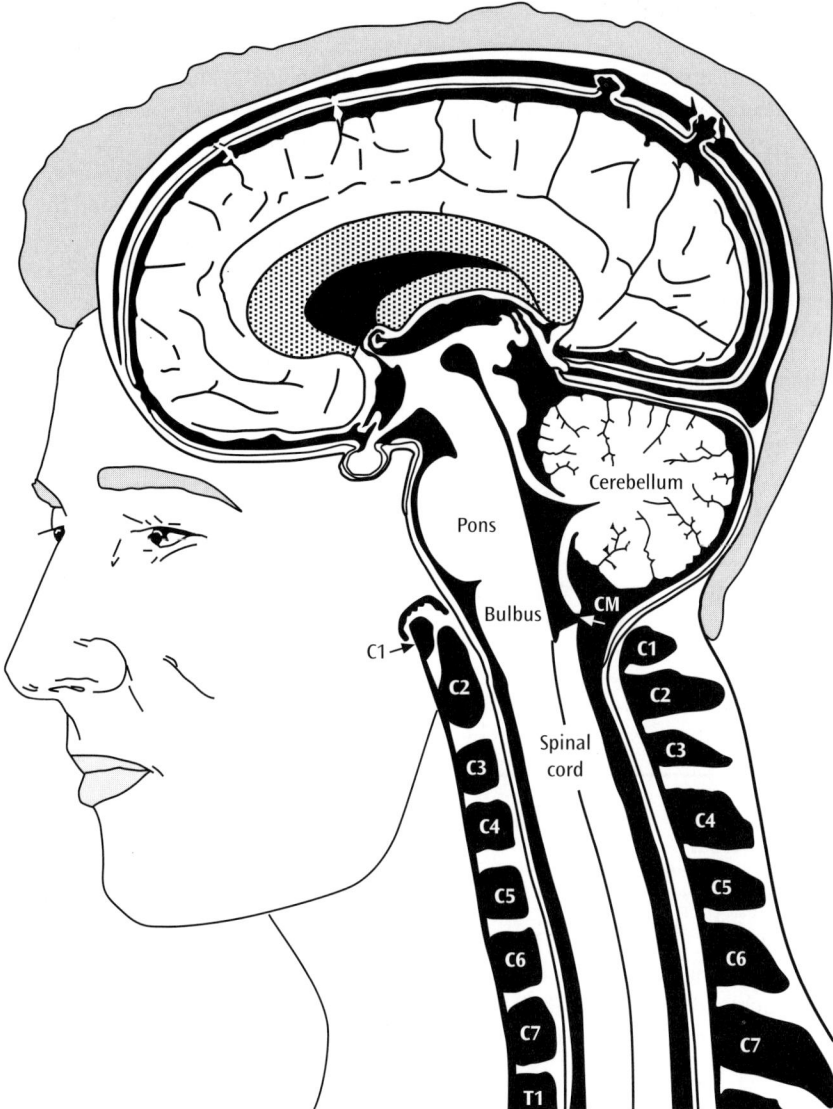

Figure 23.2 *Sketch of the cisterna magna (CM). The small arrow indicates the foramen of Magendie. Bulbus is synonymous with medulla oblongata (modified from Netter[27]).*

1 Treatment of "refractory" malignant pain:
   a Pain resistant to high doses of oral and/or parenteral morphine.
   b Types of pain inadequately relieved by epidural opioids and/or local anesthetics, or intrathecal opioids, e.g. some intermittent somatic and intermittent visceral pains, most neuropathic pains, pain due to mucocutaneous ulcers, etc.
   c Pain relieved by systemic opioids but with intolerable side-effects (nausea, vomiting, constipation, allergic reactions, etc.).
   d Pain conditions in which other therapeutic alternatives [e.g. epidural injections of butamben, dorsal column stimulation (DCS), neurolytic blockades, chordotomy, and/or other neurosurgical procedures) are not applicable or offered insufficient pain relief.

2 Treatment of "refractory" nonmalignant pain. The intrathecal treatment proved to be effective in:[12*]
   a Nociceptive musculoskeletal pain.
   b Nociceptive visceral pain.
   c Neurogenic pain (e.g. acute herpes zoster).
   d Peripheral neuropathic pain:
      i   Amyloidosis polyneuropathy.
      ii Postherpetic neuralgia.
   e Some forms of central neuropathic pain (e.g. myelosclerosis) in which intrathecal bupivacaine may relieve both refractory pain and spasticity.
   f Intractable mixed pain in the spine (e.g. that caused by vertebral compression fractures due to osteoporosis).
   g Intractable mixed pain in the extremities, e.g. from:

    i   Progressive systemic sclerosis associated with Raynaud's phenomena.

    ii   Arterial or venous insufficiency with ischemic pain and skin ulcerations in the lower extremities.

Intracisternal infusion of bupivacaine

Intracisternal infusion of bupivacaine has been successfully used in patients with:

1 "Refractory" malignant head, face, and/or neck pain conditions.
2 "Refractory" nonmalignant pain conditions, such as:
    a Trigeminal postherpetic neuralgia.
    b Chronic, refractory pain conditions from the cervical spine.

The indications for treatment of refractory nonmalignant pain conditions should be viewed with skepticism until more clinical experience is accumulated.

LIMITATIONS

Intrathecal catheterization

1 Malignant pain. Insufficient pain relief may be expected in patients with:
    a Malignant myeloma: accumulation of calcareous plaques in the subarachnoid space limits diffusion of bupivacaine and opioid to the nerve roots and spinal cord.
    b Large epidural metastases.
    c Presence of an epidural abscess and/or meningitis.
    d Presence of medullary infarction or medullary abscess.[13*]
    e Occurrence of adhesive arachnoiditis impeding diffusion of intrathecal analgesics within the subarachnoid space and through the spinal cord.
2 Nonmalignant pain. The intrathecal treatment may be unsatisfactory in:
    a Patients with complex regional pain syndrome type I (CRPS-I).
    b Some forms of central neuropathic pains (e.g. from ischemic and post-traumatic myelopathy).
    c Some forms of mixed pain in the spine, such as:
        i   Spinal/radicular pain after failed spinal surgery.
        ii   Grotesque spondylosis with arthritis.
        iii Idiopathic coccydynia.
    d All cases in which:
        i   Psychosocial factors (e.g. anxiety, hysteria, dysnosognosia, obsessive–compulsive neurosis, malingering, and alcohol and drug abuse).

        ii   Unsolved compensation claims are present, regardless of the basic pain syndrome.
3 Both malignant and nonmalignant pain. Intrathecal pain treatment at home should not be undertaken in:
    a Moribund patients.
    b Patients with overt psychoses,
    c Cases when the patient and the family do not accept the treatment.
    d Patients treated with DCS.[14]
    e Situations in which the back-up is insufficient (nurse, doctor, and hospital bed not accessible round the clock).[15***]

Intracisternal catheterization

1 Intractable pain from the shoulder and upper limb (an intrathecal catheter with the tip located at C5–C6 is preferred).
2 Presence of an intracranial metastasis with intracranial hypertension, as the subarachnoid puncture may lead to downward coning of the brainstem deprived of its hydraulic (CSF) cushion.

TECHNIQUE OF INTRATHECAL CATHETERIZATION

Preparation of patient

Preparation of the patient includes:

1 Obtaining informed consent from the patient and his/her next of kin.
2 Performing an intrathecal bupivacaine test: 2.5–15 mg (0.5–3.0 ml of iso- or hyperbaric bupivacaine) injected at an appropriate intervertebral space.
3 Giving antibiotics during the insertion procedure and for 3 days thereafter.
4 Rehydrating: an i.v. infusion with 500 ml dextran and 1,000 ml Ringer–glucose solution is started in the ward department or on the operating table.
5 Giving relatively deep sedation: i.v. titrated doses of 0.05–0.15 mg fentanyl combined with 0.5–5.0 mg midazolam, or 2.5–5.0 mg droperidol.
6 Giving oxygen: 30–40% oxygen in air by mask, or 2–3 l/min via a nasal catheter.

Equipment

1 For antisepsis and clothing:
    a DesCutan sponge (Pharmacia & Upjohn, Sverige, Solna, Sweden) impregnated with a 4% chlorhexidine solution.
    b Surgical drapes and surgical sterile tape.

2 For anesthesia:
  a A 22-gauge needle for spinal anesthesia.
  b Injection needles for filling syringes and infiltrating local anesthetic.
  c Solutions of local anesthetics: 1% mepivacaine without epinephrine (adrenaline) (Carbocaine; Astra, Södertälje, Sweden) for infiltration anesthesia at the tunnel level; 0.5% iso- or hyperbaric (heavy) solution of bupivacaine (Marcain; Astra, Södertälje, Sweden) for spinal anesthesia.
  d Narcosis apparatus available.
3 For dural puncture and intrathecal catheterization:
  a A 17-gauge (1.2–1.5 mm internal–external diameters), 9-cm-long Tuohy needle with sharp bevel; longer needles (15 or even 20 cm) should be used in obese patients.
  b A clear, nylon 18-gauge, relatively stiff catheter (Portex 100/382/116; Portex, Hythe, Kent, UK), 1.1 mm outer diameter, 900 mm long, provided with three lateral eyes, closed end, marks at 60, 70, 80, 90, 100, 150 and 200 mm from the tip, and a detachable Luer lock connection.
4 For catheter tunneling:
  a Surgical instruments: fine surgical knife with straight edges; Péan and mosquito forceps; fine surgical pincers with and without claws; small basins for isotonic saline and local anesthetic solutions.
  b A Portex tunneling instrument 04-380-999, 35 cm long (Portex, Hythe, Kent, UK).
  c Plastic glue (cyanoacrylate ester, e.g. Super Glue).[16]
5 For catheter fixation:
  a A split Silastic or rubber cuff, 1.5–2.0 cm long, with the inner diameter of 1.2 mm and the wall thickness of 2–3 mm.
  b Monofilament sutures, e.g. Novafil 00 and 000 (D & G Monofil, Manatí, Puerto Rico), mounted on atraumatic needles with a 19 mm curvature for suturing the skin.
  c Stainless-steel polyfilament threads (Stahldraht-00, Multifilament DX-4785; Dekmatel, Hamburg, Germany).
6 For dressing:
  a Mepore 4 × 4 and 9 × 15 cm absorbent, self-adhesive compresses (Mölnlycke, Mölnlycke, Sweden).
  b Pieces of self-adhesive, transparent polyurethane film 5 × 7 and 10 × 12 cm (Tegaderm, Surgical Division, St Paul, MN, USA) and 12.7 × 17.8 cm (Bioclusive; Johnson & Johnson, New Brunswick, NJ, USA).
  c Surgical, self-adhesive tape.
7 For fluoroscopic location of the intrathecal catheter tip: contrast solutions containing iodine, suitable for intrathecal administration, e.g. iohexol (Omnipaque; Nycomed, Lidingö, Sweden) containing 350 mg iodine per milliliter.

Location for catheterization procedure

Catheterization should always take place in the operating room.

Monitoring

Blood pressure, electrocardiogram, heart rate, and O_2 saturation should be continuously supervised throughout the procedure.

Imaging/location techniques

The catheter tip should be located at the level of the vertebra corresponding to the middle of the intercostal nerves from which the pain is originating. This is achieved by using the C-arm fluoroscopy apparatus and marking the respective vertebra with a lead shot, fixed with surgical tape on the patient's upwardly located costal region.

Position (patient and operator)

1 The patient:
  a "Head up" (approximately 30°), lateral, recumbent position with the painful zones (e.g. fractures of the pelvis or upper and/or lower extremities) upward. A mask is applied to the patient's face and 30–40% oxygen in air at a rate of 8–10 l/min is given (Fig. 23.3), or 2–3 l/min of humidified oxygen is administered through a nasal catheter.
  b Supine position: patients with bilateral, pelvic, and/or femoral fractures are anesthetized and intubated in the supine position and thereafter moved to the lateral recumbent position.
2 The operator sits comfortably on an operating stool, behind the patient.

Preparation of the operation site

The skin is scrubbed for 3 min with a DesCutan sponge and allowed to dry. Then, the site is draped and the drapes fastened to the skin with self-adhesive surgical tapes.

Landmarks and insertion sites

1 The landmarks are those usually used for carrying out spinal anesthesia:
  a A line uniting the posterosuperior iliac spines passes through the spinal process of the S2 vertebra, where the dural cone terminates.
  b The line uniting the highest points of the cristae iliacae crosses the L4 vertebra.

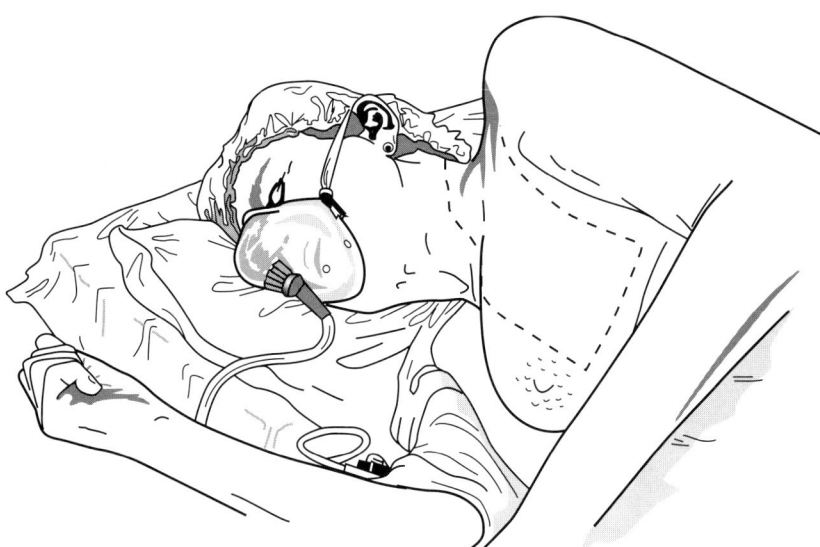

Figure 23.3 *Positioning the patient on the operating table. (Reproduced with permission from Nitescu et al.,[5] p. 147.)*

c The spinal cord ends by the conus medullaris at the height of the L2 vertebra.

d The T12 vertebral body is located in the costovertebral angle.

e The T7 vertebra is crossed by the line uniting the tips of the scapulae.

f The C7 vertebra is identified by the prominence made by its spinous process at the dorsal aspect of the base of the neck.

2 The insertion sites should be placed at distances of 10–15 cm from the intended catheter tip location, so that a length of 10–15 cm of the catheter is still in the subarachnoid space at the end of catheterization. Thereby, the risk of accidental dislocation of the catheter tip outside the dura mater is reduced.

a A lumbar insertion site (T12–L5, usually L2–L4) is chosen in patients with subdiaphragmatic pain, or when attempts to insert the catheter at medium or high thoracic levels are unsuccessful.

b A low thoracic approach (T8–T12) is used in patients with:
  i Lymphedema of the lower half of the body.
  ii Previous laminectomy in the lumbar region.
  iii Patients with pyelostomy catheters.

c A midthoracic (T4–T8) approach is used in patients with pain from the thoracic cage (e.g. rib metastases and/or fractures, mesothelioma) and lung cancer.

d A high thoracic approach (T1–T4) is used in patients with:
  i Pancoast tumors.
  ii Severe neuropathic pain from breast cancer and brachial plexopathy caused by cancer infiltration and/or radiation therapy.
  iii Refractory angina pectoris.

Anesthesia

1 Local (infiltration) anesthesia is used for:
  a Anesthesia of the interspace chosen for insertion of the intrathecal catheter.
  b Anesthesia of the skin and subcutaneous tissue along the intended tunnel course.

2 Spinal anesthesia is preferred in obese patients and in those with cardiovascular, respiratory, renal, or metabolic diseases (e.g. diabetes).

3 General anesthesia is used in patients with multiple metastases and fractures (pelvis, extremities, spine, etc.).

Dural puncture

1 Take a 17-gauge Tuohy needle with a sharp bevel.

2 Check the patency of the Tuohy needle by threading the catheter through the needle and gently withdrawing it.

3 The midline approach is preferred because the lateral approach is associated with a higher rate of accidental puncture of the epidural vessels, paresthesiae, and radicular pain.

4 The direct compared with the indirect approach:
  a Direct: without previous identification of the epidural space.
  b Indirect: the dura mater is approached after identification of the epidural space with a loss of resistance technique using a 10-ml disposable syringe half filled with air.

5 Connect (after a successful dural puncture) a 2-ml syringe to the Tuohy needle's hub in order to prevent spillage of CSF.

Inserting the intrathecal catheter

1 Check the patency of the catheter.
2 Fill the catheter with the contrast solution and clamp it with Mosquito forceps within 1 cm of its distal end.
3 Rotate the needle in order to direct the opening of its tip cranially.
4 Pass the catheter through the needle until a slight resistance is encountered at the needle tip (with a 9-cm-long needle, the graduation marked by two rings, i.e. 10 cm, reaches the needle hub).
5 Overcome the resistance by gently pushing the catheter and advancing it into the subarachnoid space under fluoroscopic control until the catheter tip reaches the height of the vertebra (previously marked by a lead shot) where the catheter tip is intended to be located.
6 Check the patency of the catheter repeatedly through the procedure (Fig. 23.4).
7 Connect the hub to the catheter and cap the hub.
8 Keep the Tuohy needle in place.

Tunneling the intrathecal catheter

1 Make an 8- to 10-mm-long transverse skin incision at the insertion site, with the Tuohy needle still in place (Fig. 23.5), and two or three other incisions along the tunnel, at 10- to 20-cm intervals. The incisions should include the whole skin thickness, up to the fascia.
2 Direct the tunneling:
   a Upwards, usually paravertebrally, over the shoulder, and further parasternally until the tunnel exit is at the level of the third chondrocostal junction (particularly indicated in patients with colostomy and/or pyelostomy).
   b Ventrally, toward the abdomen (flank, hypochondrium, iliac fossa) when the construction of a paravertebral tunnel is contraindicated (e.g.

presence of paravertebral metastases, cancerous involvement of neck structures, tracheostomy, women subjected to bilateral mastectomy and/or radiation therapy leading to "cuirass thorax").
3 Infiltrate generously the tunnel course with a local anesthetic solution, e.g. 0.5–1% mepivacaine with or without epinephrine.
4 Use a Portex 35-cm-long tunneling instrument (Fig. 23.6) provided with a central duct that opens approximately 1 cm from its pointed (javelin shaped) ends. This device is time saving and will permit tunneling in two or three steps. A short (9–12 cm), 17-gauge Tuohy needle should be used for the last step of the tunneling to leave a fine orifice at the tunnel outlet, thereby reducing a potential CSF leakage.
5 Prevent the catheter's accidental withdrawal during the tunneling: the catheter is firmly held with forceps without teeth at the incision site during its threading through the tunneling device and its passage through the tunnel (Fig. 23.7).
6 Check the patency of the catheter by the free dripping of CSF from its external end at each step of the tunneling procedure, and after its termination.
7 Turn the patient into the dorsal recumbent position. To prevent displacement of the tunnel trajectory, the last part of the tunneling (from the clavicle to the third chondrosternal junction) should be performed with the patient in this dorsal recumbent position (particularly in women with large breasts).
8 Connect the hub to the catheter and check its patency again (Fig. 23.8). This extra control is dictated by the necessity of screwing together the two pieces of the Luer connection hub rather tightly to prevent a leakage.
9 Cap the catheter hub with a Luer plug to prevent CSF spillage.
10 Secure the catheter to the hub with one or two drops of plastic glue (Super Glue) applied at the junction of the catheter with the hub.[16]

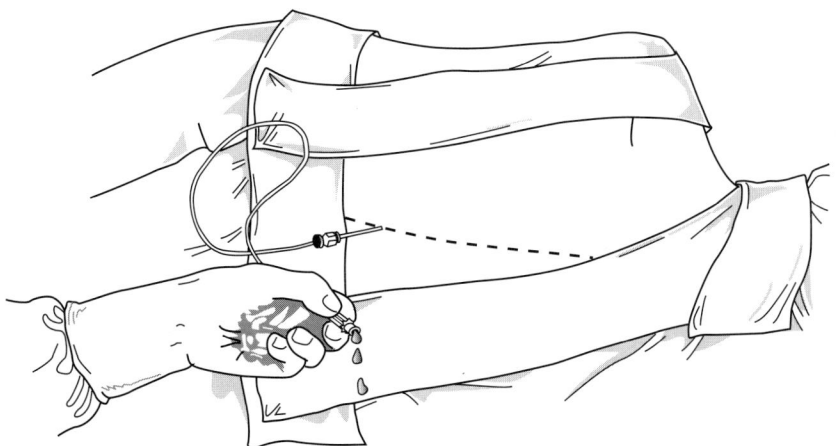

Figure 23.4 *Testing the catheter patency. (Reproduced with permission from Nitescu et al.,[5] p. 148.)*

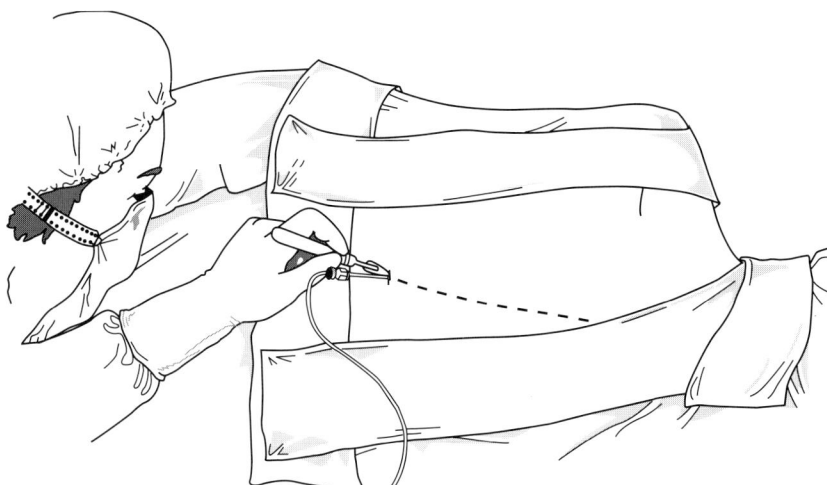

Figure 23.5 *Making a 8- to 10-mm-long, transverse skin incision at the insertion site. (Reproduced with permission from Nitescu et al.,[5] p. 148.)*

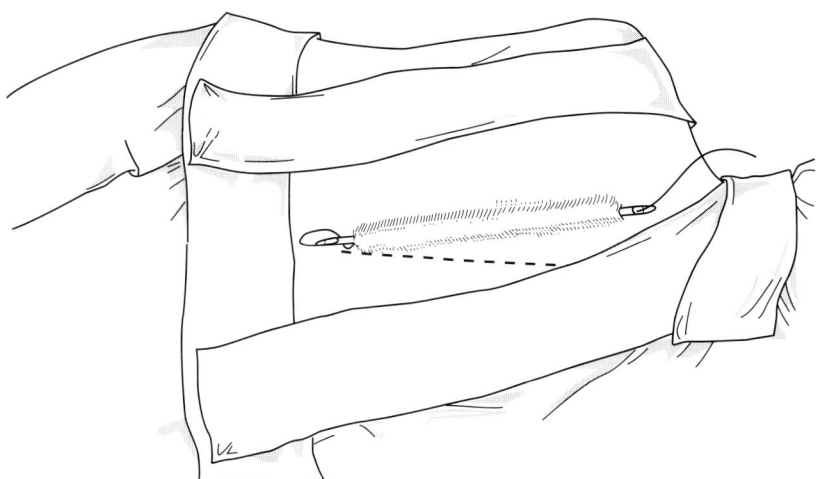

Figure 23.6 *Catheter tunneling with the Portex tunneling device. (Reproduced with permission from Nitescu et al.,[5] p. 148.)*

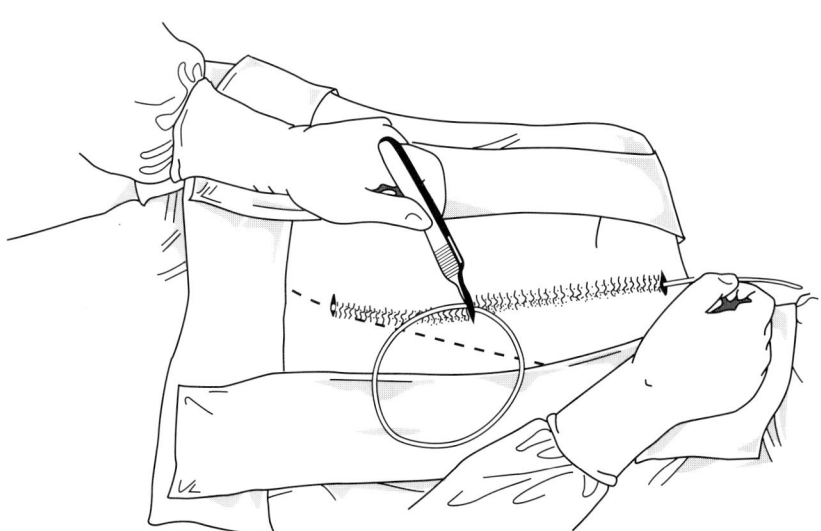

Figure 23.7 *Pulling the catheter through the tunnel: to prevent accidental catheter withdrawal, the operator holds the catheter with a fine pincer without teeth at the next nearest incision of the tunnel. (Reproduced with permission from Nitescu et al.,[5] p. 150.)*

Fixing the catheter to the skin

1 Pass a split silicone cuff around the catheter, immediately below the tunnel exit, and fixing it to the skin with two or three monofilament sutures (Novafil-00), taking a generous segment (approximately 2 cm breadth and 1 cm depth) of the integument.
2 Fasten the hub to the skin with two stainless-steel multifilament threads (Stahldraht-00), taking approximately 3 cm breadth and 1 cm depth of the skin (Fig. 23.9).
3 Close the skin incisions at the insertion site and along the tunnel with monofilament sutures (Novafil-00) mounted on atraumatic needles with a 19-mm curvature.

Substituting for the spilled cerebrospinal fluid and connecting the Millipore filter

1 Inject 10–15 ml of isotonic saline through the filter/catheter over an interval of 5 min as a prophylactic measure against occurrence of postdural puncture headache (PDPH). Thereafter, 1 ml of 0.5% bupivacaine, or 1 ml of the mixture from the pump, is injected through the hub and the catheter, and the hub plugged.
2 Fill a round (flying saucer-like, or flat), disposable, 0.22-μm, Millipore antibacterial filter, 25 mm in diameter with a surface of 2.8 cm (Vygon, Écouen, France), with the same solution as that in the pump. Connect the filter to the catheter hub, and plug its opposite end (Fig. 23.10). It is mandatory to protect the skin with a small gauze compress placed under the sharp edge of the filter.

Connecting the infusion pump

Disconnect the plug on the filter and attach the filter to an electronic infusion pump, initially programmed to deliver 4–5 ml/day. A mixture of 0.5 mg/ml morphine (or 0.015 mg/ml buprenorphine) and 4.75 mg/ml bupivacaine in a dose of 4–5 ml/day is appropriate and would give acceptable pain relief [visual analog scale (VAS) = 0–2 out of 10] in most patients at the start of the treatment.[17]*

Dressing the incisions and the tunnel exit

1 Incisions: absorbent self-adhesive compresses (Mepore 4 × 4 cm) are applied to the skin incision and their adhesion to the skin further secured by transparent self-adhesive polyurethane films (Tegaderm, 5 × 7 cm).
2 Tunnel exit: the whole tunnel exit (catheter hub, Millipore filter, and extension tube of the pump) should be covered with gauze compresses to prevent skin transpiration. A label "Warning: intrathecal catheter!" must also be applied to prevent accidental injection of unintended substances into the intrathecal catheter. Thereafter, the tunnel exit, the filter, the pump extension tubing, the gauze compresses, and the warning label are fixed to the skin with a 12.7 × 17.8 cm self-adhesive polyurethane film (Bioclusive) (Fig. 23.11).

Instructing ward personnel, the patient, and next of kin

Brief instructions containing basic information on the use of the pump, exchange of the battery, and telephone

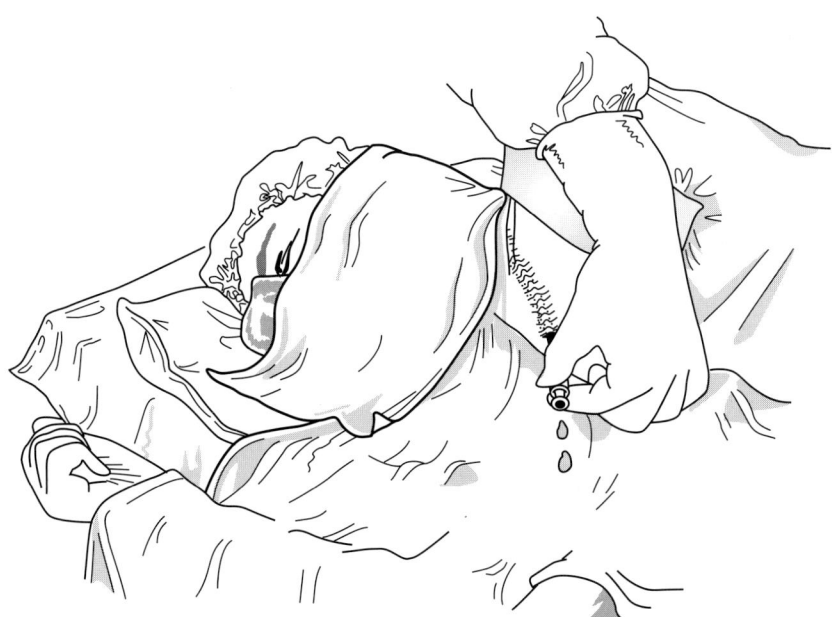

Figure 23.8 *Final check of the catheter for patency. (Reproduced with permission from Nitescu et al.,[5] p. 151.)*

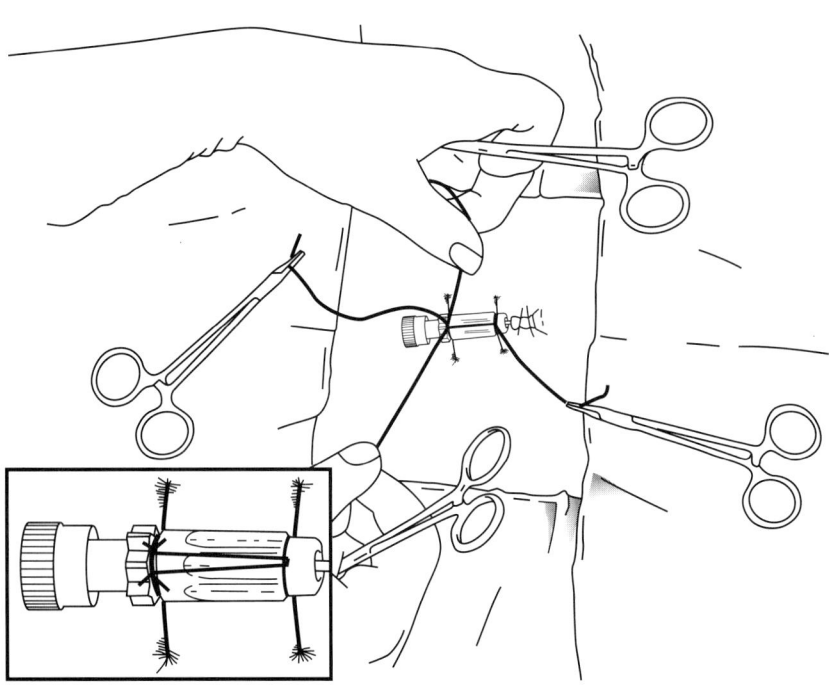

Figure 23.9 *Knotting the steel threads on the catheter hub to prevent their gliding. (Reproduced with permission from Nitescu et al.,[5] p. 151.)*

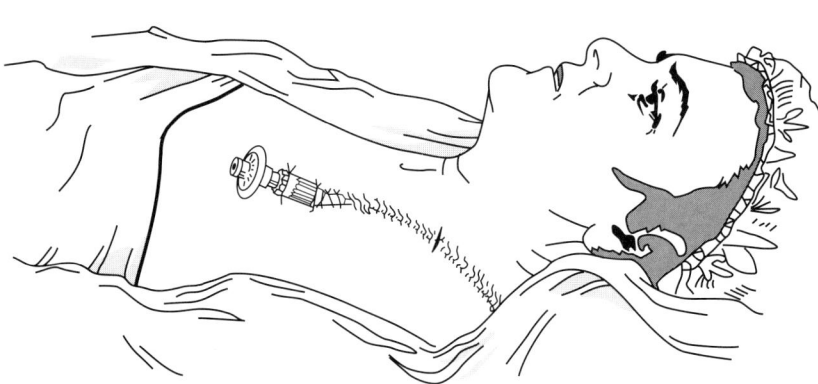

Figure 23.10 *Connecting the Millipore bacterial filter to the catheter hub. (Reproduced with permission from Nitescu et al.,[5] p. 152.)*

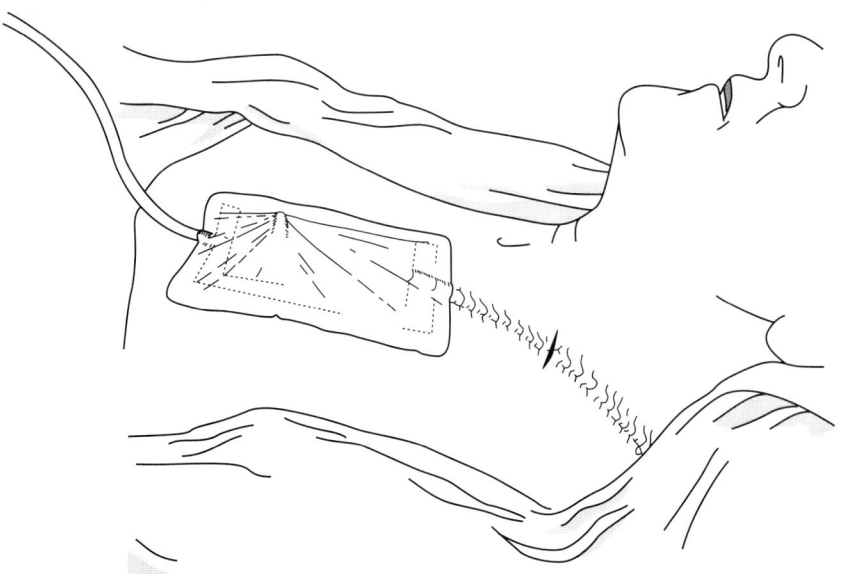

Figure 23.11 *Dressing the tunnel exit: an absorbent compress is applied to it and held in place by a self-adhesive transparent film applied over the catheter hub, Millipore filter, and extension tube of the pump. (Reproduced with permission from Nitescu et al.,[5] p. 152.)*

numbers of the nurses and doctors of the pain section should be enclosed in a hard plastic cover and placed in the pump handbag.

Postcatheterization care

1 Patients are supervised for 12 h in a postoperative care unit, and thereafter for 48–72 h in a hospital ward.
2 Antibiotics are continued for 3 days.
3 The pump delivery is adjusted (rate, intermittent dose, and lockout interval) when necessary to give the patient acceptable pain relief.
4 The first redressing of the insertion site is performed after 24–72 h.
5 The patient may take a shower after 3 days.
6 The skin sutures (except those fixing the catheter) are removed after 7–8 days.
7 The patient usually may be sent home after 48–72 h.

TECHNIQUE OF HIGH CERVICAL (INTRATHECAL) AND INTRACISTERNAL CATHETERIZATION

High intrathecal/intracisternal bupivacaine test

The high cervical intrathecal bupivacaine test consists of 2.5–5.0 mg of 0.5% isobaric bupivacaine being injected at that interspace where the catheter tip is intended to be located.

For the intracisternal bupivacaine test, 2.5–5.0 mg (0.5–1.0 ml) of 0.5% isobaric bupivacaine is injected by a direct approach into the cisterna magna at the occipital–C1 or C1–C2 interspace with the tip of the needle directed toward the patient's nose root (glabella). The puncture is safely performed under C-arm fluoroscopic control during the advancement of the needle. *The test is performed in a moderately sedated patient and with equipment for intubation at hand. A dose of 5.0 mg of bupivacaine should not be exceeded.* After the injection, some patients may experience transient (5–10 min) hoarseness and/or dysphagia, and others a transient increase in blood pressure. These symptoms usually need no treatment. In some rare cases, a sedative and/or a vasodilator should be injected. The increase of blood pressure is caused by the blockade of the vasodilator fibers of the vagal nerves by the intracisternal bupivacaine while the vasoconstrictor fibers of the cervical sympathetic chain, with their preganglionic neurons located in the spinal segments T2–T8 (and occasionally T9), remain unaffected by it. Thereby, an imbalance of the vagal/sympathetic tonus will occur.

Insertion site

The low cervical/high thoracic approach (C7–T5) with a stiff nylon catheter ensures a secure position of the catheter tip at the height of the cisterna magna (Fig. 23.12) and a low risk of accidental catheter withdrawal as a result of the inserted catheter length (15–25 cm).

The midthoracic (T7–T9) approach is used only after unsuccessful attempts to insert the catheter at the C7–T5 position. To facilitate insertion, the catheter may be provided with a guide wire. By this means, intrathecal catheters inserted at midthoracic interspaces can be advanced 28–38 cm until they reached the C1–C2 vertebrae.[8]*

Catheter direction

The cranial direction is used with all cervicothoracic approaches and semistiff nylon catheters.

Catheter endpoint

The catheter is placed at the C1–C2 vertebrae with the help of C-arm fluoroscopy (Fig. 23.13).

Intracisternal bupivacaine treatment

Continuous infusions of intracisternal bupivacaine at rates ranging from 1.0 to 3.0 mg/h apparently had no adverse effects.

Intracisternal optional bolus doses of 0.5–1.0 mg (maximum four times per hour) showed no adverse effects at a basic infusion rate of 1–3 mg/h.

INSERTION COMPLICATIONS

See Table 23.1 for potential insertion complications.

SOLUTIONS (DRUGS, CONCENTRATIONS, MIXTURES, PROPORTIONS)

Bupivacaine

Shelf solutions of bupivacaine (Marcain; Astra, Södertälje, Sweden) 5 mg/ml were used.

Morphine

Shelf solutions of morphine 10 mg/ml, with or without preservatives (sodium metabisulfite, syn. pyrosulfite,

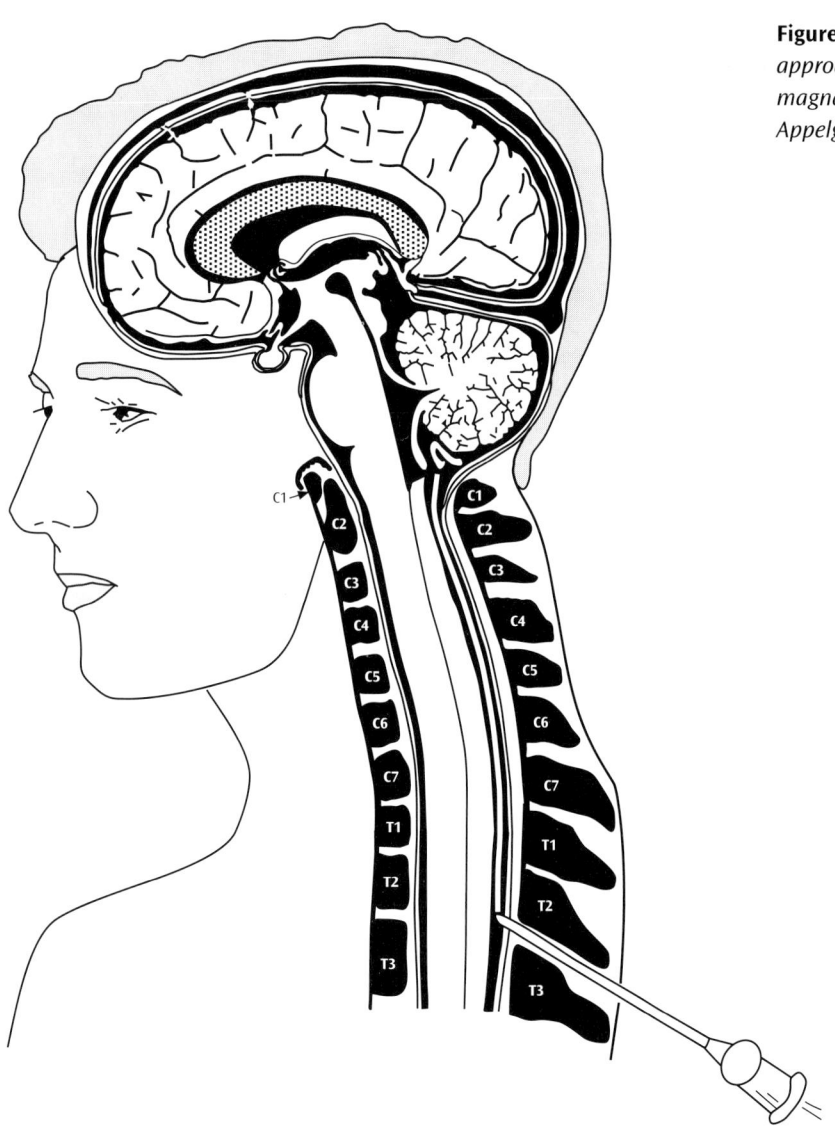

Figure 23.12 *Sketch of the high thoracic approach to catheterization of cisterna magna. (Reproduced with permission from Appelgren et al.,[8] p. 259.)*

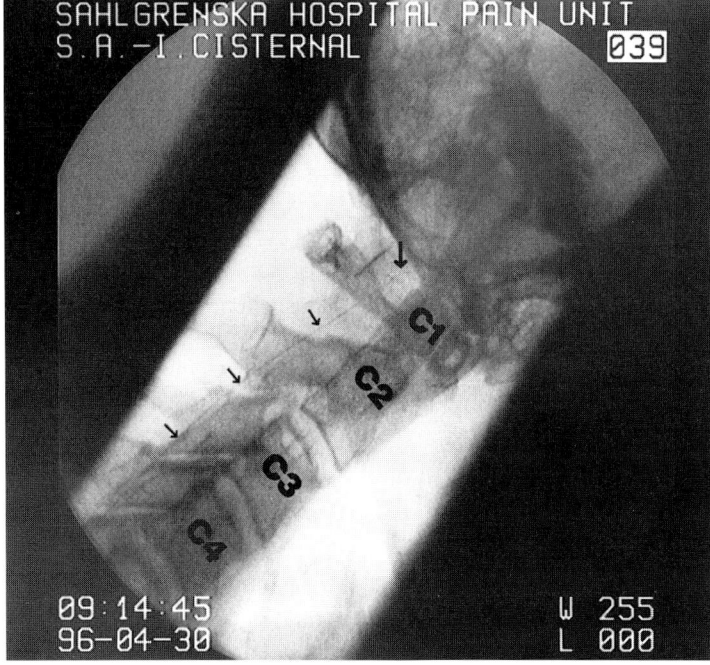

Figure 23.13 *Fluoroscopic image representing the location of the intracisternal catheter tip at the suboccipital level. Small black arrows, catheter; larger black arrow, catheter tip; C1–C4, bodies of the cervical vertebrae.*

Table 23.1 *Insertion complications*[5,12]

Type of complications and their incidence	Malignant pain[a] (%)	Nonmalignant pain (%)
During spinal dura puncture		
Unsuccessful puncture of the dura mater at the first attempt	32	28
Accidental puncture of an extradural vessel	~10	~2
Difficult dural puncture	18	14
Multiple dural punctures	14	13
Blood-stained CSF	9	4
Absence of free dripping of CSF despite successful dural puncture[b]	3	0
Radicular pain and paresthesiae on dural puncture	22	3
During advancement of the catheter		
Resistance to catheter advancement[c]	6	5
Radicular pain and paresthesiae during catheter advancement	4	~1
During catheter tunneling		
Difficult advancement of the tunneling instrument[d]	9	0
Bleeding in the tunnel	0.5	0

a. The apparently higher rates of insertion complications in patients with malignant pain were attributed to the presence of vertebral and/or epidural metastases, congestion of the epidural veins, fibrosis of the dura mater, dehydration leading to low CSF pressure, partial or total occlusion of the spinal canal, previous radiation therapy, etc.
b. Probably caused by: obstruction of the needle by a fragment of an epidural metastasis or by a dural flap; too deep advancement of the needle, which has perforated both the dorsal and the ventral dura mater during attempts at dural puncture below L2; a low CSF pressure; a lateral position of the needle bevel; extradural location of the catheter.
c. Probably caused by: partial location of the Tuohy needle's bevel in the epidural space; tilting of the catheter tip by the spinal cord, a nerve root, or the denticulate ligament; catheter curling and/or kinking; occlusion of the subarachnoid space by compression from epidural metastases or destruction of vertebral bodies.
d. In patients subjected to previous radiotherapy leading to subcutaneous fibrosis at the tunnel course.

1.0 mg/ml, and sodium edetate 0.1 mg/ml, Pharmacia & Upjohn, Solna, Sweden), were used.

Indications

Morphine is routinely added to intrathecal bupivacaine for the synergistic, antinociceptive action of spinally administered morphine and local anesthetics.

Contraindications

- Intracisternal administration (because of the strong emetic effect of morphine when it is administered in the vicinity of the emesis centrum).
- Patients reacting with severe side-effects to morphine administration, e.g. bronchospasm, clonus, seizures, urticaria, anaphylactic shock, hallucinations, severe nausea, vomiting, constipation, etc.

Buprenorphine

Shelf solutions of buprenorphine (Temgesic; Reckitt & Colman, Dansom Lane, Hull, UK) 0.3 mg/ml without preservatives were used in patients with contraindications to morphine.

Mixtures of opioid/bupivacaine

After many empirical trials, an efficient mixture was found to be 0.5 mg/ml morphine (alternatively 0.015 mg/

ml buprenorphine) and 4.75 mg/ml bupivacaine, giving the proportions ~1:10 morphine–bupivacaine and ~1:300 buprenorphine–bupivacaine. These mixtures have a pH of 4.6 and an osmolality of 282 mosmol/kg when morphine is used, and a pH of 5.03 and an osmolality of 283 mosmol/kg when buprenorphine is employed.

GUIDELINES FOR ADJUSTMENT OF THE INTRATHECAL PAIN TREATMENT

1 Place the intrathecal catheter tip in the middle of the segments of maximal pain.
2 Use a volume-programming pump for continuous infusion whenever available.
3 Titrate the intrathecal dosage individually:
   a Start with low morphine (0.5 mg/ml) and relatively high bupivacaine (4.75 mg/ml) concentrations and low volumes (4–5 ml/day).
   b Gradually increase the volumes until adequate pain relief (VAS = 0–2 out of 10) is obtained.
   c Set the incremental dose on demand below 1.25 mg of intrathecal bupivacaine. Let the intrathecal bupivacaine daily doses gradually increase in parallel with that of the intrathecal morphine, keeping the same proportions, during the course of the disease.
4 Be prepared to use higher intrathecal bupivacaine doses (per hour and on demand) in patients with deafferentation pain from the spinal cord, brachial,

and lumbosacral plexus, pain from the celiac plexus, ischemic and colicky pain, and smarting pain from large, ulcerated, mucocutaneous tumors.

5 Gradually decrease the administration of opioids given by routes other than the spinal only if this is desirable (e.g. unacceptable side-effects from the opioids). Treat possible abstinence independently of the intrathecal morphine doses.

6 Decrease (but do not interrupt) administration of sedatives if this is desirable (too deep sedation).

7 In other words, give the patients *ad libitum* access to nonopioid analgesics/sedatives and opioids administered by routes other than spinal (oral, enteral, and/or parenteral) until they obtain adequate pain (VAS = 0–2 out of 10) and anxiolytic relief.

8 Contact the patient every day and adjust the dosages when needed.

CLINICAL RESULTS

See Table 23.2 for clinical results.

Notes to table on facing page

a. Both obstruction and kinking.
b. Catheter tip outside the subarachnoid space, but still within the body.
c. Catheter tip outside the patient's body.
d. Apparently due to occurrence of adhesive arachnoiditis.
e. The patient was pain free with only systemic opioids after 332 days of intrathecal treatment.
f. Because of occurrence of paresthesiae, paresis, and/or abstinence.
g. Sepsis, caused by a postoperative infection in the spine after spinal surgery, was erroneously attributed to the intrathecal catheter.
h. Classification of pain relief: > 0–20%, minimal; > 20–40%, poor ("treatment failure"); > 40–60%, fair; > 60–80%, good; > 80–100%, excellent.
i. First series of 52 cancer patients.[6]
j. Second series of 53 patients.[17]
k. Optional bolus doses ranged from 0.5 mg (maximum four per hour) to 5 mg (once per hour) and caused no adverse side-effects at basic rates of 1–4 mg/h.
l. One milligram buprenorphine≈30 mg morphine.
m. Because of: (1) introduction of another therapy (dorsal column stimulation, DCS), ~1.0%; (2) resolution of pain, attributed to (a) amputation (25% of all patients), (b) natural evolution of the disease (acute herpes zoster, 2%), (c) withdrawal of the patients from their iatrogenic opioid addiction (~5.0%), (d) reduction of ischemia and healing of the amputation wounds (~2.0%, (e) healing of vertebral compression fractures (~2%), and (f) change of behavior after failed spine surgery (~1.0%).
n. After 3–286 days from the start of the intrathecal treatment, despite satisfactory pain relief; approximately 95% of these patients had one or more psychiatric disturbances before start of the intrathecal pain treatment.
o. All patients in this group had one or more psychiatric disturbances before the start of the intrathecal pain treatment and all of them had these disturbances throughout the treatment, e.g. severe depression, compulsive–obsessive neurosis, alcohol abuse, aggression, delirium, and compensation neurosis.
p. The first patient was a 67-year-old woman with unstable angina pectoris in whom the intrathecal pain treatment gave no more pain relief after 404 days of treatment at acceptable doses (1 mg/h) of intrathecal bupivacaine. The second patient was a 29-year-old man with post-traumatic tetraplegia due to the spinal cord injury at C6. This patient complained of inefficacy of the intrathecal pain treatment 90 days after its start and requested its arrest and reinstitution of systemic opioid therapy.
q. In the long term.
r. In the short term.
s. Lower daily doses (means ± 1 SD) were required by the patients with amyloidosis polyneuropathy (15 ± 4 mg/day) and scleroderma with Raynaud's phenomena (17 ± 11 mg/day). Higher daily doses (54 ± 11 mg) were administered to patients with post-traumatic para/tetraplegia and complex regional pain syndrome type I (54 ± 15 mg/day).
t. At the beginning of the study (1986–7). Presently, the daily doses of intrathecal opioids usually do not exceed 20 mg of parenteral morphine equivalents per day.
u. The data from the patients with nonmalignant pain conditions are too few and have therefore not been included in the table.
v. Intracisternal morphine would not be administered (risk for intractable nausea and emesis due to the vicinity of the emetic centrum).
w. Doses higher than 3 mg/h (72 mg/day) should not be administered as they are associated with occurrence of severe tiredness, faintness, and malaise.

CARE OF THE PATIENT AND OF THE INFUSION SYSTEM

Dressing the tunnel exit

1 Timing: the dressing is first changed after 24–72 h, and thereafter once or twice per week.

2 Cleanse the skin with 0.5% chlorhexidine gluconate in 70% ethyl alcohol.

3 Apply a thin layer of Inotyol (Debat Laboratories, Paris, France) over the tunnel exit and the steel suture points.

4 Insert a gauze compress between the filter and the skin and dress the tunnel exit as previously described.

Exchanging the bacterial filter

This must be carried out once a month, or even every other month.[18]*

Table 23.2 *Clinical results*[6,8,17,20]

Variables in study	Malignant pain	Nonmalignant pain
Intrathecal catheterization		
Duration of catheterization, days (*n*) (range and median)	1–575 (33)	3 to >2,500 (>60)
Catheter function (% of catheters)		
Perfect function	92.0%	99%
Catheter occlusion[a]	1.3%	1%
Catheter dislodgement[b]	1.8%	0%
Catheter withdrawal[c]	4.0%	10%
Patchy distribution of analgesia (% of patients)[d]	1.0%	0%
Reasons for interrupting the intrathecal pain treatment (% of patients)		
Patient's death	93.5%	27%
Accidental catheter withdrawal	1.5%	0%
The catheter no longer required	0.5%[e]	~38%[m]
Patient's anxiety[f]	3.5%	0%
Misinterpretation of complication[g]	0.5%	0%
Patient's refusal to continue the intrathecal pain treatment	0%	~22%[n]
Lack of cooperation on the part of the patient, the family, or the referring physician	0.5%	~9%[o]
Intrathecal pain treatment no longer efficient	0%	~2%[p]
Satisfactory pain relief[h] (% of patients) at daily doses of	85%[i] to 100%[j]	68%[q] to 95%[r]
Intrathecal bupivacaine (mg/day) (range and median)[k]	2.0–320 (34)	4.8–166 (36)[s]
Intrathecal opioid: morphine or buprenorphine (mg morphine equivalents per day; range and median)[l]	0.5–212[t] (14)	0.13–25 (33)
Opioids administered by other routes than spinal (mg of parenteral morphine equivalents per day, range and median)		
Before intrathecal treatment	7–801 (45)	5–123 (30)
During intrathecal treatment	1–620 (17)	1–71 (6)
Nonopioid analgesic and sedative drug consumption (percentage reduction)	~50%	~50%
Duration of nocturnal sleep (hours, median values) before vs. during the intrathecal pain treatment	<4 vs. 7	2 or 3 vs. >6
Gait and ambulation (before vs. during the intrathecal treatment)	Practically unchanged	Practically unchanged
Intracisternal catheterization[u]		
Duration of catheterization, days (*n*) (range and median)	3–182 (37)	–
Perfect catheter function (% of catheters)	100%	–
Satisfactory pain relief (% of patients) at daily doses of:	100%	–
Intracisternal bupivacaine,[v] range (median)	24–168[w] (36)	–
Opioids by routes other than spinal (mg morphine equivalents per day; range and median)	Decrease from 2–275 (53) mg before to 0–124 (34) mg during the intracisternal treatment	–
Nocturnal sleep increase	From 2 to 6 h	–
Gait ability pattern	No immediate, postprocedure deterioration, but deterioration over a slow, disease-related time-course	

Exchanging the infusion container (cassette)

This should be done once a month or when it is needed.

Taking a shower

Using an absorbent–impermeable dressing (see Fig. 23.11), the patient may take a shower when he or she wants, without interrupting the intrathecal infusion, giving due consideration to the following precautions:

- keep the pump in an impermeable plastic bag, away from the shower flow;
- change the dressing after taking the shower if water has infiltrated it.

SIDE-EFFECTS AND COMPLICATIONS OF INTRATHECAL PAIN TREATMENT AND THEIR MANAGEMENT

From bupivacaine

Intrathecal bupivacaine in the concentration mentioned above (4.75–5.0 mg/ml) has been associated with the following rates of transient and dose-related (> 45–90 mg/day) side-effects:[19★★★,20★★★]

- urinary retention, 33%;
- paresthesiae, 23%;
- paresis with gait impairment in 3.5% of the patients who received daily doses of 45–60 mg and in 15% of those who received > 60 mg.
- arterial hypotension (1–2%), recorded as systolic blood pressure < 100 mmHg, may occur as a brief period of orthostatic reaction after a bolus dose of 4–5 mg of intrathecal bupivacaine given in addition to the hourly dose of > 3 mg.

A dose of 60 mg of intrathecal bupivacaine per day is the level above which occurrence of side-effects is the rule rather than the exception.

From morphine

Hyperalgesia/allodynia, cerebrospinal clonus, and/or seizures are to be expected at intrathecal doses of > 60 mg/day.[6★]

From intrathecal catheterization

The rates of these complications are presented in ratio form, in which the first number refers to malignant pain and the number in brackets refers to nonmalignant pain. The complications are:

1 Dural puncture-related:
   a Accidental injury of an unknown epidural metastasis with subsequent bleeding, formation of epidural hematoma, and paraplegia: 0.3% (0%). Computed tomography (CT) or magnetic resonance imaging (MRI) scan with contrast should be performed, the suspected diagnosis confirmed, and decompressive laminectomy undertaken.
   b Paraplegia due to "medullary coning," i.e. collapse of an unknown epidural tumor against the spinal cord, caused by leakage of the CSF acting as a buffer between the spinal cord and the extramedullary tumor: ~ 1% (0%).
   c Intracranial subdural hematoma: 0% (2%), explained by CSF loss occurring after dural puncture, thereby depriving the brain of its hydraulic buffer, which leads to traction applied on the arachnoidea and its fine vessels, damage of the vessel walls, and subdural bleeding.
   d External CSF leakage: 3.5% (2%), potentially leading to PDPH, CSF pseudomeningocele, intracranial subdural hematoma, catheter track infection, epidural abscess, and meningitis. Therefore, CSF leakage must be prevented by all means and its occurrence treated immediately by:
      i Stopping CSF leakage by skin resuturing, in case of dehiscence, and local compression at the insertion for 2–3 weeks; stopping the leakage at the tunnel outlet with a purse-string suture applied around the tunnel exit and a compressive "cigar" dressing on the tunnel track; if the CSF leakage has caused PDPH, an epidural "blood patch," consisting of 20 ml of autologous blood, is applied at the interspace situated immediately below the catheter insertion site – the "blood patch" is performed with the patient in the lateral head-down (30°) position; if the epidural "blood patch" does not stop the leakage, a lumbar epidural injection of 4 ml of fibrin glue (Tissucol R, duo 500; Immuno, Austria) is given one interspace cephalad to the original puncture level.[21]
      ii Ensuring adequate pain relief: the daily doses of analgesic solutions administered intrathecally should be increased until satisfactory pain relief is obtained.
      iii Preventing occurrence of meningitis by antibiotics given parenterally.
   e PDPH: 15.5% (22%). The PDPH may be short lasting or persisting. It is treated by:
      i Intermittent injections of 15–20 ml isotonic saline administered during 5–10 minutes through the filter/catheter with a 10-ml syringe, 2–3 times/day. The injections are fol-

lowed by temporary headache relief within 5–10 minutes. Permanent relief is usually obtained within 3–5 days. To prevent pain recurrence, 2 ml of 0.5% isotonic bupivacaine is given intrathecally after injection of the isotonic saline.

ii Epidural injection of 20 ml of autologous blood ("blood patch") is performed (as previously described) when the PDPH had a duration longer than 5 days. The headache will usually disappear within 1–2 h.

Nota bene. If the PDPH does not disappear after the "blood patch," a CT or a MRI scan should be performed. This is mandatory as it may reveal an unexpected intracranial metastasis or bleeding.

f Skin breakdown at the insertion site: 2% (0%). Emergency excision and resuturing of the wound should be performed.

g Subcutaneous CSF hygroma ("pseudomeningocele"): 1.5% (0%). It presents as a visible, small, subcutaneous collection of fluid under the scar of the insertion wound in the spine, usually with no clinical significance. However, in some patients, the CSF hygroma may become sufficiently large to redistribute the analgesics infused intrathecally, thereby reducing pain relief. If skin breakdown occurs, a CSF cutaneous fistula may develop, with an increased risk of infection. The CSF hygroma is treated by:

i A simple compressive dressing at the insertion site is sometimes sufficient to cure small hygromas.

ii Aspiration and drainage may be necessary in the very rare cases of large hygromas.

iii Inoperable hygromas, complicated by a CSF fistula, require only a local, sterile, compressive dressing applied to the fistula orifice and exchanged two or three times per week.

iv Infected hygromas suggest meningitis and must be treated by hospitalization, catheter removal, and parenteral antibiotics.

2 Tunneling related: 0.5% (0%). Bleeding in the tunnel, caused by an accidental injury of a subcutaneous vessel, is treated by a compressive dressing applied for 2–4 days along the tunnel course.

3 Catheter/filter related: leakage of infusion in 1.5% (0%) of the patients. For other complications see Table 23.2.

4 Infectious complications:

a At the catheter insertion site: 0.5% (0%). The treatment consists of:

i Releasing the sutures.

ii Disinfecting the wound.

iii Applying one or two compresses imbued with fusidic acid ointment (Fucidin; Lövens, Malmö, Sweden) on the wound.

iv Covering them with gauze compresses.

v Holding them in position with a self-adhesive polyurethane film.

vi Changing the dressing every day.

vii Letting the wound heal *per secundam intentionem.*

b At the tunnel exit: 0% (1%). It is identified by presence of granulomas and *Staphylococcus*-like purulent fluid. The treatment consists of:

i Disinfecting the tunnel exit with an antiseptic solution.

ii Relieving the granulomas by diathermocoagulation.

iii Applying one or two compresses imbued with fusidic acid on the wound, covering them with dry gauze compresses, and holding them in position with a self-adhesive polyurethane film.

iv Changing the dressing as above every day.

v Giving antibiotics that are effective against *Staphylococcus*.

vi Letting the wound healing *per secundam intentionem.*

vii Withdrawing the catheter at the first sign that infection has spread to the tunnel.

c Deep catheter track infection: 0% (0.3%). It is recognized by local signs (swelling, redness, heat, tenderness) over the tunnel course, and general symptoms and signs (fever, shivering, feeling unwell). This infection is treated by:

i Giving antibiotics effective against *Staphylococcus*.

ii Opening the infected part of the tunnel by diathermic surgery, performed in narcosis.

iii Draining the pus.

iv Disinfecting the opened tunnel with an antiseptic solution.

v Withdrawing the intrathecal catheter.

vi Letting the tunnel remain open, covered with compresses soaked with fusidic acid, covering them with gauze compresses, and holding them in position with self-adhesive polyurethane film.

vii Changing the dressing once a day.

viii Applying a compressive dressing on the catheter entry site in the back.

ix Giving the patient increased doses of opioid and nonopioid analgesics (even continuous i.v. infusions, when needed).

x Allowing the wound to heal *per secundam intentionem* under the cover of parenteral antibiotics.

xi After wound healing, inserting another intrathecal catheter at a lower or higher interspace and directing its tunnel toward another region.

    xii Continuing the intrathecal pain treatment as before.

d Skin suture entry site: 4.5% (5.0%). For treatment, see above.

e Epidural abscess: 0% (?%).

f Meningitis: ~ 1% (i.e. 1:6,250 catheterization days, or 1:17 years of treatment) in patients with malignant pain compared with 4% (i.e. 1:3,717 catheterization days, or 1:10 years of treatment) in patients with nonmalignant pain.[19***,20***]

    Treatment of meningitis:

    i The intrathecal catheter is not primarily withdrawn, as it may be used for: sampling of CSF and intrathecal administration of antibiotics;[22] intrathecal administration of opioid and local anesthetics. Because of the increase in pain intensity caused by meningitis, the daily doses of the intrathecal analgesics should be increased.

    ii The intrathecal catheter must be withdrawn and another intrathecal catheter inserted if there are signs of infection at the insertion site, along the subcutaneous tunnel, or at the tunnel outlet; if the intrathecal catheter malfunctions, it must be withdrawn and replaced because the malfunctioning is usually caused by occlusion of its tip holes by fibrin plugs.

4 Intrathecal drugs related: no neuropathologic findings attributable to intrathecal morphine, preservatives, buprenorphine, or bupivacaine have been reported.[13*]

5 Death: there have been no reports of deaths caused by intrathecal treatment.

Equipment related

1 Catheter and filter leakage may occur at:

    a The tunnel outlet: the leakage may consist of edema, CSF, or infusion fluid; their differentiation may sometimes be difficult.

    b The catheter–hub connection: 0.5% (0%). Leakage can be prevented by sealing the catheter to the hub with one or two drops of a plastic-sticking glue after insertion of the catheter.[16]

2 The filter–hub connection: 1% (0%). The grooves of the filter connection may be mechanically damaged and may therefore leak.

3 The filter: 0.5% (1.0%). The leakage is caused by a crack in the filter housing as a result of mechanical damage during the manufacture or handling. Both the catheter and filter leakage are associated with the risk of infection. To prevent contamination of the CSF, cutting of the externalized end of the catheter with sterile scissors, its cleaning with an antiseptic (e.g. betadine and alcohol), and replacement of the hub and/or the filter are recommended.

4 The connection between the extension tubing and the cassette.

SIDE-EFFECTS AND COMPLICATIONS OF HIGH CERVICAL INTRATHECAL–INTRACISTERNAL PAIN TREATMENT AND THEIR MANAGEMENT

Doses of 2 mg/h in patients with poor physical condition and 3 mg/h in those with good condition appeared to be the highest permitted doses for safe intracisternal administration.

The side-effects from the intracisternal bupivacaine are:

1 Motor side-effects.

    a Impairment of the somatic fibers of the vagal nerve, expressed as hoarseness after an intracisternal injection of 5.0 mg bupivacaine.

    b Impairment of the glossopharyngeus nerve (dysphagia) after a bolus dose of 7.5 mg of intracisternal bupivacaine.

    c Light paresis of the upper extremities was observed in ~ 15% of the patients at intracisternal doses of bupivacaine of 1.5–5.0 mg/h.

    d Absence of clinical signs of gross phrenic nerve impairment is notable.

2 Sensory side-effects:

    a Feeling of coldness in the neck and skull base in ~ 8% of the patients.

    b Transient paresthesiae in the neck and upper or lower extremities in ~ 45% of the patients.

Nota bene. In patients with pain from the shoulders, the intracisternal administration of bupivacaine will give less pain relief than intrathecal administration of the same bupivacaine doses at the midcervical (C4–C5) levels. The intracisternal administration of bupivacaine does not block pain stimuli from parts of the body (upper extremities included) other than those from the head and the neck.

3 Vegetative side-effects:

    a Episodic miosis and conjunctival hyperemia were observed in ~ 8% of patients after bolus doses of 1 mg at an infusion rate of > 2 mg of intracisternal bupivacaine per hour.

    b Episodic orthostatic arterial hypotension was observed in patients with severe dysphagia and nutritional problems (dehydration and cachexia). In these patients, hypotension may occur within 5–10 min after an optional dose of 1.5 mg, given at a basic rate of > 1.5 mg/h.

4 Other side-effects:

    a Severe tiredness, faintness, and malaise were recorded in one patient at doses of intracisternal bupivacaine of ~ 3 mg/h.

    b Somnolence and sleep occurred in one patient

with severe pain and receiving 5–7 mg/h intracisternal bupivacaine. Extra doses of 5 mg intracisternal bupivacaine made the patient somnolent for approximately 30–45 min.

c Nausea, vomiting, and respiratory depression from the intracisternal bupivacaine have never been recorded.

d No deaths have been attributed to the intracisternal administration of bupivacaine.

ADVANTAGES OF THE INTRATHECAL/ INTRACISTERNAL PAIN TREATMENT

Intrathecal pain treatment

Intrathecal administration of morphine and bupivacaine in a proportion of ~ 1:10 morphine–bupivacaine has the following advantages:

- Affording the patients effective pain relief with only ~ 1/10th of the doses used for epidural treatment.
- Keeping the total opioid consumption low.
- Preventing the potential side-effects from high doses of intrathecal or systemic morphine (seizures, clonus, allodynia, hyperesthesia, respiratory depression, urinary retention, pruritus).
- Giving patients with severe pain acceptable pain relief without heavy sedation or irreversible neurologic damage from neurolytic blocks or neurosurgery.
- Adding the antimicrobial activity of the relatively high concentrations (~ 5 mg/ml) of bupivacaine to that of the preservatives in the morphine containing preservative preparations.
- Decreasing the daily volumes to be administered intrathecally usually to 4–10 ml/day (as compared with 100–360 ml in epidural administration).[20***]
- Permitting a rational utilization of home care resources: a cassette of 100 ml is sufficient for 10–25 days and a plastic polyvinyl chloride bag of 250 ml for 25–50 days. Solutions of morphine and bupivacaine in cassettes have been found to be stable for at least 30 days,[23**] and the antimicrobial barrier of the micropore filter is effective for at least 60 days.[18*] The number of home visits by the home care service nurses may be decreased to one every 7–10 days and that of the specialized pain nurses to one every 30–60 days.
- Improving the patient's quality of life by better pain relief with less sensory impairment, by better sleep in terms of hours of uninterrupted and total nighttime sleep, by increased appetite (by reduction or disappearance of nausea, vomiting, and constipation due to opioids), and by treatment in familiar (home) surroundings reduces the likelihood of depression. Most patients, except those in coma or delirium or those who are incapacitated by cancer complications and/or sequelae, can take a shower, read, watch television, listen to music, perform handicrafts, take care of their small children, take short walks, shop, garden, etc. Some patients are able to enjoy sex, traveling at home or abroad, working part time (in a car repair workshop, in a pastry shop, or doing research work), or even driving a car, despite strong recommendations not to do so.

Intracisternal pain treatment

Long-term intracisternal administration of bupivacaine may help well-selected patients with refractory pain from the head, face, and neck to obtain adequate pain relief.

ADVANTAGES OF EXTERNALIZED INTRATHECAL CATHETERS AND PUMPS OVER IMPLANTED INTRATHECAL CATHETERS AND PUMPS

Reduced rates of catheter-related complications

Catheter-related complications are reduced: occlusion rates, 1–1.3% vs. 6–12%; spontaneous dislodgement of the tip, 0–1.5% vs. 6–13%; catheter breakdown and disconnection, 0.5% vs. 12%.[19***,20***]

Reduced rates of technical failures

Technical failures are reduced to 8.5% with Portex catheters compared with 10–40% with the implanted pumps. With the latter, the failures were due to both the catheter (see above) and the pump: at 2.6–2.9 years and infusion rates of 0.9–1.7 ml/day, 33% of catheters malfunctioned and 11% of pump batteries were unserviceable.[24]

Larger reservoir volumes

Externalized pumps have larger reservoir volumes of 50–1,000 ml compared with 15–18 ml with implantable, programmable, SynchroMed pumps. The small reservoir of the SynchroMed pump has led to the use of high concentrations of infusion drugs in order to make the use of the pump efficient. High concentrations of morphine, reaching up to 40–50 mg/ml, and low infusion flows (~ 1 ml/ 24 h) are associated with a potentially higher risk of drug precipitation in the small-catheter lumen and therefore with higher rates of catheter occlusion and pump dysfunction. Further, these high concentrations may lead to severe complications in the case of even small volume overdosages: rates of 5% apneic episodes and 15% lethargy[25] have been reported. With even higher overdosages, severe respiratory insufficiency and even lethal outcomes have occurred.[26]

Presence of patient-controlled analgesia function with externalized pumps

Absence of patient-controlled analgesia (PCA) function with implantable electronic pumps does not permit a personal "tailoring" of the daily doses of the infused intrathecal drugs reported as being "efficient," as the patients will have no immediate extra control of their own pain relief.

Simplicity of conception and functioning

The SynchroMed implantable pumps are technically complicated with respect to insertion technique and programming and will require an expensive, dedicated, separate programmer.

Substantially lower cost

The programmable implantable pumps will therefore be inaccessible to most of those who might need them, in a society with more and more restricted funds for health care (see below "Efficiency of the intrathecal pain treatment").

DISADVANTAGES OF THE INTRATHECAL PAIN TREATMENT

Intrathecal compared with epidural treatment

1. Probably more cumbersome insertions.
2. Higher rates of postspinal puncture headache (10–15% vs. 0%).
3. CSF leakage: 3.5–5% vs. 0% (theoretical) and 4% (practical).
4. Meningitis: 0.5–4% vs. 0–<1%.

Externalized intrathecal catheters and pumps compared with implanted intrathecal catheters and pumps

1. Catheter outward migration: 1.5–8% vs. 0%.
2. Possibility of overdosing in patients with psychological disturbances ("placebo reactors"), who may activate the pump independently of the programmed restraints of opioid and local anesthetic.

3. Possibility of attempting suicide by releasing the cassette from the pump and trying to empty it into the intrathecal catheter.

EFFICIENCY OF THE INTRATHECAL PAIN TREATMENT

Intrathecal compared with epidural treatment

Continuous intrathecal administration of morphine and bupivacaine is more efficient than epidural administration because of:

1. Lower dosages and volumes, making it more suitable for home treatment.
2. Less expensive due to smaller doses, rarer nurse and doctor calls and visits, and use of fewer infusion containers (cassettes).
3. Improved management of pain control.
4. Exceptional catheter occlusion (1.3% vs. up to 45%) leading to
   a. Better and longer function of the infusion system.
   b. Access to the subarachnoid space for CSF sampling and injections (antibiotics, cytostatics, analgesics, etc.).

Externalized intrathecal catheters compared with implanted intrathecal catheters and pumps

1. Lower rates of complications:[19***,20***]
   a. Catheter obstruction: 1.3% vs. 6%.
   b. Catheter tip dislodgement: 1.5% vs. 6%.
   c. Catheter inward migration: 0% vs. 12%.
   d. System leakage: 1.5% vs. 25%.
   e. CSF fistula: 3.5% vs. 4%.
   f. CSF hygroma: 1.5% vs. 4%.
   g. Removal of the system: 6.5% vs. 5–50%.
   h. Infections at the catheter entry site: 0.5–7% vs. 11%.
   i. Epidural abscess: 0% vs. ?%.
   j. Systemic infection: 0% vs. 3%.
2. Less expensive:
   a. An externalized catheter system costs $4.64–6.15, plus a monthly cost of $38 to keep the system functioning.
   b. A SyncroMed electronic pump (Medtronic, Minneapolis, MN, USA) costs $6,000, to which should be added the SynchroMed Programmer (Medtronic) for external control of the implanted pump at a cost of $6,125. These comparative cost estimates do not include:
      i. Professional fees and hospital charges for the system implantation.

ii   Cost of the drugs.
iii Filling of the cassettes.
iv   Visits for exchange of the filter and the dressing or for a (re)programming of the pump.
v   Interventions to repair or replace the systems.

REFERENCES

◆ 1. Arnér S, Arnér B. Differential effects of epidural morphine in the treatment of cancer related pain. *Acta Anaesthesiol Scand* 1985; **29:** 32–6.

◆ 2. Hjortsjø CN, Lund C, Mogensen T. Epidural morphine improves pain relief and maintains sensory analgesia during continuous epidural bupivacaine after abdominal surgery. *Anesth Analg* 1986; **65:** 1033–6.

◆ 3. Kroin SJ, McCarthy JR, Penn DR, *et al*. The effect of chronic subarachnoid bupivacaine infusion in dogs. *Anesthesiology* 1987; **66:** 737–42.

◆ 4. Nitescu P, Appelgren L, Linder LE, *et al*. Epidural versus intrathecal morphine–bupivacaine: assessment of consecutive treatments in advanced cancer pain. *J Pain Symptom Manage* 1990; **5:** 18–26.

◆ 5. Nitescu P, Appelgren L, Hultman E, *et al*. Long-term, "open" catheterization of the spinal subarachnoid space for continuous infusion of opiate and bupivacaine in patients with "refractory" cancer pain. A technique of catheterization and its problems and complications. *Clin J Pain* 1991; **7:** 143–61.

◆ 6. Sjöberg M, Appelgren L, Einarsson S, *et al*. Long-term intrathecal morphine and bupivacaine in "refractory" cancer pain. I. Results from the first series of 52 patients. *Acta Anaesthesiol Scand* 1991; **35:** 30–43.

◆ 7. Crul BJ, Van Dongen RT, Snijdelaar DG. Long-term continuous intrathecal administration of morphine and bupivacaine at the upper cervical level: access by a lateral C1–C2 approach. *Anesth Analg* 1994, **79:** 594–7.

◆ 8. Appelgren L, Janson M, Nitescu P, Curelaru I. Continuous intracisternal and high cervical intrathecal bupivacaine analgesia in refractory head and neck pain. *Anesthesiology* 1996; **84:** 256–72.

◆ 9. Kunkle EC, Ray BS, Wolf HG. Experimental studies on headache: analysis of headache associated with changes in intracranial pressure. *Neurol Psychiatry* 1943; **49:** 323–58.

◆ 10. Franksson C, Gordh T. Headache after spinal anaesthesia and a technique for lessening its frequency. *Acta Chir Scand* 1946; **94:** 443–54.

◆ 11. Palma EC, Martinez RR, Garbino C. Presión intracraneana. Medida directa en la gran cisterna. *Acta Neurol Latinoam* 1979; **25:** 225–34.

◆ 12. Nitescu P, Dahm P, Appelgren L, Curelaru I. Continuous infusion of opioid and bupivacaine by externalized intrathecal catheters in long-term treatment of "refractory" nonmalignant pain. *Clin J Pain* 1998; **14:** 17–28.

◆ 13. Sjöberg M, Karlsson PÅ, Nordborg C, *et al*. Neuropathologic findings after long-term intrathecal infusion of morphine and bupivacaine for pain treatment in cancer patients. *Anesthesiology* 1992; **76:** 173–86.

◆ 14. Aldrete JA, Vascello LA, Ghaly R, Tomlin D. Paraplegia in a patient with an intrathecal catheter and a spinal cord stimulator. *Anesthesiology* 1994; **81:** 1542–5.

◆ 15. Appelgren L, Nitescu P, Curelaru I. Use of intrathecal opioids and bupivacaine in the outpatient treatment of refractory cancer pain. *Home Health Care Consult* 1996; **3:** 1A–16A

◆ 16. Aldrete JA. Securing epidural catheters to connectors. *Anesthesiology* 1995; **82:** 320.

◆ 17. Sjöberg M, Nitescu P, Appelgren L, Curelaru I. Long-term intrathecal morphine and bupivacaine in refractory cancer pain. Results from a morphine:bupivacaine regimen of 0.5:4.75 mg/ml. *Anesthesiology* 1994; **80:** 284–97.

◆ 18. De Cicco M, Mativic M, Tarabini Castellani G, *et al*. Time-dependent efficacy of bacterial filters and infection risk in long-term epidural catheterization. *Anesthesiology* 1995; **82:** 765–71.

◆ 19. Nitescu P, Sjöberg M, Appelgren L, Curelaru I. Complications of intrathecal opioids and bupivacaine in the treatment of "refractory" cancer pain. *Clin J Pain* 1995; **11:** 45–62.

◆ 20. Dahm PO, Nitescu P, Appelgren L, Curelaru I. Efficacy and technical complications of long-term continuous intraspinal infusions of opioid and/or bupivacaine in refractory nonmalignant pain: a comparison between the epidural and the intrathecal approach with externalized or implanted catheters and infusion pumps. *Clin J Pain* 1998; **14:** 4–16.

◆ 21. Gerritse BM, Dongen van RTM, Crul BJP. Epidural fibrin injection stops persistent cerebrospinal fluid leak during long-term intrathecal catheterization. *Anesth Analg* 1997; **84:** 1140–1.

◆ 22. Schoeffler P, Pichard E, Rambotiana R, *et al*. Bacterial meningitis due to infection of a lumbar drug release system in patients with cancer pain. *Pain* 1986, **25:** 75–7.

◆ 23. Nitescu P, Hultman E, Appelgren L, *et al*. Bacteriology, drug stability and exchange of percutaneous delivery systems and antibacterial filters in long-term intrathecal infusion of opioid drugs and bupivacaine in "refractory" pain. *Clin J Pain* 1992; **8:** 324–37.

◆ 24. Hassenbusch SJ, Stanton-Hicks M, Covington EC, *et al*. Long-term intraspinal infusions of opioids in the treatment of neuropathic pain. *J Pain Symptom Manage* 1995; **10:** 527–43.

◆ 25. Follet KA, Hitchon PW, Piper J, *et al*. Response of intractable pain to continuous intrathecal morphine: a retrospective study. *Pain* 1992; **49:** 21–5.

◆ 26. Groudine SB, Cresanti-Daknis C, Lumb PD. Successful treatment of a massive intrathecal morphine overdose. *Anesthesiology* 1995; **82:** 292–5.

● 27. Netter FH. Nervous system. In: *The Ciba Collection of Medical Illustrations*, vol. 1, 11th edn. Rochester, NY: The Case–Hoyt Corporation, 1975: plate 22.

24

Long-term epidural treatment of refractory malignant and nonmalignant pain using internal and external pumps

ANDREW LAWSON AND OLGA SIEMASZKO

Indications for long-term therapy	308	Selection of catheter and pumps	313
Clinical setting	308	Practical tips	315
Patient selection	310	Efficacy	316
Contraindications	310	Epidural versus intrathecal	316
Doses and regimens	311	References	316
Side-effects and their management	311		

The presence of opioid receptors in the central nervous system was first demonstrated in the 1970s,[1*] with the potent and selective effect of intrathecal opioids being demonstrated shortly afterwards.[2*] These discoveries opened the door for the use of accessible anatomical spinal compartments as routes of administration for opiate analgesics. Since that time, other spinal receptor types implicated in pain modulation have been further defined, leading to the therapeutic use of other drug classes via intraspinal routes (Table 24.1).

Of all the classes of drugs that have been used via the epidural space, the most commonly used is opioids alone or in combination with local anesthetics. Baclofen[3*] has an established place in the management of spasticity and related pain. Midazolam has been demonstrated to have analgesic properties,[4**] as has clonidine.[5**] It seems though that their principal role is as adjuvant to opioid analgesia,[6*] but there are reports of their use as sole agents.

The term "intraspinal" encompasses delivery of drugs via the epidural and the intrathecal routes. In the case of opioids, the final site of action is identical regardless of the compartment used. One of the main advantages of intraspinal administration of drugs over the intravenous route is total dose reduction and hence a potentially improved side-effect profile. To achieve the same analgesic effect, the intrathecal compartment requires one-tenth and the epidural route one-third to one-half of the intravenous dose. Provision of continuous analgesia may be achieved by catheterization of either epidural or intrathecal compartments (under a standard aseptic technique) then attachment to a pump for infusion of the desired drugs.

Many of the issues relevant to the use of epidural pumps will be equally applicable to pumps and catheters used for the intrathecal route. The principal advantages and disadvantages of each system are described in Table 24.2. The remit of this chapter is to deal exclusively and comprehensively with *epidural* drug administration, and so both external and internal pump systems will be considered. However, it should be borne in mind that, as a general principle, epidural catheters are mainly used in conjunction with *external* pumps, whereas in the case of

Table 24.1 *Drugs used via the epidural route in pain management*

Opioids
Clonidine
Midazolam
Baclofen
Local anesthetics
N-methyl-ᴅ-aspartate (NMDA) antagonists
Somatostatin analogs
Cholinesterase inhibitors
Calcium channel blockers
Nonsteroidal anti-inflammatory drugs

Table 24.2 *Epidural vs. intrathecal route*

	Advantages	Disadvantages
Epidural	Clinician familiarity with technique Equipment more readily available Dura not breached Low cost	Evidence of increased complications Occlusion and epidural fibrosis more common High dose required Possibly more side-effects Refills more common
Intrathecal	Lower dose Smaller drug volume means reduced pump refill frequency Evidence of greater efficacy	Dura breached out of necessity Increased risk of infection if external pump used CSF leakage High cost

totally implantable systems the most common practice is to utilize the intrathecal route.

INDICATIONS FOR LONG-TERM THERAPY

Long-term administration of pain relief via the epidural route can last for weeks, months, and even years depending upon the clinical situation When considering long-term epidural analgesia, the overall nature of the patient's pain and diagnosis must be considered. Pain is a biopsychosocial construct, unimodal therapy in chronic pain is less likely to succeed than multimodal therapy, and rehabilitation, physical or mental, is a vital part of chronic pain management. This is as relevant to patients receiving epidural therapy as it is to patients undergoing simple conservative treatments. Fixing on the "pump" as the golden bullet will almost invariably lead to failure. The principle should be that the epidural route is being used to produce pain relief, but that the aim is not analgesia alone. Analgesia produced should be used to facilitate rehabilitation, both mental and physical. Long-term use of epidural drug delivery systems should be seen as one part of a therapeutic algorithm (Table 24.3).

CLINICAL SETTING

Cancer pain

In approximately 80% of cancer patients, pain may be successfully managed using oral, parental, and, more recently, percutaneous opiates.[7*] Many clinicians advocate the use of escalating doses of oral medication, in particular the "gold standard analgesic" morphine, for the control of chronic malignant pain. Where opioids in combination with nonsteroidal anti-inflammatory (NSAIDs) and appropriate coanalgesics are failing to provide optimum analgesia or are producing unacceptable side-effects, then epidural drug administration may be considered. Failure of symptom control may be related to the severity of the pain or noncompliance with prescribed drugs because of unwanted side-effects. In these

selected patients the use of intraspinal opiates should be considered; however, before implementing invasive therapies it is wise to undertake further patient screening to exclude disease progression as a cause of increased pain. In addition, in a patient with cancer pain, new or deteriorating pain should not automatically be attributed to the underlying disease, as there may be a new and possibly nonmalignant pathology causing the pain.

Opioids administered epidurally will eventually bind to the μ-receptor to produce analgesia. The choice of drug is often a matter of geography as much as pharmacokinetics. The side-effect profile varies between patients, and if side-effects are intolerable with one agent then another should be used. The response of the patient to trial spinal opioids should be documented prior to implanting any permanent devices. Many physicians would wish to see both a reduction in pain intensity and functional improvement during the trial period.

Epidural opiates may be used in the terminal stages of disease, when life expectancy is short and care may be provided in the hospital or hospice setting, and also earlier in the disease process. Clonidine,[5**] NSAIDs,[8*] somatostatin,[9*] and neostigmine[10**] have all been reported to be effective when administered via the epidural route. Epidural administration should not be seen as having utility only in the last stages of life, but more as a general tool in the pain physician's armamentarium.

Nonmalignant pain

The use of long-term epidural catheterization to treat nonmalignant pain is a more controversial issue, but there are two main factors that have been the driving force behind its wider acceptance: the destigmatization of opiate use in patients and by clinicians with a concomitant reduction in fear and misconceptions surrounding opiate prescription; and the increased sophistication of catheter and reservoir technologies.

Long-term catheterization (years) is one indication for pump implantation, although patients have been managed with percutaneous access systems for periods of greater than a year. Many pain syndromes failing to respond to conventional modalities of treatment may well respond to epidural blockade (Table 24.4). Clonidine

Table 24.3 *The role of intraspinal pumps in pain management*

	Analgesics	Rehabilitation	Intervention	Surgery	Cognitive therapy
	Simple analgesics: acetaminophen (paracetamol), NSAIDs	Physiotherapy: exercise program: posture enhancement	Transcutaneous electric nerve stimulation (TENS) Acupuncture		
		Manipulation: therapeutic massage, osteopathy, chiropractic			
→	Weak opioids Co-drugs Codeine Tramadol ??Others	←	Injections: joints, somatic nerves, sympathetic nerves	Acute: decompressive	Psychology Relaxation techniques
→	Second-line drugs: antidepressant, anticonvulsant, topical capsaicin	←	←	←	←
→	Strong opioids: oral morphine, fentanyl patches	→	Denervation: joint, sympathetic nerves, intradiskal electrical thermocoagulation (IDET), cordotomy	Semiacute: fusion, reconstructive	Pain management program
→	→	→	Implantable devices: spinal cord stimulator, infusion pumps	←	←
↑	↓	↓	↓	↓	↓
↑			Pain management program		

is both sympatholytic and analgesic at the spinal cord and has been used to treat complex regional pain syndromes as well as cancer pain.[11**] Epidural opioids have been used for long-term treatment of refractory angina,[12*] failed back surgery syndrome,[13*] and peripheral vascular disease,[14*] and in combination with ketamine and bupivacaine in the treatment of complex regional pain syndromes.[15*]

Spasticity related to cerebrovascular accident or multiple sclerosis can be treated with epidural infusion of baclofen.[3*] The spasticity itself may cause secondary pain in the joints that are acted upon by the muscles in spasm. In practice, longer term treatment with spinal baclofen now invariably involves intrathecal treatment.

Other patients fall into an intermediate category, in whom temporary placement of an epidural catheter and continuous infusion may be used to break a pain cycle. The epidural catheter may be tunneled percutaneously or attached to a subcutaneous injection port. Such techniques may be particularly useful in patients with painful syndromes resulting in a significant component of

secondary immobility. Examples would be severe complex regional pain syndromes and chronic nonspecific low back pain (Table 24.5). Epidural analgesia has been used to facilitate rehabilitation in patients with severe low back pain.[16*] While experiencing pain relief the patients can undergo either active or passive movement and exercise programs to resolve some of the secondary effects of pain, including tendon and muscle shortening as well as weakness. Postherpetic neuralgia is a notoriously difficult condition to treat once established. A trial of epidurally infused local anesthetic agents over a period of

Table 24.4 *Nonmalignant pain – indications for long-term epidural treatment*

Chronic refractory angina (CRF)
Failed back surgery syndrome (FBSS)
Complex regional pain syndrome (CRPS)
Peripheral vascular disease (PVD)
Pain secondary to spasticity
AIDS-related pain

Table 24.5 *Indications for medium-term catheterization*

Chronic back pain rehabilitation
Chronic regional pain syndrome (CRPS)
Postherpetic neuralgia

weeks may prove beneficial.[17]* The pain relief obtained may continue long after discontinuation of the epidural. Similar treatments have been tried for post-thoracotomy syndromes.

PATIENT SELECTION

In general the indications for long-term epidural analgesia are:

- failure of oral, transcutaneous, and parenteral drug therapy to control symptoms;
- intractable pain unresponsive to conventional treatment;
- intolerable side-effects despite effective treatment;
- as an alternative to other more invasive and potentially destructive procedures, such as surgery and neuroablative procedures;
- absence of any contraindications.

For patients with intractable cancer pain despite the sequential use of strong opioid analgesics or unmanageable side-effects, a trial of epidural opiates is appropriate. A significant reduction in pain levels would be a suitable indication for continued epidural opiates to manage symptoms. In the case of nonmalignant pain, all conventional syndrome-specific therapies, including sequential use of strong opioid analgesics, should be attempted before a trial of spinal drug therapy. Patients with nonmalignant pain should be integrated into multidisciplinary pain management programs prior to commencement on epidural therapy, and special attention needs to be paid to psychological stability and coping mechanisms.

In general, patients with a life expectancy of less than 3 months have epidural catheters connected to external pumps and those patients with life expectancies greater than 3 months have implanted programmable infusion pumps.[18]* Table 24.6 summarizes the process of proceeding to epidural drug therapy. In general, if the six questions have been satisfied and pain is still a problem, then it would seem reasonable to proceed to a trial.

CONTRAINDICATIONS

Contraindications to epidural infusion devices can be divided into those related to the insertion of the epidural catheter (see below) and those related to running an infusion either by external or implanted pumps.

Table 24.6 *Algorithm for instituting epidural opioid therapy*

1. Does the patient still have pain despite aggressive systemic opioid therapy?
   Try changing oral opiate and/or preparation
   - Oromorph – MST – Sevredol
   - Hydromorphone – oxycodone

   Try changing route of administration
   - Transcutaneously – fentanyl patches
   - Subcutaneously – diamorphine infusion

2. Does the pain have a neuropathic element?
   Try tricyclic antidepressants – amitriptyline
   Try neuroleptic agents – gabapentin
   Try other analgesics – clonidine, tramadol

3. Are side-effects from systemic opiates the main problem?
   Are any side-effects being maximally treated?
   - Antiemetics
   - Laxatives
   - Antihistamines

4. Would a neurolytic block or surgery be contributory?

5. Is there a psychological contraindication to epidural infusion treatment?

6. If an epidural is inserted, are there adequate follow-up facilities available?
   - Medical staff
   - Nursing staff
   - Competent carer
   - Funding

MST, slow-release morphine.

Contraindications to epidural catheter

Absolute contraindications to the placement of an epidural catheter include:

- lack of patient consent;
- clotting abnormality;
- local or systemic infection.

  Relative contraindications include:

- spinal metastases;
- gross anatomical abnormality;
- extensive spinal surgery at intended site of insertion;
- insulin-dependent diabetes mellitus.

Not all of the above rule out the use of epidural catheter entirely, for example if the epidural space is obstructed by a metastatic deposit two epidural catheters may be sited, one above and one below the obstruction. Image intensification using radio-opaque dye to locate the epidural space can be used for anatomically difficult cases.

Contraindications to running an infusion

Contraindications to infusion include:

- poor patient compliance and understanding;
- lack of appropriately trained staff to insert or look after pump;
- insufficient evidence that all other methods to control pain have failed;
- psychiatric disorder or personality disorder;
- allergy to drug to be infused;
- suspected abnormal pain behavior or malingering;
- addictive personality with alcohol and/or drug abuse.

DOSES AND REGIMENS

The epidural dose of opioid required is highly variable and, in the author's experience, does not reflect a simple mathematical ratio to the pre-epidural dose. The dose of epidural morphine has been estimated as being 10–50% of the parenteral dose;[19]* the dose of other agents used epidurally is highly variable. Highly lipid-soluble drugs may have an epidural–parenteral ratio of 1:1.

Figure 24.1 shows an algorithm for epidural opioid management and introduction of other drugs. Table 24.7 shows the commonly used epidural opioids and other drugs.

Authors disagree as to the volume of solution required. In general, the higher the site, the smaller the volume required, although the addition of a low concentration of local anesthetic may necessitate higher volumes. Volumes of 5–10 ml would seem to be sufficient for cervical injections, rising to 10–20 ml for lumbar epidural injections. When instituting local anesthetic therapy, it is necessary to monitor for hypotension due to sympathetic blockade.

Key points

Ensure that the patient is hydrated.
Ensure that nursing monitoring is available for 24 h.
Check erect and supine blood pressures.
Ensure that i.v. fluids are available for a nurse to give at home if necessary.
Monitor ambulation during the first 24 h.

SIDE-EFFECTS AND THEIR MANAGEMENT

Mechanical problems and infection

Long-term use of epidural catheters can present many problems, most of which are corrected by replacing the catheter. The following are suggested remedies for problems encountered (Table 24.8).

Infection can occur with both externalized catheters and implanted systems. In one series of patients with externalized catheters in whom meticulous attention was taken to prevent infection (nursing staff follow-up for

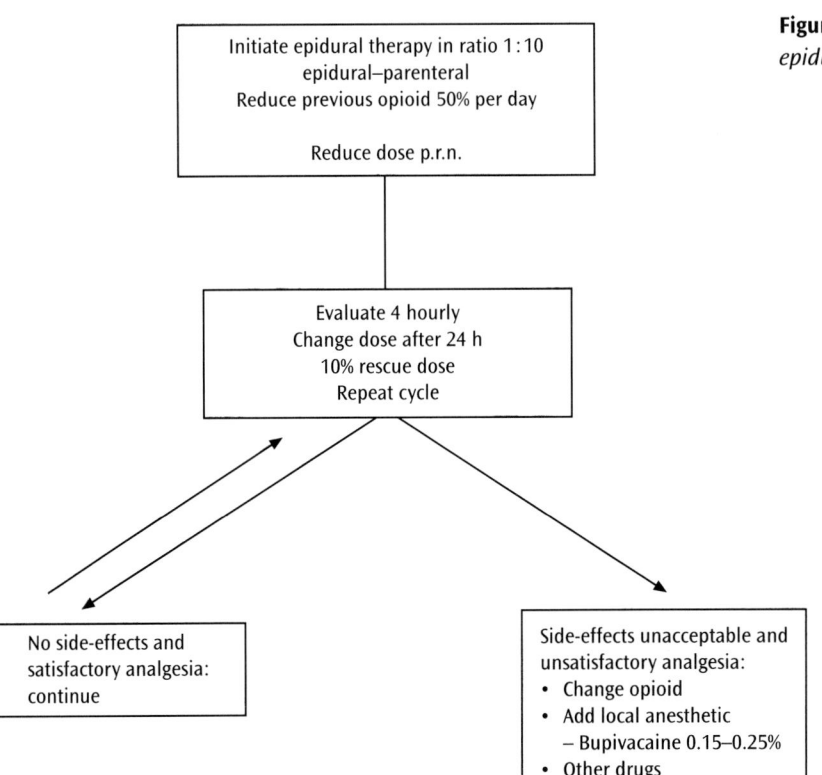

Figure 24.1 *Algorithm for instituting epidural opioid therapy.*

Initiate epidural therapy in ratio 1:10
epidural–parenteral
Reduce previous opioid 50% per day

Reduce dose p.r.n.

Evaluate 4 hourly
Change dose after 24 h
10% rescue dose
Repeat cycle

No side-effects and satisfactory analgesia: continue

Side-effects unacceptable and unsatisfactory analgesia:
- Change opioid
- Add local anesthetic
  – Bupivacaine 0.15–0.25%
- Other drugs

Table 24.7 *Dose, duration, onset, and potency of commonly used epidural drugs*

Drug	Single dose	Duration (h)	Onset	Ratio/potency to i.v.
Morphine	1–5 mg	12–24	Slow	×5–10
Hydromorphone	1–2 mg	6–12	Intermediate	×5
Methadone	1–10 mg	4–8	Rapid	Less potent
Meperidine	20–150 mg	4–8	Rapid	×1–2
Fentanyl	25–100 µg	2–4	Rapid	1:1?
Diamorphine	4–6 mg	12	Rapid	?
Midazolam	1–2 mg	?	Rapid	NA
Clonidine	50 µg/h	NA	Rapid	NA

NA, not applicable.

refills and bacterial filter changes) an infection rate of 1/7,242 treatment days was achieved.[20]*

Pharmacological side-effects

The principal side-effects are related to epidural opioid usage. Clonidine and local anesthetics have been reported to cause hypotension.

Table 24.8 *Mechanical problems and solutions with epidural catheters*

Catheter dislodgement
  Check position with radio-opaque dye, change if malpositioned

Catheter collapsing/kinking
  Flush with saline
  Pull under image intensification to straighten out
  Replace

Obstruction and occlusion
  Check filter
  Epidurography to determine site of obstruction
  Replace catheter if unable to overcome

Fibrous encapsulation
  Check with radio-opaque dye
  If entirely encapsulated then replace

Catheter migration
  Replace

Pump mechanical failure
  Change pump

Hematoma
  Drain hematoma if possible
  If epidural, urgent MRI and decompression if necessary for cord compression

Fistula formation
  Replace

Epidural abscess, cellulitis, meningitis
  CSF culture
  Antibiotic therapy

Side-effects related to epidural opiate use

Side-effects resulting from epidural opiate use may be dose dependent or dose independent, although some apparently dose-independent side-effects are in fact related to the rate of dose administration rather than total dose administered. Some of these side-effects are observed when the drug regimen is initiated, e.g. nausea, but then may subside over time.

Dose-dependent side-effects include:

- hypotension;
- central depression;
  - sedation;
  - respiratory depression;
- nausea and vomiting;
- dysphoria.

Dose-independent side-effects include:

- pruritus;
- urinary retention;
- late respiratory depression (morphine, buprenorphine);
- sedation (lipophilic opiates);
- delayed gastric emptying;
- reduced gastrointestinal absorption of drugs;
- constipation.

The advantage of administration via the epidural route over oral or parenteral administration is the improved side-effect profile. This benefit is possibly the primary reason for referral to chronic pain physicians for catheter and pump therapy.

As stated earlier, the dose required when morphine is administered by the epidural route is reduced by a factor of 10 or more. This is very important as the incidence of side-effects depends on the total dose given rather than the concentration or volume administered.[21]*

Respiratory depression
Respiratory depression may be early or late.

Early This is dependent on the amount of opioid injected, the rate of absorption into the systemic circulation, and the rates of distribution into the cerebrospinal fluid (CSF) and brainstem. It is thought to occur more often with lipophilic agents.

The likelihood of respiratory depression is increased by the coadministration of other centrally depressant drugs, such as benzodiazepines and sedative antiemetics.

Late This is seen more often with the hydrophilic opioids such as morphine and is explained by rostral spread of the drug in CSF and binding to μ-receptors in the respiratory center,

Most patients on long-term epidural opiate infusions develop tolerance to their respiratory depressant effects. In addition, the rate of infusion is slow and a steady state of drug distribution is achieved, again reducing the incidence of this potentially dangerous problem.

The occurrence of respiratory depression in a patient well established on epidural opiates may indicate migration of the catheter into the subarachnoid space (although this is more common at the time of insertion), a drug dosage error when refilling the reservoir or syringe driver, or a pump malfunction.

Hypotension

Hypotension is virtually unknown with long-term epidural opiate administration, especially if given as infusion and without local anesthetic. It is more likely to be seen when giving bolus injections or starting a new drug. Treatment includes immediate cessation of the offending drug, intravenous fluids, oxygen, and vasoconstrictors titrated to response as indicated.

Nausea and vomiting

Nausea occurs in up to 25% of patients given epidural opioids postoperatively. It is an early side-effect of chronic epidural opiate use and reduces in severity with time, usually because of the development of tolerance.[22*] In patients suffering with pain from malignancy, nausea can result from the disease itself, or from other measures aimed at treatment or palliation, such as chemotherapy. The addition of epidural opiates may contribute to the patient's symptoms, and the long-term use of antiemetics, a single agent or combination of drugs, may be required.

Pruritus

The incidence of pruritus following epidural morphine administration has been reported to be up to 70%,[23*] and the incidence is greater with epidural administration than with intravenous or intramuscular injections.

SELECTION OF CATHETER AND PUMPS

The selection of implantation device depends on the expected duration of delivery, the drug to be administered, the experience/skill of the staff inserting and maintaining the device, and cost–benefit ratio of the system.

For patients with terminal cancer who are unlikely to be returning home for any length of time, a standard nylon epidural catheter attached to an external epidural infusion pump (as used for acute postoperative pain relief) may be all that is required. The epidural catheter can be tunneled at insertion to emerge at the anterolateral aspect of the chest or abdominal wall. This provides more secure anchorage of the catheter and reduces the risk of displacement.

As the life expectancy of the patient increases, so the need for more permanent devices becomes evident. Epidural catheters made from silicone rubber with wire reinforcement are available. Du Pen added a Dacron cuff, similar to those found on tunneled feeding lines, which promotes host fibrosis around the cuff and more secure anchorage. This was followed by the introduction of the Vita cuff, which has antimicrobial properties and theoretically reduces the risk of ascending infection from the patient's skin.

Epidural catheters come as one piece (all temporary catheters and some of the longer term catheters) or as two pieces: the first part is inserted into the epidural space and the second part can be connected to a totally implantable *pump, reservoir,* or injection port.

Epidural catheters are inserted using a standard approach.

Pump classification

Classification of delivery systems for intraspinal delivery of drugs

Type 1 systems, percutaneous epidural catheters with or without subcutaneous tunneling, (e.g. Portex catheter):

- are suitable for terminal patients with short life expectancy (weeks or months);
- are associated with a high risk of infection;
- can be attached to external infusion pump;
- enable drug and dose to be altered easily;
- are similar to acute postoperative epidural infusion equipment (nursing staff are most familiar with this set-up);
- enable a trial of therapy before committing the patient to a fully implantable epidural or intrathecal system.

Type 2 systems, totally implanted epidural catheters with a subcutaneous injection port (e.g. Port-A-Cath):

- are suitable for patients with a life expectancy of several months;
- require repeated skin punctures to access the port;
- need surgical intervention for placement and removal of the port.

Type 3 systems, totally implanted epidural catheters

with implanted manually activated pump (e.g. Algomed) are suitable for:

- patients with a life expectancy of several months;
- patient-controlled administration;
- bolus administration of drugs by patient or carer.

Type 4 systems, totally implanted epidural catheters with an implanted infusion pump (e.g. Infusaid):

- are suitable for patients with a long life expectancy;
- are more expensive than types 1–3;
- require surgical skills to implant;
- can be difficult to refill.

Type 5 systems, totally implanted epidural catheters with an implanted programmable infusion pump (e.g. Synchromed):

- are suitable for patients with a long life expectancy.
- are the most expensive equipment;
- require surgical skill to implant;
- require telemetry to refill and program;
- have the greatest capabilities for personalized delivery patterns and bolus administration.

The most widely used systems are types 1 and 5, and the implantation of these will be discussed in greater detail.

Totally implanted systems

Although more expensive and requiring more experience and skill to insert, totally implantable systems provide greater sterility and freedom of movement for the patient. In one system, a subcutaneous port is attached to a tunneled epidural catheter and implanted and a needle is then passed through the skin and into the port. A drug bolus can be injected, or an external infusion pump can be set up in a similar fashion to the Port-A-Caths used for permanent intravascular cannulation.

The site of implantation is selected to provide ease of access for patient or carer, usually on the anterolateral aspect of the abdomen or lower chest. Siting the catheter on the opposite side to the patient's dominant hand makes location and needling of the port more convenient for patients who are expected to maintain and use the device themselves. However, in paraplegic patients who use external pressure to aid defecation the port should not be placed on the left.

Port-A-Cath ports are circular in design and made of a metal base and sides with a window covered by a membrane that lies flush with the skin. The membrane is durable to prevent leaking and is able to withstand repeated injections (several hundred) without deterioration. The metal rim is easy to palpate subcutaneously, and the metal base provides an endpoint to injection. A filter has been incorporated to prevent blockage of the epidural catheter, which is attached via a side-port (Fig. 24.2).

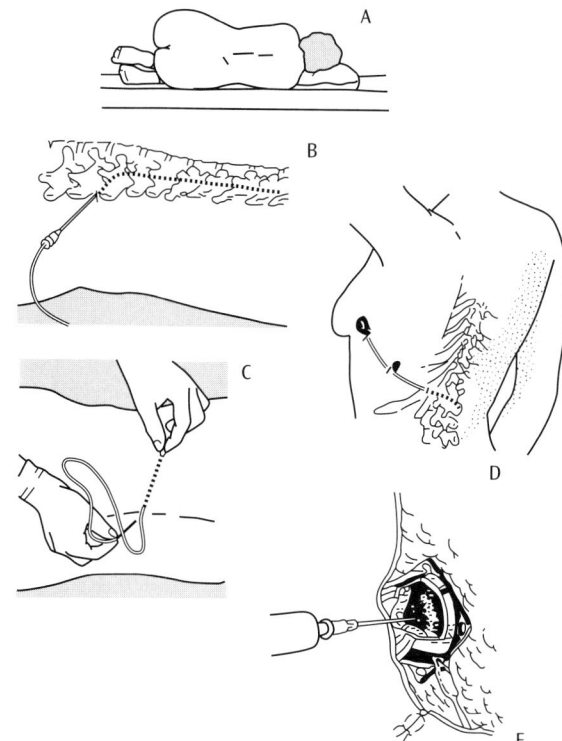

Figure 24.2 *Insertion of tunneled catheter. (A) position of the patient: insertion marked at L2. (B) Insertion of 16-gauge epidural catheter via a Tuohy needle. (C) Second incision over the 11th rib allows the catheter to be moved over the anterior chest wall. (D) Portal attached to catheter after tensioning loop and second tunnel. (E) Injection technique.*

The portal system is limited because of the need for percutaneous needling in order to deliver any drugs, and is more commonly used for intermittent bolus injections than for continuous infusions.

The Port-A-Cath system is straightforward to insert and maintain. The surgical technique is simple to learn. It may be inserted under local or general anesthesia. The patient is placed in the lateral position. An image intensifier is necessary. The epidural space is located using a loss of resistance technique and the catheter is advanced in the epidural space to the desired level. The epidural space may be dilated with saline or local anesthetic prior to insertion of the catheter. Biplanar image intensification will show whether the catheter has remained in the midline, exited through a foramen, and/or threaded up the paraspinal muscles. The catheter tip should be 3–5 cm above the desired point to allow for movement.

Once the catheter is in the desired space, an incision is made around the Tuohy needle and the remaining catheter tunneled, using a rod, to the site for the portal. To avoid passing the rod under the ribs, the tip should be continuously palpated during this process. The portal should be secured in a subcutaneous pocket. Patients should remain in bed for 24 h postoperatively to avoid excessive movement. Perioperative antibiotic cover is advisable. A small test with contrast material postoperatively will give an indication of where boluses will spread and will also confirm the integrity of the system

Other systems contain a larger reservoir with some form of pump that can be powered by a battery or expanding gas. The simpler pumps deliver at a set rate, so it is the drug dosage that is altered when the reservoir is refilled, by altering the concentration of injectate. The more sophisticated pumps are programmable via telemetry and provide a greater flexibility in drug administration regimens. Other pumps have the facility for patient-controlled administration but have not yet become commonly used.

The new generation of pumps are less bulky and have a longer battery life and more versatile programming ability.

Implanted pumps

The principles for epidural catheter insertion are the same as above. The pocket for the pump, which is usually on the lower anterior abdominal wall (above or below the belt line; avoid prostheses and wheelchair arms) is much larger than that for the Port-A-Cath. In the ambulatory patient the position of the pocket should be determined with the patient standing up preoperatively to ensure maximal comfort.

An incision is made 2–3 cm lateral to the umbilicus and the pocket fashioned with a sweeping movement of fingers, stripping subcutaneous fat away from underlying fascia. Attention to homeostasis is vital to prevent hematoma formation. Many physicians clean the pocket with peroxide prior to implanting the pump.

The IsoMed (Medtronic) continuous infusion pump (Fig. 24.3) is a circular pump with two injection ports: a central port that allows percutaneous refilling of the drug reservoir and a side-port situated close to the rim of the pump where the epidural catheter inserts into the pump. This allows aspiration of drug directly through the epidural catheter to ensure patency; in the case of intrathecal pumps, cerebrospinal fluid (CSF) may be aspirated if required. The pump is driven by an inert gas, which compresses bellows when the reservoir is filled. The pump includes a filter to prevent clogging of the catheter, and the injection ports are designed so that the central port can be filled with a 22G needle but the side port is screened so that it can only be accessed with a 25G needle. Loops enable the pump to be sutured in place. The SynchroMed (Medtronic) externally programmable pump is shown in Fig. 24.4.

The Algomed (Medtronic) patient-controlled pump consists of a reservoir, tubing attached to a patient-controlled pump, and an epidural (or intrathecal) catheter. A reservoir filling port is connected to a pumping chamber, which delivers the drug to the catheter. The pumping chamber is also connected to an activation valve;

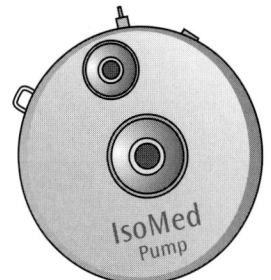

Figure 24.3 *IsoMed implantable pump.*

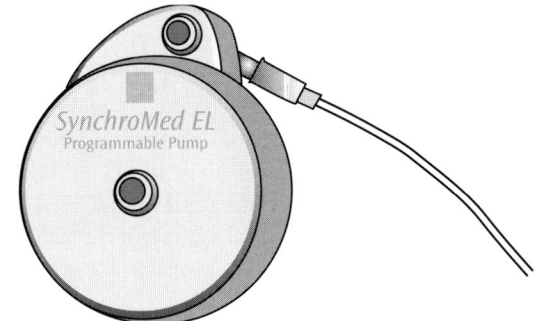

Figure 24.4 *SynchroMed externally programmable pump.*

in order to release a measured dose of drug the patient must depress buttons on both the activation valve and the pumping chamber simultaneously. Following this the pumping chamber takes 60 min to refill, constituting a "lock-out" period.

PRACTICAL TIPS

Advice to patients with implanted pumps

Before traveling, patients fitted with implanted pumps should consult their physician so that adjustments can be made to treatment regimen and follow-up can be arranged at destination if appropriate. Activities that could lead to damage to the site of implantation should be avoided. Pumps do not usually cause alarms at airport security checks, but patients should always carry pump information and an emergency card. Implantable pumps do not cause problems when using mobile phones or microwave ovens.

GAS-DRIVEN PUMPS

Snorkeling and swimming do not affect the working of pumps, but the high pressure associated with scuba diving will cause significant deviations in flow rate and therefore scuba diving is not permitted.

During air travel the infusion rate will increase slightly, but as aircraft cabins are pressurized to almost atmospheric pressure this alteration in rate is not significant.

EFFICACY

Epidural administration opiates does not necessarily provide a better quality of analgesia than delivery of opiates by any other route; however, as the site of action of opiates is in the spinal cord, the delivery of opiates as close as possible to the site of action enables a much lower dose to be administered, with a resulting lower mean plasma concentration and hence more favorable side-effect profile. The therapeutic role of epidural opiates may be justified on this basis. Although there have been few randomized controlled trials of epidural drug delivery in the management of chronic pain, many case series and reports suggest that in well-selected patients quality of life and perhaps longevity may be improved.

The success, efficacy, and cost-effectiveness of implanted epidural devices is dependent on diligent patient selection and wise choice of implantation device, taking into account the clinical setting, technical skills required, and facilities and staff available for appropriate aftercare, not forgetting the cost involved and who is responsible for funding.

EPIDURAL VERSUS INTRATHECAL

Dahm et al.[24*] studied patients with nonmalignant pain and found that the intrathecal approach using external or internal pump is associated with higher rates of satisfactory pain relief than epidural delivery. In addition, internalized epidural catheters were associated with higher rates of treatment failures, higher rates of system replacement, higher rates of system removal, and higher rates of catheter complication when compared with internalized intrathecal catheters. Nitescu et al.[25*] looked at epidural versus intrathecal administration of morphine and bupivacaine in patients with advanced cancer pain, and again intrathecal administration gave more satisfactory pain relief.

Key points

- Epidural drug delivery can improve the management of pain and reduce the frequency of unwanted side-effects.
- Epidural drug delivery can be continued for periods in excess of 1 year and is not contraindicated in patients with nonmalignant pain.
- Implantation of permanent catheters and ports is straightforward.
- Epidural drug delivery systems can be managed at home.
- Life-threatening complications are rare.
- Technical problems occur not infrequently but are not difficult to resolve.

- Lack of experience in the community should not be seen as a barrier to establishment of the technique.

REFERENCES

1. Kuhar MH, Pert CB, Snyder DH. Regional distribution and opiate receptor binding in monkey and human brain. *Nature* 1973; **245:** 447–50.
◆ 2. Cousins MJ, Mather LE, Glynn CJ, *et al*. Selective spinal analgesia. *Lancet* 1979; **1:** 1141.
● 3. Paice JA, Magolan JM. Intraspinal drug therapy. *Nurse Clin N Am* 1991; **26:** 477–98.
4. Nishiyama T, Yokoyama T, Hanaoka K. Midazolam improves postoperative epidural analgesia with continuous infusion of local anaesthetics. *Can J Anaesth* 1998; **45:** 551–5.
5. Eisenach JC, DuPen S, Dubois M, *et al*. Epidural clonidine analgesia for intractable cancer pain. The Epidural Clonidine Study Group. *Pain* 1995; **61:** 391–9.
● 6. Rawal N Spinal antinociception: clinical aspects. *Ann Med* 1995; **27:** 263–8.
● 7. Gildenberg PL. *Stereotact Funct Neurosurg* 1992; **59**(1–4): 1–8.
8. Lauretti GR, Reis MP, Mattos AL, *et al*. Epidural nonsteroidal anti-inflammatory drugs for cancer pain. *Anesth Analg* 1998; **86:** 117–18.
9. Mollenholt P, Rawal N, Gordh Jr T, Olsson Y. Intrathecal and epidural somatostatin for patients with cancer. Analgesic effects and postmortem neuropathologic investigations of spinal cord and nerve roots. *Anesthesiology* 1994; **81:** 534–42.
10. Lauretti GR, Gomes JM, Reis MP, Pereira NL. Low doses of epidural ketamine or neostigmine but not midazolam improve morphine analgesia in epidural terminal cancer patients. *J Clin Anaesth* 1999; **11:** 663–8.
11. Rauck RL, Eisenach JC, Jackson K, *et al*. Epidural clonidine treatment for refractory reflex sympathetic dystrophy. *Anesthesiology* 1993; **79:** 1163–9.
12. Blomberg SG. Long-term home self-treatment with high thoracic epidural anaesthesia in patients with severe coronary artery disease. *Anaesth Analg* 1994; **79:** 405–6.
13. Auld AW, Murdoch DM, O'Laughlin KA Intraspinal narcotic analgesia. Pain management in the failed laminectomy syndrome. *Spine* 1987; **12:** 953–4.
14. Bapat AR, Kshirsagar NA, Padmashree RB, *et al*. *J Postgrad Med* 1980; **26:** 246–9.
15. Lin TC, Wong CS, Chen FC, Lin SY, Ho ST. Long-term epidural ketamine, morphine and bupivacaine attenuate reflex sympathetic dystrophy neuralgia. *Can J Anaesth* 1998 Feb;45(2):175–7.
16. Dolin SJ, Bacon RA, Drage M. Rehabilitation of chronic low back pain using continuous epidural analgesia. *Disabil Rehabil* 1998; **20:** 151–157.
17. Tsai YC, Wang LK, Chen BS, Chen HP. Home-based

patient-controlled epidural analgesia with bupivacaine for patients with intractable herpetic neuralgia. *J Formos Med Assoc* 2000; **99:** 659–62.

18. Krames ES. Intrathecal infusion therapies for intractable pain: patient management guidelines. *J Pain Symptom Manage* 1993; **8:** 36–46.

19. Rocco AG, Iacobo C. An algorithm for the treatment of pain in advanced cancer. *Hospice J* 1989; **5:** 93–103.

20. Nitescu P, Sjoberg M, Appelgren L, Curelaru L. Complications of intrathecal opioids and bupivacaine in the treatment of "refractory cancer pain." *Clin J Pain* 1995; **11:** 45.

21. Laveaux MMD, Hasenbos MA, Harbers JB, Liem T. Thoracic epidural bupivacaine plus sufentanil: high concentration/low volume versus low concentration/high volume. *Reg Anaesth* 1993; **18:** 39–43.

22. Coombs D, Maurer L, Sanders R, Gaylor M: Outcomes and complications of continuous intraspinal narcotic analgesia for pain control. *J Clin Oncol* 1984; **2:** 1414.

● 23. Ballantyne JC, Loach A, Carr D. Itching after epidural and spinal opiates. *Pain* 1988; **33:** 149.

● 24. Dahm P, Nitescu P, Appelgren L, Curelaru I. Efficacy and technical complications of long-term continuous intraspinal infusions of opioid and/or bupivacaine in refractory non-malignant pain: a comparison between the epidural and the intrathecal approach with externalised or implanted catheters and infusion pumps. *Clin J Pain* 1998; **14:** 4–16.

● 25. Nitescu P, Appelgren L, Linder LE, *et al.* Epidural versus intrathecal morphine–bupivacaine: assessment of consecutive treatments in advanced cancer pain. *J Pain Symptom Manage* 1990; **5:** 18–26.

25

Cryoanalgesia

THOMAS A EDELL AND SOMAYAJI RAMAMURTHY

Physics and physiology of freezing	319	Cryoanalgesia in postsurgical pain management	322
Lesion size	320	Cryoneurolysis in chronic pain management	323
Duration of freeze	320	Conclusions	325
Machinery	320	References	325
Clinical applications of cryoanalgesia	322		

Cryoanalgesia, the relief of pain with the application of cold, has undoubtedly been used for millennia. Descriptions of the presurgical use of cold for operative analgesia include:[1]

- Hippocrates (460–377 BC);
- Avicenna of Persia in the Dark Ages;
- Severino of Naples during the Renaissance used ice and snow packs before surgery;
- Larré performed painless amputations on Napoleon's soldiers at subzero temperatures in the Russian winter of 1812;
- Richardson introduced ether spray for dental extractions in 1866;
- Redard developed the more easily administered ethyl chloride spray in 1891.

James Arnott, a fervent opponent of ether in the nineteenth century and the first to propose the use of cold for the treatment of cancer, touted cold application for the treatment of such maladies as headaches, skin disorders, and erysipelas. However, owing to the technical limitations of refrigeration and the further development of general and neuraxial anesthesia, cold application was little used during the first half of the twentieth century.

In 1777, Hunter reported one of the first observations of cold and tissue destruction when he noted the vascular stasis and tissue necrosis of frozen cocks' combs, as well as their favorable healing and recovery. In the 1920s, Trendelenburg studied the destructive effects on nerves, noting prolonged loss of function and regeneration without scar or neuroma formation. Smith and Fay rekindled medical interest in the use of cold therapy with the description of tumor lysis in 1939. The real advent for the use of cryoanalgesia and cryoneurolysis in modern medicine began with the introduction of the first cryoprobe by Cooper in 1961. The potential for medical uses was further enhanced when Amoils introduced the much smaller and more easily handled carbon dioxide cryoprobe in 1967.

PHYSICS AND PHYSIOLOGY OF FREEZING

The exact mechanism of freeze injury is unknown. Theories include direct ice crystal destruction, hypertonicity, protein denaturation, critical reduction of cell volume, dehydration, cell membrane rupture, ischemia, and antibody formation.[1]

Ice crystal formation is the underlying process with any type of freeze injury. It involves the removal of pure water from solution and the formation of crystals, both intra- and extracellularly. The rate of crystal formation is one of the most important aspects of the degree of cell injury. With slower rates of cooling, ice crystal formation is primarily extracellular, leading to intracellular dehydration and shrinkage but unlikely to be uniformly lethal. With more rapid rates of cooling, intracellular ice crystals form more readily, leading to cell membrane rupture and death.[1] Also, crystal size is inversely related to the rate of cooling, resulting in greater cell destruction with more rapid cooling rates.

Ice ball formation is a function of the geometry of the cryoprobe and its ability to extract heat from tissues. There is a sharp temperature gradient from the center of the ice ball outwards: approximately 10°C/mm.[1] *A temperature of –20°C must be reached in the tissues to result in uniform cell death.*[1] Therefore, one can see that, when using a gas expansion cryoprobe, which cools to –70°C (using N_2O), *the center of the ice ball must be within approximately 4–5 mm of the nerve for lethal application*. The ultimate size of the ice ball is determined by the temperature reached at the probe tip, the probe size and geometry, and the surrounding structures, i.e. thermal conductivity and vascularity.

Cryolesioning produces a *second-degree nerve injury* according to Sunderland's classification; this is in contrast to third-, fourth-, and fifth-degree injuries caused by radiofrequency, phenol, alcohol, and surgical resection.[2] In contradistinction to the more severe nerve injuries, cryoneurolysis preserves the fibrous architecture, especially the endoneurium, allowing more organized regeneration *without neuroma formation* and with a very *low incidence of neuritis*.

Freezing results in axonal disruption followed by Wallerian degeneration of the axon distal to the lesion. Nerve regeneration follows and proceeds at approximately 1–3 mm/day.[1] While return of function will depend in part on the distance of the lesion from the end-organ, functional measures can return to normal in as early as three weeks; however, electrophysiologic measurements are still diminished at 90 days, possibly due to continued decreased axonal diameter, myelin thickness, and internodal distance; nerve fiber size is not normalized until approximately one year after injury.[3] In most studies, there has been a minimal inflammatory process with complete regeneration and return of function.

LESION SIZE

The size of the cryolesion is also an important component of successful neurolysis, especially in myelinated fibers. It has been shown in cats that a lesion of 3–6 mm was sufficient to inhibit saltatory transmission of axonal impulses, whereas 4 mm was uniformly effective for rat sciatic nerves.[4] Here, again, the importance of close proximity of the ice ball and target tissue is demonstrated. The type (maximum temperature) and size of the cryoprobe are critical determinants of the size of the ice ball and thus the amount of tissue to be destroyed (see Machinery).

DURATION OF FREEZE

Gill and associates demonstrated that extending the freeze time up to 10 min and repeating the freeze–thaw cycle up to five times would produce greater lesion sizes;[5]* however, this was with temperatures ranging from –50°C to –180°C in rat livers, with the lower temperatures giving more significant results. Evans *et al.* demonstrated that, as long as the critical temperature of *< –20°C was reached for 1 min*, there is no benefit to prolonging or repeating the freezing period *in an exposed nerve*.[4]* In practice, *percutaneous applications*, with less than ideal nerve

localization, will benefit from extending the duration of cryolesioning from *2 to 4 min* and repeating the *freeze–thaw cycle two or three times*; this may enlarge the ice ball up to 15% with the gas-expansion cryoprobe, and up to 40% with the phase change cryoprobe.[1] The longer freeze time and repeat cycles are especially important when freezing nerves in close proximity to vascular structures, which act as heat sinks, e.g. intercostal nerves.

MACHINERY

As previously noted, the development of the first cryoprobe by Cooper in 1961[1] was the first step in advancing cryotherapy in modern medicine. This first cryoprobe was based upon the principle of cooling by *change of phase* from liquid nitrogen to nitrogen gas (Fig. 25.1B). In this design, liquid nitrogen passes through the inner tube within the shaft of the cryoprobe to the highly conductive tip, where it changes phase to the gas form accompanied by a rapid and significant decrease in temperature. The gas is vented via the outer tube along the shaft. The phase change probe tip can reach temperatures down to *–196°C*. This probe allowed refrigeration in a discrete fashion, such as for cataract extraction. The disadvantages of the phase change system of cooling were that it:

- was very cumbersome and expensive;
- had a slow defrost cycle;
- required handling of liquid nitrogen;
- needed separate hoses for liquid and gaseous nitrogen;
- was limited to larger diameter probes with short shafts (owing to the difficulty of forcing liquid nitrogen through a small-diameter tube).

In 1967, Amoils[6] introduced a new cryoprobe based upon the principle of high-pressure *gas expansion* through a small orifice: the Joule–Thompson effect (Fig. 25.1A). He first described the probe using high-pressure (40–50 kg/cm²) carbon dioxide gas. The gas passes through the outer tube along the probe shaft to a restriction or "expansion orifice" at the tip, after which the gas abruptly expands (with a reduction in pressure to 5.5–7.0 kg/cm²) in the tip chamber causing a rapid decrease in temperature. The low-pressure gas is then vented through the inner tube of the shaft. This probe will reach temperatures down to *–60°C to –70°C*. The advantages of the gas expansion freezing system are numerous:

- low cost, easy maintenance;
- smaller diameter probes with longer shafts;
- much less bulk, allowing greater portability;
- one long coaxial hose allowing greater distance from the machinery;
- a relatively innocuous and easily handled cooling agent;

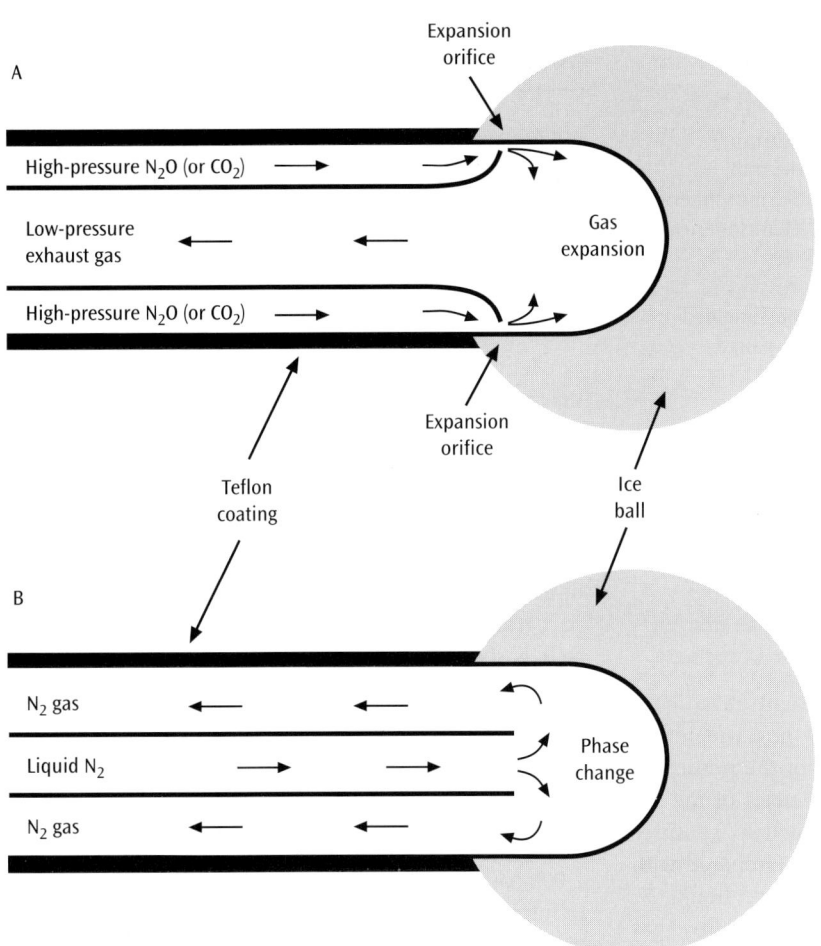

Figure 25.1 *Cross-sections of the gas expansion (A) type and the change of phase (B) type of cryogenic probes.*

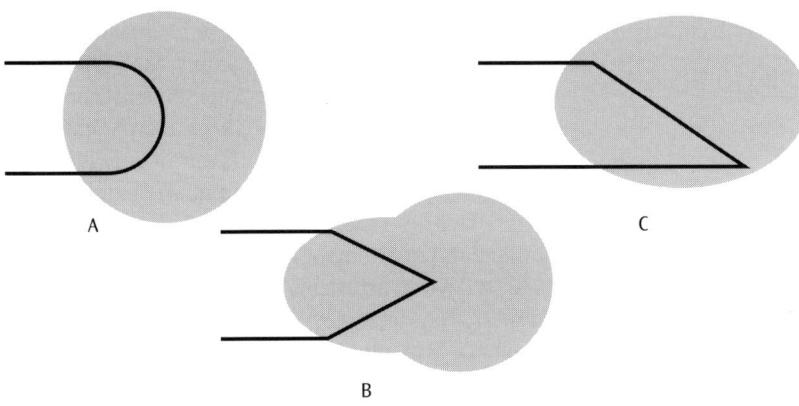

Figure 25.2 *Ice ball shapes of hemisphere- (A), trocar- (B), and bevel-shaped (C) cryogenic probe tips.*

- a foot pedal connection, which allowed rapid freezing and defrosting.

The vast majority of cryosystems in clinical use for pain management today are adaptations of Amoils' cryoprobe. Nitrous oxide gas is most often used because of its ability to be stored in liquid form at room temperature, allowing greater gas volume per tank. As well, N_2O reaches temperatures down to –70°C, whereas CO_2 freezes to –60°C. Since 1967, other important additions to the cryomachine have been:

- a thermocouple at the tip to monitor temperature;
- a nerve stimulator at the tip allowing both motor and sensory stimulation for nerve localization;
- a flow meter to monitor high-pressure gas flow;
- a pressure gauge to monitor cylinder contents;
- freeze and defrost indicators.

The gas expansion cryoprobes come in three shapes (Fig. 25.2). As seen in Fig. 25.2, the geometry of the cryoprobe tip determines the shape of the ice ball:

- The *hemispherical* tip has the most uniform ice ball.

Table 25.1 *Characteristics of two available gas expansion cryogenic probes*

Specifications	Model 2T10	Model 1H3
Length	120 mm	120 mm
Diameter	2.1 mm	1.3 mm
Ice ball diameter/length	6 mm/12 mm	3.5 mm spherical
Tip shape	Trocar	Hemispherical
Temperature indication	Yes	No
Stimulator	Yes	Yes
Cryoneedle stem insulation	Gas shielded	Gas shielded
Intravenous cannula size	12 gauge	16 gauge

Courtesy of Westco Medical Corporation.

However, this tip cannot be used alone for percutaneous techniques; rather, one must use an intravenous cannula one or two sizes larger for tissue penetration.

• The *trocar* and *bevel* tips can both be used to penetrate soft tissues. The bevel tip produces an uneven ice ball, which may effect the production of the ice ball through the desired target tissue.

The size of the cryoprobe will affect the ultimate size of the ice ball: the larger the diameter of the probe, the greater the size of the ice ball. The diameter of the gas expansion freeze-zone is approximately two or three times greater than the probe's diameter, compared with 3.5–5 times greater with the phase change liquid N_2 probe.[7] Table 25.1 compares the characteristics of two gas expansion cryoprobes currently available.

There are two companies currently producing gas expansion cryomachines in the USA:

• Westco Medical Corporation produces the "Neurostat";
• Wallach Surgical Devices produces the "Pain Blocker";

and one company in the UK:

• Spembly Medical also produces the "Neurostat."

CLINICAL APPLICATIONS OF CRYOANALGESIA

Lloyd *et al.*[8] coined the term cryoanalgesia, which is the clinical application of cryotherapy for pain management. Cryoneurolysis is essentially a prolonged somatic block. It has been used for both acute, primarily postoperative, and chronic pain conditions. In this capacity, it is principally utilized for peripheral neurolysis. As all peripheral nerves will regenerate following neurolysis, the most appropriate use of cryoanalgesia is in clinical settings where pain management is needed for weeks to months. The principal advantage of cryoneurolysis over other techniques (notably radiofrequency, chemical or surgical) is the lack of neuroma formation and the low incidence of neuritis.

CRYOANALGESIA IN POSTSURGICAL PAIN MANAGEMENT

Cryoanalgesia for postsurgical pain allows the use of the more effective open technique. The two most common uses for cryoanalgesia in postoperative pain management today are:

1 ilioinguinal nerve block for postherniorrhaphy pain;
2 intercostal nerve block for post-thoracotomy pain.

Many studies have investigated these two blocks for the management of postsurgical pain, especially intercostal cryoanalgesia. Unfortunately, these studies give conflicting results for each: some show a significant decrease in postoperative pain, whereas others show no significant difference from more conventional forms of postoperative management. Part of the problem lies in the use of different parameters to define the decrease in pain, and part results from significantly different study designs as well as surgical approaches. In addition, outcome measures, as well as the duration of follow-up, varied greatly among the different studies.

Indeed, a few studies examining the use of intraoperative cryoneurolysis for post-thoracotomy pain management actually showed an increase in post-thoracotomy neuralgia. Richardson *et al.* retrospectively reviewed 1,000 consecutive thoracotomies; they found that the use of intraoperative cryoanalgesia in 193 cases of posterolateral thoracotomies correlated with a statistically significant increase in the development of post-thoracotomy neuralgia at both 2 and 12 months.[9]*

Of special interest, both for its size and its findings, is the prospective study by Maiwand *et al.* of 600 consecutive patients undergoing thoracotomy for various reasons.[10]* In this study, 83% of the patients were free of pain postoperatively. In their pilot study of 100 patients, each patient received two freezes of 30 s duration at five intercostal levels, resulting in a mean duration of analgesia (as demonstrated by reported postoperative oral analgesic requirements) of 30 days and a mean duration of numbness of 91 days. In an attempt to decrease the duration of numbness, they decreased the freeze to one 30-s freeze in the next 600 patients. This reduction resulted in a mean duration of analgesia of 27 days and a mean duration of numbness of 38 days.

Interesting findings in this study include:

• A reduction in duration of sensory deficit with reduced freeze time, without a significant reduction in duration of analgesia.
• Sensory deficit significantly outlasting analgesia with longer freeze times.
• A significant percentage of pain-free patients, even though pain after thoracotomy usually involves nociception from muscles, ligaments, and pleura, in addition to areas directly subserved by the intercostal nerves undergoing neurolysis.

With the *open technique*, where the nerve is viewed directly, we suggest:

1 Freezing at −60°C to −70°C for 30–120 s (the longer time may be needed for the intercostal nerve, if it is not separated from the adjacent vasculature).
2 A second freeze is probably not necessary with a complete first freeze. If used, thaw until the ice ball disappears (0°C for 30–45 s) prior to refreezing.
3 *Caution: do not remove the ice ball from the frozen tissue. Wait until it has completely thawed before removing the probe.*

Of particular interest to pain clinicians is the fact that cryoneurolysis for postsurgical pain has never been shown to reduce the incidence of chronic post-thoracotomy or postherniorrhaphy pain syndromes.

CRYONEUROLYSIS IN CHRONIC PAIN MANAGEMENT

Defining the limitations of a new technique

One of the earliest case series reporting the results of cryoneurolysis for the relief of chronic pain was by Lloyd *et al.* in 1976.[8]* This study included 64 patients with intractable pain of varying etiology, including intercostal, low back, facial, cancer, and "general." Cryoanalgesia was performed with a gas expansion cryoprobe for two freeze–thaw cycles using 2-min freezes at −60°C and thawing to 0°C. Either open or percutaneous techniques, with nerve stimulation, were used. Pain relief was defined as the pain-free period. The most successful outcomes were reported with the open technique for facial pain involving either the infraorbital or mental nerves: 0/6 with no pain relief, median duration of pain relief was 21 days, and the range of pain relief was 0–112 days. The least successful results were reported using the percutaneous technique for low back pain (via sacral hiatus or foramina) or "general" (at nerve or painful foci): 9/32 with no pain relief, median duration 10 days, range 0–49 days (low back pain) to 0–224 days (general). The authors also reported that "occasionally pain relief lasted for many months despite earlier recovery of motor and sensory function."

This study illustrates the early use of a "new technique," for the relief of pain from almost any source, in order to attempt to define its limitations. In doing so, it foreshadowed dictums in use today:

1 The open technique, under direct visualization, will result in more predictable results.
2 With either technique, the duration of analgesia is unpredictable in the long term.
3 The more discrete and well defined the pathophysiology of the painful condition, the greater the likelihood for successful analgesia of any duration.

Risks of cryoanalgesia

Any nerve that can be exposed surgically or reached percutaneously with a cryoprobe can be frozen. In fact, most peripheral nerves have been frozen at one time or another in an attempt to treat chronic pain. Many clinicians will attempt cryoanalgesia just about anywhere because of the low incidence of risk, especially neuroma formation or neuritis. However, no invasive procedure is risk free. The *risks* of *cryoneurolysis* are:

- infection;
- bleeding;
- nerve damage (either from intravenous cannula trauma or from moving the probe while the ice ball is still formed);
- neuritis (low incidence generally, but possible after nerve damage);
- trauma to, or freezing of, surrounding tissues, including vascular (which could lead to thrombosis and necrosis);
- frostbite to overlying skin (more likely with superficial nerves);
- sensory deficit (expected, but intolerable for some patients);
- weakness (if motor nerves involved);
- increased pain – either immediately after an unsuccessful procedure or following regeneration of the nerve;
- no relief of pain, possibly resulting in significant patient disappointment;
- pneumothorax when used in the intercostal area, especially with the larger probes.

Patient selection

Because of the risks involved, we feel that certain steps should be taken before any neurolysis, cryoneurolysis being no exception:

1 Diagnosis of the pain syndrome.
2 Prior local anesthetic blocks, with or without steroids, both to determine that blockade of any particular nerve will result in pain relief and to ensure that the relief obtained is only temporary.
3 Sympathetic blocks, if indicated.
4 Adjuvant therapies: medications, physical therapy modalities, behavioral health, or other psychological interventions, etc.

While most peripheral nerves can be treated with cryoanalgesia, not all nerves appear to be as amenable to this treatment. The following nerves have, in our experience, been the most responsive to cryoanalgesia in chronic pain management:

- neuromas associated with scarring;
- intercostal nerves;
- medial branches of the posterior primary rami of the spinal roots.

Patient education

As with any invasive procedure in pain management, and with neurolysis in particular, patient selection and education are paramount to a successful outcome. Most clinicians advocate the use of local anesthetic blockade prior to any neurolytic to ensure adequate pain relief, except in rare circumstances such as chemical celiac plexus neurolysis for cancer pain. Prior adequate pain relief with local anesthetic blockade is *no guarantee* that a subsequent neurolysis will result in equally successful results. In fact, neurolysis can be less "dense" or "complete" than local anesthetic blockade and it is paramount that the patient be informed of this possibility. The patient must also be *made aware of the difficulty of foreseeing the actual duration of analgesia*, especially with the percutaneous technique: "weeks to months is hoped for, while no relief to days is also possible." Other important aspects of patient education and consent include:

- the temporary nature of the analgesia, in order to facilitate other modes of therapy;
- the expected presence of sensory deficit, demonstrated to the patient during local anesthetic blockade;
- the possibility of motor deficit, in some instances;
- the possibility of no pain relief;
- the possibility of increased pain following regeneration (whether true or perceived);
- the usual risks of invasive procedures (see above).

Cryoanalgesia: the percutaneous technique

We will not discuss the anatomic approaches to all of the different nerve blocks (see the appropriate sections in this book for those details); the operator's manual for the cryomachine breaks down the step-by-step process of machine check and preparation. Instead, we will summarize the process of cryoanalgesia with the percutaneous technique as it pertains to the gas expansion cryomachine:

With the *percutaneous technique*, using nerve stimulation:

1 Following placement of the cryoprobe in close prox-

imity to the nerve, maximize probe position with nerve stimulation (at = 0.5–1.0 V).

2 Freeze at –60°C to –70°C for 2–3 min (up to 4 min for intercostal nerves); repeat two or three times.

3 *Caution: do not remove the ice ball from the frozen tissue. Wait until it has completely defrosted before removing the probe.*

Key points

- Prior to skin penetration, place the intravenous (i.v.) cannula over the probe to ensure a snug fit and to measure the depth needed for a 2- to 3-mm exposure of the probe tip at the end of the cannula (surgical tape can be placed on the shaft of the probe to mark the depth).
- Have sterile, room temperature, normal saline drawn up in a syringe to drip over blanching skin for local warming.
- Choose negative polarity for more sensitive nerve stimulation.
- Check the operator's manual for the optimal gas flows for the particular cryoprobe being used: if the gas flows are too high, there will be increased freezing along the shaft; if they are too low, maximal temperature will not be reached.
- The automatic timer will begin at a preset time after gas flow has begun, regardless of whether there is sufficient gas flow for maximal freezing.
- Use great care when handling the cryoprobe to avoid damaging the insulating material on the shaft, the thermocouple, or stimulator in the tip or altering the size of the expansion orifice.

Comparisons

Cryoneurolysis versus phenol neurolysis

As stated previously, one of the greatest advantages of cryoanalgesia over other techniques of neurolysis is the lack of neuroma formation and the low incidence of neuritis. Along with radiofrequency neuroablation, it also allows a more controlled, discrete lesion potentially affording some greater measure of safety. Conversely, cryoanalgesia, like radiofrequency neurolysis, has the disadvantage of requiring more exact needle/probe placement than chemical neurolysis.

Ramamurthy *et al.* compared the use of cryoanalgesia with 6% aqueous phenol in a randomized, prospective trial in 28 patients with chronic pain of varying etiology.[11]** One or both techniques were used for the following: intercostal, tibial, supraorbital, coccygeal, or accessory nerve blocks; paravertebral somatic nerve root blocks; brachial plexus blocks; facet, neuroma, or myoneural blocks. Nerve stimulation directed localization for all blocks. Neither form of neurolysis was particularly effective for pain reduction despite previously good relief following local anesthetic blockade: only 27% obtained significant pain relief overall (although all patients experienced a significant reduction in pain for a very brief period). More patients in the phenol group experienced pain relief when comparing reductions in pain of 20% or greater; there was no significant difference when comparing higher percentages of relief. The patients were followed for 24 weeks, but there was a significant number of patients in both groups who did not experience relief beyond 2 weeks. While this study was small and the use of either of the neurolytics for any particular nerve block was much less, it demonstrates certain limitations, i.e. extent and duration of pain relief, of neurolysis for pain management in general and the poor prognostic value of local anesthetic blockade in particular. Of note, only one patient developed *neuritis* in this study, following *cryo*neurolysis of a paravertebral somatic root, perhaps as a result of the trauma of the large i.v. cannula needle tip during its initial placement.

Cryoneurolysis versus radiofrequency neurolysis

Cryoanalgesia has the advantage of a more uniform and complete regenerative process owing to a lesser degree of nerve injury, with no neuroma formation and a lower incidence of neuritis. It is also significantly cheaper ($8–10,000 vs. $20–40,000) and thus more accessible to pain clinics worldwide.

One great disadvantage is the size of the cryoprobes, leading to greater intervening tissue trauma than radiofrequency (or chemical) neurolysis. Not only are the probes much larger, but i.v. cannulas as large as 10–12 gauge are often used for tissue penetration. This is less of an issue when superficial nerves or neuromas are lesioned. However, when deeper structures are targeted, for example medial branches of the posterior primary rami or the lumbar sympathetic chain, the amount of tissue trauma is significantly greater for 14- to 16-gauge than for 22-gauge penetration.

In reality, clinicians will use whichever system is available to them, weighing the risks and benefits for each individual patient.

Duration of pain: is it a factor in outcome?

The longer a chronic pain condition persists, the greater is the possibility of central nervous system changes, i.e. plasticity, windup, or spontaneous activity. While pain relief following peripheral local anesthetic blockade would indicate the probable requirement of peripheral input to maintain the painful state, it may be that more chronic pain conditions are less responsive to the long-term somatic blockade of cryoanalgesia in certain cir-

cumstances. This may be similar to, but with the opposite result of, the phenomenon of local anesthetic somatic blockade outlasting the duration of the local anesthetic.

Wang studied the results of cryoanalgesia on peripheral neuropathies in 12 patients with chronic pain that had lasted for ≥ 1 year.[12*] All patients received only temporary relief with local anesthetic blockade. He utilized two 3-min freezes on the following nerves: ulnar, median or its palmar branch, sural, occipital, and digital. Of the patients with pain for 1.6 years, five out of six had relief for 1–12 months. Of the patients with pain lasting for 2 years, only one out of six experienced pain relief, which lasted 3 months. The presence or absence of a sympathetic component was not correlative. Of interest, the patients reported that the quality of pain relief with cryoanalgesia was superior to that with local anesthetics. While this was a very small and nonrandomized study, this disparity is striking. This aspect of cryoanalgesia for chronic pain requires further study.

CONCLUSIONS

Cryoanalgesia is a useful tool for pain clinicians. It allows complete regeneration of the nerve without neuroma formation and with a low, *but not zero*, incidence of neuritis, but the extent and duration of pain relief is often difficult to predict. The open technique with direct visualization of the nerve requires shorter freezing times and is more reliably effective than the percutaneous technique. As with any analgesic modality, patient selection is a key component to achieving positive results.

REFERENCES

● 1. Evans PJD. Cryoanalgesia: the application of low
◆   temperatures to nerves to produce anaesthesia or analgesia. *Anaesthesia* 1981; **36:** 1003–13.

2. Sunderland S. A classification of peripheral nerve injuries producing loss of function. *Brain* 1951; **74:** 491–516.

3. Kalichman MW, Myers RR. Behavioral and electrophysiological recovery following cryogenic nerve injury. *Exp Neurol* 1987; **96:** 692–702.

◆ 4. Evans PJD, Lloyd JW, Green CJ. Cryoanalgesia: the response to alterations in freeze cycle and temperature. *Br J Anaesth* 1981; **53:** 1121–6.

5. Gill W, Fraser J, Carter DC. Repeated freeze–thaw cycles in cryosurgery. *Nature* 1968; **219:** 410–13.

◆ 6. Amoils SP. The Joule Thompson cryoprobe. *Arch Ophthalmol* 1967; **78:** 201–7.

7. Arthur JM, Racz GB. Cryolysis. In: Raj PP ed. *Pain Medicine: A Comprehensive Review.* St Louis, MO: Mosby-Year Book, 1996: 297–303.

◆ 8. Lloyd JW, Barnard JDW, Glynn CJ. Cryoanalgesia: a new approach to pain relief. *Lancet* 1976; **2:** 932–4.

9. Richardson J, Sabanathan S, Mearns AJ, *et al*. Post-thoracotomy neuralgia. *Pain Clin* 1994; **7:** 87–97.

10. Maiwand MO, Makey AR, Rees A. Cryoanalgesia after thoracotomy: improvement of technique and review of 600 cases. *J Thorac Cardiovasc Surg* 1986; **92:** 291–5.

11. Ramamurthy S, Walsh NE, Schoenfeld LS, Hoffman J. Evaluation of neurolytic blocks using phenol and cryogenic block in the management of chronic pain. *J Pain Symptom Manage* 1989; **4:** 72–5.

12. Wang JK. Cryoanalgesia for painful nerve lesions. *Pain* 1985; **22:** 191–4.

26

Radiofrequency lesioning

BEN J P CRUL AND MAARTEN VAN KLEEF

Theoretical aspects of radiofrequency lesioning	327	Percutaneous radiofrequency lesioning of the dorsal root ganglion in the cervical region	334
Clinical application of radiofrequency lesioning in pain	327		
Percutaneous cervical cordotomy	328	Radiofrequency lesioning in the lumbar area	336
Radiofrequency lesioning of the Gasserian ganglion	330	Percutaneous radiofrequency lumbar facetal joint denervation	336
Radiofrequency lesioning of the sphenopalatine ganglion	331		
Radiofrequency lesioning for the treatment of vertebrogenic pain	332	Radiofrequency lesion of the dorsal lumbar root ganglion	337
Radiofrequency lesioning in the cervical area	333	Radiofrequency lesioning of the lumbar sympathetic ganglia	338
Percutaneous cervical facetal joint denervation by radiofrequency lesioning	333	References	339

Percutaneous current lesions were introduced by Kirschner[1] in 1931 for the treatment of patients with trigeminal neuralgia. The reliability and simplicity of thermocoagulation led to its widespread use in the USA and Europe. In 1953, Sweet and Mark[2] proposed the application of a high-frequency current with frequencies ranging from 300 to 500 kHz, as used in radiotransmitters. Radiofrequency lesions (RF lesions) were far more predictable than lesions produced by the earlier direct current procedures.

Another milestone was the introduction of the percutaneous cordotomy in 1965.[3] By a lateral approach through the C1–C2 intervertebral space, a heat lesion was made in the spinothalamic tract of the spinal cord. This method is mainly used in cancer patients with severe unilateral pain and remains an established technique for this indication. In 1974, after Sweet and Wepsic[4] applied RF lesioning for patients with trigeminal neuralgia, Uetmatso[5] also treated patients with spinal pain syndromes by RF lesioning. Sluijter and Metha[6] refined earlier techniques by introducing a small-diameter (22 gauge) temperature-monitoring electrode system.[7]

THEORETICAL ASPECTS OF RADIOFREQUENCY LESIONING

In RF lesioning, heat is generated in the tissue which surrounds the electrode by the radiofrequency current generated by a lesion apparatus. The RF voltage from the generator is set up between the (active) electrode and the (dispersive) groundplate, which is placed on the arm or leg of the patient. The body tissues complete the circuit and RF current flows through the tissue, resulting in an electric field.

This electric field creates an electric force on the ions in the tissue electrolytes, causing them to move back and forth at a high rate. Frictional dissipation of the ionic current within the fluid medium causes tissue heating. This is the origin of the RF lesion. Heat is generated in the tissue and not in the electrode itself, and the electrode is heated by the tissue and not the other way around. The temperature of the surrounding tissue will show a rapid decrease over the first few millimeters from the electrode tip. The size of the lesion also depends on the diameter of the electrode and the length of the uninsulated electrode tip.

The effects of RF heat on nerve fibers is still controversial, but most morphological animal studies indicate that radiofrequency current indiscriminately affects both small and large fibers. Regrettably, no morphological studies are available which imitate the conditions of RF lesions as used in actual medical practice.

CLINICAL APPLICATION OF RADIOFREQUENCY LESIONING IN PAIN

Preferably before treatment by RF lesioning is considered,

the patient is seen in a multidisciplinary setting where in addition to physicians a psychologist and physical therapist also participate. In general, RF lesioning is indicated only in patients in whom noninvasive ways of pain treatment have failed. Especially in patients with chronic non-malignant pain, it is necessary to combine RF lesioning with other measures aiming at a correction of the pain-provoking conditions. Otherwise, the beneficial effects of RF lesioning will be short-lasting. In most cases, ergonomic and psychological advice is needed. Changes in the life pattern and working habits of the patient are often necessary to prevent the recurrence of pain (Tables 26.1 and 26.2).

PERCUTANEOUS CERVICAL CORDOTOMY*

History

In 1965, Mullan et al.[3] performed their first percutaneous cervical cordotomy by a lateral approach through the C1–C2 intervertebral space. A heat lesion was made in the spinothalamic tract in the spinal cord, at first using a direct current but later a RF current. Other means of reaching the spinothalamic tract are an anterolateral approach through the intervertebral disk or a posterior approach, but these techniques have never had widespread popularity.

Applied anatomy

The spinothalamic tract, situated in the anterolateral quadrant of the spinal cord, consists of secondary nociceptive neurons conveying nociceptive stimuli from the contralateral body half. Its origin is in the dorsal horn of the spinal cord and its destination is mainly situated in the ventral posterior lateral and the central lateral nucleus of the thalamus. At the level C1–C2, the column of facetal joints is interrupted, allowing an approach to the spinal cord by a laterally introduced needle electrode.

Table 26.1 *General contraindications of radiofrequency lesioning*

Coagulopathy
Local infection
Insufficient cooperation by the patient

Table 26.2 *Equipment needed for radiofrequency (RF) lesioning*

RF lesion generator provided with impedance registration, stimulation facilities, and thermocouple lesion system
Appropriate electrode needle and corresponding electrodes
Radiographic C-arm image intensifier

Indications

Unilateral, incident, and/or neurogenic pain in advanced cancer patients resistant to other therapy. In exceptional cases, remaining pain on the contralateral side following an earlier cordotomy can be treated by a second cordotomy on the opposite site. There should be a minimum interval of 2 weeks between the interventions.

Limitations

Popularity of the intervention has decreased considerably following the introduction of rational oral analgesic therapy. A further decline in the number of patients treated occurred because of the application of continuous spinal infusion techniques. Nevertheless, the treatment still deserves an important place in the treatment of severe and resistant neurogenic pain in patients with a life expectancy of not more than 1–2 years.

Technique

It is essential that the patient is fully informed about the procedure and the sensations that he/she may experience during it. It should be stressed that his/her full cooperation is necessary to obtain an optimal result. A full neurological assessment is performed with special attention to the sensory qualities (touch, pain, temperature) and motor power functions.

The patient should be in a dorsal recumbent position. Under direct lateral vision by use of a C-arm image intensifier, a marker rule is placed on a spot midway on the antero-posterior border of the spinal canal at the level C1–C2. A 22-gauge spinal needle is inserted and advanced to reach the anterior part of the intrathecal space. To gauge the depth of insertion of the needle, lateral views can be alternated with anteroposterior projections. Once the needle is inside the intrathecal space, 3 ml cerebrospinal fluid (CSF) is aspirated into a 5-ml glass syringe. After the addition of 2 ml of contrast dye (Lipiodol Ultrafluide, a fatty iodated ester, manufactured by Guerbet Laboratoires, 93600 Aulnay-sous Bois, France), the syringe is shaken well until an emulsion appears. After intrathecal injection of the mixture, three lines become visible: the most anterior line shows the delineation of the anterior border of the spinal cord, the second line represents the dentate ligament, and the third line is the projection of the posterior dura mater (Figs 26.1 and 26.2). The target for insertion of the electrode is 1 mm anterior to the dentate ligament. A convenient trick now is to introduce a small-bore hypodermic needle through the skin projecting just anterior to the dentate ligament as a marker. At this site, a 20-gauge electrode guiding needle is pierced through the skin, and inserted in a direction perpendicular to the spinal cord. The trajectory of the needle is, therefore, in a horizontal plane. In the authors' experi-

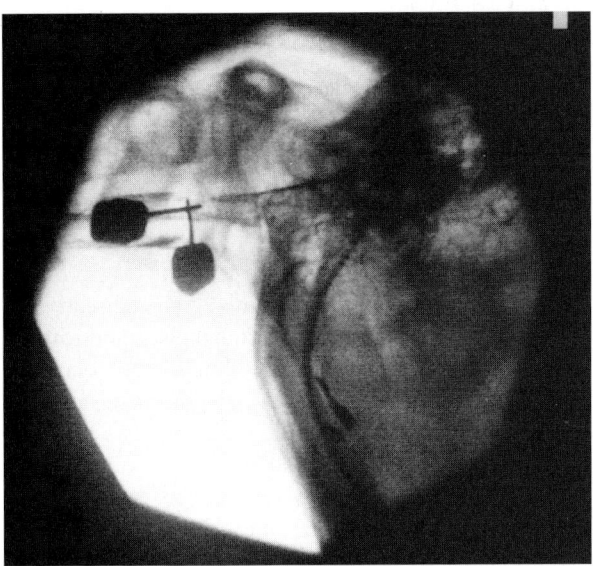

Figure 26.1 *Percutaneous cordotomy,* lateral view. *After intrathecal injection through a 22-gauge spinal needle just ventral to the spinal cord of a mixture of iodated fatty acids (Lipiodol Ultrafluide) and aspirated cerebrospinal fluid, three lines become visible: the most ventral line shows the delineation of the anterior border of the spinal cord, the second line represents the dentate ligament, and finally the third line is the projection of the dorsal dura mater. A second needle guiding the electrode is aimed at the target 1.0–1.5 mm ventral to the dentate ligament.*

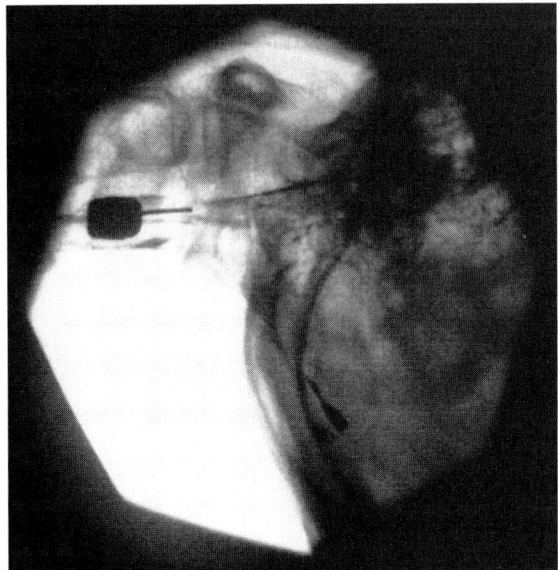

Figure 26.2 *Percutaneous cordotomy,* lateral view. *The contrast needle is removed. The electrode-guiding needle is left in place and RF lesion can be applied.*

ence, an upward (more ventral) direction carries the risk of pushing the spinal cord down by the electrode instead of the electrode entering it. During verification by alternating lateral and anteroposterior projections, the needle is advanced until the cervical dura is reached. This struc-

ture is usually rather resistant, and the utmost precaution has to be taken to prevent touching and subsequent damage of the spinal cord after an abrupt "give" of the dura. After the needle enters the intrathecal space, and after verification that its tip is just anterior to the dentate ligament, a Levin thermocouple electrode (Radionics, Burlington, MA, USA) is inserted through the needle. When the free tip of the electrode is inside the intrathecal space, the electrical impedance amounts to about 250–400 Ω. After the needle tip has been introduced into the spinal cord, the impedance rises three- to fourfold. Stimulation with 2 Hz generally provokes contractions of the longus colli musculature at 0.5–1 V. Any other contractions are an indication that the tip of the electrode is in the corticospinal (motor) tract. A lesion here would provoke a paresis of the muscles situated within the projection of the interrupted nerve fibers. Repositioning of the needle more anteriorly is needed. Sensory tracts are identified by 50 Hz stimulation. When the tip of the electrode is inside the spinothalamic tract, intensities of 0.1–0.3 V can provoke temperature sensations (warmth or cold) in the corresponding part of the contralateral body half. After meticulous assessment of the correct position of the electrode tip by repeated stimulation, a radiofrequency lesion is made, resulting in a tip temperature of 90°C for 10 s. Directly following the lesioning, pinprick tests are performed to assess the distribution of an analgesic area. Sometimes, one lesion is sufficient to attain freedom from pain. Mostly, two or three lesions are necessary with the needle tip in slightly different positions to reach this goal.

Complications

Complications are: paresis, 0.4–8%; urinary retention, 6–8% (mostly temporary); mirror pain, 6–54%; respiratory depression, 0–4%. Following a bilateral procedure, the occurrence of sleep apnea is reported.

Results

In 60–87% of the patients treated by percutaneous cervical cordotomy (PCC), pain remains under control until death.[8]

Side-effects

The known side-effects are changed body perception and loss of temperature sensation in segments under analgesia.

Discomfort of the procedure to the patient

This procedure can be very demanding for the patient, who has to be completely immobile in a supine position for 30–45 min. During assessment of the needle position and making the lesion, it is mandatory that the patient is fully aware of the procedure. Discomfort to the patient can be considerably alleviated by using repeated bolus injections or a continuous infusion of an ultra-short-acting opioid (e.g. remifentanil) during the procedure. Also, propofol can be used. Appropriate monitoring by pulse oximetry, electrocardiogram (EKG), and sphygmomanometry is mandatory.

RADIOFREQUENCY LESIONING OF THE GASSERIAN GANGLION*

History

Percutaneous electric lesioning of the Gasserian ganglion has a long history, beginning in 1931 when Kirschner[1] first described the technique. Sweet and Wepsic applied RF current and improved the procedure.[4] It is one of the techniques that has withstood the test of time. Together with microvascular decompression, RF lesioning of the Gasserian ganglion is one of the mainstays of nonpharmacological treatment of trigeminal neuralgia.

Applied anatomy

The Gasserian ganglion is situated in the middle cranial fossa, dorsal and cranial to the foramen ovale. The ophthalmic part is located medially and has the greatest distance to the foramen ovale. The maxillary cell bodies and nerve fibers are positioned centrally, whereas the mandibular section has the most lateral and superficial location. The position of the ganglion means that all parts can be reached by a needle entering through the foramen ovale.

The trigeminal nerve has a mixed composition. The motor fibers constitute the nervus intermedius, which accompanies the mandibular nerve and innervates the pterygoid, temporalis, and masseter muscles. The Gasserian ganglion contains the cell bodies of the first-order sensory neurons of the trigeminal nerve. Medially, the Gasserian ganglion is next to the carotid artery and the cavernous sinus.

Indication

This technique is indicated by trigeminal neuralgia resistant to drug treatment. In young patients who want to avoid the risk of numbness of the face and in patients with pain in the area innervated by the ophthalmic nerve, microvascular decompression may be considered.

Technique

The patient is placed in a horizontal recumbent position. The patient's head is fixed on a radiolucent head rest by an adhesive bandage. The intervention is performed under intermittent intravenous anesthesia with propofol. Great care must be taken to obtain an optimal picture of the foramen ovale. For this purpose, the C-arm of the image intensifier is placed in a caudal/cranial direction at an angle of about 45° to the horizontal plane and rotated 15–20° sideways. Consequently, a suborbital–occipital projection is obtained. The projection shows the ascending ramus and the angle of the mandible. The foramen ovale can be discerned medial to the ascending ramus. Subsequently, a marker ruler is placed on a spot on the skin overlying the projection of the foramen and an ink mark is made.

During the procedure, short periods of general anesthesia are necessary. Intermittent administration of propofol 1–1.5 mg/kg is a good choice. Under general anesthesia, a 22-gauge Sluyter–Metha (thermocouple) needle electrode with a 2-mm free tip (Radionics) is inserted at the ink-marked spot on the skin. The direction of the needle is the same as the direction of the radiation beam (tunnel-vision technique). The needle is guided through the musculature of the cheek by the left index finger, preventing piercing of the oral mucosa. If the oral mucosa is pierced, the needle has to be taken out and replaced by another sterile needle to avoid contamination of intracranial structures. Under fluoroscopic guidance, the needle is gradually pushed forward in the direction of the desired target within the foramen ovale (Fig. 26.3). Once the needle enters the foramen, a clear "give" is perceived by the operator. During lateral fluoroscopy, the penetration of the needle into the skull base is verified when the end of the needle coincides with the intersection of the clivus and the os petrosum (Fig. 26.4).

After the patient regains consciousness, electrical stimulation is applied. The patient should now feel paresthesiae in the painful area. Thresholds should be below 0.2 V. If stimulation yields a satisfactory outcome, the patient is anesthetized again and a RF lesion of 60–65°C is made of duration 60 s. After awakening, a couple of minutes later, sensibility is tested by pinprick. Hyperesthesia should be present in the previously painful area. Special attention must be paid to verifying whether pain can still be elicited by tactile stimulation of the trigger area, related to the trigeminal neuralgia. If the test results are unsatisfactory, the needle position should be adjusted. It can be necessary to reintroduce the needle, changing its direction to enter the foramen ovale at a different angle. Some authors advocate the use of a curved electrode to produce a more selective lesion and a lower complication rate.

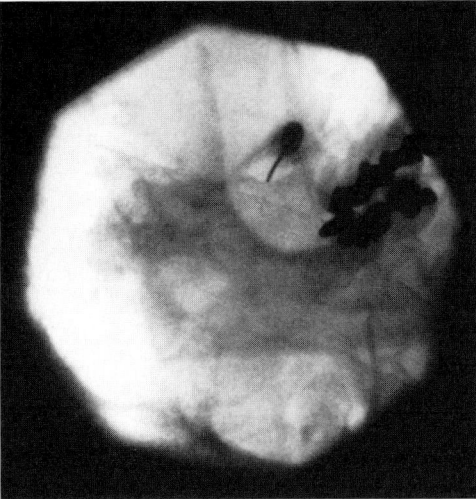

Figure 26.3 *RF lesion of the Gasserian ganglion, suborbital–occipital projection. The ascending ramus and the angle of the mandible are visible. The electrode is inside the needle, which is placed in the central part of the foramen ovale.*

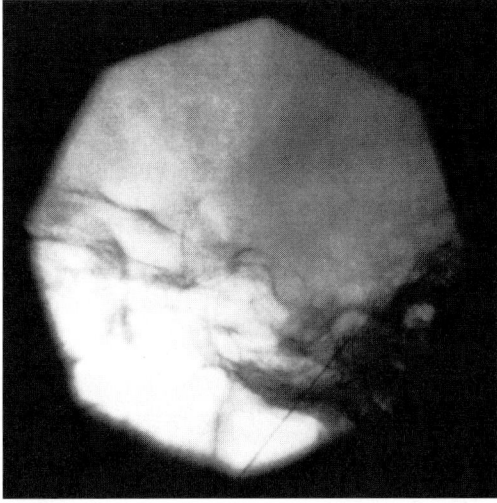

Figure 26.4 *RF lesion of the Gasserian ganglion, lateral projection. The projection of the needle–electrode coincides with the intersection of the clivus and the os petrosum.*

Results

Long-term (years) success rates vary from 80% to 90%. Sometimes, multiple treatments are necessary.[9]

Side-effects

Possible side-effects include hyperesthesia of the treated trigeminal branch.

Complications and incidence

Corneal anesthesia/hyperesthesia, 13.7%; dysesthesia in the treated area, 5–7%; masseter weakness, 1–2%.[9]

Discomfort of the procedure for the patient

The procedure can be performed during short-acting intravenous anesthesia on an outpatient basis. The procedure has a low morbidity; mortality has not been reported.

RADIOFREQUENCY LESIONING OF THE SPHENOPALATINE GANGLION*

History

Neuroablation of the sphenopalatine ganglion for the treatment of cluster headache was first reported in the early 1970s. RF procedures were reported in 1988.[10]

Applied anatomy

The sphenopalatine ganglion is an autonomous ganglion containing parasympathetic and sympathetic fibers. The ganglion is situated within the fossa sphenopalatina, just lateral to the foramen sphenopalatina, and has close relationships with the maxillary nerve and its branches (nervi alveolares). The foramen sphenopalatinum connects the fossa sphenopalatinum with the cavum nasi. The fossa can be reached by a laterally placed needle entering through the triangle formed by the zygoma and the muscular and articular processus of the mandible.

Indications

This procedure is indicated by cluster headaches that are unreactive to conservative therapy (drugs, oxygen).[10]

Technique

The patient is placed in a horizontal recumbent position. The head is fixed on a radiolucent headrest by an adhesive bandage. Although the procedure can be carried out under local anesthesia, intermittent intravenous anesthesia is preferred because the introduction of the needle is painful.

Under lateral fluoroscopic projection, the projection

of the sphenopalatine fossa can be seen in its narrow triangular form. A marker ruler is placed on the projection of the foramen sphenopalatinum and an ink dot made on the skin overlying the target.

The needle is inserted more caudally, just inferior to the zygoma, and directed medially. Often, several attempts are needed to direct the needle to the fossa, as bony structures can obstruct the passage. In our experience, it is virtually always possible to arrive at the desired target (Figs 26.5 and 26.6). It is important that the needle

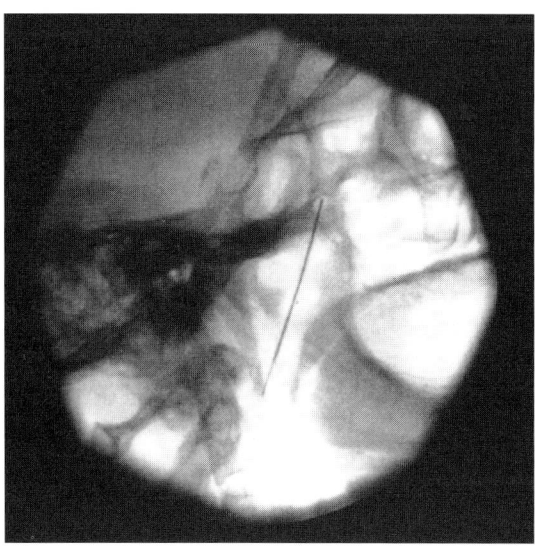

Figure 26.5 *RF lesioning of the sphenopalatine ganglion, lateral projection. The projection of the sphenopalatine fossa can be seen in its narrow triangular form. The electrode tip is positioned in the foramen sphenopalatinum.*

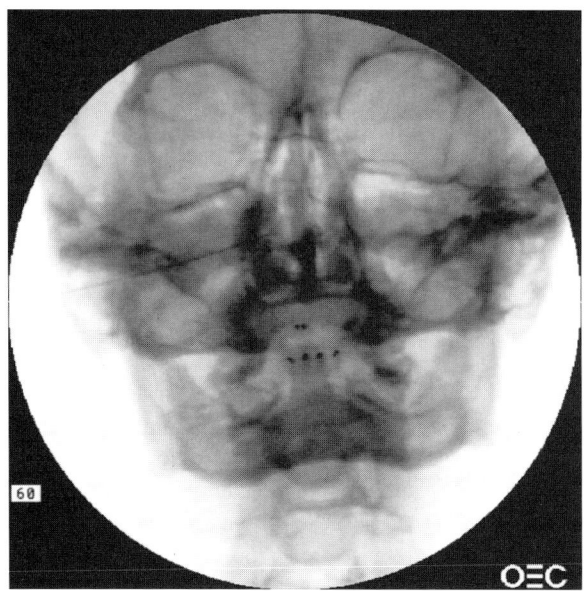

Figure 26.6 *RF lesioning of the sphenopalatine ganglion, anteroposterior projection. The tip of the electrode is projected slightly medial to the right os nasale.*

is not directed too far cranially as this risks the needle entering the dorsal part of the orbita. In the lateral fluoroscopic projection, this is at the cranial part of the fossa. In the anteroposterior fluoroscopic projection, the needle tip just projects over the ipsilateral os nasale. The target is localized about 6–7 cm under the skin.

In the awake patient, stimulation is performed using a 50-Hz current. Paresthesiae should not be felt at < 1.0V. Otherwise, the tip of the electrode is too near to the maxillary nerve. Damage to this nerve can cause numbness and dysesthesia.

When the electrode is in the correct position, a RF lesion is made at 80°C for 60 s, concluding the procedure.

Indication

The indication for this procedure is cluster headache.

Results

In episodic cluster headache, complete pain relief has been achieved in 60% of patients. In chronic cluster headache, complete relief has been achieved in 30% of patients.[10]

Complications

The following complications have been observed: hyperesthesia due to involvement of the maxillary nerve (5%), epistaxis, cheek hematomas (10%), and bleeding of the nasal mucosa (needle entering the cavum nasi via the foramen sphenoplatimum).

Efficacy of treatment

Studies on the results of the technique are scarce. Controlled studies are not available. Sanders and Zuurmond[11] reported on a series of 66 patients with cluster headache. RF lesioning of the sphenopalatine ganglion resulted in complete remission in 67% of patients, whereas partial relief was obtained in 18%.

RADIOFREQUENCY LESIONING FOR THE TREATMENT OF VERTEBROGENIC PAIN

Applied anatomy of the spine

The innervation of the spine is complex and has been well described by Bogduk.[12] The spine can be divided into dorsal and ventral compartments.

Dorsal compartment

The dorsal compartment of the spine contains the facet joints (zygapophyseal joints), the dorsal part of the dura, and intrinsic neck/back muscles and ligaments. The dorsal compartment of the spine is innervated by the posterior primary ramus, which branches off the segmental nerve immediately after it exits from its foramen. It runs in a groove formed by the superior articular and transverse processes, where it divides into a medial and a lateral branch.

Ventral compartment

The ventral compartment contains the vertebral bodies, disks, anterior and posterior longitudinal ligaments, ventral dura, and prevertebral muscles. Innervation of the ventral compartment is not related to single nerves, but more to interconnected neural networks in the anterior and posterior longitudinal ligaments and ventral dura. Fibers from the nervous plexus in the posterior longitudinal ligament innervate the outer layer of the dorsal aspect of the annulus fibrosus. This plexus is mainly formed by branches from bilateral sinuvertebral nerves. The nervous plexus in the anterior longitudinal ligament, supplied with fibers from the sympathetic, the rami communicantes, and perivascular plexuses, innervates the anterior part of the annulus fibrosus bilaterally and multisegmentally.

RADIOFREQUENCY LESIONING IN THE CERVICAL AREA

RF treatment for cervical pain syndromes is utilized for the following main diagnostic categories:

1 Cervical pain, defined as pain originating from the facet joints or from the intervertebral disk.[12,13]
2 Cervicobrachialgia, defined as pain originating from the cervical spine radiating from the neck beyond the glenohumeral joint into the upper limb with referral to a particular spinal segment.
3 Cervicogenic headache is a clinically defined headache syndrome hypothesized to originate from cervical nociceptive structures. The structures responsible for it have not been defined.[14] Each different pain syndrome may have more than one nociceptive source. As a consequence, more than one radiofrequency treatment modality may be required to relieve the patient's pain.

Two radiofrequency procedures in the cervical area are applied to reduce nociception:

1 Percutaneous cervical facetal joint denervation.
2 Radiofrequency lesion of the dorsal root ganglion.

PERCUTANEOUS CERVICAL FACETAL JOINT DENERVATION BY RADIOFREQUENCY LESIONING

Indications

- Nociceptive pain emanating from the facetal joint.
- Clinical manifestations:
  - localized cervical pain;
  - cervicogenic headache.

Technique

For a radiofrequency lesion of the medial branch of the dorsal ramus in the upper and middle cervical area, the patient is positioned prone on the operating table. The C-arm is positioned slightly oblique so that the beam of radiation is parallel to the axis of the intervertebral foramen, which is upwards and slightly caudal. In this position of the C-arm, the segmental nerves exit parallel to the line of the radiation beam. Since the electrodes will be introduced from the posterolateral side, this projection will make it easy to maintain a safe distance between the electrode tip and the exciting segmental nerve. The dorsal ramus in this projection runs over the base of the superior articular process, which is clearly visible (Figs 26.7 and 26.8). Entry points are marked posterior to the posterior border of the facetal column and slightly caudal to the target point. A Sluijter–Metha (SMK), 22-gauge, C5 cannula with a 4-mm active tip (Radionics) or alternatively a TOP XE 6 needle (COTOP International, Amsterdam, The Netherlands) is introduced and carefully advanced anteriorly and cranially until contact is made with the facetal column at the target point. The position of the C-arm is then changed to the anterior–posterior (AP) direction. This should confirm the position of the tip of the electrode adjacent to the "waist" of the articular pillars of the cervical spine at the corresponding level. At the C2 level, the electrode should be aimed at the small branches of the C2–C3 facet joint and not at the medial branch of C2, which is the greater occipital nerve. A suitable electrode placement is at the arch of C2 at the level of the upper border of foramen C3.

After this anatomical localization, electrical stimulation at a rate of 50 Hz should elicit a response (tingling sensation) in the neck at <0.5 V. On motor stimulation at 2 Hz, there must be no muscle movements in the ipsilateral shoulder/arm. However, contractions of the multifidus muscles are often visible. After this physiological control, the medial branch of the dorsal ramus is anesthetized with 1–2 ml local anesthetic solution [lidocaine (lignocaine) 10 mg/ml], and a 80°C radiofrequency thermolesion is made for 60 s at each level. When a TOP XE needle is used, 20 V over 60 s is applied, resulting in a heating of the relevant tissue to a temperature of 80°C. When

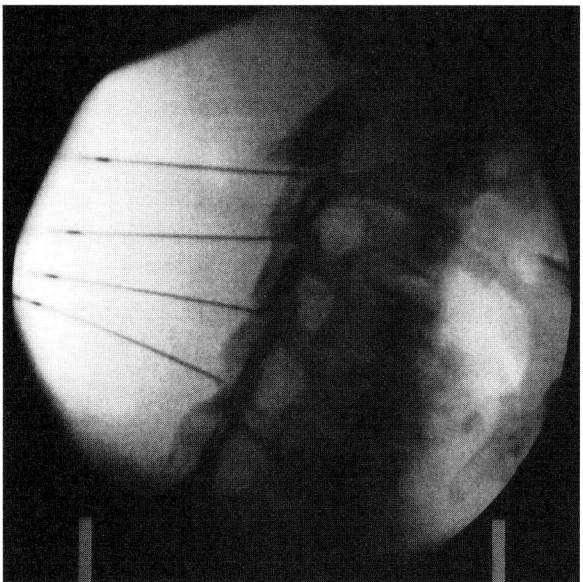

Figure 26.7 *Percutaneous cervical facetal joint denervation by RF lesioning. Oblique view. In the transverse plane, the angle of the C-arm with the horizontal is about 30° and in the sagittal plane 75–80°. The needle tips are projecting on the base of the superior articular processes.*

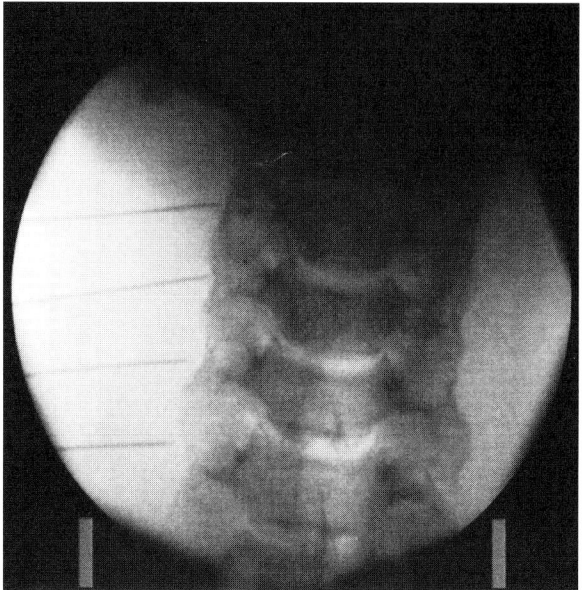

Figure 26.8 *Percutaneous cervical facetal joint denervation by RF lesioning in the anterior–posterior (AP) direction. The tips of the electrodes are adjacent to the "waist" of the articular pillars of the cervical spine at the corresponding levels.*

performing this technique, one should take care not to insert the needle too close to the mixed segmental nerve. A lesion should not be applied when muscle contractions occur at 2 Hz stimulation at a voltage less than 1.0 V.

Side-effects

There have been no reports in the literature of complications from cervical facet joint denervation when the procedure is performed as described above. There may be some postoperative burning pain in 10–20% of patients that disappears spontaneously after some weeks.

Results

In 1996, Lord *et al.* performed a randomized, double-blind, controlled trial in patients with chronic pain of the lower cervical facet joints after whiplash injury.[15] They concluded that in patients with chronic facet joint pain, confirmed with double-blind, placebo-controlled local anesthetic blocks, percutaneous RF neurotomy with multiple lesions of target nerves can provide long-lasting pain relief. Another more recent study indicated that pain relief was observed in 71% of patients after the initial procedure. The median duration of pain relief was 219 days if failures are included, but 422 days when only successful cases are considered.[16]

PERCUTANEOUS RADIOFREQUENCY LESIONING OF THE DORSAL ROOT GANGLION IN THE CERVICAL REGION**

Indication

Nociceptive pain emanating from one segment in the cervical area. Most patients present with a cervicobrachial pain or cervicogenic headache.

The level involved in the pain syndrome is selected by means of diagnostic segmental nerve blocks.

Contraindication

Sensory deficit in the painful area (neuropathic pain).

Technique

Diagnostic root blocks

For the selection of the putative pain-conducting nerve root, a series of consecutive selective root blocks is performed. In this technique, the C-arm is positioned in such a way that the direction of the radiation beam is parallel to the axis of the foramen. In the transverse plane, this axis has an angle to the horizontal of 25–35°, and in the sagittal plane an angle of 75–80° to the horizontal. With the C-arm in this position, the entry point is found by projecting a metal ruler over the caudal part of the foramen. A 50-mm, 22-gauge neurography needle (Radionics) is inserted in the direction of the radiation beam and directed to the caudal part of the foramen (Fig. 26.9). In this "tunnel-vision" projection, the needle should appear as a dot on the monitor screen. The direction of the radiation beam is than changed to anteroposterior, and the cannula is further introduced until the tip is projected just lateral from the facetal column. After identifying the segmental nerve root with 0.5 ml contrast dye (iohexol; Omnipaque 250), 0.5 ml of lidocaine 20 mg/ml is slowly injected. The position of the needle tip is critical because if the placement is too medial this results in epidural overflow, whereas if the placement is too lateral this can lead to spread of the local anesthetic into the nervous plexus, neither resulting in a selective block.[17]

Radiofrequency lesioning

After identification of the pain conduction nerve root, a radiofrequency lesion of the dorsal root ganglion (RF DRG lesion) can be performed. The same viewing technique and entry point is used as described in the diagnostic segmental root block technique.

The cannula (Radionics SMK C5 with a 4-mm exposed tip) is introduced in the direction of the radiation beam and advanced until the electrode appears on the screen

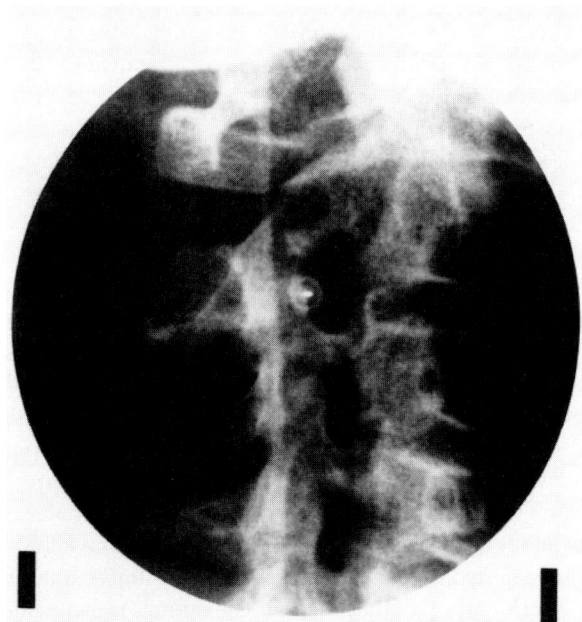

Figure 26.9 *RF lesioning of the cervical dorsal root ganglion. The C-arm is positioned in such a way that the direction of the radiation beam is parallel to the axis of the foramen. In the transverse plane, the angle with the horizontal is about 30°, and in the sagittal plane is about 15–20°. In "tunnel-vision" projection, the needle is seen as a dot on the monitor screen.*

as a dot. In practice, this dot should lie directly over the dorsal part of the intervertebral foramen at the transition between the middle one-third and the most caudal one-third. This dorsal position is chosen in order to avoid possible damage to the motor fibers of the segmental nerve and to the vertebral artery which runs anterior to the ventral part of the foramen (Fig. 26.10). The direction of the radiation beam is then changed to anteroposterior and the cannula is further advanced until the tip is projected over the middle of the facetal column (Fig. 26.11).

The stylet is now replaced by the radiofrequency (RF) electrode probe. After checking the impedance, electrical stimulation is started at a rate of 50 Hz. The patient should feel a tingling sensation at voltages between 0.4 and 0.65 V. Next, the frequency is changed to 2 Hz, and the patient is observed for muscle contractions. These should not occur below a voltage of 1.5 times the sensory threshold. Afterwards, 0.5 ml of contrast medium (Omnipaque) is injected, to exclude an accidental intradural or intravascular position of the electrode, and 2 ml of local anesthetic solution (lidocaine 20 mg/ml) is administered. A RF current is applied through the electrode in order to increase the temperature at the tip slowly to 67°C for 60 s.

Side-effects

A side-effect which is often seen (40–60%) is a mild burning sensation in the treated dermatome, which subsides spontaneously after some weeks. This burning pain is probably the result of swelling in the vicinity of the segmental nerve. A slight hypoesthesia may occur, but usually disappears after several months.

Efficacy of treatment

There are several publications in the literature evaluating the results of RF lesioning in chronic cervical pain and cervicobrachialgia using 22-gauge equipment.

Van Kleef et al.[18] showed in an open prospective study in 20 patients with chronic intractable pain in the cervical region radiating to the head, shoulder, and/or arm, an initial pain relief in 75% of patients after 3 months and in 50% of patients after 6 months.

A prospective, double-blind, randomized study comparing 67°C radiofrequency lesions adjacent to the dorsal root ganglion with sham lesions for cervicobrachial pain showed a significant alleviation of chronic cervicobrachialgia. A study comparing groups treated with 67°C and those treated with 40°C RF lesions could not demonstrate any difference.[19] A possible explanation given by the authors for lack of differences between the two groups is that a 40°C lesion is also an active treatment.

Studies about the efficacy of RF DRG in cervicogenic headache are not available.

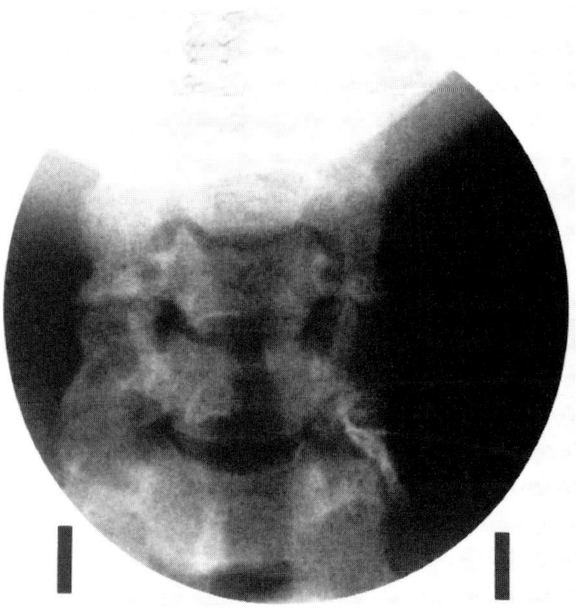

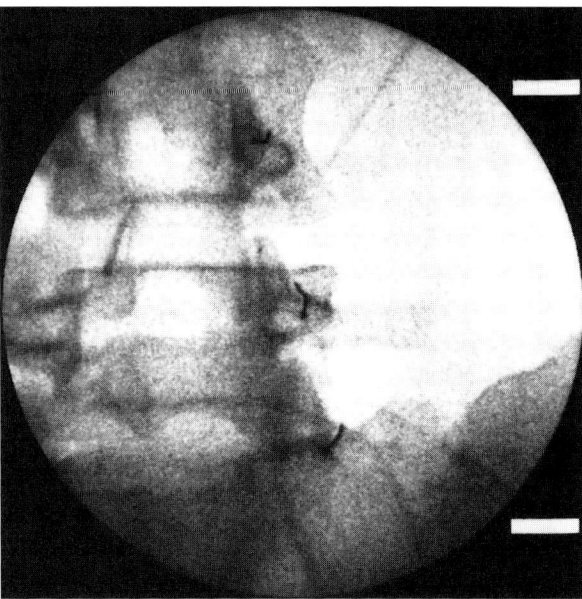

Figure 26.10 *RF lesioning of the cervical dorsal root ganglion. C-arm in the anteroposterior direction. The cannula is introduced until the tip is projected midway to the facetal column. Injection of contrast dye makes the nerve root visible.*

Figure 26.11 *RF lesioning of the lumbar dorsal root ganglion. The tip of the electrode is placed in the craniodorsal part of the foramen.*

RADIOFREQUENCY LESIONING IN THE LUMBAR AREA

Spinal pain located in the lumbar area is frequently encountered in medical practice. Some studies indicate that 70–80% of the adult working population experience lumbar pain at some stage of their life. In less than 15% of patients, specific pathology is found such as disk herniation, spondylolisthesis, spinal stenosis, or infections. In the remaining patients, the pain resolves within a few weeks, and in about 2 months 80% of patients return to normal function. In about 5–12% of this population, the complaints last for a longer period; generally, after a duration of 6 months, spontaneous relief from pain is often not complete.

PERCUTANEOUS RADIOFREQUENCY LUMBAR FACETAL JOINT DENERVATION**

Indication

Mechanical low back pain emanating from the facetal joints.

Patients are selected for the radiofrequency procedure after a positive response to a diagnostic block of the medial branch of the dorsal ramus.

Technique

With the patient prone on the operating table, the C-arm image intensifier is positioned in a slightly (10–15°) oblique position until the junction between the superior border of the transverse process and the lateral aspect of the superior articular process is clearly visible at the levels L4 and L5, and the junction of the ala of the sacrum and the articular process of the sacrum at level S1 is also visible. In these locations the medial branches of the posterior primary rami of the L3, L4, and L5 segmental nerves run in a posterior direction on their way to the groove on the posterior aspect of the base of the transverse process or of the sacral ala respectively. Entry points are marked overlying these junctions and the area is disinfected and draped. A 22-gauge SMK C10 cannula with a 5-mm active tip is introduced at each entry point in the direction of the radiation beam. Each of the three cannulas is carefully advanced, checking the proper direction following each step until the tip makes contact with bone at the posterior aspect of the junction. The cannula is then redirected in a slightly more cranial and lateral direction until contact with bone is lost. The position of the cannula is then checked on the lateral fluoroscopic projection. The depth is adjusted until the tip of the cannula is at the level of a line connecting the posterior aspects of the intervertebral foramina (Fig. 26.12).

The stylet of the cannula is replaced by a RF probe and electrostimulation at 2 Hz is carried out to confirm the proximity of the electrode to the medial branch and

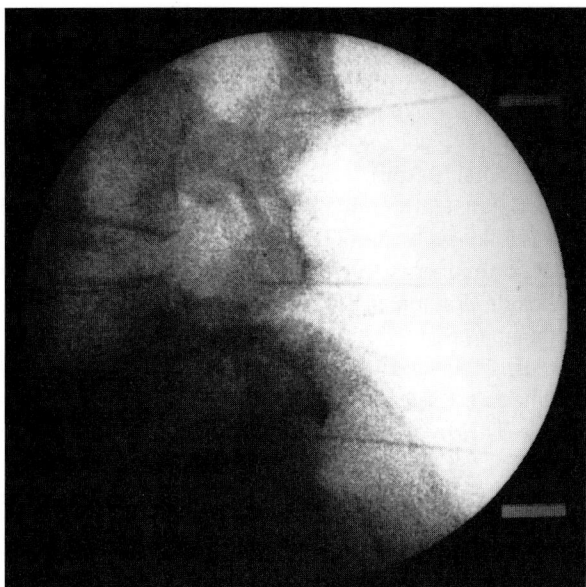

Figure 26.12 *RF lesioning of the lumbar dorsal root ganglion. In the anteroposterior projection, the tip of the electrode should be projected on a line connecting the facetal joints.*

to exclude inadvertent proximity to the exiting segmental nerve. When muscle contractions in the multifidus muscle do not occur below a voltage of 1.0 V, the cannula is repositioned. The absence of contractions of leg muscles is verified at 1.5 V. Once the position of the electrode is satisfactory, the RF probe is removed from the cannula and 1 ml of lidocaine 10 mg/ml is injected through each cannula. The RF probe is then reinserted and a 60-s 80°C lesion is made. When a TOP XE needle is used, 20 V for 60 s is applied to the electrode.

Side-effects

Although no side-effects have been reported after RF lumbar facetal joint denervation, caution should be taken that the electrode is not too close to the segmental nerve (check lateral view).

Efficacy of treatment

The first prospective, controlled, double-blind randomized study to assess the efficacy of radiofrequency facet joint denervation was conducted by Gallagher *et al.*[20] After diagnostic blocks, 41 patients were randomized as they entered the study to undergo either RF facet joint denervation or a placebo procedure, which was identical in every way apart from the heat lesion. The study showed a significant improvement in pain scores following denervation at 1 and 6 months when compared with the placebo group. A recent randomized study indicated that RF lesioning of the medial branch of the primary poste-

rior ramus results in a significant alleviation of pain and functional disability in a selected group of patients with chronic nonspecific low back pain.[21] Of the 42 patients who underwent RF treatment, 45% reported at least 50% pain relief 2 years after treatment or at the last follow-up. This relief of pain was associated with an improvement in most activities in the patient's daily life.

RADIOFREQUENCY LESION OF THE DORSAL LUMBAR ROOT GANGLION*

Indication

Radicular pain without sensory motor function disturbances.

Nerve root pain is characterized by dermatomal spread, usually into the lower leg and often into the foot. The main clinical symptoms are irradiating pain in a dermatome, and pain on straight leg raising. The diagnosis is established by pain relief after a selective nerve root block. If there is no sensory deficit, a radiofrequency lesion of the dorsal ganglion has been proposed.[22]

Contraindication

Sensory deficit in the painful area (neuropathic pain).

Technique

Diagnostic root blocks

For the selection of the putative pain-conducting nerve root, a series of consecutive selective root blocks is performed. With the patient prone on the operating table, the C-arm is positioned in the AP direction. A 100-mm 22-gauge neurography needle (Radionics) is introduced at an entry point 8 cm from the midline and 4 cm caudal to the relevant transverse process. The electrode is carefully advanced in the direction of the caudal part of the corpus vertebrae, until the tip is projected just lateral from the facetal column. After identifying the segmental nerve root with 0.5 ml contrast dye (Omnipaque 250), 0.5 ml of lidocaine 2% is slowly injected.

Radiofrequency lesion

An SMK C10 (100 mm) cannula with a 5-mm active tip is introduced at an entry point 8 cm from the midline and 4 cm caudal to the relevant transverse process. The electrode is carefully advanced to make contact with the junction of the lower border of the transverse process and the lamina. It is then manipulated slightly caudally and anteriorly until it slips into the craniodorsal part of the foramen. It is advanced until the tip is projected over the middle of the facetal column (Figs 26.13 and 26.14). Next, the posterior position in the foramen is confirmed on the transverse projection. The stylet is now replaced by a radiofrequency probe. After checking the impedance, electrical stimulation is started at 50 Hz. The patient

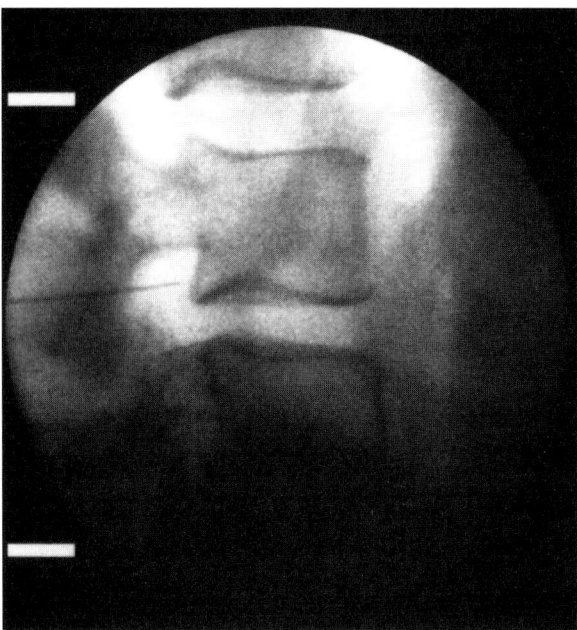

Figure 26.13 *RF lesioning of the lumbar dorsal root ganglion, lateral projection. The tip of the electrode is visible in the craniodorsal part of the foramen.*

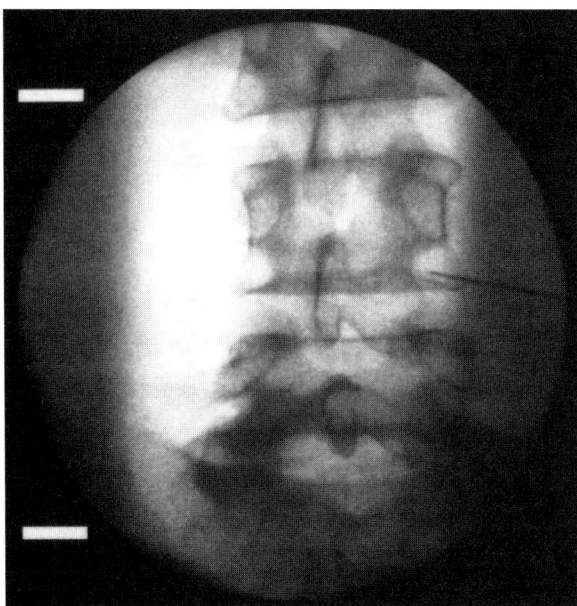

Figure 26.14 *RF lesioning of the lumbar dorsal root ganglion, anteroposterior projection. The tip of the electrode is visible medial to the lateral border of the vertebra at a line connecting the openings of the facetal joints between the first and fourth lumbar vertebra.*

should feel a tingling sensation at voltages between 0.4 and 0.65 V.

The frequency is then changed to 2 Hz and the patient is observed for muscle contractions. These should not occur below a voltage of 1.5 times the sensory threshold. Omnipaque (0.5 ml) is then injected in order to exclude an accidental intradural positioning of the electrode, and this is followed by 2 ml lidocaine 20 mg/ml.

Radiofrequency current is then applied through the electrode (Radionics RFG 3) to increase the temperature at the tip to 67°C. The temperature is maintained for 60 s.

For L5, the approach may be more difficult owing to the iliac crest. The utilization of tunnel vision is then preferable. The dorsal root ganglion of S1 cannot be reached with a straight instrument. For an RF DRG at this level, a small hole has to be drilled with a Kirschner wire into the dorsal aspect of the sacrum.

Efficacy of treatment

A recent randomized trial using as its primary outcome criteria the reduction of pain, change in physical activities, and use of analgesics could not demonstrate an efficacy of a 67°C RF lesion compared with placebo treatment.[22]

RADIOFREQUENCY LESIONING OF THE LUMBAR SYMPATHETIC GANGLIA*

Indication

Diffuse pain in the leg with autonomic dysfunction. In patients with neuropathic radicular pain, autonomic symptoms are observed quite frequently. Patients present with a nonsegmental pain in the leg in combination with diffuse sensory loss and a cold extremity. The diagnosis of sympathetically maintained pain can be asserted by diagnostic sympathetic blocks. If temporary pain relief is achieved with these blocks, radiofrequency lesioning of the sympathetic chain may be considered.

Contraindication

Following a diagnostic block, only a temperature rise of the leg is observed without a concomitant pain reduction. Here, a RF lesion can result in an increase of pain.

Technique

This block is usually performed at the L3 and L4 levels. With the patient prone on the operating table, the C-arm is positioned in an oblique direction so that the spinous processes are projected over the facetal joint column of the opposite side. An entry point is selected overlying the side of the vertebral body at the junction of the lower and middle third of the vertebra. A 20-gauge SMK C15 cannula with a 10-mm active tip is introduced under tunnel vision. It is carefully advanced, passing cranial to the segmental nerve and avoiding contact with the periosteum of the vertebral body.

The position is then checked on the transverse and AP projections. The tip should lie level with the anterior margin of the vertebra and just medial to the middle of the facetal column. This is important to avoid damage to the ilioinguinal nerve. Injection of contrast should show the typical spread of contrast. To exclude the involvement of somatic nerve structures (e.g. nervus ilioinguinalis, nervus genitofemoralis), stimulation with 50 Hz is applied. During stimulation with an intensity up to 2 V, no sensations may be felt in the distribution areas of these nerves. Subsequently, 2 ml lidocaine 20 mg/ml is injected and an 80°C RF lesioning is applied for 60 s.

Side-effects

Temporary swollen and hot foot on the treated side. Effects subside in 1–2 weeks.

Complications

Complications include neuritis of the ilioinguinal or genitofemoral nerve and complaints of burning dysesthetic pain in the inguinal region and the inner side of the thigh.

Efficacy of treatment

More than in neurolytic blocks, the exact positioning of the needle (electrode) tip is of crucial importance. Only when the needle is in the direct vicinity of the sympathetic ganglion does a lesion result in neurolysis. A study comparing the results of radiofrequency lesioning or phenol injection showed a distinct superiority of the latter.[23]

REFERENCES

1. Kirschner M. Zur Elektrochirurgie. *Arch Klin Chir* 1931; **167**: 761.
2. Sweet WH, Mark VH. Unipolar anodal electrolytic lesion in the brain of man and cat: report of five human cases with electrically produced bulbar or mesencephalic tractotomies. *Arch Neurol Psych* 1953; **70**: 224–334.
3. Mullan S, Hekmatpah J, Dobben G. Percutaneous intramedullary chordotomy utilizing the unipolar anodal electric lesion. *J Neurosurg* 1965; **22**: 548–43.
4. Sweet WH, Wepsic JG. Controlled thermocoagulation of trigeminal ganglion and rootlets for differential destruction of pain fibers. Part I. Trigeminal. *J Neurosurg* 1974; **39**:143–56.
5. Uematsu S. Percutaneous electrocoagulation of spinal nerve trunk, ganglion and rootlets. In: Schmidel H, Sweet WH eds. *Operative Neurosurgical Techniques: Indications, Methods and Results.* New York, NY: Grune and Stratton, 1982: 1171–98.
6. Sluijter ME, Metha M. Treatment of chronic back pain and neck pain by percutaneous thermal lesions. In: Lipton S ed. *Persistent Pain, Modern Methods of Treatment*, vol. 3. London: Academic Press, 1981: 141–79.
7. Stolker RJ, Vervest AC, Groen GJ. The management of chronic spinal pain by blockades: a review. *Pain* 1994; **58**: 1–20.
8. Lipton S. Percutaneous cordotomy. In: Wall PD, Melzack R eds. *Textbook of Pain*. Edinburgh: Churchill Livingstone, 1984: 632–8.
9. Taha JM, Tew JM. Treatment of trigeminal neuralgia by percutaneous radiofrequency rhizotomy. *Neurosurg Clin North Am* 1997; **8**: 31–9.
10. Sluijter ME, Vercruysse PJ, Sterk W. Radiofrequency lesions of the sphenopalatine ganglion neuralgia. *Schmerz/Pain/Douleur* 1988; **9**: 56–9.
11. Sanders M, Zuurmond WWA. Efficacy of sphenopalatine ganglion blockades in 66 patients suffering from cluster headache: a 12- to 70-months follow-up evaluation. *J Neurosurg* 1997; **87**: 876–80.
12. Bogduk N. The innervation of the lumbar spine. *Spine* 1983; **8**: 286–93.
13. Dwyer A, Aprill C, Bogduk N. Cervical zygapophyseal joint pain patterns. I. A study in normal volunteers. *Spine* 1990; **15**: 453–7.
14. Sjaastad O, Saunte C, Howdahl H, *et al*. Cervicogenic headache. An hypothesis. *Cephalalgia* 1983; **3**: 249–56.
15. Lord S, Barnsley L, Wallis B, *et al*. Percutaneous radiofrequency neurotomy for chronic cervical zygapophyseal joint pain. *N Engl J Med* 1996; **335**: 1721–6.
16. McDonald GJ, Lord SM, Bogduk N. Long-term follow-up of patients with cervical radiofrequency neurotomy for chronic neck pain. *Neurosurgery* 1999; **45**: 61–7.
17. Van Kleef M, Spaans F, Dingemans W, *et al*. Effects and side effects of a percutaneous thermal lesion of the dorsal root ganglion in patients with cervical pain syndrome. *Pain* 1993; **52**: 49–53.
18. Van Kleef M, Liem L, Lousberg R, *et al*. Radiofrequency lesion adjacent to the dorsal root ganglion for cervicobrachial pain: a prospective double blind randomized study. *Neurosurgery* 1996; **38**: 1127–32.
19. Slappendel R, Crul BJP, Braak GJJ, *et al*. The efficacy of radiofrequency lesioning of the cervical spinal dorsal root ganglion in a double blind randomized study: no difference between 40 and 67 centigrade treatments. *Pain* 1997; **73**: 159–63.
20. Gallagher J, Petricciore PL, Wedley JR, *et al*. Radiofre-

quency facet joint denervation in the treatment of low back pain: a prospective controlled double-blind study to assess its efficacy. *Pain Clin* 1994; **7:** 193–8.

◆ 21. Van Kleef N, Barendse GAB, Kessel A, *et al*. Randomized trial of radiofrequency lumbar facet denervation for chronic low back pain. *Spine* 1999; **24:** 1937–42.

◆ 22. Geurts JWM, Van Wijk RMAW, Wynne HJ, *et al*. Radiofrequency thermal lesion of the dorsal root ganglion for chronic lumbosacral radicular pain. A randomised, double blind sham-lesion controlled trial. In: Geurts JWM, Van Wijk RMAW eds. *Minimally Invasive Procedures in the Treatment of Chronic Low Back Pain*. Thesis. Utrecht: University of Utrecht, 2001.

23. Haynsworth RF, Noe CE. Percutaneous lumbar sympathectomy: a comparison of radiofrequency denervation versus phenol neurolysis. *Anesthesiology* 1991; **74:** 459–63.

PART VI

Stimulation analgesia

Transcutaneous electrical nerve stimulation

TIMOTHY P NASH

Applied anatomy	344	The trial	348
Indications	344	Setting the stimulator	348
Contraindications	345	Complications	348
Caution	345	Side-effects	349
Limitations: frequency of therapy	345	Evidence for the use of TENS	349
Equipment	346	Conclusion	352
Types of stimulation	347	References	352
Site of application	347		

Man has been aware of the effects of electricity for thousands of years. A bas relief in Egypt from 2750 BC shows an electric catfish, known as the "releaser of many" or the "shaker," amongst other fish around a dhow. About 400 BC, Hippocrates used electric fish to treat headache and arthritis, and Scribonius Largus in 46BC described the use of the electric torpedo ray by the Romans for gout and headache. The electric eel of South America was similarly used, and was studied by Baron Von Humboldt in 1800. He stood on one and experienced the development of a painful numbness up to his knees, which left him with violent pain in his knees and the rest of his joints for the remainder of the day. He prophesied that "the discoveries that will be made on the electromotive apparatus of these fish will extend to all phenomena of muscular motion subject to volition. It will perhaps be found that in most animals every contraction of a muscle fiber is preceded by a discharge from the nerve to the muscle." He also predicted that electricity is the source of life and movement in all living things.[1]

The development of the Leyden jar in 1745–6 enabled electricity to become more readily available and portable, rather than requiring a wet fish at the seaside! This led to the development of various magnetoelectric electroanesthetic equipment. In 1759, John Wesley used his electrostatic machine to treat "rheumaticky pains" in a patient "made helpless like an infant." After the second shock, he felt some change; after the third he was able to raise himself; after two more he rose and walked about the room; and before noon he was quite well. In England in 1858, Althaus described the application of his apparatus to peripheral nerves. At the same time, in Philadelphia, Francis was producing dental analgesia for extractions. Oliver in Buffalo and Garratt in Boston were similarly producing dental analgesia, and developing its use at other sites. Garratt in particular used it for dental neuralgias, hyperalgesia, tic douloureux, toothache, and jaw ache. Oliver used it also for amputation of limbs and for childbirth. The Cataphoresis machine of 1925 was used for dental analgesia and can be seen in the Charles King Collection at the Association of Anaesthetists of Great Britain and Ireland. The modern equivalent is the H-wave and Ultracalm machines.

The "gate theory" of pain[2] attempted to explain how chronic stimulation of the nervous system could be used to treat nociceptive pain, and led to the development of percutaneous stimulation of peripheral nerves and dorsal column stimulation. Transcutaneous electrical nerve stimulation (TENS) was initially introduced as a prognostic test prior to spinal cord stimulation.

Prolonged stimulation of peripheral nerves with percutaneous needle electrodes was shown in 1967 to modify the reaction of healthy human volunteers to acute noxious stimuli, without any ill effects,[3] and to inhibit the prolonged afterdischarge in the tegmentum and medulla that normally follows electrical tetanic stimulation of a peripheral nerve.[4] This confirmed clinically the spinal gate control theory of Melzack and Wall.[2] Confirmation of this effect with brief, intense transcutaneous electrical stimulations at trigger points or acupuncture points on severe clinical pain was published in 1975.[5] Such stimulation produced a decrease in pain of 60–70% depending on the type of pain, significantly higher than the strong placebo contribution.

Many different electrical stimulation therapies have now been developed, all working on the same idea. Action potential stimulation therapy mimics the action potential in its electrical waveform. Interferential therapy is a static machine used by physiotherapists, and transcutaneous spinal electroanalgesia and transcutaneous cranial electrical stimulation are claimed to produce analgesia by percutaneously stimulating the spinal cord and brain respectively. Cutaneous field stimulation uses a flexible plate with needle-like electrodes to electrically stimulate nerve fibers in the superficial skin, and has been developed to treat itch without damaging the skin.

APPLIED ANATOMY

It is still not clear how TENS and acupuncture work. Both peripheral and central neural mechanisms are involved. Acupuncture and TENS for analgesia are now considered in the light of the type of stimulus used. Conventional TENS is a high-frequency, low-intensity stimulus, and acupuncture and acupuncture-like TENS is a low-frequency, high-intensity stimulus.

The low-intensity (TENS) stimulus is considered to activate large muscle (type I) and large skin (Aβ) fibers. This produces gating by segmental inhibition of the central afferents of the polymodal C pain fibers within the substantia gelatinosa, possibly through interneurons with γ-amino-butyric acid receptors. The Aβ-fibers pass in the dorsal columns to produce descending inhibition via the periaqueductal gray matter. The analgesia is often of rapid onset and short duration, and tolerance can develop from continuous therapy. At least part of TENS-mediated hypoalgesia is a consequence of a direct peripheral effect of TENS.[6]

Low-frequency, high-intensity stimulation (acupuncture) is considered to act by stimulating small muscle afferents (type III, Aδ-fibers) to produce both segmental and suprasegmental inhibition via endorphinergic and serotoninergic pathways. Segmental inhibition is produced by presynaptic inhibition via interstitial enkephalinergic fibers in the substantia gelatinosa. The central afferents of the Aδ-fibers pass in the spinothalamic tract to the hypothalamus, and again can produce suprasegmental inhibition via endorphinergic and serotoninergic pathways. The analgesia produced has slow onset and long duration, and 30-min treatments do not produce tolerance.

INDICATIONS

TENS is used widely. In Canada, 93% of hospitals use it for acute pain, 43% for labor and delivery, and 96% for chronic pain, amounting to an estimated 450,000 hospital uses of TENS per year.[7]

TENS can be used for localized, mild, superficial pain of somatic or neurogenic origin, but is less useful for widespread, severe, deep-seated pain. It may be useful for visceral pain, especially angina pectoris.

Acute pain

Most acute pain is due to trauma, and settles sufficiently quickly to render TENS unnecessary. Sports injuries, however, including back sprains, torn ligaments, and pulled muscles, can respond usefully. Major trauma usually includes multiple injuries, and will produce pain that is widespread and severe. TENS is unlikely to be of any value in this situation.

TENS may also be valuable for the pain of fractured ribs, acute orofacial inflammatory pain (periodontal infections and pulpal inflammation), acute rheumatoid arthritis, myalgia, and myofascial pain. Postoperative pain has also been treated, with the electrodes applied adjacent to the incision by the surgeon at the end of surgery. TENS has also been used to reduce postoperative nausea and vomiting, and found to be equivalent to commonly used antiemetic drugs.

TENS can also be used to provide analgesia for procedures such as dental treatment and lancet-induced trauma to the fingertip, and has become popular in relieving the pain of labor. During labor, two sets of electrodes are used: one pair at T10–L1 for the first stage and a second at S2–S4 for the second stage. Primary dysmenorrhea may also respond.

Chronic pain

TENS is associated with improvement on multiple outcome variables in addition to pain relief for chronic pain patients, and can be effective long term.

Myofascial/musculoskeletal/spasticity

TENS can be useful in myofascial or muscular pain, and has been used instead of the Milwaukee brace in managing idiopathic scoliosis. TENS can also be effective in reducing spinal spasticity.

Neuropathic

TENS has been used successfully for the pain of peripheral diabetic neuropathy, and also for phantom limb pain, when it can be usefully applied to the contralateral leg. Other neuropathic pains such as brachial plexus avulsion and postherpetic neuralgia can also respond, provided the electrodes can be positioned on the skin with sufficient sensation to produce paresthesiae in the painful area.

Visceral

TENS is useful for angina pectoris, providing an increased work capacity, reduced frequency of anginal attacks, and reduced consumption of short-acting nitroglycerine, all because of a decreased afterload resulting from systemic vascular dilatation. Lactate metabolism is reduced and there is less pronounced ST segment depression with an increased coronary flow to ischemic areas in the myocardium. TENS has also been shown to have an effect on lowering blood pressure and may decrease the sympathetic activity either directly or indirectly as a consequence of pain inhibition.

TENS can also improve tissue perfusion and ulcer healing in peripheral vascular disease, leprosy, and in skin flaps with deficient circulation after reconstructive surgery. TENS can also be useful in thrombophlebitis.

TENS may be a useful treatment for noncardiac chest pain of esophageal origin, and can decrease lower esophageal sphincter pressure in patients with achalasia. It can also reduce perception of gut distension without interfering with local and reflex gut responses.

TENS has been shown to produce prompt onset of analgesia with no significant effect on uterine activity in patients with primary dysmenorrhea. It may also have a role in the treatment of detrusor instability and urinary urgency.

TENS has also been successfully used for antiemesis in cancer therapy.

Evidence in brief for TENS

- Not effective for acute pain.
- Not effective for labor pain.
- Lack of evidence of efficacy in chronic pain.
- No evidence in favor of any one type of stimulation.
- As good as aspirin in myofascial pain.
- Some evidence for phantom limb pain.
- Can reduce postoperative nausea.
- Positive physiological effects in angina.
- Can reduce health care costs by 55% for medication and 66% for physiotherapy or occupational therapy.

CONTRAINDICATIONS

- Broken/dysesthetic/numb skin.
- Application to front of neck.
- Stimulation over fetus.

Application of the electrodes to broken or dysesthetic skin will be poorly tolerated, and application to numb areas will be unsuccessful. It is essential that paresthesiae

can be generated in the region of the pain or within the same or closely related dermatome.

The electrodes should never be applied to stimulate over the anterior part of the neck, as the laryngeal muscles and carotid sinus may be stimulated.

Except in labor, it is probably sensible to avoid stimulation over the pregnant uterus, and especially during the first trimester, as electrical fields may have an effect on the development of the fetus. If premature labor and miscarriage occur while TENS is being used, the treatment is likely to be blamed, despite its application well away from the uterus. No reports exist in the literature, however.

CAUTION

- Cardiac pacemaker.
- Driving/operating machinery.
- Senility/low intelligence quotient (IQ).

Caution should be exercised in the presence of a cardiac pacemaker, although it is not uncommon to use it in the presence of a fixed rate pacemaker, with the agreement of the cardiologist in charge of the patient. Patients with cardiac pacemakers should not be excluded from the use of TENS, but careful evaluation and extended cardiac monitoring should be performed.[8,9] It is our practice to give the patient an initial trial in the day-ward with electrocardiographic monitoring prior to discharging them with a unit.

It is unwise to use TENS in senile patients, children, or those with a low IQ, as they need a good understanding of how to apply and use the unit.

Caution should be observed while driving or operating machinery, as transient disconnection of the electrodes can cause a surge of current on reconnection that could startle the patient and cause gross sudden movement, with the consequent dangers.

LIMITATIONS: FREQUENCY OF THERAPY

The use of TENS for acute pain depends on the availability to the patient of both the unit and the education on its use.

For it to be effective in postoperative pain, sterile electrodes must be applied alongside the incision and underneath the dressings, preferably by the surgeon. The site of application must not have been denervated by the surgery.

For chronic pain, TENS must be used for at least 30 min twice a day and for at least 1 month before any effect may be felt. About half the patients using TENS can reduce their pain by more than 50%, and the analgesia is rapid both in onset (less than 0.5 h in 75% patients) and in offset (less than 0.5 h in 51% patients). One-third of patients generally use TENS for over 61 h/week.[10]

EQUIPMENT

- TENS stimulator.
- Electrode leads.
- Electrodes:
  - carbon–rubber, with electrode gel and fixative;
  - disposable.

Transcutaneous electrical nerve stimulation is normally provided by a portable, battery-operated, transistorized pulse generator connected via leads to electrodes applied to the skin. Generally, it has the following controls:

1 Combined on/off and amplitude (intensity) control.
2 Frequency control (from around 2 Hz to over 100 Hz or even to 250 Hz).
3 Mode selector to select between continuous and pulsed stimulation, sometimes with a further choice to modulate the stimulation giving a slow increase then decrease in amplitude or frequency to produce a sensation similar to stroking. Modulated or pulsed output reduces the development of tolerance to the stimulation.
4 Width control (varying the width of the electrical pulse, usually between 40 and 500 μs).
5 Multichannel units will have a separate amplitude switch for each channel.

There are also stimulators that produce complex waveforms to achieve deeper stimulation (LIKON) or further reduce the development of tolerance by utilizing multiple electrodes activated randomly (CODETRON). A new nonportable stimulator, action potential stimulation therapy, uses a waveform that mimics the action potential. It is generally used with below-threshold stimulation.

A pair of insulated wires with a small jack plug at one end connects to the stimulator, and separate plugs at the other end connect to the electrodes. The leads are the weakest link in the circuit, and frequently fracture at the junction with the plugs at either end. The more supple the leads, the less likely they are to fracture, and the more comfortable to wear.

The electrodes are generally either carbon–rubber (conductive) or disposable self-adhesive electrodes. The carbon–rubber electrodes require electrode gel applying between the electrode and the skin, and fixing in place with adhesive tape. Alternatively, karaya pads, made from conductive karaya gum and adhesive on both sides, may be used. The self-adhesive electrodes require no fixative or gel, becoming adhesive with wetting of the surface of the electrode that is applied to the skin.

Some older machines may have sponge or cotton wool pads that require wetting, and may be fixed in place with velcro bands. Larger electrodes require greater voltage output but less pulse-charge density than the smaller electrodes, and evoke significantly greater nonpainful and maximally tolerated painful muscle torques for high-threshold stimulation.[11]

Electrode position

The electrodes are used in pairs. To avoid short circuiting between them, they should never be positioned with less than 1 cm between their edges. The electrodes should be positioned to lie over, and along the line of, the nerves supplying the area to be treated (Fig. 27.1). Consequently, the electrodes should be applied longitudinally on the limbs, and along the main axis of the nerves or dermatomes on the trunk.

Connect the electrodes to the leads before applying to the skin. The skin should be clean and dry and free from grease or powder. If not, the electrical conductivity will be affected, and self-adhesive electrodes will become soiled and lose their adhesiveness. Electrodes should not stay on the skin for more than 24 h.

Carbon–rubber electrodes

Carbon-rubber electrodes are applied to the skin after smearing a layer of conductive gel over the skin surface of the electrode, and then placing it in the required position and fixing it in position with adhesive tape. Saline jelly is advisable to give good electrical conductivity between the skin and the electrode, normally in a strength of 2% sodium chloride and containing a bactericide. Electrocardiograph (EKG) jelly contains a much higher concentration of saline, which will irritate the skin if left on for the usual time for TENS therapy. It should therefore be avoided. KY Jelly, although not an electrode gel, in practice does provide adequate conductivity, and may be useful when allergies develop to the normal electrode gels. Once applied, the electrode is fixed in position with adhesive tape. The most suitable is Micropore because it does not usually cause skin irritation and is easy to apply.

Self-adhesive electrodes

The electrode is normally stored on a backing sheet of either wax or polythene. It should be peeled off the backing sheet, moistened, and applied evenly to the skin. To remove it, it should be peeled off the skin from one corner and immediately applied to the backing sheet to prevent drying.

Connection to the stimulator

The electrodes are then connected to the stimulator via the leads. *The stimulator must be switched off at the time of connection.* The stimulator is then switched on and adjusted appropriately.

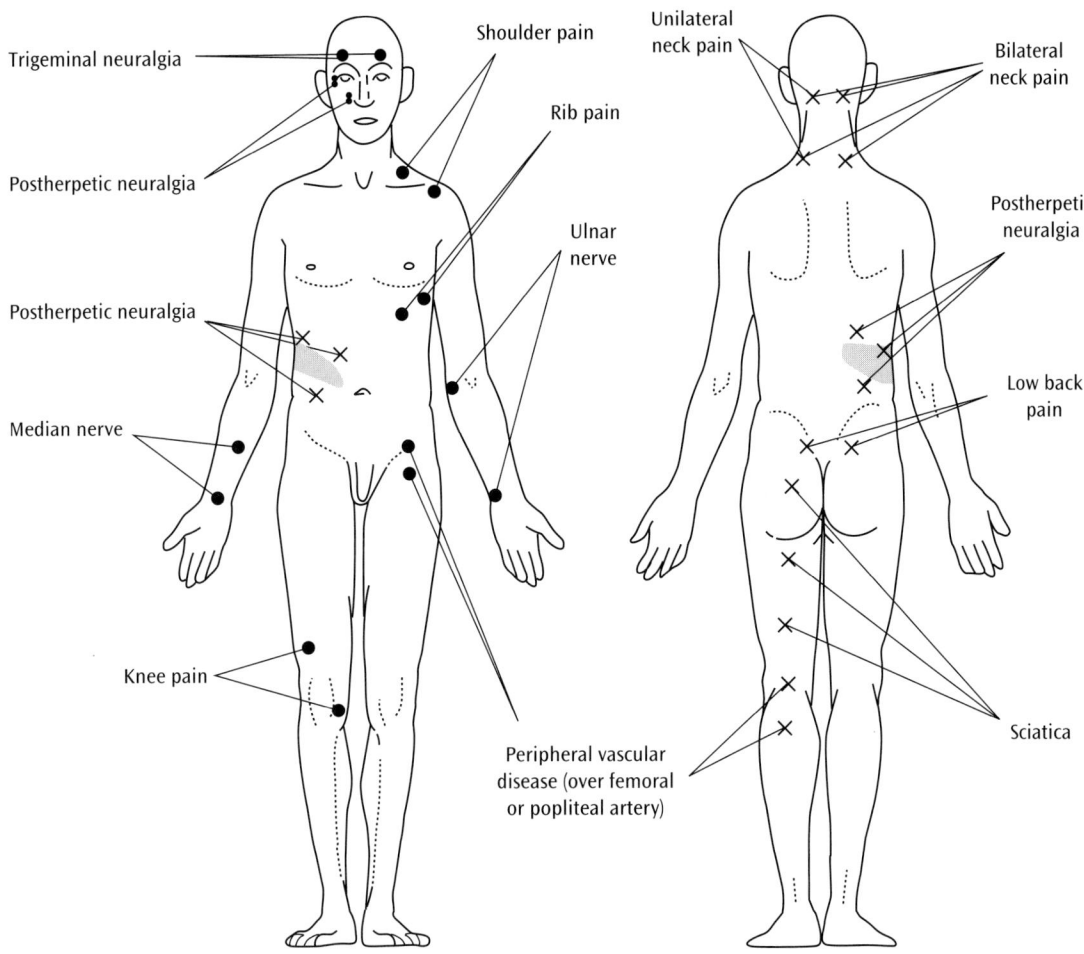

Figure 27.1 *Useful TENS electrode application points.*

TYPES OF STIMULATION

TENS can be used in three different types of stimulation modality:

1 Continuous (conventional); high frequency (40–150 Hz); low intensity (10–30 mA).
2 Pulsed (burst); low frequency (bursts of 100 Hz at 1–2 Hz); low intensity (10–30 mA).
3 Acupuncture-like (Acu-TENS); low frequency (bursts of 100 Hz at 1–2 Hz); high intensity (15–50 mA).

Application

- Clean skin well before application.
- Check stimulator is switched off.
- Apply electrodes to skin with normal sensation.
- Position electrodes with their adjacent edges at least 2 cm apart.
- Position along direction of nerves or dermatomes supplying the painful area.
- Connect electrodes to stimulator.

- Select stimulation mode (continuous, pulsed, modulated).
- Turn stimulator on and increase amplitude to maximum comfortable.
- Increase frequency to maximum comfortable.
- Increase pulse width to maximum comfortable.
- If using acupuncture-like TENS, increase amplitude to produce muscle twitches in muscles between electrodes.

SITE OF APPLICATION

The rationale of use is to apply the electrodes to the skin to stimulate along the general direction of the nerves supplying the area to be treated. Thus, when treating the limbs, the electrodes should be applied longitudinally; on the trunk, they should be placed along the course of the nerves or the dermatomes. Whichever stimulation modality is used, the stimulation sensation should be directed into the painful part and should be strong but comfortable.

When conventional or pulsed stimulation is used, muscle twitching should not be produced, but acupuncture stimulation should be adjusted to be strong enough to produce muscle twitching. Large areas of pain will require two or more pairs of electrodes, by using either a double adaptor lead with a single channel unit or a dual channel stimulator with two leads.

In angina pectoris, the electrodes are applied to the dermatome where the pain is felt. Thus, stimulation of the cutaneous afferents from that dermatome will enter the cord at the same or closely related level as that of the visceral afferents producing the pain.

THE TRIAL

It is normal to have a trial period of treatment to ensure that the pain is not aggravated by TENS, to teach the patient how to use the system, and to give a guide as to the likelihood of the pain responding to treatment. However, initial poor response does not mean that long-term use will not achieve some benefit. At least 1 h of stimulation is required in the first instance. It should then be used regularly for at least 1 h three times each day for a minimum of 14 days. The frequency of use should be adjusted according to need and response. The patient should use TENS as much as they wish, and be encouraged to compare the effects of all modalities. This will enable them to choose the modality most effective for them, or the most effective at particular times, using all types of stimulation as necessary. They should be told that a period of post-stimulation analgesia may occur.

The patient should be reviewed regularly over the first year, and thereafter as required, if they continue to use TENS.

SETTING THE STIMULATOR

Continuous (conventional) stimulation

All the controls should be set at zero, and the mode switch set at continuous. The amplitude should then be increased slowly to the maximum comfortable level, i.e. strong but comfortable, and then the pulse frequency increased to the maximum comfortable level. If there is a pulse width control, this should also be increased to again the maximum comfortable level.

Pulsed (burst) stimulation

All controls should be set at zero, and the mode switch set to pulsed mode. The amplitude, pulse frequency, and pulse width are adjusted as in continuous stimulation.

Acupuncture-like TENS (Acu-TENS)

Adjust the stimulator as for pulsed stimulation, but increase the amplitude to produce muscle twitches in the muscles beneath the electrodes. These muscle twitches should not be so strong that they are painful.

Sequential stimulation

Sequential TENS involves two periods of stimulation with different parameters. If conventional TENS is used initially, this may enable burst stimulation to be better tolerated, with the possibility of greater efficacy and more prolonged effect.[12]

Choice of stimulation modality

Patients will choose the most suitable settings for their own pain by trial and error. There is no evidence in favor of any particular settings for any particular condition.

COMPLICATIONS

1 Skin irritation occurs in 30% of patients, and is usually due to inadequate technique. The commonest cause is failure to clean carbon–rubber electrodes after use; these must be removed from the skin at least once in every 24 h. Electrodes should not be applied to the same area of skin every day, but an adjacent position on fresh skin should be used.
2 Allergic reactions are uncommon, but may occur to the electrode, the jelly, or the fixative (tape or gum). When this does occur, a different type of jelly, tape, or electrode should be used. Thus, carbon–rubber electrodes can be replaced by self-adhesive electrodes; TENS saline jelly can be replaced by KY Jelly (practically, KY Jelly works, although it is theoretically not conductive!); Micropore tape can be replaced by some other suitable tape (even Sellotape!).
3 Electrical skin burn can occur, particularly if excessive current is applied to denervated or poorly innervated areas of skin which are numb or partially numb. Before using TENS, always check that there is normal sensation where the electrodes are being applied.
4 There may be failure of various parts of the equipment. The most common parts to fail are the leads, which may fracture where they connect to the plugs. The plugs themselves may become dirty, corroded, or heavily oxidized. The battery may fail, or be inserted incorrectly. If rechargeable batteries are used, the charger itself may be at fault.
5 Tolerance may develop to the analgesic effect, and occurs in about 30% of patients, developing slowly

over time. Apparent tolerance may be due to a worsening of the pain. This may be reversed by temporary withdrawal of TENS or by changing the pulse pattern (perhaps from continuous to pulsed).

6 A case of respiratory arrest, explained by the production of tetanic stimulation of the intercostal muscles of a patient using TENS for angina, has been described.[13]

SIDE-EFFECTS

Only 47% of patients considered the TENS sensations to be consistently pleasant. Forty-six percent suffered side-effects:[14]

1 Sensations at the site of TENS application (18%). The sensations felt included:
   a pins and needles;
   b soreness;
   c tingling;
   d itching;
   e prickling;
   f numbness;
   g shaking;
   h burning;
   i stabbing;
   j a new "pulling" pain.
2 Sensations at a distance to site of application (12%).
3 Headaches (8%).
4 Increased pain (8%).
5 Muscle aches (6%).
6 Nausea (3%).
7 Bad temper (3%).
8 Dizziness (1%).

EVIDENCE FOR THE USE OF TENS

Experimental evidence

Evaluating TENS in randomized, double-blind trials is not easy. TENS can almost never be properly blinded. This leads to bias that can exaggerate the estimate of treatment effect by up to 17%. Trials that are not randomized or are inadequately randomized exaggerate the estimate of treatment effect by up to 40%.[15] This has to be taken into account when reviewing the evidence of efficacy of TENS or any of its stimulation modalities.

The effect of TENS appears to be similar to that produced by other nonpharmacological analgesic manipulations such as counterirritation and changes in attention.[16]** Like counterirritation, it needs to be felt to be effective, as shown by a trial where subthreshold TENS had no effect on myofascial pain syndromes when com-

pared with placebo in a single-blind trial.[17]** This confirms the need to produce paresthesiae within the painful area to provide analgesia.

TENS is associated with improvement on multiple outcome variables in addition to pain relief for chronic pain patients who are long-term users. Also, for some patients, long-term TENS use continues to be effective.[18]*

Acupuncture and acupuncture-like TENS produce stimulation, either mechanical or electrical, at low frequencies (below 10 Hz) given at an intensity that produces muscle contractions which extend to the whole muscle group (high-intensity, low-frequency stimulation), with TENS producing high-frequency, low-intensity stimulation (Table 27.1).

Considerable experimentation has been performed in animals, human volunteers, and in the clinical arena. Despite this, no one stimulation modality (acupuncture like or conventional) has been proven better than any other in any particular situation. Stimulation modality is therefore chosen on the basis of patient preference or prolongation of battery life.

There has been the suggestion from nonblinded studies that high-frequency TENS, continuous or pulsed, may be more effective than low-frequency TENS in rheumatoid arthritis patients with severe wrist pain.[19]** Again, nonblinded studies have suggested that acupuncture-like TENS is more effective in neurogenic pain.[20]**

However, there was no significant difference in efficacy between continuous 100 Hz, pulsed 100 Hz, continuous 10 Hz, or pulsed 10 Hz in a randomized, double-blind study comparing the four different stimulation modalities in 200 patients (Fig. 27.2). Combining groups also gave no significant difference between pulsed and continuous stimulation or low and high frequency, although there was a trend for a speedier response with pulsed high-frequency acupuncture-like TENS. Half of the patients found TENS reduced their pain by more than 50%, and there was a steady increase in the number achieving a 50% reduction in pain with time (Fig. 27.3).[21]**

Indeed, patients choose frequencies and patterns of stimulation according to reasons of comfort that may not be related to mechanisms specific to the pain system.*[22] In

Table 27.1 *The different qualities of conventional TENS (TENS) and acupuncture/acupuncture-like TENS*

	TENS	Acupuncture
Frequency	40–100 Hz	1–4 Hz
Intensity	Low	High
Sensations	Tingling, vibration	Teh Chi, close to pain, beating
Induction time	Short	Long
Pain threshold effect	Transient	Long lasting
Distribution	Segmental	Segmental and nonsegmental

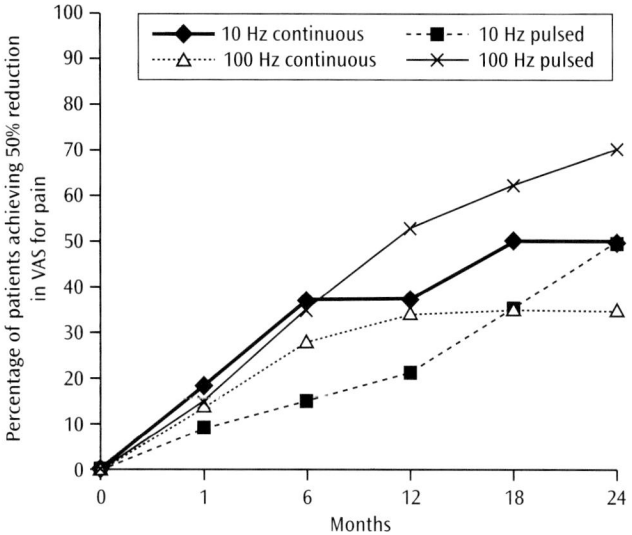

Figure 27.2 *Percentage of patients over time achieving 50% reduction in VAS for pain according to stimulation modality.*

one study, they preferred modulated stimulation modes such as frequency modulation and burst rather than conventional constant mode.[23*,24*] A recent prospective continuous sample of 154 patients referred to the TENS clinic showed that 59% used conventional TENS as this gave the best reduction in patient's pain, and a 50% reduction in pain was found in 44% of patients. Those with neuropathic pain tended to have a greater effect ($P = 0.17$), and it was less beneficial in the over 60 years age group. The average time for those who gained benefit for TENS to start to reduce pain was 26 min, and relief continued for 77 min after switching off the machine.[14]

Acute pain

In a systematic review of TENS for acute postoperative pain,[25***] TENS was judged by the reviewers to be no better than placebo in 15 out of 17 randomized studies. The two positive trials showed a reduced analgesic consumption, one after total hip replacement and the other after abdominal and thoracic surgery.

A more recent study of TENS applied at the dermatomal level of the skin incision in a randomized controlled trial of hysterectomy or myomectomy patients found TENS to be as effective as Zusanli acupoint stimulation, and both treatments were more effective than stimulation at a nonacupoint (shoulder) location.[26**]

Neither indomethacin nor TENS reduced the postoperative opiate requirement after cholecystectomy.[27] *However, TENS has been shown to significantly reduce the pain of lancet-induced trauma to the fingertip.[28*] In a further study, 78% of children preferred electrodental anesthesia to local anesthesia for dentistry.[29*]

TENS has also been used to reduce postoperative nau-

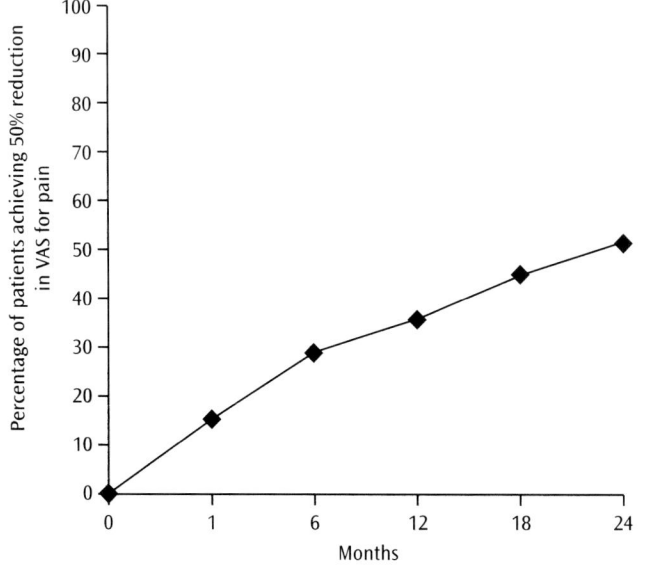

Figure 27.3 *Total percentage of patients achieving 50% reduction in VAS for pain over time.*

sea and vomiting, and found to be equivalent to commonly used antiemetic drugs. The incidence of vomiting postoperatively was significantly less in the TENS-treated group than in the control group.[30]**

Pain of labor

Similarly, TENS has not been shown to have any value in labor pain and the pain of delivery in any randomized controlled trials. Indeed, in one randomized controlled trial, intracutaneous sterile water injections were found to be more effective than standard care (back massage, bath, and mobilization) or transcutaneous electrical nerve stimulation for relieving low back pain during labor. Randomized controlled trials provide no compelling evidence for TENS having any analgesic effect during labor. Weak positive effects in secondary (analgesic sparing) and tertiary (choosing TENS for future labors) outcomes may be the result of inadequate blinding causing overestimation of treatment effects.[31]***

Chronic pain

TENS has been a successful analgesic treatment for 58.6% of 1,582 patients attending a UK clinic over a period of 10 years. TENS for chronic pain requires to be used for at least 30 min twice a day, and for at least 1 month before any effect may be felt. One-third of patients utilized TENS for over 61 h/week.[32]* Pulse frequencies between 1 and 70 Hz were utilized by 75% of patients, and 44% of patients benefited from burst mode stimulation.[10]*

In chronic pain, there is a lack of evidence of efficacy, rather than a lack of efficacy. There is evidence that TENS should be used for at least 30 min twice a day for at least 1 month to obtain any effect and this effect may be progressive, with 51% of patients reducing their visual analog scale (VAS) score for pain by over 50% at 2 years.[21]*** None of the randomized trials used TENS for an equivalent duration to that of either Johnson et al.[22]*** or Nash et al.,[21]*** stimulation being for fewer than 4 weeks in 83% of the trials and for fewer than 10 h per week in 85% of the trials. Sixty-seven percent of the patients had fewer than 10 total sessions of TENS. McQuay and Moore[33] therefore concluded that TENS may be useful in chronic pain, although the evidence is not conclusive.

Myofascial/musculoskeletal/spasticity

One randomized controlled trial of acupuncture against TENS in elderly back pain patients in general practice showed TENS to be of similar efficacy for pain, but not for increased flexibility of the spine. Systematic reviews of acupuncture have shown an effect, which could suggest that TENS does have an effect in chronic pain, although a more recent Cochrane review has suggested a lack of effect from acupuncture in low back pain.[34]***

Vibratory stimulation and TENS are as efficient, and in some patients more efficient, pain suppressive measures as aspirin in myofascial or muscular pain. It is suggested on the basis of these findings that vibratory stimulation

and TENS merit consideration in the choice of treatment of myofascial or musculoskeletal pain.[35]**

TENS also appears to be effective in reducing spinal spasticity, as measured clinically.[36]* Repeated applications of TENS can reduce clinical spasticity and improve control of reflex and motor functions in hemiparetic subjects. Furthermore, the underlying mechanisms may be due partly to an enhancement in presynaptic inhibition of the spastic plantarflexor, and partly to a possible "disinhibition" of descending voluntary commands to the paretic dorsiflexor motor neurons.[37]*

Electrical stimulation is similar to the Milwaukee brace in managing idiopathic scoliosis.[38]**

Neuropathic pain

Transcutaneous electrical nerve stimulation is useful for neuropathic pain, including postherpetic neuralgia, painful peripheral neuropathies (especially if sufficient sensation is retained in the area of pain), and phantom limb pain.

TENS applied to the contralateral leg in phantom limb pain has been shown to be significantly more effective than when applied to the outer ear, and skin conductance variations correlated well with stump sensations.[39]**

Visceral

Transcutaneous electrical nerve stimulation appears to reduce esophageal pain sensitivity and thus may be a useful treatment for noncardiac chest pain of esophageal origin.[40]* It has been shown to decrease lower esophageal sphincter pressure in patients with achalasia.[41]* Also, somatic stimulation reduces perception of gut distension without interfering with local and reflex gut responses.[42]*

TENS has been shown to produce prompt onset of analgesia with no significant effect on uterine activity in patients with primary dysmenorrhea, possibly by reducing uterine ischemia, or by spinal or supraspinal inhibition of pain transmission.[43]**,[44]**,[45]**

However, TENS does significantly increase uterine contractions when applied to post-term pregnant women.[46]*

Transcutaneous electrical nerve stimulation may also have a role in the treatment of detrusor instability and urinary urgency.[47]***,[48]*,[49]*

Intractable angina

TENS can be very useful in intractable angina. It produces an increased tolerance to pacing, improved lactate metabolism, and less pronounced ST depression. In the long term, there is an increase in work capacity, reduced frequency of anginal attacks, and reduced consumption of short-acting nitroglycerine, all due to a decreased afterload resulting from systemic vascular dilatation.[50]*,[51]* There is also an increased coronary flow to ischemic areas in the myocardium. TENS has been shown to have an effect on lowering blood pressure at low frequencies (2 Hz). TENS may decrease the sympathetic activity either directly or indirectly as a consequence of pain inhibition. This hypothesis is supported by the fact that arterial levels of epinephrine (adrenaline) and nor-epinephrine (noradrenaline) dropped during TENS in TENS responders.[52*]

Peripheral ischemia

The subjective pain assessment and the maximum pain tolerance produced by ischemic pain after a submaximal effort tourniquet test were significantly modified by peripheral electrical stimulation at non-noxious intensities.[53*]

There is also evidence that it can improve tissue perfusion and ulcer healing in peripheral vascular disease[54*,55*] and leprosy.[56*]

The most useful stimulation modalities for ischemic pain, as for other pain states, are still under discussion. High-intensity, low-frequency TENS has been shown to prevent cooling of the hand in a controlled comparison with high-frequency, low-intensity stimulation and placebo.[57] Stimulation of 4 Hz had a significantly greater hypoalgesic effect on experimentally induced ischemic pain,[58] although in a further study looking purely at femoral arterial blood flow in normal subjects the flow rate was directly proportional to the frequency of stimulation.[59] Transcutaneous electrical nerve stimulation appears, therefore, to have a mild inhibitory action on the sympathetic nervous system and this is more apparent when the stimulation may be greater, as during isometric exercise.[60]

Blood flow in skin flaps with deficient circulation after reconstructive surgery can be significantly increased by TENS (P-value less than 0.001), but not by placebo TENS.[61*,62*]

TENS can also be useful in thrombophlebitis.[63*]

CONCLUSION

Transcutaneous electrical nerve stimulation (TENS) has been shown not to be effective in postoperative and labor pain. In chronic pain, there is evidence that TENS effectiveness increases slowly, and that large doses need to be used. There is a lack of evidence for the effectiveness of TENS in chronic pain, rather than evidence for lack of efficacy.[64***] However, cost simulations of medication and physiotherapy or occupational therapy indicate that, with long-term TENS use, costs can be reduced by up to 55% for medications and by up to 69% for physio- or occupational therapy.[65***]

REFERENCES

1. Nash TP. Development of medicine and stimulation produced analgesia. *Pain Clin* 1992; **5:** 181–5.

◆ 2. Melzack R, Wall PD. Pain mechanisms: a new theory. *Science* 1965; **150:** 971–9.

◆ 3. Wall PD, Sweet WH. Temporary abolition of pain in man. *Science* 1967; **155:** 108–9.

4. Shealy CN, Taslitz N, Mortimer JT, Becker DP. Electrical inhibition of pain: experimental evaluation. *Anesth Analg* 1967; **46:** 299–305.

◆ 5. Melzack R. Prolonged relief of pain by brief, intense transcutaneous somatic stimulation. *Pain* 1975; **1:** 357–73.

6. Walsh DM, Lowe AS, McCormack K, *et al.* Transcutaneous electrical nerve stimulation: effect on peripheral nerve conduction, mechanical pain threshold, and tactile threshold in humans. *Arch Phys Med Rehabil* 1998; **79:** 1051–8.

7. Reeve J, Menon D, Corabian P. Transcutaneous electrical nerve stimulation (TENS): a technology assessment. *Int J Technol Assess* 1996 **12:** 299–324.

8. Chen D, Philip M, Philip PA, Monga TN. Cardiac pacemaker inhibition by transcutaneous electrical nerve stimulation. *Arch Phys Med Rehabil* 1990; **71:** 27–30.

9. Rasmussen MJ, Hayes DL, Vlietstra RE, Thorsteinsson G. Can transcutaneous electrical nerve stimulation be safely used in patients with permanent cardiac pacemakers? *Mayo Clin Proc* 1988; **63:** 443–5.

◆ 10. Johnson MI, Ashton CH, Thompson JW. An in-depth study of long-term users of transcutaneous electrical nerve stimulation (TENS). Implications for clinical use of TENS. *Pain* 1991; **44:** 221–9.

11. Alon G. High voltage stimulation. Effects of electrode size on basic excitatory responses. *Phys Ther* 1985; **65:** 890–5.

● 12. Sandkuhler J. Long-lasting analgesia following TENS and acupuncture: spinal mechanisms beyond gate control. In: Devor M, Rowbotham MC, Wiesenfeld-Hallin Z eds. *Proceedings of the 9th World Congress on Pain, Progress in Pain Research and Management*, vol. 16. Seattle, WA: IASP Press, 2000.

13. Mann CJ. Respiratory compromise: a rare complication of transcutaneous electrical nerve stimulation for angina pectoris. *J Accident Emerg Med* 1996; **13:** 68.

14. Richardson C, MacIver K, Wright M, Wiles JR. Patient reports of the effects and side-effects of TENS for chronic non-malignant pain following a four week trial. *Pain Clin* 2002; **13:** 265–76.

◆ 15. Deyo RA, Walsh NE, Schoenfeld LS, Ramamurthy S. Can trials of physical treatments be blinded? The example of transcutaneous electrical nerve stimulation for chronic pain. *Am J Phys Med Rehabil* 1990; **69:** 6–10.

16. Marchand S, Bushnell MC, Duncan GH. Modulation of heat pain perception by high frequency transcutaneous electrical nerve stimulation (TENS). *Clin J Pain* 1991; **7:** 122–9.

17. Kruger LR, van der Linden WJ, Cleaton-Jones PE. Transcutaneous electrical nerve stimulation in the treatment of myofascial pain dysfunction. *S Afr J Surg* 1998; **36:** 35–8.

18. Fishbain DA, Chabal C, Abbott A, *et al*. Transcutaneous electrical nerve stimulation (TENS) treatment outcome in long-term users. *Clin J Pain* 1996; **12**: 201–14.

◆ 19. Mannheimer C, Carlsson CA. The analgesic effect of transcutaneous electrical nerve stimulation (TNS) in patients with rheumatoid arthritis. A comparative study of different pulse patterns. *Pain* 1979; **6**: 329–34.

◆ 20. Eriksson M, Sjolund B. Acupuncture-like electroanalgesia in TNS-resistant chronic pain. In: Zotterman Y ed. *Sensory Functions of the Skin*. Oxford: Pergamon Press, 1976: 575–81.

◆ 21. Nash TP, Williams JD, Machin D. TENS: does the type of stimulus really matter? *Pain Clin* 1990; **3**: 161–8.

22. Johnson MI, Ashton CH, Thompson JW. The consistency of pulse frequencies and pulse patterns of transcutaneous electrical nerve stimulation (TENS) used by chronic pain patients. *Pain* 1991; **44**: 231–4.

23. Tulgar M, McGlone F, Bowsher D, Miles JB. Comparative effectiveness of different stimulation modes in relieving pain. Part I. A pilot study. *Pain* 1991; **47**: 151–5.

24. Tulgar M, McGlone F, Bowsher D, Miles JB. Comparative effectiveness of different stimulation modes in relieving pain. Part II. A double-blind controlled long-term clinical trial. *Pain* 1991; **47**: 157–62.

● 25. Carroll D, Tramèr M, McQuay H, *et al*. Randomization is important in studies with pain outcomes: systematic review of transcutaneous electrical nerve stimulation in acute postoperative pain. *Br J Anaesth* 1996; **77**: 798–803.

26. Chen L, Tang J, White PF, *et al*. The effect of location of transcutaneous electrical nerve stimulation on postoperative opioid analgesic requirement: acupoint versus nonacupoint stimulation. *Anesth Analg* 1998; **87**: 1129–34.

27. Laitinen J, Nuutinen L. Failure of transcutaneous electrical nerve stimulation and indomethacin to reduce opiate requirement following cholecystectomy. *Acta Anaesthesiol Scand* 1991; **35**: 700–5.

28. Webster DP, Pellegrini L, Duffy K. Use of transcutaneous electrical nerve stimulation for fingertip analgesia: a pilot study. *Ann Emerg Med* 1992; **21**: 1472–5.

29. teDuits E, Goepferd S, Donly K, *et al*. The effectiveness of electronic dental anesthesia in children. *Pediatr Dent* 1993; **15**: 191–6.

30. Fassoulaki A, Papilas K, Sarantopoulos C, Zotou M. Transcutaneous electrical nerve stimulation reduces the incidence of vomiting after hysterectomy. *Anesth Analg* 1993; **76**: 1012–14.

● 31. Carroll D, Tramer M, McQuay H, *et al*. Transcutaneous electrical nerve stimulation in labour pain: a systematic review. *Br J Obstet Gynaecol* 1997; **104**: 169–75.

32. Johnson MI, Ashton CH, Thompson JW. Long term use of transcutaneous electrical nerve stimulation at Newcastle Pain Relief Clinic. *J R Soc Med* 1992; **85**: 267–8.

33. McQuay H, Moore A. Transcutaneous electrical nerve stimulation (TENS) in chronic pain. In: McQuay H, Moore A, eds. An evidence-based resource for pain relief. Oxford, Oxford University Press, 1998: 205–211.

● 34. van Tulder MW, Cherkin DC, Berman B, *et al*. The effectiveness of acupuncture in the management of acute and chronic low back pain. A systematic review within the framework of the Cochrane Collaboration Back Review Group. *Spine* 1999; **24**: 1113–23.

35. Lundeberg T. The pain suppressive effect of vibratory stimulation and transcutaneous electrical nerve stimulation (TENS) as compared to aspirin. *Brain Res* 1984; **294**: 201–9.

36. Goulet C, Arsenault AB, Bourbonnais D, *et al*. Effects of transcutaneous electrical nerve stimulation on H-reflex and spinal spasticity. *Scand J Rehabil Med* 1996; **28**: 169–76.

37. Levin MF, Hui-Chan CW. Relief of hemiparetic spasticity by TENS is associated with improvement in reflex and voluntary motor functions. *Electroencephalogr Clin Neurophysiol* 1992; **85**: 131–42.

38. Fisher DA, Rapp GF, Emkes M. Idiopathic scoliosis: transcutaneous muscle stimulation versus the Milwaukee brace. *Spine* 1987; **12**: 987–91.

39. Katz J, France C, Melzack R. An association between phantom limb sensations and stump skin conductance during transcutaneous electrical nerve stimulation (TENS) applied to the contralateral leg: a case study. *Pain* 1989; **36**: 367–77.

40. Borjesson M, Pilhall M, Eliasson T, *et al*. Esophageal visceral pain sensitivity: effects of TENS and correlation with manometric findings. *Dig Dis Sci* 1998; **43**: 1621–8.

41. Guelrud M, Rossiter A, Souney PF, Sulbaran M. Transcutaneous electrical nerve stimulation decreases lower esophageal sphincter pressure in patients with achalasia. *Dig Dis Sci* 1991; **36**: 1029–33.

42. Coffin B, Azpiroz F, Malagelada JR. Somatic stimulation reduces perception of gut distention in humans. *Gastroenterology* 1994; **107**: 1636–42.

43. Milsom I, Hedner N, Mannheimer C. A comparative study of the effect of high-intensity transcutaneous nerve stimulation and oral naproxen on intrauterine pressure and menstrual pain in patients with primary dysmenorrhea. *Am J Obstet Gynecol* 1994; **170** (1 Pt 1): 123–9.

44. Kaplan B, Peled Y, Pardo J, *et al*. Transcutaneous electrical nerve stimulation (TENS) as a relief for dysmenorrhea. *Clin Exp Obstet Gynecol* 1994; **21**: 87–90.

◆ 45. Dawood MY, Ramos J. Transcutaneous electrical nerve stimulation (TENS) for the treatment of primary dysmenorrhea: a randomized crossover comparison with placebo TENS and ibuprofen. *Obstet Gynecol* 1990; **75**: 656–60.

46. Dunn PA, Rogers D, Halford K. Transcutaneous electrical nerve stimulation at acupuncture points in the induction of uterine contractions. *Obstet Gynecol* 1989; **73**: 286–90.

47. Bower WF, Moore KH, Adams RD, Shepherd R. A urody-

namic study of surface neuromodulation versus sham in detrusor instability and sensory urgency. *J Urol* 1998; **160** (6 Pt 1): 2133–6.

48. Okada N, Igawa Y, ogawa A, Nishizawa O. Transcutaneous electrical stimulation of thigh muscles in the treatment of detrusor overactivity. *Br J Urol* 1998; **81** (4): 560–4.

49. Nakamura M, Sakurai T, Tsujimoto Y, Tada Y. Bladder inhibition by electrical stimulation of the perianal skin. *Urol Int* 1986; **41** (1): 62–3.

50. Mannheimer C, Carlsson CA, Emanuelsson H, *et al*. The effects of transcutaneous electrical nerve stimulation in patients with severe angina pectoris. *Circulation* 1985; **71**: 308–16.

51. Mannheimer C, Carlsson CA, Vedin A, Wilhelmsson C. Transcutaneous electrical nerve stimulation (TENS) in angina pectoris. *Pain* 1986; **26**: 291–300.

52. Emanuelsson H, Mannheimer C, Waagstein F, Wilhelmsson C. Catecholamine metabolism during pacing-induced angina pectoris and the effect of transcutaneous electrical nerve stimulation. *Am Heart J* 1987; **114**: 1360–6.

53. Woolf CJ. Transcutaneous electrical nerve stimulation and the reaction to experimental pain in human subjects. *Pain* 1979; **7**: 115–27.

◆ 54. Kaada B. Promoted healing of chronic ulceration by transcutaneous nerve stimulation (TNS). *VASA* 1983; **12**: 262–9.

55. Debreceni L, Gyulai M, Debreceni A, Szabo K. Results of transcutaneous electrical stimulation (TES) in cure of lower extremity arterial disease. *Angiology* 1995; **46**: 613–18.

56. Kaada B, Emru M. Promoted healing of leprous ulcers by transcutaneous nerve stimulation. *Acupunct Electrother Res* 1988;**13** (4): 165–76.

57. Scudds RJ, Helewa A, Scudds RA. The effects of transcutaneous electrical nerve stimulation on skin temperature in asymptomatic subjects. *Phys Ther* 1995; **75**: 621–8.

58. Walsh DM, Foster NE, Baxter GD, Allen JM. Transcutaneous electrical nerve stimulation. Relevance of stimulation parameters to neurophysiological and hypoalgesic effects. *Am J Phys Med Rehabil* 1995; **74**: 199–206.

59. Zicot M, Rigaux P. Effect of the frequency of neuromuscular electric stimulation of the leg on femoral arterial blood flow. *J Mal Vasc* 1995; **20**: 9–13.

60. Sanderson JE, Tomlinson B, Lau MS, *et al*. The effect of transcutaneous electrical nerve stimulation (TENS) on autonomic cardiovascular reflexes. *Clin Auton Res* 1995; **5** (2): 81–4.

61. Kjartansson J, Lundeberg T. Effects of electrical nerve stimulation (ENS) in ischemic tissue. *Scand J Plast Reconstr Surg Hand Surg* 1990; **24** (2): 129–34.

62. Kjartansson J, Lundeberg T, Samuelson UE, Dalsgaard CJ. Transcutaneous electrical nerve stimulation (TENS) increases survival of ischaemic musculocutaneous flaps. *Acta Physiol Scand* 1988; **134**: 95–9.

63. Roberts HJ. Transcutaneous electrical nerve stimulation in the symptomatic management of thrombophlebitis. *Angiology* 1979; **30**: 249–56.

● 64. McQuay HJ, Moore RA, Eccleston C, *et al*. Systematic review of outpatient services for chronic pain control. *Health Technol Assess* 1997; **1** (6): i–iv and 1–135.

65. Chabal C, Fishbain DA, Weaver M, Heine LW. Long-term transcutaneous electrical nerve stimulation (TENS) use: impact on medication utilization and physical therapy costs. *Clin J Pain* 1998; **14**: 66–73.

28

Acupuncture

CYNTHIA M KAHN AND JONATHAN AMMEN

Yin and yang	355	Insertion	357
Treatment	356	Complications	357
Point location	357	References	358
Needles	357	Appendix	358

Acupuncture is a form of energetic medicine that has been used in China for over 3,000 years. It is used to treat a variety of medical conditions and is particularly effective in the treatment of pain problems. Acupuncture is based on the theory that energy (qi) flows along invisible channels that affect every organ and cell in the body. There are 14 main channels and over 400 acupuncture points that lie along the channels (Figs A28.1–A28.3). The channels are given the names of the organs upon which they appear to act or are given the name of the function they perform. The channels are surface representations of ways to access deeper organs and functions.

Much of the practice of Chinese acupuncture evolved within the conceptual framework of Taoism, and, as such, the logic employed is nonlinear and holistic. Chinese acupuncture is based on identification of complex patterns through tongue and pulse diagnosis as well as an extensive medical history. When illness or pain occurs, it is believed to be due to the imbalance or obstruction of the flow of energy along the channels. Once the pattern of imbalance is identified, a treatment is designed to help correct the imbalance and to promote the smooth flow of energy along the channels. Insertion of hair-thin needles into specific points along the channels can help correct the balance of energy, thereby promoting resolution of illness and decreasing pain.

YIN AND YANG

Fundamental to Oriental medicine, the concept of yin and yang describe the interdependent opposing forces of nature at work in all living systems. Growth and decay, hot and cold, active and sedentary – all are yang/yin polarities. Yin refers to cooler, darker, quiescent, more fluid, and substantial objects and processes. Yang refers to warmer, brighter, more active, dry, and energetic objects and processes. Yin and yang cannot exist without each other. Together, the complex of opposites creates a whole. Healthy living systems are well balanced in their yin and yang attributes. Clinically, pain in an individual whose condition is more yang than yin tends to be more acute, severe, and rapid in onset. Yin pain is characterized as more diffuse and nagging, often chronic, with a cold component that is responsive to heat.

As mentioned earlier, qi can be conceptualized as energy flowing along the acupuncture channels. However, it is also used to describe a range a dynamic physiological processes. It can describe organ or system function, and it is responsible for the growth, development, and all physiologic activity of an organism. Deficiency or excess of qi can result in abnormal physiologic function (i.e. pain or illness). A patient who has deficient qi is generally weak, sensitive to cold, pale, and may have a depressed, withdrawn, or flat affect. A patient who has excess qi is more robust, less sensitive to cold, tends more toward agitation and anxiety rather than withdrawal and depression, and tends to be more functional than a deficient person with the same problem. Stagnation of the flow of qi may cause pain that varies in location and quality, but is often associated with muscle tension or palpable muscle spasm. As qi flows through the channels continuously, it can be accessed at acupuncture points to relieve obstruction of qi or to redirect qi flow in order to restore balance, decrease pain, and eliminate illness. Normal and excess-type patients respond to moderate or strong stimulation of acupuncture points and placement of a greater number of needles than deficient patients to achieve similar results.

Other types of painful conditions are also described in Oriental medicine. Pain can be due to blood stagnation. Just as qi is flowing in the body, so is blood, and if the flow is obstructed the pain that occurs is described as more fixed in location than with qi stagnation, often having a stabbing quality. Red or purple discoloration of the painful area may occur. Pain can also be associated with a heat condition. The patient will report a warm sensation, with worsening symptoms the hotter they feel. Swelling, warmth, and redness may be present in the painful area, although not necessarily so. Pain associated with a cold condition worsens when the patient is exposed to cold and improves when heat is applied. The patient may complain of feeling cold, or that the painful area feels cold, although on examination of the painful area the temperature may be normal. Dampness can also cause pain. Pain due to a damp condition is a duller but more constant pain, often worse in damp weather or having an onset associated with extended exposure to dampness. There may be local or systemic edema.

Viewed from the western medical perspective, extensive research into the mechanisms of acupuncture analgesia has revealed that there is a neurohumoral response when an acupuncture point is stimulated.[1] When the point is stimulated, sensory afferents are activated and messages are sent to the brain to release endorphins. The endorphins block the transmission of painful stimuli at the level of the spinal cord, periaqueductal gray neurons in the midbrain, the pituitary, the thalamus, and the hypothalamus. In 1990, acupuncture was endorsed by the World Health Organization for the treatment of over 40 ailments, including painful conditions such as osteoarthritis and rheumatoid arthritis.[2] In 1997, the National Institutes of Health Consensus Statement endorsed the use of acupuncture for postoperative pain and nausea. It was also found to be helpful in the treatment of fibromyalgia and other musculoskeletal conditions, without the side-effects associated with nonsteroidal anti-inflammatory drugs and steroid injections.[3]

Our goal is to provide a basic introduction to acupuncture that will allow the safe exploration of its possibilities as an adjunctive treatment for many acute and chronic pain conditions. We hope that the few basic techniques described in this chapter will stimulate a desire to learn more about acupuncture and the ways in which it may be integrated into treatment algorithms for many pain syndromes. We strongly encourage that, initially, these techniques should be practiced under the supervision of a trained acupuncturist.

TREATMENT

During the first acupuncture treatment, a practitioner trained in traditional Chinese medicine will take an extensive health history and may examine the tongue, abdomen, face, voice, posture, and pulse of the patient. The information obtained will be used to identify the pattern of imbalance. A treatment plan is designed, consisting of a series of acupuncture points chosen because of their particular characteristics and their ability to move energy along the affected channels. Treatment should occur in a comfortable, quiet setting with an ambient temperature of 72–77°F. The treatment table should be 75–80 cm (30–32 inches) wide with an adjustable face rest for the prone position. Once the patient is comfortable, hair-thin needles are then inserted at the chosen points, and are usually retained for 10–20 min. During that time, the needles may be stimulated by manual twirling or lifting and thrusting techniques, by gentle electrical current, or by application of heat via a burning herb called moxa (*Artemesia vulgaris*) to promote the flow of energy (qi) along the channels. Treatment success is affected by point selection, needle angle, needle depth, and degree of stimulation at the points. The patient may feel a tingling, heaviness, aching, or warm sensation associated with the flow of energy (the qi response). A profound sense of relaxation may occur, allowing the patient to fall asleep during the treatment. After the needles are removed, the patient usually continues to feel relaxed. However, some patients may experience transient dizziness, weakness, and fatigue. If this occurs, subsequent treatments should employ fewer needles with little or no stimulation after insertion and a shorter needle retention time. Occasionally, a patient will complain of worsening of their usual symptoms for 12–36 h after the first or second acupuncture treatment. This reaction should resolve with further treatment. If not, a less stimulating treatment should be given, using fewer needles and a shorter retention time. It is important that patients avoid coming to treatments hungry, after a heavy meal, or after drinking alcohol. Between 1 and 3 h of low-stress or relaxing activity should follow each treatment. Some patients experience immediate benefit from the treatment, whereas others require several sessions before improvement is noted. Chronic conditions tend to take longer to respond.

An initial treatment test period of three to five visits within 2 weeks is recommended. A majority of patients with painful conditions who are likely to respond to acupuncture will do so during this test period. If there is no therapeutic result in three to five treatments, this may indicate that acupuncture will not benefit the patient at all or that a more comprehensive treatment plan including acupuncture may be required. Patients with chronic conditions should expect to undergo a lengthy course of treatment. Therapeutic gains should be made slowly and steadily during the course of treatment, although specific symptoms may wax and wane. For best results, patients should continue to be treated two to three times weekly to obtain the maximum benefit in the shortest period of time. If sessions occur once a week or less, progress can be made, although at a slower rate. Treatment should be continued for one to three visits after the best expected gains are achieved in order to sustain the beneficial effects of the course of acupuncture. The degree of treatment success varies considerably from patient to patient.

In order that the reader may be able to use a few basic acupuncture techniques in their practice, we have "translated" some traditional Chinese medical diagnostic patterns into western medical diagnoses. This will allow the identification of patients who are appropriate candidates for acupuncture and will help in the selection of appropriate acupuncture points for the treatment of common pain conditions. Point formulae for the treatment of many common painful conditions will be presented.

POINT LOCATION

Acupuncture points are described as being a certain distance of "body inches," or *cun*, from an anatomic landmark such as a bony prominence or crease of a major joint. One cun is equal to the distance between the interphalangeal creases of the middle finger (Fig. A28.4) Another useful measurement is the width of the second through fifth fingers, which is equal to 3 cun (Fig. A28.4) The distance between the elbow and the wrist is 12 cun, and the distance between the elbow and the axilla is 9 cun. These and other important proportional measurements are shown in Figs A28.4 and A28.5. Acupuncture points are identified by the meridian on which they lie and by number. They are also given Chinese names that describe their function or emphasize a particular characteristic of the point. In this chapter, the meridian and number will be used to identify acupuncture points. The abbreviations used to identify the meridians are listed in Table A28.1.

The points used in the recommended treatments are described in Table A28.2 and are also illustrated in Figs A28.6–A28.21. You will note that some points selected to treat a particular pain condition are located close to the affected body part, whereas others are distant from it. The best combination of points is one that treats the underlying disharmony as well as working to treat the local symptoms. Point combinations have been selected that will allow the reader to provide safe and effective treatment. Please refer to Table A28.3 for acupuncture point prescriptions used to treat a variety of common painful conditions.

NEEDLES

We recommend 32- to 36-gauge, sterile, disposable, stainless-steel, single-use needles that are 1–4 cm (0.5–1.5 inch) long. Longer needle lengths of 5–15 cm (2–6 inches) can be used at specific acupuncture points. Many brands come with an insertion tube. This can preserve sterility and decrease the discomfort associated with piercing the skin during insertion. Japanese (Seirin) needles can also be used. Recommended gauges include Seirin 00, 1, 2, and 3 in 15-mm to 30-mm lengths.

INSERTION

After the acupuncture point has been located, the area should be swabbed with isopropyl alcohol and the insertion tube placed over the point. The entire needle should be within the insertion tube except for a small part that extends above the top of the tube. While pressing the tube gently into the skin, quickly and lightly tap the needle so that it penetrates the skin. Then, remove the insertion tube and gently guide the needle to the recommended depth. If the needle has been placed correctly and is at the right depth, the patient may note "the arrival of qi" and feel a dull ache, a distending feeling, or an electric sensation that often travels along the course of the channel on which the point lies. Care should be taken to avoid paresthesiae or puncture of vessels during needle insertion.

COMPLICATIONS

Acupuncture is usually a very safe form of therapy. However, because needles are inserted at various depths into the body, bleeding, hematomata, organ puncture, or infection may occur. There have been rare cases of pneumothorax, pneumoperitoneum, hemothorax, cardiac tamponade, and perforation of the kidney and bladder. Osteomyelitis, thrombophlebitis, endocarditis, and hepatitis B have also been associated with the use of acupuncture needles, especially in cases where needles have been reused. No cases of human immunodeficiency virus (HIV) transmission have been documented to date. Needles may fracture – surgical removal may be required. Contact dermatitis can occur in patients who are sensitive to the nickel, zinc, or chromium in stainless steel. Nerve injury and compartment syndrome have also occurred. These severe complications are very rare (reference 4, pp. 54–6). With vigilance and careful attention to technique, acupuncture remains one of the safest medical treatments in use today. The most common complication you are likely to see will be a small bruise associated with capillary bleeding after the needle has been removed.

It is important to use single-use needles and to follow universal precautions for all patients. Special care should be used when treating patients who are anticoagulated, pregnant, or who have a cardiac pacemaker. Careful avoidance of deep needle insertion and close monitoring for bleeding is important when treating an anticoagulated patient. Some acupuncture points (spleen 6, stomach 36, large intestine 4, bladder 67 – see Table A28.2 for location of points) can stimulate uterine activity. These points should be used very cautiously in pregnant women. If you use electrical stimulation of the acupuncture needles, it is important to avoid electrical stimulation on or across the chest, especially in patients with cardiac pacemakers.

Approximately 5% of patients will have a vasovagal reaction to needling (reference 4, pp. 294–6). This phenomenon is called "needle shock." Patients complain of lightheadedness, nausea, general malaise, and anxiety. They may break out in a cold sweat and even faint in extreme cases. The needles should be removed immediately. Needle shock occurs most often during the first or second visit. It is recommended that patients be treated in the supine or prone position for the first few visits. The seated position can be used if it is more comfortable for the patient during subsequent visits when they are less prone to needle shock. If it occurs when the patient is in the seated position, it is important to remove the needles as quickly as possible and place the patient in the supine position. The airway and vital signs should be monitored closely. Appropriate resuscitative efforts should be undertaken as required by the patient's clinical condition. Most often, symptoms resolve spontaneously after the needles are removed.

We hope that this basic introduction to acupuncture will stimulate readers to learn more about it and to be able to integrate it into their practice of pain medicine. There are a number of publications that supplement the theoretical and practical knowledge outlined in this chapter.[5-7] Most importantly, we encourage the observation of experienced acupuncturists and that readers should undergo treatment to enhance their understanding of acupuncture and its effect on the human body.

REFERENCES

1. Stux G, Pomeranz B. *Basics of Acupuncture*, 4th edn. Berlin: Springer-Verlag, 1997: 7–23.
2. World Health Organization Executive Board Eighty-seventh Session. *Traditional Medicine and Modern Health Care*, EB87/11. Geneva: WHO, October 1990: 5–6.
3. National Institutes of Health Consensus Development Statement. Acupuncture. November 3–5, 1997: 1–19; http://odp.od.nih.gov/consensus/statements/cdc/107/107_stmt.htm
4. Helms J. *Acupuncture Energetics: A Clinical Approach for Physicians*. Berkeley, CA: Medical Acupuncture Publishers, 1995.
5. Deadman P, Al-Khafaji M, Baker K. *A Manual of Acupuncture*. East Sussex, UK: Journal of Chinese Medicine Publications, 1998.
6. Filshie J, White A. *Medical Acupuncture: A Western Scientific Approach*. Edinburgh: Churchill Livingstone, 1998.
7. Stux G and Pomeranz B (1997) Basics of Acupuncture, 4th Edition. Springer-Verlag, Berlin, Germany.

APPENDIX

The figures and tables can be found on the following pages.

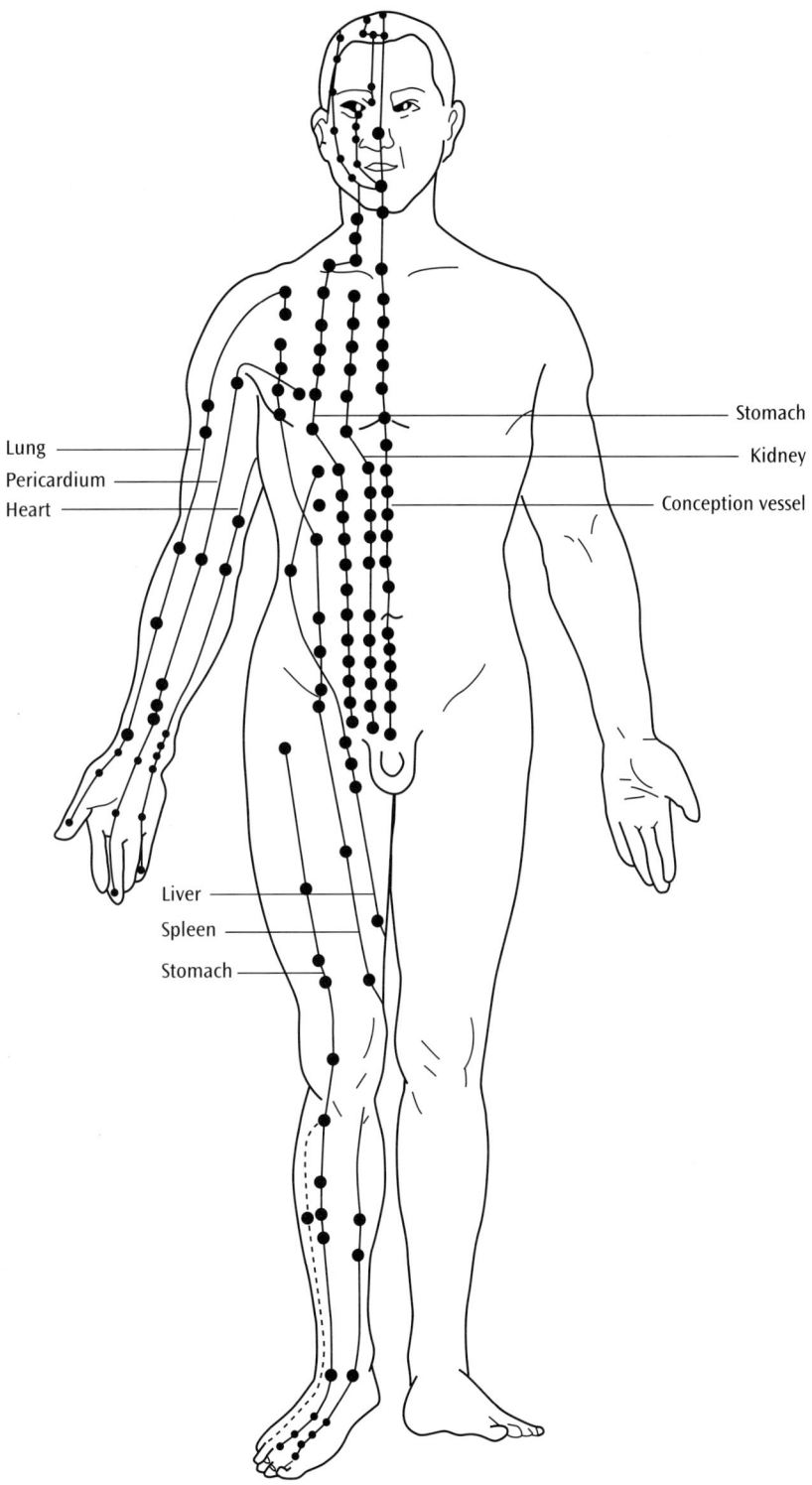

Figure A28.1

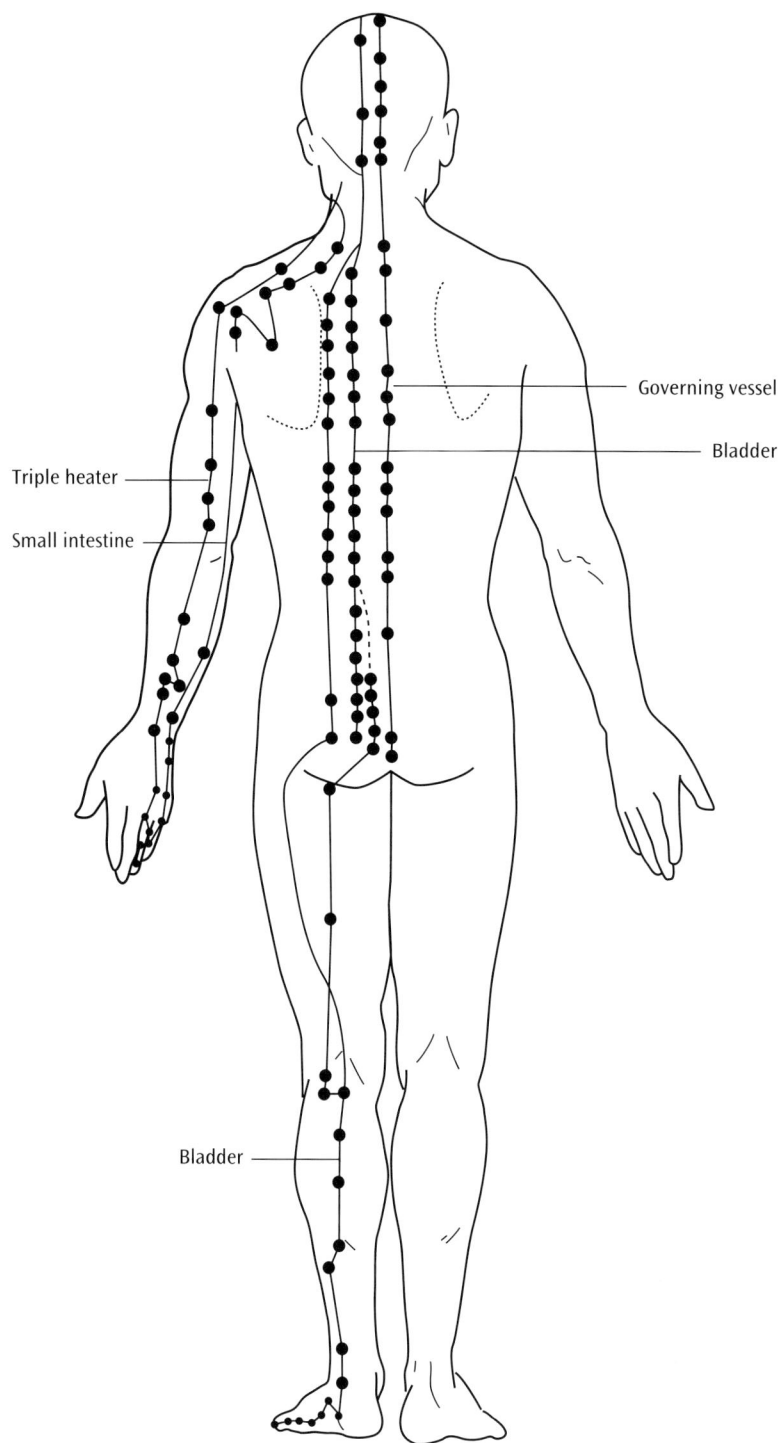

Governing vessel

Bladder

Triple heater

Small intestine

Bladder

Figure A28.2

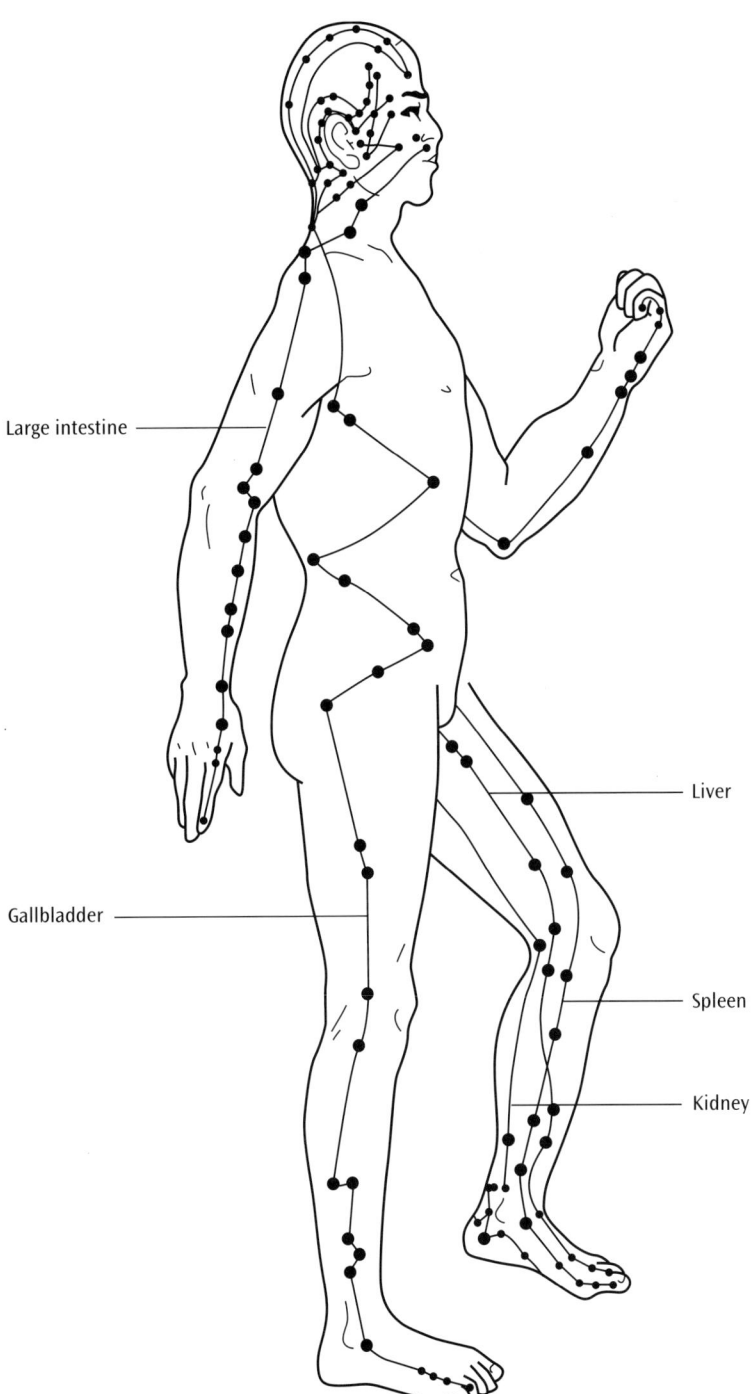

Large intestine

Gallbladder

Liver

Spleen

Kidney

Figure A28.3

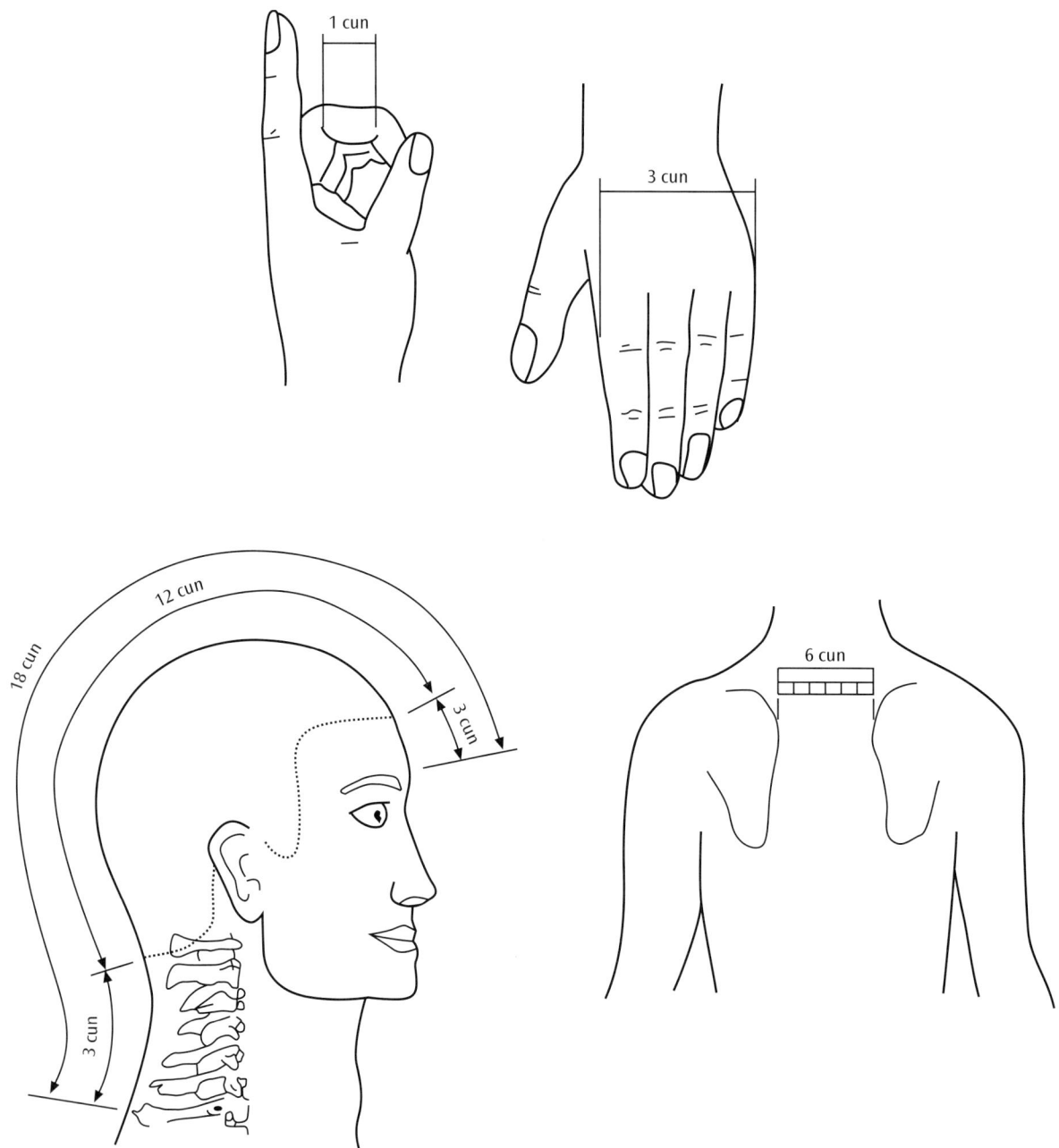

Figure A28.4

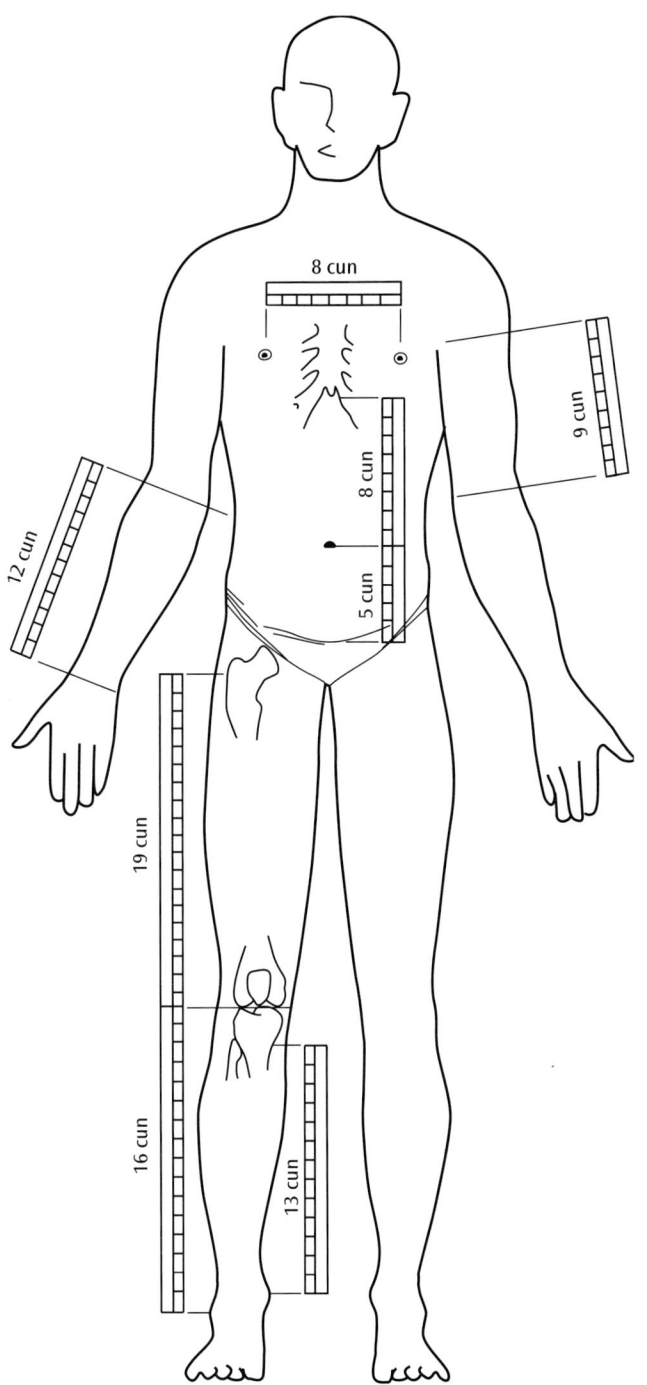

Figure A28.5

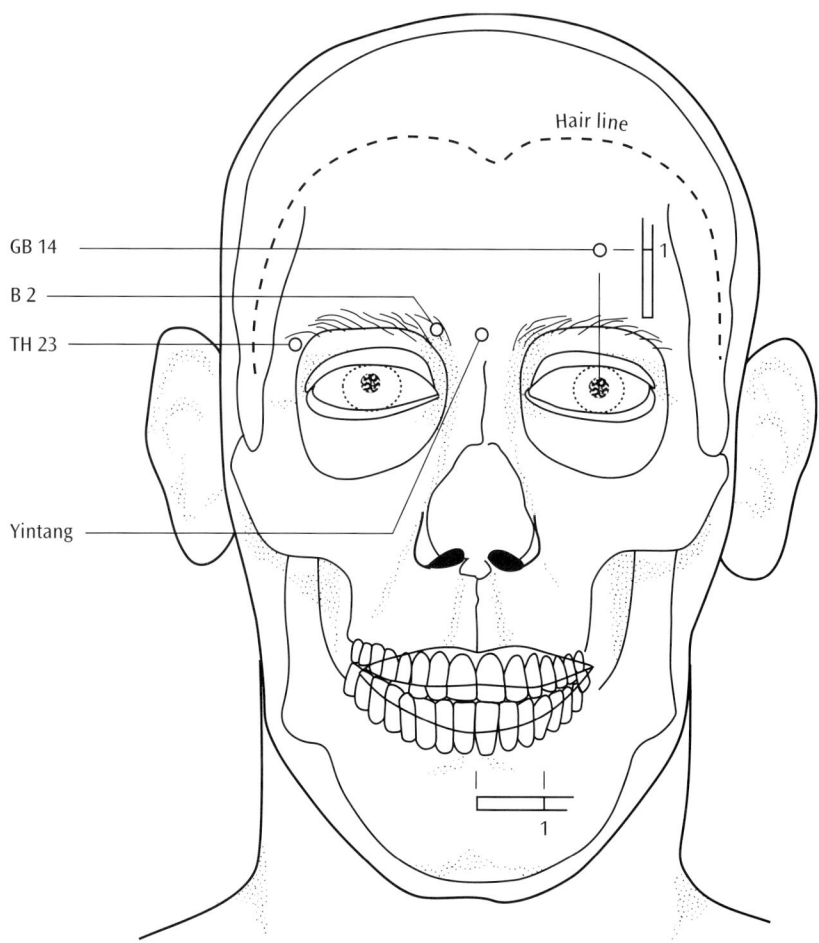

Figure A28.6

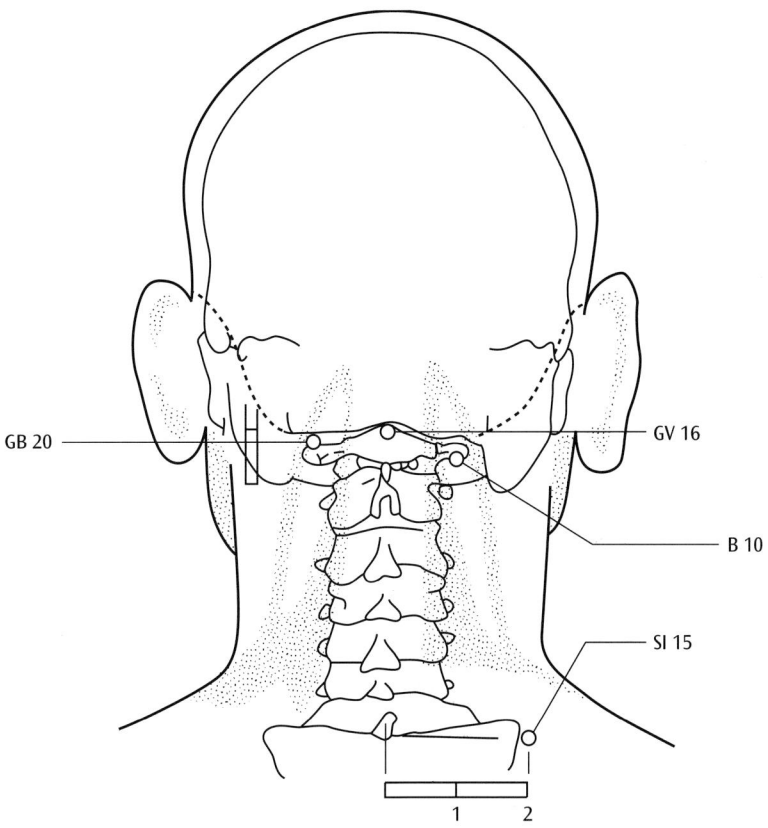

Figure A28.7

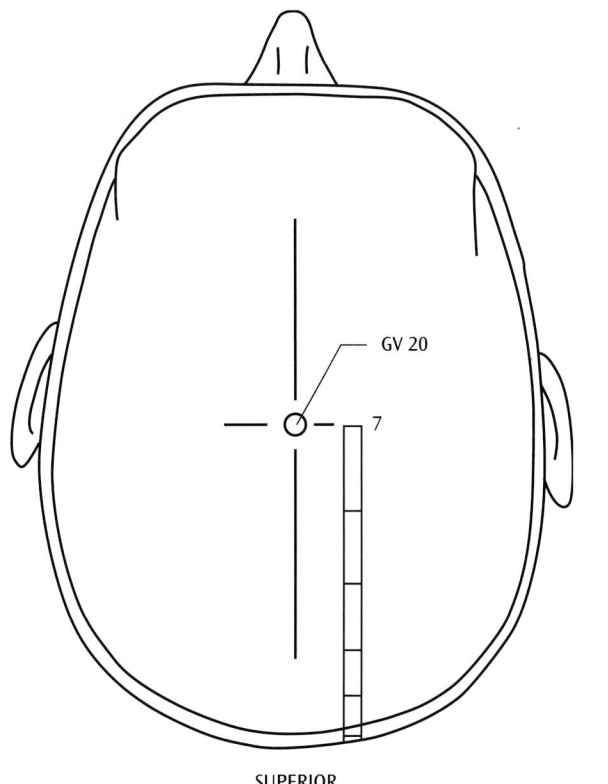

Figure A28.8

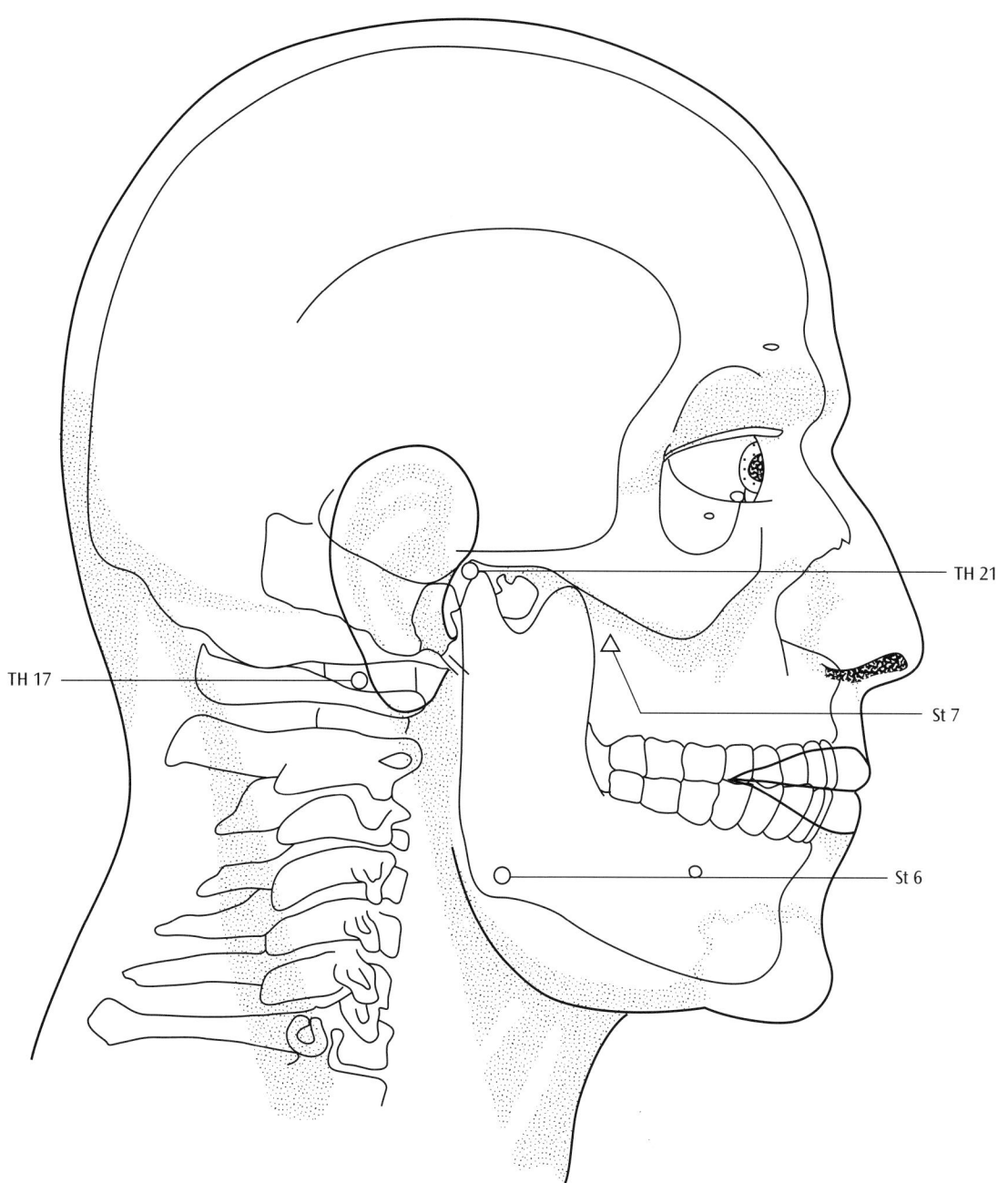

TH 21

TH 17

St 7

St 6

Figure A28.9

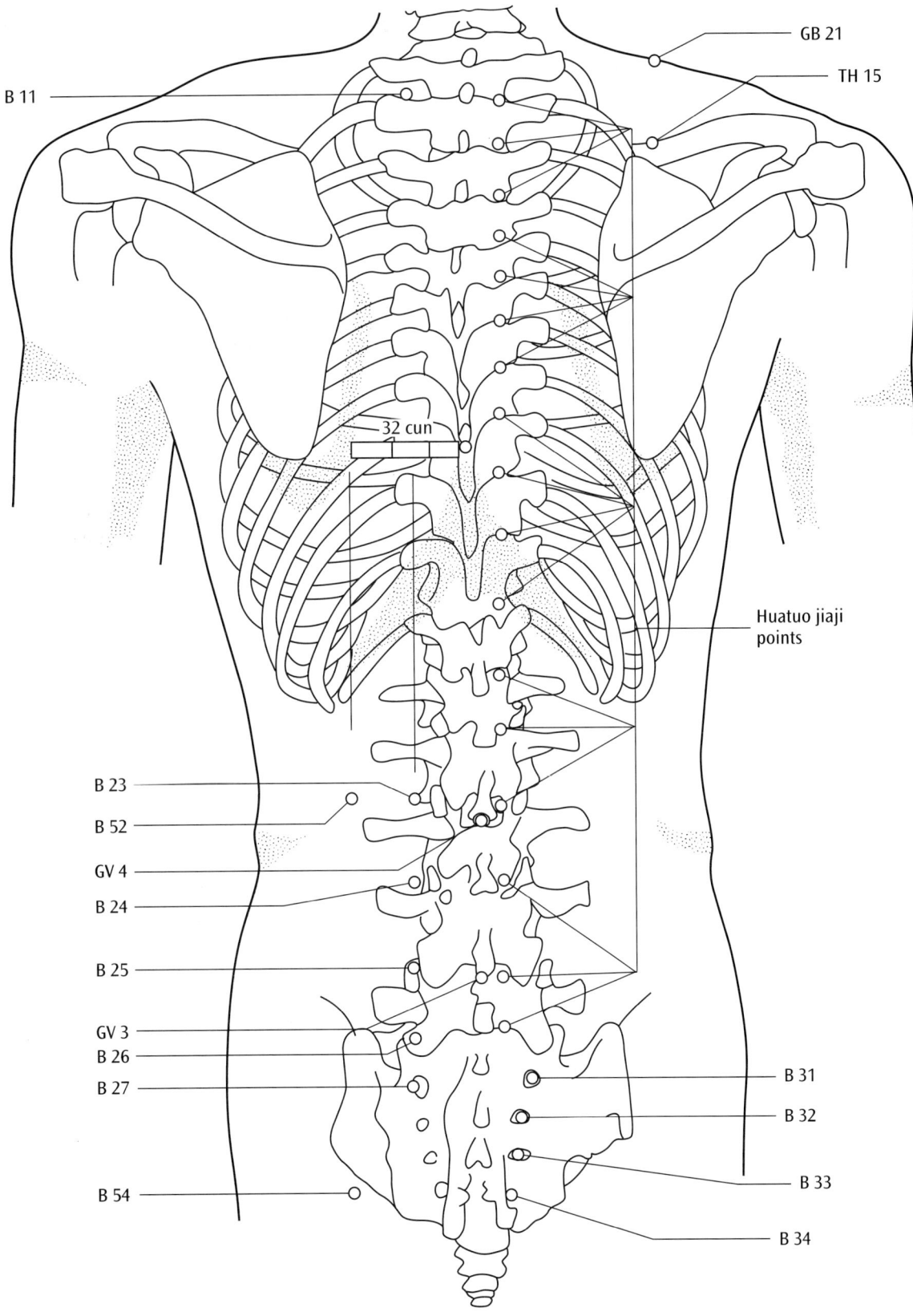

Figure A28.10

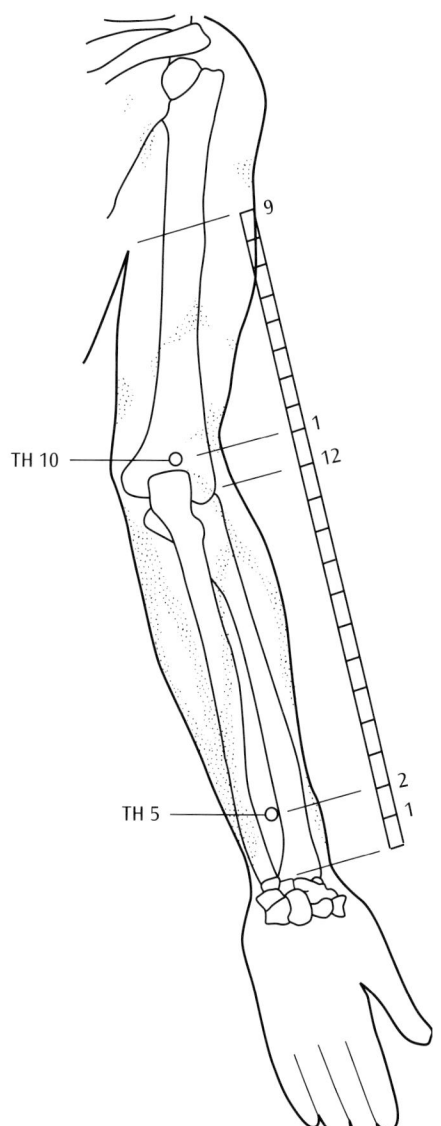

Figure A28.11

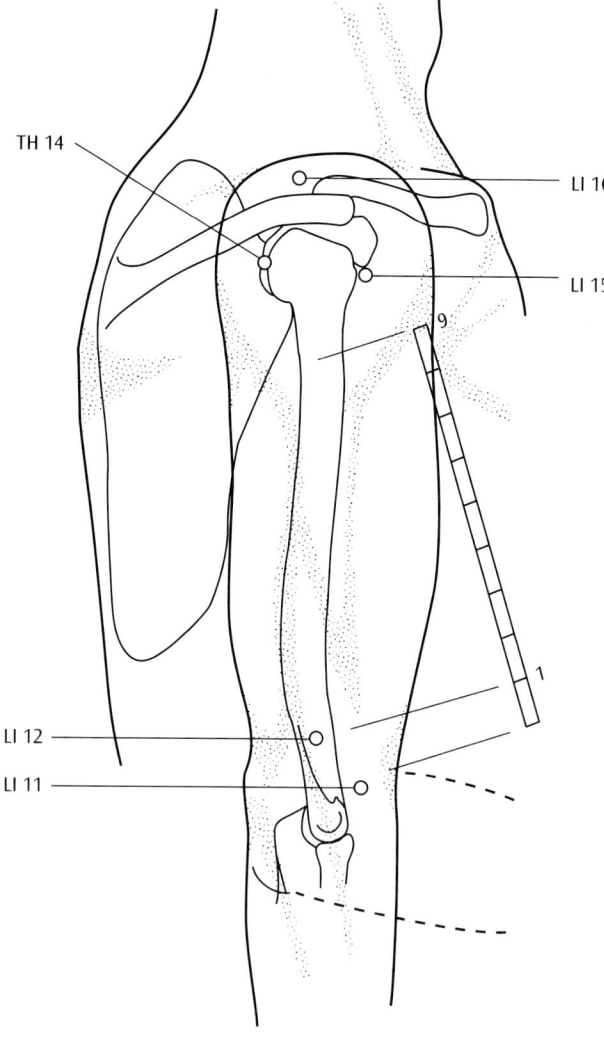

Figure A28.12

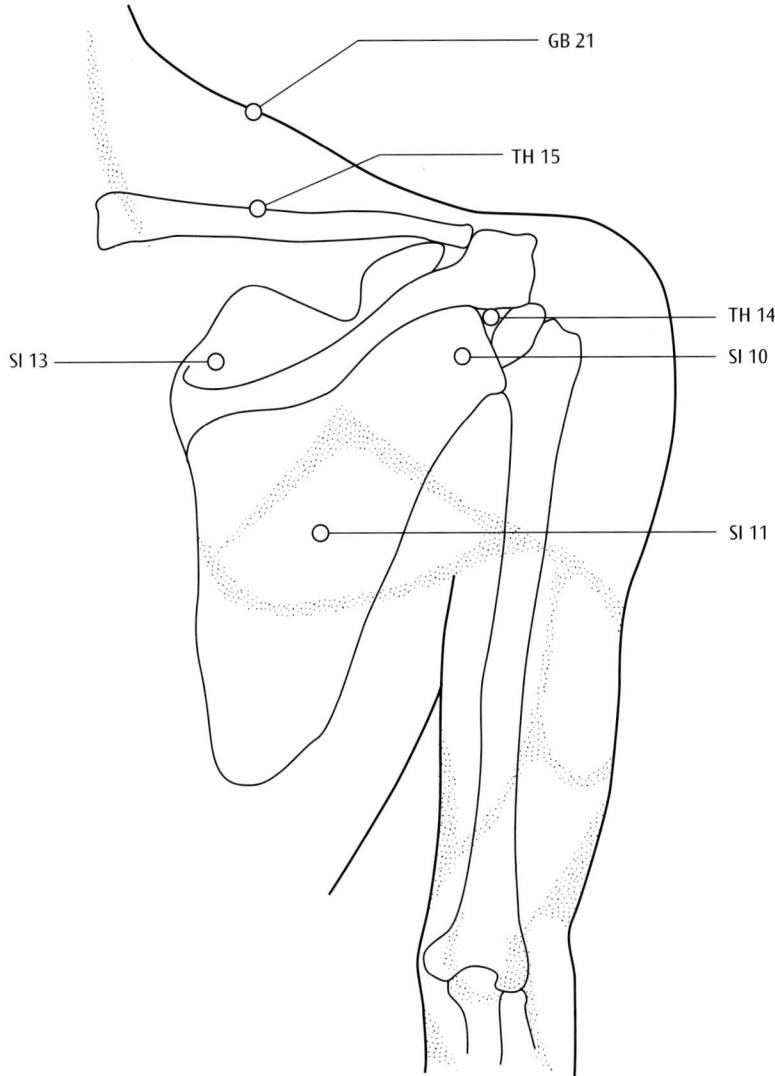

Figure A28.13

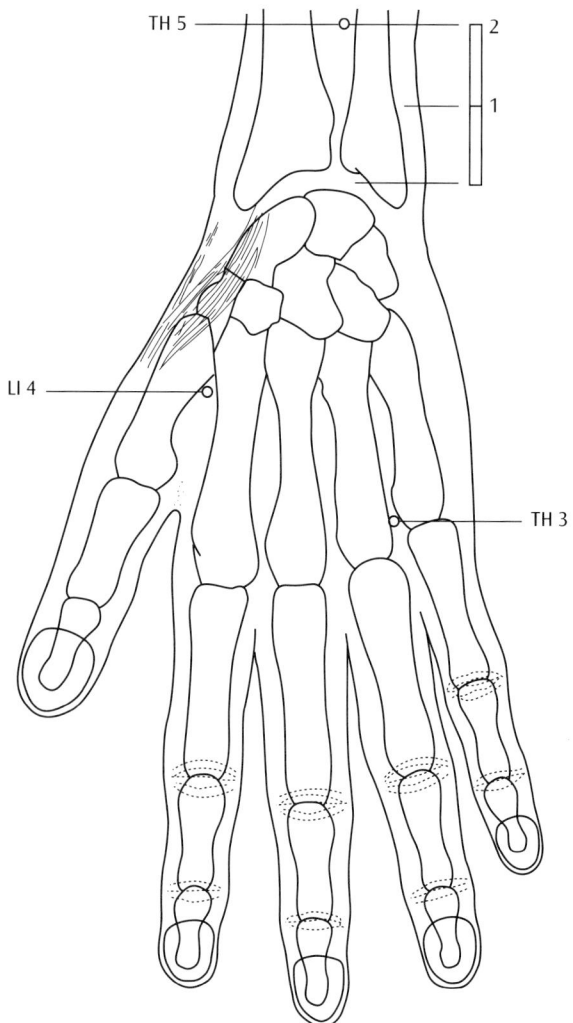

Figure A28.14

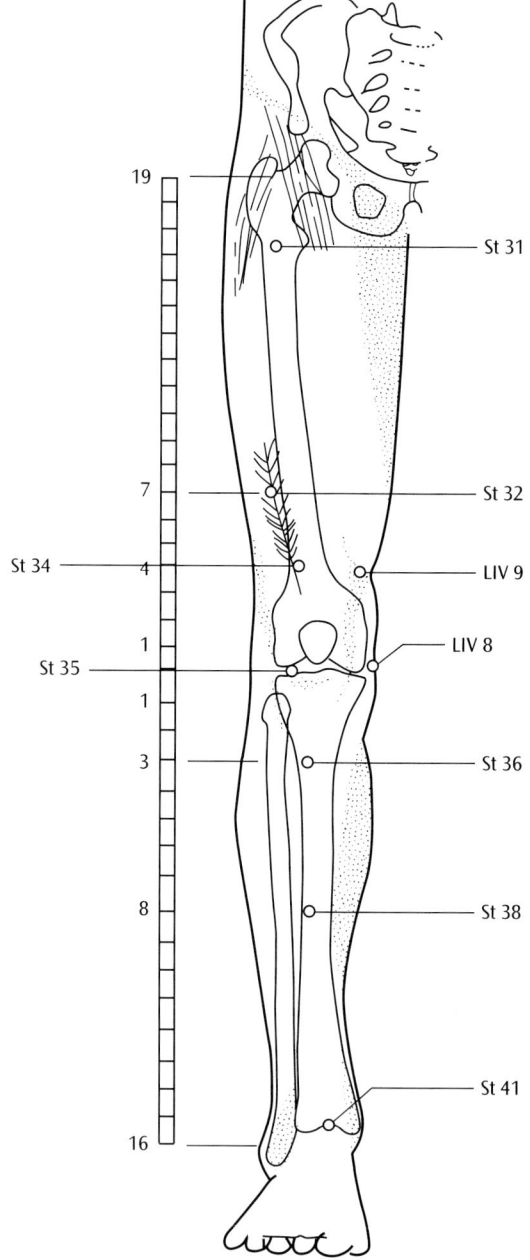

Figure A28.15

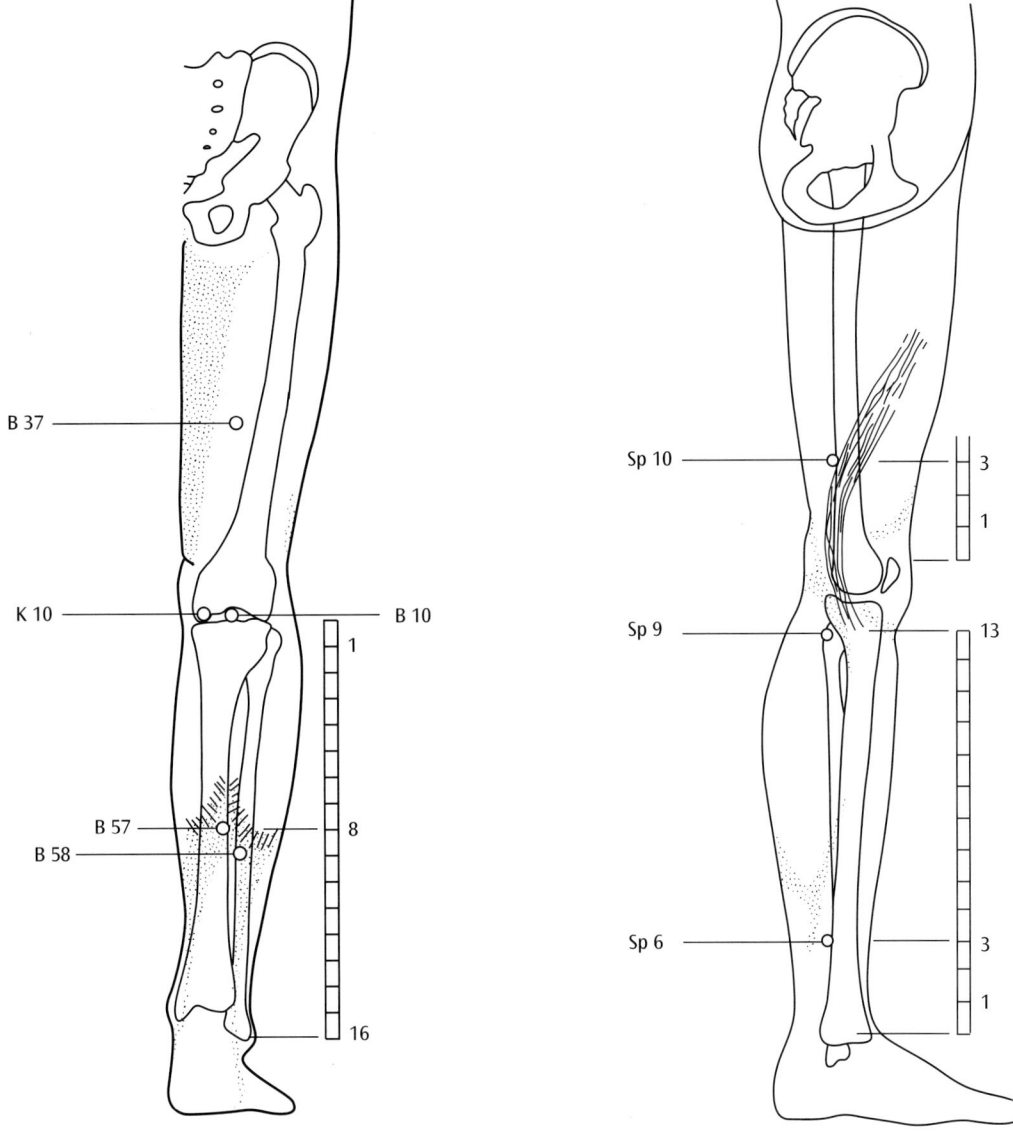

Figure A28.16

Figure A28.17

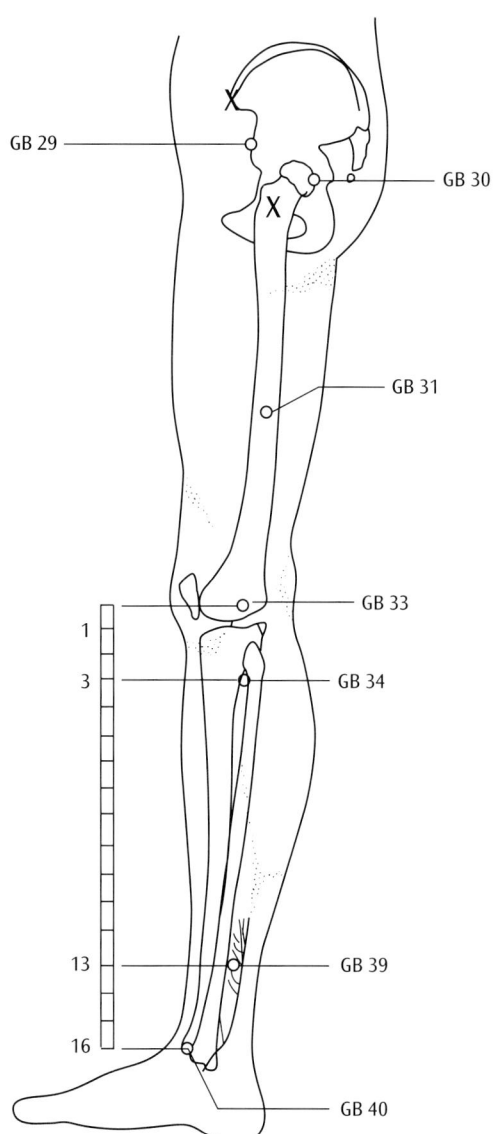

GB 29

GB 30

GB 31

GB 33

1

3

GB 34

13

GB 39

16

GB 40

Figure A28.18

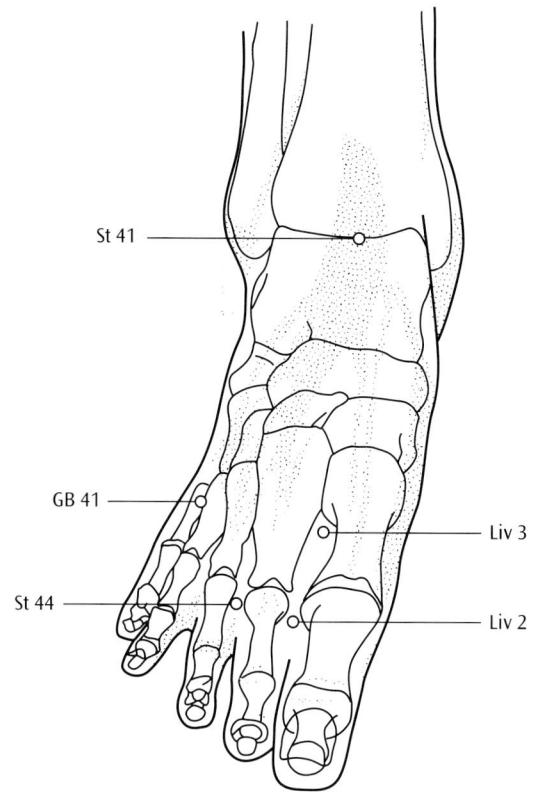

St 41

GB 41

St 44

Liv 3

Liv 2

Figure A28.19

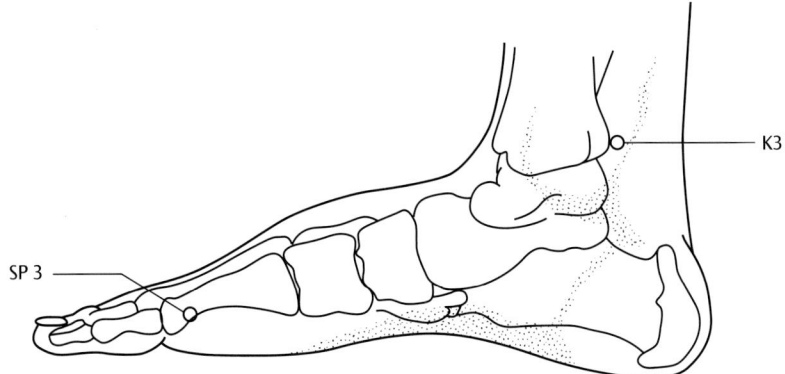

Figure A28.20

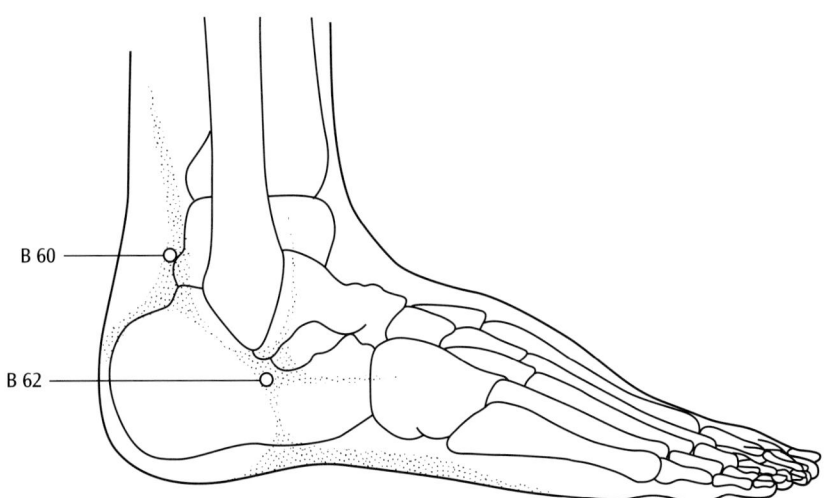

Figure A28.21

Table A28.1

Sp	Spleen	St	Stomach
K	Kidney	B	Bladder
Liv	Liver	GB	Gallbladder
CV	Conception vessel	GV	· Governing vessel
Pc	Pericardium	TH	Triple heater
Lu	Lung	LI	Large intestine
Hrt	Heart	SI	Small intestine

Table A28.2

Point	Chinese name	Location	Depth of insertion	Indications, special notes
Large intestine meridian				
LI 4	Hegu	Dorsal surface of the hand, in the thumb at the highest point of the thumb web	1 cun	General pain, headache, neck pain
LI 11	Quchi	With the elbow flexed, palm on chest, at the lateral end of the transverse cubital crease	1–1.5 cun	Elbow pain
LI 12	Zhuoliao	With the elbow flexed, palm on chest, 1 cun superior and lateral to LI 11	0.3–0.5 cun	Elbow pain
LI 15	Jianyu	Just anterior and inferior to the acromion, in the middle of the upper portion of the deltoideus muscle	0.6–1.2 cun	Shoulder pain
LI 16	Jugu	On the upper aspect of the shoulder in the depression between the acromial extremity of the clavicle and the scapular spine	0.5–1 cun	Shoulder pain, biceps tendinitis
Stomach meridian				
St 6	Jiache	In the depression one fingerbreadth anterior and superior to the lower angle of the mandible	0.3–0.5 cun	Toothache, jaw pain
St 7	Xiaguan	In the depression at the lower border of the zygomatic arch, anterior to the condyloid process of the mandible	0.3–0.5 cun	Toothache, jaw pain
St 31	Biguan	Directly inferior to the anterior superior iliac spine, level with the lower border of the pubic symphysis, in the depression lateral to the sartorius muscle	1–1.5 cun	Thigh pain, lower leg pain
St 32	Futu	6 cun above the laterosuperior border of the patella on a line between the anterior superior iliac spine and the lateral patellar border	1–1.5 cun	Leg pain
St 34	Langqiu	2 cun above the laterosuperior border of the patella	0.5–1 cun	Leg pain, knee pain – angle toward pain area; breast pain – angle upward
St 35	Dubi	With knee flexed, in the depression below the patella and lateral to the patellar ligament	0.7–1 cun	Leg pain, knee pain. Angle obliquely upward and slightly toward patellar midline
St 36	Zusanli	3 cun below ST 35 and one fingerbreadth lateral to the anterior crest of the tibia	0.5–1.3 cun	Important tonic point. Knee pain, leg pain, gastric and abdominal pain, and digestive disorders
St 38	Tiaokou	8 cun below St 35, 3 cun below St 37, one fingerbreadth lateral to the anterior crest of the tibia	0.5–1 cun	Shoulder pain – treat with B 57 while patient moves shoulder/ arm
St 41	Jiexi	Between the tendons of the extensor digitorum longus and hallucis longus at the junction of the leg and dorsal foot	0.5–0.7 cun	Ankle pain, foot pain
St 44	Neiting	In the depression distal and lateral to the second matatarsodigital joint between the second and third toes, proximal to the web margin	0.3–0.5 cun	Toothache

Table A28.2 *Continued*

Point	Chinese name	Location	Depth of insertion	Indications, special notes
Spleen meridian				
Sp 3	Taibai	Just proximal and inferior to the head of the first metatarsal bone at the junction of the red and white skin	0.3–0.5 cun	Leg pain, foot pain
Sp 6	Sanyinjiao	3 cun above the tip of the medial malleolus, posterior to the tibia	0.5–1.5 cun	Meeting of liver, spleen and kidney meridians
Sp 9	Yinlingchuan	With knee flexed, point is in the depression between the inferior margin of the medial condyle of the tibia and m. gastrocnemius	1–3 cun	Knee pain, pain behind the heterolateral eye
Sp 10	Xuehai	With knee flexed, point is 2 cun above the mediosuperior border of the patella on the medial bulge of the quadriceps femoris muscle	0.7–1.3 cun	Knee pain, thigh pain, dysmenorrhea
Small intestine meridian				
SI 10	Naoshu	With the arm adducted the point is approximately 2 cun above the end of the axillary fold, in the depression inferior and lateral to the scapular spine	0.8–1 cun	Shoulder pain
SI 11	Tiansong	In the infrascapular fossa, one-third of the way down from the scapular spine to the inferior angle of the scapula	0.5–1 cun	Shoulder pain, bursitis
SI 15	Jianzhongshu	2 cun lateral to the lower border of the spinous process of the seventh cervical vertebra	0.3–0.6 cun	Neck pain, shoulder pain
Bladder meridian				
B 11	Dashu	1.5 cun lateral to the lower border of the spinous process of the first thoracic vertebra 1.5 cun (approximately two fingerbreadths) lateral to the midline	0.25–0.5 cun	Use caution, pneumothorax risk with deep insertion. Angle obliquely downward or medially. Influential point of the bones
B 2	Zanzhu	At the medial end of the eyebrow, or on the supraorbital notch	0.3–0.5 cun	Needle obliquely downward or laterally
B 10	Tianzhu	1.3 cun lateral to the midline of the neck just below the occiput, on the ridge of the trapezius	0.5 cun	Neck pain, headache, shoulder pain, back pain
B 23	Shenshu	1.5 cun lateral to the lower order of the spinous process of the second lumbar vertebra	1–1.5 cun	Lumbar pain, chronic knee pain
B 24	Qihaishu	1.5 cun lateral to the lower border of the spinous process of the third lumbar vertebra	1–1.5 cun	Lumbar pain
B 25	Dachangshu	1.5 cun lateral to the lower border of the spinous process of the fourth lumbar vertebra	1–1.5 cun	Lumbar pain, sciatica
B 26	Guanyuanshu	1.5 cun lateral to the lower border of the spinous process of the fifth lumbar vertebra	0.7–1 cun	Lumbar pain

Table A28.2 *Continued*

Point	Chinese name	Location	Depth of insertion	Indications, special notes
B 27	Xiaochangshu	1.5 cun lateral to the midline of the back, at the level of the first posterior sacral foramen	0.5–1 cun	Lumbar pain
B 31	Shangliao	In the first posterior sacral foramen, about midway between the posterior superior iliac spine and the midline	0.7–2 cun	Lumbar pain, sciatica. Angle obliquely upward for deeper insertion
B 32	Ciliao	In the second posterior sacral foramen. approximately midway between the inferior border of the posterior superior iliac spine and the midline	0.7–2 cun	Lumber pain, sciatica, and lower extremity pain. Angle obliquely upward for deeper insertion
B33	Zhongliao	In the third posterior sacral foramen	0.7–2 cun	Lumbar pain, sciatica, dysuria, Angle obliquely upward for deeper insertion
B 34	Xialiao	In the fourth posterior sacral foramen	0.5–2 cun	Lumbar pain, sciatica, hypogastric pain. Angle obliquely upward for deeper insertion
B 37	Yinmen	On the posterior midline of the thigh 6 cun below the lower crease of the buttocks	0.7–1.5 cun	Low back pain, sciatica, leg pain
B 40	Weizhong	Center of popliteal crease	0.75–1.5 cun	Knee pain, lumbar pain
B 52	Zhishi	3 cun lateral to the lower border of the spinous process of the second lumbar vertebra	0.7–1 cun	Lumbar pain
B 54	Zhibian	3 cun lateral to the midline at the level of the fourth sacral foramen	1–2 cun	Sciatica, lumbar pain
B 57	Chengshan	8 cun below knee crease, inferior to the belly of the gastrocnemius	1–1.5 cun	Back pain. Shoulder pain (with St 38), lower leg pain
B 58	Feiyang	7 cun above tip of lateral malleolus on the posterior border of the fibula 1 cun inferior and lateral to B 57	0.7–1.5 cun	Luo point. Alternative to B 57 if more tender
B 60	Kunlun	In the depression between the external malleolus and the Achilles tendon, at the level of the malleolar prominence	0.75 cun	Neck pain, back pain, lower leg pain
B 62	Shenmai	In the depression just inferior to the external malleolus	0.3 cun	Leg pain, ankle pain, acute back strain
Kidney meridian				
K 3	Taixi	In the depression midway between the tip of the medial malleolus and the calcaneus tendon.	0.25–1 cun	Lower leg pain, ankle pain, Achilles tendinitis, and chronic lumbar pain
K 10	Yingu	At the medial end of the popliteal fossa between the tendons of the semitendinosus and semimembranosus muscles with the knee flexed	0.5–0.8 cun	Knee pain, medial leg pain, hernia
Triple heater meridian				
TH 3	Zhongzhu	On the dorsal hand in the depression between the fourth and fifth metacarpal bones, proximal to the metacarpophalangeal joint	0.3–0.5 cun	Temporal headache

Table A28.2 *Continued*

Point	Chinese name	Location	Depth of insertion	Indications, special notes
TH 5	Waiguan	On the posterior aspect of the forearm 2 cun proximal to the wrist crease, between the radius and ulna	0.3–0.5 cun	Headache
TH 10	Tianjing	With elbow flexed, point is in depression 1 cun superior to the olecranon	0.3–0.5 cun	Elbow pain
TH 14	Jianliao	Posterior, inferior aspect of the acromion process at the level of LI 15	0.7–1.25 cun	Neck pain
TH 15	Tianliao	Posterior to GB 21 on the superior margin of the scapula	0.3–0.5 cun	Neck pain, shoulder pain
TH 17	Yifeng	Posterior to the ear lobe in the depression between the mandible and the mastoid process	1 cun	Neck pain, jaw pain
TH 21	Ermen	In the depression anterior to the supratragic notch, slightly superior to the condyloid process of the mandible	0.3–0.5 cun	Needle with the mouth open. Toothache
TH 23	Sizhukong	In the depression at the lateral end of the eyebrow	0.3 cun	Needle obliquely posteriorly. Headache
Gall bladder meridian				
GB 14	Yangbai	On the forehead, 1 cun above the eyebrow on the pupil line	0.3–0.5 cun	Angle downward horizontally under the skin. Headache
GB 20	Gengchi	In the posterior neck just below the occiput, in the depression lateral to the trapezius	0.5–1 cun	Headache, neck pain, eye pain, sinus pain, shoulder pain
GB 21	Jianjing	Midway between the acromion and the lower border of the seventh cervical vertebra, on the most superior line of the shoulder	0.5 cun	Use caution in patients with heart condition
GB 29	Juliao	Midway between the anterior superior iliac spine and the highest point of the greater trochanter of the femur	1–2 cun	Hip pain
GB 30	Huantiao	One-third distance between greater trochanter and hiatus of sacrum with patient in lateral recumbent position with leg flexed	1.5–2.5 cun	Add second needle at nearby pain sites if found. Sciatica, leg pain
GB 31	Fengshi	On the midline of the lateral thigh 7 cun above the transverse popliteal crease. With patient standing, hands close at sides point location level with tip of middle finger	0.75–1.5 cun	Puncture perpendicularly or angled toward pain. Leg pain, sciatica, back pain
GB 33	Xiyangguan	With the knee flexed, 3 cun superior to GB 34, lateral to the knee joint, in the depression between the tendon of biceps femoris muscle and the femur	0.5–0.75 cun	Knee pain with iliotibial band involvement, sciatica
GB 34	Yanglingquan	In depression anterior and inferior to the small head of fibula	1–1.5 cun	Master point of the sinews. Leg pain, knee pain, sciatica, epigastric pain

Table A28.2 *Continued*

Point	Chinese name	Location	Depth of insertion	Indications, special notes
GB 39	Juegu	3 cun superior to the upper margin of the external malleolus in the depression between the posterior border of the fibula and the peroneus longus and brevis tendons	0.4–0.5 cun	Ankle pain, lateral neck stiffness and pain, sciatica
GB 40	Qiuxu	Inferior and anterior to the external malleolus in the depression lateral to the tendon of extensor digitorum longus muscle	0.3–0.5 cun	Ankle pain, leg pain, sciatica
GB 41	Linqi	Lateral to the tendon of extensor digiti minimi muscle, in the depression distal to the meeting of the fourth and fifth metatarsal bones	0.5–0.5 cun	Temporal headache
Liver meridian				
Liv 2	Xingjian	Just proximal to the web between the first and second toes	0.5 cun	Vertex headache. Needle obliquely upward
Liv 3	Taichong	In depression distal to junction of first and second metatarsals	0.5–0.75 cun	General pain point. Headache, foot pain
Liv 8	Ququan	With knee flexed, just above the medial end of the transverse popliteal crease	0.5–1 cun	Knee and medial thigh pain, genital pain, lower abdominal pain
Liv 9	Yinbao	4 cun above the medial epicondyle of the femur, between the vastus medialis and sartorius muscles	0.5–0.75 cun	Used for hip joint referring pain to the groin
Governing vessel meridian				
GV 3	Yaoyangguan	On the midline of the back, below the spinous process of the fourth lumbar vertebra	0.5–1 cun	Lumbosacral pain, chronic knee and lower extremity pain
GV 4	Mingmen	On the midline of the back, below the spinous process of the second lumbar vertebra	0.5–1 cun	Lumbar pain
GV 16	Fengfu	Just inferior to the occipital protuberance in the depression on the midline	0.5–1 cun	Neck pain
GV 20	Baihui	7 cun above the posterior hairline, on a line between the tips of the ears.	0.3–0.5 cun	Needle horizontally along the skin, angle toward pain area
Extraordinary and nonmeridian points				
	Yintang	On the midline of the face between the medial ends of the eyebrows	0.3–0.5 cun	Angle horizontally downward along the skin. Frontal headache, relaxation
	Huatuo jiaji	Group of bilateral points at the lateral and inferior borders of each spinous process from T1 to L5	0.5–1 cun	Local pain

Table A28.3 *Acupuncture treatment prescriptions*

Ankle pain	St 41, B 60, GB 39, GB 40, SP 5, SP 6
Lower leg pain	Choose points in the pain area and both proximally and distally on the same meridian: B 57, B 60, K3, St 38, GB 34, GB 39, B 58, Sp 6, B 40, Liv 3
Leg pain	Choose points in the pain area and both proximally and distally on the same meridian: St 31, St 32, St 34, St 35, St 36, Sp 3, Liv 3, GB 30, GB 31, GB 34, GB 39, GB 40, B 62
Knee pain	St 34, St 36, The eyes of the knee, SP 10 Sp 9, Liv 8, GB 33, GB 34, B 11, B 40, K 10, GV 3
Joint-related hip pain	GB 30, GB 31, GB 34, GB 29, Liv 9
Sciatic pain	Select points along the pain trajectory: GB 30, GB 31, GB 34, GB 39, B54, B 25, B 26, B 31, B 32, B 33, B 34, B 37, B 40, B 54, tender lumbar Huatuo jiaji points
Lumbar pain	Select points in the pain area B 23, B 24, B 25, B 27, B 31, B 32, B 40, B 51, GV 3, GV 4, tender Huatuo jiaji points
Elbow pain	Locate the most tender point on the elbow. Needle this point in combination with distal and proximal points on the same meridian which are also tender. Also choose from the following for lateral aspect pain: LI 11, LI 12, TH 10, GB 34
Neck pain	Use *ashi* (local tender points) and choose from: GV 16, SI 15, TH 15, TH 17, LI 4, B 10, B 60, GB 20, GB 21
Shoulder pain	Use *ashi* (local tender points) and choose from: St 38, LI 15, SI 10, LI 11,GB 34, SI 11, LI 16, TH 14
Toothache	St 44, K 3, B 23
	Upper: LI 4, St 7, TH 21
	Lower: LI 4, St 6
Headache	Combine local points in the pain area with distal points. Use caution in stimulating points on the head General points: LI 4, Liv 3, TH 5, GV 15, GV 20, GB 20, B 60, Yintang Frontal pain: Yintang, GB 14, LI 4, B 2, Lu 7, St 8, GB 20 Occipital pain: GB 20, GB 21, GV 15, B 10, B 60, LI 4 Temporal pain: LI 4, TH 23, TH 5, TH 3, Taiyang, GB 20, GB 41 Vertex pain: GV 20, B 60, Liv 2, Liv 3

These acupuncture prescriptions may be used in conjunction with *ashi* (local tender) points.

29

Spinal cord stimulation

JOHN R WEDLEY

Applied anatomy	381	Implantation	384
Contraindications	381	Complications	388
Limitations	382	Programming	388
Indications	382	References	388
Preparation	382		

Spinal cord stimulation was originally called dorsal column stimulation, reflecting its assumed mode of action. It began as a neurosurgical procedure,[1,2] and the indications for its use were unclear. To begin with, single electrodes were implanted surgically; later, multiple single electrodes were implanted both percutaneously and by laminotomy at varying sites as dictated by the location of pain. However, initial encouraging results were not sustained over a 2-year follow-up.

Long-term results have improved because of a better understanding of the need for precise electrode placement to give stimulation in the painful area, because of better patient selection, and because of the increasing use of multiple small electrodes on a single lead (usually four or eight electrodes; Fig. 29.1) with varying patterns of stimulation to target the painful area.

Good axial stimulation is harder to obtain than stimulation in the limbs. Stimulation in a single limb is usually easily obtained by placing a single lead on one side of the midline of the spinal cord. A single lead placed precisely on the physiological midline will produce good bilateral stimulation.

Axial stimulation (e.g. in the lower back) usually requires two leads with multiple electrodes placed on either side of the midline of the cord. Some patients may require different levels and patterns of stimulation over different areas of the spinal cord to prevent unacceptably strong stimulation in the normal areas. This can now be achieved with the ANS Dual Stim and Genesis systems or the Medtronic Synergy system.

APPLIED ANATOMY

Anesthesiologists are familiar with inserting catheters into the epidural space, often in less than optimal circumstances. The percutaneous technique for insertion of an electrode lead is much the same. The electrode is inserted through a Tuohy needle and the epidural space is located by loss of resistance. The same care is needed in advancing the lead as when advancing a catheter. The use of radiographic screening to visualize the position of the lead means that it is also available during the insertion of the Tuohy needle into the epidural space. Screening makes this part of the procedure safer and easier.

Neurosurgeons perform a limited laminotomy and dissect down to the dura, and then apply flat plate electrodes directly to it (Fig. 29.2).

Key points

- This open technique is not to be undertaken by anyone who does not have the appropriate surgical training.
- Only the insertion of percutaneous leads is described.

CONTRAINDICATIONS

- *Local sepsis.* The electrode lead should never be inserted through or in close proximity to an area of skin sepsis.
- *Systemic infection.* Bacteria in the blood stream will readily colonize any implanted foreign material. Patients with chronic or recurrent infections, for example urinary tract infections, will from time to time experience bacteremia that may invade the spinal cord stimulator system, requiring it to be removed.

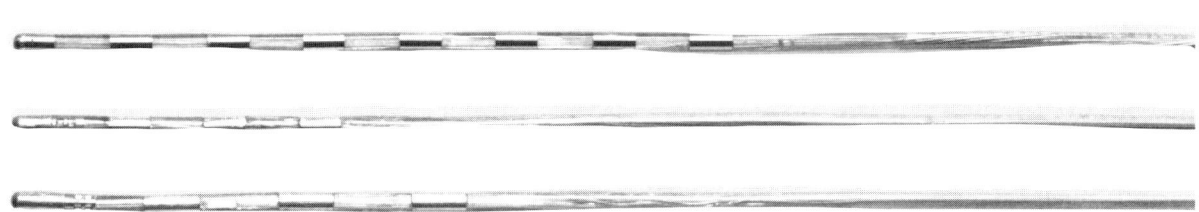

Figure 29.1 *Percutaneous electrodes.*

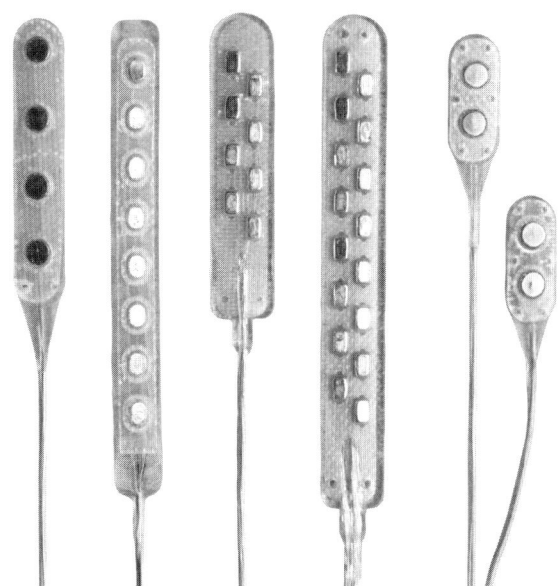

Figure 29.2 *Neurosurgical electrodes.*

- *Bleeding disorders.* Any condition that would increase the risk of spontaneous hemorrhage in the epidural space. The Liverpool Intractable Angina group implants patients on warfarin, but first converts them to intravenous (i.v.) heparin for the implantation procedure.
- *Scarring in the epidural space.* As a result of either previous interventions or infection.
- *Patients with implanted cardiac pacemakers.* Radiofrequency (RF) systems are contraindicated. Care is required with totally implantable systems (seek the manufacturer's advice).

LIMITATIONS

Patient selection

Spinal cord stimulation (SCS) is an invasive and expensive form of treatment that is not without complica-

tions. The most common complications are infection and movement of the electrode lead. Both of these complications may require repeated insertion or even removal of the system. Because this treatment is not suitable for everyone, patients need to be carefully selected beforehand.

Patients with chronic pain are less active and lose their fitness levels. They become depressed and develop abnormal patterns of behavior such as fear/avoidance, leading to further inactivity. The outcome following SCS treatment is better in individuals who are less depressed and have higher energy levels.[3*]

Key points

- All patients should have a multidisciplinary assessment before implantation.
- A treatment plan should be agreed to address any abnormal behavior patterns, depression, and poor fitness levels.

INDICATIONS

- Ischemic limb pain.[4*,5*]
- Failed back surgery syndrome.[6,7***,8*,9]
- Refractory angina pectoris.[10,11**]
- Complex regional pain syndromes [CRPS I and II; regional pain syndrome (RSD); causalgia].[12,13*]
- Peripheral neuropathic pain.[6,14*]
- Phantom limb pain.
- Raynaud's disease.[15*]

PREPARATION

Equipment

Two systems are available for spinal cord stimulation.

A totally implantable system

This system has its own internal power source – an implantable pulse generator (IPG). The IPG looks like a cardiac pacemaker (Fig. 29.3) and is based on pacemaker technology. Improvements in battery technology and programming techniques enable this system to drive complicated patterns of stimulation using multiple electrode arrays (the Medtronic Synergy system and the ANS Genesis system), but it remains limited by its inability to produce a large power output over a prolonged period of time. It is not suitable when wide pulse widths (450 μs) and rapid frequencies (130 Hz) are required to stimulate multiple electrodes.[4-6] These are the requirements for stimulation often seen in patients with failed back surgery syndrome. A rechargeable totally implantable system has long been promised and is eagerly awaited.

The simplest system (Medtronic Itrel II) provides the patient with two levels of stimulation. The stronger stimulation is usually used when the patient is ambulant. The lower level of stimulation is accessed using a magnet and is used when the patient is sitting or lying in a position where the electrode is pushed into closer contact with the spinal cord. The magnet can also be used to switch the stimulation on or off. Patients need to be warned to take care where they place the magnet as it will wipe credit cards clean.

A system that allows the patient to alter their stimulation within preset limits (Medtronic Itrel III) using their own miniprogrammer is more suitable for patients with electrodes implanted at the cervical level because movement of the head alters the level of stimulation.

A radiofrequency (RF)-coupled system

Instead of an IPG, a radioreceiver (Fig. 29.4) connected to the electrodes is implanted below the skin. An external transmitter unit (Fig. 29.5) that is small enough to be worn on a belt or waistband provides the stimulation.

The transmitter can be programmed to give different patterns of stimulation to different combinations of electrodes. When the patient wants to use the stimulator, an antenna from the transmitter is placed on the skin over the receiver site. It can be held in place by disposable double-sided self-adhesive patches. The coupling between the antenna and the receiver is by means of a radiofrequency signal. The batteries in the transmitter can be changed easily as often as necessary.

Key points

- RF systems are most suitable for multiple electrode stimulation, but require a large power output to provide adequate stimulation.

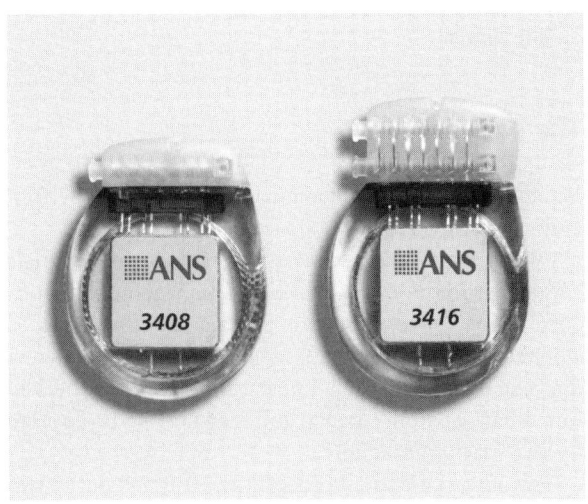

Figure 29.4 *Implantable radioreceivers.*

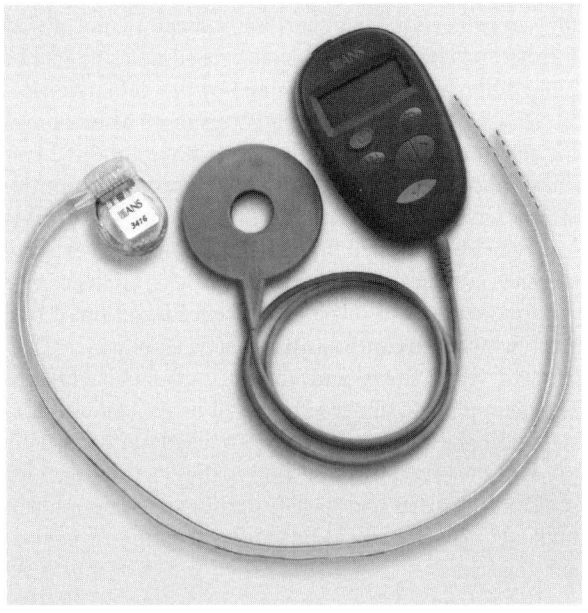

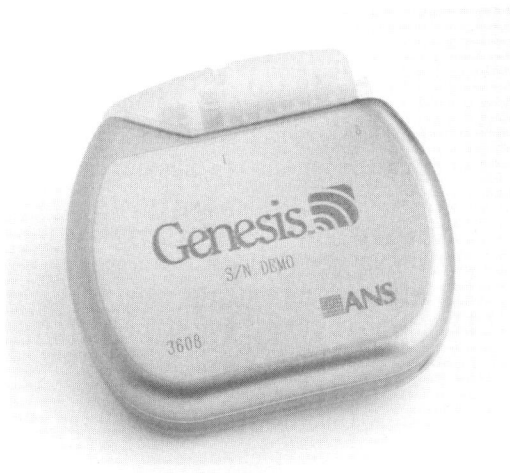

Figure 29.3 *Implantable pulse generator.*

Figure 29.5 *External transmitter and antenna.*

- Totally implantable systems with their own miniprogrammer are more suitable where there is significant electrode movement.
- Systems with magnets may be impractical for some people.

Both totally implantable systems and RF systems can be used to power single leads with four or eight electrodes, or two leads with four electrodes. Only RF systems can be used to power two leads with eight electrodes on each (ANS Dual Octrode systems).

Having selected the patient and chosen the most appropriate system, the next stage is to proceed to implantation of the electrode lead.

Key point

- Choose the appropriate system before embarking on any surgery.

The patient

Patients with intractable angina and those with peripheral vascular disease who are taking anticoagulants usually have the whole system implanted during a single surgical procedure. This makes the management of anticoagulation easier as the oral anticoagulant needs to be stopped before the procedure and restarted the following day. The patient's coagulation status needs to be checked immediately before surgery, and they need to be covered by i.v. heparin throughout.

For other patients, the procedure is carried out in two stages. In the first stage, the electrode lead is inserted into the epidural space and externalized to a screener unit. Some physicians use cheap leads with single electrodes for screening. This has the disadvantage of not giving targeted patterns of stimulation. The stimulation will be quite different from that obtained by the definitive electrodes and will give false-negative results. It also requires the electrode screening lead to be removed and the epidural space to be further invaded to insert the definitive electrodes. All of the commercially available electrode leads can be connected through extensions to an external screener. If pain relief is achieved, the extensions can be removed without disturbance of the leads for the second stage, which is to convert to a permanent system.

Both RF systems and totally implantable systems can be implanted under either local or general anesthesia. Local anesthesia with or without sedation is usually used for the first stage (insertion of the electrode lead for screening). The second stage (insertion of the permanent implant) may be carried out under sedation or general anesthesia.

The patient's preference for the position of the IPG or receiver should be determined before the commencement of any surgery as it may dictate the patient's position on the operating table. The IPG or receiver is best placed on the opposite side to the patient's dominant hand, so that the patient can easily place the antenna or miniprogrammer over it. In the UK, the preferred site is usually beneath the skin of the abdominal wall. In patients with flat abdomens, between the beltline and the lower ribs is suitable providing the patient is tall enough to prevent the device digging into their lower ribs when they sit down. In patients with rounded abdomens, the level of the umbilicus is better as it coincides with the maximum convexity of the abdomen; below this line, the devices tilt forward, and above this line they tend to tilt backwards. An alternative site is over the lower ribs in the anterior axillary line, but patients need to be tall enough for there to be enough space for the device not to interfere with their underwear. In patients less than 5 ft 2 in (158 cm) tall, it can be quite difficult to find a suitable site that the patient is comfortable with. In the USA, the upper outer quadrant of the buttock is sometimes used, but this is not an easy place for the patient to reach.

Key point

- Determine the patient's preference for the site of the IPG or receiver before commencing any surgery.

IMPLANTATION

Implantation is a sterile procedure and must be performed in a suitable sterile environment. A C-arm is required for radiographic screening.

Most physicians give i.v. antibiotics for the implantation stages. Opinions differ about the use of oral antibiotics afterwards.

First stage

The patient is positioned on a radiotranslucent operating table with the C-arm aligned for screening in the anteroposterior plane. The preferred position is prone, with the spine slightly flexed by means of a pillow under the abdomen.

An alternative position is to have the patient lying on their side with the nondominant side uppermost. This may be preferred when both stages are to be carried out at the same time, otherwise the patient will need to be turned after insertion of the electrode leads to allow insertion of the IPG or receiver.

The image intensifier is used to identify the desired level of entry into the epidural space, which is then marked on the skin. The skin is then cleaned and draped. The entire area must be prepared, including the receiver site if it is to be a one-stage procedure.

- For pain in the legs, the epidural space should be

entered at L1/2 or below, and the lead should be threaded up so that the electrodes lie between T9 and T12.

- For back pain, the best results are obtained with two octrapolar leads, the electrodes being positioned on either side of the midline in the lower thoracic region.
- For anginal pain, the epidural needle should be inserted at T5/6 or below and threaded up to lie between C6 and T2.
- For upper limb pain, the epidural needle is inserted at T3/4 or below and the lead is threaded up so that the electrodes lie between C4 and T1.

Enough lead should be inserted into the epidural space to allow fixation by the tissues. At least three clear vertebral levels are required from the entry point to the tip of the lead to give stability.

Sedation is not always necessary for the first stage, but movement of the electrode lead in the epidural space may provoke muscle spasm sufficient to prevent it being placed in the appropriate area. Either sedation or light anesthesia is, therefore, usually used. A separate suitably qualified anesthesiologist must provide this.
There is no place for the operator/anesthesiologist.

1 Infiltration with bupivacaine 0.25% with epineph-rine (adrenaline) will make it more comfortable for the patient during the awake stimulation phase, and the vasoconstriction will give a clearer operative field when the incision is made.
2 At the beginning of the procedure, make a paraverte-bral incision and insert an anchor stitch with a non-absorbable suture (such as 2/0 silk) into the deep tissues and clip the ends ready for later use. It is eas-ier to do this now, and avoids the risk of damaging the lead with the suture needle if it is done later.
3 Most physicians have their own preferred technique for identifying the epidural space. Using a pediat-ric i.v. positioning set filled with saline attached to the Tuohy needle and opened to full flow improves the accuracy of this part of the procedure. Flow will cease as the muscle is traversed, and will sud-denly recommence as the epidural space is entered. A Tuohy needle with a modified tip (Fig. 29.6) is used to prevent damage to the electrode lead while it is being maneuvered through the needle. Flow may therefore begin when the hole at the end of the needle is only part way into the epidural space. It should be carefully advanced until continuous flow is obtained. A shallow (30–40° to the skin) paraverte-bral approach allows an oblique entry into the epidu-ral space, which makes the electrode easier to thread up to the desired level and prevents kinking. The needle tip should be as close to the epidural anatom-ical midline as possible.
Never inject local anesthetic through the Tuohy nee-dle, as this will prevent test stimulation and exact placement of the electrodes.

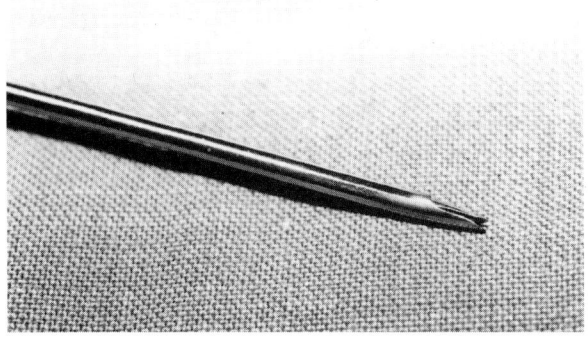

Figure 29.6 *Modified tip of Tuohy needle.*

4 Confirm that the epidural space has been entered by gently passing a guide wire through the needle while screening with the image intensifier. This must never be a forced maneuver. The guide wire can easily pierce the dura. For this reason, it is safest to advance the guide wire with the patient awake to avoid undue pressure on the dura or nerve roots. The patient will complain of pain and you will know when to stop; however, this may also provoke muscle spasm, pre-venting you manipulating the guide wire any further. The golden rule is to manipulate the guide wire gen-tly and never exert undue pressure.
5 The ANS guide wire is quite floppy and is mounted over a rigid stylet. The tip of the stylet can be bent to enable the guide wire to be manipulated in the desired direction. If you wish to have a straight guide wire again, simply cut off the bent tip of the stylet and an equal length of the floppy guide wire at the bottom end.
6 Introducing the guide wire into the epidural space will create a track ready to accept the electrode lead. When the guide wire reaches the desired level, remove it and quickly insert the lead through the track created for it.
7 The ANS system now allows the Tuohy needle to be withdrawn and a flexible introducer to be threaded over the guide wire. This prevents damage to the electrode lead during subsequent maneuvers.
8 The Medtronic leads come ready mounted on a stiff stylet with a curved tip. An alternative straight sty-let is also provided. The ANS leads do not have a sty-let, but have greater intrinsic stiffness. When using the ANS system, bending the tip of the guide wire to enable it to be manipulated into the desired position can create the desired track.
9 Remove the guide wire from the Tuohy needle and insert the electrode lead. Repeated screening with the image intensifier will reveal the direction that the lead is taking. Advance the lead to the desired verte-bral level. Repeat the process to insert a second lead if required.

Never exert undue force when manipulating a lead or guide wire.

10 Connect the proximal end of the lead that protrudes through the Tuohy needle or introducer to a sterile screening cable. The other end of this cable is passed out of the sterile field and is connected to an external screening stimulator.

Performing test stimulation

1 You will need an assistant to alter the settings on the external transmitter.

2 The patient must be completely awake for this part of the procedure. If sedation or anesthesia have been used earlier, you must allow time for them to wake up completely. Benzodiazepines can severely alter the patient's perception of stimulation.

3 You may need to test various electrode combinations with different stimulation parameters (rate, amplitude, and pulse width) in order to achieve paresthesiae at the target site. Manipulation of the lead to different vertebral levels may be necessary.

4 Uncomfortable stimulation, particularly if accompanied by muscle twitching, would imply anterior placement of the lead. This can be confirmed by lateral radiographic screening. It can be avoided by:

   a Making sure the tip of the Tuohy needle is as close to the anatomical midline in the epidural space as possible.

   b Using frequent or continuous screening with the image intensifier to monitor and adjust the position of the lead while it is being advanced in the epidural space.

5 When you are satisfied with the final position of the lead, turn off the screening transmitter and disconnect the screening cable from the lead. If desired, the patient can be resedated or anesthetized. If the lead has a stylet, remove it carefully so as not to disturb the position of the lead. Use the image intensifier to help you while doing this. Next remove the Tuohy needle, taking care not to pull out the lead, in the same way as you would remove a Tuohy needle from around an epidural catheter. Again, use the image intensifier to show you the effect on the position of the lead as you withdraw the Tuohy needle and adjust your manipulation appropriately. The bevel of the Tuohy needle is constructed to prevent shearing of the lead as the needle is gently pulled out of the epidural space.

6 Slide the anchoring device over the end of the lead and pass the suture that was inserted earlier into the deep fascia around the device and through its eyelet. Tie this firmly.

7 The end of the lead now needs to be joined to an extension cable if an external screening trial is to take place. The connector between the lead and the extension cable needs to be buried subcutaneously.

This can be done either by undercutting the lateral side of the existing incision to form a pouch or by making a new separate more lateral incision to house the connector. The advantage of this latter approach is that the midline incision does not need to be disturbed when converting the external screening system to a totally implantable one at a later date. The separate lateral incision needs to be made at a distance that is a few inches less than the proximal end of the lead. If this is made right at the end of the lead, it is very difficult to apply the boot. The boot is a plastic sleeve that is slid over the connecter to protect it from body fluids. Having made the lateral incision, the Tuohy needle is now reused. It is pushed subcutaneously from the lateral incision so that the point emerges in the midline incision. The proximal end of the lead is now inserted into the point of the needle as far as possible. Removing the Tuohy needle will leave the end of the lead lying in the lateral incision. *When using the Tuohy needle to tunnel the lead, always pass the Tuohy needle from the lateral incision to the midline incision – NOT the other way round.*

8 Clean any blood off the lead and connector with water before making the connection and applying the boot. Chloride in the blood will cause the stainless steel to slowly corrode and the wire will break after some months if blood is left in contact with it. *Use water to clean off any blood – NOT saline.*

9 The boot must be slid over the end of the lead sufficiently far to allow the connection to be made between the lead and the extension cable. The boot is then slid back over the connector and a nonabsorbable suture is tied around both ends to seal them. *Do not forget to slide the boot over the lead BEFORE making the connection with the extension cable.*

10 The manufacturers will provide a tunneling device to enable you to pass the extension subcutaneously to a stab wound in the flank, where it will emerge to be connected to the external transmitter. They vary in design so *follow their instructions.*

Screening trial

Opinions differ about the desirable level of activity of the patient immediately after a lead has been implanted. In the past, patients were sometimes confined to bed for days on end. There is no evidence that this prevents movement of the lead, and most physicians now allow their patients to mobilize at will. It is quite likely that most leads that move soon after implantation do so while the patient is being lifted off the operating table and turned into the recovery position.

Opinions also differ on the desirable length of the external screening trial period. The longer the trial, the greater the risk of infection. Most patients are able to tell almost immediately whether they are getting worthwhile pain relief. External screening for a week rarely causes any problems. A few patients may need longer to decide whether they want to proceed to a permanent implant. A trial period of 2 weeks usually does not cause any problems; by 3 weeks, the risk of infection increases markedly. It is doubtful whether patients benefit from longer periods to make their decision.

Microbiologists frown upon oral antibiotics during the trial period. They increase the risk of MRSA (methicillin-resistant *Staphylococcus aureus*) developing.

If the wounds are covered by a transparent waterproof dressing before the patient leaves the operating room, there is no reason why they should be disturbed during the trial screening period. The patient may take a shower after the first 24 h, provided the screening cable is disconnected from the external transmitter and securely protected in a polythene bag.

Second stage

Before embarking on the second stage, remove all dressings. Next, take hold of the screening cable and pull gently, thus exposing a length of sterile wire as it exits through the stab incision. Cut this sterile wire with a sterile pair of scissors.

If the trial is unsuccessful

If there has been no benefit from the trial stimulation, the lead will have to be removed:

- Clean and drape the patient's skin.
- Open the lateral incision to expose the connector and the midline incision to expose the anchoring device.
- Cut the suture that holds the anchoring device to the deep fascia. Pull the lead out of the back and remove the anchoring device. Pulling on the connector can now pull out the remains of the extension screening cable and the lead through the lateral incision.
- Suture the lateral pouch and central incision.

If the trial is successful

If the patient has benefited from the trial of stimulation, a permanent system will need to be implanted. The type of system will depend on the number of electrodes and the parameters used to obtain good stimulation. An RF system should be chosen if (1) more than three electrodes have been used, (2) the amplitude for adequate stimulation exceeds 3 V, or (3) a fast rate (> 100 Hz) with a wide pulse width (> 250 μs) has been required.

Key point

- If in doubt, it is better to choose an RF system.

Implantation of a permanent system is best carried out with the patient in the lateral position.

1 Clean and drape the whole operative area, including the receiver/IPG site.
2 Many physicians prefer to make the pouch for the receiver/IPG first as this allows more time to achieve hemostasis. The position for the pouch will have already been decided in discussion with the patient. If the pouch is too deep then adequate RF coupling will not occur. This will prevent stimulation by interfering with power transfer from the RF transmitter antenna and will prevent programming by interfering with data transfer to an IPG. The pouch should be of an even depth of less than half an inch (1.25 cm). This is particularly important with an RF system as it allows the receiver and antenna to lie parallel with each other. Hemorrhage is less troublesome if blunt dissection is used to form the pouch. The skin incision to form the pouch should be parallel with the skin creases and should not overlie the edge of the implanted device (this can cause problems with the scar at a later date); about a quarter of the way down from the upper (cephalad) edge of the device is a good position. The pouch must be large enough to accommodate the device, but not so large that the device is able to move around inside it. *Do not implant the receiver/IPG too deep.*
3 Open up the incision over the connector and lift it out. Cut the sutures on either end of the boot and slide the boot back over the lead. Undo the connector and remove it along with the remains of the screening extension cable. Use the manufacturer's tunneling device: for a Medtronic system to tunnel a new extension from the receiver/IPG pouch to the lead; for an ANS system to tunnel the lead around to the receiver/IPG pouch. *There are important differences between the Medtronic and ANS tunneling systems.*
4 The Medtronic tunneling device has a removable arrowhead and must be pushed from the lead *toward* the receiver/IPG pouch. The arrowhead is then removed and replaced by a carrier, which holds the connector end of the new extension. This is then pulled back to the end of the lead, where it can be connected in the same way as the original extension. *Do not forget to put the boot on the lead before connecting up the Medtronic extension. Use water, not saline, to clean off any blood before making the connections.*
5 The ANS system is different. The tunneling rod can be passed in any direction. It is encased in a plastic tube, which remains in the wound when the metal rod is removed. The lead can then be threaded through the tube, which can be removed leaving the end of the lead to be connected directly to the receiver/IPG.

6 It may be easier to pass the tunneling tool around the chest wall in two stages. An additional incision can be made in the flank and the tunneling tool passed to this first.

7 With the Medtronic system, it is necessary to pass the tunneling device from the flank incision to the receiver/IPG pouch first. Pull the extension connector end back to the flank incision and then repeat the maneuver from the lead end to the flank incision.

8 Once the tunneling is completed, the extension lead (Medtronic) or the lead end (ANS) can be connected to the IPG or RF receiver.
   Do not forget to put the boot on the lead before connecting up the ANS receiver or IPG.
   Use water, not saline, to clean off any blood before making the connections.

9 Secure the receiver/IPG to the deep tissue with a suture through its available slot.

10 Suture all your incisions.

COMPLICATIONS

- *Infection.* This is always a potential problem. With time, the fat layer disappears over subcutaneous, implanted foreign material. Ulceration of the skin can provide a portal of entry for bacteria. Once infected, the only solution is to remove the foreign material – in this case the implant. Patients must be warned to seek help as soon as any skin ulceration occurs. The danger of the spread of infection to the meninges is ever present.

- *Movement of the electrode lead.* This is a particular problem for patients moving to their car from a wheelchair and vice versa. Advising patients to avoid any activity does not reduce the incidence. Patients should be encouraged to be as active as possible.

- *Dural tap.* Cerebrospinal fluid (CSF) leak may occur when the Tuohy needle is introduced into the epidural space or as a result of manipulating the guide wire or electrode lead. It is more likely to occur when there is scarring in the epidural space as a result of previous surgery or arachnoiditis. It may be possible to successfully implant a lead by entering the epidural space at a higher level. Multiple attempts should be avoided. In cases where extensive scarring is known to exist, the risks should be discussed in detail with the patient before deciding to proceed. It is often wiser to refer these patients to a neurosurgeon for consideration of implanting a lead at open operation.

- *Subdural hematoma.* This is fortunately an extremely rare occurrence. It must be suspected wherever there is any sign of increasing loss of sensation or weakness. Loss of bowel or bladder control demands emergency decompression. Time is of the essence. There may only be hours to prevent permanent neurological damage.

Key point

- Seek urgent neurosurgical help if a subdural hematoma is suspected.

PROGRAMMING

- Good stimulation requires an understanding of programming. This has been a much neglected area in the past.

- In bipolar stimulation, stimulation is always greater at the negative electrode. A screened cathode (+ – + configuration) gives a softer edge to the stimulation and increases patient acceptance. Increasing the pulse width recruits more fibers and may make the stimulation spread. It may also make the stimulation become unpleasantly strong. Conversely, reducing the pulse width may focus the stimulation more precisely into the desired area and make the stimulation softer and more acceptable.

- When dual leads with multiple electrodes are used, programming becomes more difficult and complex and the aid of computer technology is being sought (e.g. the ANS "Pain Doc").

REFERENCES

1. Nashold Jr BS, Friedman H. Dorsal column stimulation for the control of pain. Preliminary report on thirty patients. *J Neurosurg* 1972; **36:** 590–7.

2. Shealy CN, Mortimer JT. Dorsal column electro analgesia. *J Neurosurg* 1970; **32:** 560–4.

◆ 3. Olsen KA, Bedder MD, Anderson VC, *et al.* Psychological variables associated with outcome of spinal cord stimulation trials. *Neuromodulation* 1998; **1:** 6–13.

4. Jacobs MJHM, Jorning PJG, Beckers RCY, *et al.* Foot salvage and improvement of micro vascular blood flow as a result of epidural spinal cord electrical stimulation. *J Vasc Surg* 1990; **12:** 354–60.

5. Jacobs MJHM, Jorning PJG, Joshi SR, *et al.* Epidural spinal cord stimulation improves microvascular blood flow in severe limb ischemia. *Ann Surg* 1988; **207:** 179–83.

● 6. Simpson BA. Spinal cord stimulation. *Pain Rev* 1994; **1:** 199–230.

7. Turner JA, Loeser JD, Bell KG. Spinal cord stimulation for chronic low back pain: a systematic literature synthesis. *Neurosurgery* 1995; **37:** 1088–95.

8. De La Porte C, Van de Klefte E. Spinal cord stimulation in failed back surgery syndrome. *Pain* 1993; **52:** 55–61.

● 9. North RB, Guarino AH. Spinal cord stimulation for failed back surgery syndrome: technical advances, patient selection and outcome. *Neuromodulation* 1999; **2:** 171–8.

● 10. Dejongste MJL. Efficacy, safety and mechanisms of spinal cord stimulation used as an additional therapy for patients suffering from chronic refractory angina pectoris. *Neuromodulation* 1999; **2:** 188–92.

11. Mannheimer C, Eliasson T, Augustinsson L-E, *et al.* Electrical stimulation versus coronary bypass surgery in severe angina pectoris. *Circulation* 1998; **97:** 1157–63.

● 12. Stanton-Hicks M. Spinal cord stimulation for the management of complex regional pain syndromes. *Neuromodulation* 1999; **2:** 193–201.

13. Bennett DS, Alo KM, Oakley J, Feler CA. Spinal cord stimulation for complex regional pain syndrome I (RSD): a retrospective multicentre experience from 1995–1998 of 101 patients. *Neuromodulation* 1999; **2:** 202–10.

14. Tesfaye S, Watt J, Benbow SJ, *et al.* Electrical spinal-cord stimulation for painful diabetic peripheral neuropathy. *Lancet* 1996; **348:** 1698–701.

15. Robaina FJ, Dominguez M, Diaz M, *et al.* Spinal cord stimulation for relief of chronic pain in vasospastic disorders of the upper limb. *Neurosurgery* 1989; **24:** 63–7.

PART VII

Patient-controlled analgesia

30

Intravenous and subcutaneous patient-controlled analgesia: practical points and protocols

RICHARD BARRETT

Background	393	Subcutaneous patient-controlled analgesia	395
Guidelines	394	Monitoring	395
Patient information	394	Management of common side-effects of	
Equipment and drugs	394	patient-controlled analgesia opioids	398
Staffing and training	394	Conclusion	398
Setting up the patient-controlled analgesia	394	References	399
Intravenous patient-controlled analgesia	395		

Patient-controlled analgesia (PCA) is a well-established technique for managing acute pain, especially postoperative pain. Its true merit, measured in terms of patient benefit[1*,2] and when compared with intramuscular (i.m.) opioids given according to an algorithm,[3*] is a source of some controversy. However, if PCA is prescribed for the well-informed patient, it confers the advantage of allowing the patient to achieve a level of comfort "on demand" as well as providing analgesia in anticipation of discomfort or pain, for example intentional movement, or for interventions such as physiotherapy or surgical dressing changes.

The use of an opioid PCA should not be considered as the sole means of managing acute pain; adjuncts such as nonsteroidal anti-inflammatory drugs (NSAIDs) and nonopioid analgesics, for example acetaminophen (paracetamol), provide a more balanced approach[4**] and the potential for opioid sparing when administered concurrently.[5**,6**] In addition, the use of local anesthesia is to be encouraged either as wound infiltration at operation – pre- or postoperatively – or for regional techniques.[7*]

Although the subcutaneous (s.c.) route has aroused interest recently,[8**,9*] intravenous (i.v.) PCA is the more commonly used approach. There is a wide range of opioids, nonopioids, and NSAIDs in current PCA usage. To cover every agent is beyond the scope of this chapter. The following provides an outline of basic principles that can be applied to either route.

BACKGROUND

The PCA delivery system is a sophisticated, tamper-proof, programmable electronic pump that drives either a syringe or an infusion bag. In common with many other interventions, it is a system that relies upon accuracy in its programming and a clear understanding by the supervisor of its many functions. A continuous process of education of all the medical and nursing staff who will be caring for the patient using PCA is a *sine qua non*. Subsequently, its safe operation is dependent upon four criteria:

- A comprehensive guideline should exist for the safe and effective use of PCA (including the management of complications), and this must be followed at all times. The guideline must reflect best practice and should be validated by the hospital's risk management committee or its equivalent.
- The patient must understand the correct operation of the PCA equipment and be able to operate it successfully. Modifications, such as a mouthpiece and "blow-pipe" to replace the pushbutton, extend the use of the PCA to patients unable to operate it by hand.

- Only trained staff should program the PCA equipment, and trained staff must monitor its use in the clinical environment.
- The PCA system must be stored securely when not in use and regularly maintained and serviced.

GUIDELINES

In the absence of a national framework from which to work, and possibly to adapt for local conditions, it becomes the remit of the acute pain management team to construct and disseminate PCA guidelines – their importance cannot be overemphasized. Critically:

- the guideline is evidence based and should follow "best practice;"
- the document is clear and concise;
- a comprehensive and stepwise approach is adopted when setting up and initiating the PCA;
- required monitoring standards and observations are detailed;
- the recognition and management of side-effects and complications are made particularly clear;
- simple "troubleshooting" advice is given;
- 24-h contact numbers for advice and assistance are provided;
- the guideline is reviewed at least annually.

PATIENT INFORMATION

An information leaflet, also prepared by the acute pain management team and given to the patient in advance of surgery, perhaps at the preoperative assessment or in the outpatient clinic, can allay anxieties about the technique which might, at first glance, seem intimidating. Written with the lay public in mind, it should be clear and should answer commonly asked questions and concerns, such as "Can I overdose myself?" and "Will I become addicted to the morphine?"[10*]

The leaflet provides the opportunity to address issues such as alternatives and adjuncts to PCA, and advice on "comfort" measures that can be employed following surgery.

Currently, there is no requirement for obtaining written consent from the patient for PCA; however, it would seem prudent that a record is made in the notes that discussion has taken place with the patient regarding its use. Other methods of pain relief, including regional analgesia and oral or rectal NSAIDs and/or acetaminophen, and their benefits and disadvantages should also be discussed preoperatively.

EQUIPMENT AND DRUGS

Because safe practice is of paramount importance, standardization of equipment – PCAs, opioid solutions, and "disposables" – is essential. Ideally, the opioid solutions should be supplied by the hospital pharmacy and delivered to the patient through a sterile, sealed system. There is little to be gained here by discussing the relative merits and disadvantages of all the opioids that are in current use or have been used in the past.

STAFFING AND TRAINING

Before opioid PCAs can be introduced into the clinical environment, a carefully structured program of education and training is necessary. Once the guidelines for the use of the PCA have been tested for clarity, relevance, and ease of application, they can form the basis of training and the regular staff updates that should follow. The emphasis in PCA education is on familiarity with the equipment, "troubleshooting," monitoring the patient, and recognizing signs and symptoms of opioid side-effects and overdose and managing these complications.

Education and training should be seen as *the* major roles of the acute pain management team and can be conducted as formal lectures, as a part of acute pain management study days, tutorials, or as "one-to-one" teaching at the patient's bedside.

SETTING UP THE PATIENT-CONTROLLED ANALGESIA

Before initiating the PCA, adequate analgesia should be established by the use of i.v. boluses of opioid. After the opioid solution has been installed in the pump, the PCA program must be checked. Although the format will vary according to the manufacturer, the principal keys, and therefore the variables, will be similar:

- clear memory function;
- bolus dose (μg/ml or mg/ml);
- solution concentration (μg/ml or mg/ml);
- rate of injection (ml/h);
- lock out (min);
- successful attempts;
- solution remaining (μg/ml or mg/ml);
- background infusion.

Background infusions of opioid have been used with success in pediatric PCA pain management.[11**] However, in adult patients, a background infusion is recognized as a contributing factor to postoperative hypoxemia and a cause of respiratory depression, without conferring analgesic advantage over the use of PCA alone.[12*,13*] Therefore, in the interests of patient safety, its use cannot be recommended.

The inclusion of an antiemetic in the PCA opioid solution has been studied and benefits have been claimed of reduced nausea and vomiting associated with opioids;

meta-analysis has shown that droperidol is the agent of choice.[14***] However, the disadvantages of this practice are that the patient may feel nauseated despite the presence of the antiemetic (which may not achieve satisfactory plasma levels through lack of PCA triggering) and may be deprived of "escape" antiemesis. Second, the patient may not experience opioid-induced nausea and yet will receive an antiemetic unnecessarily and with it the risk of unwanted side-effects (for the management of postoperative nausea and vomiting, see below).

INTRAVENOUS PATIENT-CONTROLLED ANALGESIA

For intravenous PCA, an indwelling i.v. cannula is connected to a thin-walled catheter and Luer locked to the opioid-containing syringe or infusion bag delivery system. If the PCA and an existing intravenous infusion are to be conjoined, a "Y" connector with a nonreturn valve, to avoid reflux, must be used in-line and care must be taken to avoid "siphoning." Siphonage can occur through malposition of the pump above the level of the patient together with an incorrectly filled syringe containing a small volume of air or with a leaking plunger or barrel.[15]

Small bolus doses are used with a short lockout period, e.g. morphine 1 mg available at 5-min intervals.

For simplicity and therefore safety of titration, solution concentrations, for example morphine 1 mg/ml, are used in the adult patients.

Potentially, a rapid rate of injection (100 ml/min) could induce sensations of light-headedness and nausea, although in practice this has not been verified.[16*]

Advantages of intravenous patient-controlled analgesia

- Easy titration of opioid against pain.
- Rapid analgesic response.
- Intravenous access is made available.
- Well-established application of PCA.

Disadvantages of intravenous patient-controlled analgesia

- Small bolus doses may necessitate frequent button-pressing to achieve acceptable analgesia.
- Opioid-induced nausea or dysphoria may be linked to bolusing by the patient – leading to dissatisfaction with, and abandonment of, the technique.
- Diminishing plasma levels of opioid may lead to poor sleep patterns postoperatively.
- Continuous patent i.v. access is essential – "tissuing" of the i.v. infusion can lead to loss of analgesic control.

- Increased incidence of opioid-induced pruritus by the i.v. route (cf. the s.c. route).

SUBCUTANEOUS PATIENT-CONTROLLED ANALGESIA

For s.c. PCA, an indwelling 23-gauge cannula is inserted in an area of skin that is both comfortable for the patient and accessible, e.g. overlying deltoid. This is connected to a thin-walled catheter and, again, Luer locked to the opioid infusion in the PCA. A clear dressing over the skin puncture site allows easy inspection and the cannula can be resited if local inflammation occurs.

In the well-perfused patient receiving s.c. PCA, the rate of absorption appears to be a predictable pharmacokinetic profile of the opioid.[9*]

Volumetrically, similar sized boluses are used (1 ml) with a concentration of opioid, typically heroin (diamorphine) around 2.5 mg/ml, and an extended lock-out period, for example 20 min, that can be modified according to the patient's analgesic requirements.

Advantages of subcutaneous patient-controlled analgesia

- Larger opioid doses are available in each bolus, helping to achieve satisfactory analgesia.
- Less patient association of opioid bolus delivered with opioid-induced nausea or dysphoria.
- Better postoperative sleep patterns than i.v. PCA.[17**]
- Resiting a s.c. cannula is relatively straightforward.
- A patent i.v. infusion is not essential while the s.c. PCA is in use.

Disadvantages of subcutaneous patient-controlled analgesia

- The immediate titration of opioid dose against pain is not as easy as with i.v. PCA.
- The longer lock-out period precludes "instant" analgesia in response to unexpected pain stimuli.

MONITORING

The PCA should neither create a barrier between the patient and the nurse caring for that patient nor become an excuse for suboptimal monitoring and supervision. The ventilatory depressant effect of opioids is well recognized, and in the context of opioid PCA has been the subject of investigation.[18**] There is debate about the role of pulse oximetry while PCA is in use;[19*,20] paradoxically, pulse oximetry is not routinely used when i.m. opioids are given unless the patient's condition demands it.

Signature ————————————————— Bleep or contact no. —————

Pain Management Team bleep. Anesthetist on call bleep

Observations (as often as patient's condition dictates – a minimum of 4 hourly)

Date	Time (24 h)	Resps	Pulse	BP	Temp.	O$_2$ sat. %	Epidural rate ml/h (please initial changes)	Pain (0–10) on movement	Nausea (0–10)	Sedation (0–3/S)	
											Urinary retention (requiring catheter) Please tick box ☐
											Pruritus requiring treatment please tick box ☐
											Respiratory depression requiring treatment please tick box ☐
											Hypotension requiring treatment please tick box ☐
											Inadequate analgesia requiring change in treatment please tick box ☐
											Any other comments?

Pain score:

Figure 30.1 *Sample Acute Pain Control chart, Salisbury District Hospital, UK.*

```
0                                          10
No pain                                    Worst pain
```

Nausea score

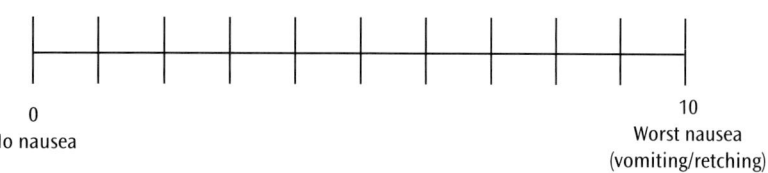

```
0                                          10
No nausea                                  Worst nausea
                                           (vomiting/retching)
```

Sedation score

0 = awake, alert
1 = occasionally drowsy, easy to rouse
2 = frequently drowsy
3 = somnolent, difficult to rouse
s = asleep, easy to rouse

Analgesic guidelines

Prescribe acetaminophen and NSAID (unless contraindicated) <u>regularly</u> for 4 days. Supplement with dihydrocodeine if necessary.

Antiemetic guidelines for PONV

i.m. Cyclizine 50 mg × 6 hourly   = give regularly for 24 h and review
i.m. Prochlorperazine 12.5 mg × 8 hourly = give regularly for 24 h and review
i.m. Metoclopramide 10 mg × 6 hourly   = give regularly for 24 h and review

NB A combination of the above may be given if required, i.e. insufficient to control PONV. This may increase sedation scores.

Uncontrolled, severe PONV

As above **and add:**

i.m. Ondansetron 4 mg (or i.v. ondansetron up to 8 mg slowly) × 6 hourly
i.v. Dexamethasone 8 mg i.v. stat.

Bridging the gap

After cessation of PCA/epidural, prescribe Oramorph 30 mg × 4 hourly or 10 mg i.m. hourly PRN via i.m. cannula if nil-by-mouth. Ensure adequate alternative simple analgesia is prescribed.

Figure 30.1 *Continued.*

Likewise, although there is no consensus on the frequency of observations, the PCA should not be viewed as a "fire and forget" intervention, handing total analgesic responsibility to the patient. The potential exists either for mishap or for the patient not to make sensible use of the PCA.

Regular observations

- Pain assessment by visual analog score (VAS) or numerical rating scale (NRS) of 0–10.
- Nausea score (VAS/NRS 0–10).
- Sedation score (observer, 0–3; concession may be made for "asleep").
- Systemic blood pressure, heart rate, respiratory rate, body temperature.
- Other opioid side-effects: pruritus, confusion, urinary retention, and constipation.
- Inspection of cannula site.

In recording these observations, the nursing staff should be aware of previously defined parameters outside of which action (according to the guidelines) is taken, e.g. a lower limit for respiratory rate or a high VAS/NRS pain score.

Using a specially designed and easily interpreted form

(Fig. 30.1) that incorporates all these observations, which is then examined alongside the fluid balance chart, can create a more complete picture of the postoperative progress of the patient.

Good analgesic management is an important aspect of postoperative care, but it is only one of several components that can optimize the patient's recovery.

MANAGEMENT OF COMMON SIDE-EFFECTS OF PATIENT-CONTROLLED ANALGESIA OPIOIDS

At the risk of repetition, staff caring for patients using opioid PCA must be able to recognize the common side-effects and complications and respond in accordance with the PCA guidelines. Resuscitation facilities (including naloxone) must be available nearby and staff training must include familiarization with these facilities and techniques.

Respiratory depression

- Determine the patient's respiratory rate and consciousness level.
- Summon assistance.
- Give minimum 40% oxygen by mask.
- Support ventilation as necessary.
- Administer i.v. naloxone 0.2 mg and repeat as necessary to establish an acceptable respiratory rate and level of consciousness.
- Adopt a higher level of observation of the patient, including pulse oximetry.
- Reconsider the use of opioid PCA in that patient; consider analgesic alternatives to opioids.

Sedation

- Establish the level of consciousness.
- If opioid central depression can be established as the cause, manage as for respiratory depression.
- Exclude other causes of excessive sedation.

Nausea and vomiting

- Give prescribed antiemetics regularly, e.g. cyclizine 50 mg i.m. 6 hourly (maximum 150 mg/24 h).
- Add antiemetics "step-wise" in accordance with postoperative nausea and vomiting (PONV) guidelines, e.g. ondansetron 4 mg i.m./i.v.
- Reassure the patient.
- If PONV persists, consider using analgesic alternatives to opioids.
- Consider other causes of nausea and vomiting.

Pruritus

- Reassure the patient.
- Give i.m. naloxone 0.1 mg, and repeat as necessary to control symptoms.
- If persistent, consider using analgesic alternatives to opioids.

A regular review of the use of PCA can demonstrate those situations when it is most effective and others in which it is less so. The use of a form, such as that described in Fig. 30.1, can make analysis of such effectiveness considerably easier to interpret when scanned into a database and can be used to direct future practice.

Untoward events, other than opioid side-effects, must be recorded on the chart or in the patient's notes. This is necessary not only in the interests of improving the safety of the service provided, i.e. risk management, but also in anticipation of an incident inquiry (and potential litigation).

A comprehensive annual review of PCA interventions should be a basic requirement for a pain management team.

CONCLUSION

The PCA represents a significant advance in the management of acute pain. The achievements of producing inexpensive, accurate, and portable infusion pumps that are easily programmed have meant that this mode of analgesic delivery is widely available, however this should not give rise to complacency. Patient safety is the first priority.

The potential for mishap such as opioid overdose or, at the other extreme, inadequate analgesia must not be overlooked. A system is only as good or as safe as its weakest component. Familiarity with this technique is not an excuse to hand over analgesia completely to the patient under any circumstances; emphasis must be placed on careful explanation to the patient beforehand and regular supervision and close monitoring while the PCA is in use.

The successful and safe use of PCA opioids depends on the provision of guidelines that must be properly constituted and disseminated.

Before establishing PCA in clinical practice, education of the staff caring for these patients is mandatory. Thereafter, the introduction of PCA on a restricted basis at first (e.g. to a single ward or clinical area) allows initial "teething problems" to be overcome, as well as inspiring confidence among the clinical staff supervising its use. A continuous program of education and audit must follow this in order to maintain the highest standards of care and patient comfort.

REFERENCES

1. Taylor NM, Hall GM, Salmon P. Patients' experiences of patient controlled analgesia. *Anaesthesia* 1996; **51:** 525–8.
2. Hall GM. Editorial. Patient-controlled analgesia – who benefits? *Anaesthesia* 1997; **52:** 401–2.
◆ 3. Gould TH, Crosby DL, Harmer M, *et al*. Policy for controlling pain after surgery: effects of sequential changes. *Br Med J* 1992; **305:** 1187–93.
4. Montgomery JE, Sutherland CJ, Kestin IG, Sneyd JR. Morphine consumption in patients receiving rectal paracetamol and diclofenac alone and in combination. *Br J Anaesth* 1996; **77:** 445–7.
5. Schug SA, Sidebotham DA, McGuinnety M, *et al*. Acetaminophen as an adjunct to morphine by patient-controlled analgesia in the management of acute postoperative pain. *Br J Clin Pharmacol* 1998; **45:** 57–62.
6. Cobby TF, Crighton IM, Kyriakides K, Hobbs GJ. Rectal paracetamol has a significant morphine-sparing effect after hysterectomy. *Anesth Analg* 1999; **88:** 1354–61.
7. Dahl JB, Moiniche S, Kehlet H. Wound infiltration with local anesthetics for postoperative pain relief. *Acta Anaesthesiol Scand* 1994; **38:** 7–14.
8. Gopinathan C, Sockalingham I, Fung MA, *et al*. A comparative study of patient-controlled epidural diamorphine, subcutaneous diamorphine and an epidural diamorphine/bupivacaine combination for postoperative pain. *Eur J Anaesthesiol* 2000; **17:** 189–96.
9. Semple TJ, Upton RN, MacKintyre PE, *et al*. Morphine blood concentrations in elderly postoperative patients following administration via an indwelling subcutaneous cannula. *Anaesthesia* 1997; **52:** 318–23.
10. Chumbley GM, Hall GM, Salmon P. Why do patients feel positive about patient-controlled analgesia? *Anaesthesia* 1999; **54:** 386–9.
11. Doyle E, Harper I, Morton NS. Patient-controlled analgesia with low dose background infusion after lower abdominal surgery in children. *Br J Anaesth* 1993; **71:** 818–22.
12. Russell AW, Owen H, Ilsley AH, *et al*. Background infusion with patient-controlled analgesia: effect on postoperative oxyhaemoglobin saturation and pain control. *Anaesth Intensive Care* 1993; **21:** 174–9.
● 13. Sidebotham D, Dijkhuizen MRJ, Schug SA. The safety and utilization of patient controlled analgesia. *J Pain Symptom Manage* 1997; **14:** 202–9.
● 14. Tramer MR, Walder B. Efficacy and adverse effects of prophylactic anti-emetics during patient-controlled analgesia therapy: a quantitative systematic review. *Anesth Analg* 1999; **88:** 1354–61.
15. Wallace PGM. Editorial. Infusion systems. *Anaesthesia* 1996; **51:** 613–14.
16. Woodhouse A, Mather LE. The effect of dose delivery with patient-controlled analgesia on the incidence of nausea and vomiting after hysterectomy. *Br J Clin Pharmacol* 1998; **45:** 57–62.
17. Dawson L, Brockbank K, Carr ECJ, Barrett RF. Improving patients' postoperative sleep: a randomized control study comparing subcutaneous with intravenous patient-controlled analgesia. *J Adv Nurs* 1999; **30:** 875–81.
18. Wheatley RG, Somerville ID, Sapsford DJ, Jones JG. Postoperative hypoxaemia: comparison of extradural, intramuscular and patient-controlled opioid analgesia. *Br J Anaesth* 1990; **64:** 267–75.
◆ 19. Tsui SL, Irwin MG, Wong CM, *et al*. An audit of the safety of an acute pain service. *Anaesthesia* 1997; **52:** 1042–7.
20. Rowlingson JC. Just when we thought we understood patient controlled analgesia. *Anesth Analg* 1999; **89:** 3–6.

31

Alternative opioid PCA delivery systems – transcutaneous, nasal, and others

GUNNVALD KVARSTEIN

Applied anatomy	401	Summary	404
Contraindications and limitations	404	References	405

A high percentage of patients still complain about insufficient postoperative pain relief. This can hardly be due to the lack of potent analgesics, but may reflect improper administration and dosage.[1]* Published and unpublished audits suggest that intramuscular opioid injections are still the mainstay in postoperative pain management.[2]* Intramuscular absorption is highly dependent on local perfusion. Intramuscular administration is therefore associated with undesirable peaks and troughs of drug concentration in the effector organ. For the individual patient, a preset dose may just as easily represent an overdose as an underdose. Patient-controlled analgesia (PCA), however, allows opioid titration until the desired level of analgesia is achieved, which is essential in order to provide adequate pain management. Safety is assured by technical devices that limit the total dosage.

Advances in pharmaceutical technology, together with a more profound understanding of dermal physiology and the pharmacokinetics of opioids, have made transdermal and transmucosal administration a promising field. Even though the products are still in their infancy, the alternative PCA therapies appear to be more convenient than conventional analgesic therapy (conventional i.v. PCA) for both patient and nursing staff (Table 31.1). Patient-controlled epidural analgesia is discussed in Chapter P32.

APPLIED ANATOMY

The transdermal route

The skin is an important protective barrier. However, it may also be an effective and noninvasive route for drug administration, and transdermal delivery seems to provide stable plasma concentrations. Under normal conditions, changes in skin blood flow appear not to be a clinical problem.[4]

The oral and nasal transmucosal route

The buccal, sublingual, and nasal mucosa have an abundant blood flow and excellent lymphatic drainage and represent a more permeable barrier than skin. Accordingly, the mucosa allows rapid absorption of lipophilic drugs, facilitating dose titration.[3] However, buccal administration of *hydrophilic* drugs, such as morphine, is more unpredictable.

Both patient- and drug-related factors have been shown to influence the bioavailability of nasally administered drugs. The patient-related factors include mucosal blood flow, secretion, and ciliary activity as well as site of drug deposition and head position. The drug-related determinants are lipophilicity, molecular size, and pK and pH of the solution, as well as drug concentration, dose volume, and droplet size. For example, smaller droplets lead to more prolonged and higher drug levels.

The inhalation route

The vascular tracheal mucosa should theoretically be an effective route for drug administration, and studies with fentanyl have shown useful analgesia despite low serum concentrations. A different mode of analgesia compared with i.v. administration has therefore been suggested.[5]** However, the reports are far from conclusive. Other data

Table 31.1 *Alternative PCA delivery systems*

Transdermal
Iontophoretic/electromotive devices for drug administered
  through skin

Transmucosal
Nasal aerosol sprays
Buccal aerosol sprays
Drug-impregnated "lollipops"[3]

suggest that fentanyl administered by inhalation is no more effective than when administered by other parenteral routes.[6]**

The oral/gastrointestinal route

In acid environments, opioids are highly ionized and unable to penetrate gastric mucosa. Even though absorption is favored in the more alkaline environment of the small intestines, a large portion is still metabolized in the liver (the first-pass effect). Thus, the bioavailability of orally administered opioids is low and unpredictable. However, for drugs that are metabolized into more potent substances, such as morphine, codeine, or tramadol (but not in slow metabolizers), the first-pass effect may be an advantage.

Transdermal opioid delivery

For transdermal administration fentanyl is the prototypical drug, providing plasma concentrations as stable as those obtained by intravenous infusion.[7]* Within the commercially available delivery system Duragesic® (Jansen Pharmaceuticals, Titusville, NJ, USA), fentanyl is stored in a gel matrix and separated from the patient by a rate-controlling membrane.

Postoperative use has led to a reduction in supplementary opioids and even improved respiratory function.[8]** Some clinical data indicate that transdermal fentanyl is a convenient, effective, and safe method for controlling moderate to severe postoperative pain.[9]** On the other hand, the stable plasma opioid concentration provided by dermal patches is not always the best method of controlling acute pain whose intensity varies over time. According to other studies, the combination of transdermal opioid delivery systems with i.v. PCA does not seem to be better than i.v. PCA alone.[10]** Because of the risk of overdose as pain subsides, the transdermal fentanyl patch is not recommended in the management of postoperative pain.

To manage acute pain, an iontophoretic, on-demand system has therefore been developed. Examples include E-TRANS® (model 4502; ALZA Corporation, Palo Alto, CA, USA) and TRANSFENTA® (Jansen Pharmaceuticals). The system combines the benefit of transdermal patches with those of a PCA pump by electrical field-promoted delivery. The device is applied to the skin like a fentanyl patch, but differs in one way: the patient must activate an electrical current by pushing a button in order to receive a bolus. Fentanyl is not absorbed without an applied current.[9]** A bolus dose of fentanyl (40 µg) is delivered over 10 min and may be repeated six times per hour. The maximum dose per hour is 240 µg. This bolus of 40 µg fentanyl has been shown to be effective without serious side-effects.[9]**

A basal current of 100 µA seems to provide adequate serum levels (1–3 ng/ml).[9]** The amount of fentanyl absorbed increases proportionally with the amount of current delivered, and the serum level seems to be determined by the product [current × duration].[9]*,[11]** However, when the current is increased to 170 µA, the bolus of 40 µg fentanyl is absorbed independently of the delivery time (2.5, 5.0, or 10.0 min).[11]**

Differences in serum concentration between male and female volunteers or among various anatomic locations of the system have not been found.[12]* As the system delivers a maximum of 80 doses, a new delivery system, applied at a different skin site, is recommended every 24 h (Table 31.2).

Transmucosal opioid delivery

Opioids can be effectively administered via both nasal and oral mucosa. Bioavailability[13,14] following transmucosal administration is the same or even better than after oral or intramuscular delivery. When used by the patient it is superior to customary p.r.n. therapy administered by nursing staff. Likewise, intranasal and i.v. PCA give equivalent pain control and patient satisfaction[15]** with an onset of action that is nearly as fast as that for i.v. therapy.[15]**

Sufentanil

Sufentanil is the most investigated intranasal drug. It is highly lipophilic and therefore an ideal drug for intranasal administration, with a bioavailability of approximately 70%. The onset time is about 10 min.

Table 31.2 *E-TRANS® and TRANSFENTA® characteristics*

Bolus dose: 40 µg
Lock-out time 10 min
An electrical field promotes transdermal delivery of the
  drug
Standard electrical current: 170 µA over 10 min (may vary)
No fentanyl is absorbed when current is not applied
Pain control equivalent to i.v. PCA:
High global satisfaction assessment score
Side-effects are similar to i.v. and tolerable

Fentanyl

Fentanyl is pharmacokinetically much like sufentanil and is also well suited for intranasal administration. Significant pain reduction has been reported after 10 min, and within 20 min the efficacy equals that of i.v. fentanyl.[15]** With a bioavailability of around 70%, an equipotent intranasal dose is 1.3–1.5 times the i.v. dose. There have been reports that intranasal fentanyl administration has led to improved quality of life in patients with chronic pain.[16]*

Meperidine

Postoperatively, meperidine (pethidine) administered by intranasal PCA provides better analgesia than similar s.c. doses and is equally as effective as i.v. meperidine.[17]** To achieve the same degree of pain relief, the intranasal dose has to be 1.36 times the i.v. dose.

Butorphanol

Butorphanol is a mixed agonist/antagonist, and is rapidly absorbed by the vascular nasal mucosa. Equivalent analgesic efficacy compared with i.v. butorphanol[18]** is achieved within 15 min and lasts for 4.5 h. Systemic availability varies from 70% to 48% in elderly women. However, the age- and sex-related changes are not large enough to necessitate dosage differences.

One spray is applied into one nostril every 3 h as needed for pain. Two milligrams seems to be the optimal dose, but it is better tolerated when divided into 1-mg increments given 1 h apart. The system has been applied successfully in children as young as 6 years old with doses of 25 µg/kg. Intranasal butorphanol is also used to manage migraine attacks. However, abuse problems are considerable.

Properties of the ideal transdermal and transmucosal drug are shown in Table 31.3.

Patient-controlled intranasal analgesia (PCINA) devices

A nasal aerosol spray with a premetered dose of 0.09 ml has been tested for both fentanyl and meperidine (pethidine). The device does not provide any lock-out time.

The Baxter PCINA on-demand system consists of a mechanically driven infusor, a flow restrictor tube, and a patient-controlled module for bolus administration. The product is a modification of the intravenous Baxter PCA system. The delivered bolus volume is accurate and the device is easy to use.[19]* A bolus volume of 0.5 ml (= 25 µg fentanyl) is injected through a 26-gauge plastic cannula with the needle tip removed. The flow restrictor provides a flow rate of 2 ml/h or 5 ml/h and the lock-out interval equals 6 or 15 min.[19]*

Another PCINA device (Therapeutic Goods Administration approval number 54005, Go Medical, Subiaco, 6008 Western Australia) is now commercially available.[16]* (Fig. 31.1A and B). The bottle is filled with 200 µg (4 ml) of fentanyl or 200 mg (4 ml) of meperidine. One bolus dose equals 9 µg fentanyl or 9 mg meperidine. The patient should therefore be carefully instructed that repeated doses are required for pain control. Every 4 min fentanyl or meperidine may be aspirated from the reservoir bot-

Table 31.3 *Properties of the ideal transdermal and transmucosal drug*

Highly potent
Highly water and lipid soluble
Not irritating to skin, mucosa, or cilia
Unaffected by enzymes in the epidermis and mucosa
Stable at room temperature[4]

A

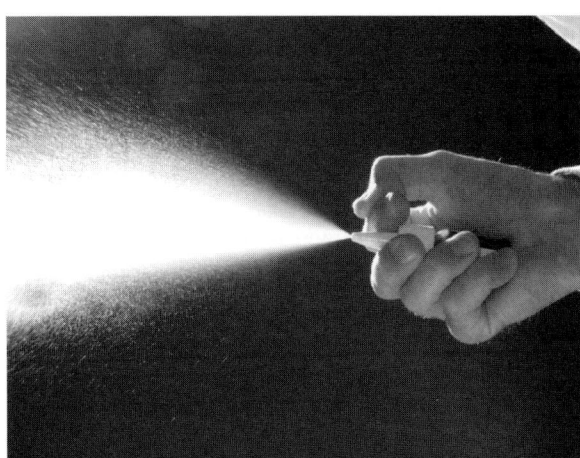

B

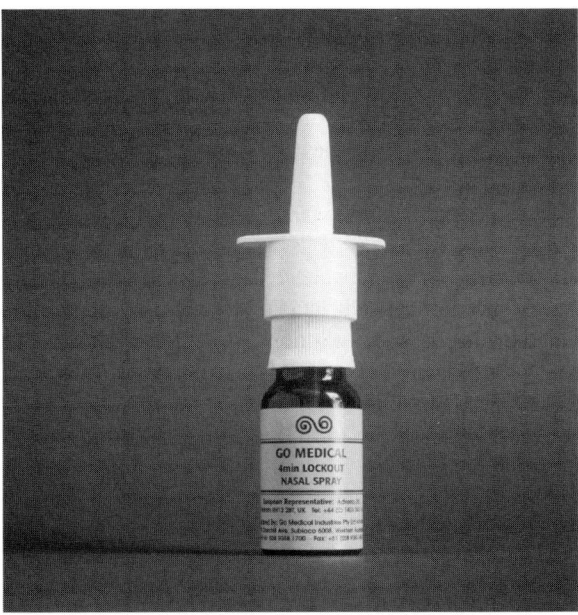

Figure 31.1 *Intranasal PCA (PCINA) gives equivalent pain control and patient satisfaction to i.v. administration. PCINA devices are now commercially available.*

tle through a resistance tube into a chamber of 0.18 ml with a maximal filling rate of 0.19 ml per 4 min. With frequent pressing of the button (i.e. more than 15 demands per hour) the maximum hourly dose may reach 142.5 mg meperidine or 142.5 µg fentanyl. The safety features seem to be similar to those of i.v. PCA. A special screw top demonstrates whether the bottle has been opened or tampered with. The device provides finer droplets at 80 µm, which improve the bioavailability and reduce the incidence of bitter and burning taste after meperidine administration. The Go Medical PCINA device may be stored in a standard locked cupboard (Table 31.4).

Buccal and sublingual delivery systems

A new delivery system for fentanyl was introduced in 1992; oral transmucosal fentanyl citrate (OTFC) ("lollipop"). The active drug is incorporated into a dissolvable matrix on a stick. OTFC provides rapid and noninvasive analgesia with an onset time of 5–15 min. Bioavailability is greater and absorption more rapid than with oral administration.[20*] Doses of 0.5–1 mg or 15–20 µg/kg provide adequate analgesia in adults. One milligram of OTFC is equivalent to 5 mg of morphine i.v.[20*] OTFC in units containing 200, 400, 600, 800, 1,200, or 1,600 µg of fentanyl citrate (Oralet® and Actiq®) is rapidly gaining in popularity. In cancer patients on controlled-release opioids, OTFC may act as a PCA treatment for "breakthrough pain"[21**] (Fig. 31.2).

Oral bedside PCA

The issues of autonomy and control are equally important for patients receiving traditional oral opioids. A bedside reservoir of analgesics ("oral bedside PCA") may indeed provide more autonomy and improved analgesia for selected patients in the late postoperative period.[22*]

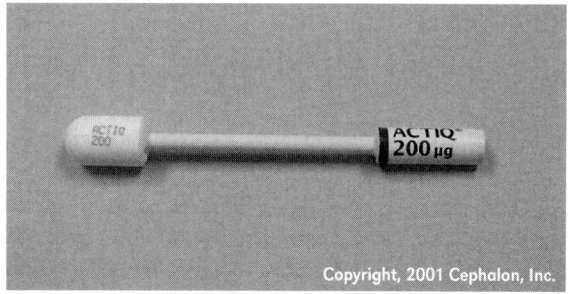
Copyright, 2001 Cephalon, Inc.

Figure 31.2 *A new delivery system for oral transmucosal fentanyl administration (Actiq®). The active drug is incorporated into a dissolvable matrix on a stick.*

CONTRAINDICATIONS AND LIMITATIONS

Previous allergic and serious adverse reactions exclude transdermal and transmucosal delivery. To minimize the risk of intentional and accidental overdose, the monitoring should be the same as for i.v. PCA. Whether an intravenous line is necessary is controversial[23*] (Table 31.5). Make sure that Actiq® and more lollipop-like devices are kept out of the reach of children.

SUMMARY

Both the skin and the mucosa are promising routes for drug administration. New transdermal and transmucosal delivery systems have been shown to provide postoperative pain relief with adverse effects similar to those of i.v. administration. It should be borne in mind that a bedside reservoir of analgesics ("oral bedside PCA") may provide autonomy and adequate analgesia in the later postoperative period.

Table 31.4 *PCA system characteristics*

Baxter PCINA device
Bolus volume: 0.5 ml = 25 µg fentanyl
Lock-out interval: 6 or 15 min
To avoid cross-infection the device is for single-patient use only
The bottle must be kept vertical for 5 min after use to ensure refilling

Go Medical PCINA device
Bolus volume: 0.18 ml (9 µg fentanyl, 9 mg meperidine)
Lock-out interval: 4 min
Repeated doses are required for pain control

Table 31.5 *Adverse reactions to and complications of transdermal, intranasal, and oral transmucosal opioid administration*

The incidence of adverse events is similar to that of i.v. opioid therapy[15**]
Skin reactions after transdermal administration are mild and seem to be well tolerated[9**]
Clinically relevant respiratory depression is rare[9**]
Higher doses of intranasal meperidine are associated with a bitter taste[17]
No significant changes in nasal mucosa are observed[24*]
The most important side-effects include pruritus, nausea, vomiting, dizziness, dry mouth, respiratory depression

REFERENCES

1. Cohen FL. Postsurgical pain relief: patients' status and nurses' medication choices. *Pain* 1980; **9:** 265–74.

2. Lehmann KA, Henn C. Status of postoperative pain therapy in West Germany. Results of a representative survey. *Anaesthesist* 1987; **36:** 400–6.

● 3. Stanley TH. New routes of administration and new delivery systems of anesthetics. *Anesthesiology* 1988; **68:** 665–8.

● 4. Biddle C, Gilliland C. Transdermal and transmucosal administration of pain-relieving and anxiolytic drugs: a primer for the critical care practitioner. *Heart Lung* 1992; **21:** 115–24.

5. Worsley MH, MacLeod AD, Brodie MJ, *et al.* Inhaled fentanyl as a method of analgesia [see comments]. *Anaesthesia* 1990; **45:** 449–51.

6. Higgins MJ, Asbury AJ, Brodie MJ. Inhaled nebulised fentanyl for postoperative analgesia. *Anaesthesia* 1991; **46:** 973–6.

7. Duthie DJ, Rowbotham DJ, Wyld R, *et al.* Plasma fentanyl concentrations during transdermal delivery of fentanyl to surgical patients. *Br J Anaesth* 1988; **60:** 614–18.

8. Rowbotham DJ, Wyld R, Peacock JE, *et al.* Transdermal fentanyl for the relief of pain after upper abdominal surgery. *Br J Anaesth* 1989; **63:** 56–9.

◆ 9. Gupta SK, Bernstein KJ, Noorduin H, *et al.* Fentanyl delivery from an electrotransport system: delivery is a function of total current, not duration of current. *J Clin Pharmacol* 1998; **38:** 951–8.

10. Sevarino FB, Paige D, Sinatra RS, Silverman DG. Postoperative analgesia with parenteral opioids: does continuous delivery utilizing a transdermal opioid preparation affect analgesic efficacy or patient safety? *J Clin Anesth* 1997; **9:** 173–8.

11. Nimmo WS. Fentanyl, absorption from Transfenta® on-demand doses delivered by various currents in healthy volunteers [Abstract]. Annual Scientific Meeting of the American Pain Society, San Diego, 1998.

12. Gupta SK. Transdermal electrotransport system appears feasible in feeding fentanyl. *Anesthesiology Topics.* ASTRA Professional Science Distribution 1998; **17** (3).

13. Bell MD, Murray GR, Mishra P, *et al.* Buccal morphine – a new route for analgesia? *Lancet* 1985; **1:** 71–3.

14. Scavone JM, Greenblatt DJ, Friedman H, Shader RI. Enhanced bioavailability of triazolam following sublingual versus oral administration. *J Clin Pharmacol* 1986; **26:** 208–10.

◆ 15. Striebel HW, Pommerening J, Rieger A. Intranasal fentanyl titration for postoperative pain management in an unselected population. *Anaesthesia* 1993; **48:** 753–7.

◆ 16. O'Neil G, Paech M, Wood F. Preliminary clinical use of a patient-controlled intranasal analgesia (PCINA) device. *Anaesth Intensive Care* 1997; **25:** 408–12.

◆ 17. Striebel HW, Bonillo B, Schwagmeier R, *et al.* Self-administered intranasal meperidine for postoperative pain management. *Can J Anaesth* 1995; **42:** 287–91.

18. Abboud TK, Zhu J, Gangolly J, *et al.* Transnasal butorphanol: A new method for pain relief in post-cesarean section pain. *Acta Anaesthesiol Scand* 1991; **35:** 14–18.

19. Striebel HW, Romer M, Philippi W, Schwagmeier R. A device for patient-controlled intranasal analgesia (PCINA). *Schmerz* 1995; **9** (2): 84–8.

20. Stanley TH, Hague B, Mock DL, *et al.* Oral transmucosal fentanyl citrate (lollipop) premedication in human volunteers. *Anesth Analg* 1989; **69:** 21–7.

◆ 21. Portenoy RK, Payne R, Coluzzi P, *et al.* Oral transmucosal fentanyl citrate (OTFC) for the treatment of breakthrough pain in cancer patients: a controlled dose titration study. *Pain* 1999; **79:** 303–12.

22. Litman RS, Shapiro BS. Oral patient-controlled analgesia in adolescents. *J Pain Symptom Manage* 1992; **7** (2): 78–81.

23. Joly LM, Lentschener C, Benhamou D. Patient-controlled intranasal analgesia. *Anesth Analg* 1997; **85:** 465.

24. Hermens WA, Merkus FW. The influence of drugs on nasal ciliary movement. *Pharm Res* 1987; **4:** 445–9.

PART VIII

Epidural and spinal analgesia – protocols and charts

Epidural analgesia for acute pain, including patient-controlled epidural analgesia

HARALD BREIVIK

Thoracic or lumbar epidural catheter?	409
Risks to the patient from epidural analgesia	410
Optimizing efficacy and safety of epidural analgesia	410
Epinephrine markedly increases the effectiveness of the epidural analgesic infusion	412
Epinephrine markedly increases safety of bupivacaine and fentanyl epidural analgesia	412
Epidural epinephrine does not decrease spinal cord blood flow	412
Epinephrine is of utmost importance in the efficacy and safety of prolonged postoperative epidural analgesia	413
Prescription for safe and effective epidural analgesia and patient-controlled epidural analgesia for postoperative pain relief	413
Necessary requirement for a successful postoperative pain management program	414
Alternative epidural analgesic mixtures	415
Epidural analgesia after abdominoperineal or lower limb surgery	415
References	415

The outcome after major surgery can be improved by relieving dynamic pain. The intense pain provoked by deep breathing, coughing, or moving a body part affected by surgery can be relieved effectively only with continuous neuraxial or peripheral nerve blocks. This enables patients to breathe deeply and cough, thereby preventing retention of secretions and development of atelectasis, pneumonia, and sepsis. Reducing dynamic pain will also enable the patients to perform active movements of limbs after orthopedic surgery, hastening rehabilitation of normal function. Thus, continuous cervical/brachial plexus blockade with catheter techniques and infusions of local anesthetics provides excellent analgesia and improves circulation and mobility of the upper extremity after shoulder, arm, or hand surgery.[1] Epidural or continuous femoral nerve block enables patients to move their lower limbs more during the early days after major knee surgery.[2**] This results in a more rapid rehabilitation than with intravenous (i.v.) patient-controlled analgesia (PCA) with morphine.[2**] Epidural analgesia as well as intercostal nerve blocks improve pulmonary function and reduce pulmonary complications after thoracic and upper abdominal surgery.[3***]

Epidural analgesia with a local anesthetic is the most effective. Epidural local anesthetics, with or without opioids, decrease the risk ratio of developing postoperative pulmonary complications such as atelectasis and pneumonia by 50–70% compared with systemic opioids.[3***] Epidural opioids alone do not always reduce the risk of postoperative pulmonary complications.[3***,4***] Thus, it is important to realize that a local anesthetic is needed in an epidural infusion in order to improve pulmonary functions after major surgery.

This is also true for gastrointestinal motility after abdominal surgery: an epidural local anesthetic (and an epidural local anesthetic with an opioid) shortens the time of intestinal paralysis after surgery compared with i.v. morphine PCA or epidural morphine alone.[4**,5,6**,7]

THORACIC OR LUMBAR EPIDURAL CATHETER?

It is now well established that a thoracic epidural is beneficial for patients who are at high risk of cardiac or pulmonary complications after thoracic or major abdominal surgery.[3***,5,8,9] Postoperative myocardial infarction, respiratory and renal failure, stroke, and mortality were reduced by perioperative thoracic epidural analgesia,[4] but not by lumbar anesthesia and analgesia.[10–13] A recent double-blind comparison of thoracic epidural (bupivacaine plus fentanyl) and i.v. fentanyl PCA did not find any differences in dynamic pain or outcome after abdominal aortic aneurysm surgery, but nor did it document (owing to the blinding procedure) that the catheter remained in the epidural space.[14] Even in the best of hands, there is at least a 10% catheter failure rate, which may be as high as 50% during the first few days after surgery.[15] The authors also used a low thoracic position (T10–11) of the epidural catheter, which does not give optimal myocardial protection.

Thoracic epidural analgesia containing a local anesthetic:[9]

- dilates stenotic coronary arteries and increases myocardial oxygen supply;
- decreases myocardial oxygen consumption;
- decreases myocardial ischemic events and postoperative myocardial infarction;
- improves lung function and oxygenation;
- improves gastrointestinal motility.

On the other hand, lumbar epidural analgesia with a local anesthetic:[9]

- dilates arteries of the lower part of body;
- constricts coronary arteries;
- decreases myocardial oxygen supply;
- causes leg weakness and urinary retention;
- does not improve gastrointestinal motility.[7]

Thus, a lumbar epidural may even increase the cardiac risk and does not improve either pulmonary function or gastrointestinal motility. Lack of awareness of these important differences between thoracic/thoracolumbar and lumbar epidural analgesia is one obvious reason for the confusion and conflicting opinions regarding the effects of epidural analgesia on outcome after surgery.[8-13,15-17]

RISKS TO THE PATIENT FROM EPIDURAL ANALGESIA

Even with the epidural catheter in a low thoracic or thoracolumbar area, if an excessive dose of a local anesthetic is administered epidurally, the patient may develop:

- orthostatic hypotension;
- motor blockade;
- urinary retention.

If an excessive dose of an opioid is administered epidurally, the following may occur:

- respiratory depression (immediate as well as late);
- increased incidence and severity of itching;
- nausea.

Rare, but potentially catastrophic complications are:

- epidural bleeding;
- epidural infection.

Leg weakness and back pain are early warning symptoms of impending catastrophic complications. It is essential to have a regular monitoring regime to detect changes in leg weakness. Excessive doses of local anesthetic should be avoided in the lumbar or thoracolumbar epidural as motor blockade may occur, concealing early signs of spinal cord compression/ischemia.[18,19]

OPTIMIZING EFFICACY AND SAFETY OF EPIDURAL ANALGESIA

The efficacy and safety of epidural analgesia is optimized by exploiting the principle of synergy[20,21]*** in combining two or more drugs with different mechanisms of analgesia and different side-effect profiles.

For more than a decade, we have successfully managed over 13,000 patients who underwent major surgery[21] using a combination of the following low concentrations of drugs:

- a local anesthetic (bupivacaine 1 mg/ml);
- an opioid (fentanyl 2 µg/ml);
- an adrenergic agonist [epinephrine (adrenaline) 2 µg/ml].

These three drugs cause spinal cord analgesia by three separate mechanisms acting on the pain impulse transmission process in the spinal cord. Fentanyl and epinephrine (like clonidine) act on pre- and postsynaptic opioid receptors and α_2-receptors, respectively, to inhibit pain impulse transmission from the primary afferent nociceptive neurons to the interneurons and transmission neurons in the dorsal horn of the spinal cord. Subanesthetic doses of bupivacaine inhibit excitatory synaptic mechanisms in the same area of the spinal cord.

Exploiting their synergistic antinociceptive effects, concurrent administration of these three pain-inhibiting drugs allows a reduction in the dose of each drug (Figs 32.1 and 32.2).[22**,23**,24*] The three drugs have different side-effects. Therefore, the overall risks of adverse effects are reduced. This is true for respiratory depression, nausea, itching, decreased gastrointestinal motility, sedation, hypotension, urinary retention, motor blockade, and leg weakness.[21,22,23**,24**]

- Nurses on the surgical wards titrate the infusion rate of the epidural analgesic mixture.
- Patients, when awake and coherent, with stable cardiorespiratory functions, are allowed to use the dose administration button of the patient-controlled infusion pump to give themselves boluses when needed.

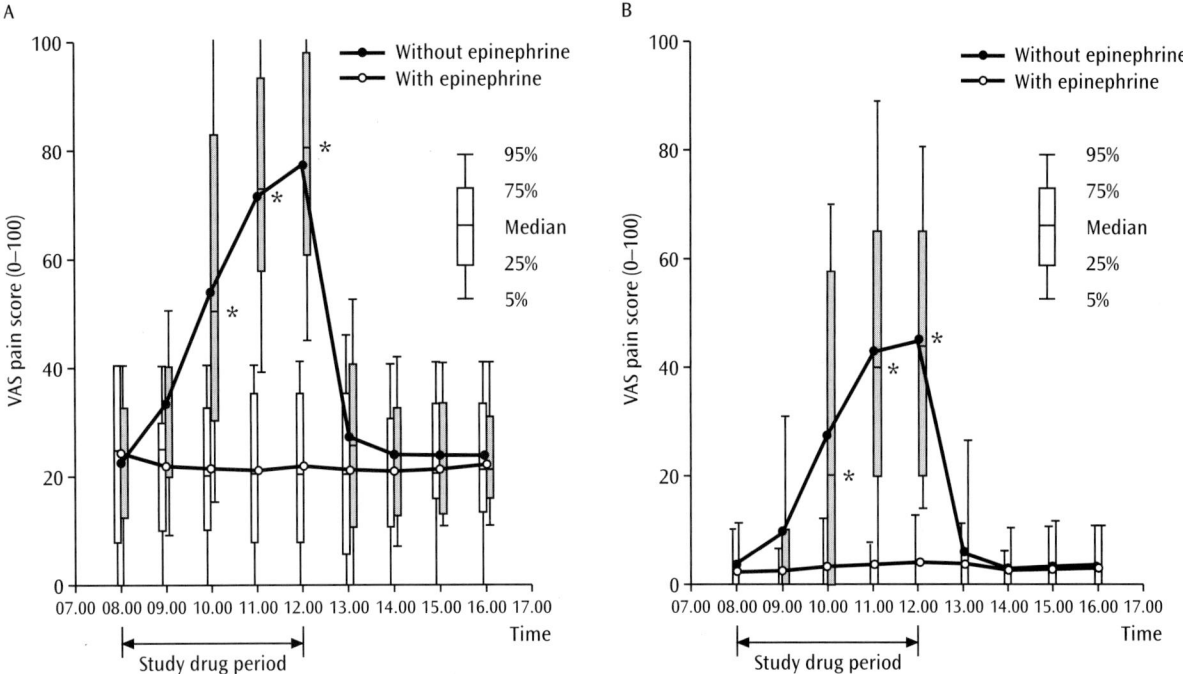

Figure 32.1 *Double-blind, crossover study documenting the marked potentiation by epinephrine (adrenaline) of epidural analgesia from bupivacaine and fentanyl. Visual analog scale (VAS) scores of pain intensity when coughing (A) and pain at rest (B) after major thoracic or abdominal surgery during infusion of epidural analgesic mixture containing bupivacaine 1 mg/ml and fentanyl 2 µg/ml with or without epinephrine 2 µg/ml. Reproduced with permission from Niemi and Breivik.[22]*

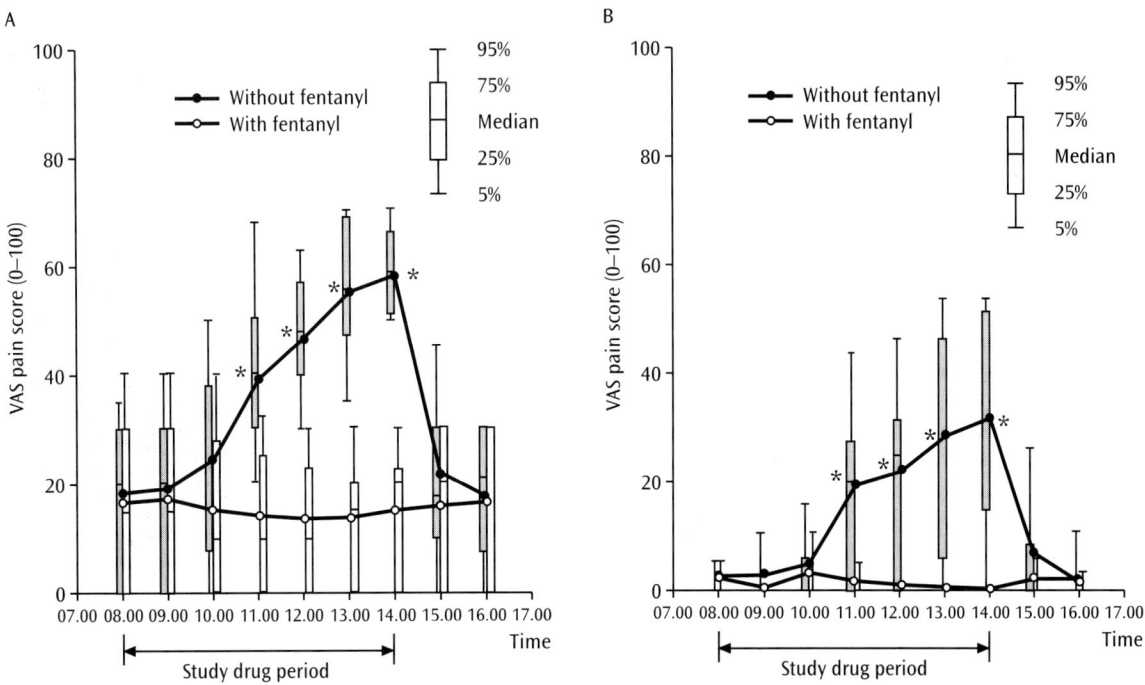

Figure 32.2 *Double-blind, crossover study documenting the marked potentiation by fentanyl of epidural analgesia from bupivacaine and epinephrine (adrenaline). Visual analog scale (VAS) scores of pain intensity when coughing (A) and pain at rest (B) after major thoracic or abdominal surgery during infusion of epidural analgesic mixture containing bupivacaine 1 mg/ml and epinephrine 2 µg/ml with or without fentanyl 2 µg/ml. Reproduced with permission from Niemi and Breivik.[23]*

EPINEPHRINE MARKEDLY INCREASES THE EFFECTIVENESS OF THE EPIDURAL ANALGESIC INFUSION

Epinephrine has been administered with opioids and local anesthetics for epidural analgesia for vaginal and surgical deliveries.[25**,26**] We have used epinephrine in our standard epidural regimen to reduce the dose of local anesthetics with fentanyl. In a randomized, double-blind, crossover study, we documented the powerful effects of epinephrine in this regard.[22**] Pain intensity was practically zero during rest after major abdominal or thoracic surgery with this triple mixture of bupivacaine, fentanyl, and epinephrine (Fig. 32.1). When epinephrine was removed from the mixture, pain increased and, in spite of more patient-administered bolus epidural doses, i.v. rescue morphine was needed. When our standard mixture with epinephrine was reintroduced, pain relief again became optimal.

Similarly, pain during coughing was only mild after major thoracic and upper abdominal surgery when the triple mixture was infused (Fig. 32.1). When epinephrine was removed from the mixture, pain during deep breathing/coughing increased to severe intensity, but adding epinephrine again reduced cough-provoked pain to only mild pain (Fig. 32.1). In a study to establish optimal doses, we documented that epinephrine 0.5 μg/ml and 1.0 μg/ml had less effect on the efficacy of the analgesic mixture than did 1.5 μg/ml, which had almost the same effect as 2.0 μg/ml.[27]

Exactly the same findings have been reproduced in a recently completed randomized, double blind, crossover study of thoracic epidural analgesia with ropivacaine 1 mg/ml with fentanyl 2 μg/ml with or without epinephrine 2 μg/ml.[28]

EPINEPHRINE MARKEDLY INCREASES SAFETY OF BUPIVACAINE AND FENTANYL EPIDURAL ANALGESIA

Epinephrine is important for safety of prolonged epidural infusion of the analgesic mixture because absorption of fentanyl (and bupivacaine) into the systemic circulation is reduced. This is shown by a significantly lower serum concentration of fentanyl when epinephrine is added to the epidural infusion. With adrenaline 2 μg/ml, fentanyl is almost undetectable in serum.[22**] When epinephrine is removed from the epidural infusion, the serum fentanyl concentration increases and patients experience adverse effects from systemic absorption: sedation, nausea, and pruritus.[22**] Human error in programming epidural infusion pumps has occurred, with 10 times the prescribed infusion rate (80 ml/h instead of 8 ml/h) being administered to a patient for 3 h before the error

was detected. Besides a profound analgesia and weak legs, no systemic adverse effects occurred (G. Niemi and H. Breivik, personal communication). Epinephrine, unlike the more specific α₂-receptor agonist clonidine, does not cause sedation or hypotension;[29] furthermore, again unlike clonidine, it causes epidural vasoconstriction and less systemic resorption of concurrently administered drugs.[22,30]

EPIDURAL EPINEPHRINE DOES NOT DECREASE SPINAL CORD BLOOD FLOW

Epidural epinephrine 2 μg/ml at 5–15 ml/h does not decrease spinal cord blood flow. The potent constrictive action of epinephrine on vessels outside the central nervous system has led to misunderstanding and unfounded concern about the blood supply to the spinal cord when administering epinephrine-containing epidural infusions. There are, however, no human data supporting this concern, only misinterpreted case histories in which a temporal association with epidural or subarachnoidal administration of epinephrine has been interpreted as the cause of spinal cord ischemia.[31]

Epinephrine has been used with spinal anesthetics for decades without any clinical spinal cord dysfunction being observed.[31***,32***] In 20 patients undergoing gynecological laparoscopy under selective spinal anesthesia with lidocaine (lignocaine) 10 mg and sufentanil 10 μg with and without epinephrine 50 μg, spinal cord function (spinothalamic, dorsal column, and motor) was well preserved, with or without epinephrine.[33**] Several animal studies have shown that administering subarachnoid epinephrine (up to 200-μg bolus) does not decrease spinal cord blood flow in cats or dogs.[34**,35**,36**] A recent study in dogs using a spinal-window preparation demonstrated a modest reduction (10.6%) in spinal pial vessel diameter produced by epinephrine 5 μg/ml – a small change that did not lead to a critical decrease in spinal cord blood flow.[37**]

However, epinephrine administered epidurally reduces the epidural blood flow markedly.[34**] Concentrations of epinephrine from 0.5 to 5 μg/ml have been found to be safe in epidural infusions.[26**,38**,39**,40**]

In a dose-determining study, we documented that epinephrine concentrations of 0.5 μg/ml or 1.0 μg/ml were less effective than 1.5 and 2 μg/ml in potentiating epidural analgesia from bupivacaine and fentanyl. There was no significant difference between 1.5 and 2 μg/ml (G. Niemi and H. Breivik, personal communication). Therefore, we chose a concentration of epinephrine of 2 μg/ml to minimize any unknown spinal cord adverse effects related to a continuous epidural epinephrine infusion. With this background and our own extensive clinical experience with epinephrine in our standard triple-component epidural analgesic infusion,[21*,41*] we are convinced that the minute dose of epinephrine (about 20 μg/h) is not only advantageous for its analgesic effect but is also very safe in this respect.

EPINEPHRINE IS OF UTMOST IMPORTANCE IN THE EFFICACY AND SAFETY OF PROLONGED POSTOPERATIVE EPIDURAL ANALGESIA

There are several positive interactions which occur between epinephrine and the two other components:

- Epinephrine reduces systemic absorption of opioids and local anesthetics, thereby decreasing the systemic adverse effects of fentanyl and bupivacaine. More of these two drugs may therefore pass through the meninges to the cerebrospinal fluid (CSF) and spinal cord, where important aspects of analgesic action occur.
- Epinephrine, being an α_2-agonist, has an analgesic effect of its own in the spinal cord.[42]**
- Epinephrine synergistically potentiates the analgesic effect of bupivacaine and fentanyl.

PRESCRIPTION FOR SAFE AND EFFECTIVE EPIDURAL ANALGESIA AND PATIENT-CONTROLLED EPIDURAL ANALGESIA FOR POSTOPERATIVE PAIN RELIEF

Our prescriptions for safe and effective epidural and patient-controlled epidural analgesia, which we have practiced now for more than a decade at the University Clinic Pain Services of Rikshospitalet, Oslo, Norway, and Inselspital, Berne, Switzerland, are summarized below. More details and background can be found in several key references.[21–24,41,43,44]

Epidural analgesia

- Use a thoracic or thoracolumbar epidural catheter for major thoracic and abdominal surgery.
- Use a triple-component analgesic mixture with low doses of a local anesthetic, an opioid, and an adrenergic agonist:
  - bupivacaine 1 mg/ml;
  - fentanyl 2 μg/ml;
  - epinephrine 2 μg/ml.
- Use a closed system with a 550-ml bag and a remote administration set in an electronically controlled and driven, tamper-proof, PCA infusion pump (Fig. 32.3).
- Use nurse-adjusted epidural analgesia infusion rates of 5–10 ml/h and patient-controlled rescue bolus injections (4 ml up to twice per hour), but only when the patient is alert, coherent, and has stable cardio-respiratory vital functions. The infusion rate and catheter site determine the segmental spread of the epidural analgesia. Epidural bolus doses will only deepen and strengthen the intensity of analgesia.
- The nurses on the surgical wards monitor and record the following every 4 h:
  - sensory levels – upper and lower (using cold stimuli, e.g. ice cube in plastic glove);
  - motor function (any leg weakness?);
  - pain intensity during rest and movement (using a five-point verbal categorical rating scale);

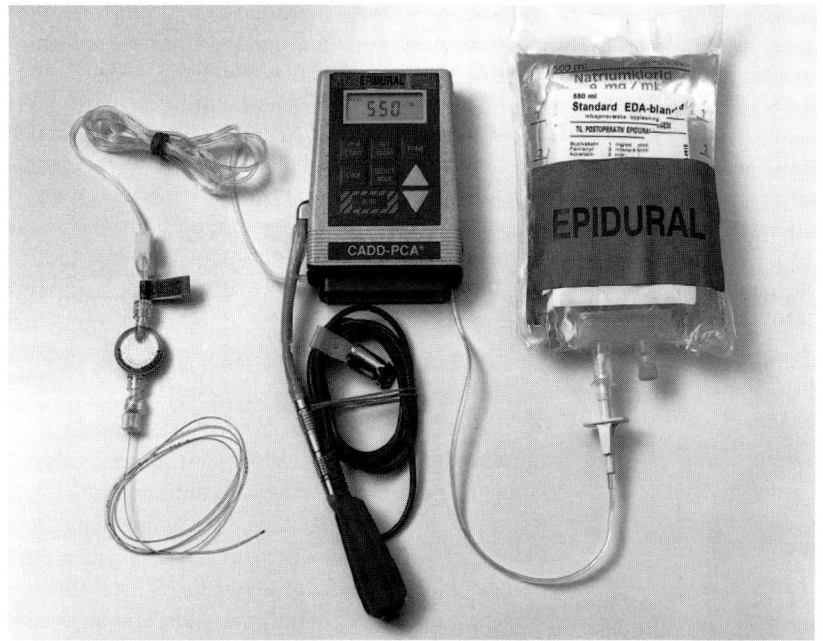

Figure 32.3 *A closed system for delivering the epidural analgesic mixture. A 550-ml bag prepared by our hospital pharmacy and Fresenius-Kabi, Halden, Norway, contains bupivacaine 1 mg/ml, fentanyl 2 μg/ml, and epinephrine (adrenaline) 2 μg/ml. This solution is stable for several months.*[44] *The epidural analgesic mixture is delivered at a constant infusion of 5–10 ml/h, titrated by the nurses on the surgical ward through a Deltec CADD pump. If more analgesia is required, the patient is allowed to self-administer a rescue analgesic bolus dose of usually 4 ml, up to twice per hour. This is possible only when the patient is awake, clear-headed, and has stable cardiorespiratory vital signs.*

– sedation;
– respiratory rate;
– systolic blood pressure;
– drug consumption;
– occurrence of any side-effects.
• Nurses pay strict attention to sterile technique in caring for epidural catheters and line connections.

With our reliable, closed infusion pump system, adverse effects such as major respiratory depression and hypotension (in normovolemic patients) are practically eliminated. There is only minimal motor block in a few patients with low thoracic or lumbar catheters. *However, epidural bleeding and infection are always potential risks:* [18,19]

• Everyone involved in the care of these patients must be prepared to look for *early signs of infection or hematoma in the epidural space:*
  – new backache;
  – leg weakness.
  or increasing leg weakness in the few cases with some motor blockade from the epidural bupivacaine in low thoracic or lumbar segmental epidural catheters (usually erroneously too low).
• Everyone involved in the care of postoperative epidural analgesia patients should have a *high awareness of the need for urgent magnetic resonance imaging (MRI) or computed tomography (CT) scan* to verify diagnosis if there is any suspicion of spinal canal bleeding or infection and the need to expedite appropriate intervention. [18,19]

Outcome

By the end of 2001, we had prospectively followed more than 13,000 patients having epidural analgesia after major surgery for more than 55,000 postoperative patient–days.

• Approximately 90% of the patients have been satisfied with the pain relief they received.
• Technical problems with the epidural catheter are reasons for unsatisfactory results in about 10% of patients. This varies considerably with the experience of the anesthesiologist placing the epidural catheter and the pain nurse and anesthesiologist monitoring the postoperative epidural analgesia.
• We have had 11 potentially serious complications, i.e. less than one per 1,000 patients and less than one per 5,000 patient–days. These were:
  – Bleeding in one patient in whom the epidural catheter was removed (on direct orders from the surgeon) about 2 h after low-molecular-weight heparin was given subcutaneously.
  – Epidural abscess in one patient, a paravertebral abscess in another patient, and epidural catheter

tract infections without abscess formation in eight patients.

All of these were discovered early, treated successfully, and none of the patients had permanent neurological complications. We have had no patients with severe respiratory depression during epidural analgesia using our protocol. However, one patient had an i.v. morphine PCA line erroneously connected to an epidural catheter, and another patient had fentanyl 100 μg epidural bolus doses erroneously prescribed by a junior doctor. These two patients developed respiratory depression as a result of human errors; however, both were discovered early and were successfully treated with repeated naloxone injections.

Thus, the way we are monitoring patients having epidural analgesia has proved effective in busy wards and our protocol appears to ensure the patient's safety.

NECESSARY REQUIREMENT FOR A SUCCESSFUL POSTOPERATIVE PAIN MANAGEMENT PROGRAM

One important lesson from the last decade of experience with acute postoperative pain relief, using epidural analgesia as well as intravenous opioid patient-controlled analgesia and upgraded "low-technology" traditional pain relief, is that in order to have a successful postoperative epidural pain management service, the following factors need to be taken into account:

• A minimum number of dedicated pain personnel: at least one pain nurse supported by an anesthesiologist who is able to spend most of his/her time on postoperative pain management.
• Through an – always ongoing – educational program, the nurses on the surgical wards have to learn, and relearn, how to monitor and manage pain. There should be standard orders on how to adjust treatment, how to look out for early symptoms of potentially harmful adverse effect, and how to prevent and treat such adverse effects.
• This is an instrument for continuous quality improvement, such that all patients will have better pain control, i.e. not only those who benefit from high-skill, high-technology, postoperative epidural analgesia or i.v. opioid PCA but also those who require only low-technology approaches. [21]
• To exploit fully the beneficial effects of optimal epidural analgesia on outcome of major surgery, only a labor-intensive monitoring and continuous quality improvement regimen will secure ongoing dynamic pain relief for 4–7 days after surgery; [10,21] a failure rate of the epidural catheter of 43% before 3 days' after surgery is definitely not optimal epidural analgesia. [45]

ALTERNATIVE EPIDURAL ANALGESIC MIXTURES

There are many alternative recipes for postoperative epidural analgesia. Ropivacaine[28] is an alternative to bupivacaine, being less cardiotoxic but more expensive. When coadministering bupivacaine with fentanyl and epinephrine for epidural infusion analgesia, very low doses are required so that cardiotoxicity is not an issue.[21]

Sufentanil is more potent than fentanyl, it is well documented and approved for epidural administration in several countries. With epinephrine and bupivacaine, sufentanil appears to function as well as fentanyl.[26] It is more expensive than fentanyl and our hospital pharmacy is still not able to obtain sufentanil (or ropivacaine) in dry form for our triple-component epidural mixture.

Morphine or diamorphine and bupivacaine, with or without epinephrine, may be a bit less sensitive to optimal segmental siting of the epidural catheter, but nausea and pruritus often reduce the quality of analgesia.[15]

EPIDURAL ANALGESIA AFTER ABDOMINOPERINEAL OR LOWER LIMB SURGERY

Prolonged epidural analgesia after lower abdominal or abdominoperineal surgery or major orthopedic surgery of the lower limb requires balancing the composition of the epidural analgesic mixture with segmental siting of the epidural catheter. A lumbar epidural catheter with a local anesthetic-containing epidural infusion will easily cause cauda equina nerve root anesthesia with motor blockade and leg weakness. For opioid and adrenergic components to affect dorsal horn pain transmission, the catheter has to be placed above L2 for a low-dose infusion to reach the spinal cord.

With our standard triple-component epidural solution, we have obtained the best results (best analgesia with least leg weakness) for perineal pain by placing the catheter at the thoracolumbar or upper lumbar levels.[24]

REFERENCES

1. Brown DL, Bridenbaugh LD. The upper extremity. Somatic block. In: Cousins MJ, Bridenbaugh PO eds. *Neural Blockade in Clinical Anesthesia and Management of Pain*, 3rd edn. Philadelphia, PA: Lippincott-Raven, 1998: 345–71.

2. Capdevila X, Barthelet Y, Biboulet P, *et al*. Effects of perioperative analgesic technique on the surgical outcome and duration of rehabilitation after major knee surgery. *Anesthesiology* 1999; **91**: 8–15.

3. Ballantyne JC, Carr DB, deFerranti S, *et al*. The comparative effects of postoperative analgesic therapies on pulmonary outcome: cumulative meta-analyses of randomized, controlled trials. *Anesth Analg* 1998; **86**: 598–612.

4. Park WY, Thomson JS, Lee KK. Effect of epidural anesthesia and analgesia on perioperative outcome. A randomized, controlled veterans affairs cooperative study. *Ann Surg* 2001; **234**: 560–71.

5. Wattwil M, Thoren T, Hennerdal S, Garvill J-E. Epidural analgesia with bupivacaine reduces postoperative paralytic ileus after hysterectomy. *Anesth Analg* 1989; **68**: 353–8.

6. Liu SS, Carpenter RL, Meal JM. Epidural anesthesia and analgesia: their role in postoperative outcome. *Anesthesiology* 1995; **82**: 1474–506.

7. Liu SS, Carpenter RL, Mackey DC, *et al*. Effects of perioperative analgesic technique on rate of recovery after colon surgery. *Anesthesiology* 1995; **83**: 757–65.

8. Steinbrook RA. Epidural anesthesia and gastrointestinal motility. *Anesth Analg* 1998; **86**: 837–44.

9. Van Aken H, Gogarten W, Rolf N. Epidural anesthesia in cardiac risk patients. *Anesth Analg* 1999; 89 (Review Course Suppl.): 104–10.

10. Breivik H. Postoperative pain management: why is it difficult to show that it improves outcome? *Eur J Anaesthesiol* 1998; **15**: 748–51.

11. Rodgers A, Walker N, Schug S, Kehlet H. Reduction of postoperative mortality and morbidity with epidural or spinal anaesthesia: results from overview of randomised trials. *Br Med J* 2000; **321**: 1493–7.

12. Beatty WS, Badner NH, Choi P. Epidural analgesia reduces postoperative myocardial infarction: a meta-analysis. *Anesth Analg* 2001; **93**: 853–8.

13. Scott NB, Turfrey DJ, Ray DAA, *et al*. A prospective randomized study of the potential benefits of thoracic epidural anesthesia and analgesia in patients undergoing coronary artery bypass grafting. *Anesth Analg* 2001; **93**: 528–35.

14. Norris EJ, Beattie C, Perler BA, *et al*. Double-masked randomized trial comparing alternative combinations of intraoperative anesthesia and postoperative analgesia in abdominal aortic surgery. *Anesthesiology* 2001; **95**: 1054–67.

15. Wheatley RG, Schug SA, Watson D. Safety and efficacy of postoperative epidural analgesia. *Br J Anaesth* 2001; **87**: 47–61.

16. Stenseth R, Bjella L, Berg EM, *et al*. Thoracic epidural analgesia in aortocoronary bypass surgery: hemodynamic effects. *Acta Anaesthesiol Scand* 1994; **38**: 826–33.

17. Stenseth R, Berg EM, Bjella L, *et al*. Effects of thoracic epidural analgesia on coronary hemodynamics and myocardial metabolism in coronary artery bypass surgery. *J Cardiothorac Vas Anesth* 1995; **9**: 503–9.

18. Breivik H. Neurological complications in association

with spinal and epidural analgesia – again. *Acta Anaesthesiol Scand* 1998; **42:** 609–13.

● 19. Breivik H. Infectious complications of epidural anaesthesia and analgesia. *Curr Opin Anaesthesiol* 1999; **12:** 573–7.

● 20. Berenbaum MC. What is synergy? *Pharmacol Rev* 1989; **41:** 93–141.

● 21. Breivik H. *Progress in Pain Research and Management.* Seattle, WA: IASP Press, 2000: 787–807.

◆ 22. Niemi G, Breivik H. Adrenaline markedly improves thoracic epidural analgesia produced by a low-dose infusion of bupivacaine, fentanyl and adrenaline after major surgery. *Acta Anaesthesiol Scand* 1998; **42:** 897–909.

◆ 23. Niemi G, Breivik H. Epidural fentanyl markedly improves thoracic epidural analgesia in a low-dose infusion of bupivacaine, adrenaline and fentanyl. A randomized, double-blind crossover study with and without fentanyl. *Acta Anaesthesiol Scand* 2001; **45:** 221–32.

◆ 24. Breivik H, Niemi G, Haugtomt H, Högström H. Optimal epidural analgesia: importance of drug combinations and correct segmental site of injection. *Bailliere's Clin Anaesthesiol* 1995; **9:** 493–512.

◆ 25. Cohen S, Armar D, Pantuck CB, *et al.* Epidural patient-controlled analgesia after cesarean section buprenorphine–0.015% bupivacaine with epinephrine versus fentanyl–0.015% bupivacaine with and without epinephrine. *Anesth Analg* 1992; **74:** 226–30.

◆ 26. Cohen S, Armar D, Pantuck CB, *et al.* Postcesarean delivery epidural patient-controlled analgesia. Fentanyl or sufentanil? *Anesthesiology* 1993; **78:** 486–91.

27. Niemi G, Breivik H. The minimally effective concentration of adrenaline in a low-dose thoracic epidural infusion of bupivacaine and fentanyl after major thoracic and abdominal surgery. A randomised, double-blind dose-finding study. *Acta Anaesthesol Scand* 2002 (in press).

28. Niemi G, Breivik H. Epinephrine markedly improves thoracic epidural analgesia produced by a small-dose infusion of ropivacaine, fentanyl, and epinephrine after major thoracic or abdominal surgery: a randomized, double-blind crossover study with and without epinephrine. *Anesth Analg* 2002; **94:** 1598–605.

● 29. Paech MJ, Pavy TJ, Orlaikowski CE, *et al.* Postoperative epidural infusion: a randomized, double-blind, dose-finding trial of clonidine in combination with bupivacaine and fentanyl. *Anesth Analg* 1997; **84:** 1323–8.

◆ 30. Verborgh C, Van der Auwera C, Noorduin H, Camu F. Epidural sufentanil for postoperative pain relief: effects of adrenaline. *Eur J Anaesthesiol* 1988; **5:** 183–91.

● 31. Bromage PR. Neurologic complications of epidural and spinal techniques. *Bailliere's Clin Anaesthesiol* 1994; **7:** 793–815.

● 32. Hodgson PS, Neal JM, Pollock JE, Liu SS. The neurotoxicity of drugs given intrathecally (spinal). *Anesth Analg* 1999; **88:** 797–809.

◆ 33. Vaghadia H, Solylo MA, Henderson CL, Mitchell GW. Selective spinal anesthesia for outpatient laparoscopy. II. Epinephrine and spinal cord function. *Can J Anaesth* 2001; **48:** 261–6.

◆ 34. Kozody R, Palahniuk RJ, Wade JG, *et al.* The effect of subarachnoid epinephrine and phenylephrine on spinal cord blood flow. *Can Anaesth Soc J* 1984; **31:** 503–8.

◆ 35. Porter SS, Albin MS, Watson WA, *et al.* Spinal cord and cerebral blood flow responses to subarachnoid injection of local anesthetics with and without epinephrine. *Acta Anaesthesiol Scand* 1985; **29:** 330–8.

◆ 36. Dohi S, Takeshima R, Naito H. Spinal cord blood flow during spinal anesthesia in dogs: the effects of tetracaine, epinephrine, acute blood loss, and hypercapnia. *Anesth Analg* 1987; **66:** 599–606.

◆ 37. Iida H, Ohata H, Iida M, *et al.* Direct effects of alpha1- and alpha2-adrenergic agonists on spinal and cerebral pial vessels in dogs. *Anesthesiology* 1999; **91:** 479–85.

◆ 38. Baron CM, Kowalski SE, Greengrass R, *et al.* Epinephrine decreases postoperative requirements for continuous thoracic epidural fentanyl infusions. *Anesth Analg* 1996; **82:** 760–5.

◆ 39. Lysak SZ, Eisenach JC, Dobson CE. Patient-controlled epidural analgesia during labor: a comparison of three solutions with a continuous infusion control. *Anesthesiology* 1990; **72:** 44–9.

◆ 40. Sakaguchi Y, Sakura S, Shinzawa M, Saito Y. Does adrenaline improve epidural bupivacaine and fentanyl analgesia after abdominal surgery? *Anaesth Intensive Care* 2000; **28:** 522–6.

◆ 41. Breivik H, Högström H, Niemi G, *et al.* Safe and effective post-operative pain-relief: introduction and continuous quality-improvement of comprehensive post-operative pain management programmes. *Bailliere's Clin Anaesthesiol* 1995; **9:** 423–60.

◆ 42. Collins JG, Kitahata LM, Suzukawa M. Spinally administered epinephrine suppresses noxiously evoked activity of WDR neurons in the dorsal horn of the spinal cord. *Anesthesiology* 1984; **60:** 269–75.

● 43. Breivik H. Benefits, risks and economics of post-operative pain management programmes. *Bailliere's Clin Anaesthesiol* 1995; **9:** 403–22.

◆ 44. Kjønniksen I, Brustugun J, Niemi G, *et al.* Stability of an epidural analgesic solution containing adrenaline, bupivacaine and fentanyl. *Acta Anaesthesiol Scand* 2000; **44:** 864–7.

45. Rigg JRA, Jamrozik K, Myles PS, *et al.* Epidural anaesthesia and analgesia and outcome of major surgery: a randomized trial. *Lancet* 2002; **359:** 1276–82.

Epidural steroid injections for back pain and sciatica

EDWARD WALSH

Applied anatomy	417	Imaging techniques	422
Indications	418	Drugs used for epidural steroid injections	422
Contraindications	419	Complications	423
Number and frequency of injections	419	Evidence for a particular therapy or drug	424
Preparation	419	References	425
The technique of epidural steroid injection	420		

Epidural local anesthetics without steroids have been used since about 1903 for back pain and sciatica. Steroids, such as hydrocortisone, were added empirically to the local anesthetic in the 1950s because they were known to relieve joint pains. After 1972, depot steroids, such as methylprednisolone, became more widely used. Only later was a reason sought to explain the apparent beneficial action of steroids in the epidural space. As steroids have an anti-inflammatory effect, it was considered that they relieved some painful inflammatory process in the epidural space. This hypothesis has never been confirmed but it is now known that degenerative disks release inflammatory enzymes and chemicals into the epidural space and onto nerve roots and other sensitive tissues.[1] However, the exact mechanism of spinal nerve root pain is still poorly understood.

The first case report of an epidural steroid injection for sciatica was published by Robecchi and Capra[2] in 1952. Lievre et al.[3] published the first series of 20 patients in 1953. Many reports of epidural steroids followed in the world literature. The first publications in the English literature were in 1960.[4,5]

The first attempt at a randomized controlled double-blind trial of epidural steroids was carried out in 1973 by Dilke et al.[6] Since then, about 15 randomized, controlled trials of widely varied quality have been published. Not until 1997, 45 years after the first published epidural steroid injection, was a properly conducted randomized controlled trial carried out by Carette et al.[7]** using an imaging technique to confirm herniated disks.

Key points

- Epidural steroids have been used for nerve root pain for almost 50 years.
- Steroids were used empirically as nerve root inflammation was assumed.
- Only recently, have studies been carried out on patients with confirmed herniated disks.

APPLIED ANATOMY

A knowledge of the anatomy of the epidural space is assumed (see Preparation below). The relevant aspects of applied anatomy for epidural steroid injections are:

1. If the dura mater is punctured accidentally, it is possible that an inadvertent injection of the steroid preparation into the intrathecal space might occur, which might increase the risks of intrathecal toxicity and infection.
2. Steroid can be delivered at the level of disk herniation, usually L3/4 to L5/S1 by the lumbar approach. As the dura mater lies just anterior to the epidural space at these levels, careless technique can easily lead to dural

puncture. But, the presence of the herniated disk at the level of injection is thought unlikely to increase the risk of dural puncture as there is a segmentally occuring pyramidal space occupied by epidural fat lying beneath the ligamentum flavum.[8]

3 With the caudal approach, there is a reduced risk of dural puncture as the dura mater is some distance from the sacral hiatus. However, there is still a possibility of dural puncture, as anatomical variations do occur in the relation of the dura mater to the cephalad part of caudal epidural space.[8] By this route, the steroid is delivered further away from the lesion, so a larger volume may be needed. The site of entry for the caudal approach is nearer to the anus and perineum, both sources of potential infection.

4 Once in the epidural space, the steroid has to reach the site of the pathological process, namely the degenerating, herniated, or sequestered disk or the inflamed or compressed nerve root. These are situated anteriorly and laterally to the point of entry of the needle to the epidural space in the case of the lumbar route and anteriorly and superiorly in the caudal route. The steroid gets to the site of the lesion by virtue of the volume of the injectate and the pressure used. However, adhesions and septa may prevent the spread of steroid to the target site.

5 When the steroid does arrive at the site of the lesion, it may still have problems transferring across the poorly permeable anterior longitudinal ligament and other membranes that separate the epidural space from the affected disk or nerve root.

6 More is now known about the anatomy of the lumbar and caudal epidural space because of studies using magnetic resonance scans.[9,10] Such knowledge may help operators to reduce the risk of inadvertent intrathecal injection.

7 Also, more is known about the innervation of the lumbar dura mater and posterior longitudinal ligaments, which may explain why radicular-type pain may occur without a significantly herniated disk.[11]

Key points

- A knowledge of spinal and epidural anatomy is essential for safe practice.
- It is important to know the relations of the dura mater to avoid dural puncture and inadvertent intrathecal injection of the steroid preparation.

INDICATIONS

The only widely accepted indication is sciatica,[12,13] defined as a constant or intermittent pain in one or both legs, radiating below the knee, preferably with:

1 signs of nerve root irritation – a positive straight leg raising test (production or exacerbation of sciatica by raising the leg); *and/or*

2 signs of nerve root compression – motor, sensory, or reflex deficits; *and*

3 computed tomography (CT) or magnetic resonance imaging (MRI) scan evidence of a herniated disk at a level corresponding to the symptoms and clinical findings.

It is difficult to make a confident clinical diagnosis of nerve root pain as none of the tests that are part of the history and physical examination has high diagnostic accuracy.[14] An MRI scan can help in reaching a diagnosis of nerve root pain, but only to support clinical observations. About 20% of nonsymptomatic patients under 60 years and 36% of those over 60 years have herniated disks on MRI scanning.[15] Therefore, the presence of a prolapsed disk on MRI does not always mean that the disk is the cause of a patient's sciatic-type pain, especially if the symptoms and signs do not correlate with the MRI findings. An MRI scan may rule out other causes of spinal pathology, but these causes are rare and so this may not justify the additional expense.[8] There is also a poor correlation between MRI findings and response to epidural steroids.[8]

The following are not indications:

1 *Mechanical back pain.* Nerve root pain does not manifest itself as back pain alone. There is little to support the use of epidural steroids in this condition. None of the proposed mechanisms can logically explain how such spinal pain could be relieved by epidural steroids. Not all back pain has a spinal origin.

2 *Spinal stenosis.* In theory, epidural steroids may relieve some of the effects of spinal stenosis, but the underlying lesion is bony, joint, or ligamentum flavum overgrowth, which epidural steroids cannot be expected to resolve. The literature does not support epidural steroids for this indication.[16**,17**]

3 *Epidural fibrosis.* Much has been written about the use of epidural steroids in epidural fibrosis, but there is no good evidence to support their use. The hydrostatic effect of a large volume injection on the symptom of sciatica in epidural fibrosis may have more effect than the steroid.[18**,19**]

Attempts have been made to try to predict which patients are more likely to respond to epidural steroid injections.[20] Factors such as nonradicular pain, injury at work, and a long history of sciatica suggested a negative response.

Key points

- The only indication for epidural steroid injection is nerve root pain.

- Back pain alone is not an indication.

CONTRAINDICATIONS

The absolute and relative contraindications for epidural steroid injection can be divided into those relating to:

1 The epidural injection
   a Absolute
      i Preexisting infection at or near the injection site: risk of epidural sepsis.
      ii Bleeding disorder: risk of epidural hematoma and resultant compression of spinal cord or cauda equina.
      iii Anticoagulants if given in a therapeutic dose: risk as in a-ii.
   b Relative
      i Unusual anatomy: increased risk of dural tap and nerve damage.
      ii Previous spinal surgery at level of proposed injection: possible increased risk of dural tap and nerve root damage owing to distorted anatomy.
      iii Anticoagulants if given in a thromboprophylactic dose: risk as in a-ii.
      iv Medications affecting coagulation, e.g. aspirin: risk as in a-ii.
2 The local anesthetic (if used)
   a Absolute
      i Allergy to local anesthetics – risk of allergic reaction.
   b Relative: nil
3 The steroid
   a Absolute
      i Uncontrolled sepsis local or distant to the injection site: risk of exacerbating the infection and spread to the epidural space.
      ii History of tuberculosis: risk of reactivation.
   b Relative
      i Preexisting fluid retention where steroid-induced fluid retention might exacerbate heart failure: risk of increased congestive cardiac failure.
      ii Insulin-dependent diabetes mellitus: possible increased risk of infection.[21]
      iii Systemic steroids: possible increased risk of infection.[22]
      iv Where an increased stress is expected soon after a series of injections, for example major surgery, especially if a large dose of steroid is to be used (see complications): risk of hypotension secondary to steroid-induced adrenal suppression.
      v Pregnancy.

Key point

- A careful assessment must be made of the patient to be sure that there are no contraindications to epidural injection and use of steroids.

NUMBER AND FREQUENCY OF INJECTIONS

No optimal number or frequency of injection has been established.

Commonly, one to three injections are performed at weekly or 2-weekly intervals, as the effect of the steroid may persist for 10–14 days after each injection. For safety reasons, it is best not to exceed three injections in any one treatment series, so as to reduce the total period that the adrenal cortex may be depressed.

If the first injection provides no benefit or if the patient's symptoms are worse, then a second injection is unlikely to help.

Key point

- The optimal number and frequency of epidural steroid injections are not known.

PREPARATION

The patient

Before the day of injection

Epidural steroid injection remains a controversial treatment because its efficacy is unproven and the duration of benefit, safety, risks, side-effects, and complications are uncertain. It can also be difficult to be sure a patient's pain is really a nerve root pain. Furthermore, in this technique, a depot steroid is given for an indication and by a route not recommended in the product information sheet. It is necessary, therefore, for doctors carrying out epidural steroid injections to:

1 obtain a more informed consent from patients;
2 treat patients extra carefully;
3 realize that the manufacturer has no liability for any complications related to the steroid preparation. Operators, therefore, have to assume liability and should discuss this with their employer and/or insurers.

The following measures are recommended in preparing a patient for this treatment. They should be taken *before* the day of the procedure so that the patient has sufficient time to consider the information.

1 Ensure that the patient has an accepted indication for epidural steroid injection (see above).
2 If epidural steroid injections are to be used for other low back pain and leg pain conditions, they should preferably be given as part of a research project approved by an ethics committee.
3 The operator should:
   a have received training in the technique of epidural injection and specifically in the administration of epidural steroids;
   b be competent and practised in this technique – at least 20 epidural injections each year can be considered a minimum for safe practice;
   c be familiar with the literature on epidural steroids so that proper information can be given to the patient;
   d if he or she is a trainee, be supervised by a staff member who works to the above recommendations;
   e be competent in resuscitation, especially if local anesthetic is used epidurally.
4 The operator should personally:
   a record the patient's history and examination, especially the neurological status of the lower limbs;
   b give the patient verbal and written information on the technique, on its efficacy, likely outcome, and duration, and on the risks, possible side-effects, and complications of epidural steroids;
   c make it clear to the patient that the steroid is being used for an indication and by a route not recommended in the product information sheet and therefore complications may be less predictable;
   d obtain written consent in which the patient not only consents to the procedure but also states that the above information has been given.

On the day of the injection

1 The injection should be carried out in a clean area using a sterile technique with monitoring and full resuscitation facilities available especially if local anesthetic is to be used epidurally.
2 Special precautions should be taken to ensure that the steroid is not injected into the cerebrospinal fluid.
3 Facilities should be available to monitor the patient during the procedure and for at least an hour afterwards.

After the injection

1 The operator should arrange to see the patient as an outpatient at least once after the injection and not later than 6 weeks.
2 In the meantime, if a problem arises, the patient should be able to contact the operator through the clinic where the injection was carried out.

The equipment

The following equipment should be made ready:

1 A trolley or other surface for the patient to lie or sit on that can be adjusted for height and be put in the Trendelenburg position if necessary.
2 Resuscitation equipment and drugs.
3 Monitoring equipment suitable for the patient's medical condition.
4 Operating room clothes, hat, mask, and sterile gloves for the operator.
5 A trolley covered with a sterile drape for the epidural equipment.
6 Solution for sterilizing the skin – such as chlorhexidine in spirit.
7 Swabs and forceps for applying the sterilizing fluid to the injection site.
8 A sterile drape with a central aperture for covering the patient's back and allowing access to the injection site.
9 Hypodermic needles and syringe for infiltrating the tissues with local anesthetic.
10 Filter needle for drawing up local anesthetic from glass ampoules (if used).
11 Needles and syringes for drawing up the steroid and the local anesthetic.
12 A 16- or 18-gauge epidural needle.
13 A loss-of-resistance syringe.
14 Sterile swabs.
15 Single use only ampoules of local anesthetic, sodium chloride, and the steroid.

The following monitors should be available:

1 noninvasive blood pressure;
2 pulse oximetry;
3 electrocardiograph.

Key points

- Epidural steroid injections should be carried out carefully by an experienced operator.
- Extra care and precautions should be taken because steroid preparations are not licensed for nerve root pain or epidural administration.

THE TECHNIQUE OF EPIDURAL STEROID INJECTION

It is assumed that the operator is familiar with and experienced in the standard technique of lumbar and caudal epidural injection.[23] The suggestions made here are specifically to aid experienced epiduralists who have the knowledge, skills, and attitudes needed for carrying out standard "single-shot" epidural steroid injections.

There is no good evidence for any particular aspect of the technique or for the caudal over the lumbar route or vice versa.[24] The following suggestions are made to aid efficiency and safety.

General

1 The patient should be fully conscious during the procedure to warn of any trauma to, or irritation of, nerves or their roots.
2 The patient should be warned of possible discomfort on entry into the epidural space and when the local anesthetic (if used) and steroid are injected.
3 When the epidural space is entered, the needle should be left without the syringe on for a few moments to check for cerebrospinal fluid, in case an accidental dural puncture has been made.
4 Local anesthetic or sodium chloride 0.9% can be used to dilute the steroid preparation. The advantage of using local anesthetic is that if, after the epidural injection, the sciatic pain resolves for at least the duration of the effect of the local anesthetic, then the steroid may be assumed to have reached its target. However, use of local anesthetic increases the risks of the procedure.
5 If local anesthetic is used, it should be injected into the epidural space as a test dose of 2–3 ml first. The syringe may be left on for a test period of 2–3 min, during which time an inadvertent intrathecal injection may manifest itself by lower limb anesthesia. Blood pressure should be monitored.
6 The diluted steroid may then be injected. As the solution is particulate, the injectate should be kept mixed to ensure even dispersal of the drug in the diluent.
7 Position of the patient during and after the injection may affect the spread of the injected steroid suspension by gravitational sedation. Therefore, experienced pain clinicians place the patient in the lateral position with the affected side down during injection of the epidural steroid solution.
8 Very special attention should be paid to reducing the risks of infection.

Lumbar route

1 The patient can lie on one side or sit up. Sitting up helps with identifying the midline and confirming that the level selected corresponds with the level of the lesion. A line between the iliac crests may pass through L3/4, but this is an unreliable sign.
2 An epidural needle should be used.
3 A loss-of-resistance syringe should be used to confirm entry into the epidural space.
4 There is an increased risk of dural puncture and inad-

vertent intrathecal injection as the dura mater is just beyond the lumbar epidural space.
5 In the non-obese patient, lumbar injections can be accurately placed without X-ray screening.

Caudal route

1 The patient can lie on one side or on his/her front with hips supported by a pillow. In the latter position, turning the toes inwards can help to expose the sacral hiatus area.
2 A 3.8-cm (1.5 inch) 18-gauge needle can be used.
3 A loss-of-resistance syringe should be used to confirm entry into the epidural space.
4 There is a reduced risk of dural puncture and inadvertent intrathecal injection as the dura mater is above the caudal epidural space, but anatomical variations do occur in the relation of the dura mater to the cephalad part of caudal epidural space.[9]
5 The use of an imaging technique should be considered, as it is more difficult to place the needle accurately in the epidural space by this approach irrespective of the weight of the patient.[25]

Other techniques

As well as the standard midline and lateral approaches to the epidural space, the techniques of perineural and periradicular (transforaminal) injection have also been proposed.[26,27] In these methods, steroid is delivered directly onto the nerve root, either by a posterior transmidline approach from the opposite side or through the intervertebral foramen on the affected side.

If such accurate delivery is important for a good result, then results of these techniques should be much better than those of the standard technique. Insufficient studies have been published so far to be sure that these techniques are better and safer than the ordinary technique.

Steroids can be delivered accurately on to the supposed site of the lesion by means of an epiduroscope.

Monitoring

1 During the procedure, regular measurements of blood pressure and oxygen saturation should be made, especially if epidural local anesthetic has been used.
2 After the procedure, regular measurements of blood pressure and pulse rate should be made and the patient's lower limb motor power and ability to pass urine should be assessed prior to discharge, especially if epidural local anesthetic has been used.

Key points

- There are several ways of carrying out epidural steroid injections.
- It is essential that whatever technique is used it should be designed to limit risk, especially of dural puncture and intrathecal injection.

IMAGING TECHNIQUES

Most standard epidural steroid injections are carried out worldwide without the use of an imaging technique.

However, if imaging facilities are available, they could be used with contrast to ensure:

1   The needle enters the epidural space. It is estimated that about 25% of caudal and 30% of lumbar epidural injections of steroid do not end up in the epidural space.[24] It is thought that in the non-obese patient lumbar epidural injections can be placed accurately without X-ray screening, but caudal epidural injections, to be placed accurately, require X-ray screening no matter what the weight of the patient.
2   The needle does not enter the intrathecal space.
3   The injectate spreads anteriorly around the dura mater to the site of the lesion, namely the degenerating, herniated, or sequestered disk and the affected nerve root.
4   Correct placement of 20-gauge Tuohy needles. These are more difficult to place than 17- or 18-gauge needles, especially in elderly men, and may need fluoroscopy to confirm placement.[32]

To avoid failure resulting from the steroid not reaching the lesion, various measures have been recommended:

1   The use of an image intensifier and contrast medium.[33] Its usefulness in complicated cases has been questioned.[34] The use of contrast medium may introduce its own problems, such as allergic reactions, possible chemical interaction with the steroid preparation, and increased osmolarity of the injectate.
2   The use of CT scan.[35]
3   Perineural or transforaminal injection using an image intensifier. This can ensure that the needle is as close to the affected nerve root as possible.[26,27,35]
4   Application of the steroid by direct vision onto the affected nerve root using an epiduroscope.[36]

Key point

- Imaging during epidural steroid injection may improve safety and demonstrate that the steroid has reached the intended target area.

DRUGS USED FOR EPIDURAL STEROID INJECTIONS

During an epidural steroid injection, the operator can inject the steroid preparation on its own or mixed with either local anesthetic or sodium chloride 0.9%.

The steroid

Steroid preparations commonly used in epidural steroid injection contain either methylprednisolone or triamcinolone. The use of betamethasone and hydrocortisone has also been reported in the literature.

The two most commonly used steroid preparations in the UK contain the following constituents:

1	Lederspan (Wyeth)	Triamcinolone hexacetonide 20 mg/ml Polyethylene glycol 3% Polysorbate 0.2% Benzyl alcohol 0.9% Sodium chloride 0.9%
2	Depo-Medrone (Pharmacia Upjohn)	Methylprednisolone acetate 40 mg/ml Polyethylene glycol 3% Myristyl picolinic acid 0.2% Sodium chloride 0.9%

Similar steroid preparations are used worldwide.

The optimum dose of steroid has not been established. Smaller doses seem to work as well as larger ones with less risk of steroid-related complications. Assuming equipotent anti-inflammatory activity, a dose of 20–40 mg of triamcinolone or methylprednisolone seems reasonable.

The local anesthetic

The commonly used local anesthetics are:

1   lidocaine (lignocaine) hydrochloride 0.5–1.0%;
2   bupivacaine hydrochloride 0.125–0.25%.

The injectate

A total volume of the steroid and local anesthetic or sodium chloride of up to 10 ml is desirable for the lumbar route, as the injectate will be delivered more locally to the site of the suspected lesion. For caudal injections, a larger final volume of 15–20 ml is necessary to ensure that the steroid reaches the target site. Large volumes, for example 40 ml, can be painful and produce adverse mechanical effects if injected rapidly and forcibly.

Key points

- Methylprednisolone and triamcinolone are commonly used in epidural steroid injections.
- A small dose should be used to limit unwanted steroid effects.
- The steroid is often used mixed with local anesthetic.

COMPLICATIONS

Types of complications

The complications of epidural steroid injection can be related to:

1 the mechanical aspects of the procedure;
2 the effects of the drugs used:
   a the steroid itself;
   b the additives (vehicle) in the steroid preparation;
   c the local anesthetic (if used);
3 misplacement of the drugs.

The mechanical aspects

The main complication is dural puncture, which may lead to postdural puncture headache. The incidence is at least as great as for nonsteroidal epidural injections and may be greater. Access to the epidural space may be more difficult in patients having epidural steroid injections since they may not be able to bend their backs adequately and may have had surgery at the site of the injection.

Large volume epidural injection (greater than 40 ml) may lead to disturbed vision and retinal hemorrhages.[37] Epidural injection of volumes of 10–20 ml may increase intrathecal pressure for 10 min.[38] It is thought that the raised intrathecal pressure may result in increased intracranial and retinal venous pressure. If severe, the retinal veins may rupture.

If the dura is punctured, some of the injectate may be forced into the intrathecal space following a subsequent correctly sited epidural injection.

The steroid itself

1 If an excessive, repeated dose of steroid is given, it may cause adrenal suppression.[39] Smaller doses may still have a depressant effect on the adrenal glands, which may only be manifested if the patient has a subsequent stress, such as a major infection or surgery.
2 There is a moderate risk that bacterial infections may worsen after steroid injections as a result of the steroid's anti-inflammatory effects. Diabetic patients may be at extra risk in this respect.[40] Latent tuberculous infections may be reactivated.

3 There is no definite evidence that the steroid has a toxic effect in the epidural space. Two studies in animals showed no short- or long-term toxic effects:
   a Delaney et al.[33] examined the toxicity of epidural triamcinolone in 48 cats. They compared triamcinolone plus lidocaine with lidocaine (lignocaine) alone, lidocaine plus vehicle, and no intervention. Light and electron microscopy showed slight inflammation in all four groups at 30 days, but only in one cat in the lidocaine alone group and in another cat in the lidocaine plus steroid group at 120 days. Meningeal thickening occurred in two cats in the lidocaine plus vehicle group at 30 days but not at 120. All effects were mild and transient and did not lead to adhesions or neural toxicity.
   b Cicala et al.[41] looked at epidural methylprednisolone for toxicity in 36 rabbits. They compared the effects of methylprednisolone plus lidocaine with Ringer's solution and with sodium chloride plus talc at 10 days. They found that neither methylprednisolone plus lidocaine nor Ringer's solution caused any inflammation or thickening of the meninges or nerve roots at 10 days, whereas talc did.

The additives in the steroid preparation

There are no known complications of the additives in the steroid preparations following epidural injection. In the complete steroid preparation, they do not seem to be toxic.[40,41]

Of the individual additives, most is known about polyethylene glycol, which is present at 3% in both preparations shown above. In rabbit nerve preparation, Benzon et al.[42] found that 20% or more of polyethylene glycol is needed before even reversible toxic effects are produced.

In clinical practice, the undiluted preparation is rarely given. Usually, it is given mixed with local anesthetic or sodium chloride, with each 1 or 2 ml of the steroid preparation diluted to 10 ml. In effect, this reduces the concentration of polyethylene glycol from 3% to at least 0.6%, well below the 20% threshold for even transient toxicity.

The local anesthetic (if used)

Complications related to the local anesthetic should not be greater than for nonsteroid epidural injections that include local anesthetic. They are:

1 Allergic reactions, leading to cardiorespiratory collapse.
2 Overdose of local anesthetic in the epidural space, leading to hypotension and motor block, possibly affecting the respiratory nerves.
3 Inadvertent injection of local anesthetic into the intrathecal or subdural space, leading to cardiorespiratory collapse and paralysis.

Misplacement of drugs

Serious complications may result if the drugs are inadvertently injected into the intrathecal space or the subdural space (see above). These complications are related to the effect of the local anesthetic (if used).

There has been much concern over possible toxic effects of an inadvertent intrathecal injection of the steroid preparation on the tissues in the intrathecal space. Two studies in animals have examined this:

1 Abram et al.[43] looked at the effects on the intrathecal space and its contents of a triamcinolone-containing preparation compared with sodium chloride in rats at 1 day and 20 days of treatment. They found that there were no histological changes even after 20 days of treatment.
2 Latham et al.[44] gave 23 sheep intrathecal injections of either various volumes of sodium chloride or 1 ml, 2 ml, or more of betamethasone. After 6 weeks, there were no toxic effects seen in the spinal cords, meninges, or nerve roots of sheep which had sodium chloride or 1 ml (5.7 mg) betamethasone. Effects were seen consistently in sheep that had had more than 2 ml. The authors concluded that given that the volume of cerebrospinal fluid in the sheep is approximately one-third of that in humans, small volumes (up to 2 ml) of betamethasone injected intrathecally in humans are unlikely to cause arachnoiditis, but that the risk of this complication increases substantially with higher doses.

Nevertheless, all possible care should be taken to avoid accidental injection of steroid into the intrathecal space.

Depo-steroids, when mixed with local anesthetic, may form aggregates. If these aggregates find their way into blood vessels, either in or outside the epidural space, they could pose a hazard.

Incidence of complications

One way of looking at complications is to examine all the complications mentioned in the literature on epidural steroid series. Abram and O'Connor[38] looked at 53 papers on epidural series between 1960 and 1991. Thirty

of these papers looked specifically for complications in 3,800 patients.

Twenty-two of these 30 series listed short-term complications in 142 patients (3.7%). The commonest was headache (44 patients in eight series), followed by temporary worsening of the pain (28 patients in 11 series).

Longer term complications were seen in 39 patients in 14 series (1%). These were almost entirely the symptoms of dural tap (37 patients).

Another way of looking at complications is to examine the literature written specifically on complications of epidural steroids. Abram and O'Connor[45] examined 12 such papers (Table 33.1). These complications can be divided according to their likely causes. They can be largely avoided if a proper technical procedure is observed. There were no reports of arachnoiditis.

Key points

- When carried out properly, epidural steroid injection has a low incidence of complications.
- The commonest complications are similar to those seen after ordinary epidural injections.
- There is no clear evidence that the steroids used have a toxic effect in the epidural space.

EVIDENCE FOR A PARTICULAR THERAPY OR DRUG

There is no good evidence that any steroid preparation is more effective than another. Of more concern is whether epidural steroids are effective in alleviating sciatica. The evidence is not very extensive, good, or clear. Relatively few randomized, double-blind, controlled trials (RCTs) have been carried out and several are not of very high quality. Two major meta-analyses have been made:

1 Koes et al.[46]*** examined 12 RCTs carried out between 1971 and 1992. He scored them out of 100 according to four categories of quality and compared the conclusions in each paper with its quality score. Three of these studies can be excluded as they do not address primary nerve root pain or the qual-

Table 33.1 Complications of epidural steroids

		Number of patients with complication
Related to adrenal function	Cushing's symptoms	3
	Adrenal suppression	12
Infection	Bacterial meningitis	2
	Epidural abscess	2
Technique	Chronic dural leak	1
	Intracranial air	3
Hypersensitivity	Allergy	1
Chemical irritation	Transient aseptic meningitis	1

ity score was too low. Of these three studies, only the poorest quality one showed steroid to be better than control.

The results showed that only four out of nine studies had quality scores of more than 60 and that even in these best studies, as well as overall in the totals, there was no clear difference between patients who had had a good response to epidural steroids and those who had not.

2 Watts and Silagy[47]*** examined 11 studies from 1971 to 1994. They looked at the additional benefit relative to controls produced by epidural steroids in the short term, 60 days, and in the longer term, 1 year. They looked for patients who had had at least a 75% benefit after 60 days or any improvement at 1 year.

In the short term, the odds ratio for epidural steroids was 2.61(1.80–3.77), and at 1 year was 1.87(1.31–2.68). These odds ratios for short- and longer term benefits have been converted into numbers needed to treat (NNT), giving 6 and 11 respectively.[48] The authors pointed out that an NNT of 6 in the short term was acceptable for a chronically painful condition.

Why a systematic review and meta-analysis of basically the same studies can reach different conclusions is explored by Hopayian and Mugford.[49]

3 Since 1995, there have been a few randomized controlled trials, the best of which was carried out by Carette et al.[8] They studied 158 patients with radiologically proven herniated disks. Patients in the active group received up to three epidural injections of methylprednisolone. The main outcome measure was the Oswestry Disability Score adapted for sciatica, but leg pain, finger–floor distance, sensory deficit, and analgesic intake were also noted.

At 3 weeks, and indeed thereafter, there was no difference in the Oswestry score between epidural steroid patients and controls. There were significant improvements in finger–floor distance and sensory deficit at 3 weeks and in leg pain at 6 weeks, but no difference in any measure thereafter or at 1 year. The number of patients subsequently requiring surgery was also not different.

4 In a smaller study of 36 patients with confirmed prolapsed intervertebral lumbar disks, Buchner et al.[50] compared three injections of methylprednisolone and bupivacaine, but not bupivacaine alone, against conservative noninjection treatment. The outcome measures were visual analog pain scale, straight leg raising test, and functional status at 2, 6 and 24 weeks.

The epidural steroid group only showed a statistically significant difference in improved straight leg raising test at 2 weeks but not for pain or function at any time. Karppinen et al.[29] carried out a double-blind, randomized controlled trial on 160 patients with herniated nucleus pulposus. Eighty were treated with periradicular injection of methylprednisolone and pupivacaine and the controls with sodium chloride 0.9%. The steroid group had significantly less leg pain, more lumbar flexion, and greater patient satisfaction at 2 weeks, whereas the saline group had less back pain at 3 and 6 months and less leg pain at 6 months. The effect of steroid and pupivacaine, as in the case of standard epidural steroid injections, seems to be short lived.

The results of the studies performed by Carette et al.[8] and Buchner et al.[50] would further increase the short and longer term NNTs for epidural steroids that were calculated from Watts and Silagy's meta-analysis. In other words, more patients would need to be treated before one patient benefited.

Key points

- Epidural steroids have been used for nerve root pain for almost 50 years.
- The only generally approved indication for this treatment is nerve root pain.
- Steroids are not licensed for this indication or for the epidural route, so special precautions must be taken.
- The evidence for efficacy is equivocal or better for radicular pain. There is no evidence for effect in "low back" pain.
- If injected properly, epidural steroids are safe in the epidural space and have a low incidence of complications.

REFERENCES

1. Lee HM, Weinstein JN, Meller ST, et al. The role of steroids and their effects on phospholipase A_2. An animal model of radiculopathy. Spine 1998; 23: 1191–6.

2. Robecchi A, Capra R. L'idrocortisone (composto F). Prime esperienze cliniche in campo reumatologico. Minerva Med 1952; 2: 1259–63.

3. Lievre JA, Block-Michel H, Pean G, Uro J. L'hydrocortisone en injection locale. Rev Rheum 1953; 20: 310–11.

4. Goebert HW, Jallo SJ, Gardner WJ, et al. Sciatica: treatment with epidural injections of procaine and hydrocortisone. Cleveland Clin Q 1960; 27: 191–7.

5. Brown JH. Pressure caudal anesthesia and back manipulation. Conservative method for treatment of sciatica. Northwest Med (Seattle) 1960; 59: 905–9.

6. Dilke TF, Burry HC, Grahame R. Extradural corticosteroid injection in the management of lumbar nerve root compression. Br Med J 1973; 2: 635–7.

● 7. Carette S, Leclaire R, Marcoux S, et al. Epidural corticosteroid injections for sciatica due to herniated nucleus pulposus. N Engl J Med 1997; 336: 1634–40.

8. Abram SE. Need for precise diagnosis prior to epidural steroids: in reply. Anesthiology 2000; 93: 565–6.

9. Crighton IM, Barry BP, Hobbs GJ. A study of the anatomy of the caudal space using magnetic resonance imaging. Br J Anaesth 1997; 78: 391–5.

10. Westbrook JL, Renowden SA, Carrie LE. Study of the anatomy of the extradural region using magnetic resonance imaging. *Br J Anaesth* 1993; **71**: 495–8.

11. Kallakuri S, Cavanaugh JM, Blagoev DC. An immunohistochemical study of innervation of lumbar spinal dura and longitudinal ligaments. *Spine* 1998; **23**: 403–11.

● 12. Abram SE. Treatment of lumbosacral radiculopathy with epidural steroids. *Anesthesiology* 1999; **91**: 1937–41.

13. NHMRC Working Party. The value of epidural steroids in the management of diverse conditions causing back pain. In: *Epidural Use of Steroids in the Management of Back Pain*. Canberra: National Health and Medical Research Council of Australia, 1994: 24–5.

14. Andersson GB, Deyo RA. History and physical examination in patients with herniated lumbar discs. *Spine* 1996; **21**: 10S–18S.

15. Boden SD, Davis DO, Dina TS, *et al*. Abnormal magnetic-resonance scans of the lumbar spine in asymptomatic subjects. A prospective investigation. *J Bone Joint Surg (Am)* 1990; **72**: 403–8.

16. Rivest C, Katz JN, Ferrante FM, Jamison RN. Effects of epidural steroid injection on pain due to lumbar spinal stenosis or herniated disks: a prospective study. *Arthritis Care Res* 1998; **11**: 291–7.

17. Fukusaki M, Kobayashi I, Hara T, Sumikawa K. Symptoms of spinal stenosis do not improve after epidural steroid injection. *Clin J Pain* 1998; **14**: 148–51.

18. Revel M, Auleley GR, Alaoui S, *et al*. Forceful epidural injections for the treatment of lumbosciatic pain with post-operative lumbar spinal fibrosis. *Rev Rheum Engl Ed* 1996; **63**: 270–7.

19. Meadeb J, Rozenberg S, Duquesnoy B, *et al*. Forceful sacrococcygeal injections in the treatment of postdiscectomy sciatica. A controlled study versus glucocorticoid injections. *Joint Bone Spine* 2001; **68** (1): 43–9.

20. Hopwood MB, Abram SE. Factors associated with failure of lumbar epidural steroids. *Reg Anesth* 1993; **18**: 238–43.

21. Knight JW, Cordingley JJ, Palazzo MG. Epidural abscess following epidural steroid and local anesthetic injection. *Anaesthesia* 1997; **52**: 576–8.

22. Ngan Kee WD. Steroid therapy and extradural analgesia. *Br J Anaesth* 1992; **69**: 423.

23. Brown DL, Wedel DJ. Introduction to regional anesthesia. In: Miller RD ed. *Anesthesia*, 3rd edn. New York, NY: Churchill Livingstone, 1990: 1395–9.

24. McGregor AH, Anjarwalla NK, Stambach T. Does the method of injection alter the outcome of epidural injections? *J Spinal Disorders* 2001; **14**: 507–10.

25. Price CM, Rogers, PD, Prosser AS, Arden NK. Comparison of the caudal and lumbar approaches to the epidural space. *Ann Rheum Dis* 2000 **59** (11): 879–82.

26. Kraemer J, Ludwig J, Bickert U, *et al*. Lumbar epidural perineural injection: a new technique. *Eur Spine J* 1997; **6**: 357–61.

27. Lutze M, Stendel R, Vesper J, Brock M. Periradicular therapy in lumbar radicular syndromes: methodology and results. *Acta Neurochir (Wien)* 1997; **139**: 719–24.

28. Botwin KP, Gruber RD, Bouchlas CG, *et al*. Complications of fluoroscopically guided transforaminal lumbar epidural injections. *Arch Phys Med Rehabil* 2000; **81**: 1045–50.

● 29. Karpinnen J, Malmivaara A, Kurunlahti M, *et al*. Periradicular infiltration for sciatica: a randomized controlled trial. *Spine* 2001; **26**: 1059–67.

30. Richardson J, mcGurgan P, Cheema S, *et al*. Spinal endoscopy in chronic low back pain with radiculopathy. A prospective case series. *Anaesthesia* 2001; **56**: 454–60.

31. White AH, Derby R, Wynne G. Epidural injections for the diagnosis and treatment of low-back pain. *Spine* 1980; **5**: 78–86.

32. Liu SS, Melmed AP, Klos JW, Innis CA. Prospective experience with a 20-gauge Tuohy needle for lumbar epidural steroid injections: Is confirmation with fluoroscopy necessary? *Reg Anesth Pain Med* 2001 **26** (2): 143–6.

33. el-Khoury GY, Ehara S, Weinstein JN, *et al*. Epidural steroid injection: a procedure ideally performed with fluoroscopic control. *Radiology* 1988; **168**: 554–7.

34. Fredman B, Nun MB, Zohar E, *et al*. Epidural steroids for treating "failed back surgery syndrome": is fluoroscopy really necessary? *Anesth Analg* 1999; **88**: 367–72.

35. Schmid G, Vetter S, Gottmann D, Strecker EP. CT-guided epidural/perineural injections in painful disorders of the lumbar spine: short- and extended-term results. *Cardiovasc Intervent Radiol* 1999; **22**: 493–8.

36. Johnson BA, Schellhas KP, Pollei SR. Epidurography and therapeutic epidural injections: technical considerations and experience with 5334 cases. *Am J Neuroradiol* 1999; **20**: 697–705.

37. Purdy EP, Ajimal GS. Vision loss after lumbar epidural steroid injection. *Anesth Analg* 1998; **86**: 119–22.

38. Usubiaga JE, Usubiaga LE, Brea LM, Goyena R. Effect of saline injections on epidural and subarachnoid space pressures and relation to postspinal anesthesia. *Anesth Analg* 1967; **46**: 293–6.

39. Jacobs S, Pullan PT, Potter JM, Shenfield GM. Adrenal suppression following extradural steroids. *Anaesthesia* 1983; **38**: 953–6.

● 40. Delaney TJ, Rowlingson JC, Carron H, Butler A. Epidural steroid effects on nerves and meninges. *Anesth Analg* 1980; **59**: 610–14.

● 41. Cicala RS, Turner R, Moran E, *et al*. Methylprednisolone acetate does not cause inflammatory changes in the epidural space. *Anesthesiology* 1990; **72**: 556–8.

42. Benzon HT, Gissen AJ, Strichartz GR, *et al*. The effect of polyethylene glycol on mammalian nerve impulses. *Anesth Analg* 1987; **66**: 553–9.

● 43. Abram SE, Marsala M, Yaksh TL. Analgesic and neurotoxic effects of intrathecal corticosteroids in rats. *Anesthesiology* 1994; **81**: 1198–205.

44. Latham JM, Fraser RD, Moore RJ, *et al*. The pathologic effects of intrathecal betamethasone. *Spine* 1997; **22:** 1558–62.

● 45. Abram SE, O'Connor TC. Complications associated with epidural steroid injections. *Reg Anesth* 1996; **21:** 149–62.

46. Koes BW, Scholten RJ, Mens JM, Bouter LM. Efficacy of epidural steroid injections for low-back pain and sciatica: a systematic review of randomized clinical trials. *Pain* 995; **63:** 279–88.

47. Watts RW, Silagy CA. A meta-analysis on the efficacy of epidural corticosteroids in the treatment of sciatica. *Anaesth Intensive Care* 1995; **23:** 564–69.

48. McQuay HJ, Moore A. Epidural steroids for sciatica. *Anaesth Intensive Care* 1996; **24:** 284–5.

49. Hopayian K, Mugford M. Conflicting conclusions from two systematic reviews of epidural steroid injections for sciatica: which evidence should general practitioners heed? *Br J Gen Pract* 1999; **49** (438): 57–61.

● 50. Buchner M, Zeifang F, Brocai DR, Schiltenwolf M. Epidural corticosteroid injection in the conservative management of sciatica. *Clin Orthop* 2000; **375:** 149–56.

PART IX

Pediatric techniques

34

Procedures for pediatric pain management

RICHARD HOWARD

General considerations	431	Local anesthetic techniques	439
Systemic analgesia for infants and children older than 6 months	434	Conclusion	443
		References	443
Analgesia for neonates and infants aged 6 months or younger	438		

The management of pain in children is a relatively new and developing clinical science, and health workers and parents are often anxious about the appropriate treatment of pain and understandably fearful of the side-effects of analgesics. Because of this, safe and effective analgesia can only take place if an appropriately supportive clinical environment exists, including accessible background information and clear guidance on the assessment of pain, the prescription and administration of analgesics, and the appropriate use of other treatments for pain.

GENERAL CONSIDERATIONS

Planning

In many acute pain situations, for example postoperative pain, the degree of pain and its likely progression can be fairly accurately predicted, allowing standardization of treatment and anticipation of adverse effects. Standardization of pain management using protocols and guidelines not only ensures uniformity of care but also simplifies education of patients, parents, and staff members and allows easier and meaningful audit of outcomes. The overall responsibility for pain management should rest with designated personnel, and expert help should be readily accessible. The virtues of an organized pain management service are obvious in this respect and are frequently recommended, but the lack of such a facility should not prevent the institution of the proper care.[1]

Developmental level

Analgesia must be appropriate to the developmental level of the child, and analgesic protocols must be flexible enough to encompass the range of patients encountered. For example, very young children will not be able to understand the concept of patient-controlled analgesia (PCA) and some older children cannot operate the handset because of delayed development or disability. Neonates are an important group whose vulnerability to dangerous side-effects can sometimes lead to inappropriate analgesic management. Selection of analgesia also requires an understanding of the developmental pharmacology of analgesics, and the influence of important interactions between child, family, and health professionals, which is more fully discussed in Chapter A25.

The assessment of pain

There is an enormous literature on pediatric pain assessment. Numerous pain assessment tools have been devised in order to facilitate both behavioral and self-report measures in children at all stages of development and in different settings. Once the validity of a tool for the age and situation for which it is to be used has been established, choosing an assessment tool depends on user preference as much as anything else. In general, self-report should be considered for children older than 4 years, and observer/behavioral measures for younger children or those unwilling or unable (e.g. neurodevelopmental delay or depressed consciousness) to participate in pain assessment.

Self-report of pain

Self-assessment of pain is generally regarded as the preferred method where possible. In general, although children of 4 years have the cognitive ability to quantify pain ("a little," "a lot"), the use of linear visual analog scales or pain rating tools (e.g. the poker chip tool,[2] which requires the child to select a number of wooden chips representing the intensity or amount of pain) requires levels of cognitive development which are sometimes achieved later. In practice, each child is encouraged to self-assess where appropriate and other methods substituted when necessary. Of the many "child-friendly" self-assessment tools available, face scales such as the Oucher, Wong and Baker, or Bieri models are popular and well validated.[3**,4**,5**]

Behavioral measures

Evaluation of observational approaches to pain assessment is notoriously difficult: behaviors are obviously very age dependent and no behavioral tool exists which claims to be valid for all age groups. Preterm neonates particularly are known to have very limited and sometimes contradictory responses to pain, and will almost certainly need separate evaluation. Table 25.1 in Chapter A25 lists tools available for postoperative and procedural pain assessment in neonates and infants. Those with the widest applicability include the children's postoperative pain scale (CHIPPS), valid for postoperative pain from term neonate to 5 years, and the "COMFORT scale," which was not originally developed as a pain tool specifically but was recently shown to be valid over the 0–3 years age range in critical care.[6**,7**,8**,9**]

Figure 34.1 shows a practical example of a pain measurement system that is suitable for all ages as it uses a behavioral method for the youngest children and a faces scale or linear visual analog scale for those able to self-report. By utilizing different components of the chart, a common "pain score" for different ages can be achieved. Pain assessment should clearly link with care, such that high scores are quickly and appropriately treated with analgesics or other measures. An example of a simple protocol is shown in Table 34.1.

Routes of analgesia

The route of delivery of analgesia is the point of interface with the patient and is a particularly important issue for children. For example, the technique of intramuscular injection of opioids, which was the mainstay of postoperative analgesia for many years, often failed in pediatric practice. This was because many children would rather endure significant pain than be subjected to a distressing and possibly painful needlestick, and nurses were understandably reluctant to administer such treatments to unwilling children.

Oral

When it is available, the oral route is the route of choice for analgesia and other drugs, and most children will take analgesia orally. Some infants and young children will not accept tablets or capsules but liquid formulations or elixirs are available; otherwise, analgesics can sometimes be dissolved or mixed with something more palatable such as a favorite drink or flavor.

Rectal

Rectal drug administration is very popular in pediatric practice. Easy administration and slow absorption kinetics are convenient and will allow analgesic plasma levels to be maintained with relatively infrequent dosing. Acetaminophen (paracetamol) and the nonsteroidal anti-inflammatory drugs (NSAIDs) are very often given this way, particularly in the perioperative period; suppositories suitable for most ages are widely available. The pharmacokinetics of rectal acetaminophen has been well investigated in infants and children. Relatively high doses are required to achieve adequate plasma levels initially and the dosing interval depends on the clearance of the drug, both of which are age dependent.[10*,11*] Codeine, morphine, and many other potent analgesics have also become available as rectal formulations. Drawbacks are that rectal absorption may be erratic and unpredictable for some drugs, leading to uncertainty about the correct dose and redosing interval, and that some children or their families perceive it to be unpleasant or unacceptable.[12*]

Intravenous

Potent analgesia is frequently infused intravenously in severe acute pain because of its rapid onset and efficacy. Intravenous access may be difficult in children and is most conveniently obtained after topical local anesthesia of the skin (or better still while under general anesthesia for postoperative pain). Two infusions or access sites are sometimes established, one for analgesic infusion and a second for maintenance of fluid therapy and other drugs. Intravenous opioid infusions, intravenous PCA, and nurse-controlled analgesia (NCA) have all been described in children.[1,13] The NSAID ketorolac is available as an intravenous formulation, and propacetamol, an intravenous acetaminophen prodrug, has also been used in pediatric practice.[14]

Subcutaneous

Subcutaneous infusion of opioids is as effective as other parenteral routes, and both subcutaneous PCA and NCA have been described. The pharmacokinetics of subcutaneous infusion have not been well investigated in children, but bioavailability and rates of absorption seem to be predictable. Subcutaneous access is much easier to establish than intravenous and can last up to 10 days

- **Assess pain**   Using one of the following score systems
- **Plan**   Is an intervention required? If so, what?
- **Implement**   Implement intervention(s)
- **Evaluate**   Rescore at an appropriate interval to evaluate effectiveness

FLACC   **Behavioral pain assessment**

CATEGORIES	SCORING		
	0	1	2
Face	No particular expression or smile	Occasional grimace or frown, withdrawn, disinterested	Frequent to constant quivering chin, clenched jaw
Legs	Normal position or relaxed	Uneasy, restless, tense	Kicking, or legs drawn up
Activity	Lying quietly, normal position, moves easily	Squirming, shifting back and forth, tense	Arched, rigid, or jerking
Cry	No cry (awake or asleep)	Moans or whimpers, occasional complaint	Crying steadily, screams or sobs, frequent complaints
Consolability	Content, relaxed	Reassured by occasional touching, hugging or being talked to, distractible	Difficult to console or comfort

Each of the five categories (F) face, (L) legs, (A) activity, (C) cry, and (C) consolability is scored from 0 to 2, which results in a total score of between 0 and 10

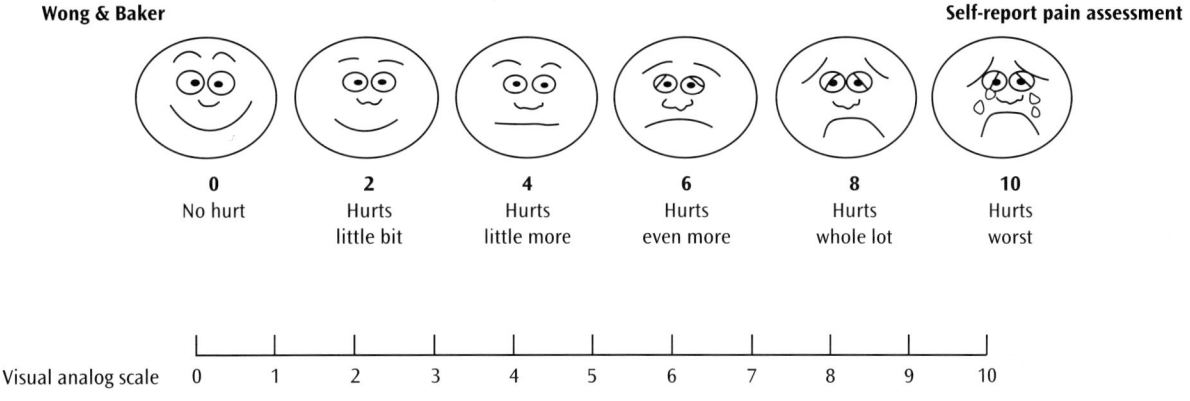

Wong & Baker   **Self-report pain assessment**

0	2	4	6	8	10
No hurt	Hurts little bit	Hurts little more	Hurts even more	Hurts whole lot	Hurts worst

Visual analog scale   0   1   2   3   4   5   6   7   8   9   10

Figure 34.1 *Behavioral and self-report pain measurement tools. Adapted from Wong and Baker[4] and Merkel* et al.[6]

before resiting of a cannula is necessary. Local anesthetics, particularly bupivacaine, are often infiltrated subcutaneously into surgical wounds and lacerations, normally under general anesthesia, and may provide effective postoperative analgesia for many hours (see Chapter A25).

Intramuscular

The intramuscular route was briefly mentioned above. It is mostly regarded as painful and unsuitable for the majority of children. However, this route may still have a place in pediatric acute pain management, particularly in the anesthetized or heavily sedated child, as a predictable and convenient short-term solution. Intramuscular absorption of opioids is complete and predictable and is an effective method of analgesia delivery with a longer dosing interval than intravenous administration. An intramuscular injection, given under general anesthesia, may provide several hours of analgesia until such time as oral or rectal analgesics become effective.

Epidural

Local anesthetics, opioids, and other analgesics are frequently given epidurally, particularly in the postoperative period. The epidural space in children is easily accessed by the caudal route and lumbar and thoracic intravertebral epidurals have become increasingly popular. Catheters located in the epidural space allow drugs to be infused for several days if necessary (see below).

Inhalational

Nitrous oxide has analgesic properties and can be inhaled as a 50% mixture with oxygen using special apparatus. It is particularly suitable for fairly brief painful procedures, such as dressing changes, removal of sutures or chest tubes, joint injections, and many other painful diagnostic and therapeutic procedures.[15] Nitrous oxide is usually self-administered with trained supervision and is there-

Pain score		
P = 0	No pain[a]	Reassess frequently
P = 1–3	Mild pain[a]	Review analgesia: NCA – give bolus (10 min before activity) PCA – encourage bolus (10 min before activity) Epidural – increase rate
P = 4–7	Moderate pain[a]	Give analgesia: NCA – give bolus PCA – encourage bolus Epidural – contact pain service to review
P = 8–10	Severe pain[a]	Give analgesia: NCA – contact pain service PCA – contact pain service Epidural – contact pain service

Table 34.1 *Pain score–pain management action plan*

a. Ensure supplementary analgesia is given (acetaminophen plus an NSAID if appropriate).

fore suitable for children older than 5–6 years who are able to understand and cooperate.

Novel routes of analgesia may also be considered for special situations, including transdermal, intranasal, and transmucosal.[16,17]

SYSTEMIC ANALGESIA FOR INFANTS AND CHILDREN OLDER THAN 6 MONTHS

Analgesics for mild to moderate pain

The detailed pharmacology of individual drugs is discussed elsewhere. Table 34.2 lists the drugs and doses of commonly used analgesics for mild/moderate pain in pediatric practice. Local drug-licensing restrictions may mean that some analgesics are unavailable in some countries or that doses and indications may vary. The analgesics are grouped into three classes; acetaminophen, NSAIDS, and opioids; drugs from different classes are often used together as part of a multimodal technique. This approach has a number of advantages as it improves analgesia while reducing side-effects and the interval between doses. In the presence of pain, analgesics should be given at regular intervals rather than *pro re nata* (p.r.n.) and the quality of analgesia assessed concurrently. If analgesia must be prescribed p.r.n., the indications for administration should be clearly established. Monitoring for unwanted and adverse effects should be routine, together with strategies to minimize and treat them should they occur.

Acetaminophen (paracetamol)

This is a low-potency analgesic when used alone, but is much more effective in combination with NSAIDs and/ or opioids. Hepatotoxicity is the principal adverse effect. Doses less than 150 mg/kg/day have only rarely been

associated with toxicity, but the use of maximum doses for more than 5 days is not recommended.[18]

Nonsteroidal anti-inflammatory drugs

Although there may be some interindividual differences in the response to NSAIDs, these drugs are largely used interchangeably for acute pain. The choice of NSAID depends on availability and convenience, some drugs in this group being easily obtainable in child-friendly formulations and presentations. NSAIDs are not used in the neonatal period nor for some months beyond. There is very little information available regarding toxicity of NSAIDs in early life, but after 6 months of age they appear to have a similar side-effect profile to that in older children. Caution has been advised when using NSAIDs in the presence of renal impairment, bleeding tendency, and peptic ulceration. They should not be used in the presence of aspirin-induced asthma, but are probably safe in asthma arising from other causes.[19]

Codeine

Codeine is a low-potency opioid, the efficacy of which appears to largely depend on its metabolism to morphine. The enzyme systems responsible for this are both genetically and developmentally regulated, which means that a significant number of children may derive little benefit from the drug (see Chapter A25). Nevertheless, codeine has an excellent safety record in pediatric practice and can be used if reliable methods of pain assessment are also employed.[20]

Oxycodone and hydrocodone

These are semisynthetic opioids with similar, or slightly greater, efficacy than codeine. They are available in oral formulations, both tablets and liquid, and have been recommended for use in children.[21] Both of these agents are

Table 34.2 *Drugs and doses of commonly used analgesics for mild/moderate pain in pediatric practice*

Drug	Class of analgesic	Oral/rectal/intravenous	Doses	Notes
Acetaminophen	Antipyretic–analgesic	Oral	90 mg/kg/day (15–20 mg/kg q.i.d.)	Loading dose may be required
Ibuprofen	NSAID	Oral	20 mg/kg/day (5 mg/kg q.i.d.)	Maximum 800 mg/day
Diclofenac	NSAID	Oral Rectal	3 mg/kg/day (1 mg/kg t.i.d.) 3 mg/kg/day (1 mg/kg t.i.d.)	Maximum 150 mg/day
Ketorolac	NSAID	Oral Intravenous	0.5–1 mg/kg q.i.d. 0.5 mg/kg q.i.d.	Dosage restrictions apply in some countries Maximum dose 40 mg/day
Codeine	Opioid	Oral Rectal	1 mg/kg q.i.d. 1 mg/kg q.i.d.	
Oxycodone	Opioid	Oral	0.2 mg/kg q.i.d.	
Hydrocodone	Opioid	Oral	0.2 mg/kg q.i.d.	
Tramadol	Opioid Intravenous	Oral 1 mg/kg q.i.d.	1 mg/kg q.i.d. Novel mode of action	

Acetaminophen (paracetamol).
NSAID, nonsteroidal anti-inflammatory drug; q.i.d., four times daily; t.i.d., three times daily.

available in combination formulations with NSAIDs and acetaminophen.

Tramadol

Tramadol is a novel analgesic with opioid receptor-mediated, serotoninergic, and adrenergic mechanisms of action. It is available in oral and parenteral formulations and, so far as it has been evaluated in children, appears safe.

Analgesics for moderate to severe pain

Opioids

As pain intensity increases, so analgesics of increasing potency can be combined. Moderate and severe pain will usually require the addition of potent opioid analgesics, their efficacy can be further increased by combination with acetaminophen and NSAIDs. Table 34.3 lists the high-potency opioid drugs and doses most commonly used in pediatric practice.

Morphine

Morphine is the opioid drug of choice – it is the best investigated in children and has been used the most extensively at all ages. Morphine is safe and inexpensive, administration is flexible, it is well absorbed orally, it can be given parenterally, it is effective in the epidural space, and is also sometimes given intrathecally. The efficacy of morphine for acute pain is limited only by its side-effects, which must be carefully monitored and treated (see Tables A25.5 and A25.6). The opioids have a predictable dose-dependent side-effect profile producing respiratory depression, sedation, nausea and vomiting, itching, and constipation. Effective treatments for all these exist,

and opioids are very safe when they are used appropriately for acute pain. Tolerance and physical dependence also occur with prolonged use and these drugs should not be abruptly withdrawn after more than 5 days of administration, especially if high doses have been given (see below).

Morphine infusion

Regimens for the use of morphine (outside the neonatal period) are given in Table A25.4 and below. Intravenous morphine by repeated injection, infusion, or a combination of both is very effective for acute pain. Onset of analgesia is rapid (within minutes) after intravenous injection of morphine and therefore it is suitable for the pain of trauma, brief procedures, and after surgery, particularly in the postanesthesia recovery room. For more persistent acute pain, analgesia is maintained by infusing the drug either intravenously or subcutaneously, adjusting the rate of infusion according to the response (see Table A25.3). More flexible but complex techniques such as patient-controlled analgesia (PCA) and nurse-controlled analgesia (NCA) can also be used.

Patient-controlled analgesia

Popular in adult practice, PCA has similar advantages and indications in children. PCA can be considered for children of 6 years and above provided they are able to understand the concept and physically able to press the handset. PCA pump programming is recommended for children (Table 34.4). In practice, children younger than 12 years are likely to need special help in the form of preuse education, frequent reeducation encouragement, and reminders, if the technique is to work satisfactorily. It is important to emphasize that the safety of PCA depends on self-administration and therefore only the patient should press the handset. A small continuous

Table 34.3 *Opioid: dosage/administration**

Drug	Route	Dose	Note
Morphine	Oral	0.2–0.4 mg/kg q.i.d.	Long-acting preparations available
	Intravenous	0.05 mg/kg	Incremental/loading dose
	Subcutaneous	0.05 mg/kg	Incremental/loading dose
	Epidural	0.02–0.05 mg/kg	Incremental/loading dose
Fentanyl	OTFC (oral–transmucosal)		See relevant product
	Transdermal		See relevant product
	Intravenous	0.0005 mg/kg	Incremental dose, infusion preferred
	Epidural	0.001 mg/kg	Infusion preferred
Meperidine	Oral	2 mg/kg q.i.d.	
	Intravenous	0.5–1 mg/kg	Incremental/loading dose
	Subcutaneous	0.5–1 mg/kg	Incremental/loading dose
Hydromorphone	Oral	0.06 mg/kg q.i.d.	
	Intravenous	0.005–0.015 mg/kg	Incremental/loading dose
	Subcutaneous	0.005–0.015 mg/kg	Incremental/loading dose
	Epidural	0.001–0.003 mg/kg	Incremental dose infusion preferred
Methadone	Oral	0.2 mg/kg t.i.d.	
	Intravenous	0.1–0.2 mg/kg	Incremental/loading dose

*NB Respiration ALWAYS monitored.
Meperidine (pethidine). OTFC, oral transmucosal fentanyl citrate.

("background") infusion is safe and may improve night-time sleeping in children.

Nurse-controlled analgesia

The flexibility of a simple morphine infusion can be improved by using a programmable PCA pump so that the primary nurse is able to conveniently give supplementary doses of analgesia using the handset.[1] Typically, a continuous infusion of 10–20 µg/kg/h of morphine is supplemented by up to three extra doses of 20 µg/kg/h at the patient's request or caregiver's discretion (Table 34.4). Advantages of NCA are flexibility to treat rapidly changing analgesic requirements, accuracy, and convenience. NCA is suitable for children who are too young or who are unable to use PCA, or in situations where frequent potentially painful procedures are carried out.

Fentanyl

Fentanyl is an extremely potent rapidly acting opioid which is very lipid soluble. It may have less effect on the pulmonary vasculature than morphine and is therefore sometimes used in the presence of pulmonary hypertension. Oral–transmucosal preparations of fentanyl are available in some countries and they may be useful for procedural pain. Transdermal fentanyl has been used for cancer pain; it may also have potential advantages for acute pain, but has been little investigated. The most common use of fentanyl is by intravenous or epidural (see Local anesthesia) infusion. Owing to its high potency and efficacy, intravenous fentanyl is only used in situations where respiration is supported or where high levels of monitoring are available (Table 34.5).

Meperidine (pethidine)

Traditionally, meperidine has been used after hepatobiliary surgery and in pain due to pancreatitis as it was thought to have less effect on intrabiliary pressures than other opioids – this is probably not true. It has also been used for acute pain associated with sickle hemoglobinopathy. Meperidine probably offers little advantage over morphine; additionally, prolonged infusion is associated with accumulation of a neurotoxic metabolite – normeperidine (norpethidine) – which may cause muscle twitching or convulsions.

Hydromorphone and methadone

Hydromorphone is a highly lipid-soluble morphine derivative with a long duration of action. Its high lipid solubility has made it popular for epidural use and it has been used extensively for cancer pain. Methadone, like hydromorphone, has a very long duration of action and for this reason has been traditionally used in the management of opioid withdrawal and in addiction states. It has sometimes been suggested for acute pain, the principal advantage being intravenous dose intervals of up to 4 h.

Side-effects of opioid analgesia

The adverse effects of opioid analgesics are predictable and (mostly) dose related (see above). The most dangerous side-effects are easily treated with the opioid antagonist naloxone, although of course analgesia will also be reversed. Opioid partial agonists are sometimes used to treat opioid side-effects; but little investigation has been done in children.

Table 34.4 *Protocols for intravenous morphine administration*

Morphine infusion		
Preparation	Morphine sulfate 1 mg/kg in 50-ml solution	
Concentration	20 μg/kg/ml	
Initial dose	2.5–5.0 ml (50–100 μg/kg)	
Infusion	0.5–1.5 ml/h (10–30 μg/kg/h)	
PCA		
Preparation	Morphine sulfate 1 mg/kg in 50-ml solution	
Concentration	20 μg/kg/ml	
Initial dose	2.5–5.0 ml (50–100 μg/kg)	
Programming	Background infusion:	0–0.2 ml/h (0–4 μg/kg/h)
	PCA dose:	0.5–1.0 ml (10–20 μg/kg/h)
	Lockout interval:	5 min
NCA		
Preparation	Morphine sulfate 1 mg/kg in 50-ml solution	
Concentration	20 μg/kg/ml	
Initial dose	2.5–5.0 ml (50–100 μg/kg)	
Programming	Background infusion:	0.5–1.0 ml/h (10–20 μg/kg/h)
	NCA dose:	0.5–1.0 ml (10–20 μg/kg/h)
	Lockout interval:	20 min
Subcutaneous morphine		
Preparation	Morphine sulfate 1 mg/kg in 20-ml solution	
Concentration	50 μg/kg/ml	
Initial dose	1–2.0 ml (50–100 μg/kg)	
Programming	Infusion:	0.2–0.4 ml/h (10–20 μg/kg/h)

PCA, patient-controlled analgesia; NCA, nurse-controlled analgesia.

Nausea and vomiting

Nausea and vomiting can sometimes be reduced by manipulating dosing regimens, for example by decreasing the duration of PCA and NCA doses, or more commonly by antiemetic drugs. Antiemetics causing extrapyramidal side-effects are generally avoided in children. 5-Hydroxy-tryptamine (5-HT) antagonists, antihistamines, and corticosteroids (dexamethasone) are used alone or in combination. Recommended treatments and doses are shown in Table 34.6.

Respiratory depression

Slowing of respiratory rate is common during acute opioid treatment and is usually accompanied by sedation. Reduction in the rate of infusion or dose of opioid when this occurs is usually sufficient to prevent dangerous respiratory depression. Safe management depends on experienced staff, suitable monitoring, and frequent pain assessments. If potentially life-threatening respiratory depression does occur, naloxone should be administered. Naloxone should be prescribed for each patient receiving opioid infusion, and the circumstances under which it should be given should be stated.

Monitoring for patients on systemic opioid infusions

It is widely accepted that morphine infusion analgesia can be safely managed in general ward areas provided a suitable standard of monitoring is used and dosages and infusion rates are carefully titrated against response. Analgesia is usually achieved before sedation occurs, and this precedes respiratory depression in most children. Table 34.7 shows suggested monitoring; the assessment of analgesia has been discussed, examples of sedation and nausea and vomiting scales are also shown. Respiration can be monitored by counting respiratory rate and by pulse oximetry while breathing air, which is a sensitive measure of hypercarbia and respiratory depression.

Other drugs for moderate/severe pain

Ketamine

N-Methyl-D-aspartate (NMDA) antagonists are interesting in acute pain management because of the important role of the NMDA receptor in the generation of postinjury hypersensitivity or hyperalgesia. Ketamine is the most widely available drug of this class. Low-dose ketamine has been shown to be useful in postoperative

Table 34.5 *Protocol for intravenous fentanyl infusion (with respiratory support)*

Preparation	Fentanyl 0.1 mg/kg in 50-ml solution
Concentration	2 μg/kg/ml
Initial dose	2.5–5.0 ml (5–10 μg/kg)
Infusion	0.5–2 ml/h (1–4 μg/kg/h)

Table 34.6 *Drug treatment of opioid side-effects*

Drug	Dose	Route
Respiratory depression		
Naloxone	4 µg/kg	Intravenous
Nausea and vomiting		
Cyclizine	1 mg/kg	Oral/intravenous (maximum 50 mg)
Ondansetron	100 µg/kg	Oral/intravenous (maximum 8 mg)
Metoclopramide	150 µg/kg	Oral/intravenous (maximum 10 mg)

pain in the adult and, although few studies exist in children, the available evidence suggests at least similar efficacy.[22**,23**] Ketamine can be combined with opioid, typically morphine (Table 34.8), in order to improve efficacy, although the evidence to support this in children is mainly anecdotal.[24]

Clonidine

Oral and intravenous clonidine has been used for analgesia in children and also for preanesthetic medication.[25,26] Clonidine can be given orally, intravenously, and epidurally; analgesia is prolonged (up to 12h), but may be accompanied by unpredictable sedation and hypotension. The usual clonidine dosage in children is 1–2 µg/kg intravenously or epidurally, or 2–4 µg/kg orally.

ANALGESIA FOR NEONATES AND INFANTS AGED 6 MONTHS OR YOUNGER

Neonates and young infants are a special group of patients because the immaturity of many physiological mechanisms complicates both the response to pain and the effects of analgesics (see Chapter A25). Pain assessment is particularly difficult at this age and has been the subject of considerable interest. Pain assessment tools that are appropriate and valid to both the infant's stage

Table 34.7 *Suggested monitoring for children receiving opioids*

Analgesia	Validated pain score
Sedation	Sedation scale
Respiration	Respiratory rate, pulse oximetry (in air)
Cardiovascular	Heart rate/blood pressure
Nausea and vomiting	Nausea scale

Table 34.8 *Protocol for ketamine–morphine infusion*

Preparation	Ketamine 2 mg/kg and morphine 1 mg/kg in 50-ml solution
Concentration	40 µg/kg/ml ketamine; 20 µg/kg/ml morphine
Initial dose	2.5–5.0 ml (100–200 µg/kg ketamine)
Infusion	0.5–1.5 ml/h (20–60 µg/kg/h ketamine; 10–30 µg/kg/h morphine)

of development and the situation in which they are to be used must be chosen – many are listed in Table A25.1 i.

High standards of care are necessary if pain is to be managed safely in early life. Special training and skills are a prerequisite for staff prescribing and delivering care, and facilities should meet the potential need for supportive therapy should it be necessary. In practice, this means that inpatient care is usually necessary, often at high-dependency or intensive care levels provided in specialized units with multidisciplinary support.

Systemic analgesia

The choice of analgesics is very limited in the neonate. So little is known about the effects of many drugs during the phase of rapid development up to 6 months of age that each patient must be considered individually and closely monitored as responses are often unpredictable.

Acetaminophen and nonsteroidal anti-inflammatory drugs

NSAIDs are traditionally not prescribed below the age of 6 months except in unusual circumstances. In fact, very little is known of the effects of NSAIDs in the immature, but the important role of prostaglandins in autoregulation of organ perfusion, particularly cerebral and renal, has discouraged their use.

Acetaminophen has been used extensively at all ages as both an analgesic and an antipyretic. It is widely considered to be a safe analgesic, although efficacy studies are lacking. Acetaminophen is probably a weak analgesic in the neonate; used alone, it was ineffective at reducing the pain response to heel lance in term neonates.[27***] The pharmacokinetics of acetaminophen have been fairly well studied in the neonate, although data must be interpreted with some caution owing to the low numbers of subjects in most studies. Plasma levels and elimination are very dependent on route of administration – high initial doses being required when given rectally. Potential hepatotoxicity should limit treatment at full doses to 5 days or fewer; recommended maximum daily doses are also sometimes reduced to 60 mg/kg/day.[28]

Opioids

Depression of respiration is the principal effect which

limits opioid analgesia in the neonate and infant. If respiration is supported, high doses are well tolerated, otherwise responses are difficult to predict and the therapeutic ratio appears small. Codeine phosphate and morphine have been used widely in the neonate and infant:

1　Codeine has a good safety record and a single dose of 1 mg/kg is unlikely to depress respiration in a healthy neonate. Codeine is metabolized to morphine, and indeed all or some of its effects may be caused by morphine. Further doses of codeine might therefore be expected to lead to opioid side-effects due to either compound. Codeine cannot be given intravenously as severe hypotension has been reported, presumably because of histamine release.[29]

2　Morphine has principally been used intravenously when respiration is supported in the neonate (Table 34.9). The pharmacokinetics of morphine indicate that after a loading dose infusion rates should be lower than those normally used for older children, although substantial interpatient variation may be expected.[30-32] NCA, as described previously, is suitable for neonates, combined with frequent pain assessments and monitoring for side-effects. At present, opioid infusion can only be recommended in intensive care areas.

Local anesthetics

Local anesthesia avoids many of the complications of systemic analgesics in the neonate. Toxicity may be more likely in early life – some authorities would therefore recommend reduced doses, particularly if infusions are used. Plasma levels of bupivacaine certainly seem to rise dramatically after 48 h of epidural infusion at a constant rate in the neonate. Ropivacaine and levobupivacaine have not yet been well evaluated, but their lower toxicity

would clearly be advantageous in this vulnerable group.[33] Topical local anesthesia is suitable for procedures in the neonate, lidocaine (lignocaine)–prilocaine cream is safe provided the dose is proportionately limited according to size (see Chapter A25).

Local anesthetic blocks are described in detail in the next section. The most useful in the neonate are listed in Table 34.10. Following major surgery, epidural analgesic infusion has been described using the caudal approach to the epidural space.[34] As the spine is shorter and straighter in early life, a catheter can reliably be threaded to lumbar or thoracic sites through a Tuohy needle or intravenous cannula inserted through the sacrococcygeal membrane. The principal advantage is the relative ease and safety of the approach in comparison with direct lumbar or thoracic placement, the skin–epidural distance in a neonate being 0.5 cm or sometimes less. Opioid–local anesthetic solutions have not been extensively used in the neonatal period.

LOCAL ANESTHETIC TECHNIQUES

Children dislike needles and will not usually cooperate with uncomfortable or prolonged procedures; consequently, with a few exceptions, local anesthetic techniques can only be performed in children while under general anesthesia. This limits their utility mostly to the post-surgical period, which is their commonest indication. Evidence for efficacy of local anesthesia is discussed in Chapter A25. Blocks are performed using full asepsis and with monitoring commensurate with the potential risks. Local anesthetic techniques are suitable for all ages with low morbidity, provided recommended doses are not exceeded and a suitable environment is available for placement and aftercare.[35,36] For convenience, techniques using local anesthetics with adjunctive compounds, for example opioids, clonidine, and ketamine, are also described here.

Table 34.9 *Suggested morphine infusion protocols in the neonate*[a]

Neonatal morphine infusion	
Preparation	Morphine sulfate 1.0 mg/kg in 50-ml solution
Concentration	20 µg/kg/ml
Initial dose	0.5–5.0 ml (10–100 µg/kg)
Infusion	0.1–0.6 ml/h (2–12 µg/kg/h)
Neonatal NCA	
Preparation	Morphine sulfate 1 mg/kg in 50-ml solution
Concentration	20 µg/kg/ml
Initial dose	0.5–5.0 ml (10–100 µg/kg)
Programming	Background infusion: 0.0–0.5 ml/h (0–10 µg/kg/h)
	NCA dose: 0.5–1.0 ml (10–20 µg/kg/h)
	Lockout interval: 20 min

a. With full cardiorespiratory monitoring in intensive care areas.
NCA, nurse-controlled analgesia.

Table 34.10 *Useful local anesthetic blocks in the neonate*

Block	Procedure
Penile	Circumcision Meatoplasty
Ilioinguinal	Inguinal herniorrhaphy Orchiopexy
Umbilical	Umbilical hernia
Caudal	Surgery below level of T12
Thoracic/lumbar epidural (caudal approach)	Major surgery

Peripheral nerve blocks

Dorsal nerves of penis

Anatomy

The two dorsal nerves supply the distal two-thirds of the penis. They arise as terminal branches of the pudendal nerves and can be blocked as they emerge from under the pubic bone in the subpubic space at the base of the penis. The nerves then run close to the dorsal penile arteries and veins on the corpora cavernosa of the penis. The subpubic space is covered anteriorly by the skin and the superficial and deep layers of fascia of the anterior abdominal wall. It is divided into two compartments (each containing a nerve and vessels) by the suspensory ligament of the penis.

Method

Injections are made lateral to the symphysis pubis on both sides at the base of the penis. After antisepsis, a short-beveled 22-gauge regional block needle is inserted posteriorly through the two fascial layers, which can be felt as separate slight reductions in resistance about 0.5 cm or more from the skin. After gentle aspiration, 0.1 ml/kg of local anesthetic solution is injected on either side.

Local anesthetic solutions

Only plain (no vasoconstrictor) solutions of local anesthetic should be used; 0.5% bupivacaine is suitable.

Complications

Hematoma owing to puncture of vessels or corpora cavernosa is possible. Compression due to large hematoma may cause edema or swelling of the penis.

Ilioinguinal/iliohypogastric nerves

Anatomy

The ilioinguinal and iliohypogastric nerves supply the inguinal region. They arise from the lumbar plexus and lie conveniently close together medial to the anterior–superior iliac spine (ASIS). The ilioinguinal nerve and a third nerve – the genital branch of the genitofemoral nerve – also supply the skin of the scrotum on that side. The ilioinguinal and iliohypogastric nerves lie beneath the external oblique aponeurosis between the internal oblique and the transversus abdominis muscles.

Method

A short, beveled 22-gauge regional block needle is inserted one child's finger's breadth medial to the ASIS. The needle is advanced until a change in resistance is felt as it passes through the external oblique aponeurosis, sometimes described as a "click" or "pop." The position can be confirmed by observing the needle supported by the fascia moving with respiration when it is released. After gentle aspiration, the local anesthetic is injected – 0.2–0.5 ml/kg. If the scrotum is also to be anesthetized,

the genital branch of the genitofemoral nerve can be blocked by injecting close to the pubic tubercle on that side – 0.1–0.2 ml/kg.

Local anesthetic solution

Bupivacaine 0.25% up to a maximum dose of 2.5 mg/kg (1 ml/kg).

Complications

Unwanted motor block of the femoral nerve producing leg weakness.

Fascia iliaca compartment block[37]

The femoral nerve, obturator nerve, and lateral cutaneous nerve of the thigh can be blocked together by injecting local anesthetic into the confined space of the fascia iliaca compartment in which they lie.

Anatomy

The nerves arise from the lumbar plexus and run beneath the inguinal ligament deep to the fascia iliaca, which is itself continuous with the deep layers of the ligament. In the thigh, the fascia iliaca lies beneath the fascia lata and forms the roof of the "compartment." Inferior to the inguinal ligament, the fascia iliaca forms the roof of a space known as the "lacuna musculorum," which is continuous with the fascia iliaca compartment above. Local anesthetic injected into the lacuna musculorum spreads to block the nerves as they pass through the compartment.

Method

A 22-gauge, short, beveled regional block needle is inserted 0.5 cm below the inguinal ligament two-thirds of the distance laterally from the pubic tubercle. The needle is advanced at an angle of 60° to the skin in a cephalad direction using a saline-filled syringe to detect loss of resistance, which is detected twice as the needle tip penetrates the fascia lata and the fascia iliaca. After gentle aspiration, the local anesthetic solution is injected.

Local anesthetic solution

Bupivacaine 0.25% at a dose of 0.5 ml/kg (0.7 ml/kg) has been recommended for children < 20 kg.

Infraorbital nerve

The nerve supplies the skin and mucous membrane of the upper lip and lower eyelid and the skin between. It has been particularly advocated for cleft lip repair and is also suitable for surgery of the supplied area of the face and to the maxillary incisors, canine, and premolar teeth.

Anatomy.

The infraorbital nerve, which runs in the infraorbital canal, emerges through the infraorbital foramen of the maxilla, which is palpable below the midpoint of the infraorbital margin. The foramen is located approximately half-way between this point and the angle of the mouth and medial (at least 0.75 cm) to the nasal alar base.

Method

The nerve is blocked either percutaneously or intraorally through the labial sulcus. The intraoral technique utilizes the dentition as a landmark and is therefore more suitable for the older child.

Percutaneous technique

The needle is introduced perpendicular to, and through, the skin at the site of the infraorbital foramen. It is advanced until bony resistance is established and then slightly withdrawn and the local anesthetic injected.

Intraoral technique

The midpoint of the infraorbital ridge is palpated externally with the index finger. The infraorbital foramen is then identified as a bony depression just below this point with the fingertip. Using the thumb of the same hand, the upper lip is retracted and the needle advanced through the labial sulcus opposite the first premolar or first primary molar. Infiltration of local anesthetic below the palpating index finger will be felt as a slight swelling at that point.

Local anesthetic solution

Bupivacaine 0.5% at a dose of 0.5–0.75 ml with epinephrine (adrenaline) is injected.

Brachial plexus

The nerve supply to the upper limb is provided by the brachial plexus formed from the nerve roots of the fifth cervical (C5) to first thoracic (T1) spinal nerves with variable contributions from C4 and T2. The nerves of the plexus pass through the neck and below the midpoint of the clavicle into the axilla. Many methods of blocking the plexus have been described using both supraclavicular and infraclavicular approaches, and they are described in the specialist texts on the subject that may be consulted. Supraclavicular approaches to the brachial plexus have been little used in children except in expert hands because of the need to inject in close proximity to the pleura and vital structures of the neck. The axillary approach is safer, and hence the method of choice where practical, and will provide analgesia to forearm and hand.

Axillary approach
Anatomy

The three composite cords of the brachial plexus are closely related to the axillary artery in the axilla. The nerves and artery are ensheathed in fascia forming a number of compartments which are discontinuous with those above the clavicle, limiting spread of the local anesthetic solution.

Method

In the supine position, the arm is abducted to 90° with the elbow flexed. The axillary artery is palpated with the index finger, high in the axilla and overlying the humerus against which it can be compressed. The finger is moved along the artery to the midpoint of the axilla and the needle (attached to a short extension tube) is inserted just above this point toward the artery until it enters the fascial sheath, identifiable by a sudden reduction in resistance. The location is confirmed by observing pulsations of the unsupported needle and failure to aspirate blood before injection. A catheter can also be located in this position to allow reinjection or infusion of local anesthetic. If the artery is unintentionally entered, it should be transfixed and two injections made: one on either side followed by compression of the vessel to avoid hematoma formation.

Local anesthetic solution

Bupivacaine 0.25% at a dose of 0.5 ml/kg followed by further injections or an infusion not exceeding recommended doses of local anesthetic.

Intercostal nerves

Cutaneous segmental sensory innervation in the thorax and upper abdomen is supplied by consecutive intercostal nerves which may be individually blocked by one or more injections or, more commonly, by the use of catheters in various sites in order to provide more extensive and continuous analgesia. These techniques are to be compared with epidural block in terms of ease and safety of insertion technique and the quality of analgesia.

Intercostal block

Classical approaches to the intercostal space have been used successfully in children. The midaxillary line approach is the most commonly chosen. A slightly modified technique of needle insertion has been advocated in children, possibly reducing the likelihood of pneumothorax as the needle enters the intercostal space parallel to the rib.[38]

Catheter techniques
Subcostal block

A catheter placed in one or more intercostal spaces allows infusion of local anesthesia, as described previously in children.[39]

Paravertebral block

Local anesthesia in the paravertebral space, which exists between T1 and T12 where it is obliterated by the psoas muscle, allows unilateral multiple spinal segments to be blocked by a single injection. Catheters in the paravertebral space allow infusion of local anesthetic and extended analgesia that may be similar to epidural blockade.[40]

Anatomy

As in the adult, the paravertebral space in children is a potential space communicating from T1 to T12 lateral to the thoracic vertebral bodies. Dorsally, the space is limited by the transverse process of the vertebra and the costotransverse ligament; anterolaterally, it is limited by the parietal pleura. The space contains the intercostal nerve and thoracic sympathetic chain as well as the intercostal vessels.

Method

In the lateral decubitus position, a Tuohy needle is inserted about 1 cm lateral to the vertebral spinous process and advanced perpendicularly until contact is made with the transverse process. The needle is withdrawn slightly and then "walked" along the transverse process either above or below where it is advanced close to the bone. The paravertebral space is detected by loss of resistance on piercing the costotransverse ligament and injection made and a catheter inserted. For thoracotomy, puncture should be at T5/6; for abdominal surgery (unilateral incision), puncture should be at T9/10. A catheter can also be placed directly in the paravertebral region during thoracic surgery.

Local anesthetic solution

Bupivacaine 0.25% at a dose of 0.5 ml/kg followed by infusion of 0.2 ml/kg/h.

Epidural analgesia

In comparison with other techniques, local anesthetics given into the epidural space can provide analgesia to relatively extensive areas of the body as a function of the total drug dosage. Catheters are also easily placed into the epidural space and considerable experience of prolonged epidural local anesthetic infusion in children is available. Other drugs are effective at lower doses than required for systemic administration: opioids, ketamine, and clonidine can be used alone or in combination with local anesthetics in the epidural space.

Caudal approach

The indications for caudal analgesia are very wide and have been discussed previously in Chapter A25. Pain following almost all surgery involving an incision below the level of the umbilicus (T10) can be reduced or abolished using a caudal method of drug administration.

Anatomy

Ossification of the five sacral vertebral segments begins with the two lowest at the age of about 18 years and is complete by the end of the third decade. The sacral hiatus is a defect in the fifth vertebra and is covered by ligaments, subcutaneous fat, and skin. The size of the hiatus decreases with maturity and may become ossified in the adult. The sacral canal contains the distal (caudal) epidural space, cauda equina, and dura extending to S3 at birth and S2 in childhood. Identification of the sacral hiatus is usually easy in infancy and childhood. It is palpable as a soft depression between the sacral cornua of S5. It is also located at the apex of an equilateral triangle, the base of which is between the posterior iliac spines. An alternative approach with the child in the lateral position is to find the hiatus at the midline intersection of a line drawn perpendicularly from the greater trochanter of the femur when the leg is flexed at the hip.

Method

Once the hiatus is located, under aseptic conditions, a needle is inserted through the skin in the midline at an angle of 45° aiming cranially. There is a sudden change in resistance as the needle passes through the relatively dense membrane and into the space. Intravascular or intradural location of the needle are excluded by gentle aspiration on the needle and by removing the syringe from the needle for 30 s or longer. An intravascular cannula (22 gauge) can also be used, which is gently advanced over the needle for 2–3 cm once the space is entered. Alternatively, a catheter can also be advanced into the space, and for some considerable distance higher if it is desired to reach lumbar or thoracic epidural segments. The extent of local anesthetic block depends on the volume of solution injected (see Table A25.6). Other analgesics used alone or in combination with caudal local anesthetic include: clonidine, 1–2 µg/kg; ketamine, 0.5 mg/kg; and opioids, e.g. morphine 20–50 µg/kg in preservative-free solutions.

Lumbar and thoracic epidural analgesia

Anatomy

The principal surface landmarks and technique of epidural analgesia are similar at all ages, except that distances are much smaller in early life and ligaments softer and less easily identified. The vertebral column is also less curved in early life and this combined with the shorter distances involved mean that catheters can easily be threaded from one spinal segment to another.

Technique

In children, general anesthesia is a prerequisite with full cardiorespiratory monitoring. An 18-gauge Tuohy epidural needle is suitable for all ages, and shorter versions of the needle are available for children less than 10 kg (1 year) of age. Also available are 19-g needles, which are preferred by some practitioners for very small infants and neonates, but the fine 23-gauge epidural catheter which must be used with this needle is prone to technical problems.[41]

Identification of the epidural space

A technique of loss of resistance to continuous pressure on a syringe of saline (as described elsewhere) is preferred. Air is not recommended to detect loss of resistance in children because of the risk of venous air embolus, unblocked dermatomes due to air pockets in the epidural space, and a possible association with neurological damage.[42] Dural tap or accidental penetration of the dura has been reported in children, but the incidence is very low if the above technique is used to locate the space. The use of epidural test doses is controversial; epinephrine-containing solutions may also detect intravascular injection, but high rates of false-positive and false-negative tests have been reported. Prior estimation of the depth of the epidural space may be helpful, and a number of formulae have been suggested; however, interindividual variation is common.[43,44] In the neonate, the lumbar epidural space is between 0.4 and 1.5 cm from the skin, depending on approach. Below 6 months, there is little correlation between depth, age, and weight. In older infants and children between 6 months and 10 years, 1 mm/kg is a good approximation,[44] or depth (cm) = 1 + 0.15 × age (years) and depth (cm) = 0.8 + 0.05 × weight (kg) respectively.[43]

Epidural catheters

An epidural catheter, if indicated, is placed through the needle. A minimum length of 4 cm is normally left in the space as this reduces the chances of dislodgment of the catheter because of movement.[41] The catheter should be fixed at the skin using a clear plastic dressing such that the entry site can easily be inspected later; it is usually also taped to the child's back as far as the shoulder. Minor technical complications are common, particularly occlusion and kinking of fine catheters; disconnection and dislodgment also occur more frequently in pediatric practice.[45] The use of larger catheters where possible, experience, and improved fixation technique should reduce these to a minimum. Retrograde leakage of the infusate back to the insertion site also occurs, but does not usually reduce efficacy. The infection rate of epidural catheters is low even when located below the "nappy line."[46] Slight redness at the insertion site is common; inflammation with redness and swelling or visible pus is an indication for removal of the catheter, skin swab culture, and appropriate antibiotic therapy if indicated.

Epidural drugs and infusions

Drugs, doses, and infusion rates for epidural analgesia are given in Table 34.11. An initial dose of local anesthetic with or without opioid is followed by a continuous infusion of the solution. For intraoperative use, concentrated local anesthetic solutions are usually required initially to establish a sensory motor block; for postoperative or other acute pain, analgesia can be provided by

Table 34.11 *Drugs doses and infusion rates for epidural analgesia*

Bupivacaine–morphine	
Initial dose	Bupivacaine 0.25% 0.5–0.75 ml/kg
Infusion	Bupivacaine 0.125% with preservative-free morphine 0.001%
Rate	0.1–0.4 ml/h
Bupivacaine–fentanyl	
Initial dose	Bupivacaine 0.25% 0.5–0.75 ml/kg
Infusion	Bupivacaine 0.125% with fentanyl 1–2 µg/ml
Rate	0.1–0.4 ml/h
Ropivacaine[a]	
Initial dose	Ropivacaine 0.2% 0.5–0.75 ml/kg
Infusion	Ropivacaine 0.2%
Rate	0.1–0.4 ml/h

a. See references 47 and 48.

more dilute solutions. Augmentation of analgesia using opioids is common – morphine, hydromorphone, and fentanyl are all popular. Complications of local anesthesia include accidental intravascular injection, unwanted motor block, and toxicity due to accidental overdose or accumulation after prolonged infusion. Meticulous technique, monitoring, and frequent review of infusion rates should minimize these problems.

Inadequate analgesia may be the result of a poorly located catheter or inadequate spread of local anesthetic; tachyphylaxis also occurs. Relocation of the catheter by judicious withdrawal of a short (1 cm) length, increasing the volume or strength of the analgesic infusion, or the addition of adjunctive analgesics may overcome these problems.

Epidural local anesthetic–opioid combinations remain popular, but improvements in analgesia are at the expense of opioid-related complications. Sedation, respiratory depression, and itching can be treated with small doses of naloxone; nausea and vomiting is managed with antiemetics as with systemic administration (see Table 34.6).

Retention of urine

This bothersome complication of epidural analgesia occurs more frequently when opioids are used, when thoracic dermatomes are blocked, and in older children. Prophylactic urinary catheterization is indicated for high-risk groups, otherwise urine output is monitored.

CONCLUSION

Substantial planning and expertise are needed to implement safe and effective analgesia in neonates, infants, and children. The number of established treatments for pain in children remains relatively small and may be inadequate for some circumstances. Much more investigation into the effects of development on pain and analgesia are required in order to better evaluate the effectiveness of treatments in pediatric practice. Substantial progress has been made in the last few years, and the subject is at least given much greater priority than before. Pediatric pain management still does not feature prominently in the basic education and training of many health professionals. Until this occurs, progress in the field is likely to remain slow.

REFERENCES

◆ 1. Lloyd-Thomas AR, Howard RF. A pain service for children. *Paediatr Anaesth* 1994; **4:** 3–15.

2. Hester NO. The preoperational child's reaction to immunizations. *Nurs Res* 1979; **28:** 250–5.

◆ 3. Beyer JE, Denyes MJ, Villaruel AM. The creation, validation and continuing development of the oucher: a measure of pain intensity in children. *J Paediatr Nurs* 1992; **7**: 335.

◆ 4. Wong DL, Baker CM. Pain in children: comparison of assessment scales. *Okla Nurs* 1988; **33**: 8.

5. Bieri D, Reeve RA, Champion GD, *et al*. The Faces Pain Scale for the self-assessment of the severity of pain experienced by children: development, initial validation, and preliminary investigation for ratio scale properties. *Pain* 1990; **41**: 139–50.

6. Merkel SI, Voepel-Lewis T, Shayevitz JR, Malviya S. The FLACC: a behavioral scale for scoring postoperative pain in young children. *Pediatr Nurs* 1997; **23**: 293–7.

◆ 7. Buttner W, Fincke W. Analysis of behavioural and physiological parameters for the assessment of postoperative analgesic demand in newborns, infants and young children. *Paediatr Anaesth* 2000; **10**: 303–18.

8. Ambuel B, Hamlett KW, Marx CM, Blumer JL. Assessing distress in pediatric intensive care environments: the COMFORT scale. *J Pediatr Psychol* 1992; **17**: 95–109.

9. van Dijk M, de Boer JB, Koot HM, *et al*. The reliability and validity of the COMFORT scale as a postoperative pain instrument in 0 to 3-year-old infants. *Pain* 2000; **84**: 367–77.

◆ 10. Anderson BJ, Woollard GA, Holford NH. A model for size and age changes in the pharmacokinetics of paracetamol in neonates, infants and children. *Br J Clin Pharmacol* 2000; **50**: 125–34.

◆ 11. van Lingen RA, Deinum JT, Quak JM, *et al*. Pharmacokinetics and metabolism of rectally administered paracetamol in preterm neonates. *Arch Dis Child (Fetal Neonatal edn)* 1999; **80**: F59–63.

12. Seth N, Llewellyn NE, Howard RF. Parental opinions regarding the route of administration of analgesic medication in children. *Paediatr Anaesth* 2000; **10**: 537–44.

◆ 13. Bray RJ. Postoperative analgesia provided by morphine infusion in children. *Anaesthesia* 1983; **38**: 1075–8.

14. Granry JC, Rod B, Monrigal JP, *et al*. The analgesic efficacy of an injectable prodrug of acetaminophen in children after orthopaedic surgery. *Paediatr Anaesth* 1997; **7**: 445–9.

15. Bruce E, Franck L. Self-administered nitrous oxide (Entonox) for the management of procedural pain. *Paediatr Nurs* 2000; **12**: 15–19.

16. Striebel HW, Oelmann T, Spies C, *et al*. Patient-controlled intranasal analgesia: a method for noninvasive postoperative pain management. *Anesth Analg* 1996; **83**: 548–51.

17. Ashburn MA, Lind GH, Gillie MH, *et al*. Oral transmucosal fentanyl citrate (OTFC) for the treatment of postoperative pain. *Anesth Analg* 1993; **76**: 377–81.

18. Howell TK. Paracetamol-induced fulminant hepatic failure in a child after 5 days of therapeutic doses. *Paediatr Anaesth* 2000; **10**: 344–35.

◆ 19. Short JA, Barr CA, Palmer CD, *et al*. Use of diclofenac in children with asthma. *Anaesthesia* 2000; **55**: 334–7.

● 20. Williams DG, Hatch DJ, Howard RF. Codeine phosphate in paediatric medicine. *Br J Anaesth* 2001; **86**: 413–21.

● 21. Tobias JD. Weak analgesics and nonsteroidal anti-inflammatory agents in the management of children with acute pain. *Pediatr Clin North Am* 2000; **47**: 527–43.

● 22. Schmid RL, Sandler AN, Katz J. Use and efficacy of low-dose ketamine in the management of acute postoperative pain: a review of current techniques and outcomes. *Pain* 1999; **82**: 111–25.

23. Marcus RJ, Victoria BA, Rushman SC, Thompson JP. Comparison of ketamine and morphine for analgesia after tonsillectomy in children. *Br J Anaesth* 2000; **84**: 739–42.

24. Javery KB, Ussery TW, Steger HG, Colclough GW. Comparison of morphine and morphine with ketamine for postoperative analgesia. *Can J Anaesth* 1996; **43**: 212–15.

25. Reimer EJ, Dunn GS, Montgomery CJ, *et al*. The effectiveness of clonidine as an analgesic in paediatric adenotonsillectomy. *Can J Anaesth* 1998; **45**: 1162–7.

● 26. Nishina K, Mikawa K, Shiga M, Obara H. Clonidine in paediatric anaesthesia. *Paediatr Anaesth* 1999; **9**: 187–202.

◆ 27. Shah V, Taddio A, Ohlsson A. Randomised controlled trial of paracetamol for heel prick pain in neonates. *Arch Dis Child (Fetal Neonatal edn)* 1998; **79**: F209–11.

● 28. Southall D. *Prevention and Control of Pain in Children – a Manual for Health Care Professionals*. London: BMJ Books, 1997: 56.

29. Shanahan EC, Marshall AG, Garrett CPO. Adverse reactions to intravenous codeine phosphate in children. A report of three cases. *Anaesthesia* 1983; **38**: 40–3.

● 30. Kart T, Christrup LL, Rasmussen M. Recommended use of morphine in neonates, infants and children based on a literature review. Part 1. Pharmacokinetics. *Paediatr Anaesth* 1997; **7**: 5–11.

31. Lynn A, Nespeca MK, Bratton SL, *et al*. Clearance of morphine in postoperative infants during intravenous infusion: the influence of age and surgery. *Anesth Analg* 1998; **86**: 958–63.

◆ 32. Lynn AM, Nespeca MK, Bratton SL, Shen DD. Intravenous morphine in postoperative infants: intermittent bolus dosing versus targeted continuous infusions. *Pain* 2000; **88**: 89–95.

33. Kanai Y, Katsuki H, Takasaki M. Comparisons of the anesthetic potency and intracellular concentrations of S(–) and R(+) bupivacaine and ropivacaine in crayfish giant axon in vitro. *Anesth Analg* 2000; **90**: 415–20.

34. Bosenberg AT, Bland BA, Schulte-Steinberg O, Downing JW. Thoracic epidural anesthesia via caudal route in infants. *Anesthesiology* 1988; **69**: 265–9.

35. Dalens B. Peripheral nerve blockade in the management of postoperative pain in children. In: Schecter NL, Berde CB, Yaster M eds. *Pain in Infants, Children and Adolescents*. Baltimore, MD: Williams and Wilkins, 1993: 261–80.

36. Giaufre E, Dalens B, Gombert A. Epidemiology and morbidity of regional anesthesia in children: a one-year prospective survey of the French-Language Society of Pediatric Anesthesiologists. *Anesth Analg* 1996; **83:** 904–12.

◆ 37. Dalens B, Vanneuville G, Tanguy A. Comparison of the fascia iliaca compartment block with the 3-in-1 block in children. *Anesth Analg* 1989; **69:** 705–13.

38. Shelly MP, Park GR. Intercostal nerve blockade for children. *Anaesthesia* 1987; **42:** 541–54.

39. Cooper MG, Seaton HL. Intra-operative placement of an intercostal catheter for post thoracotomy pain relief in a child. *Paediatr Anaesth* 1992; **2:** 165–7.

40. Lonnqvist PA, Richardson J. Use of paravertebral blockade in children. *Techniques Reg Anaesth Pain Manage* 1999; **3:** 184–8.

41. Sage FJ, Lloyd Thomas AR, Howard RF. Paediatric lumbar epidurals: a comparison of 21-G and 23-G catheters in patients weighing less than 10 kg. *Paediatr Anaesth* 2000; **10:** 279–82.

42. Sethna NF, Berde CB. Venous air embolism during identification of the epidural space in children. *Anesth Analg* 1993; **76:** 925–7.

43. Hasan MA, Howard RF, Lloyd-Thomas AR. Depth of epidural space in children. *Anaesthesia* 1994; **49:** 1085–107.

44. Bosenberg AT, Gouws E. Skin–epidural distance in children. *Anaesthesia* 1995; **50:** 895–7.

45. Wood CE, Goresky GV, Klassen KA, *et al*. Complications of continuous epidural infusions for postoperative analgesia in children. *Can J Anaesth* 1994; **41:** 613–20.

46. Strafford MA, Wilder RT, Berde CB. The risk of infection from epidural analgesia in children: a review of 1620 cases. *Anesth Analg* 1995; **80:** 234–8.

47. Moriarty A. Postoperative extradural infusions in children: preliminary data from a comparison of bupivacaine/diamorphine with plain ropivacaine. *Paediatr Anaesth* 1999; **9:** 423–7.

48. Ivani G, Lampugnani E, De Negri P, *et al*. Ropivacaine vs bupivacaine in major surgery in infants. *Can J Anaesth* 1999; **46:** 467–9.

Clinical trials

35

Clinical trials: acute and chronic pain

AUDUN STUBHAUG

The clinical trial	449	Pain intensity	455
Explanatory and pragmatic attitudes	449	What is a clinically important reduction in pain intensity?	455
What is the purpose of the study?	450		
Choose a primary efficacy variable	450	Repeated measurements: create a summary measure such as SPID or TOTPAR	456
Study design	450		
Assay sensitivity	450	Consumption of rescue analgesia	456
Choice of treatments and controls	450	Onset of analgesia	456
Why is knowledge of the placebo response essential in studies of pain?	453	Remediation time	457
		Global assessment	457
Placebo treatment is not unethical	454	Evoked pain	457
Method of randomization	454	Outcomes that can easily be extracted for use in meta-analysis	457
Inclusion of patients: inclusion based on pain mechanisms?	454		
		Long-term trials: assessment of quality of life	457
Blinding and unblinding: active placebo	454	Statistical issues	458
Parallel or crossover studies?	454	Publish your trial	458
More about outcomes in trials of pain treatment	455	References	458

A clinical trial is a planned experiment designed to assess the efficacy of a treatment by comparing the outcomes in a group of patients treated with a test treatment with those observed in a similar control group of patients. The patients should normally be assigned to one of the groups by a randomization procedure, and enrolled and followed over the same time period. Thus, studies using historical controls do not qualify as clinical trials. Even if most published clinical trials assess drug treatment, effects of other kinds of interventions can, and should, be tested in the same way, e.g. surgical procedures, physical therapy, nursing procedures, and patient information. This chapter will specifically address trial methodology in assessment of analgesic drugs, but most issues are relevant for other interventions as well.

THE CLINICAL TRIAL

1 Define the purpose of the study. Perform a thorough literature search. State specific hypotheses.
2 Define clearly main outcome(s), classification variables, and confounding variables.

3 Design the study. Controls. Placebo? Blinding. Calculate sample size.
4 Apply for approval from ethical committee and drug regulatory authorities (when applicable).
5 Use an adequate randomization method and maintain allocation concealment.
6 Conduct the trial. Make sure there is no unmasking of patient or observer blinding.
7 Analyze the results. Use descriptive statistics, test the hypotheses, and estimate treatment effect size.
8 Draw conclusions with care. Be careful with a posteriori hypotheses.
9 Publish the results in sufficient detail to permit an informed judgment of the validity of your conclusions.

EXPLANATORY AND PRAGMATIC ATTITUDES

Schwartz and Lellouch[1] have made an informative distinction between explanatory and pragmatic orientations in the design of a clinical trial. *Explanatory studies* seek to find a causal relationship that has general validity out-

Table 35.1 *Explanatory versus pragmatic attitudes*

Design issue	Explanatory	Pragmatic
Main question	General biological principle, e.g. can presurgical treatment prevent postoperative hypersensitivity?	What is the best treatment in clinical practice? For example, acetaminophen with or without NSAID
Patient selection	Selective	Inclusive
Treatments	Specific actions (e.g. selective receptor agonists/antagonists)	Clinical favorites, including combinations
Controls	Placebo	Other active medication
Dose	High, often fixed	Titrate as in clinic
Treatment conditions	Optimal	Corresponding to clinical practice
Outcomes	Biologically meaningful	Clinically relevant
Analysis	Per protocol	Intention to treat

Acetaminophen (paracetamol).
NSAID, nonsteroidal anti-inflammatory drug.

side the particular clinical situation studied – a biological principle. A strict study design may be necessary to obtain a precise answer to a specific question. *Pragmatic studies*, on the other hand, seek to find the best way to treat patients in specific clinical situations. The results are not necessarily valid for other populations than the one studied. Most clinical trials have elements of both these orientations. However, it is useful to be aware of the difference. Too often, general conclusions are drawn from pragmatic studies, or limitations of the study are not sufficiently emphasized. Table 35.1 summarizes typical differences regarding trial design issues between explanatory and pragmatic studies.

WHAT IS THE PURPOSE OF THE STUDY?

A thorough literature search in the field is necessary. On the basis of this search, you should be able to define the purpose of the study clearly. How will the proposed research advance the literature and potentially lead to improved patient care? If this is difficult to clarify in the early stage, it will probably not become easier at a later stage.

CHOOSE A PRIMARY EFFICACY VARIABLE

If many efficacy variables are measured, a statistical problem arises. Even if there is no true difference between two treatments, the probability (P) of finding a statistically significant difference at the 0.05 level if 10 different independent variables are tested is $1 - 0.95^{10} = 0.40$ (i.e. 40%). To avoid this problem, a *primary efficacy variable* should be chosen before the start of the study. This primary efficacy variable should be the basis for the *sample size determination*. Ideally, the primary efficacy variable should be a biologically or clinically meaningful outcome. However, sometimes a *surrogate endpoint* must be used. A surrogate endpoint can be defined as an observed variable that relates in some way to the variable of primary interest.

Outcomes used in studies in pain relief are discussed in more detail later.

STUDY DESIGN

The randomized, double-blind, placebo-controlled trial has become the standard in investigation of new analgesics. Several authors have shown that, in general, inadequately controlled clinical trials yield larger estimates of treatment effects than adequately controlled ones.[2] Thus, proper randomization and blinding is essential. It is also of crucial importance that the study is designed so that it is capable of finding a real difference. The study must have *assay sensitivity*.

ASSAY SENSITIVITY

Demonstration of assay sensitivity means that a study is able to show a significant difference between a standard analgesic and placebo, between two active drugs, or between two different doses of an active drug. One classical pitfall is to compare two active drugs, find no difference, and conclude that the two drugs are equally effective (see Equivalence trial). Assay sensitivity can be divided into *upside sensitivity* (the ability to discriminate between two active drugs) and *downside sensitivity* (the ability of a study to discriminate between an active drug and placebo). The score of placebo and standard active drug in a pain model decides upside and downside sensitivity in that pain model (symptomresearch.com). In general, it is difficult to have both high upside sensitivity and high downside sensitivity in the same trial.

CHOICE OF TREATMENTS AND CONTROLS

The number of treatment groups necessary depends on the aim of the study. The aim could be to demonstrate:

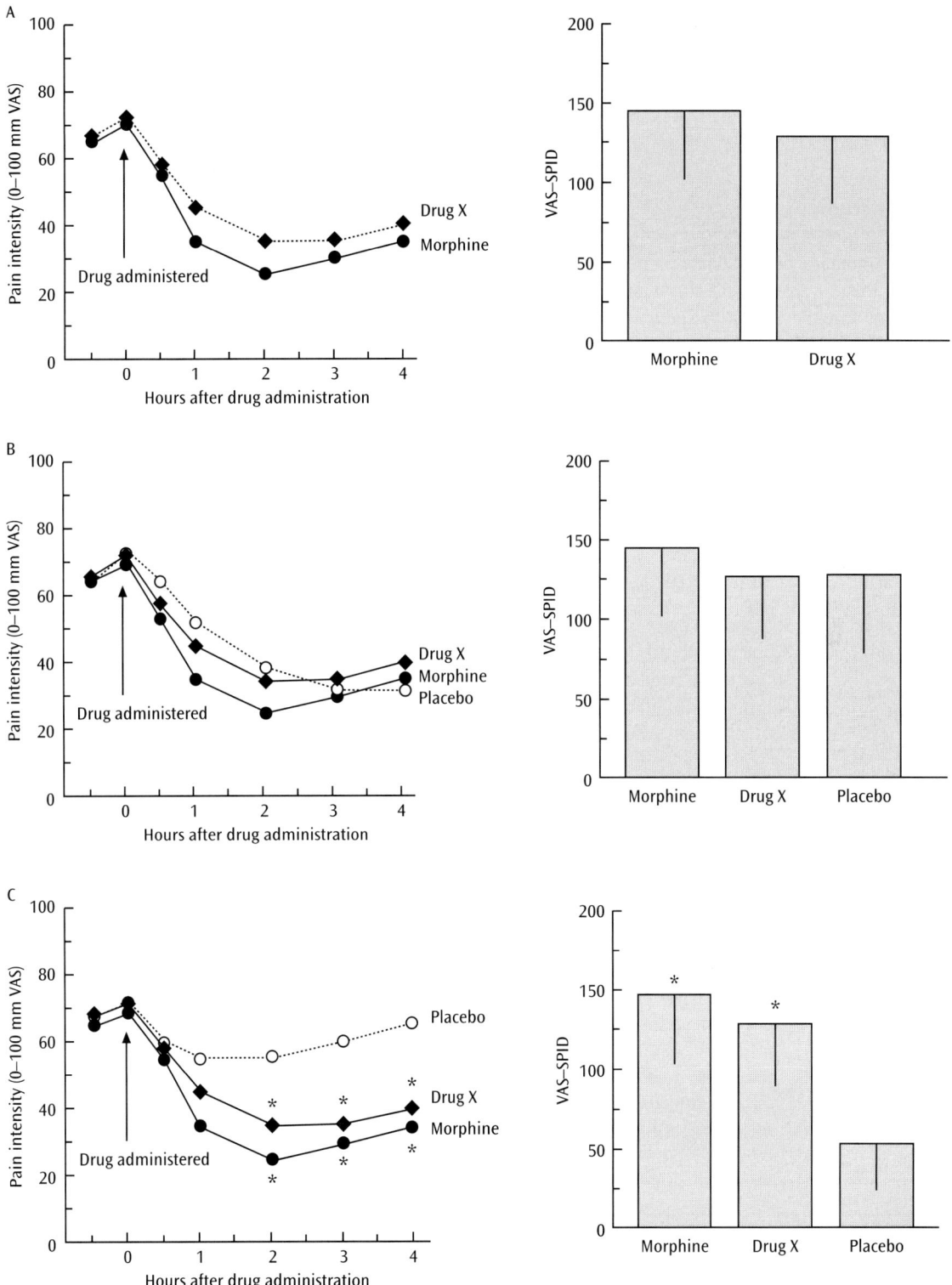

Figure 35.1 *The pain intensity (left) and the corresponding summed pain intensity differences (SPID; right) are based on pain intensity (visual analog scale – VAS). Pain intensity difference (PID) is the pain intensity at drug intake minus the pain intensity at a given time point. SPID is the area under the curve multiplied by the trapezoid rule (see Fig. 35.4). Asterisk, significantly different from placebo. A, B, and C show three different results. A, No difference between drug X and the standard active drug. Possible interpretations: 1, the drugs are equally effective; 2, study methods are insensitive. B, Study methods are insensitive to the analgesic effect of the standard analgesic. Assay sensitivity is not demonstrated. No conclusions can be drawn. C, Assay sensitivity is demonstrated – the study can detect the analgesic effect of the standard. Drug X is superior to placebo. Upside sensitivity is not tested. (Reproduced with permission from Stubhaug and Breivik.[1])*

- superiority;
- equivalence;
- the relative potency;
- additive effect;
- synergy.

Superiority studies

A typical example is a pivotal trial of a new analgesic. As a minimum, the new drug in one single dose is compared with placebo, and the aim is to show superiority over placebo. To help in interpretation, at least a third group should be added, using a standard analgesic drug (Fig. 35.1). For a complete discussion of design and interpretation of superiority studies, see Max and Lynn.[3]

Equivalence trials

The aim of an equivalence study is to show that one active drug [e.g. a new cyclo-oxygenase 2 (COX-2) antagonist] has equal efficacy to a standard drug (e.g. a nonselective COX antagonist). The problem with this kind of study is that huge numbers of subjects are needed to prove that there is no clinically significant difference. If the two drugs are truly equivalent and give 75% overall treat-ment success, and we want to prove that the two treatments do not differ with more than 10% success rate, we will need 232 patients in each group to find this with 80% confidence ($\alpha = 0.05$). Underlying the interpretation of any equivalence trial is the assumption that the standard therapy is effective under the experimental conditions of the study. This is not necessarily true and is a threat to the validity of such trials. Assay sensitivity is not proven unless a third group is added. Another problem is to know what a clinically important difference is under the specific conditions of the trial. A third group receiving placebo could both serve as a yardstick in judgment of what difference is clinically significant and prove presence of assay sensitivity.[5-7]

Relative potency

To find the relative potency, i.e. the relative size of a standard drug necessary to produce an effect equivalent to a test drug unit, at least four groups are needed. With two groups of standard and test drugs, there must be linearity and overlap in effect size to be able to calculate relative potency (Fig. 35.2). Several doses of each drug would be preferable. As shown in Fig. 35.2, relative potency may vary depending on whether peak analgesia or total analgesia over a time period is used for analysis if the drugs have different kinetics.

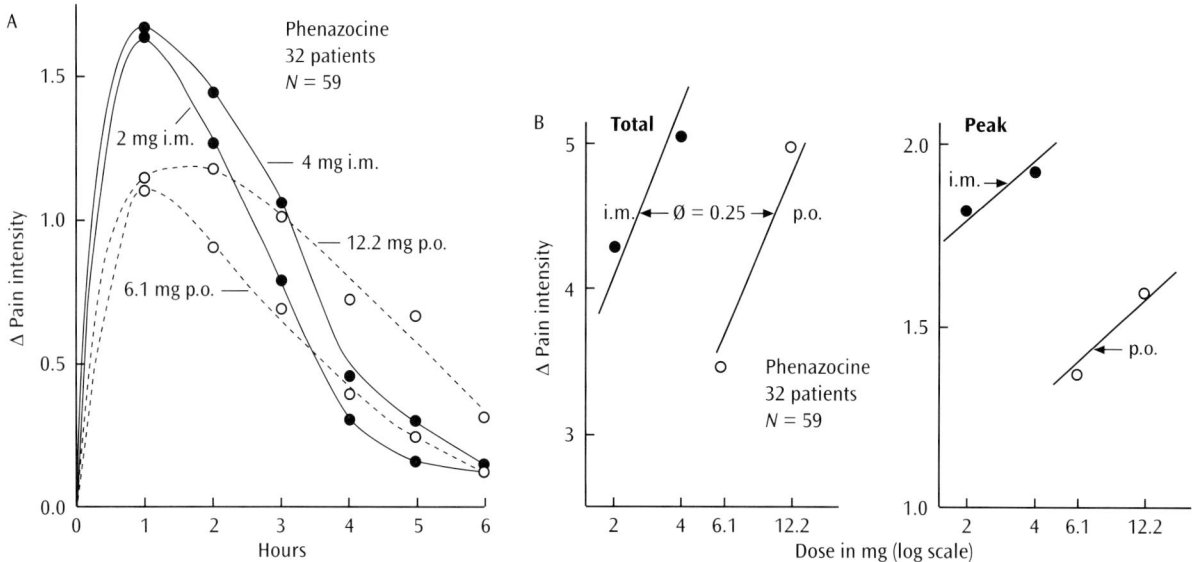

Figure 35.2 *Four-point relative potency assay. A, Time–effect curves for intramuscular (i.m.; filled circles and solid lines) and oral (p.o.; open circles and dashed lines) phenazocine. Change in pain intensity is shown against time in hours. Note the difference in the time-courses of analgesia between the two routes. Estimates of relative potency will vary depending on which criterion is used: peak effect, total effect after 3 h, total effect after 6 h, or effect at a specified time. B, Dose–effect curves for i.m. (filled circles) and p.o. (open circles) phenazocine. Total (left) and peak (right) change in pain intensity is plotted against dose in milligrams on a log scale. For total scores (6 h), the arrows indicate equieffective doses of p.o. and i.m. phenazocine; ⌀ = 0.25, indicating the relative potency of the two routes of administration of the drug. Note that the relative potency calculated for total scores will change according to the duration of the study. For peak scores, there is no overlap between the levels of the response seen with the two routes, and no relative potency can be calculated. (Reproduced with permission from Beaver et al.[8])*

During recent years, some studies have aimed at deciding relative potency by use of the patient-controlled analgesia (PCA) technique. This technique relies on a number of assumptions. The principle of PCA is that each patient will be able to titrate his plasma concentration and effect an organ concentration that lies constantly around the MEAC (minimum effective analgesic concentration). By comparing drug consumption, one should, in theory, be able to calculate relative potencies of different opioids.

Objections to the validity of PCA comparisons are, however, numerous. The pharmacokinetic profiles of the drugs being compared should be similar. If the duration of analgesia differs, the relative potency calculated is influenced by the duration of the study period. The PCA drug (e.g. morphine) may relieve one component of the pain experience (e.g. acute nociceptive pain) but not another pain component (e.g. acute neuropathic pain). Especially in such situations, the severity of pain is not the only factor that determines whether or not the patient will push the dose-demand button. Patients may choose not to push the demand button because they have the impression that the drug gives rise to side-effects such as unpleasant cognitive dysfunction, sedation, and nausea, and a patient may prefer some pain to these side-effects. Thus, both analgesic profile and side-effect profile of the drugs being compared should also be similar when the PCA technique is used to explore relative potency between analgesic drugs. In addition, groups of patients receiving the same drug in different bolus sizes should be included as a test of assay sensitivity of the method.[9]

Additive effects

To document the additive effects of treatments is of interest when two drugs examined represent different classes of drugs with different side-effect profiles. A typical design would then have four groups: placebo, each of the drugs separately, and a fourth group with the combination of both drugs. Ideally, it should also have groups with high doses of the single drugs. This would ideally prove that the combination of smaller doses of both drugs is beneficial compared with a higher dose of either single drug owing to fewer side-effects or to a limiting ceiling effect of analgesia of the single drugs.

Synergy

To distinguish between additive and synergistic combinations requires more advanced designs and statistical expertise. Several doses of each drug and the combination are needed.[10] A graphical presentation as an isobologram is easily interpreted (Fig. 35.3). If the combination (with confidence limits) lies below the line of additivity, synergy has been proven.

WHY IS KNOWLEDGE OF THE PLACEBO RESPONSE ESSENTIAL IN STUDIES OF PAIN?

One problem in trials of pain relief is that we do not know how large the spontaneous reduction of pain without any treatment at all would be. The spontaneous reduction of pain intensity with time can represent a major problem in studies of acute postoperative pain. For ethical reasons, we are unable to measure it. A placebo group receiving placebo treatment and an adequate rescue drug when needed is the closest we can get. The placebo response, measured as the reduction of pain after placebo treatment, is of course also part of the active drug response. Thus, knowledge of the placebo response in a study helps with interpreting the active drug response. As there are huge differences in the placebo response between studies,[11] use of historical data on placebo response is worthless. This must be kept in mind when evaluating trials that have included only active drugs.

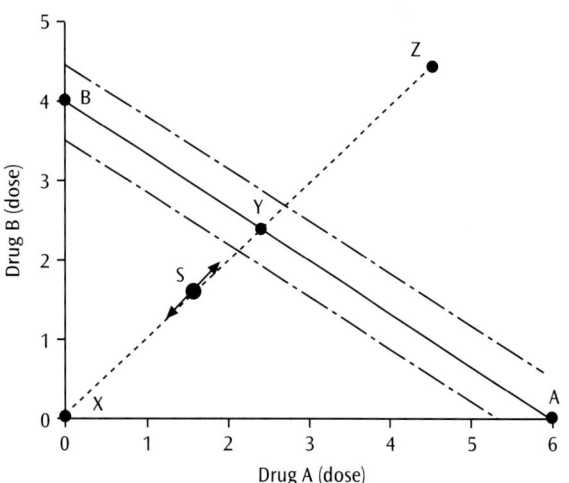

Figure 35.3 *Isobologram showing doses of drugs A and B that have been calculated to give, for example, a 50% reduction in pain intensity (points A and B are calculated by regression from groups receiving escalating doses of A and B as single drugs). With simple additive effect, the doses of a combination of A and B necessary to give a 50% reduction in pain lie along the line A–B (shown with the confidence interval as dashed lines). Several groups receiving escalating doses of the combination in a defined dose relation (in this case 1:1) have been tested. Line X–Z indicates the possible mixtures of this combination. The doses necessary to give 50% pain relief are calculated by regression. Point Y represents a simple additive effect; points along the line X–Y show synergism; points along line Y–Z show antagonism. If the calculated dose of the combination lies along X–Y and confidence limits do not cross the confidence limits for line A–B, the synergism has been proven, as indicated by point S (arrows represent the confidence interval for S).*

PLACEBO TREATMENT IS NOT UNETHICAL

Is the clinical trial necessary, and is it ethical to randomize patients and to give placebo treatment? The answer to these questions depends on what we know about the treatments in question. In medical practice, potentially harmful treatments are often given without any documentation of effect. The major ethical question is to evaluate the balance between the importance of the objective of the study and the inherent risk to the participating subject. The degree of risk and discomfort must be favorably balanced by the probability of benefit to the patient or to patients in general. Participation in a clinical trial may have several advantages for the patient. However, even a modest additional discomfort or risk would be unethical if the study was designed in a way to preclude useful conclusions, or if the results for some reason are withheld from publication. Thus, proper study design, including placebo when relevant and publication of the results, are important ethical imperatives.

METHOD OF RANDOMIZATION

As previously mentioned, randomization is crucial. Randomization is an insurance against imbalance between treatment groups with respect to important but not necessarily known confounding factors. Variables that are known to affect results can be controlled for by *stratified randomization* (e.g. sex, age).

Proper randomization minimizes systematic allocation bias, but with small sample sizes randomization does not prevent random imbalance, which must be tested for. The exact method used for production of the treatment allocation list should be chosen carefully (e.g. envelope method, computer generation, use of lists of random numbers, randomization in blocks etc.).[12,13]

After proper randomization, adequate allocation concealment must be continued. Proper allocation concealment prevents those who admit participants to the trial from knowing the upcoming assignments.[14] Thus, quasirandomization, such as allocating to active or placebo, alternating weeks, or allocation by day of birth, is not acceptable.

INCLUSION OF PATIENTS: INCLUSION BASED ON PAIN MECHANISMS?

A careful description of the population under study is important. The protocol must define clearly the *inclusion criteria* and the *exclusion criteria*. Normally, a *baseline pain* above a certain level will increase the sensitivity. If patients with a low baseline pain are included, the potential treatment effect may be small compared with random fluctuations in pain intensity.

There is now a trend toward a mechanism-based pain diagnosis and treatment. Inclusion criteria based on an understanding of the pain mechanism should be considered in clinical pain trials.[15] In chronic pain trials, a screening period before a patient is randomized to treatment is usually necessary. Sometimes, an *enriched enrolment* procedure is indicated to exclude nonresponders. If, for example, a new oral *N*-methyl-D-aspartate (NMDA) receptor antagonist is to be tested against neuropathic pain but is expected to help only a small subgroup of patients that are difficult to define on the basis of clinical judgment, it may be acceptable to include only patients who respond to an intravenous (i.v.) infusion of ketamine. Such an enriched enrolment strategy is meant to increase sensitivity and to reduce the risk of type II error (see below), but it may easily introduce bias and problems with the interpretation of the results.

BLINDING AND UNBLINDING: ACTIVE PLACEBO

Blinding of treatment is especially important when subjective responses are measured. A double-blind procedure means that neither the patient nor the observer can identify the assigned treatment. A randomized, double-blind technique is a "gold standard" that should be used whenever possible. It is important to be aware that the possibility of unblinding of patient and observer is a serious threat to the validity of the study. The risk of unblinding increases with the duration of the study, and especially with crossover designs. After several weeks on an active drug, both patients and investigators often correctly guess the treatment allocation. *Active placebo* aims to mimic typical side-effects of active drugs such as sedation and dry mouth without having any direct pharmacodynamic effect on pain. Drugs such as benzotropine and benzodiazepines have been used to reduce the risk of unblinding.

PARALLEL OR CROSSOVER STUDIES?

This is often an important question. A parallel design is never wrong, but will often require a much higher number of patients to answer the question than a crossover design. Parallel studies are preferred by regulatory agencies for pivotal trials of new drugs. Single centers may be forced to use a crossover design to be able to include a sufficient number of patients to answer the research question. Whereas a parallel study is easy to analyze, the crossover design has several possible pitfalls.

The most serious problem with crossover designs is the interaction between treatments (*carryover effects*). This means that the effects of a treatment persist into the subsequent period. A *period effect* means a systematic difference between periods, irrespective of the treatment. Other problems with the crossover design include an increased length of study with more variation in pain, loss of data as a result of more dropouts than in parallel studies, and an increased risk of unblinding.

Parallel studies are by far the most common in postoperative analgesic trials: each patient is allocated to receive only one of the treatments tested. Parallel studies are the most straightforward, are easy to analyze, and are preferred by the majority of clinical trialists.[16] If the study population of a parallel trial is very heterogeneous, the problems that are likely to arise include variability of results, overlap between groups, and a low test power; no difference between drugs can be demonstrated even if a true difference exists. If the treatment effect is clinically meaningful, but nevertheless is small compared with interindividual variance, statistical power can be increased considerably by use of a crossover design.

It is important to remember that period effects and carryover effects exist, having both pharmacological and psychological reasons. To reduce the influence of these effects, a balanced design is necessary. Patients are randomized to predefined sequences (Tables 35.2–35.4). Carryover effects and period effects can also be calculated and accounted for in the efficacy analysis. However, both design and analysis of such studies are much more complicated than in parallel studies, and should be avoided if statistical expertise is not available. For a thorough discussion of crossover designs, see Jones and Kenward.[17]

MORE ABOUT OUTCOMES IN TRIALS OF PAIN TREATMENT

What is a meaningful endpoint?

As discussed above, the answer to this may differ according to the study. In a recent qualitative study in chronic pain patients on opioid treatment, the patients chose the most meaningful endpoints to be (in descending order of importance): decreased pain, decreased frequency of scheduled doses, decreased opioid dose, decreased constipation, decreased drowsiness, improved sleep, improved activity of living, and improved concentration.[18] This demonstrates that simply assessing pain intensity may be an oversimplification. Similarly, important outcomes in acute pain include the ability to mobilize, to take deep breaths, and the absence of distressing side-effects.

PAIN INTENSITY

Pain intensity is most commonly evaluated by a four- to five-point categorical verbal rating scale (VRS) (e.g.

Table 35.2 *Typical two-treatment crossover design*

Sequence	Treatment	
	Period 1	Period 2
1	A	B
2	B	A

Table 35.3 *A three-group, complete crossover design*

Sequence	Treatment		
	Period 1	Period 2	Period 3
1	A	C	B
2	B	A	C
3	C	B	A
4	A	B	C
5	B	C	A
6	C	A	B

Table 35.4 *Four-group complete crossover as a reduced, balanced, Latin square design*

Sequence	Treatment			
	Period 1	Period 2	Period 3	Period 4
1	A	D	B	C
2	B	A	C	D
3	C	B	D	A
4	D	C	A	B

This Latin square ensures that (1) each subject has all treatments, (2) each treatment occurs with equal frequency in each period, and (3) that each treatment pair (e.g. A followed by D) occurs with equal frequency

0 = no pain, 1 = weak pain, 2 = moderate pain, 3 = strong pain, 4 = very severe pain), by a visual analog scale (VAS) (100-mm scale anchored at the two ends by the descriptors "no pain" and "worst pain imaginable"), or by an 11-point numerical rating scale NRS (0–10; 0 = no pain, 10 = worst pain imaginable). Both the VAS and the 11-point NRS are proven to discriminate better than the five-point VRS in acute and chronic pain.[19] For a thorough discussion on pain intensity measurement, see Chapter P2.

WHAT IS A CLINICALLY IMPORTANT REDUCTION IN PAIN INTENSITY?

Two recent studies by Farrar et al.[20,21] concluded that an approximate reduction of 30% in pain intensity corresponds well with the patient's experience of clinically meaningful pain relief. Thus, if pain intensity is the main outcome, it seems reasonable to design a study that is large enough to be able to detect a 30% reduction in pain intensity.

REPEATED MEASUREMENTS: CREATE A SUMMARY MEASURE SUCH AS SPID OR TOTPAR

Pain intensity and pain relief are usually measured repeatedly in studies on acute pain. Very often, there are different time intervals between the measurements. In such cases, it is a good idea to create a summary measure for a study-relevant time period and use this as the main efficacy variable. Summed pain intensity difference (SPID) (Fig. 35.4) is an example of one such summary measure. Note that it is not simply a sum of measurements, but an area under the curve (AUC) that takes time intervals between measurements into account. Correspondingly, TOTPAR is the AUC for pain relief (categorical scale) multiplied by time data.

CONSUMPTION OF RESCUE ANALGESIA

In many studies, in both acute and chronic pain, patients are offered a rescue drug when needed. This is often necessary for ethical reasons. In such cases, group differences after the primary intervention will be divided into two outcomes: pain and rescue drug consumptions. As shown in Fig. 35.5, this may reduce the sensitivity of each of the two outcomes, but can be compensated for by increasing the number of patients included.[22] The PCA consumption as the single main outcome has weaknesses that have been discussed above (see Relative potency).

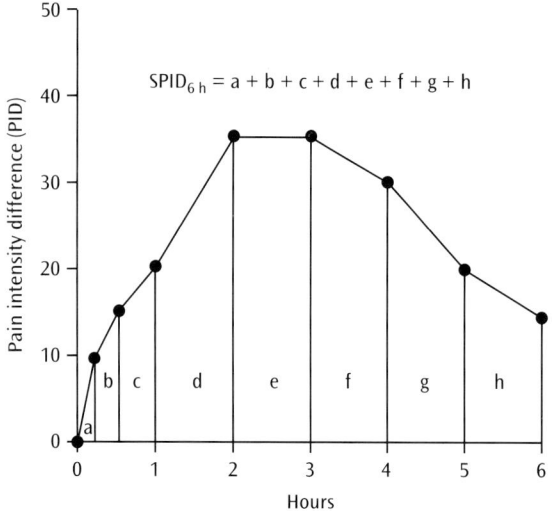

Figure 35.4 *Graphical display of individual pain intensity differences in a study of acute pain. Pain intensity difference (PID) is pain intensity at drug intake minus pain intensity at a given time point. SPID is the area under the curve multiplied by the PID curve calculated by the trapezoid rule. In this case, pain intensity is measured after 15 min, 30 min, 1 h, 2 h, 3 h, 4 h, 5 h, and 6 h. SPID corresponds to the areas a + b + c + d + e + f + g + h.*

ONSET OF ANALGESIA

There is no generally accepted definition of how the onset of analgesia should be assessed clinically in acute pain. Onset can be described in terms of both the probability of obtaining onset and, for patients who obtain onset, the distribution of time to onset. One relatively new method is the use of patient-operated stopwatches. The watches are started when the trial drug has been administered. The patient is instructed to stop one watch the moment a defined clinically significant amount of pain relief is first experienced, e.g. when the *first perception of pain relief* is present or when *meaningful pain relief* is first experienced.[23] For many patients, the *first perception of pain relief* is *not* followed by a lasting *meaningful pain relief*. *Time to meaningful pain relief* seems more robust against placebo onset than *time to first perception of pain relief*.

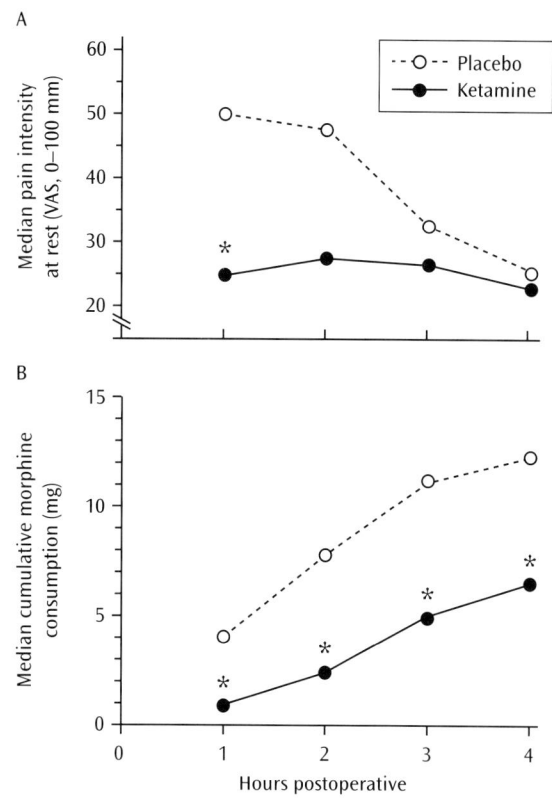

Figure 35.5 *Difference in pain intensity and morphine consumption (PCA) for the first postoperative 4 h between a group receiving a low dose of ketamine and placebo. Note that an initial difference in pain intensity at 1 h leads to a higher opioid consumption in the group with more pain. This leads to reduced pain but never a full compensation. The initial group difference in pain intensity is divided between the two variables of pain intensity and opioid consumption. After 4 h, no group difference is present (data not shown). (Reproduced with permission from Stubhaug et al.[22])*

Onset can also be derived from the pain relief readings at prefixed time points. A common estimate of onset is the midpoint of the time interval between the first interview at which the patient reported onset and the preceding interview. This derived onset variable is a calculated value, not a measured one, and is often unable to discriminate between active drugs and placebo even if the active drugs are superior in other efficacy measures.

Regardless of method, it will be difficult to calculate one single value to characterize onset: for example, how should one correct for patients who do not experience onset before they receive rescue drug? Laska *et al.* have proposed a clinically useful way to express relief and onset characteristics of a drug using a set of percentiles.[23] A hypothetical example could read as follows: "For patients whose pain is similar to that experienced by patients examined in this study, it may be expected that 80% will experience an effect from the drug. Of those who have an effect, 25% will feel that they are obtaining meaningful relief by 10 min or sooner, 50% by 20 min or sooner, 75% by 40 min or sooner, and almost all who obtain an effect will have obtained it by 60 min."

Similar to measurement of onset, the patient can be asked to stop a second watch when the clinically significant pain relief is no longer felt (offset).

REMEDICATION TIME

In trials where a single dose is given, the time when a rescue drug is needed and the subsequent response to the rescue drug should be recorded.

This remediation time is a useful summary score,[16] and the response to a standard rescue drug gives important additional information.

GLOBAL ASSESSMENT

A global question such as "What is your overall satisfaction with the treatment?" is an important question at the end of the study because it gives the patient an opportunity to evaluate the positive effects (analgesia, better sleep, etc.), the negative drug effects (side-effects), and the comfort and feasibility of the method employed. A patient with total analgesia but unacceptable side-effects may choose to give a low score on the global assessment. Global assessment scales should have options for both improvement and worsening.

EVOKED PAIN

Our understanding of pain mechanisms has changed. Instead of simply assessing the complex composite mea-

sure "pain at rest," additional information can be achieved by using several types of stimuli to evoke pain. Mechanical (Table 35.5), thermal, and electrical stimuli can be used to measure pain thresholds and to assess response to suprathreshold stimuli. Likewise, a standardized body movement can be a clinically meaningful stimulus (e.g. coughing).

In a postoperative study, a low dose of ketamine was shown to block the development of static hyperalgesia (measured with von Frey filaments) around a nephrectomy incision, although it had only a minor effect on pain at rest.[22] Correspondingly, in a dental model, Gilron and colleagues found that an AMPA/kainate glutamate receptor antagonist (LY 293558) had only a minimal effect on resting pain, but had a robust effect on pain evoked by mouth opening.[24] This demonstrates that simply testing new drugs for their effect on pain intensity at rest may falsely lead to the conclusion that they are without efficacy.

In trials on chronic pain patients, use of thermal, mechanical, and electrical stimuli have produced interesting new information about disease mechanisms and treatment effects.[25–27]

OUTCOMES THAT CAN EASILY BE EXTRACTED FOR USE IN META-ANALYSIS

With the increased focus on systematic reviews, there has been a call for standardization of outcomes and reporting in trials in pain relief to make it easier to compare and reproduce research results.

Quantitative data have been dichotomized into *success* or *failure* before data from several studies are combined. Until now, the fraction of patients achieving > 50% of the maximum possible pain relief has most frequently been extracted from acute pain trials, and the fraction achieving an estimation of 50% pain relief has been extracted from studies in chronic pain.[28] A significant change in the mean may be the result of both a moderate change in many patients and a major change in a small number of patients. Therefore, extraction of data should ideally be based on individual data of a standard dichotomous or dichotomizable outcome.

LONG-TERM TRIALS: ASSESSMENT OF QUALITY OF LIFE

There is a huge lack of long-term trials in chronic pain. Most trials last at the most a few weeks. Longer term trials are necessary to assess whether treatment effects are lasting and, most importantly, to assess the impact of treatment on a patient's global situation, taking into account side-effects and measures of quality of life (QOL).

Table 35.5 *Evoked mechanical pain: nature of stimuli and proposed research tools*

Nature of mechanical stimulus	Research tool
Static	
Punctate	von Frey filaments
Blunt	Pressure algometer
Dynamic	
Spatial distribution	Artist's brush
	Cotton wool swab
	Toothbrush
Temporal distribution	Repetitive von Frey filament stimulation, e.g. 2 Hz

STATISTICAL ISSUES

It is beyond the scope of this chapter to cover statistical issues in any detail. Statistical planning before the start of the study is very important: if you think you will need help with the statistics, this is the time to seek it.

One critical aspect in the planning of a clinical study is to estimate the sample size required. The number of subjects necessary to obtain a certain power depends upon the magnitude of the difference that is considered interesting to detect and the variance of the variable under study in the population. It follows that knowledge about the variation is critical. Sample size calculations based on pilot results are generally more reliable than results from the literature. The purpose of the sample size determination is to avoid both false-positive (type I error) and false-negative (type II error) results (Table 35.6).

PUBLISH YOUR TRIAL

The revised CONSORT statement presents a checklist of 22 items that should be properly reported and a flow diagram to show the passage of patients through a randomized controlled trial.[29] There is no reason not to use these guidelines when applicable. According to the revised Helsinki Declaration, all results should be published, and the Medical Editors' Trial Amnesty (META) gives no excuse for trials remaining unregistered.[30]

REFERENCES

1. Schwartz D, Lellouch J. Explanatory and pragmatic attitudes in therapeutical trials. *J Chronic Dis* 1967; **20**: 637–48.

◆ 2. Schulz KF, Chalmers I, Hayes RJ, Altman DG. Empirical evidence of bias. Dimensions of methodological quality associated with estimates of treatment effects in controlled trials *JAMA* 1995; **273**: 408–12.

● 3. Max MB, Lynn J. Symptom research. An interactive textbook. Available at http://www.symptomresearch.com/

● 4. Stubhaug A, Breivik H. Post-operative analgesic trials: some important issues. In: Breivik H ed. *Post-operative Pain Treatment. Baillière's Clin Anaesthesiol* 1995; **9**: 569–98.

● 5. Tramer MR, Reynolds DJ, Moore RA, McQuay HJ. When placebo controlled trials are essential and equivalence trials are inadequate. *Br Med J* 1998; **317**: 875–80.

● 6. Landow L. Current issues in clinical trial design: superiority versus equivalence studies. *Anesthesiology* 2000; **92**: 1814–20.

7. Stubhaug A. Comparison of tramadol with morphine for post-operative pain following abdominal surgery. *Eur J Anaesth* 1996; **13**: 416–17.

8. Beaver WT, Wallenstein SL, Houde RW, Rogers A. A clinical comparison of the effects of oral and intramuscular administration of analgesics: pentazocine and phenazocine. *Clin Pharmacol Ther* 1968; **9**: 582–97.

● 9. Max MB. Divergent traditions in analgesic clinical trials. *Clin Pharmacol Ther* 1994; **56**: 237–41.

● 10. Tallarida RJ, Stone DJ, Raffa RB. Efficient designs for studying synergistic drug combinations. *Life Sci* 1997; **61**: 417–25.

● 11. Turner JA, Deyo RA, Loeser JD, *et al*. The importance of placebo effects in pain treatment and research. *JAMA* 1994; **271**: 1609–14.

● 12. Meinert, CL. *Clinical Trials. Design, Conduct and Analysis*. New York, NY: Oxford University Press, 1986.

● 13. Pocock SJ. *Clinical Trials. A Practical Approach*. New York, NY: John Wiley & Sons, 1983.

14. Schulz KF. Randomised trials, human nature, and reporting guidelines. *Lancet* 1996; **348**: 596–8.

◆ 15. Woolf CJ, Max MB. Mechanism-based pain diagnosis: issues for analgesic drug development. *Anesthesiology* 2001; **95**: 241–9.

Table 35.6 *Cells A–D show four possible results of a clinical trial; small sample sizes increase the risk of the results shown in cells B and C*

		Objective truth	
		Difference between treatments	No difference between treatments
Conclusion of the clinical trial	Difference between treatments	A: Correct conclusion of the clinical trial (true positive)	C: Incorrect conclusion (false positive); type I error
	No difference between treatments	B: Incorrect conclusion (false negative); type II error	D: Correct conclusion of the clinical trial (true negative)

16. Sriwatanakul K, Lasagna L, Cox C. Evaluation of current clinical trial methodology in analgesimetry based on experts' opinions and analysis of several analgesic studies. *Clin Pharmacol Ther* 1983; **34:** 277–83.

17. Jones B, Kenward MG. *Design and Analysis of Cross-Over Trials*. London: Chapman and Hall, 1989.

18. Casarett D, Karlawish J, Sankar P, *et al*. Designing pain research from the patients perspective: what trial end points are important to patients with chronic pain? *Pain Med* 2001; **2:** 309–16.

19. Breivik EK, Bjornsson GA, Skovlund E. A comparison of pain rating scales by sampling from clinical trial data. *Clin J Pain* 2000; **16:** 22–8.

20. Farrar JT, Portenoy RK, Berlin JA, *et al*. Defining the clinically important difference in pain outcome measures. *Pain* 2000; **88:** 287–94.

21. Farrar JT, Young Jr JP, LaMoreaux L, *et al*. Clinical importance of changes in chronic pain intensity measured on an 11-point numerical pain rating scale. *Pain* 2001; **94:** 149–58.

22. Stubhaug A, Breivik H, Eide PK, *et al*. Mapping of punctuate hyperalgesia surrounding a surgical incision demonstrates that ketamine is a powerful suppressor of central sensitization to pain following surgery. *Acta Anaesthesiol Scand* 1997; **41:** 1124–32.

23. Laska EM, Siegel C, Sunshine A. Onset and duration: measurement and analysis. *Clin Pharmacol Ther* 1991; **49:** 1–5.

24. Gilron I, Max MB, Lee G, *et al*. Effects of the AMPA/kainate antagonist LY293558 on spontaneous and evoked postoperative pain. *Clinical Pharmacol Ther* 2000; **68:** 320–7.

25. Attal N, Brasseur L, Parker F, *et al*. Effects of gabapentin on the different components of peripheral and central neuropathic pain syndromes: a pilot study. *Eur Neurol* 1998; **40:** 191–200.

26. Sjolund KF, Belfrage M, Karlsten R, *et al*. Systemic adenosine infusion reduces the area of tactile allodynia in neuropathic pain following peripheral nerve injury: a multi-centre, placebo-controlled study. *Eur J Pain* 2001; **5:** 199–207.

27. Jørum E, Warncke T, Stubhaug A. Cold allodynia and hyperalgesia in neuropathic pain: the effect of *N*-methyl-ᴅ-aspartate (NMDA) receptor antagonist ketamine; a double blind, cross-over comparison with alfentanil and placebo. *Pain* (in press).

● 28. McQuay H, Moore A. *An Evidence-based Resource for Pain Relief*. Oxford: Oxford University Press, 1998.

◆ 29. Moher D, Schulz KF, Altman DG. The CONSORT Statement: revised recommendations for improving the quality of reports of parallel-group randomised trials. *JAMA* 2001; **285:** 1987–91.

30. Roberts I. An amnesty for unpublished trials. One year on, many trials are unregistered and the amnesty remains open. *Br Med J* 1998; **317:** 763–54.

36

Clinical trials: dental pain

ELSE K BREIVIK

Advantages of the dental pain model	462	Baseline pain intensity as a confounding factor	465
Limitations of the dental pain model	462	Downside assay sensitivity	465
The protocol and good clinical trial practice	462	Upside assay sensitivity	465
Patient information, consent, and monitoring	463	Placebo control?	466
Operative procedures	463	Rescue analgesic drug	466
Patient understanding of instructions and compliance		Practical tips	467
with protocol	463	References	467
Improving and documenting assay sensitivity	464		

Surgical removal of impacted or incompletely erupted third molars in ambulatory patients is a common procedure both in general dental practice and in oral surgery practice (Fig. 36.1). The procedure results in hyperalgesia 2–4 h later, with cardinal signs of inflammation (rubor, calor, tumor, dolor, functio laesa) involving the extraction socket, surrounding mucosa, and masticatory organs. The study of pain and pain relief after this type of oral surgery is often referred to as "the dental pain model." The postoperative pain experienced varies from mild to severe following dissipation of the local anesthetic block, reaching its peak within the first 12 h. Following this initial period, acute pain abates and the patient requires less analgesic medication.[1] Although the duration of pain and discomfort may last for more than 4 postoperative days, it is usually transient and is limited to 1–3 postoperative days.[2] Other sequelae, such as trismus with reduced mouth opening and facial swelling, may also appear gradually, peaking at between 48 and 72 h.[3]** The majority of these patients are healthy young adults (18–30 years old) without former experience of oral disability or consuming medication that may influence pain assessment or that may interact with the analgesic under study. This chapter will predominantly address trials for the relief of postoperative pain after third molar surgery and only briefly discuss other acute dental pains that have been employed for the evaluation of analgesics.

Using the dental pain model, Lökken and coworkers published the first study on acute pain and inflammation following third molar removal in 1975,[4]** and in the subsequent decade they published several clinical studies which examined the efficacy of oral analgesics using this model.[5] A crossover design was originally used in patients who required bilateral surgical removal of third molars, with each patient undergoing unilateral surgery on two separate occasions and receiving alternate

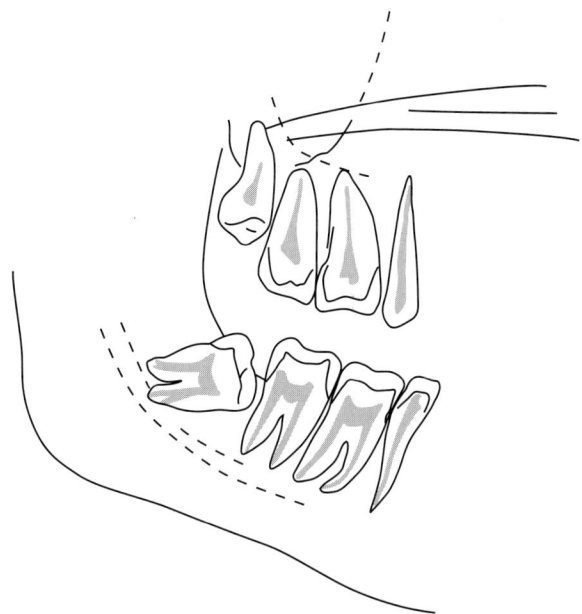

Figure 36.1 *Surgical removal of impacted third molars is a useful setting for acute postoperative pain trials. The impacted third molar in the lower jaw requires surgical removal, a procedure that will be associated with postoperative pain of moderate to severe intensity in about 50% of patients.*

interventions on each. However, this crossover design has lost some of its popularity because of the limited number of test drug groups possible in this design (see Improving and documenting assay sensitivity) and because of a potential carryover effect when each patient acts as his or her own control. The parallel group design is now more common, in which each patient undergoes one operation and receives a single treatment only. The parallel design also enables more than two test drugs to be examined, and carryover effects are absent because each subject participates only once. However, a drawback of the parallel design is a greater variation in assessments between patients than in the assessments from each patient on two separate occasions using the crossover design. The dental pain model has been extensively used in the evaluation of the pain-relieving effects of nonsteroidal anti-inflammatory drugs (NSAIDs), acetaminophen (paracetamol), opioids, local anesthetics, and combinations of these given before, during, or after surgery.[1] Not only traditional and new analgesic and anti-inflammatory drugs, but also antibiotics, corticosteroids, homeopathic treatment, low-energy-level laser, and complementary healing have been evaluated using the dental pain model.[1,6**,7**,8,9**,10,11**]

ADVANTAGES OF THE DENTAL PAIN MODEL

The dental pain model is generally considered to be sensitive in documenting whether the analgesic effectiveness of "mild" analgesics is superior to that of placebo,[12**] as well as in discriminating between analgesic drugs of differing analgesic potencies.[13] In oral maxillofacial surgical units, there is an abundance of otherwise healthy young adult patients undergoing third molar surgery, of whom about half will require analgesia. Most patients are willing to participate and, being young adults, will understand instructions and comply with protocol requirements when well informed by the investigator. The surgical procedure is usually elective and postoperative pain is confined to one area of the body. The large number of patients undergoing third molar surgery at oral maxillofacial surgical units means that an adequate supply of patients can be found within a reasonable time frame for trial execution. Thus, the readily available patients, the relative simplicity of the procedure, and the immediate pain experienced create an ideal setting for analgesic trials.[14**]

LIMITATIONS OF THE DENTAL PAIN MODEL

The natural course of postoperative pain following third molar surgery is fairly short. Time to peak pain intensity after removal of impacted wisdom teeth is about 6h after surgery.[15*] Therefore, trials can only be of limited duration, ideally taking place within the first 6–11 postoper-

ative hours. Variation in baseline pain after third molar surgery is large,[16**] with only 40–60% of patients reporting moderate to severe pain.[17**,18**,19**] The dental pain model has been recommended only for single-dose studies owing to this variability among patients.[20] Only 20–40% of patients undergoing unilateral mandibular third molar surgery have been reported to experience pain and discomfort during the first 3 postoperative days,[21*] whereas 37–75% of patients undergoing surgical removal of all four third molars experience pain and discomfort during the first 3 postoperative days.[22*] Owing to this variation of pain intensity during the first postoperative days, repeated dose analgesic trials lasting more than 11 h may thus not have sufficient assay sensitivity for differences to be detected between analgesic test drugs.

Surgical removal of third molars is usually performed on outpatients under local anesthesia, but occasionally general anesthesia is employed. Recovery from general anesthesia is often complicated by side-effects which may hinder pain intensity evaluations. The postoperative facilities at the oral maxillofacial surgical units may also be insufficient for pain assessment.

THE PROTOCOL AND GOOD CLINICAL TRIAL PRACTICE

The study of subjective experience such as pain is notoriously subject to bias. Meticulous protocol design and subsequent close adherence to it and monitoring improves the quality of the trial. Analgesic trials using the dental pain model should adhere to the general rules of good clinical trial practice,[23] which demand not only high ethical and scientific standards but also meticulous conduct, recording, terminating, and reporting of trials according to preestablished criteria in the study protocols. Inadequate methodological standards correlate with bias in estimation of treatment effect, and blind assessments of analgesics produce significantly lower and more consistent measurements than open assessments.[24] Analgesic trials therefore require strict adherence to the principles of randomized controlled trials (RCTs).[24,25]

The essence of good clinical trial design and execution is to:

- Define a clear purpose and hypothesis.
- Describe the effect variables and how they will be measured.
- Describe any known confounding variables and control for them by exclusion criteria or by stratified randomization.
- Justify study design: parallel groups or crossover; single dose or multiple repeated doses of test drug. Control group(s): standard active, one or more doses, and placebo.
- Calculate sample size to achieve sufficient statistical power. If necessary, perform pilot study to be able to estimate variation and sample size.

- Receive ethical committee approval prior to starting the trial.
- Randomize using accepted methodology.
- Mask test drugs and secure blinding of patients and observer.
- Receive oral and written informed patient consent.
- Guide, inform, and support patients to ensure protocol compliance and to ensure that there is no unblinding of patients nor of observers.
- Ensure blinding of patients and observers *throughout* the study period and *beyond* evaluation of effect variables measured in each patient (= double blind).
- Analyze data using descriptive statistics and test statistics. Estimate treatment effects with confidence intervals.
- Make conclusions based on findings and statistical analysis.
- Record details of dropouts, missing data, rescue treatment.
- Publish the study according to The CONSORT Statement, allowing the reader to evaluate the validity of your findings.[25]

PATIENT INFORMATION, CONSENT, AND MONITORING

Asking eligible patients to participate in analgesic trials is preferably done at the first visit, when the criteria for inclusion have been checked but before the patient has been given an appointment for surgery. The principles of the Declaration of Helsinki should be adhered to. Thus, patients should be informed of the basis for conducting the trial, the stage of test drug development, the expected test drug efficacy, and the expected side-effects of active control groups and placebo when included. Patients should be informed that they do not have to give a reason for not participating in the trial and that their consent to participate or refuse will not affect the standard of clinical care that they will receive.

Our experience is that the majority of patients do not decline when asked to participate, and, if they do, the usual reason is the inconvenience of staying in the clinic for baseline pain assessments and instructions. This refusal is less often the case if they have been informed of trial procedures at an earlier visit. In trials in which placebo is included, however, more patients are reluctant to participate, despite the availability of rescue medication. Written informed consent must be obtained prior to surgical procedure.

OPERATIVE PROCEDURES

To reduce variability in pain due to surgical trauma, the surgical technique should be strictly standardized and the operation preferably performed by a single surgeon.[26]** Surgical removal of impacted third molars is usually performed under local anesthesia using lidocaine (lignocaine) 20 mg/ml and epinephrine (adrenaline) 12.5 µg/ml (Xylocain–Adrenaline, AstraZeneca, Sweden). This technique allows evaluation of baseline pain about 3 h later.[27]** A 3- to 4-cm soft-tissue incision is performed and the mucoperiosteum reflected to visualize the tooth. Cortical alveolar bone is then removed by burr under saline irrigation and the impacted tooth is sectioned and elevated. Finally, the mucoperiosteal flap is repositioned with sutures and an inlay of a 2 × 1 cm gauze drain saturated with 3% chlortetracycline ointment (Aureomycin, Wyeth Lederle, USA) is left in the wound opening.[28]** No other antibiotics, sedatives, or other drugs are administered to the patients eligible for trial participation. The procedure should be performed in the morning, so that assessments are taken during the afternoon and early evening for all patients.

PATIENT UNDERSTANDING OF INSTRUCTIONS AND COMPLIANCE WITH PROTOCOL

To adequately measure the baseline pain intensity of trial participants, patients should remain in the clinic until full recovery from the local anesthetic block is clearly evident. One investigator has the responsibility for patient surveillance. Patients are instructed to rate their present pain intensity half-hourly after surgery or extraction on a visual analogue scale (VAS), or a numerical rating scale (NRS). A categorical verbal rating scale has been demonstrated to be a less sensitive measure of pain intensity and is no longer used in our department.[29]**,[30]** After dissipation of the effects of the local anesthetic, patients who do not report a pain intensity of more than 50 mm on a 100-mm VAS are excluded and discharged from the clinic with routine postoperative instructions; routine analgesics are prescribed. The duration of the conduction block (inferior alveolar nerve block) with lidocaine 20 mg/ml with epinephrine 12.5 µg/ml is on average 85 min for the dental pulp and 190 min for the oral soft tissue.[27] In our studies, patients did not experience moderate to severe pain until 3–3.5 h after injection of local anesthesia.[19]**,[29]**

Patients who do report a pain intensity equal to or greater than 50 mm on a 100-mm VAS are randomized, given the test drug, and asked to remain for a further 0.5 h in order to rate pain relief on a five-point verbal pain relief scale (PAR). Patients then record the remaining pain intensity assessments after they have left the clinic. By now, the observer will have an impression of the patient's ability to understand instructions and use the VAS and the PAR.

Since most of the pain diaries will be attended to after

the patients have left the clinic, the patients must be contactable by the investigator or monitor to ensure the quality of the trial data. Contacting participants by telephone in the afternoon increases patient compliance, reminds patients of their obligations as trial participants, and serves as an extra service for the patient if they have questions regarding their postoperative course, assessments in their home diary, or rescue drug intake. Overall ratings of drug efficacy and side-effects are performed at the end of the observation period as a global score on a VAS or a categorical scale. The home diary is returned on the seventh postoperative day when sutures and chlortetracycline gauze are removed.

Inclusion criteria for trial participants prior to drug administration

- Indications for surgical removal of third molars are present[31] (Box 36.1).
- Either sex, between 18 and 40 years old.
- No history of chronic pain.
- Asymptomatic third molar on the day of operation (no symptomatic pericoronitis or pulpitis).
- Baseline pain intensity (i.e. pain at drug intake) of predetermined magnitude (see Baseline pain as a confounding factor).

Exclusion criteria for trial participants prior to drug administration

- Concomitant medication (except oral contraceptives).
- Systemic steroid treatment during the last month.
- Known hypersensitivity to the test drugs.
- Bronchial asthma or gastrointestinal ulcerative disease (if test drug is an NSAID).
- Inflammatory gastrointestinal disease (Crohn's disease or ulcerative colitis).
- Hepatic or renal disease.

Box 36.1 *Report of a workshop on the management of patients with third molar teeth*[31]

Indications for third molar removal according to The National Institute of Health (NIH), USA:

- One or more episodes of pericoronitis.
- Unrestorable caries in the third molar tooth.
- Distal caries in the adjacent tooth.
- Periodontal disease (resulting in bone destruction).
- Evidence of follicular enlargement.
- Resorption of the third molar or adjacent tooth.

- Pregnant or lactating women.
- Anxiety related to dental treatment.
- Alcohol consumption 1 day or less preoperatively.
- Deviation from surgical procedure as specified in the protocol.
- No pain or inadequate pain intensity level after offset of local anesthesia (baseline pain).
- When motivation and compliance with protocol is questionable.

IMPROVING AND DOCUMENTING ASSAY SENSITIVITY

The objectives of comparative analgesic trials are to demonstrate that the effectiveness of one treatment is significantly better than another, or that a new drug is superior to placebo and at least as effective as a "standard" analgesic. Interpretation problems arise when no difference is revealed between the treatments in a trial that does not embody placebo or standard analgesic comparators.[32] As a result, it cannot be ascertained whether the outcome for the test drug indicates that it is equally effective or whether the assay sensitivity is inadequate. Study error could occur, for example, because patients were too stressed in the clinical setting to respond normally to medication or to understand properly the pain questionnaires/pain diaries. The procedure or the information from the clinical investigator could be insufficient, or contain confounding factors, or data could vary merely because of random variation. Selection of adequate control groups (standard analgesics in two doses, or placebo, or both) is therefore essential to verify and document that the study methodology can distinguish between degrees of analgesic effectiveness. Testing the analgesic drug against a placebo control will detect whether it is an analgesic. Testing the analgesic drug against a standard analgesic control, for example acetaminophen, can indicate how much of the pain relief is caused by placebo effects.[32]

The importance of documenting assay sensitivity was well illustrated in another dental test model for the evaluation of oral analgesics: acute apical periodontitis or acute apical abscess causes moderate to severe odontalgia. The dental treatment is usually pulpectomy and analgesics are usually prescribed for the management of postoperative pain. In patients with moderate to severe baseline pain, pulpectomy combined with placebo medication resulted in a 50% reduction in pain during the first 24 h.[33]** This means that most of these patients get pain relief from the dental treatment alone. Analgesic trials performed on endodontic emergency patients must therefore also have test drug comparators that enable assay sensitivity to be controlled. Assay sensitivity was documented by Doroschak and coworkers through the superior analgesic effect of the combination flurbiprofen plus tramadol compared with placebo on endodontic pain.[33]**

BASELINE PAIN INTENSITY AS A CONFOUNDING FACTOR

Adequate and homogeneous baseline pain intensity is an important factor in determining the outcome of a trial of analgesic drugs.[34] Even in standardized forms of surgery such as the surgical removal of impacted third molars, patients vary tremendously in their reported discomfort.[16**] Mild pain may be sufficient in a trial where the aim is to document that a weak analgesic drug is superior to placebo.[16**] However, patients who enter the study suffering from severe pain have a greater potential for pain relief, as measured by the decrease in pain intensity, than patients who enter the study with a lower pain intensity. Thus, in trials designed to document whether two or more analgesic drugs are significantly different from each other, at least moderate to strong pain intensity is required.[19**,34**]

It is well documented that postoperative pain intensity after third molar surgery increases with the extent of the surgical intervention.[2,35*,36*] This was confirmed in a trial of 293 patients who were stratified into groups according to the extent of trauma of third molar removal: extraction of one upper third molar, surgical removal of one mandibular impacted third molar, or surgical removal of two ipsilateral impacted third molars.[16**] Although baseline pain intensity was related to the extent of surgical trauma, the variation in pain intensity experienced by patients with similar degrees of surgical trauma was large (Fig. 36.2). The duration and degree of surgical trauma are thus only partly responsible for the postoperative pain intensity. In a follow-up study in which patients were screened for their baseline pain before leaving the clinic, one in two patients did not reach a postoperative pain intensity of 50 mm or above on a 100-mm VAS after local anesthetic offset.[19**] In a follow-up study, 46 of 166 patients (38%) experienced less pain intensity than 50 mm on a 100-mm VAS after surgical removal of impacted third molars.[29**]

Similarly, Desjardins[37**] reported that a substantial proportion (30–50%) of patients undergoing extraction of erupted third molars did not develop postoperative pain. Patients undergoing more extensive procedures involving mucoperiostal flaps and removal of alveolar bone (e.g. periodontal surgery or surgical removal of impacted third molars) less frequently had no or little postoperative pain (10–20%).[38**] Hansson et al.[17**] found that 14 of 100 patients did not report any pain at all and 40 patients (40%) did not use any analgesics during the 70-h observation period following surgical removal of third molars. Nörholt[18**] stated that 34% of patients after surgical removal of third molar(s) reported no pain or only mild pain. Therefore, in the dental pain model, pain intensity varies substantially irrespective of the extent of surgery, and a predetermined intensity of baseline pain should be met before patients are finally included in the trial.[39,40]

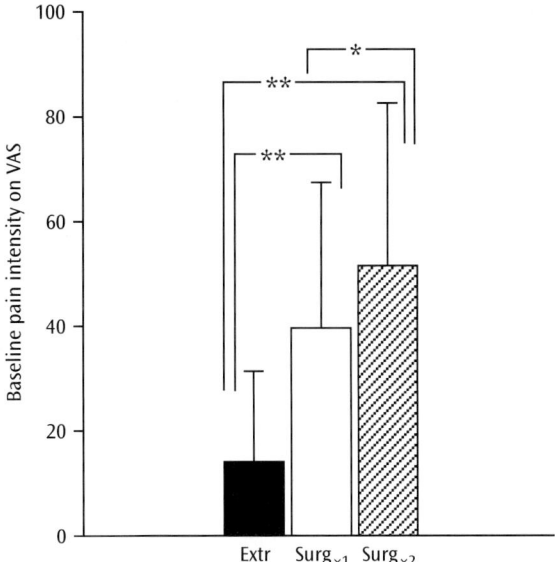

Figure 36.2 *Mean (standard deviation) baseline pain intensity in the three clinical groups following third molar removal. Ex, extraction of one fully erupted maxillary third molar (n = 100); Surg$_{X1}$, surgical removal of one impacted mandibular third molar (n = 95); Surg$_{X2}$, surgical removal of two ipsilateral impacted third molars (n = 98); VAS, visual analog scale (0–100 mm). *P < 0.05; **P < 0.01 (Kruskal–Wallis). (Source: Breivik and Bjornsson.[16])*

Despite efforts to include only patients with a certain degree of pain intensity, there might be upper outliers of baseline pain that need adjusting for. Adjusting for baseline pain intensity as a covariant should thus be part of the statistical analysis of the outcome data.

DOWNSIDE ASSAY SENSITIVITY

It is vital that the study is designed so that a clinically meaningful and statistically significant difference between placebo and the active drug can be measured, particularly for the study of analgesics of modest efficacy. This is called downside assay sensitivity, which can be quantified by the inclusion of a standard analgesic and placebo arm in the protocol.[20] An example of this is a single-dose study designed to compare a novel analgesic (FS 205-397) with aspirin 650 mg as a standard and with placebo following oral surgery. As the standard analgesic (aspirin) was associated with significantly better pain relief than placebo, it was possible to conclude that the study design was of sufficient downside sensitivity.[41**]

UPSIDE ASSAY SENSITIVITY

When a new drug is compared with a standard active analgesic drug only (without a placebo control group), the study must document upside assay sensitivity.[20]

This means that the study must be able to show clinically meaningful and statistically significant differences between two standard analgesic drugs of differing efficacy, or between two doses of a known standard analgesic drug.[22,32] An example of this is a single-dose study designed to compare diflunisal with acetaminophen with or without codeine following oral surgery in which acetaminophen with codeine afforded significantly more pain relief than acetaminophen alone.[42**] Consequently, sound conclusions can be drawn from the analysis of efficacy data of diflunisal in that the study design demonstrated sufficient upside sensitivity.

PLACEBO CONTROL?

Although the inclusion of a placebo arm in dental pain trials is desirable, its omission can be occasionally justified, e.g. when the use of a placebo group is ethically difficult (e.g. evaluation in children) or when placebo has previously been compared with an active standard analgesic comparator. Instead, a second dose level of the standard analgesic will ensure that meaningful interpretation of the analgesic assay data is possible.[32]

An inert placebo arm or an active comparator is mandatory in RCTs to demonstrate the efficacy of a test drug,[32] and withholding an active treatment is unlikely to result in serious harm in short-term analgesic trials. Nevertheless, the Declaration of Helsinki states that "every patient should be assured of the best proven, diagnostic and therapeutic method"; therefore, efforts should be made to limit the number of trials which include placebo

controls. However, placebo control is necessary when one needs to establish whether the test drug is an active analgesic in the study population. Inclusion of a placebo arm is also required when there is reason to doubt whether a dental pain model has satisfactory downside assay sensitivity. This was not the case in a dental pain study designed to investigate whether the efficacy of two standard analgesics (acetaminophen 1 g and acetaminophen 1 g plus codeine 60 mg) differed. A placebo arm was not included as the downside assay sensitivity had previously been established in an identical dental pain study, and therefore the use of placebo might be considered unethical.[19**] Adequate upside assay sensitivity was documented in another study by including two standard analgesics arms (acetaminophen 1 g and acetaminophen 1 g plus codeine 60 mg), the results demonstrating that acetaminophen plus codeine was superior to acetaminophen alone for pain relief (Fig. 36.3).[29**]

RESCUE ANALGESIC DRUG

Whenever a placebo treatment or a test drug of uncertain analgesic efficacy is included in a clinical trial, the provision of rescue analgesia is mandatory.[32] In practice, this means that such analgesic trials must ensure that a rescue analgesic of proven efficacy is available to all patients included in the study. This can be accomplished by giving all participants rescue medication in sealed envelopes with written instructions, or prescriptions of a standard rescue analgesic, or both.

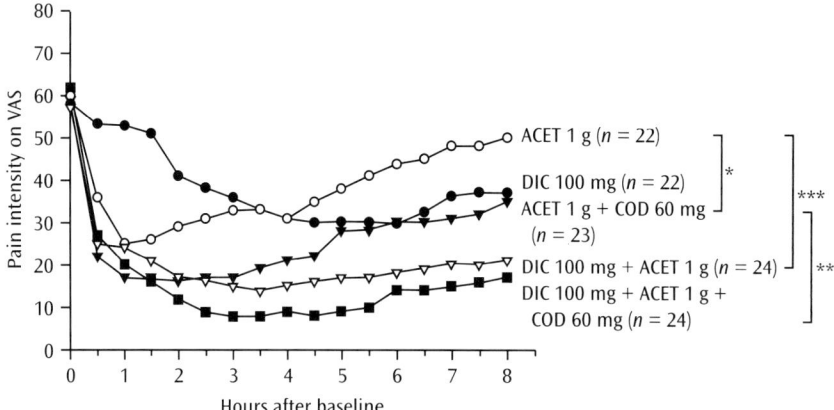

Figure 36.3 *Comparison of mean pain intensity ratings on a 100-mm visual analog scale (VAS) when various analgesic combinations are taken after surgical removal of third molars. In a randomized, double-blind study, 120 patients with moderate to strong pain after surgery received in a single oral dose combinations of diclofenac (DIC; enteric coated tablets), acetaminophen (ACET), and codeine (COD). Diclofenac plus acetaminophen with or without codeine was superior to diclofenac alone or acetaminophen alone (***P < 0.01). Diclofenac plus acetaminophen plus codeine was superior to acetaminophen plus codeine (**P = 0.01). Adequate upside assay sensitivity was documented as acetaminophen plus codeine was superior to acetaminophen alone (*P < 0.05) (GLM). (After Breivik et al.[29])*

PRACTICAL TIPS

- The visual analog scale (VAS) should be printed, not copied, to avoid distortion of size when copying the sheet.
- The direct assessment of change in pain intensity in patients reporting similar baseline pain intensity should be the primary outcome measure in an analgesic trial on acute postoperative pain.
- Recovery rooms for trial participants and patients being screened for trial participation should be separate from the other patients at the clinic.
- A simple screening procedure at the end of the studies, such as asking the participants what test drug they thought they had been given, will document that a double-blind procedure was not inadvertently unblinded during the trial, e.g. by side-effects or other cues.[43★★,44★★]

The postsurgical dental pain model used for analgesic efficacy evaluation has many advantages, such as pain confined to one area of the body and young and healthy patients largely unencumbered by concurrent disease and thus concomitant medication. The potential study population is large, and therefore studies of sufficient power can be conducted. Limitations of the dental pain model are the relatively transient duration of pain and the large interindividual variation in pain experienced following the oral surgical procedure. However, adherence to the principles of protocol design, meticulous planning, protocol compliance, and trial execution will result in reliable data when using this pain model.

REFERENCES

- 1. Seymour RA, Walton JG. Pain control after third molar surgery. *Int J Oral Surg* 1984; **13:** 457–85.
2. Szmyd L, Shannon IL, Mohnac AM. Control of postoperative sequela in impacted third molar surgery. *J Oral Ther Pharmacol* 1965; **1:** 491–6.
3. Troullos E, Hargreaves KM, Butler DP, Dionne RA. Comparison of nonsteroidal anti-inflammatory drugs, ibuprofen and flurbiprofen, with methylprednisolone and placebo. *J Oral Maxillofac Surg* 1990; **48:** 945–52.
- 4. Lökken P, Olsen I, Norman-Pedersen K. Bilateral surgical removal of impacted lower third molar teeth as a model for drug evaluation: a test with ibuprofen. *Eur J Clin Pharmacol* 1975; **8:** 209–16.
5. Lökken P, Skjelbred P. Aspirin or paracetamol? *Lancet* 1981; **8259:** 1346–7.
6. Baxendale BR, Vater M, Lavery KM. Dexamethasone reduces pain and swelling following extraction of third molar teeth. *Anaesthesia* 1993; **48:** 961–4.
7. Fernando S, Hill CM, Walker R. A randomised double blind comparative study of low level laser therapy following surgical extraction of lower third molar teeth. *Br J Oral Maxillofac Surg* 1993; **31:** 170–2.
- 8. Meechan JG, Seymour RA. The use of third molar surgery in clinical pharmacology. *Br J Oral Maxillofac Surg* 1993; **31:** 360–5.
9. Wirth DP, Brenlan DR, Levine RJ, Rodriguez CM. The effect of complementary healing therapy on postoperative pain after surgical removal of impacted third molar teeth. *Complement Ther Med* 1993; **1:** 133–8.
- 10. Urquhart E. Analgesic agents and strategies in the dental pain model. *J Dent Res* 1994; **22:** 336–41.
11. Lökken P, Straumsheim PA, Tveiten D, Skjelbred P. Effects of homeopathy on pain and other events after acute trauma: placebo controlled trial with bilateral oral surgery. *Br Med J* 1995; **319:** 1439–42.
- 12. Cooper SA. Models for clinical assessment of oral analgesics. *JAMA* 1983; **75:** 24–9.
- 13. Forbes JA. Oral surgery. In: Max M, Portenoy R eds. *Advances in Pain Research and Therapy*, vol. 18. New York, NY: Raven Press, 1991: 347–74.
- 14. Cooper SA, Beaver WT. A model to evaluate mild analgesics in oral surgery. *Clin Pharmacol Ther* 1976; **20:** 241–50.
15. Fisher SE, Frame JW, Rout PGJ. Factors affecting the onset and the severity of pain following the surgical removal of unilateral impacted mandibular third molar teeth. *Br Dent J* 1988; **164:** 351–4.
16. Breivik EK, Björnsson GA. Variation in surgical trauma and baseline pain intensity: effects on assay sensitivity of an analgesic trial. *Eur J Oral Sci* 1998; **106:** 844–52.
17. Hansson P, Ekblom A, Thomsson M, Fjellner B. Pain development and consumption of analgesics after oral surgery in relation to personality characteristics. *Pain* 1989; **37:** 271–7.
- 18. Nörholt SE. Thesis. Treatment of acute pain following removal of mandibular third molars. *Int J Oral Maxillofac Surg* 1998; **27** (Suppl. 1): 16.
19. Breivik EK, Haanæs HR, Barkvoll P. Upside assay sensitivity in a dental pain model. *Eur J Pain* 1998; **2:** 179–86.
- 20. Cooper SA. Single dose analgesic studies: the upside and downside of assay sensitivity. In: Max M, Portenoy R, Laska E eds. *Advances in Pain Research and Therapy*, vol. 18. New York, NY: Raven Press, 1991: 117–23.
21. Berge TI, Bøe OE. Predictor evaluation of postoperative morbidity after surgical removal of mandibular third molars. *Acta Odontol Scand* 1994; **52:** 1–8.
22. Shugars DA, Benson K, White RP, *et al.* Developing a measure of patient perceptions of short-term outcomes of third molar surgery. *J Oral Maxillofac Surg* 1996; **54:** 1402–8.
- 23. Meinert CL. *Good Clinical Trial Practice*. Nordic Guidelines, Upsala: Nordic Council of Medicine, 1989.
24. Jadad RA, Moore RA, Carroll D, *et al.* Assessing the quality of reports of randomized clinical trials: is blinding necessary? *Controlled Clin Trials* 1996; **17:** 1–12.
- 25. Moher D, Schultz, KF, Altman DG. The CONSORT state-

ment: revised recommendations for improving the quality of reports of parallel-group randomised trials. *Lancet* 2001; **357**: 1191–4.

26. Bjørnsson GA, Bjørnland T, Skoglund LA. Reproducibility of postoperative courses after surgical removal of symmetrically impacted wisdom teeth. *Methods Find Exp Clin* 1995; **17**: 345–56.

27. Yagiela JA. Local anesthetics. In: Dionne RA, Phero JC eds. *Management of Pain and Anxiety in Dental Practice*. Amsterdam: Elsevier Science Publishers BV, 1993: 109–34.

28. Skjelbred P, Løkken P. Paracetamol versus placebo: effects on post-operative course. *Eur J Clin Pharmacol* 1979; **15**: 27–33.

29. Breivik EK, Barkvoll P, Skovlund E. Combining diclofenac with paracetamol or paracetamol–codeine after oral surgery: a randomised, double blind, single oral dose study. *Clin Pharmacol Ther* 1999; **66**: 625–35.

30. Breivik EK, Björnsson GA, Skovlund E. A comparison of pain rating scales by sampling from clinical trial data. *Clin J Pain* 2000; **16**: 22–8.

31. Anonymous. Report of a workshop on the management of patients with third molar teeth. *J Oral Maxillofac Surg* 1994; **52**: 1102–12.

◆ 32. Max MB, Laska EM. Single-dose analgesic combinations. In: Max M, Portenoy R eds. *Advances in Pain Research and Therapy,* vol. 18. New York, NY: Raven Press, 1991: 55–95.

33. Doroschak AM, Bowles WR, Hargreaves KM. Evaluation of the combination of Flurbiprofen and Tramadol for management of endodontic pain. *J Endodontics* 1999; **25**: 660–3.

◆ 34. Lasagna L. The psychophysics of clinical pain. *Lancet* 1962; **572**: 637–9.

35. Houmes RJ, Voets MA, Verkaaik A, *et al*. Efficacy and safety of tramadol versus morphine for moderate and severe postoperative pain with special regard to respiratory depression. *Anesth Analg* 1992; **74**: 510–14.

36. Oikarinen K. Postoperative pain after mandibular third molar surgery. *Acta Odontol Scand* 1991; **49**: 7–13.

37. Desjardins PJ. Analgesic efficacy of piroxicam in postoperative pain. *JAMA* 1988; **84** (Suppl. 5A): 35–41.

38. Jorkjend L, Skoglund L. Effect of non-eugenol- and eugenol-containing periodontal dressing on the incidence and severity of pain after periodontal soft tissue surgery. *J Clin Periodontol* 1990; **17**: 341–4.

39. Sriwatanakul K, Lasagna L, Cox C. Evaluation of current clinical trial design methodology in analgesimetry based on experts' opinions and analysis of several studies. *Clin Pharmacol Ther* 1983; **34**: 277–83.

40. Breivik EK. Analgesic trials in oral surgery. Methodological aspects of the dental pain model with special emphasis on assay sensitivity and effects of combining paracetamol with codeine and/or diclofenac. Doctoral thesis. Oslo, Norway, University of Oslo, 1999.

41. Mehlisch DR, Sterling WR, Mazza FA, Singer JM. A single-dose study of the efficacy and safety of FS 205-397 (250 mg or 500 mg) versus aspirin and placebo in the treatment of postsurgery dental pain. *J Clin Pharmacol* 1990: **30**: 815–23.

42. Forbes JA, Beaver WT, White EH, *et al*. Diflunisal. A new oral analgesic with an unusually long duration of action, *JAMA* 1982; **248**: 2139–42.

43. Hughes JR, Krahn D. Blindness and the validity of the double-blind procedure. *J Clin Psychopharmacol* 1985; **5**: 138–42.

44. Carroll KM, Rounsville BJ, Nich C. Blind man's bluff: effectiveness and significance of psychotherapy and pharmacotherapy blinding procedures in a clinical trial. *J Consult Clin Psychol* 1994; **62**: 276–80.

37

Clinical trials: cancer pain

ULF E KONGSGAARD

Analgesic requirements	469	Inclusion criteria and accretion of patients	475
Pain instability	470	Size and duration of study	475
Pain assessment in cancer pain trials	471	Factors difficult to control in cancer pain trials	476
Polypharmacy as a problem for cancer pain trials	471	Special problems in cancer pain trials	477
Requirements of appropriate clinical trials in cancer pain	472	Ethical issues	478
Issues of study design in cancer pain trials	472	Summary	479
Selection and stratification of patients with cancer pain	474	References	479

Cancer is a common cause of death in our society, and pain caused by a cancer or as a complication of cancer therapy occurs frequently. Many epidemiological surveys have demonstrated that approximately 25% of patients with localized disease report pain, and that the prevalence of pain can be as high as 90% in patients with advanced cancer.[1] A large proportion of patients with metastatic cancer have pain long before the terminal stage of their illness. Recent studies have reported that adequate pain control can be achieved in up to 88% of patients with cancer-related pain,[2*] however many patients still have inadequate pain management.[3*] Unrelieved pain impairs functional status, compromises quality of life, and may interfere with anticancer treatment.

Patients with advanced cancer may present complex dispositions of symptoms, of which pain is the most prevalent. Furthermore, the patients suffering from pain from a variety of tumors, often with unstable disease, regularly present extremely heterogeneous pain profiles.[3*] The study of pain control in this population has in the past often been ignored. Pain treatment has been mostly empirical, incomplete, and possibly resulted in unnecessary suffering for many patients.

The following causal categories of pain are associated with cancer:

- caused by cancer itself;
- related to cancer and/or debility;
- caused by treatment;
- caused by concurrent disorders.

Cancer patients have pain that has both acute and chronic features. The acute pain can be subdivided into subacute pain, episodic pain, and intermittent pain, whereas chronic pain should include baseline pain as well as breakthrough pain. These distinctions can influence the therapeutic choices and consultant's recommendations, the aggressiveness of the therapy, and the very expectations of it. Different categories of pain can have practical value because they capture the multidimensional aspects of cancer pain. However, the clinical and pathological characteristics of cancer pain and its response to analgesic treatment have not been firmly established, which necessitates evaluations of the effectiveness and safety of old and new drugs and of routes of administration as well as of invasive procedures.

Furthermore, we need to know more about the characteristics of pain in cancer patients from specific subgroups of the population, including cultural and racial minorities and the economically disadvantaged.

ANALGESIC REQUIREMENTS

An important factor complicating the study of pain in cancer patients is the remarkable variability in dose and response to analgesics. Variability relates to characteristics inherent in pain; however, real individual requirements vary from patient to patient and also within patients. In clinical practice as well as in scientific studies, there is a difference between analgesic efficacy and the possibility for effective treatment. Confusion in the terms of efficacy and responsiveness has contributed to the controversy of opioids in pain conditions. The term efficacy points to the receptor occupancy, but does not consider the emergence of side-effects. Effective pain treatment considers a favorable balance between pain relief and undesirable side-effects without indicating a possible maximal effect. To clarify this nomenclature, Portenoy et al.[4]* have introduced the term responsiveness to characterize the degree of analgesia achieved at a dose associated with intolerable and unmanageable side-effects, i.e. maximal efficacy. This implies individual dose titration aiming at equilibrium between satisfactory pain relief and tolerable side-effects and ensuring that a sufficient dose reaches the site of action with adequate absorption and distribution. This emphasizes the analgesic response as a relative phenomenon that accounts for interindividual variability and the occurrence of dose-dependent analgesia.

The emergence of tolerance is another factor to consider regarding opioid responsiveness. Tolerance is a complex phenomenon, which has led to some controversy as to how often it occurs with systemic opioids in the clinical management of cancer pain. Chronic opioid exposure leads to adaptations at the receptor level in processes mediating acute actions of opioids as well as to adaptations in the regulation in the longer term of the function of neurons. In the clinical setting, dose escalation is used to assess the presence or absence of tolerance. Surveys using this criterion indicate that the rate and extent of tolerance differ dramatically among cancer patients.[5] It seems, however, that the most common reason for dose escalation in patients with cancer pain is disease progression. Even if tolerance does not appear to have major clinical consequences in most patients, it cannot be neglected in assessment of analgesic requirements in a clinical trial.

Variability in response may also be associated with pharmacokinetic factors. Renal impairment enhances opioid toxicity, probably because some of the opioids have active metabolites dependent upon renal excretion. Recent data indicate that genetic variability may be responsible for individual differences in the potency of the antinociceptive effects of morphine.[6]* Other factors also have to be considered, such as patient age, emotional reactions of fear, anxiety, and reactive repression.

Elements of variability in analgesic requirements

- Variation of individual requirements.
- Variation within patient groups.
- Variation relating to type of pain.
- Tolerance.
- Pharmacokinetics:
  - renal failure;
  - hepatic failure.
- Emotional, spiritual, and psychological factors.

PAIN INSTABILITY

Patients with chronic cancer-related pain usually experience fluctuations in pain intensity. When these episodes of increased pain intensity are clinically significant and interrupt a background pain that is otherwise controlled and tolerated, they are commonly described as breakthrough pain. Breakthrough pain is extremely heterogeneous,[7]* and may vary in frequency, onset and duration, severity, quality, etiology, pathophysiology, and impact.[8]* The few existing studies of breakthrough pain indicate that it is a common phenomenon associated with adverse outcomes. Bruera et al.[9]* demonstrated that the presence of breakthrough pain reduces the likelihood of a satisfactory response to opioid therapy. An oral transmucosal formulation of fentanyl in a matrix (OTFC) that dissolves when rubbed against the buccal mucosa has been developed specifically for breakthrough pain. Although efficacy and patient preference for this formulation has been demonstrated,[10]** an expected relationship between the OTFC and the total daily opioid dose was not found.[11]**

The lack of data may relate to the difficulties in defining and measuring subtypes of pain. The methodological challenge in studying a highly variable subjective phenomenon that may or may not occur during any planned assessment period is evident. Assessment of breakthrough pain is difficult, given the heterogeneity and lack of predictability. It is also difficult to interpret measures of pain intensity combined with analgesic consumption. Breakthrough pains must be distinguished from recurrent acute pains and other clinically insignificant fluctuations in the intensity of chronic pain. This demands a clearer definition of the phenomenon – one which can distinguish different types of pain according to intensity and temporal characteristics. Background pain intensity may also vary during the day with particular individual patterns. Baseline drift (natural fluctuations of symptons not associated with the intervention) is important in respect to both symptons and the pharmacological actions from analgesics. This should engage measurements of pain intensity at several specific periods of the day. Studies are needed to clarify the true effectiveness of the conventional therapeutic approaches to breakthrough pain, e.g. by comparing escalation of the baseline dose with optimal use of rescue dose as alternative interventions for breakthrough pain. Additional studies that evaluate the size and timing of the rescue dose are needed.[11]*

Temporal aspects of pain

- Background pain.
- Pain fluctuations.
- Recurrent pain.
- Breakthrough pain.
- Incident pain.

PAIN ASSESSMENT IN CANCER PAIN TRIALS

Cancer pain is a complex experience. It involves personality, learning, and situational components. Severity as well as the degree of interference with function is crucial to the adequate assessment of pain. The changing expression of cancer pain demands repeated assessment, as new causes for pain can emerge rapidly. In advanced cancer cases, pain from multiple etiologies may be the rule and not the exception. These elements are critical for studies of the epidemiology of pain and for studies of treatment outcomes and encompass a requirement of a multidimensional assessment of the pain syndrome, including patients' clinical, psychological, and psychiatric characteristics and a number of social and family variables. Furthermore, a comprehensive assessment of the patient with cancer pain can have important clinical implications in recognizing disease progression.

Although animal experiments have been momentous for the understanding of pain mechanisms and analgesia, extrapolating data of animal experiments to human pain perception may be an important source of contradictory evidence concerning opioid responsiveness in the cancer pain population. Animal experiments assess nociception rather than pain. In analyzing pain in the cancer patient, it is important to distinguish the terms nociception, pain, and suffering. Nociception is defined as the activity in the nervous system following tissue damage. Pain is the perception of this activity, including cognitive and affective processes in the brain. Pain may or may not be the result of active tissue damage. Suffering may be defined as a threat to the integrity of the personality. Suffering in the cancer patient affects the quality of life (Fig. 37.1). Although pain has an important influence on suffering, other factors such as anxiety, depression, dependence, physical immobility, and social isolation also affect quality of life.

There are numerous ways to categorize the types of pain that occur in cancer patients. These include definitions based on the neurophysiologic mechanisms of pain, its temporal aspects, its intensity, the categories of cancer patients with pain, and the specific pain syndromes that occur in this population. It is important to acknowledge the wide disagreement on the choice of the best outcome measures for pain clinical trials.[12]** Several tools, however, are available for pain assessment and measurement. They can be divided into two main categories: intensity scales and questionnaires intended to capture multidimensionality of cancer pain. Among intensity scales, the most used methods are visual analog scales (VASs), numerical scales (NRSs), and verbal rating scales (VRSs). VASs can be difficult to use with less educated patients and with the elderly, whereas 0–10 NRSs seem to have common meaning across cultures while keeping some desirable psychometric properties if compared with VRSs. However, we cannot rely on pain intensity measures alone to evaluate

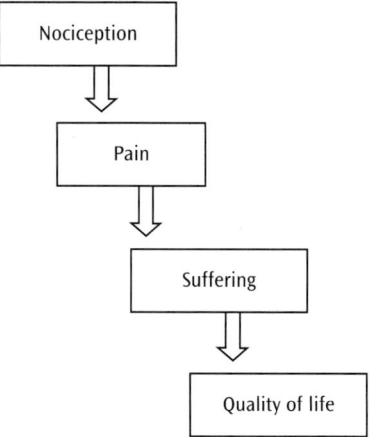

Figure 37.1 *The pain experience: steps in the production and perception of pain.*

treatment efficacy, and therefore a series of currently validated assessment instruments is available for the multidimensional evaluation of cancer pain.

Validated assessment instruments for multidimensional evaluation of cancer pain

- McGill Pain Questionnaire.[13]
- Brief Pain Inventory.[14]
- Memorial Pain Assessment Card.[15]

In general, four criteria are important in choosing a measure appropriate for clinical practice as well as for clinical trials:[16]***

- *Validity*. It is important to measure what you think you are measuring.
- *Reliability*. If staff change, it is important that the measurement does not.
- *Responsiveness*. Clinically important changes should be detectable.
- *Appropriateness*. Patients, families, and staff should feel comfortable using the measure in this setting, should not be burdened by it, and should find it clinically useful.

POLYPHARMACY AS A PROBLEM FOR CANCER PAIN TRIALS

A large number of cancer pain patients will eventually be treated with adjuvant analgesics – other drugs to control distressing symptoms as well as drugs to combat the disease itself. This practice of polypharmacy may confound the interpretation of clinical trials. A study of 676 patients with advanced cancer found widespread use of adjuvant drugs for symptom control; the adjuvants most frequently used were phenothiazines, night sedatives, and antiemetics.[17] Daytime sedatives, nonsteroidal anti-inflammatory drugs, antidepressants, and anticonvulsants were also used. The concomitant use of this heterogeneous group of drugs may affect the pharmacokinetics or pharmacodynamics of opioids. The true influence of these drugs on opioid effects, however, may be difficult to determine. Besides drug interactions, the side-effects of adjuvant drugs may confound the side-effects, such as sedation and confusion, of the trial medications.

Improvement in pain treatment is likely to require drug combinations, however few analgesic combinations have been studied, particularly in chronic dosing trials. Controlled clinical trials of such combinations present particular challenges.

Drug interactions (therapeutic effects as well as side-effects)

- Additive effects.
- Synergistic effects.
- Antagonistic effects.

Randomized clinical trials of blind dose titration are required in order to establish the efficacy and safety of a new analgesic drug. When comparing efficacy or when changing from one opioid agonist to another, equianalgesic conversion tables are generally being used. However, there is still a surprising lack of consensus over appropriate conversion tables for these drugs. A unique characteristic of methadone is that the equianalgesic dose ratio increases in patients exposed to higher doses of opioids. This is different from other opioid agonists in which the equianalgesic ratio appears to be independent of the opioid exposure. These findings suggest that there is only partial cross-tolerance between opioid agonists.[18*] Switching from one route of drug administration to another requires other conversion tables that are influenced by a number of variables. Furthermore, ethical reasons dictate a ready availability of rescue medication at all times for breakthrough pain. The potential limitations of the use of an additional dose of rescue medication as an outcome measure must also be considered. Factors other than pain level may play a role in the patient's decision-making about taking an additional rescue dose.[12**] Using several opioid agonists simultaneously could influence interpretation of analgesic requirements and drug-induced toxicity. Authors have reported significant improvement or complete disappearance of opioid side-effects with both opioid rotation and dose reduction,[19*] probably because of a decrease in the circulating levels of the active metabolites or parent compound responsible for the side-effects.

REQUIREMENTS OF APPROPRIATE CLINICAL TRIALS IN CANCER PAIN

Some results are so highly dramatic that no comparison group is needed. Successful results of this magnitude, however, are rare. Given the wide spectrum of the natural history of cancer in general and cancer pain specifically, and even the variability of an individual patient's response to any intervention, the need for a defined control or comparison group is obvious.

Several research projects designed to investigate clinical cancer pain syndromes have been based on conclusions from research conducted with normal subjects experiencing experimental pain. Furthermore, clinical studies on drugs for cancer pain are often performed on patients with an early stage of cancer. The studies often define several exclusion criteria, selecting patients without any confounding factors, and the results are extrapolated to the terminally ill cancer pain population.[20*] This can avoid confounding factors and have an expected survival that outlasts the planned duration of a study; however, the clinician must be aware of the limited generalizability. Sound methodology is a prerequisite to balance the credibility, reliability, and applicability of clinical research. It is important to understand the pitfalls and constraints of relevant research methods to appreciate historical and current practical limitations. Ideal designs of trials present real challenges and sometimes prohibitive problems that can at worst lead to misinterpretations of results and faulty conclusions. It is apparent that the design of reliable and meaningful clinical trials is becoming more, rather than less, difficult.

ISSUES OF STUDY DESIGN IN CANCER PAIN TRIALS

Historical control study designs

The simplest approach to evaluating a new treatment is to compare a single group of patients given the new treatment with a group previously treated with an alternative regimen. The argument for using a historical control design is that all new participants can receive the new intervention, which makes recruitment easy and fast. Historical control studies have undoubtedly contributed to medical knowledge, however the studies have important limitations. They are particularly vulnerable to bias due to other factors apart from treatment that have changed over time.[21*] Sacks et al.[22***] compared trials of the same treatments in which randomized or historical controls were used and found a consistent tendency for historically controlled trials to yield more optimistic results than randomized trials. The historical control study may still have a place in scientific investigation despite its limitations. As a rapid, relatively inexpensive method of obtaining initial impressions regarding a new therapy, such studies can be important.

The use of historical controls can furthermore be justified in controlled situations of relatively rare conditions, such as in evaluating treatments for refractory pain symptoms in advanced cancer. In such situations, randomization is not always possible. The goal should, nevertheless, be to retain all the methodological features of a well-conducted trial other than the randomization.

Sequential trials

A sequential trial depends at any stage on the results so far obtained. The results during the course of the trial determine the number of observations made. Since patients are started on treatment serially and not simultaneously, it is possible to assess the response to treatment as it becomes available in sequential order. This conveys an ethical advantage, with the possibility of terminating the trial quickly when one intervention is an important new advance. A sequential trial is most appropriate when the response is obvious soon after treatment is started. These trials may prove economical and helpful as a pilot to determine the variance of the measurements.

Randomized controlled trials

The randomized controlled trial (RCT) has become the ideal standard for clinical investigations and provides the essential background to practicing evidence-based medicine. A randomized controlled trial should, nevertheless, only be used when there is genuine doubt about the efficacy of the treatments and the investigator cannot know whether or not patients will suffer.

Advantages of the randomized design

- Removes the potential of bias in the allocation of participants.
- Facilitates blinding.
- Tends to produce comparable groups.
- Validity of statistical tests of significance is guaranteed.

Investigators should carefully weigh the advantages and disadvantages of crossover versus parallel study designs to ensure validity without compromising effectiveness. Although certain situations will provide preferences, both designs can at times be employed, as illustrated by Deschamps et al.[23**] and Parris et al.,[24**] who conducted trials comparing immediate release analgesics with controlled release analgesics.

Parallel study designs

The standard parallel study design is the one most commonly used and has the advantage of simplicity in that a single treatment or combination of treatments is given to each group and a fixed number of patients are involved (Fig. 37.2). Parallel designs are less dependent on assumption about disease progression. They are more appropriate for patients whose condition may change over the longer period needed by a crossover study. They should also be used when there is a possibility of significant carryover effects. Furthermore, parallel study designs are considered where it is reasonable to assume baseline homogeneity between treatment groups, or when precautions such as stratification and blocking have been taken to attain it. In cancer patients, this last condition may be difficult to accomplish; moreover, a large number of patients may be needed to obtain the desired statistical power. However, the duration of the study need not be as long as in a crossover study and the dropout rate may be smaller.[25***] In a parallel-group trial, precision may be increased when the within-subject variance is lower than that of the between-subject variance and baseline measurements are employed to provide within-subject data.

When to consider using the standard parallel study design

- The duration of treatment has to be long.
- The effect of one treatment is different when it follows another treatment.
- There are chances of significant carryover effects.
- A large number of treatments are to be compared.
- The number of subjects available for the trial is unlimited.

Crossover study designs

Crossover designs are used to increase the sensitivity of a study by using each patient as his own control (Fig. 37.3). This increases validity and reduces the sample size required compared with parallel group studies with the same statistical power. A crossover design is only achievable for a chronic condition that reverts to its original state with the cessation of treatment. This is not the typical situation in long-term studies of patients with advanced cancer, the majority of whom continue to have underlying disease progression. Therefore, crossover designs are mostly applicable for studies of relatively short duration. Crossover trials may be recommended when the therapeutic effects of the medication cease soon after it is discontinued during a washout period and its effects would not differ whether it was given first or last. A difference between treatment effects may be the result of the carryover effect of one treatment into the next period

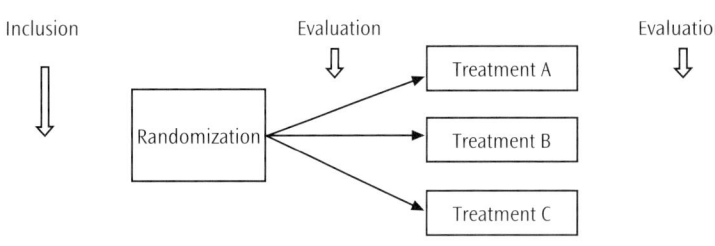

Figure 37.2 *Standard parallel designs to assess the effects of three treatments (A, B, and C).*

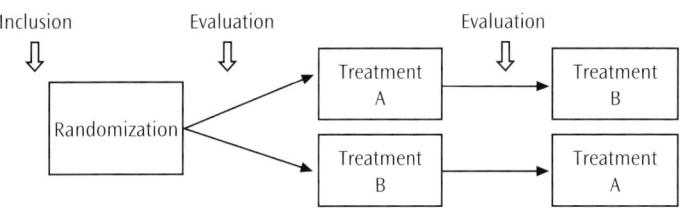

Figure 37.3 *Crossover design to assess the effects of two treatments (A and B).*

or of an influence of the time of assessment from the beginning of the trial – a so-called order effect. In cancer patients receiving narcotics, a washout period is not always possible since it would be unethical to abruptly withdraw or withhold analgesic medication during the washout phase.

When to consider using the crossover trial

- A baseline measurement cannot be made.
- Any carryover effect is of short duration.
- Extending the treatment period does not alter the difference between the treatment effects.
- Prolongation of the trial will not result in a large increase in dropout.
- Within-subject variation is restricted.
- An order effect is absent or can be balanced out.

Addition of other treatment sequences or a third treatment period offer possible unbiased estimates of treatment effects even in the presence of various types of carryover effects (Fig. 37.4).

Enriched enrollment study designs

A variant of the crossover design, the enriched enrollment design, may be useful in studying treatments to

which only a minority of patients respond.[26]** However, these designs are open to criticism that prior exposure to the treatment may defeat the double-blind procedures and may sometimes result in spurious positive results.

Cluster-randomized trials

Cluster-randomized trials represent an important experimental design, supplementing ordinary randomized clinical trials.[27] They are particularly relevant when evaluating interventions at the level of clinic, hospital, district, or region. Sample sizes need to be greatly increased, and an adequate number of clusters is essential. One should rigorously guard against selection bias.

SELECTION AND STRATIFICATION OF PATIENTS WITH CANCER PAIN

Although the early stages of protocol development may proceed with only a rough outline of the intended type of patient, the final protocol must include a detailed specification. The objective is to guarantee patients to whom the findings of the trial may be applied. Furthermore, it is important to focus on the type of patient considered most likely to benefit from the new intervention under

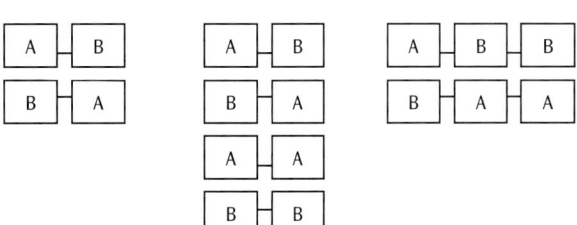
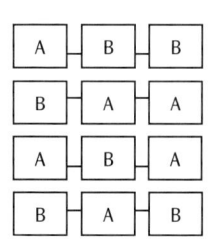

Figure 37.4 *Examples of different crossover designs used to compare two treatments (A and B). The three more complex designs on the right are more able to distinguish treatment from carryover effects.*

investigation. Patients are usually chosen from a study population defined by eligibility criteria. As long as selection of participants into a trial occurs, they must be regarded as special. Therefore, investigators may have the problem of generalizing from participants actually in the trial to the study population, and then to the population with the condition.

The variability in cancer pain patients requires that strategies must be used to reduce heterogeneity of treatment groups in clinical trials. One strategy would be to select patients with specific characteristics, such as type of tumor, pain syndrome, pain category, or functional status. This would increase the validity of the study, but at the risk of the trial remaining small and its findings lacking generalizability. While stratification provides a better balance between treatment groups, it increases the complexity of the trial and the need for a larger sample size and reduces the degrees of freedom. Moreover, extended subset analyses increase the risk of dubious results produced by chance effects alone. An alternative approach to reduce stratification to a manageable size would be to categorize patients into a confined number of strata on the basis of a configuration of variables. A standardized staging system of cancer pain that could be used for such purposes, similar to those developed to classify various malignancies, is needed. Bruera et al.[9]* have assessed the accuracy of a staging system for cancer pain which included the assessment of pain, previous opioid dose, cognitive function, psychological distress, tolerance, and past history of alcohol or drugs. They found the staging system highly accurate in predicting patients with good prognosis, but patients with "poor prognosis" were still able to achieve good pain control in more than 50% of cases.

INCLUSION CRITERIA AND ACCRETION OF PATIENTS

Any clinical trial requires a precise definition of which patients are eligible for the inclusion. Investigators often study patients who are more stable than those who could eventually benefit from the new treatment regimens. Ideally, strategies should be undertaken to guarantee that the sample population studied corresponds to patients clinically most likely to benefit from the intervention. This is not, however, always possible with cancer patients. Many trials of controlled release opioid preparation have used stable patients requiring a moderate dose of narcotics. The results from these studies may not always be relevant for patient groups with severe pain, who require much higher doses of opioids or need alternative routes of administration because of impairment of gastrointestinal mobility.

Participating in a drug trial will frequently demand that the patients refrain from taking part in any other investigational drug trial during the study or a fixed number of days prior to inclusion. At university hospitals, in particular, a large number of patients will be encouraged to take part in a variety of protocols, thus limiting the potential number of patients available for a cancer pain study.

Patients participating in clinical trials must meet inclusion criteria that necessitate the exclusion of those with significant organ dysfunction. Thus, many patients who initially may meet inclusion criteria but are at or near borderline may rapidly deteriorate during the study and have to be withdrawn from the trial. This might limit the relevance of the results obtained when applied to patients with advanced cancer. To make the results of trials more generalizable, it may be necessary to extend the range of acceptable values for patient inclusion into these trials. However, decisions regarding the level of clinical dysfunction at which patients are still eligible for participation in clinical trials rely on the clinical judgment of researchers and are a source of bias.[27] Investigators study only those participants available to them. Participants must demonstrate performance standards that may be too rigorous for many patients at this stage of their illness. Patient selection would also rule out a large proportion of terminal cancer patients who may not be able to respond to the demands of a clinical trial because of impaired cognitive function or affective disorders. As these disorders are often found in indirect form and misdiagnosed as depression, their prevalence is difficult to assess. Depression is common in cancer patients and its severity may increase as the disease progresses.[28]* There is also a correlation between pain intensity and psychomotor impairment, as well as a relationship between pain intensity and fatigue and vigor.

Problems with inclusion criteria and accretion of patients

- Unstable pain.
- Impaired cognitive function.
- Depression.
- Metabolic disturbances.
- Organ dysfunction.
- Participation in other trials.

SIZE AND DURATION OF STUDY

A trial must be large enough to detect clinically important differences between treatments. As pointed out previously, strict inclusion criteria are important; however, one does not wish to be so restrictive about patient entry that the trial remains small and thus its findings lack generality. Despite detailed criteria and adequate protocol adherence, differences in study conditions could possibly vary in a multicenter, multinational trial with a large number of investigators. Such a study design can, on the other hand, be necessary to provide larger groups of patients in order to account for the large biological variability in humans.

In deciding the number of patients to include in a clinical study, the researcher must consider the statistical implications of sample size. The risk of obtaining misleading results increases with small samples. At least 5% of small trials will yield differences significant at the 0.05 level by chance alone when there are no true differences in treatment efficacy. Obviously, studies of cancer pain must be large enough to control for factors likely to confound results.[25]***

Factors influencing the number of subjects required in a study

- The objectives defined for the trial.
- The level of significance that must be achieved if the objective is reached.
- The confidence with which a result will be reported if the objective is not reached.
- The variability of the endpoint measurements.

Researchers must also consider how many potentially eligible patients can be included in the trial within a reasonable time frame. The achievable accrual rate of patients is often less than half what is estimated.

Factors causing a decreased accrual rate

- Investigators may be overenthusiastic in their assessment.
- Some patients will not be eligible for the trial.
- Some eligible patients may not enter the trial.
- Some patients may not be evaluable.

The absence of a critical mass of qualified researchers and of a central institution able to coordinate trials in this area are important constraints for patient accrual.[29] Another dimension is the selected nature of patients who may agree to take part in such studies. Consent rates of only one in seven to about one in 12 or 13 eligible patients may be likely.[30]

The duration of intervention may be fixed for all patients or be dependent on each patient's progress. The former is easier to interpret but sometimes fails to incorporate sufficient flexibility to handle therapy in each patient's best interest. Short, fixed periods of therapy are often satisfactory for phase II trials of short-term efficacy. However, for trials of more long-term effects, the duration of therapy may require a more complex definition that incorporates plans for dealing with side-effects, dose modification, and patient withdrawal. Treatment periods should be long enough that patients will approach maximal response. Too short a period may not be adequate to demonstrate the efficacy or safety of the medication or delivery system tested.

FACTORS DIFFICULT TO CONTROL IN CANCER PAIN TRIALS

Cancer pain comprises a group of heterogeneous disorders characterized by variable responses to treatment. Few of the experimental conditions used in chronic pain models or animal research are representative of the patient with cancer and pain. Therefore, a number of factors difficult to control can influence clinical trials in cancer pain patients.

The incidence of side-effects

Accurate data concerning the incidence of side-effects are difficult to attain in cancer patients owing to ancillary treatment. There is, in any case, little agreement about what constitutes acceptable versus unacceptable side-effects. Ultimately, the patient must be regarded as the final authority on when a side-effect is sufficiently disagreeable. There is a paucity of sensitive tools to accurately characterize these effects, and their apparent incidence and seriousness will naturally differ with changes in the methods used to characterize them.

Two dimensions need to be considered when evaluating the severity of side-effects: intensity and duration. Deschamps et al.[23]** employed an index that took into account both the intensity and duration of side-effects to measure toxicity. In addition to the descriptive statistics provided, this index had the advantage of allowing comparison of the relative importance of each side-effect. Side-effects can indicate whether the drug has reached its site of action. Therefore, the capacity for nonresponders to achieve complete pain relief with less than optimal doses cannot be determined. Accumulation of opioid metabolites may result in excitatory toxicities such as myoclonus/seizures, hyperalgesia, and hyperactive delirium/hallucinations. A number of psychoactive drugs, including midazolam, barbiturates, and baclofen, have been tried for the management of opioid neurotoxicity, however these drugs are likely to increase sedation and to decrease cognitive abilities. The route of administration of opioids, either oral or spinal, also influences the dose at which side-effects would emerge.

Patient compliance

A protocol for the therapy must remain sufficiently straightforward to be followed without confusion or inconvenience. All clinical studies are inundated with problems of noncompliance, but in pain studies of patients with advanced cancer these problems are even more complex and challenging. Assuming adequate instrumentation to assess pain, the procedure chosen for pain data collection may not be sensitive enough to detect swings in pain that may occur throughout the day. Some patients report more pain in the morning than during the rest of the day. However, the reverse may be true in other patients.[25]*** Cancer patients often have reservations about using opioids because they fear the psychoactive components of opioids such as toxicity, addiction, and mental confusion. Furthermore, myths regarding addiction and the stigma of using controlled substances still occur in patients' perceptions and may compromise patients' compliance in clinical trials. In addition, patients may fail to comply because they are concerned that using opioids too early will endanger pain relief when they have more pain, or because they fear that being placed on opioids signals that death is near. A number of patients may also underreport the severity of pain and the lack of adequate pain relief because of a variety of reasons, such as not wanting to acknowledge disease progression, not wanting to divert the physician's attention from treatment of the disease, and not wanting to tell the physician that pain treatments are unsuccessful. Weiss *et al.*[31]* showed that a large proportion of patients with pain chose to tolerate pain instead of increasing pain therapy.

Patient withdrawals

Loss of patients may be significant in long-term studies. Cognitive impairment and progressively limited physical mobility may interfere with data acquisition during clinical trials. Ideally, patients should not be selected for participation in clinical trials at late stages of their illness. However, prediction of life expectancy in patients with cancer is notoriously inaccurate.[32]* Many patients entering clinical trials are likely to die or deteriorate significantly enough during the trial to compromise data collection. In a study by Kongsgaard and Poulain[33]** evaluating the efficacy and safety of transdermal fentanyl in chronic cancer pain, 138 patients were recruited and began the dose-titration phase. Owing to disease progression and inadequate symptom control, only 72 patients completed the double-blind study. Even studies of short duration may experience significant patient losses: in a placebo-controlled drug trial in cancer patients, 90% of the placebo group withdrew in the first day.[34]** Loss to follow-up is one of the significant reasons for exclusions after randomization. At times, participants lost to follow-up could still be included in the analysis if outcome information could be obtained from another source. Such opportunities, however, seldom arise. In any case, exclusions, withdrawals, and losses to follow-up should always be reported in clinical studies.

Supplementary treatment

Psychological interventions to reduce anxiety, depression, and pain have been shown to reduce aggravating symptoms and improve quality of life for cancer patients.[35]** Important supplementary treatment of this type may influence the nature of the study, introduce bias, and interfere with the correct interpretation of results in clinical trials. Nevertheless, confining such ancillary initiatives as well as other treatment measures, for example palliative radiation therapy and chemotherapy, in cancer patients already participating in a study would be unethical, irrespective of ideal requirements of clinical trials.

SPECIAL PROBLEMS IN CANCER PAIN TRIALS

In patients with advanced cancer, a willingness to address pain and other intolerable symptoms is a medical and moral imperative, irrespective of scientific, clinical, or economic impediments.

Persistent cancer pain: intractable cancer pain

Persistent pain is rarely a problem before metastatic cancer is present. Both the presence and severity of pain are dictated by several factors, including the primary site of the disease and the sites of metastases. The fear of uncontrolled pain is a key motivator behind a growing movement to legalize euthanasia for terminally ill patients. Interventional techniques continue to play an important role in the management of cancer pain. They should not be considered as an isolated treatment but as a component of general therapeutic guidelines. Although such guideline recommendations are consistent with common clinical practice and are supported by substantial anecdotal confirmation of effect, the evidence is lacking in sufficient weight and consistency regarding patients with refractory pain problems. Nevertheless, we must continue providing care for patients with pain that is refractory to pharmacological management, especially given the availability of treatments that appear to be effective. The provision of clinical care must thus proceed in parallel with an increased focus on the development of research initiatives.[36]

Celiac plexus blocks represent an example of the problems related to the evolving role of interventional strategies. An 85–94% incidence of good to excellent relief of pain has been obtained in large series of patients receiving one or more neurolytic celiac blocks for pain from pancreatic cancer. In a series of 136 patients, analgesia was present until the time of death in 75% of cases, and in an additional 12.5% of patients pain relief was maintained for more than 50% of survival time.[37]* However, this case series contains retrospective data and illustrates that what can be inferred from reports documenting outcomes for celiac plexus neurolysis is inadequate, despite this intervention being the single procedure with perhaps greatest consensus regarding claims for efficacy. A recent meta-analysis of 59 papers on celiac neurolysis for cancer pain found that only two involved randomization, and only one of these employed a control group.[38***] One important conclusion was that treated patients experienced not only improved pain control, reduction in opioid use, and improved function but also statistically significant improvement in survival. Designing clinical trials for the variety of available invasive therapies may for ethical reasons challenge and entirely frustrate efforts to randomly allocate patients into placebo control groups. Generally, the only justification for performing such invasive procedures, especially the ones that are irreversible, is a reasonable expectation that they will work, coupled with a lack of reasonable alternatives. There are, however, few clinically analogous animal models that can serve as testable bases for the requirement of "reasonable expectation" of therapeutic efficacy. Direct comparisons with noninvasive therapies, which are necessary to justify the usually higher risk and costlier invasive interventions, do not offer patients a sufficiently similar experience upon which to make fair assessments or draw conclusions.[39]

Assessment of analgesic cost

Several methods are available to evaluate the economic costs and health benefits of health care interventions:[40]

- Cost-minimization analysis determines which interventions have the minimum cost under the assumption that all interventions yield the same clinical outcome.
- Cost–benefit analysis incorporates and converts all outcomes into a certain currency. Interventions are considered to be cost-effective if the sum total of the benefits is greater than the sum total of the costs.
- Cost–consequence analysis uses the outcome measure currency per unit of clinical outcome, such as dollars per millimeter of blood pressure change or dollars per life saved.
- Cost–utility analysis is the method of economic evaluation of health care programs that incorporates utilities for health states, such as dollars per quality-adjusted life year.

If we have an intervention that both saves money and improves health, then we have an obvious choice. Comparing two interventions becomes difficult if one intervention costs money and improves health. However, to properly evaluate a health care intervention, we need to know its alternative. In cancer pain patients, we clearly have to consider the ethical side. Still, estimation of the gains of quality-adjusted life expectancy using new pain

treatments compared with standard of care must be performed.

ETHICAL ISSUES

Ethical conduct, which should be a self-evident element of any clinical trial, means treating the patient with the intervention believed to be the best. However, the reason that a clinical trial is being considered at all is that there is uncertainty about the potential benefits of a new treatment. The inclusion of untreated controls does not obviate treatment effects and introduces bias because there is no blinding. How should informed consent be performed? Are the ethical aspects of randomization discussed? Are placebo controls necessary, possible, ethical, and interpretable?

Individual versus collective ethics

Volunteer studies present obvious ethical and experimental constraints, and interventional approaches are rarely, if ever, the only choice for pain and symptom control. Direct comparison with noninvasive therapies, which are necessary to justify the usually higher risk and costlier invasive interventions, do not offer patients a sufficiently similar experience upon which to make failed assessments or to draw firm conclusions.[39] Thus, provisions of adequate yet ethical controls are often impossible. Individual ethics mean that each patient should be given that treatment which is thought to be most beneficial to control the symptoms. Collective ethics are concerned with achieving medical progress as efficiently as possible so that all patients may subsequently benefit from superior therapy. Most people feel instinctively that we should pay exclusive attention to individual ethics. Individual ethics must be compromised to some extent since otherwise patients would be exposed to improvised therapy based on clinical opinion and insubstantial evidence. Each clinical trial requires a balance between individual ethics and collective ethics. The society as a whole and the laws on medical ethics have perhaps not fully appreciated the reality of clinical trials.

Placebo treatment

Placebos in medical practice are given with the expectation that patients will benefit from nonspecific effects, so efforts are made to maximize these effects. In clinical trials, placebo effects should be minimized to allow the specific effect to show. However, a placebo cannot be employed if there is definite evidence that withholding standard treatment would be detrimental to the patient. Although it would be unethical to withhold an active analgesic for a prolonged period, administration may be delayed for a short interval, e.g. in postoperative pain. If pain relief is not achieved at the end of that period, active treatment can then be given; thus, arguments for using a placebo in this situation can be made provided that the patient has given an informed consent and rescue medication is available whenever the patient should request it.

Generally, chronic administration of a placebo cannot easily be justified in pain syndromes that normally respond to established therapy. In these situations, the only feasible way to conduct placebo-controlled trials may be to give both placebo and active treatment groups access to a standard analgesic rescue dose in spite of the challenging interpretation of analgesic requirements and drug-induced toxicity, as outlined earlier. In such studies, rescue analgesic becomes another important outcome measure. Both pain report and rescue analgesic consumption should be examined as primary outcome measures. The use of a placebo to demonstrate efficacy of a new drug or drug formulation could be unethical in trials with cancer patients and comparison should have to be made with an analgesic standard. However, unless the drug tested represents a major breakthrough in the treatment of pain, a very large patient sample would be needed to demonstrate a clear-cut superiority over the standard. More likely, the differences between treatments would be relatively modest in comparison with the variability between patients and would therefore remain undetected. If the use of placebo group is difficult, an alternative approach is to use a second dose level of the standard analgesic.

Patient information and consent

The usual trial design requires consent to be obtained prior to randomization, but Zelen[41] has suggested that randomization can precede informed consent so that only those allocated to the new treatment are asked to consent. Even if this strategy does increase recruitment, the approach is impossible in double-blind or single-blind trials and there will always be a risk of systematic bias. Overreliance, on the other hand, is another facet of the problem. As numerous studies have demonstrated, subjects rarely display an adequate understanding of consent forms[42*,43*] and often do not even understand the meaning or implications of randomization.[44] Dying patients are especially vulnerable, and balancing research and clinical roles is difficult.[45*] Patients suffering from a terminal illness or refractory symptoms may pay little attention to the informed consent process if they perceive enrollment in a clinical research protocol as their last hope for effective treatment. Patients as well as physicians have been shown to overestimate the potential benefit they will receive from enrollment, which can blur the line between enrollment in research and receiving medical treatment.

Despite increasing international collaboration, cross-cultural knowledge, and competency, different countries have adopted widely divergent attitudes to informed consent for every patient entering a clinical trial. In multi-center, multinational trials, this could influence results in spite of detailed criteria and adequate protocol adherence.

When preparing a clinical trial for publication, attention should be paid to the guidelines set out in the revised CONSORT statement, paticularly with regard to the inclusion of a flow diagram in the manuscript. These guidelines also provide a useful point in the design stages of a trial.[46]

SUMMARY

More research in cancer pain is needed to improve current techniques because even established treatment programs cannot always relieve pain at the end of life. This research should identify, using anatomical, pathophysiological, or mechanistic approaches, groups of patients at risk for unrelieved pain. Relevant trials in cancer pain patients are therefore badly needed, using sound methodology balancing the credibility, reliability, and applicability of clinical research. However, since the armamentarium of the clinical investigator today is very different from that of 50 years ago, there is a tendency to a transition away from observational bedside clinical research to more molecular and systematic approaches based on the biochemical and cellular events leading to pathology. The current models for clinical pain research address many shortcomings of the past. Most analgesics have been evaluated using the acute, postoperative analgesic assay. Far fewer studies are performed on cancer patients, and these studies are often of the acute assay type. While you cannot extrapolate from acute pain studies, there are still lessons to be learned. Directly related to the cost–benefit question is the concern that many of our models of assessing pain relief over time are inadequate. Many studies in the past have failed to capture the true clinical dimensions of cancer patients, including restriction of time in respect of a potentially terminal disease. In the future, we need to further develop research methodology, validated instruments, and assessment tools that more clearly define these dimensions.

REFERENCES

1. Jacox A, Carr DB, Payne R. New clinical-practice guidelines for the management of pain in patients with cancer. *N Engl J Med* 1994; **330**: 651–5.
2. Zech DF, Grond S, Lynch J, *et al*. Validation of World Health Organization Guidelines for cancer pain relief: a 10-year prospective study. *Pain* 1995; **63**: 65–76.

◆ 3. Caraceni A, Portenoy RK. An international survey of cancer pain characteristics and syndromes. *Pain* 1999; **82:** 263–74.

4. Portenoy RK, Foley KM, Inturrisi CE. The nature of opioid responsiveness and its implications for neuropathic pain: new hypotheses derived from studies of opioid infusions. *Pain* 1990; **43:** 273–86.

5. Portenoy RK. Tolerance to opioid analgesics: clinical aspects. *Cancer Surv* 1994; **21:** 49–65.

6. Elmer GI, Pieper JO, Negus SS, Woods JH. Genetic variance in nociception and its relationship to the potency of morphine-induced analgesia in thermal and chemical tests. *Pain* 1998; **75:** 129–40.

◆ 7. Portenoy RK, Hagen NA. Breakthrough pain: definition, prevalence and characteristics. *Pain* 1990; **41:** 273–81.

8. Zeppetella G, O'Doherty CA, Collins S. Prevalence and characteristics of breakthrough pain in cancer patients admitted to a hospice. *J Pain Symptom Manage* 2000; **20:** 87–92.

9. Bruera E, Schoeller T, Wenk R, *et al.* A prospective multicenter assessment of the Edmonton staging system for cancer pain. *J Pain Symptom Manage* 1995; **10:** 348–55.

10. Coluzzi PH, Schwartzberg L, Conroy JD, *et al.* Breakthrough cancer pain: a randomized trial comparing oral transmucosal fentanyl citrate (OTFC®). *Pain* 2001; **91:** 123–30.

◆ 11. Portenoy RK, Payne D, Jacobsen P. Breakthrough pain: characteristics and impact in patients with cancer pain. *Pain* 1999; **81:** 129–34.

12. Farrar JT, Portenoy RK, Berlin JA, *et al.* Definin the clinically important difference in pain outcome measures. *Pain* 2000; **88:** 287–94

13. Melzack R. The McGill Pain Questionnaire: major properties and scoring methods. *Pain* 1975; **1:** 277–99.

14. Daut RL, Cleeland CS, Flanery RC. Development of the Wisconsin Brief Pain Questionnaire to assess pain in cancer and other diseases. *Pain* 1983; **17:** 197–210.

15. Fishman B, Pasternak S, Wallenstein SL, *et al.* The Memorial Pain Assessment Card. A valid instrument for the evaluation of cancer pain. *Cancer* 1987; **60:** 1151–8.

● 16. Ramsay M, Winget C, Higginson I. Review: measures to determine the outcome of community services for people with dementia. *Age Ageing* 1995; **24:** 73–83.

17. Walsh TD. Adjuvant analgesic therapy in cancer pain. In: Foley KM, Bonica JJ, Ventafridda V eds. *Advances in Pain Research and Therapy.* New York, NY: Raven Press, 1990: 155–69.

18. Bruera E, Pereira J, Watanabe S, *et al.* Opioid rotation in patients with cancer pain. A retrospective comparison of dose ratios between methadone, hydromorphone, and morphine. *Cancer* 1996; **78:** 852–7.

19. de-Stoutz ND, Bruera E, Suarez AM. Opioid rotation for toxicity reduction in terminal cancer patients. *J Pain Symptom Manage* 1995; **10:** 378–84.

20. Kaasa S, DeConnon F. Palliative care research. *E J Cancer* 20001; **37** (Suppl. 8): 5153–9.

21. Grimes DA, Schulz KF. Bias and causal association in observational research. *Lancet* 2002; **359:** 248–52.

22. Sacks H, Chalmers TC, Smith H. Randomized versus historical controls for clinical trials. *Am J Med* 1982; **72:** 233–40.

23. Deschamps M, Band PR, Hislop TG, *et al.* The evaluation of analgesic effects in cancer patients as exemplified by a double-blind, crossover study of immediate-release versus controlled-release morphine. *J Pain Symptom Manage* 1992; **7:** 384–92.

24. Parris WC, Johnson-BW J, Croghan MK, *et al.* The use of controlled-release oxycodone for the treatment of chronic cancer pain: a randomized, double-blind study. *J Pain Symptom Manage* 1998; **16:** 205–11.

● 25. Kerr IG. Clinical trials to study pain in patients with advanced cancer: practical difficulties. *Anticancer Drugs* 1995; **6** (Suppl. 3): 18–28.

26. Byas SM, Max MB, Muir J, Kingman A. Transdermal clonidine compared to placebo in painful diabetic neuropathy using a two-stage "enriched enrollment" design. *Pain* 1995; **60:** 267–74.

27. Portenoy RK. Cancer pain general design issues. In: Max M, Portenoy R, Laska R eds. *Advances in Pain Research and Therapy.* New York, NY: Raven Press, 1991: 233–66.

28. Spiegel D, Sands S, Koopman C. Pain and depression in patients with cancer. *Cancer* 1994; **74:** 2570–8.

29. MacDonald N, Bruera E. Clinical trials in cancer pain research. In: Foley KM, Bonica JJ, Ventafridda V eds. *Advances in Pain Research and Therapy.* New York, NY: Raven Press, 1990: 443–9.

30. Stambaugh JE. Commentary: issues for chronic pain models with specific emphasis on the chronic cancer pain model. In: Max M, Portenoy R, Laska R eds. *Advances in Pain Research and Therapy.* New York, NY: Raven Press, 1991: 287–9.

31. Weiss SC, Emanuel LL, Fairclough DL. Understanding the experience of pain in terminally ill patients. *Lancet* 2001; **357:** 1311–5.

32. Banning A, Sjogren P, Henriksen H. Pain causes in 200 patients referred to a multidisciplinary cancer pain clinic. *Pain* 1991; **45:** 45–8.

33. Kongsgaard UE, Poulain P. Transdermal fentanyl for pain control in chronic cancer pain. *Eur J Pain* 1998; **2:** 54–61.

34. Stambaugh JEJ, Drew J. The combination of ibuprofen and oxycodone/acetaminophen in the management of chronic cancer pain. *Clin Pharmacol Ther* 1988; **44:** 665–9.

35. Syrjala KL, Donaldson GW, Davis MW, *et al.* Relaxation and imagery and cognitive–behavioral training reduce pain during cancer treatment: a controlled clinical trial. *Pain* 1995; **63:** 189–98.

36. Patt RB. The current status of anesthetic approaches to cancer pain management. In: Payne R, Patt RB, Strat-

ton Hill C eds. *Assessment and Treatment of Cancer Pain.* Seattle, WA: IASP Press, 1998: 195–211.

37. Brown DL, Bulley CK, Quiel EL. Neurolytic celiac plexus block for pancreatic cancer pain. *Anesth Analg* 1987; **66:** 869–73.

◆ 38. Eisenberg E, Carr DB, Chalmers TC. Neurolytic celiac plexus block for treatment of cancer pain: a meta-analysis. *Anesth Analg* 1995; **80:** 290–5.

39. Clark PI, Leaverton PE. Scientific and ethical issues in the use of placebo controls in clinical trials. *Annu Rev Public Health* 1994; **15:** 19–38.

40. Detsky AS, Naglie IG. A clinician's guide to cost-effectiveness analysis. *Ann Intern Med* 1990; **113:** 147–54.

41. Zelen M. A new design for randomized clinical trials. *N Engl J Med* 1979; **300:** 1242–5.

42. Lavelle JC, Byrne DJ, Rice P, Cuschieri A. Factors affect-ing quality of informed consent. *Br Med J* 1993; **306:** 885–90.

43. Joffe S, Cook EF, Clearly PF, *et al.* Quality of informed consent in clinical cancer trials: a cross-sectional survey. *Lancet* 2001; **358:** 1772–7.

44. Snowdon C, Garcia J, Elbourne D. Making sense of randomization; responses of parents of critically ill babies to random allocation of treatment in a clinical trial. *Soc Sci Med* 1997; **45:** 1337–55.

45. Casarett DJ, Karlawich JHT. Are ethical guidelines needed for palliative care research? *J Pain Symptom Manage* 2000; **20:** 130–9.

46. Moher D, Schulz KF, Altman DG. The CONSORT statement: revised recommendatons for improving the quality of reports of parallel-group randomized trials. *JAMA* 2001; **285:** 1987–91.

38

Clinical experimental pharmacological protocols: how to evaluate the use of a new drug

MÄRTA SEGERDAHL

Experimental background research	483	Clinical studies in chronic pain patients	489
Animal data	483	Techniques and considerations in study design	489
Pharmacology	484	Interpreting data: pitfalls	490
Safety perspectives	484	Ethical, regulatory, and financial considerations	491
Clinical experimental protocols	485	References	492
Clinical randomized controlled trials in acute pain	487		

This chapter covers:

- How to scientifically address a problematic clinical issue.
- The importance of defining the clinical problem, e.g. burn injury, postoperative pain, neuropathic pain.
- Breaking down the problem and setting up a hypothesis, e.g. "adenosine reduces secondary hyperalgesia."
- Designing a method to answer the specific questions "What variables are the most suitable?" "Is there an appropriate model?" Decide on a primary (and maybe a secondary) endpoint.
- How to go about the task and what to consider: flow chart, pharmacokinetics, medical products agency, ethical review board.

It will also address issues on developing a new pharmacological treatment regimen, which scientific and strategic steps to take, and how to make a research plan for the development of a new pain treatment. Adenosine treatment for pain relief will be used as a practical example.

Issues on pharmacology, animal, and human research data together with their interpretations will be presented; these questions will of course vary depending on the drug under study, especially with regard to pharmacokinetics and dose finding. Several aspects of performing human experimental studies, such as pain models, pharmacological treatment, and study design, will be discussed.

EXPERIMENTAL BACKGROUND RESEARCH

If your aim is to evaluate a new or old compound for pain treatment, it is essential to have all the latest animal data relevant to efficacy and toxicology. In order to study drug effects in humans, it is necessary to have toxicology data from short- and long-term administration in at least two species, one of which should be a large animal, e.g. dog or sheep. Also, data on the intended mode of administration is required in order to obtain approval from your national medical products agency (MPA); for efficacy, see below (Interpretations).

ANIMAL DATA

The effects of adenosine and adenosine analogs are well documented in animal research.[1] In different species, mainly rodents, numerous studies have shown a delay in withdrawal thresholds for noxious heat stimuli in normal tissue (the hotplate test, tail immersion test). In rodents, acute peripheral inflammation, such as in the formalin and writing tests of pain behavior, has been reduced by adenosine analogs. In experimental surgery in anesthetized rabbits and dogs, double-blind studies have shown reduced nociceptive reflexes during adenosine infusion. After peripheral nerve injury using the Bennett, Chung, and Gazelius models, adenosine receptor stimulation by adenosine and its analogs has been shown to reduce pain behavior, increase thermal and tactile thresholds (in presumably allodynic areas), and reduce substance P levels.[2] In a model of chronic allodynia induced by a spinal cord lesion, intrathecal (i.t.) administration of the adenosine analog R-PIA increased the vocalization threshold to tactile stimuli.[2,3]

In this experimental study of rats, adenosine or its analogs were administered systemically or intrathecally. The reduction on pain behavior induced by adenosine lasted for 5–7 h, a markedly long duration considering the short half-life of the compound.

Adenosine combinations with other analgesics

There are data supporting the involvement of adenosine mechanisms in several different pain-modulating systems.[1,4,5] Cui et al.[4] have shown that rats not responding to dorsal column stimulation can become responders by adding i.t. adenosine at a low dose. In a recent study in rats, i.t. adenosine by itself was found to be ineffective in increasing the withdrawal threshold to heat stimuli in normal skin, whereas adenosine combined with i.t. clonidine enhanced the antinociceptive effect of clonidine. No interactions were found between anticholinergic mechanisms and adenosine.[6] Lavand'homme and Eisenach have also found that exogenous and endogenous adenosine enhanced the spinal antiallodynic effect of morphine in rats with peripheral nerve damage.[5] These indications of a synergistic action between adenosine and dorsal column stimulation, clonidine, and opioids may in the future yield additional information on the mechanism of antinociception exerted by adenosine. An unspecific interaction with the N-methyl-D-aspartate (NMDA) receptor complex has also been suggested.[1]

General interpretation

Experimental data do not fulfill the criteria to permit their direct clinical applications. There are several reasons for this. The most important is that antinociception (neurophysiological or behavioral) in rodents cannot be interpreted as the equivalent to pain relief in humans. Furthermore, species differences exist in pharmacology, drug tolerance, and dose requirements. Often, the border between antinociception, motor impairment, and sedation is difficult to establish. Analog compounds are often used in animals, and their effects may differ from the effects of the clinically available compounds in both action and duration. It is important to consider animal models in comparison with their possible clinical parallel with a critical eye. Nevertheless, there is enough experimental evidence of antinociception to support further investigations of potential adenosine-mediated pain relief in humans.

PHARMACOLOGY

Of course, the pharmacology of the substance is of great importance when studying the actions and estimating the future clinical applicability of pharmacologically active compounds, and it is essential to study these in detail. All compounds vary in their bioavailability, adverse effects, and toxicology.

The endogenous compound adenosine is present in all living cells and tissues under normal physiological conditions. It has numerous functions, with the most important being the intracellular binding site for phosphate ions to provide adenosine triphosphate (ATP). Adenosine also has several extracellular regulatory functions that are related to energy turnover, thrombocyte aggregation, inflammatory response, etc. Adenosine exerts its action mainly via cell-surface-bound receptors – A_1, A_{2a}, A_{2b}, and A_3. Of these, the A_1 and A_{2a} receptors are involved in the nociceptive system.[7***] Normally, drug metabolism is an important issue when developing new compounds for the modulation of pain. Regarding the endogenous compound adenosine, the metabolism is totally independent of liver and kidney function and thus quite different from what we normally have to consider. However, as mentioned below, there are other problems related to adenosine metabolism. Pharmacological data exist on "normal" levels of adenosine in blood and in the cerebrospinal fluid for both animals and humans. Normal physiological levels are well established and are stable under normal conditions. During pathophysiological conditions, local levels may rise by a couple of orders of magnitude, e.g. during severe ischemia. Local blood levels of adenosine may then vary considerably because adenosine is released from the tissue following intracellular energy depletion. Adenosine, endogenous as well as exogenously administered, is eliminated from the blood mainly by uptake in endothelial and red blood cells with a plasma half-life of only a few seconds. Studying adenosine plasma levels is thus technically difficult. This very rapid cell uptake, as well as its coexistence with the endogenously formed adenosine, must also be taken into account when designing studies and interpreting results.

Levels of adenosine can be altered by adenosine reuptake blockers, such as dipyridamole, which will result in considerably elevated plasma levels and thus give rise to adverse effects. Also, all effects of adenosine may be blocked by methylxanthines, which are unspecific adenosine receptor blockers, e.g. theophylline and caffeine – well-known and easily available drugs.[7***]

SAFETY PERSPECTIVES

In studies focusing on safety evaluation, preclinical as well as human phase I studies, there are toxicological and dose-related effects related to the drug class and the specific compound that must be considered.[8]

Regarding adenosine in animals, a dose-dependent and reversible motor impairment by various adenosine analogs has frequently been observed, but no motor impairment has been reported after adenosine administration in mice or rats.[9] Toxicity after chronic i.t. administration of adenosine in rats has been evaluated with regard to behavior, spinal cord morphology, and cell count and was not associated with detectable neurotoxicity.[10] In a chronic toxicity screen in dogs, no behavioral or histological evidence of neurotoxicity was found.[6]

In humans, adenosine is a licensed drug for intravenous (i.v.) administration, and its cardiovascular safety is well documented.[11]* Intravenous bolus doses will give a transient AV nodal block. Doses of 150–500 µg/kg/min have been given to anesthetized patients to produce controlled hypotension.[12] In conscious humans, an i.v. infusion at a dose of 70 µg/kg/min may be associated with chest tightness and cutaneous flush, whereas 50 µg/kg/min reduces these symptoms. Intra-arterial infusion will induce pain. The half-life in cerebrospinal fluid (CSF) after i.t. administration is 10–20 min.[13] Constipation is a common adverse effect in pain therapy, however adenosine does not influence the rate of gastric emptying.[12] After i.t. administration in healthy volunteers (1,000–2,000 µg), no sedation, motor deficiencies, or disturbances in extremity reflexes, balance, or voiding was observed. In volunteers as well as in patients, a dose of 1,000–2,000 µg may give rise to a transient (30–60 min) dose-dependent pain in the lumbar region.[13*,14*] The mechanism is unknown, but local vasodilation leading to a migraine-like pain is possible; this is supported by animal data.[12] The pain could, however, be prevented by coadministration of a nonmotor blocking dose of local anesthetic.

CLINICAL EXPERIMENTAL PROTOCOLS

Background

Applying the line of thinking initiated by Woolf,[15] the nociceptive system can have four different states or "modes":

- Healthy tissue, where a low-intensity stimulus is innocuous and a high-intensity stimulus results in pain.
- Tissue damage has activated central descending inhibition together with local segmental inhibition at the spinal level.
- Prolonged nociceptive input has increased the excitability of the dorsal horn neurons, i.e. central sensitization. This manifests as a reduction in threshold, increased responsiveness, an expansion of the extent, and recruitment of novel inputs from receptive fields.

All of these factors contribute to clinical nociceptive pain. These altered states of neural transmission include functional plasticity and are reversible.

- The nervous system may however become permanently damaged and constitute the pathology of chronic pain where this functional plasticity is disturbed.

All of these states need to be studied to conclude the therapeutic value of a new compound for analgesic use.

Different pain types, such as cutaneous pain, deep somatic pain from musculoskeletal tissue, and visceral pain, also have their specific characteristics in neuro-anatomy, physiology, and vulnerability to adverse effects that demand differentiation in their treatment. Therefore, these facets must be studied separately, and interpretations of analgesic effects in clinical trials must be limited to the specific component of pain studied. This is a prerequisite for mechanism-based analgesic therapy. A summary of possible assessments in different modalities is presented in Table 38.1.

Adenosine

Normal state

In two single-blind, parallel group, placebo-controlled studies on normal hairy skin of healthy volunteers an infusion of adenosine 35–70 µg/kg/min was given, either alone or with morphine and ketamine as active controls (Table 38.2). In these studies, only adenosine increased the heat pain threshold (C-fiber mediated), with no effect on cold (Aδ-fiber mediated) or warmth (C-fiber mediated) perception nor on suprathreshold pain provocation. Also, there was no augmentative effect of the combination of adenosine with morphine (0.1 mg/kg) nor any effect by morphine alone on thermal perception. These studies lend support to a selective influence of adenosine on thermal C-fiber-mediated nociceptive transmission in the normal nonsensitized state, but without influence on thermal non-noxious threshold perception.[12] These results were repeated when adenosine was administered by i.t. injection (500, 1,000, or 2,000 µg) in an open label safety and dose escalation study. In the latter study, suprathreshold cold pain was also induced, using the cold immersion test (holding the foot in an ice-water bath for 1 min). In this experiment, no effect of i.t. adenosine on pain intensity was found compared with the control situation or with repeated immersions in untreated controls.[13]* This evidence mitigates against a centrally mediated modulating effect by adenosine on continuous cold pain (Aδ-fiber mediated).

Acute tissue damage

The tourniquet method has been used to induce continu-

Table 38.1 *Examples of documented qualitative and quantitative sensory assessments in experimental pain models*

Types and modes of pain	What can be determined	Modality-specific assessments
Cutaneous pain		
Normal tissue	Perception thresholds	Mechanical stimulation, cold, warmth
	Pain thresholds	Mechanical stimulation, heat, cold
	Pain at threshold and suprathreshold stimulation	Mechanical stimulation, heat, cold
Nociceptive pain/primary hyperalgesia	Spontaneous pain	
	Perception thresholds	Mechanical stimulation, cold, warmth
	Pain thresholds	Mechanical stimulation, heat, cold
	Evoked pain at threshold and suprathreshold stimulation	Mechanical stimulation, heat, cold, repetitive mechanical stimulation
Central sensitization/secondary hyperalgesic area	Area determinations	Dynamic (soft brush) and static (pinpoint) mechanical stimulation
	Perception thresholds	Mechanical stimulation, cold, warmth
	Pain thresholds	Mechanical stimulation, heat, cold
	Evoked pain at threshold and suprathreshold stimulation	Repetitive mechanical stimulation, heat
Deep somatic pain		
Normal tissue	Pain threshold	Pressure algometry, electric stimulation
Nociceptive pain	Spontaneous pain	
	Pain threshold	Pressure algometry, electric stimulation
	Pain at threshold and suprathreshold stimulation	Pressure algometry, electric stimulation, hypertonic saline injection
	Pain at continuous stimulation	Ischemia, hypertonic saline
Central sensitization/secondary hyperalgesia	Spontaneous pain	
	Area determination of referred pain	Dynamic and static mechanical stimulation, hypertonic saline
	Perception thresholds	Mechanical stimulation, cold, warmth
	Pain thresholds	Mechanical stimulation, heat, cold
	Evoked pain at threshold and suprathreshold stimulation	Repetitive mechanical stimulation, heat, electric stimulation, hypertonic saline

ous ischemic pain – a mainly C-fiber-mediated nociceptive type pain (Table 38.3).[12] This pain resembles clinical postoperative deep somatic pain. The subjects rated pain [visual analog scale (VAS) 0–100] up to 30 min and the VAS scores were then added to a sum of pain scores (SPS), which is equal to an "area under the curve" (AUC) measurement. The study design was randomized, double-blind, and crossover. Adenosine infusion (70 μg/kg/min) reduced the SPS by 30% compared with placebo. In addition, it was found that the combined administration of a clinical dose of morphine (0.1 mg/kg) or a low dose of ketamine (0.1 mg/kg) increased pain tolerance – expressed as the number of subjects not reaching a VAS score of 100 within the 30 min of provocation time. This is thought to indicate that exogenous adenosine exerts an inhibitory effect on some pain processing at a level proximal to the occluded arm, and that this action has a positive interaction with clinical doses of morphine or ketamine. Rae *et al.* later confirmed the analgesic effect of adenosine on tourniquet pain.[16]** In an open label safety and dose escalation study, the tourniquet test results were similar when adenosine was given as an i.t. injection. This tourniquet technique is thus a reproducible method that is valid for evaluating the analgesic effects of adenosine as well as morphine and ketamine.

Experimental methods illustrating central sensitization

In other experimental models, inflammatory pain was induced by topical application of either mustard oil (MuO) or a Peltier thermode at 46–47°C for 7 min, resulting in first-degree skin burns (Table 38.3).[12]** These stimuli are associated with an inflammatory noxious stimulus that is sufficient to activate nociceptive afferent C-fibers and induce a surrounding area of secondary allodynia/hyperalgesia (SH) as an expression of central sensitization. In these models, double-blind, placebo-controlled, crossover studies of i.v. infusion and an open label study of the effects of i.t. administration have been

Table 38.2 *Pain-reducing effects by adenosine in clinical volunteer and patient models*

	Intravenous	Intrathecal
Volunteers; cutaneous nociception	HPT ↑	No change
Volunteers; central sensitization	Area ↓ ~40%	Area ↓ 50%
Volunteers; ischemic	SPS ↓ ~30% Increased pain tolerance	SPS ↓ 16%
Patients; acute superficial	Anesthetic requirement ↓ Pain at emerging from anesthesia ↓ Morphine consumption ↓ by 25%	No data
Patients; acute deep somatic	Anesthetic requirement ↓	No data
Patients; acute visceral	Anesthetic requirement ↓ 60% Morphine requirement ↓ 20–45%	No difference from placebo
Patients; neuropathic pain	Spontaneous pain ↓ 30–50% Evoked pain ↓ 45% von Frey pain threshold ↑ twofold Allodynic area ↓ (not quantified)	Spontaneous pain ↓ 61% Evoked pain ↓ 70% Allodynic area ↓ 77%

Table 38.3 *Effect of intravenous adenosine infusion, 50–100 μg/kg/min, and 500–1,000 μg intrathecal adenosine injection on the development of secondary allodynia (brush and von Frey area) and on the sum of pain scores (SPS) in response to ischemic tourniquet pain*

Pain model	Adenosine route	Pain (SPS)	von Frey area	Brush area
MuO	i.v.		−30 to 40%	−22 to −75%
	i.t.		−50%	−
Thermal burn	i.v.		−55%	−
Tourniquet pain	i.v.	−30 to 40%		
	i.t.	−16% (NS)		

MuO, mustard oil; i.v., intravenous; i.t., intrathecal; NS, not statistically significant.

performed in healthy volunteers, revealing that adenosine (50–60 μg/kg/min i.v. or 500–2,000 μg i.t.) can attenuate development of the areas of tactile allodynia by 30–50%. This applied to both dynamic (Aβ stimulation; MuO) and static (Aδ- and C-fiber stimulation; MuO and burn injury models) allodynia. Although adenosine, as an i.v. infusion or administered i.t., reduced the area of secondary allodynia, there was no reduction in tactile pain threshold within the remaining SH area. Thus, all experimental studies in healthy volunteers suggest that adenosine infusion primarily counteracts the mechanisms involved in the development of central sensitization.

In healthy subjects, 500, 1,000, or 2,000 μg of adenosine was injected i.t. at the lower lumbar level. In agreement with previous studies performed during i.v. adenosine administration, i.t. adenosine reduced the area of secondary allodynia that developed after mustard oil application without influencing the tactile pain thresholds in the remaining secondary allodynic area.[12]* Ischemic pain ratings in the tourniquet test were not significantly reduced and cold pain was unaffected. Again, this implies that i.t. administration of adenosine primarily counteracts the pain symptoms related to central sensitization.

Correlation between animal experimental models and the clinical problem or situation

A human experimental model that corresponds as closely as possible to a documented animal model should be sought. The same state and mode of pain should be used, and roughly the same time frame. If these criteria are fulfilled, one may cautiously draw conclusions regarding the mechanism of the compound (Fig. 38.1).

CLINICAL RANDOMIZED CONTROLLED TRIALS IN ACUTE PAIN

Intravenous administration

Inflammatory pain

In a randomized controlled trial (RCT) of 72 patients suffering from acute epicondylalgia that measured the primary endpoint of long-term analgesic effect (5–30 days) following a 1-h infusion of adenosine, there was no difference between adenosine and placebo groups. The

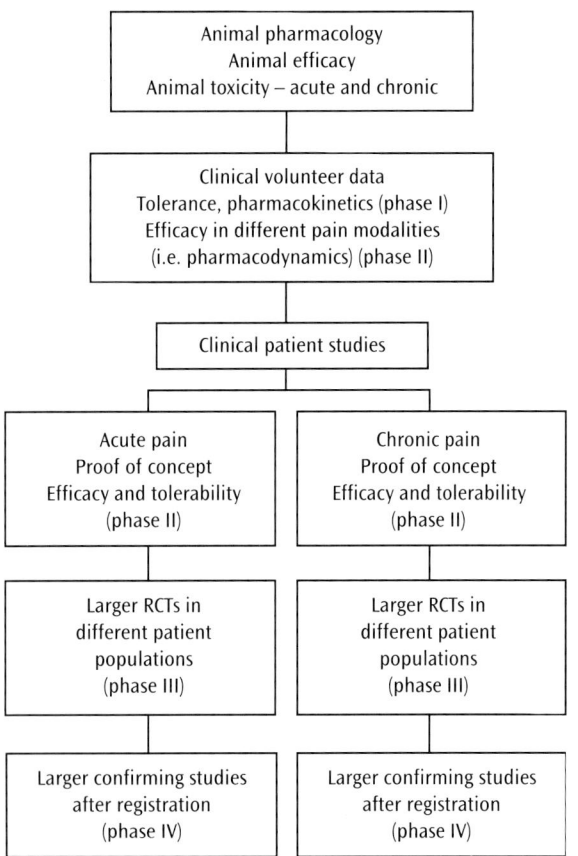

Figure 38.1 *Development of novel drugs from compound to analgesic, schematic overview of experimental line.*

recovery rate in the study population group was similar to that expected from results of other studies (unpublished data).

Mechanistic interpretation

Adenosine does not have a long-term analgesic effect in an established acute pain condition with an ongoing noxious (inflammatory) focus.

Perioperative pain

In three clinical, randomized, double-blind, placebo-controlled, parallel group studies of pain associated with shoulder surgery (30 patients), breast surgery (72 patients), and hysterectomy (41 patients),[12**] representing deep somatic, cutaneous/subcutaneous, and visceral pain, anesthetic requirements and postoperative analgesic requirements were analyzed. Anesthetic requirements were significantly reduced during surgery, especially during visceral surgery. Also, after breast surgery, fewer patients (8/31 versus 19/32) perceived pain immediately when regaining consciousness after surgery in the adenosine group than in the placebo group. Thus, antinociception is a likely explanation for the reduced anesthetic requirement during adenosine infusion. In another study, Zaraté et al.[17**] reported on 32 women undergoing major gynecological surgery who received adenosine or remi-

fentanil (an ultra-short-acting opioid) intraoperatively in a randomized double-blind manner. Intraoperative hemodynamic data were analyzed and control of blood pressure in the adenosine-treated groups was more stable than in the placebo/remifentanil groups in all four studies.

Mechanistic interpretation

Intraoperative i.v. infusion of adenosine has antinociceptive effects.

Postoperative analgesia

In the study by Zarate et al.,[17**] the 0- to 2-h morphine requirement was 45% lower in the adenosine group. After surgery in all four studies, the 24-h opioid requirement after intraoperative adenosine infusion was reduced by approximately 20–27%.[12,17**] This indicates an extended pain-reducing effect by adenosine.

Mechanistic interpretation

Intravenous adenosine infusion in conjunction with surgery has antinociceptive effects lasting for at least 24 h postsurgery. Is this a preemptive effect?

Intrathecal administration

If i.v. adenosine is effective in reducing perioperative pain, and the mechanism of action is hypothesized to be that central sensitization is being reduced at the spinal cord level, the following question arises: "Can we increase the efficacy by administering adenosine closer to the target organ?" In order to determine whether i.t. adenosine administration could reduce intraoperative anesthetic and postoperative analgesic requirements, 40 women undergoing elective hysterectomy received 500 μg of adenosine or placebo intrathecally in a randomized, double-blind, placebo-controlled study.[18**] After i.t. adenosine administration, anesthetic requirements and postoperative 24-h opioid requirements were not reduced. Since i.t. administration of adenosine, as shown in healthy volunteers, is associated with a marked elevation of CSF adenosine levels, at least during the period of surgery (approximately 1 h), the study suggests that lumbar spinal mechanisms are not primarily responsible for the antinociceptive effect of intraoperative adenosine administration. It is therefore possible that the perioperative pain-reducing effect of i.v. adenosine infusion is mediated either by peripheral anti-inflammatory actions or by some supraspinal site of action not readily accessible via i.t. adenosine injection.

Mechanistic interpretation

Intrathecal adenosine injection was not as effective as i.v. adenosine administration when associated with visceral surgery. This may be due to pharmacokinetic differences or to differences in central and peripheral effects.

CLINICAL STUDIES IN CHRONIC PAIN PATIENTS

Intravenous administration

In one report, two patients suffering neuropathic pain were treated with a low-dose adenosine infusion that resulted in alleviation of pain.[12]* In one of these patients, 45 min of infusion of adenosine 50 μg/kg/min, but not placebo, abolished the preexisting allodynia to touch and warmth and dysesthesia to cold, increased the tactile pain threshold, and normalized the tactile perception and heat pain threshold. The duration of total pain relief was 6 h, after which time pain gradually returned and reached habitual levels after 48 h. These observations initiated a randomized double-blind, placebo-controlled, crossover study in seven patients suffering chronic neuropathic pain.[12]** These patients had allodynia and hyperalgesia. Quantitative sensory testing was performed before and immediately after completed study treatment. Patients received adenosine 50 μg/kg/min i.v. for 45–60 min. In all of the six patients suffering from spontaneous pain, baseline pain intensity ratings were reduced by 50%. Also, tactile pain thresholds in the neuropathic areas were elevated, indicating reduced hypersensitivity. Apart from this, the duration of the perceived pain relief extended from 6 h to 4 days, by far outlasting any direct action of the infused compound. Recently, a multicenter, randomized, double-blind, crossover study in 26 patients with intractable neuropathic pain of post-traumatic origin confirmed the earlier results.[19]** In this study, the areas of allodynia were significantly reduced by adenosine treatment.

Intrathecal administration

The first clinical case report on i.t. adenosine receptor agonist administration to a pain patient relates to R-PIA.[12]* The pain-reducing and antiallodynic effects of a single spinal injection (50 μg) of the weak A$_1$-receptor-selective agonist lasted for several months. In an open label tolerability study in 14 patients suffering intractable chronic neurogenic pain with tactile hyperphenomena, 500 or 1,000 μg of adenosine was injected spinally at the lumbar level.[12]* A majority of patients demonstrated a reduction of > 50% in spontaneous and evoked pain, including an increased tactile pain threshold to von Frey stimulation. Areas of tactile hyperphenomena were also markedly reduced by 30–100% (median 77%) (Table 38.1). The median duration of pain reduction was 24 h. Thus, in this patient population, i.t. adenosine administration reduces various aspects of pain, primarily via adenosine receptor activation at the spinal level.

These data from the first pilot efficacy study indicate that animal data on experimental neuropathy models may be prognostic of clinical effects. However, further controlled and blinded studies are warranted before the use of i.t. adenosine for the treatment of neuropathic pain can be promoted for routine clinical use.

TECHNIQUES AND CONSIDERATIONS IN STUDY DESIGN

Study design basics: blinding, randomization, placebo control, and internal positive drug control

From the perspectives of your hypothesis and your model, decide on the study design (Figs 38.2 and 38.3). Is your number of possible inclusions large or small? A prospective, randomized, double-blind design will give you the least biased results, i.e. it is the most robust. The question is then whether you should have two or more parallel groups – receiving different treatments – or whether each volunteer/patient should receive all treatments – a crossover design. Statistically, a parallel group study is the least complicated. It is commonly used in clinical trials, where a large potential study population is available. However, in clinical volunteer studies, many of the sensory testing variables show a greater variability between individuals than between treatments. Thus, in the healthy volunteer situation, where there is an opportunity to study the same phenomenon repeatedly with basically the same background situation, a crossover design is more robust. Also, many chronic pain states vary greatly from individual to individual when it comes to underlying pain mechanisms, which will lead to a certain proportion of responders and a certain proportion of nonresponders. In these cases, and when the number of patient inclusions is difficult to predetermine, a number-of-one design can be utilized (*n* of 1).

When designing study protocols, it is essential to include a sufficiently large study population that statistical power in excess of 80% is obtained. The medical risks to which the subjects will be exposed is also an important consideration when determining the population size for a study.

When designing the study protocol and flow chart (an example is shown in Fig. 38.4), there are numerous details to consider. The pharmacology of the compound needs to comply with the experimental pain model you plan to use, i.e. adjustment of the trauma and assessment point to the maximum effect of the study drug. It is tempting to try to attempt to gather excessive data during the experimental period. For scientific and logistical reasons, choose your effect parameters with care.

Gender aspects

When recruiting volunteers, consider whether the gender distribution of the study population is appropriate.

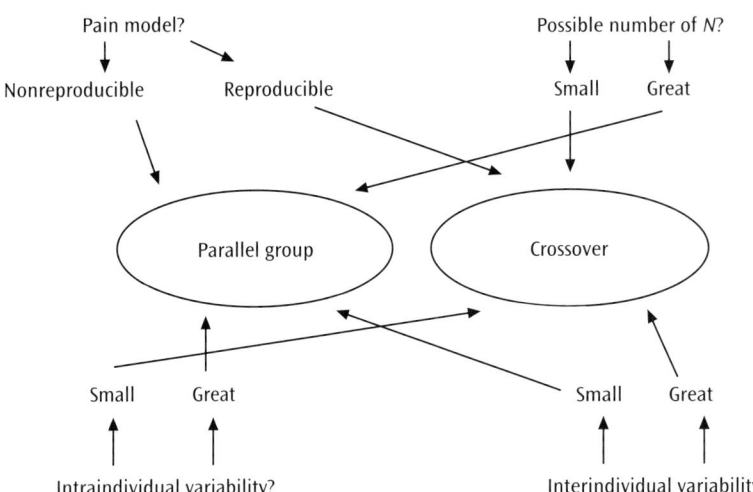

Figure 38.2 *Parallel groups or crossover?*

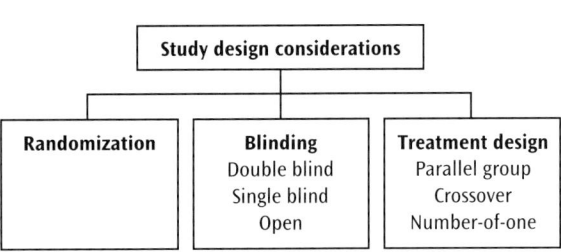

Figure 38.3 *There are three important decisions to make on the study design, based on your group of subjects and the planned interventions. Randomization is essential to reduce bias. Double-blinding is gold standard, but safety and ethical issues may force you to renounce to single-blind or open design. The treatment design is further addressed in Fig. 38.2. Number-of-one can be used in single case studies and under special circumstances.*

The question of gender differences in pain perception and tolerance has been widely investigated, but the matter is still controversial. Lately, studies have shown a lower pain threshold and tolerance to heat and electrical stimulation, with higher between-session discrimination in females.[20**,21*,22*] There is no evidence that hormone levels interfere with the stability of the method in females, even though it is not yet established whether cyclic hormonal variation mirrors psychophysical testing. Nevertheless, as the analgesic you intend to study is probably not aimed at a single-sex clinical population, an appropriate mix of gender in the study population will minimize the impact of gender differences on whole group treatment results.

INTERPRETING DATA: PITFALLS

Why does your study not yield the expected results? There may be a number of reasons for unexpected drawbacks

and misinterpretations.[23–25] For example, if you study a clinically well-documented analgesic, for instance morphine, in a human experimental model, it may appear to be without effect despite the subjects/patients reporting drug-related (in this case opioid) side-effects. First, you may have chosen a clinical pain model that is more or less sensitive to opioid mechanisms. In animals (as this type of study is not easily performed in humans), μ-receptors are shown to be present mostly on the afferent nerve terminals of the first-order neurons; in primates, these receptors are mainly on C-fiber terminals but sparsely on Aδ-fiber terminals.[26,27] Thus, it is possible that the opioid effect is more pronounced in tonic C-fiber-induced pain and less pronounced in conditions of phasic pain.[12**,28**] This is, in fact, seen also in a clinical setting, where severe intermittent (labor) pain is known to respond poorly to morphine.[29**]

Second, the dose of drug used may simply be too low or the time from drug dosage to pain assessments be too long or too short relative to the pharmacokinetics of the drug. Third, the degree of experimental trauma may exceed the efficacy of the drug being studied. Fourth, the study design or group size may lack sufficient power to answer the experimental question. There is statistical computer software that includes power calculations, but the expected relevant treatment effect may be difficult to predict. However, human experimental pain studies with relevant protocols are needed to bridge the gap between laboratory data and clinical practice. They may reduce the number of inappropriate clinical trials by providing an indication of appropriate models for clinical trials in patients with negative results due to irrelevant clinical pain models. However, clinical trials in acute and chronic pain will always be necessary to determine the efficacy, tolerability, and safety of a novel analgesic treatment.

When taking further steps toward investigating clinical applicability and efficacy, other issues impact upon the successful development of a clinically useful analgesic, for example:

• Possible different modes of administration. Does the

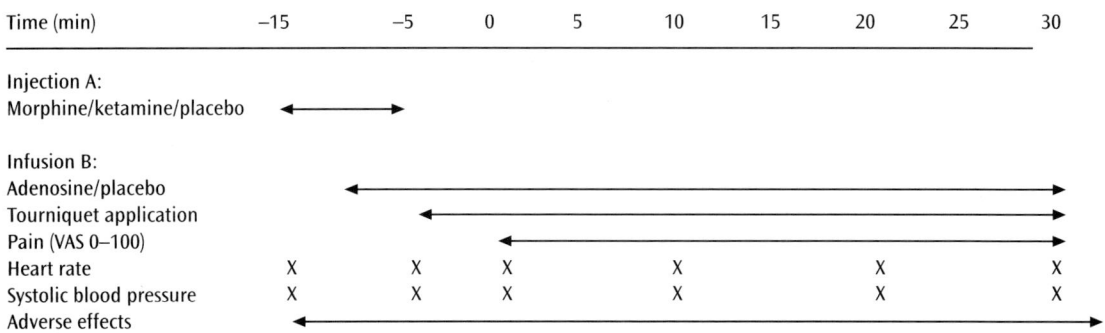

Figure 38.4 *An example of a flow chart for a clinical study protocol on human experimental pain, illustrating all interventions and assessment time points. Note the importance of being explicit when defining what is considered 'time 0", preferably at the time when your pain stimulation begins. Also, be sure there is enough time to perform each pain assessment.*

compound have different effects when given i.v., i.t., or orally?

- Analgesics aimed at alleviating chronic pain. Is the oral bioavailability sufficient? What are the long-term side-effects? Does tolerance develop?

The endogenous compound adenosine is well known pharmacologically and is safe in animal toxicology studies.[6,10] However, adenosine has no effect when given orally as it is reabsorbed and degraded before it reaches its target organ. Intravenous and i.t. administration are impractical in clinical practice. An implantable pump system is one possibility that could be utilized, but it is technically demanding and requires stand-by resources for maintenance. There is also the question of tolerance. Adenosine is an endogenous receptor antagonist, and like other receptor agonists, for example opioids, tolerance will develop over time.

ETHICAL, REGULATORY, AND FINANCIAL CONSIDERATIONS

Prior to any study in human beings, the study protocol must be reviewed by a research ethical committee or ethi-

cal review board (ERB). If the study is to be performed with a novel drug, or examines a new indication for an old drug, the study protocol will also need to reviewed by a medical products agency (MPA). The protocol must also adhere to good clinical practice (GCP)[30] and will be performed in accordance with the Declaration of Helsinki.[31] Adherence to the ethical guidelines for pain research of the International Association for the Study of Pain (IASP) are also important.[32]

When contacting your national medical products agency (MPA) and ethical review board (ERB), it is essential to declare all financial arrangements relevant to the study. When setting up a budget for the study, or a contract, be careful to make an appropriate estimate of the costs. The cost of laboratory and other clinical investigations, such as radiographs and blood samples, are often easy to estimate. What is difficult and takes time and experience is making a proper estimate of the financial cost: the time needed for everybody involved, such as nurses and investigators (including all preparation work and study report), rental costs of facilities, institutional overheads, etc. are also important issues. Do not hesitate to ask for independent help in setting up contracts, e.g. the research contracts of your hospital or university. Most universities and hospitals will have a special core

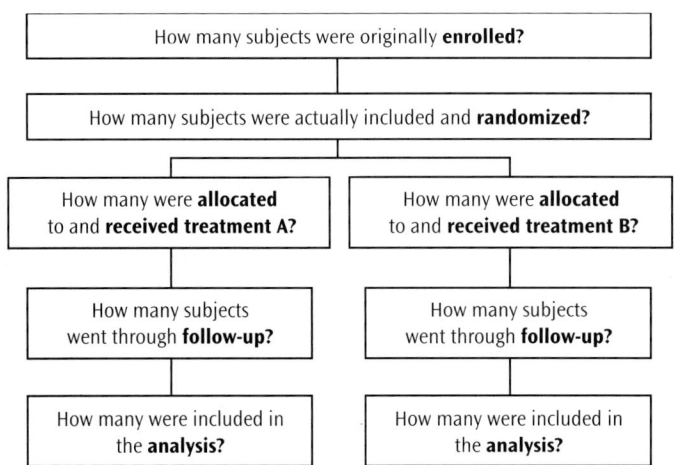

Figure 38.5 *Flow chart for evaluating the steps of randomized controlled trials (freely interpreted and abbreviated from the CONSORT Group[33]).*

facility that can supply you with a template for this purpose. Avoid making this a strenuous part of your scientific work!

A description of how to present scientific data is not the aim of this chapter. However, it should be noted that the MPA will require a scientific report from your study. The revised CONSORT (Consolidated Standards of Reporting Trials) statement gives guidelines for good-quality reporting that are also useful for preparing manuscripts as well as evaluating study reports produced by other groups (Fig. 38.5).[33]

REFERENCES

● 1. Sawynok J. Adenosine receptor activation and nociception. *Eur J Pharmacol* 1998; **347:** 1–11.

2. Sjölund KF, von Heijne M, Hao JX, *et al.* Intrathecal administration of the adenosine A1 receptor agonist R-phenylisopropyl adenosine reduces presumed pain behaviour in a rat model of central pain. *Neurosci Lett* 1998; **243:** 605–10.

3. von Heijne M, Hao JX, Sollevi A, Xu XJ. Effects of intrathecal morphine, baclofen, clonidine and R-PIA on the acute allodynia-like behaviours after spinal cord ischaemia in rats. *Eur J Pain* 2001; **5:** 1–10.

4. Cui JG, Meyerson BA, Sollevi A, Linderoth B. Effect of spinal cord stimulation on tactile hypersensitivity in mononeuropathic rats is potentiated by simultaneous GABA(B) and adenosine receptor activation. *Neurosci Lett* 1998; **247:** 183–6.

5. Lavand'homme PM, Eisenach JC. Exogenous and endogenous adenosine enhance the spinal antiallodynic effects of morphine in a rat model of neuropathic pain. *Pain* 1999; **80:** 31–6.

6. Chiari A, Yaksh TL, Myers RR, *et al.* Preclinical toxicity screening of intrathecal adenosine in rats and dogs. *Anesthesiology* 1999; **91:** 824–32.

● 7. Pelleg A, Porter RS. The pharmacology of adenosine. *Pharmacotherapy* 1990; **10:** 157–74.

◆ 8. Narang PK, Bianchine JR. Phase I studies. Initial evaluation of drug toxicity, dose response, and efficacy. In: Max M, Portenoy R, Laska E eds. *Advances in Pain Research and Therapy*, vol.18. New York, NY: Raven Press, 1991: 49–53.

9. von Heijne M, Hao JX, Sollevi A, Xu XJ. Intrathecal adenosine does not relieve allodynia like behavior in spinally injured rats. *Neuroreport* 1999; **10:** 3247–51.

10. Rane K, Karlsten R, Sollevi A, *et al.* Spinal cord morphology after chronic intrathecal administration of adenosine in the rat. *Acta Anaesthesiol Scand* 1999; **43:** 1035–40.

11. Cerqueira MD, Verani MS, Schwaiger M, *et al.* Safety profile of adenosine stress perfusion imaging: results from the Adenoscan Multicenter Trial Registry. *J Am Coll Cardiol* 1994; **23:** 390–2.

● 12. Segerdahl M, Sollevi A. Adenosine and pain relief – a clinical overview. *Drug Res Dev* 1998; **45:** 151–8.

13. Rane K, Segerdahl M, Sollevi A. Intrathecal adenosine administration. A phase 1 clinical safety study in healthy volunteers, with additional evaluation of its influence on sensory thresholds and experimental pain. *Anesthesiology* 1998; **89:** 1108–15.

14. Belfrage M, Segerdahl M, Arner S, Sollevi A. The safety and efficacy of intrathecal adenosine in patients with chronic neuropathic pain. *Anesth Analg* 1999; **89:** 136–42.

15. Woolf CJ. The dorsal horn: state-dependent sensory processing and the generation of pain. In: Wall PD, Melzack R eds. *Textbook of Pain*, 3rd edn. London: Churchill Livingstone, 1994: 101–12.

16. Rae CP, Mansfield MD, Dryden C, Kinsella J. Analgesic effect of adenosine on ischemic pain in human volunteers. *Br J Anaesth* 1999; **82:** 427–8.

17. Zaraté E, Sa Rego MM, White PF, *et al.* Comparison of adenosine and remifentanil infusions as adjuvants to desflurane anesthesia. *Anesthesiology* 1999; **90:** 956–63.

18. Rane K, Sollevi A, Segerdahl M. Intrathecal adenosine administration in abdominal hysterectomy lacks analgesic effect. *Acta Anaesthesiol Scand* 2000; **44:** 868–72.

19. Sjölund K-F, Belfrage M, Karlsten R, *et al.* Systemic adenosine infusion reduces the area of tactile allodynia in neuropathic pain following peripheral nerve injury: a multi-center, placebo-controlled study. *Eur J Pain* 2001; **5:** 199–207.

20. Feine JS, Bushnell MC, Miron D, Duncan GH. Sex differences in the perception of noxious heat stimuli. *Pain* 1991; **44:** 255–62.

21. Fillingim RB, Maixner W, Kinkaid S, Silva S. Sex differences in temporal summation but not sensory–discriminative processing of thermal pain. *Pain* 1998; **75:** 121–7.

22. Walker JS, Carmody JJ. Experimental pain in healthy human subjects: gender differences in nociception and in response to ibuprofen. *Anesth Analg* 1998; **86:** 1257–62.

23. Gracely RH. Experimental pain models. In: Max M, Portenoy R, Laska E eds. *Advances in Pain Research and Therapy*, vol. 18. New York, NY: Raven Press, 1991: 33–47.

◆ 24. Cooper SA. Commentary. Single-dose analgesic studies: the upside and downside of assay sensitivity. In: Max M, Portenoy R, Laska E eds. *Advances in Pain Research and Therapy*, vol. 18. New York, NY: Raven Press, 1991: 117–24.

◆ 25. Chapman CR. Experimental pain models and analgesic efficacy. In: Max M, Portenoy R, Laska E eds. *Advances in Pain Research and Therapy*, vol. 18. New York, NY: Raven Press, 1991: 49–53.

26. Yaksh TL. Pharmacology and mechanisms of opioid analgesics activity. *Acta Anaesthesiol Scand* 1997; **41:** 94–111.

27. Zhang X, Bao L, Shi TJ, *et al*. Down-regulation of mu-opioid receptors in rat and monkey dorsal root ganglion neurons and spinal cord after peripheral axotomy. *Neuroscience* 1998; **82:** 223–40.

28. Cooper BY, Vierck Jr CJ, Yeomans DC. Selective reduction of second pain sensations by systemic morphine in humans. *Pain* 1986; **24:** 93–116.

29. Olofsson C, Ekblom A, Ekman-Ordeberg G, *et al*. Lack of analgesic effect of systemically administered morphine or pethidine on labour pain. *Br J Obstet Gynaecol* 1996; **103:** 968–72.

◆ 30. Dixon Jr JR. The International Conference on Harmonization Good Clinical Practice guideline. *Quality Assurance* 1998; **6:** 65–74.

◆ 31. World Medical Association Declaration of Helsinki. Ethical principles for medical research involving human subjects. *Bull World Health Organ* 2001; **79:** 373–4.

◆ 32. Charlton E. Ethical guidelines for pain research in humans. Committee on Ethical Issues of the International Association for the Study of Pain. *Pain* 1995; **63:** 277–8; http://www.iasp-pain.org/ethicopen.html

◆ 33. Moher D, Schulz KF, Altman D. The CONSORT statement: revised recommendations for improving the quality of reports of parallel–group randomized trials. *JAMA* 2001; **285:** 1987–91.

Techniques of systematic reviews and meta-analysis in pain research

ANNA D OLDMAN AND LESLEY A SMITH

Framing the question	496	Qualitative reviews	501
Finding the evidence	496	Conclusion	503
Appraising the evidence	497	References	504
Meta-analysis	498		

What we call scientific knowledge today is a body of statements of varying degrees of certainty. Some of them are most unsure; some of them are nearly sure; but none is absolutely certain.

How you get to know is what I want to know.

Richard Feynman[1]

A systematic review can be defined as a review of a particular subject undertaken in such a way that the risk of bias is reduced. This involves searching for all published (and sometimes unpublished) information on a topic, sifting through this mass of information, and distilling it through quality filters. A review is only as good as the trials available to the reviewer – trials in poorly researched areas are likely to produce inaccurate estimates of efficacy.

Clinicians and policy-makers have ever increasing amounts of information to digest merely to keep up with new research findings. Trials often give conflicting results and, with time pressure, it can be almost impossible to assimilate and assess all of the available information in a given area. Systematic reviews, at their best, provide clear, evidence-based statements about the efficacy of interventions and, where possible, how different interventions compare. They can be useful tools for practitioners of evidence-based medicine when used alongside clinical knowledge that takes into account the patient's unique biology and circumstances (Fig. 39.1).

Large, well-designed, randomized, controlled trials can also provide reliable sources of evidence. Together, these constitute the best chance we have of getting to the truth of whether an intervention is effective or not. Box 39.1 illustrates a hierarchy of evidence.

The aim of this chapter is to provide a step-by-step guide to carrying out quantitative (meta-analysis) and qualitative systematic reviews in pain. To successfully incorporate the findings of systematic reviews into the decision-making process, it is important to understand how the conclusions of a review have been reached. We have therefore aimed to provide an overview of the main processes involved in carrying out systematic reviews to assist the reader in critically appraising the conclusions drawn by the authors of published reviews. We illustrate each step using a worked example. The review process comprises the three main steps illustrated in Fig. 39.2.

It is easy to underestimate the time and resources required to complete a review. Each stage requires much painstaking work, and a review is likely to take months to complete rather than weeks.

This chapter does not aim to provide definitive answers on how to do a systematic review. Evidence-

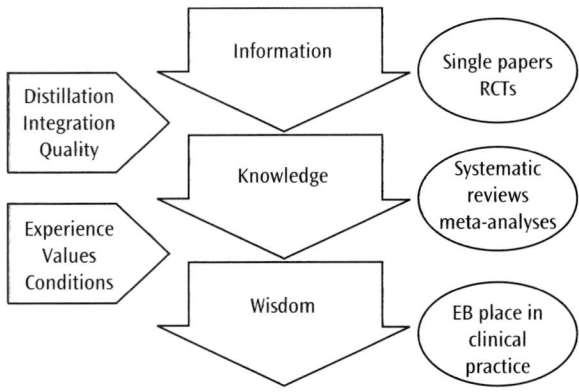

Figure 39.1 *Evidence-based medicine in practice.*

Box 39.1 *Hierarchy of evidence*

Type and strength of evidence

I Strong evidence from at least one systematic review of multiple, well-designed, randomized, controlled trials.

II Strong evidence from at least one properly designed, randomized, controlled trial of appropriate size.

III Evidence from well-designed trials without randomization, single-group pre–post, cohort, time series, or matched case-controlled studies.

IV Evidence from well-designed, nonexperimental studies from more than one center or research group.

V Opinions of respected authorities, based on clinical evidence, descriptive studies, or reports of expert committees.

based medicine is an evolving science, and a number of methodologies have been adopted. Our experience lies predominantly in the field of acute pain and interventions for which randomized controlled trials exist. Our approach is to assess whether an intervention is effective based on statistical significance, and then whether this difference is of clinical relevance.

FRAMING THE QUESTION

Before starting the process of a systematic review, it is important to define the main question you want the review to answer. It is too easy to measure what is measurable, and perhaps less straightforward to measure what is important. A good systematic review does not unthinkingly accept outcomes with limited scientific or clinical relevance. Is a particular outcome worthwhile to patients, carers, or to society as a whole? The more specific and clinically relevant the question, the more useful the review will be. It may be necessary to impose values on a group of trials rather than taking the outcomes that the authors have used.

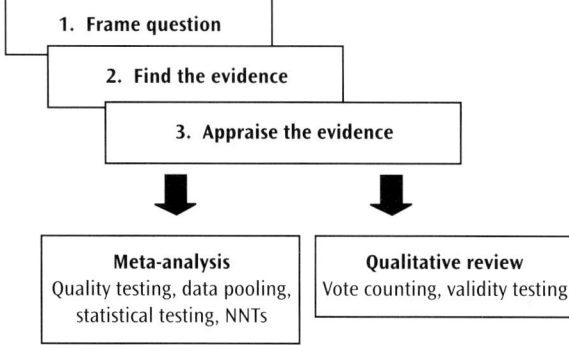

Figure 39.2 *The review process.*

If we are interested in the efficacy of, for example, aspirin or acupuncture, our review questions might be: "Is single-dose oral aspirin effective in relieving postoperative pain in adults?" or "Is acupuncture effective in relieving acute and chronic back or neck pain?"

There are six main considerations to framing your question. Table 39.1 illustrates these for the examples given above.

FINDING THE EVIDENCE

Which trials to include?

The gold standard for any review must be one that includes the highest quality evidence available to answer the question. What constitutes good evidence? The best evidence comes from large, well-designed, randomized, controlled trials that are double blind. Lack of randomization, inadequate blinding, and small trials all risk overestimation of treatment effects.[2–4] For example, trials that are not randomized can lead to overestimation of treatment effects by up to 40%.[2] This is illustrated clearly in a systematic review of transcutaneous electrical nerve stimulation (TENS) for postoperative pain, in which the randomized trials overwhelmingly showed that it does not work whereas the nonrandomized trials showed that it does.[3] Although there are therapeutic areas where randomization is notoriously difficult, such as treatments for cancer and palliative care, systematic reviews using nonrandomized trials are problematic. This chapter therefore concentrates on systematic reviews of randomized trials.

A criticism sometimes leveled at systematic reviews is that lumping together information from different trials gives unreliable results. It is legitimate to combine information as long as care is taken to ensure that this is carried out in a way that makes sense. Trials must be as similar as possible, especially if data are to be pooled. This includes type of:

- patients (diagnosis, age, sex);
- pain (type, severity);
- comparison groups;
- dose, route of administration, and formulation of drug;
- outcomes (outcome measures, time points);
- blinding of patients and investigators.

If these factors vary across trials, then it may be more appropriate to carry out subgroup analyses, for example of different doses or different patient groups, or to consider a qualitative review. For example, a review of epidural corticosteroids for sciatica[5] carried out subgroup analyses based on the time at which pain relief was measured: short-term (1–60 days following epidural) and long-term (12–52 weeks) pain relief. It is not useful to carry out a subgroup analysis based on inadequate

Table 39.1 *The review question*

	Aspirin	Acupuncture
1 What kind of studies?	Randomized, double-blind, controlled trials	Randomized controlled trials
2 What type of intervention?	Single oral standard doses of aspirin	Any type of acupuncture, single or multiple sessions
3 What type of pain?	Acute, postoperative pain	Acute or chronic pain (nonmalignant)
4 Which outcomes?	Pain relief over 0–4 h, adverse effects	Pain relief – early and late outcomes
5 What types of patients?	Adult	Adult
6 Which comparison groups?	Placebo	Placebo

amounts of patient data. In this case, a qualitative review may be more appropriate (see Qualitative reviews).

Having framed the review question, it is important to look for all studies that could possibly answer it. A review can only be considered as systematic when it includes a thorough search of all of the available evidence.

How to search

There are two main approaches to planning a search strategy. In all cases, a search should include every likely variant of a term, and include the wild card (*) to cast the net as wide as possible:

High sensitivity, high yield

The aim of this approach is to identify as many references as possible in order to minimize the chances of missing relevant trials. A highly sensitive search for randomized, controlled trials (RCTs) would include any terms that might uncover an RCT, such as "trial" and "study" and "random*" rather than "random*" alone. With this approach, there is a higher risk of identifying and retrieving studies that do not meet the inclusion criteria, but there is less likelihood of missing trials inadequately indexed on the databases.

High precision, low yield

The aim of this approach is to target the clinical trials more specifically. This search will be labor saving: it will generate fewer hits and a greater proportion of them will be relevant. The risk of this approach is that some trials may be missed, something to consider if there is a paucity of trials in the area being reviewed.

We recommend a sensitive search strategy, together with a broad free text search (i.e. one that searches all fields in the database). The following databases are recommended for searching (as relevant):

- MEDLINE   http://research.bmn.com/medline
- EMBASE   www.bids.ac.uk/embase.html
- Cochrane Library
  www.update-software.com/clibhome/clib.html
- Biological Abstracts www.biosis.org/index.html
- CINAHL (nursing and allied health)
  www.cinahl.com/prodsvcs/prodsvcs.html

- PsycLIT   www.apa.org/psycinfo/accesspi.html
- AMED (allied and complementary medicine)
  www.bl.uk/services/stb/amed.html
- PUBMED   www.ncbi.nlm.nih.gov/PubMed

Examples of sensitive search strategies are shown in Box 39.2.

APPRAISING THE EVIDENCE

How many trials meet your inclusion criteria? A balance needs to be struck between adhering to tightly defined inclusion criteria (and rejecting many trials) and broadening out the criteria to let more trials in. This balance will depend on how many trials are available. Are there enough trials with similar patients, outcomes, etc.? (see Table 39.1). For example, our review of aspirin for postoperative pain yielded 72 trials meeting very tightly defined criteria, all with similar patients, similar pain, outcomes, control group, etc., enabling data pooling (meta-analysis).[6] In contrast, the 13 trials included in the acupuncture review studied acupuncture given in different ways, at different sites, different numbers and lengths of sessions, different control groups and outcomes, and different degree of blinding (double, single, and nonblinded).[7] Here, data

---

Box 39.2 *Sensitive search strategies*

Acupuncture for neck or back pain
(acupuncture or electro-acupuncture or electroacupuncture or laseracupuncture or laser-acupuncture) *and* (back* or lumb* or sciatic* or myofasci* or radicul* or spondyl* or neck* or cervic* or whiplash).

Aspirin for postoperative pain
(aspirin or "acetylsalicylic acid" or "acetyl salicylic acid" or "acetyl-salicylic acid" or aspirine or aspirina or aspirinetta) *and* (surg* or post-surg* or postsurg* or dental or molar or extract* or operat* or post-operat* or postoperat* or "acute pain") *and* (random* or doubleblind or double-blind or "double blind" or trial* or double-dummy or "double dummy" or "clinical study").

pooling was not possible, and a qualitative methodology was adopted.

Should qualitative or quantitative reviews be carried out when very few trials exist or trials are of poor quality? A review is a comprehensive and unbiased way of interpreting and summarizing research findings. A conclusion that there is no evidence, or that the evidence is not sufficient to establish efficacy (poor-quality or insufficient data), is useful to policy-makers, practitioners, and patients.

The following section covers the main approaches to data analysis.

META-ANALYSIS

Quality control

Once you have found all reports of trials relevant to your review question, the next step is to confirm that these reports meet minimum quality standards. The quality standards that you set may be different for each review as RCTs may not be available for all clinical questions. However, for systematic reviews of pain, using only RCTs makes sense as (1) there are many RCTs for pain interventions, and (2) when subjective outcomes such as pain are used, it is especially important to have a high minimum quality standard.

Here, we define quality as a study design that reduces the likelihood of bias. It is important to eliminate trials that may introduce bias into the systematic review. Table 39.2 shows the Oxford Quality Rating Scale, which can be used to score trials for quality.[8] Instructions are in Box 39.3. The scale is simple, short, reliable, and valid. It can be used to assess the scientific quality of any clinical trial in which pain is an outcome measure or in which analgesic interventions are compared for outcomes other than pain (e.g. adverse effects). The maximum score a trial can have is five (two for randomization, two for blinding, and one for withdrawals and dropouts). For a trial to be included in a meta-analysis, we suggest a minimum score of two, with at least one point for randomization and one for blinding.

The choice of whether to assess the reports blind or open is down to the resources available to you. Blind assessment (not knowing the author, journal, year of publication, etc.) will produce more consistent and lower quality scores.[8] If more than one person independently scores the trials for quality, results are more likely to be consistent.

Analyzing the data

Data extraction should include information to verify that trials meet the inclusion criteria as well as the data

Table 39.2 *Oxford Quality Rating Scale*

	Score
Was the study randomized?	
Yes	1
Appropriate?	
Yes	1
No	−1
Was the study double blind?	
Yes	1
Appropriate?	
Yes	1
No	−1
Were withdrawals and dropouts described?	
Yes	1

required for statistical analysis. The strength of meta-analysis comes from the pooling of similar trials with similar patients and similar outcomes, generating a large pool of patients upon which to calculate efficacy. Care must therefore be taken when pooling data to ensure that like is compared with like. For example, the meta-analysis of aspirin for postoperative pain[6] was based on adult patients who all had pain of moderate to severe intensity with pain measured over 0–4 or 0–6 h using standardized pain scales, where aspirin was compared with placebo. When meta-analyses are carried out using trials with the same comparison group (e.g. placebo), treatments can be ranked against each other on a particular outcome.[9] Combining data from trials is hazardous when comparison groups are not the same.

In a meta-analysis, efficacy data can be presented diagrammatically, statistically, and in terms of clinical relevance. There are many ways of doing this, and the most useful are described below.

L'Abbé plots

A paper by Kristen L'Abbé and colleagues[10] describes a simple graphical representation of the information from trials. Each point on a L'Abbé scatter plot is one trial in the review. The proportion of patients achieving the outcome with the experimental intervention is plotted against the proportion of patients achieving the outcome with the control intervention (Fig. 39.3).

For *treatment*, trials in which the experimental intervention was better than the control will be in the upper left of the plot, between the *y*-axis and the line of equality. If experimental was no better than control, the point will fall on the line of equality; if control was better than experimental, the point will be in the lower right of the plot between the *x*-axis and the line of equality.

For *prophylaxis*, this pattern will be reversed. Because *prophylaxis* reduces the number of bad events – such as preemptive analgesia to prevent postoperative pain – we expect a smaller proportion to be harmed with treatment than with control. So if experimental is better than con-

---

Box 39.3 *Scoring the items of the Oxford Quality Rating Scale*

Question 1
- Give one point if the study was described as randomized (this includes words such as randomly, random, and randomization).
- Give an additional point if the method of randomization was described and it was appropriate (e.g. table of random numbers, computer-generated numbers, coin-tossing). A randomization method is appropriate if it allowed each patient to have the same chance of receiving each treatment, and the investigators could not predict which treatment was next.
- Deduct one point if the method of randomization was described but was inappropriate (e.g. alternate allocation to treatment group, or according to date of birth, hospital numbers, etc.).

Question 2
- Give one point if the study was described as double blind, or if it was implied that neither care-giver nor patient could identify the treatment being assessed.
- Give an additional point if the method of double blinding was described and was appropriate (e.g. identical placebo, double-dummy pill, etc.).
- Deduct one point if the study was described as double blind but the method of double blinding was inadequate (e.g. different colored pills, patient or care-giver could identify treatment, etc.).

Question 3
- Give one point if there was a description of withdrawals and dropouts. The numbers and the reasons must be stated. If there were no withdrawals, it must be stated.
- Score zero if there was no statement on withdrawals and dropouts.

---

trol, the cluster of trial points should be between the *x*-axis and the line of equality.

The important point about a L'Abbé plot is that it shows *all* of the extant data on one piece of paper. When combined with numbers in the trial, and a summary measure such as number needed to treat (NNT), it is a concise way of summarizing lots of information. An example from the meta-analysis of aspirin is given in Fig. 39.4.

Statistical significance

There are several statistical tests used in meta-analysis to determine whether treatment is different from control. Choice very often seems to be governed by custom and practice rather than by any inherent intellectual advan-

tage, and the debate about which test is most appropriate continues. A good review will give sufficient detail so that when the dust has settled calculations can be redone according to the prevailing opinion. For pain interventions, event rates usually occur frequently (e.g. approximately 50% of patients improve with treatment). In this

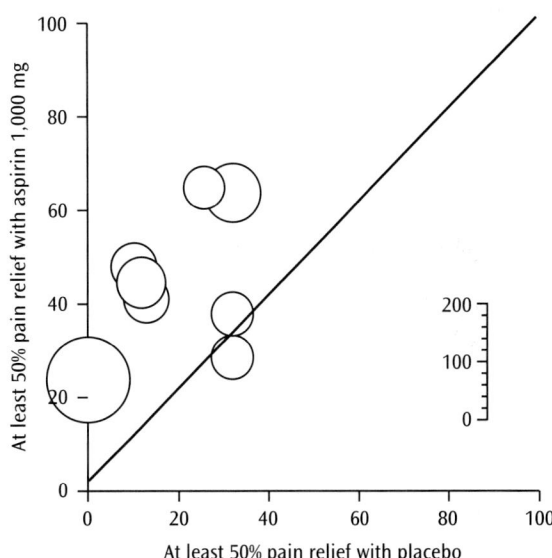

Figure 39.4 *L'Abbé plot of aspirin showing the proportion of patients in each study achieving at least 50% pain relief over 4–6 h for aspirin 1,000 mg. All trials were randomized, and double blind and baseline pain was of at least moderate intensity. Point size is linearly proportional to the total number of patients in each trial.*

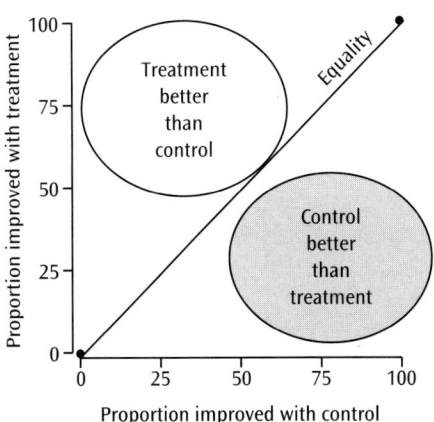

Figure 39.3 *L'Abbé plot.*

situation, the relative benefit (RB) is a robust measure of statistical significance. A method for calculating RB with a 95% confidence interval (CI) is given by Gardner and Altman.[11] When the CI of the RB does not cross 1, then the intervention is statistically different from control.

The most popular alternative to calculating RB is the odds ratio.[12] The odds ratio of an outcome is the ratio of the probability of the outcome occurring to the probability of it not occurring. Here, statistical significance is assumed when the lower 95% CI of the odds ratio is less than 1. The odds ratio can give a distorted impression when analyses are conducted on subgroups that differ substantially in baseline risk.[13] Where control even rates are high (certainly when they are above 50%), odds ratios should be interpreted with caution.

Heterogeneity

Statistical testing for heterogeneity is often recommended in meta-analysis. This intends to assess how similar the component trials of the meta-analysis were. However, all of these tests lack power, so that although a positive test for heterogeneity suggests that trials were not similar a negative test does not provide complete reassurance that there is no heterogeneity.[14]

Where care has been taken to avoid pooling trials of disparate design, with different patients and different outcomes, the main reason for apparent heterogeneity in meta-analysis is the random play of chance.[4] Small trials are subject to wide variations in control and experimental event rates. When calculating the RB, a fixed effects or a random effects model must be chosen.[15] A random effects model is more conservative, and assumes that heterogeneity exists. A fixed effects model is more appropriate when the assumption is that heterogeneity does not exist.

How well does the intervention work?

While the RB is an indication that an intervention works, a statistical output is of limited help when trying to determine how well it works – its clinical relevance. A number of methods exist to express clinical significance. Traditionally, the effect size is estimated using the standardized mean difference.[16] The advantages of this approach are that data obtained with different measurement scales, and continuous data, can be pooled, The z-score output is in standard deviation units, and is therefore scale free. However, the disadvantage of effect size is that it is difficult to interpret and is not intuitive for clinicians or patients.

Number needed to treat

The number needed to treat is a popular measure of clinical relevance in meta-analysis. It is the reciprocal of the change in absolute risk brought about by an intervention, and is calculated using dichotomous data according to the equation:

$$\text{NNT} = 1/(\text{IMP}_{act}/\text{TOT}_{act}) - (\text{IMP}_{con}/\text{TOT}_{con})$$

where IMP_{act} is the number of patients given active treatment achieving the outcome; TOT_{act} is the total number of patients given the active treatment; IMP_{con} is the number of patients given a control treatment achieving the outcome; TOT_{con} is the total number of patients given the control treatment.[17]

Different NNTs can be calculated for an intervention based on different outcomes of interest. For example, we may be interested in a range of outcomes for acute interventions for migraine. NNTs can be calculated for the number of patients who have mild or no pain at 2 h, or the harder outcome of mild or no pain at 24 h following treatment. Table 39.3 provides examples of NNTs based on different outcomes.

The NNT should always be calculated together with its CI.[17] The lower the NNT, the better the treatment. Because few treatments are 100% effective and because few controls have no effect (even placebo or no treatment), NNTs of effective treatments are usually in the range 2–4. It is important to remember that the NNT is always relative to the comparator and applies to a particular clinical outcome. The duration of treatment necessary to achieve the target should also be specified. For example, the NNT for at least 50% pain relief over 4–6 h for patients with moderate to severe postoperative pain for aspirin 1,000 mg compared with placebo is 4.0 (95% CI 3.2–5.4). An NNT of 4 means that for every four patients treated with aspirin 1,000 mg one patient will improve who would not have done so if treated with placebo.

For prophylaxis, where fewer events occur in the treated group than in the control group, NNTs with negative signs will be produced using the equation above. The NNT number is correct and can be used. Alternatively, to produce NNTs with a positive sign, you can switch the active and control groups around (1/proportion benefiting from control intervention minus the proportion benefiting from the experimental intervention).

Where trials do not report dichotomous data, it is possible to convert continuous data (such as mean pain relief or mean pain intensity values) to dichotomous data.[21–23] For example, mean SPID (sum of pain intensity difference), mean TOTPAR (total pain relief), or their equivalents based on a visual analog scale can all be converted to produce similar dichotomous data for meta-analysis. A meta-analysis in postoperative pain might set the dichotomous hurdle as 50% pain relief. Mean SPID and TOTPAR values can all be converted to express the proportion of patients achieving this outcome, thus enabling the data to be pooled.

Confidence intervals

The 95% CI of the NNT is an indication that 19 times out of 20 the "true" value will be in the specified range. If the RB is not statistically significant, the CI of the NNT

Table 39.3 *Examples of NNTs from systematic reviews*

Reference	Condition	Treatment	Comparator	Outcome and when assessed	NNT (95% CI)
18	Migraine	Sumatriptan 100 mg	Placebo	Mild or no pain at 2 h	3.0 (2.8 to 3.4)
9	Postoperative pain	Ibuprofen 400 mg	Placebo	At least 50% pain relief at 4–6 h	2.7 (2.5 to 3.0)
19	Recent soft-tissue injury, sprains, strains, or trauma	Topically applied ketoprofen	Placebo	At least 50% pain relief at 1 week	2.6 (2.3 to 3.2)
20	Dysmenorrhea	Naproxen (550 mg or 275 mg, four times daily: 3–5 days per cycle)	Placebo	At least moderate pain relief	2.6 (2.0 to 3.4)

is infinite, indicating that treatment is no different from control. An NNT with an infinite CI is then but a point estimate, and it may be inadvisable to quote the NNT. However, opinion is divided because a point estimate may still have clinical importance as a benchmark until further data are available, and decisions should take this into account. Altman[24] suggests a way to improve the presentation of the CI around the NNT in this situation.

Clearly, an important factor in determining the range of the confidence interval is the amount of patient data available. In general, the more patients included in the analysis, the tighter the confidence interval will be. For instance, using the example of a standard analgesic intervention for acute pain to assess the direction and magnitude of the effect reliably (i.e. CI of NNT within ±0.5 of its true value), at least 500 patients per group are required.[4] Less patient information is required to calculate statistical significance, but it is important to consider whether failure to demonstrate a difference is due to lack of effect or a lack of data.

Limitations of the number needed to treat

One disadvantage of the NNT approach is that it needs dichotomous data. Furthermore, because of the way the NNT is calculated, it is sensitive to trials with high control event rates. As the control event rate increases, the potential for treatment-specific improvement decreases and higher (and apparently less effective) NNTs result. So, as with any summary measure from a meta-analysis, NNTs need to be treated with caution when control event rates are high.

How safe is the intervention?

An important part of clinical decision-making is knowing how likely a treatment is to cause harm. A systematic review is more useful if it can provide estimates of harm as well as efficacy. However, information on adverse effects is often collected and reported inadequately, making reliable estimates of harm difficult.

Number needed to harm

The number needed to harm (NNH) is calculated in the same way as the NNT, and the same rules on data pooling apply. When the incidence of adverse effects is low, it is likely that only a point estimate of harm will be generated as the CI will be infinite. A review can calculate estimates of minor and major harm, where major harm can be defined as any adverse effect causing the patient to withdraw from the study and minor harm as unpleasant adverse effects that do not cause study withdrawal.

QUALITATIVE REVIEWS

A qualitative review is one in which no pooling of data is possible. Combining data is not possible if there is no quantitative information on the individual trials of the review. Second, combining data may not be sensible if the trials are not similar enough, e.g. with different interventions, different patients, outcomes, etc.

Appraising the evidence

Quality control

Do your trials meet a basic quality standard? We suggest that included trials should be:

- randomized;
- group sizes of at least 10 patients;
- double or single blind (as the intervention allows).

In most cases, trials that do not meet these criteria should be excluded from a review. Where blinding is not possible or extremely difficult, a more flexible approach is required. Similarly, when very few trials pass the quality hurdle, inclusion criteria may need to be reassessed. For example, a review of TENS for chronic pain found that true blinding of TENS was not possible, and included trials that were defined as unblind or single blind.[9] Including trials of poor quality will weaken the review conclusion, but this may be the best evidence available.

Assessing efficacy and reaching a conclusion

There are two main approaches to qualitative reviews – vote counting and vote counting where trial validity is taken into consideration. Each approach has different strengths and weaknesses. A vote-counting exercise (how many trials say the intervention works versus how many say it does not work) provides a simple conclusion. The weakness of this approach is that it does not take into account the validity of each trial nor the robustness of each trial conclusion. A review that takes trial validity into account is likely to provide a more accurate conclusion.

Vote counting

How many of the included trials say that the intervention works, and how many that it does not? A vote-counting exercise, based on the number of positive versus the number of negative trials, provides a simple estimate of efficacy. An example of a vote-counting review has been carried out for intravenous regional sympathetic blocks (IRSBs) in patients with reflex sympathetic dystrophy (RSD, also known as complex regional pain syndrome).[25] Eight trials met inclusion criteria and, of these, two concluded that IRSB showed some advantage over the control treatment and six showed no benefit. On this basis, authors were able to conclude which drugs were effective and how strong or weak the evidence for this was (i.e. how many data were available to support the conclusion). A useful way of diagrammatically expressing results is with the L'Abbé plot (Fig. 39.3).

Vote counting based on trial validity

The findings of individual trials carry more weight in a qualitative review than in a data-pooling exercise. For example, a small trial will carry the same weight as a large trial. Furthermore, qualitative reviews are more likely to be carried out in areas where trial methodology is poor, or few trials exist. Broader inclusion criteria are therefore necessary to find suitable numbers of trials. In these circumstances, it is possible that a double-blind trial may sit alongside a nonblinded trial. Here, as for size, these trials will be given equal weighting in a vote-counting exercise. One way of overcoming this flaw is to take the validity of each trial into consideration, and to give more weight to the trials of highest validity when drawing an overall conclusion. A useful diagrammatic way of expressing this kind of finding is with a scatter diagram.

There is no single recognized way of assessing trial validity. However, we know that trials can report inaccurate or misleading results when the methodology is biased or inadequate. Double-blind trials with large groups, standardized outcome measures, sensitive designs, and appropriate methodologies are less biased than those without. The checklist in Table 39.4 will help when ranking trials according to validity. For each trial, the more times you are able to tick item 1 for each section, the more valid the trial.

What is the evidence that these items are important in pain trials?

- *Blinding.* A trial should be adequately blinded to eliminate observer and patient bias. Blinding is especially important when outcomes are subjective (e.g. pain, nausea) rather than objective (e.g. death, vomiting).
- *Group size.* Trials with small group sizes are unreliable.[4] As a yardstick, a typical effective treatment for acute or chronic pain has an analgesic response rate of approximately 50%, and placebo response rate of 20% for an outcome of pain half gone. In this case, to be 95% confident that a statistically significant difference could be demonstrated, at least 40 patients per group would be needed.
- *Outcome measures.* Poor outcome measures give unreliable findings. Standard pain intensity or pain relief measures, rated by the patient, are the most reliable estimate of efficacy. Other outcome measures such as physician or carer ratings are less valid and may overestimate treatment effect. In most cases, analgesic consumption is not a sensitive measure of pain relief.
- *Baseline pain.* A trial with no or little pain at baseline cannot measure a reduction.
- *Internal sensitivity.* A trial that cannot demonstrate that it is sensitive enough to measure an effect is of limited validity. Does a negative result mean the intervention does not work, or that the trial failed to measure the effect? For trials that do not have a placebo group, an additional active control group of an intervention with proven efficacy is an important way of demonstrating that the trial is sensitive enough to measure an effect.

Data analysis

- *Definition of outcomes.* A trial with unclear definitions of outcomes such as "clinical improvement" or "successful treatment" is less valid than one with clear definitions.
- *Presentation of data.* Papers should support their findings by presenting mean or median data with dispersion values (standard deviation, interquartile range) or dichotomous data. Without this information, it is difficult to see how authors have reached their conclusions.
- *Statistical tests.* Reports should choose the correct tests, not do too many of them (data trawling), and correct for multiple testing. Any single statistical significance that is the result of multiple testing, and that emerges among many negatives, lacks credibility.
- *Handling of dropouts.* A trial that does not report dropout rates, or does not adequately handle dropouts in the efficacy analysis, is less valid. Studies

Table 39.4 *Assessment of trial validity*

Blinding	1 Was the trial convincingly double blind?
	2 Was the trial convincingly single blind?
	3 Was the trial either not blind or the blinding unclear?
Size of trial groups	1 Was the group size ≥ 40?
	2 Was the group size 30–39?
	3 Was the group size 20–29?
	4 Was the group size 10–19?
Outcomes	Look at outcomes relevant to the review question:
	1 Did the trial include standard outcome measures, and use the outcome appropriately?
	2 Did the trial include nonstandard outcomes and/or use the outcome inappropriately?
Trial design	Baseline pain
	1 For all treatment groups, were baseline levels sufficient for the trialist to be able to measure a change following the intervention (i.e. there was enough baseline pain to detect a difference between baseline and post-treatment levels)?
	2 For all treatment groups, were baseline levels insufficient to be able to measure a change following the intervention, or, was it not possible to assess baseline levels?
	Internal sensitivity
	1 Did the trial demonstrate internal sensitivity?
	2 Did the trial fail to demonstrate internal sensitivity?
Data analysis	Definition of outcomes
	1 Did the paper define the relevant outcomes clearly, including, where relevant, exactly what "improved," "successful treatment," etc. represented?
	2 Did the paper fail to define the outcomes clearly?
	Data presentation: location and dispersion
	1 Did the paper present mean data with standard deviations, or dichotomous outcomes, or median with range, or sufficient data to enable extraction of any of these?
	2 Did the paper fail to present the above?
	Statistical testing
	1 Did the trialist choose an appropriate statistical test, with correction for multiple tests where relevant?
	2 Did the trialist choose inappropriate statistical tests and/or multiple testing was carried out, but with no correction, or were no statistical tests carried out?
	Handling of dropouts
	1 Was the dropout rate ≤ 10%, or was it > 10% but dropouts were included in an intention-to-treat analysis?
	2 Was the dropout rate > 10% and dropouts were not included in the analysis, or was it not possible to calculate a dropout rate from data presented in the paper?

may lose patients for many different reasons. Unless high dropout rates make good clinical sense, a rule of thumb can be that when the proportion of lost patients and data exceeds 10% the validity of the data declines unless an intention-to-treat analysis has been used.

A number of rating scales measure aspects of trial validity. The items covered here form the basis of a new scale – The Oxford Pain Validity Scale.[7]

An example of a review that includes an assessment of trial validity is one of acupuncture for back and neck pain.[7] Thirteen trials were identified, of which five concluded that acupuncture was effective and eight that it was not. Does this mean that the intervention works? In a simple vote-counting exercise it would be difficult to draw a

conclusion. However, when trials were ranked according to validity, it was found that the more valid trials were less likely to show a positive finding. The overall conclusion was that there is no convincing evidence for the analgesic efficacy of acupuncture for neck or back pain. Figure 39.5 shows the results for the acupuncture review.

CONCLUSION

In summary, although a range of methods exists for meta-analysis and systematic reviews, we have aimed to provide a framework for carrying out a review taking into account the most important methodological issues. The most useful reviews pay careful attention to trial qual-

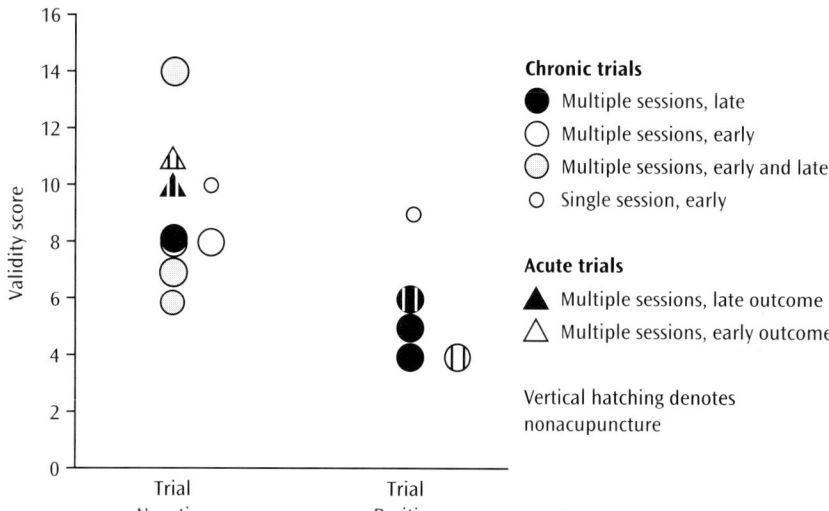

Figure 39.5 *Efficacy of acupuncture.*

ity and validity, report on outcomes which are clinically meaningful, and express results in a clear and clinically useful way.

Acknowledgments Henry McQuay, Andrew Moore, Eija Kalso, and Geoff Gourlay provided many useful suggestions and ideas in the writing of this chapter.

REFERENCES

1. Feynman RP. *The Meaning of it All.* London: Penguin Books, 1999; 27.

2. Schulz KF, Chalmers I, Hayes RJ, Altman DG. Empirical evidence of bias: dimensions of methodological quality associated with estimates of treatment effects in controlled trials. *JAMA* 1995; **273:** 408–12.

● 3. Carroll D, Tramer M, McQuay H, *et al.* Randomization is important in studies with pain outcomes: systematic review of transcutaneous electrical nerve stimulation in acute postoperative pain. *Br J Anaesth* 1996; **77:** 798–803.

◆ 4. Moore RA, Gavaghan D, Tramer MR, *et al.* Size is everything – large amounts of information are needed to overcome random effects in estimating direction and magnitude of treatment effects. *Pain* 1998; **78:** 209–16.

● 5. Watts RW, Silagy CA. A meta-analysis on the efficacy of epidural corticosteroids in the treatment of sciatica. *Anaesth Intensive Care* 1995; **23:** 564–9.

● 6. Edwards JE, Oldman A, Smith L, *et al.* Oral aspirin in postoperative pain: a quantitative systematic review. *Pain* 1999; **81:** 289–97.

● 7. Smith LA, Oldman AD, McQuay HJ, Moore RA. Teasing
◆ apart quality and validity in systematic reviews: an example from acupuncture trials in chronic neck and back pain. *Pain* 2000; **86:** 119–32.

◆ 8. Jadad AR, Moore RA, Carroll D, *et al.* Assessing the qual-

ity of reports of randomized clinical trials: is blinding necessary? *Controlled Clin Trials* 1996; **17:** 1–12.

● 9. McQuay HJ, Moore RA. *An Evidence-based Resource for*
◆ *Pain Relief.* Oxford: Oxford University Press, 1998.

10. L'Abbé KA, Detsky AS, O'Rourke K. Meta-analysis in clinical research. *Ann Intern Med* 1987; **107:** 224–33.

11. Gardner MJ, Altman DG. Confidence intervals rather than P values: estimation rather than hypothesis testing. *Br Med J* 1986; **292:** 746–50.

12. Armitage P, Berry G. *Statistic Methods in Medical Research.* Oxford: Blackwell Scientific Publications, 1994.

13. Sinclair JC, Bracken MB. Clinically useful measures of effect in binary analyses of randomized trials. *J Clin Epidemiol* 1994; **47:** 881–9.

14. Gavaghan DJ, Moore RA, McQuay HJ. An evaluation of homogeneity tests in meta-analyses in pain using simulations of individual patient data. *Pain* 2000; **85:** 415–24.

15. Lau J, Ioannidis JPA, Schmid CH. Summing up evidence: one answer is not always enough. *Lancet* 1998; **351:** 123–7.

16. Glass GV. Primary, secondary, and meta-analysis of research. *Educ Res* 1976; **5:** 3–8.

17. Cook RJ, Sackett DL. The number needed to treat: a clinically useful measure of treatment effect. *Br Med J* 1995; **310:** 452–4.

● 18. Tfelt-Hansen P. Efficacy and adverse events of subcutaneous, oral, and intranasal sumatriptan used for migraine treatment. A systematic review based on number needed to treat. *Cephalalgia* 1998; **18:** 532–8.

● 19. Moore RA, Carroll D, Wiffen PJ, *et al.* A systematic review of topically-applied non-steroidal anti-inflammatory drugs. *Br Med J* 1998; **316:** 333–8.

20. Zhang WY, Li Wan Po A. Efficacy of minor analgesics in primary dysmenorrhoea: a systematic review. *Br J Obstet Gynaecol* 1998; **105:** 780–9.

● 21. Moore A, McQuay H, Gavaghan D. Deriving dichotomous outcome measures from continuous data in randomised controlled trials of analgesics. *Pain* 1996; **66:** 229–37.

22. Moore A, McQuay H, Gavaghan D. Deriving dichotomous outcome measures from continuous data in randomised controlled trials of analgesics: verification from independent data. *Pain* 1997; **69:** 127–30.

23. Moore A, Moore O, McQuay H, Gavaghan D. Deriving dichotomous outcome measures from continuous data in randomised controlled trials of analgesics: use of pain intensity and visual analogue scales. *Pain* 1997; **69:** 311–15.

24. Altman DG. Confidence intervals for the number needed to treat. *Br Med J* 1998; **317:** 1309–12.

● 25. Jadad AR, Carroll D, Glynn CJ, McQuay HJ. Intravenous regional sympathetic blockade for pain relief in reflex sympathetic dystrophy: a systematic review and a randomized, double-blind crossover study. *J Pain Symptom Manage* 1995; **10:** 13–20.

PART XI

Other issues

40

The expert medicolegal report

PETER J D EVANS

Why do people complain?	510	Preparation of the report	514
What do they complain about?	510	History	514
What should concern the expert?	510	The examination	515
Clinical governance	512	The conclusion and opinion	515
Legal standing	512	References	516

There is little doubt that most of us practice in increasingly litigious societies and whereas some may argue that this is a bad thing the reality is that complaints tend to lead to a more questioning behavior in medical practice. The negative side is that it can lead to a practice that is defensive and driven by a need to do "no harm." In medicine, serendipity has been a critical factor in some changes of practice. The current role of acetyl salicylic acid against thromboembolism is just one such example. It is possible that such approaches may be stifled because of a more restrictive practice.

The Cochrane Collaboration[1] has been an important development in the approach to best medical practice and, although not established as a result of litigation, it offers a way to look more critically at what we do. The concept of the evidence-based review and the meta-analysis distilling the international experience on a treatment helps to provide a sound basis for clinical care. It is not the only approach, and others advocate a graded scale to measure efficacy.[2] There are also many situations where the gold standard (the double-blind, placebo-controlled study) cannot be applied. This is often the case with the nuances of surgical practice, where there is a need for rigorous clinical audit as an alternative strategy.

In the UK over the past few years there have been a number of high-profile cases involving lapses of medical practice. These have influenced public opinion adversely and undermined confidence in medical practice. Doctors have, publicly, been shown to have variable standards of care. Sadly, the many are implicated by the few, and the profession is under great pressure to reduce poor practice and improve performance. Within the practice of pain management, there are many situations that could give rise to litigation (Table 40.1).

The UK has enjoyed a privileged position with a relatively low level of medical litigation. However, patients are more readily going to court to settle grievances or to seek financial compensation.[3] It has long been recognized that within medicine the surgical disciplines of obstetrics and anesthesia have carried greater risk of litigation.[4] Pain management is also becoming an area of concern. This reflects a greater recourse to invasive or destructive procedures (spinal cord stimulation, radiofrequency lesioning) as well as increased expectation by the patient of what should or can be achieved.

The introduction of clinical governance and revalidation are major steps in the right direction. What these provide is the basis from which reasoned judgment can be applied. There is little point in even considering giving an opinion on a problem if one is standing on the extreme right or left of the common standard or has little exposure to the treatment or type of problem that forms the basis of the litigation. The "expert" value of the opinion will carry very little weight in a court of law.

Table 40.1 *Potential sources for medical litigation*

Acute pain	Chronic pain
Lack of consent	Personal injury
Complication of therapy	Inadequate preparation
Inappropriate treatment	Medical negligence
Assault	Work compensation
	Informed consent
	Unlicensed preparations

WHY DO PEOPLE COMPLAIN?

In an ideal world, all treatment would be successful and no complications would occur. In general, the public accept that life is imperfect and mistakes and errors occur. They see imperfection in every aspect of daily life and most are happy to accept that some problems and side-effects may occur as a result of medical treatment. However, it is when they feel that an injustice has been done that they choose to complain. Over 57% of patients take an action because they just want an answer. They feel that, for whatever reason, "the facts" have been hidden, obscured, or suppressed. They may also feel that the clinician is not sincere in his explanation.

Too often, doctors provide overoptimistic projections with regard to outcomes and can minimize the risks associated with procedures. So it is not surprising that a significant number of patients use the courts as means of financial redress.

A review of 227 patients who were claiming negligence highlighted some important issues.[5] Over 70% of the respondents had been seriously affected by the incidents leading to the litigation. The events had created long-term effects on work and social life. Often, the decision that finally determined legal action was the poor communication and insensitive handling of the original injury. Where explanations had been given, less than 15% were considered satisfactory. Four themes emerged from the analysis:

- concern with standards of care – to prevent future events occurring;
- an explanation – to know how and why the event happened;
- compensation for loss – pain, suffering, income, and future care;
- accountability – admission of fault, honesty.

WHAT DO THEY COMPLAIN ABOUT?

Motor vehicle accident and work-related injury represent the largest number of cases that involve persistent pain as a primary component (Table 40.2). The majority of these claims are settled "out of court," but nevertheless the process can be drawn out. Often, liability is admitted early on but agreeing the quantum can take many years. The defendants will always wish to leave a protracted period so that the maximum recovery will take place and disability will be minimized. The plaintiff may resist attempts to respond early, as it may appear to weaken their case.

It is now recognized that prolonged litigation leads to chronicity for both pain and disability.[6] Furthermore, the concept of "compensation neurosis" is ill founded because the emotional distress caused by the compensation process can produce long-term damage.[7]

Table 40.2 *Types of litigation: as presented to the author (1997–2000)*

Problem	Incidence	%
Work-related injury	32	37
Road traffic accident	16	18
Medical negligence		
Acute pain	14	16
Chronic pain	21	24
Lack of consent	1	1
Lack of care/treatment	3	3

WHAT SHOULD CONCERN THE EXPERT?

Standards of care

It should seem obvious that maintaining the highest standard of care would be normal. But, often, lapses in care, failure to carry out the expected preparatory work, failure to adhere to normal care pathways, and failure to even examine the patient have led to incidents occurring. Often, the doctor concerned knew what should have been done, but failed in the implementation. The expert in a report should seek to understand how the injury or event occurred and what omissions or failures by the doctor contributed to the event. However, this is not an opportunity for the expert to pursue a personal crusade or individual philosophy on a pattern of care. At all times, the expert has to acknowledge that reports are addressed to the courts and should always be impartial.

Personal loss and suffering

In an expert report, it will be necessary to assess the impact of the injury on the loss or distress experienced by the patient. The financial value of such a loss is for the court to determine. Nevertheless, it is reasonable to suggest how life has altered and what limitation is imposed on daily existence because of the personal injury. This may be a big concern where the symptoms and loss of mobility are great yet the physical findings are limited.

The subjective nature of pain may require a greater reliance on secondary characteristics such as anxiety and depression, avoidance behavior, elaborated responses, post-traumatic stress disorders, and sickness records for those who remain in employment.

Where an individual has become disabled, it will be important to bring out the impact that "carers" have on the home environment and activities. Likewise, it will be important to address the impact that the patients may have on the health provision service, such as the National Health Service (NHS) in the UK, and other social services.

Probably the most difficult area to assess is the impact

that the perception or symptom of pain has on functional capacity. Most chronic pain suffers will indicate that they do not undertake actions or tasks because doing so triggers or aggravates their pain. Often, the tasks may be very basic or trivial such as brushing teeth, combing hair, or putting on clothes. Such limitation in activity may prove difficult to explain in the absence of any recorded muscular or neurological disease. It will be necessary to explore with the patient, and record, all restrictions.

Nevertheless, the courts are well aware of the development of "illness behavior," and it is perfectly acceptable to link impaired functioning to the original injury or accident.

The competence or otherwise of the clinician

When one is assessing events it will be an important consideration to investigate the skill of the doctor in relation to specific treatments. If an adverse event occurs and the doctor is found to have undertaken only one or two such procedures then the background becomes important. One might wish to consider the training previously undertaken as well as any other supportive evidence of competency.

The suitability of the treatment that is planned or undertaken

In the UK, the advent of clinical governance and the establishment of NICE (National Institute for Clinical Excellence) altered the basis on which clinical decision-making is achieved. In the past, the "Bolam" concept[8] acknowledged that there could be differing clinical opinions. However, today, much greater emphasis will be placed upon what is felt to be the most appropriate course of action. When forming an opinion, all available resources will be studied, and it will be expected that the clinicians involved will have made themselves aware of the same information.

The only caveat to this view is that every opinion must be considered in the light of the information that was available at the time the injury to the plaintiff occurred. Over the period that a negligence claim may be pursued, opinions and information may change, and it would be unfair to review competence or treatment by present-day standards.

The nature of the incident or complication

All treatments carry a risk, and part of the process of informed consent is to identify as far as possible the known risks. If a complication is rare but has been described, it is less likely that claims for negligence will

arise unless it can be shown that the risk was increased because of a poor technique or because the treatment itself was inappropriate.

Where the complication is quite common, claims may arise because of the way that the problem was managed rather than for the event itself.

Informed consent

This is an issue that applies to both acute and chronic pain management. The difficulty for the clinician is to decide what level of detail should be provided to inform but not frighten patients. However, it has a wider remit than this. For a patient to make a valued judgment, he/she needs to know not only what can go wrong but also what the likelihood is that a particular treatment will prove efficacious. For example, to advise a patient that, following an epidural block with steroids (for back pain), there is a 1: 10,000 chance of a serious adverse event has a very different weighting from stating that only one in four patients will derive improvement not achieved by other means. A process of shared decision-making offers one method of improving consent.[9]

The assessment of risk, or more precisely the risk–benefit ratio, of treatment being worthwhile has yet to be fully evaluated. Systematic reviews and randomized controlled trials undoubtedly provide guidance. Unfortunately, many treatments for chronic pain have never been subjected to rigorous analysis. Sometimes, it is difficult to establish a control group (e.g. acupuncture); sometimes, because the control arm also involves an invasive procedure (e.g. radiofrequency lesion generation), it may not be possible to run a true double-blind study.

A recent document from the Department of Health provides a detailed analysis of how consent should be sought and also the issues relating to young people and those without independent capacity.[10]

Lack of consent

Most written consent forms that are signed by patients carry a caveat to "include all necessary procedures at the time of surgery." This is not an opportunity for clinicians to disregard their expected responsibilities. Issues can arise out of seemingly straightforward pain-relieving procedures.

One example might be the role of neural blockade in the anesthetized patient. If a block is performed after the patient has been put to sleep, although the laudable principle of providing perfect pain relief is commendable, such a technique may not be considered part of the basic anesthetic, which has already commenced. If the patient suffers nerve injury or finds the postoperative paralysis and anesthesia unacceptable, there are potentially grounds for complaint. Obtaining consent, written if necessary, in advance of the event will provide the only safe form of defense.

If nerve injury alone is the issue, occurring after a block performed on the conscious or unconscious patient, greater weight will be given in support of a technique involving stimulation and adherence to sound anatomical principles.[11]

Problems may also arise if a drug is used outside its "product license" and no advice to this effect has been given to the patient. Although it is recognized that a large number of older drugs are routinely given in this manner for the treatment of chronic pain, newer compounds cannot enjoy this "wide exposure" privilege.

Malingering: false claims

A small percentage of patients will exaggerate claims for the benefit of financial gain. This is more common in claims related to work injury and road traffic accidents. If the plaintiff feels aggrieved because a job has been lost, the injury was not their fault, or the employer made unreasonable demands or provided inadequate support and protection, one can understand how this emotional trigger will influence symptoms and behavior. This is the common presentation.

It is most unusual to see plaintiffs who clearly have "made the whole thing up." Insurance companies are always looking for these scenarios and invest considerable resources in investigating claimants. Video evidence is being used increasingly to observe claimants and defendants in their home environment. The findings can surprise even the most experienced medical examiner and can, on occasion, cause an expert to appear ill informed.

Sadly, this type of pernicious investigation of claimants only adds to the distress of the genuine plaintiff. It is a necessary consequence of any form of compensation process. Experts will be expected to view video evidence and provide suitable commentary.

CLINICAL GOVERNANCE

Clinical governance has a broad remit and covers all aspects of current medical practice. Its introduction has changed the way medicine is delivered. In time, it should help to clarify one of the key elements – "best practice." It is within this context that one should seek to look at the medicolegal basis upon which claims are based.

- Was there a duty of care?
- Upon whom did that duty lay?
- Was there a failure to fulfill that duty?
- Did actual harm occur?
- If there was a breach of duty, did it cause the damage?

Improving standards is a slow process and involves both willingness and a commitment by all staff to make the change. There are some useful drivers of change.

A complaints procedure

The establishment of a complaints procedure is a healthy sign. It encourages openness in practice, exposes shortcomings, and highlights failure in service. Learning from errors can lead to improvements, if positive changes in practice are adopted.

Not all complaints are valid, and the majority never result in litigation. Addressing issues early and expressing honest responses will defuse most situations. Such action will certainly aid in greater understanding and communication between the patient and the health care team, even if issues cannot be resolved.

Best practice

Best practice is an attempt to discover the consensus within a discipline or specialty for a particular practice or procedure. The strength of evidence to support a view can be determined. A systematic review, for example, would have high weighting. Such studies have their limitations, and sometimes when the evidence is in short supply it may be impossible to make a valued judgment on efficacy. A number of other measures need to be considered. Useful tools include clinical audit, complication rates, outcome studies, personal series, and individual case reports. All these help to generate a picture of the relevance of a particular treatment, and will enable the determination of indexes such as the NNT (number needed to treat) and NNH (number needed to harm).[12]

Clinical guidelines

Finally, it is possible to approach best practice by looking at clinical guidelines and trying to develop a process and pathway by which a treatment can be introduced or maintained within given parameters. This practice must also involve disregarding therapies that no longer have a place or have been shown to have extremely limited efficacy.

LEGAL STANDING

For many years, the basis on which medical negligence was assessed was based on the case Bolam v. Friern Barnet.[8] However, such an approach has been challenged and there have been recent changes in the law.

Bolam

The determination of negligence is for the courts. It is not the role of the clinician to apportion blame or culpability. The medical expert should attempt to give a balanced view of what is current best practice and what is perhaps appropriate for the level of skill and training of the doctor involved in litigation. It is acknowledged that the skill employed by a trainee doctor would in normal circumstances be less than that displayed by a consultant.[13]

Sometimes, it may be difficult to define an absolute course of action and the expert must give an opinion as to what he or she would have done in the same circumstances. Evidence to support such opinions is normally derived from published articles, although personal extensive experience with a procedure is always of additional merit.

It is easy to reflect on a particular event and be critical, however it is less easy to be analytical during the course of such an event.

Where the body of medical opinion supports a particular action, there is little difficulty. The problems tend to occur if less conventional approaches are adopted and something goes wrong. Then the decision might be to decide whether the issue was one of mishap or negligence.

To succeed in litigation, the plaintiff must be able to demonstrate that the defendant owed a legal duty of care. Furthermore, it must be demonstrated that such care fell below the standard required by the law and that the defendant could reasonably have foreseen that the careless behavior in question could have damaged the plaintiff. Damage must have occurred and a causal link between behavior and damage must be proved.

Nevertheless, "A doctor is not negligent, if he is acting in accordance with a practice accepted as proper by a reasonable body of medical men skilled in that particular art, merely because there is a body of such opinion that takes a contrary view."[8]

Consequently, it may prove difficult to demonstrate that a negligent act has occurred, although there are numerous areas for potential concern. Such a situation may result where a treatment performed to relieve pain has led to a serious or untoward complication. A claim could also result when the treatment itself is subject to debate or inadequate consent has been obtained.

Woolf recommendations

Since April 2000, the conduct of medical litigation has changed dramatically. It has been acknowledged that the process of "going to court" has become extremely costly. In the UK, the NHS has to put aside many millions of pounds to cover the cost of current cases trawling through the courts.

Lord Woolf[14] chaired a number of working parties on the subject of negligence in the UK. The groups concluded that the civil justice system had become excessively adversarial, slow, complex, and expensive. This was particularly true of medical negligence. There were five areas of great concern:

1　The relationship between the costs of the litigation and the amount involved was particularly disproportionate. The costs were particularly excessive in low-value cases.
2　The delay before claims were resolved was unacceptable.
3　Unmeritorious cases were pursued and clear-cut claims defended for longer than happens in other areas of litigation.
4　The success rate was lower than in other personal injury litigation.
5　The lack of cooperation between the parties to the litigation and the mutual suspicion as to the motives of the opposing party was frequently more intense than in other classes of litigation.

As a result of the working parties, a number of changes have been introduced, the effect of which has been to change and speed up the process:

1　The introduction of "fast track" mechanisms for minor cases.
2　Restrictions in the application of legal aid.
3　The development of mediation as an alternative to court.
4　The imposition of strict timetables by the courts on all aspects of cases.
5　The reduction in the number of expert witnesses that can be called.
6　The alternative use of a single "joint medical expert" by both parties.
7　Conferences of medical experts to agree the medical findings to minimize the need for court attendances.

Far too few treatments for chronic pain have been subjected to rigorous analysis, hence the risk for litigation is greater. In order to explore the likely areas of concern, it is appropriate to look at a range of common issues and cite examples. The majority of claims result from personal injury and loss of income from work-related incidents (Table 40.2). Nevertheless, claims for medical negligence are increasing.

The clinician may also become involved in assessing pain as part of a claim for personal injury or when determining the prognosis and future management of a patient suffering pain and disability from a work-related injury.

Acute pain management is not exempt either. Litigation may result from intraoperative pain procedures such as injections or blocks. It could also result from a failure to consent and has led on occasion to charges of assault. Claims may also arise because of ongoing symptoms following an otherwise normal procedure. Examples might include postspinal headache and low back pain following epidural anesthesia (Table 40.1). The presented cases demonstrate different facets of patient care, but the essential element is the evaluation of the validity of the treatment in the context for which it is being used.

PREPARATION OF THE REPORT

There are three principal elements to a report: (1) the history, (2) the physical and other finding, and (3) the comment and opinion.

Most medical reports are structured in this format. The content may well run to several thousand words, so it is important that the report is annotated effectively. This can be by paragraph, but it is often easier to number each individual statement or comment. Of course, one should use an easy-to-read type face and a font size that is appropriate. Double line spacing also adds to clarity.

Preparing a useful medical report involves time and deliberation. It is necessary to assess the injury and the circumstances around the event. Reference to General Practitioner (GP) records will give insight into the patient's past behavior and previous relevant problems. The history should be extensive – details of all relevant problems, events, investigations, treatments, and responses should be recorded. Consistency of these facts across all medical reports strengthens the plaintiff's or defendant's case.

The examination should be an opportunity to substantiate the patient's claims. Observing patients while they are waiting and as they undress are useful points. Invariably, lawyers will want assessments on disability and the duration of problems before recovery. These are often the most difficult estimates to make and largely depend on the personal experience of the examiner.

The inclusion of recognized scales can be useful:

- Depression (Beck)[15]
- Disability (Roland–Morris)[16]
- Health status (SF 36)[17]

When preparing the report, it is important to evaluate the validity of claims and the opinions of other experts. Reference to published studies is always extremely valuable. When drawing a conclusion, it is useful to record the initial problems and level of disability and to relate that to the recovery made up to the time of the examination. Giving a prognosis is difficult, and it is often more relevant to provide advice on further lines of support or treatment. However, when the prospects of further improvement are slim, this should be clearly stated.

HISTORY

The history is an opportunity to explore the background to the problem. The expert should gather as much infor-

mation as possible relating to the problem (Table 40.3). This is a time-consuming activity, but provides great understanding of the patient and the problem. Information should be recorded in chronological manner, and particular reference made to relevant issues. It is not appropriate to be judgmental. However, in a patient making a claim for a work-related back injury, it is essential to record past episodes of back pain – even previous claims. One will be asked to give an opinion as to the relative impact of past disease on the present complaint.

Previous behavior can provide an illuminating background on the patient. A history of relevant psychiatric disease or affective disorder will give an insight into the ability of the patient to manage "life events." Similarly, patients who are failing to cope will tend to consult their GPs frequently, often for relatively trivial concerns.

The sickness record is also an indicator to recovery. Patients who maintain a work ethic, even if the scale of duties is reduced, have a better prognosis. Those who remain off sick for 2 years or more are unlikely to return to useful employment.

The impact of previous treatment needs to be recorded.

The social and domestic framework in which the patient exists should be included. If the patient has been significantly disabled by the injury or condition, the social impact may be considerable (Table 40.4). There is often major disruption to life styles, there may be role reversal by family members, support needed for children,

Table 40.3 *Source information for medical reports*

GP records
Hospital notes
Nursing reports
Therapy reports (physiotherapy, occupational, etc.)
Accident and emergency records
Previous medical reports
Written correspondence
Social service reports

Table 40.4 *Social impact of injury*

Loss of employment	Income reduction
	Care assistants
Benefits cycle	Driving support
	Domestic cleaning
	Care facilities for children
	Meals preparation
	Bathing aids
	Boredom and depression
	Social isolation
	Family conflict
	Recrimination and anger
	Inability to enjoy social pleasure
	Dining, theatre, sports
	Impaired sexual relationships

and the individual may become socially isolated and depressed. All of these factors should be recorded in the body of the history.

THE EXAMINATION

This is the most critical part of the whole process and generally provides "the substance" to the claim. Here, there can be a factual representation of the plaintiff's problems.

A full physical examination is required, but emphasis must be placed on the musculoskeletal and neurological systems.

Neurological examination

One is looking for evidence of loss of function, including obvious sensory changes, failure of coordination, and any dissociative losses. One should observe the usual parameters, including reflexes, coordination, position sense, gait, and overall fitness.

Particular attention should be paid to the areas of distribution of the changes and whether they are consistent with nerve injury. The use of pain drawings can assist. Likewise, the availability of electromyograph (EMG) reports will add support to any conclusions.

The presence of altered sensation (allodynia and hyperalgesia) is very important, particularly when one is assessing neuropathic or complex regional pain syndromes. It may be necessary to resort to qualitative sensory testing to confirm the nature of small-fiber damage or sympathetic fiber impairment and the exact areas of distribution.

A simpler approach can be to measure the impairment of the sympathetic systems by testing the responses to heat and cold.

When there are advanced changes (e.g. Sudeck's atrophy), photographic evidence is invaluable.

Musculoskeletal system

One is obviously looking for physical deformity, loss of joint range, and evidence of disuse such as muscle wasting.

Simple measurement observations can be used to record the degree of restriction, such as flexion, extension, or rotation. Measuring muscle girth can assess evidence of muscle wasting. The more subjective measures of muscle power and muscle spasm should be recorded. There are a number of mechanical grip strength recorders available and these can be used. Various categorical scales are used to assess lumbar muscle spasm, but they remain very subjective.

It is necessary to differentiate whether or not the restrictions in movement are the result of the onset of pain or a consequence of a fixed deformity. One should look for inappropriate signs; these are particularly relevant in managing back-related problems.[18]

As many patients suffer from limited mobility, it is important to observe their locomotion and, in particular, how patients manage changes in posture, e.g. getting onto an examination couch or out of a chair,

Likewise, valuable information can be gleaned by the way the patient sits during the history-taking. Is there evidence of rigid posture, fidgeting, position changing, or other feature indicative of discomfort? In assessing illness behavior, is the plaintiff displaying evidence of elaborated responses, movements, or posture and using any support such as a splint, crutch, or corset?

THE CONCLUSION AND OPINION

The purpose of the report is to present to the court an analysis of the plaintiff's condition that is structured around the history and physical examination. It is then necessary to form an opinion as to how the present state arose and whether or not such a condition can be linked to any antecedent event. At all times, the report should be objective and succinct. It is often worthwhile attaching explanations for common conditions, such as illness behavior and neuropathic pain, by way of explanation.

If one is of the opinion that the plaintiff has suffered injury, it is imperative that one presents a suitable case by drawing out the salient facts and demonstrating a causal link. One should not only explore one's own personal experience but seek to back up any comment or view by reference to the published medical literature. It may also be relevant to include recommendations from professional bodies, such as national and professional medical societies.

Increasingly, the courts are requesting that medical experts meet after reports have been exchanged so that a joint statement can be produced identifying the areas of commonality and disagreement in the evidence.

Although this can help to reduce the attendance of experts in court, which is to be encouraged, it does sometimes diminish the possibility of a fuller explanation of events in the court.

Cases in which the primary complaint is pain are often the most difficult to present. The lack of physical signs and the subjective nature of symptoms can add to the confusion. Nevertheless, more reliance is now given to the behavioral aspects of cases, and psychologists are frequently consulted to add weight to the observation of the pain clinician. Likewise, the concept of post-traumatic stress disorder and somatoform pain disorder are more readily accepted.

Frequently, one is asked to give recommendations as to the prognosis and the eventual return of the plaintiff to a

Table 40.5 *Predicted work time loss after injury in years*

Condition	Persistent pain	Functional recovery	Full recovery
Simple fracture	No	1	1
Neuropathic pain	Yes	2	5
Low back pain	Yes	2	3–5
Acute sciatica	No	1	1
Back pain on benefit	Yes	10	?
Neuropathy	Yes	?	?
Fibromyalgia	No	3–5	5–7
Nerve entrapment	No	1–2	1–2

Functional recovery reflects the time period in which the plaintiff should be able to return to former or equivalent employment.

more normal existence. There are no hard rules and, frequently, the conclusion is based on the experience of the clinicians and their own clinical practice (Table 40.5).

Finally, it must be remembered that anything ones writes in a medical report may be studied very closely by lawyers for either party. Therefore, one must always be certain to check all direct statements for clarity and ensure that all opinions can be substantiated.

REFERENCES

1. Cochrane Collaboration. UK Cochrane Centre. *Bandolier* 1995; **16:** 7–8.
2. *Bandolier*. Evidence based everything. *Bandolier* 1995; **12:** 1.
◆ 3. Aikenhead AR. The pattern of litigation against anaesthetists. *Br J Anaesth* 1994; **73:** 10–21.
4. Coleman NA. Litigation in anaesthesia. *Br J Hosp Med* 1996; **55:** 62–4.
◆ 5. Vincent C, Young M, Phillips A. Why do people sue doctors? A study of patients and relatives taking legal action. *Lancet* 1994; **343:** 1609–13.
6. Mendelson G. Compensation and chronic pain. *Pain* 1992; **48:** 121–3.
7. Guest HG, Drummond PD. Effects of compensation on emotional state and disability in chronic back pain. *Pain* 1992; **48:** 125–30.
8. Bolam v. Friern Barnet. HMC 1957; 2 AER 118.
9. Charles C, Gafni A, Whelan T. Shared decision-making in the medical encounter: what does it mean? *Soc Sci Med* 1997; **44:** 681–92.
10. Department of Health. *Reference Guide to Consent for Examination or Treatment*. London: HMSO; 2001.
11. Chambers WA. Peripheral nerve damage and regional anaesthesia. *Br J Anaesth* 1992; **69:** 429–30.
12. Moore RA, McQuay HJ. Getting NNTs. *Bandolier* 1997; **36:** 1–3.
13. Dawson J. *Rights and Responsibilities of Doctors*. London: British Medical Association, 1998.
● 14. Woolf, Lord. Medics, lawyers and the courts. *J R Coll Phys* 1997; **31:** 686–93.
15. Richter P, Werner J, Heerlein A, *et al*. On the validity of the Beck Depression Inventory, a review. *Psychopathology* 1998; **31:** 160–8.
16. Stratford PW, Binkley J, Solomon P, *et al*. Defining the minimum level of detectable change for the Roland–Morris questionnaire. *Phys Ther* 1996; **76:** 359–65.
17. Ruta DA, Hurst NP, Kind P, *et al*. Measuring health status in British patients with rheumatoid arthritis: reliability, validity and responsiveness of the short form 36-item health survey (SF-36). *Br J Rheumatol* 1998; **37:** 425–36.
◆ 18. Waddel G, McCulloch JA, Kummel E, Venner RM. Non-organic physical signs in low back pain. *Spine* 1980; **5:** 117–25.

Index

Page numbers in **bold** refer to tables or boxes; page numbers in *italic* refer to figures. Abbreviations: PCA, patient-controlled analgesia; RCTs, randomized controlled trials; TENS, transcutaneous electrical nerve stimulation.

abdomen peripheral nerve blocks 215–218
    see also individual types
abdominal aortic dissection, celiac plexus block
    complications 250
abdominoperineal surgery, postoperative epidural analgesia 415
abnormal temporal summation, testing 34
acetaminophen (paracetamol), in children
    analgesia for patients 6 months or younger 438
    analgesia for patients over 6 months 434
    doses **435**
    rectal administration 432
acetylsalicylic acid, L'Abbé plot *499*
action potential stimulation therapy 344
acupuncture 355–379
    abbreviations to identify meridians **373**
    complications 357–358
        needle shock 357–358
    cun 357
        lengths *362–363*
    efficacy assessment in systematic review *503*
    endorsements in medicine 356
    energy (qi) 355
        channels 355
        deficiency 355
        excess 355
    mechanism of action 344
    needles 357
    neurohumoral response 356
    points **374–378**
        ankle *372, 373*
        anterior view of whole body *359*
        arm *368*
        elbow *368*
        face/head *364*
            anterior view *364*
            lateral view *366*
            posterior view *365*
            top of *365*
        foot *372, 373*
        hand *370*
        hip *372*
        knee *370, 371, 372*
        lateral view of whole body *361*
        leg *370, 371, 372*
        location 357
        neck *365*
        posterior view of whole body *360*
        scapula *369*
        shoulder *368, 369*
        spine *367*
        thigh *371*
        upper body *367*
    stimulation characteristics **349**
    treatment 356–357

        frequency of sessions 356
        needle insertion 356, 357
        patient assessment 356
        prescriptions **379**
        stimulation of needles 356
        symptom worsening after 356
        test period 356
    yin and yang 355
acute pain
    clinical RCTs 487–488
        see also clinical experimental pharmacological protocols
    neurophysiological mechanisms 27–28
        nociceptor activation 27
        sensitization of C-nociceptors 28
    opioids *see* opioids, acute pain management
    TENS indications 344
        experimental evidence 350–351
adaptation, biofeedback psychophysiological assessment 122
addiction, in opioid therapy 80
adenosine
    in experimental protocols 485–486
        acute tissue damage 485–486
        animal data 483–484
        combinations with other analgesics 484
        effect on allodynia development and pain scores **487**
        inflammatory pain RCTs 487–488
        intrathecal administration RCTs 488, 489
        intravenous administration RCTs 487–488, 489
        normal state 485
        pain-reducing effects **487**
        perioperative pain RCTs 488
        safety perspectives 485
    pharmacology 484
adenosine analogs, in experimental protocols, animal data 483–484
adrenaline *see* epinephrine
adrenal suppression, epidural steroid injection complication 423
affect, pain measure 5
age
    of children and analgesics *see* children
    effect on opioid pharmacokinetics 64
alcohol, neurolytic agent 198
alfentanyl 67–68
    intravenous, doses and paradigms 45
    pharmacokinetics 68
algometer, pressure threshold determination 32
allergic reactions, TENS complication 348
allodynia 28
ambulatory infusion of opioids, cancer pain management 71
amitriptyline, treatment schedule *103*
analgesia
    caudal *see* caudal analgesia
    in cryotherapy *see* cryoanalgesia
    development of novel drug from compound *488*

epidural *see* epidural analgesia
intraspinal *see* intraspinal analgesia
lumbar *see* lumbar analgesia
stimulation induced *see* stimulation-induced analgesia
subcutaneous infusions **89**
anesthesia
intrathecal catheterization 290
local *see* local anesthetics
angina pectoris, TENS 345
electrode positioning 348
experimental evidence 351–352
ankle
intra-articular injections 261, *262*
nerve blocks 229–230
anatomical aspects 229
complications 230
indications 229
landmarks and practical steps *229*
see also individual types
antiarrhythmics 108–109
adverse effects 109
contraindications 108
dosing and treatment schedule 108, **109**
pretreatment safety measures **109**
antidepressants 101–104
adverse effects 103–104
contraindications 102
dosing and treatment schedule 102
indications 101
see also individual types
antiemetics
inclusion in PCA solution 394–395
subcutaneous infusions **89**
antiepileptics 104–108
adverse effects 107–108
contraindications 105
dosing and treatment schedules 105–107, **106**
indications 104–105
pretreatment safety measures **106**
antisecretory agents, subcutaneous infusions **90**
antispasmodics, subcutaneous infusions in cancer pain
control 92
anxiety
cognitive theory 164
effect on pain perception 15–16, 114
in children 149
pain measure 5
relaxation induced 130
anxiolytics, subcutaneous infusions in cancer pain control 92
aorta dissection, celiac plexus block complications 250
arthropathy, exacerbation by intra-articular injections 259
articular cartilage, deterioration by intra-articular injections 259
aspirin, L'Abbé plot *499*
attention regulation in chronic pain 135–146
clinical case example 144–146
development of purposeful attention 145–146
phase I – reconceptualizing pain experience 136
acknowledging pain 137–138
complications 139
context 138–139
establishing rationale for self-management 138
giving difficult messages 138
reconceptualizing pain experience 138
understanding patient's expectations and pain
experience 138
phase II – developing awareness through objective
observation 136
clinical tools **141**

complications 140
delivery stages 139
practical tips 139
phase III – reengagement of attention to ability 136
clinical tools **142**
complications 140–141
delivery stages 140
practical tips 139, 140
phase IV – development of purposeful attention 136–137
clinical tools **142**
complications 143–144
delivery process 143
practical tips 141, 143
phase V – generalization and maintenance 137
clinical tools **143**
complications 144
delivery process 144
practical tips 144
treatment phases 136–137
application 137–144
avoidance, pain response 163
axillary block 208–210
in children 441
anatomical aspects 441
local anesthetic solution 441
method 441
landmarks and practical steps 208–210, *209, 211*

back pain
celiac plexus block complications 250
epidural steroid injection *see* epidural steroid injections
low *see* low back pain
bacterial infections, epidural steroid injection complication 423
bed rest 184
behavioral measures
child pain assessment 432, *433*
in pain-related fear *see under* pain-related fear
biliary tract, opioids' pharmacological effects 63
biofeedback 117, 121–133
in children 155–160
components of training 155–156
discern–control–generalize 156–157
integrated approaches 157–159
limitations 159–160
parental involvement 156
physiological modality 156
potential nonspecific pain control mechanisms 161
potential specific pain control mechanisms 160–161
practice 155–156
psychophysiologic profile 157
schedule 155
technique 156
training and professional certification 161
definition 121
evidence-based reviews 131–132
general approach 121–122
assumptions 121–122
indirect approaches 124
meta-analyses 131
average improvement rates **131**
modalities and abbreviations **155**
operations 121
psychophysiological assessment 122
adaptation 122
baseline 122
components 122–124, **123**
muscle discrimination 123–124
muscle scanning 123

reactivity 122–123
recommendations **124**
recovery 123
relaxation aid 124–125
electromyograph-assisted relaxation 124–125
skin conductance-assisted relaxation 125
skin temperature-assisted relaxation 125
select treatment considerations 125–130
autogenic training 127
coaching model 125–126
components of session 126
diaphragmatic breathing 127
education of patient 125
goals 126
imagery 126
learning and practicing skills 126
progressive muscle relaxation training 127–130, **128**
see also progressive muscle relaxation training
specific approaches 122–124, 130
headaches 130
bladder, opioids' pharmacological effects 63
bleeding disorders, spinal cord stimulation contraindication 382
Botox (BTX-A) 277
dosing guidelines for spasticity treatment **281**
preparation 278, **279**
botulinum toxin injections 277–283
additional treatments and outcomes 280
BTX-A Botox see Botox (BTX-A)
BTX-B Myobloc 277
contraindications **279**
dose selection 280
dosing guidelines for spasticity treatment **281**
duration of benefit 280
equipment and patient considerations 278–279
adverse effects 279, **279**
explanation of injections 279
requirements for EMG-guided injections **279**
topical anesthetic creams 278–279
historical aspects 277
mechanism of action 277–278, *278*
neuromuscular conduction inhibition 278
preparation 278, **279**
suboptimal response or treatment failure 280, 282
causes 280
guidelines for reducing resistance risk **282**
neutralizing antibody formation 280, 282
serological tests 282
test dose injections 282, *282*
techniques 279–280
EMG guidance 279–280
nontarget muscle testing 280
steps to ensure correct needle placement **280**
brachial plexus block 204–210
anatomical aspects 205–206, *206*
in children 441
complications **211**
indications 205
testing of four main peripheral nerves **207**
see also individual types
bradycardia, opioid induced 62
breakthrough pain
in cancer patients 470
in opioid therapy 80
oral transmucosal fentanyl citrate (OTFC) 470
breathing, diaphragmatic see diaphragmatic breathing
bubble blowing, in children 150
buccal delivery route in patient-controlled analgesia (PCA) 404
bupivacaine

alternative epidural analgesia 415
intracisternal infusion, indications for refractory pain 288
intrathecal administration
adverse effects 300
indications for refractory pain 286–288
peripheral nerve block agent 198
potentiation of epidural analgesia by epinephrine *411*
potentiation of epidural analgesia by fentanyl *411*
buprenorphine 68
butorphanol 68
transmucosal delivery in PCA 403

cancer pain
analgesia requirements 469–470
responsiveness 470
tolerance 470
variability 469–470
clinical trials see cancer pain clinical trials (below)
epidural treatment of refractory pain 308
instability 470
opioids see opioids, cancer pain management
pain intensity measurements 23
for patients with persistent pain 23
persistent 477–478
subcutaneous infusions 85–99
advantages 85
analgesia choice 88
assumptions 86
complications 96–98
drug reactions 97
equipment malfunction 96
prescribing errors 97–98
reactions at injection site 96–97
contraindications 86
drug combinations 92, **93–94**
drugs administered 88, **89–90**
drugs to be mixed with normal saline **92**
indications 86, **86**
initiation 95
managerial issues 98–99
guidelines 98
policies 98
procedures 98
protocols 98
standards 98–99
monitoring 95–96
nonopioid analgesics 91–92
opioids see opioids, subcutaneous infusions in cancer pain control
preparation of infusion 95
prescribing 95
priming and siting 95
syringe drivers 85
see also syringe drivers
temporal aspects 470
visceral, neurolytic blocks 247–253
see also individual types
cancer pain clinical trials 92, 95, 469–481
comparison groups 472
ethical issues 478–479
individual versus collective ethics 478
patient information and consent 479
placebo treatment 478–479
factors difficult to control 476–477
incidence of adverse effects 476
patient compliance 476–477
patient withdrawals 477
supplementary treatment 477

inclusion criteria and accretion of patients 475
  organ dysfunction patient exclusion 475
  problems 475
  terminal patient exclusion 475
pain assessment 471
  animal experiments 471
  evaluation instruments 471
  pain categories 469, 471
  pain experience *471*
  terminology 471
pain instability 470
polypharmacy as problem 471–472
  adjuvant analgesics 471–472
  drug interactions 472
requirements 472
selection and stratification of patients 474–475
  heterogeneity reduction strategies 475
  staging system 475
size and duration of study 475–476
  factors causing decreased accrual rate 476
  factors influencing number of subjects required 476
specific problems 477–478
  assessment of analgesic cost 478
  methodological 92, 95
  persistent/intractable cancer pain 477–478
study design issues 472–474
  cluster-randomized trials 474
  crossover designs 473–474, *474*
  enriched enrollment study designs 474
  historical control study designs 472–473
  parallel designs 473, *474*
  randomized controlled trials 473
  sequential trials 473
variability in analgesic requirements 469–470
carbamazepine
  adverse effects 107
  contraindications 105
  dosing schedule and pretreatment safety measures 105, **106**
cardiac arrhythmia, intravenous regional sympathetic block complication 245
cardiovascular system, opioids' pharmacological effects 62
caudal analgesia
  in children 442
  epidural steroid injections 418, 421
celiac plexus block 248–251
  anatomical aspects 248
  complications 249–250
    abdominal aortic dissection 250
    backache 250
    diarrhea 249, 250
    malposition of needle 250
    orthostatic hypotension 249, 250
    paraplegia and transient motor paralysis 250
    retroperitoneal hemorrhage 250
  drugs and dosing 249
  efficacy 250–251
  indications 248
  new perspectives 251
  persistent cancer pain 477–478
  technique 248–249
    needle placement and contrast medium spread *249*
central nervous system (CNS), opioids' pharmacological effects 62, 63
central sensitization 28
  experimental models illustrating 486–487, **487**
cerebrospinal fluid (CSF), production and loss 286
cervical hematoma, stellate ganglion block complication 239
cervical plexus block 203

anatomical aspects *204*
deep 203
  anatomical aspects 203
  complications 203
  landmarks and practical steps 203, *205*
indications 203
superficial 203
  anatomical aspects *204*
  landmarks and practical steps 203, *204*
cervical spine, radiofrequency lesioning 333
cervical zygapophyseal (facet) joints
  blocks 272–274
    evidence for use of 274–275
    intra-articular blocks 272–273
    medial branch blocks 273–274
    needle positioning *275*
    positioning of C-arm *274*
  denervation with radiofrequency lesioning 333–334
    adverse effects 334
    indications 333
    results 334
    technique 333–334, *334*
  dysfunction 190
    accompanying myofascial pain 190
    etiology 190
    referred pain 190
  pain 270
cervicothoracic sympathetic chain 237, *238*
  block *see* stellate ganglion block
chest wall rigidity, opioid induced 63
children
  analgesia for patients 6 months or younger 438–439
    systemic analgesia 438–439
    see also individual drugs
  analgesia routes 432–434
    epidural 433
    inhalation 433–434
    intramuscular 433
    intravenous 432
    oral 432
    rectal 432
    subcutaneous 432–433
  biofeedback *see* biofeedback, in children
  developmental issues 147–148
  hypnosis *see* hypnosis, in children
  intra-articular injections, evidence for use 256
  local anesthetic techniques 439–443
    epidural analgesia *see* epidural analgesia, in children
    in patients aged 6 months or younger 439–443
    peripheral nerve blocks **439,** 440–442
    see also individual blocks
  opioid analgesia *see* opioids, in children
  pain intensity assessment 21
  pain score–pain management action plan **434**
  procedures for pain management 431–445
    developmental level 431
    general considerations 431–434
    pain assessment 431–432
      see also pain assessment, in children
    planning 431
  relaxation *see* relaxation, in children
  self-regulation skills *see* self-regulation skills training, in children
  systemic analgesia for patients over 6 months 433–438
    adverse effects of opioid analgesia 436–437
      see also opioids, adverse effects
    alternative drugs for moderate to severe pain 437–438
    analgesics for mild to moderate pain 433–435, **435**

analgesics for moderate to severe pain 435–436
    systemic opioid infusions monitoring 437, **438**
    see also individual drugs
chronic pain
    attention regulation *see* attention regulation in chronic pain,
        phase I
    clinical pattern 135–136
    clinical RCTs 489
        see also clinical experimental pharmacological protocols
    cryoanalgesia 323–325
        duration of pain 325
        limitations 323
        patient education 324
        patient selection 323–324
        percutaneous technique 324
        risks 323
    distraction unsuitability for patients 135, 136
    opioids *see* opioids, chronic pain management
    pain intensity measurements 23
    TENS indications 344–345
        experimental evidence 351
    treatment protocols *see* opioids, in chronic nonmalignant
        pain (protocols)
circadian variation, effect on pain perception 16
cisterna magna 286, *287*
civil justice system 513
    areas of concern 513
    changes to speed up process 513
    see also medicolegal aspects
climatic conditions, effect on pain perception 16
clinical experimental pharmacological protocols 483–493
    acute pain studies 487–488
        inflammatory pain 487–488
        intrathecal administration 488
        intravenous administration 487–488
        perioperative pain 488
        postoperative analgesia 488
    adenosine 485–486
        see also adenosine
    animal data 483–484
        adenosine and adenosine analogs 483–484
        adenosine combinations with other analgesics 484
        general interpretation 484
    background 485
        research 483
    central sensitization models 486–487, **487**
    chronic pain studies 488
        intrathecal administration 488
        intravenous administration 488
    correlation between animal models and clinical problem 487
    development of novel drugs from compound to analgesic *488*
    ethical, regulatory and financial considerations 491
        flow chart for evaluation of RCTs *491*
    interpreting data 490–491
    pharmacology of substances 484
    pitfalls in results 490–491
    qualitative and quantitative sensory assessments **486**
    safety perspectives 484–485
    study design techniques and considerations 489–490, *490*
        basics 489
        gender aspects 489–490
        parallel groups or crossover *490*
        substances *491*
    see also clinical trials
clinical governance *see under* medicolegal aspects
clinical neurophysiology *see* neurophysiological techniques
clinical trials 449–459
    analgesia onset 456–457

assay sensitivity 450
blinding and unblinding of treatment 454
cancer pain *see* cancer pain clinical trials
crossover designs 454–455, 473–474, *474*
    four-group complete **455**
    problems 454–455
    three-group complete **455**
    typical two-treatment **455**, *474*
dental pain 462–463
    see also dental pain model
evoked pain 457
    nature of mechanical stimulus and proposed research
        tools **458**
experimental pharmacological protocols *see* clinical
    experimental pharmacological protocols
explanatory and pragmatic studies 449–450, **450**
global assessment 457
inclusion of patients 454
long-term trials 457
outcomes for use in meta-analysis 457
outcomes of pain treatment trials 455
    meaningful endpoints 455
pain intensity *451,* 455
    clinically important reduction 455
    difference (PID) *456*
    summed difference (SPID) *451,* 456
parallel design 454–455, 473
    three-treatment assessment *474*
placebo
    active 454
    cancer pain and ethical issues 478–479
    dental pain model 466
    essentiality of knowing response 453
    treatment ethicality 454
primary efficacy variable choice 450
publishing 458
purpose of study 450
quality of life assessment 457
randomization 454
remedication time 457
repeated measurements 456
rescue analgesia consumption 456
    difference in pain intensity and morphine
        consumption *456*
result possibilities **458**
statistical issues 458
study design 450
    balanced design 455
    parallel or crossover studies 455–456, *490*
treatments and controls choice 450–453
    additive effects 453
    equivalence trials 452
    isobologram *453*
    relative potency *452,* 452–453
    superiority studies *451,* 452
    synergy 453
clonidine, analgesia for children over 6 months 438
cluster headache, radiofrequency lesioning indication 331
cluster-randomized trials, in cancer pain clinical trials 474
Cochrane Collaboration 509
codeine 66
    in children
        analgesia for patients 6 months or younger 439
        analgesia for patients over 6 months 434
        doses **435**
    synthetic derivatives 67
        see also oxycodone; tramadol
cognitive measures of pain 5–6

cold
  pain condition 356
  physiotherapy agent 185
communication, in physiotherapy 179–180
complex regional pain syndromes
  intravenous phentolamine indication 42
  sympathetic block indication 235–236
concurrent validity, pain measure 10
confrontation, pain response 163
constipation, opioid induced 63
convulsions, opioid induced 62
coping, pain measure 6
cordotomy, percutaneous cervical see percutaneous cervical
  cordotomy
cortical pain modulation 113–114
  inhibition of pain response 114
corticosteroids
  historical aspects 255
  intra-articular administration see intra-articular injections
  subcutaneous infusions in cancer pain control **90,** 92
cough, opioid induced 62
crossover studies see under clinical trials
cryoanalgesia 185, 198–199, 319–326
  chronic pain see under chronic pain
  clinical applications 322
  comparisons 324–325
    phenol neurolysis 324–325
    radiofrequency neurolysis 325
  duration of freeze 320
  historical aspects 319
  lesion size 320
  machinery 320–322
    see also cryoprobes
  percutaneous technique 324
  physics and physiology of freezing 319–320
    cryolesioning 320
    ice ball formation 319–320
    ice crystal formation 319
    nerve regeneration 320
  postsurgical see under postoperative pain management
cryoneurolysis 322
cryoprobes 320–322
  change of phase type 320, 321
  gas expansion type 320–322, 321
    characteristics **322**
    ice ball shapes 321
    tip geometry 321–322
cutaneous field stimulation 186, 344
cutaneous nerve blocks
  lateral see lateral cutaneous nerve
  medial see medial cutaneous nerve
  posterior see posterior cutaneous nerve

dampness, pain condition 356
dental pain model 461
  advantages 462
  clinical trials 461–468
    baseline pain intensity as confounding factor 465, 465
    downside assay sensitivity 465
    exclusion criteria 464
    improving and documenting assay sensitivity 464
    inclusion criteria 464
    operative procedures 463
    pain intensity rating comparisons between analgesics 466
    patient compliance with protocol 463
    patient information, consent, and monitoring 463
    patient understanding of instructions 463

placebo control 466
    practical tips 467
    protocol and good trial practice 462–463
    rescue analgesic drug 466
    upside assay sensitivity 465–466
  crossover design 461–462
  limitations 462
  parallel group design 462
  surgical removal of impacted third molars 461, 461
    indications **463**
depression
  effect on pain perception 16, 114
  pain measure 5
diamorphine 66–67
  alternative epidural analgesia 415
  pharmacokinetics 67
diaphragmatic breathing
  biofeedback component 127
  in children 149–150
diarrhea, celiac plexus block complications 249, 250
diclofenac, in children, doses **435**
disease interactions, effect on opioid pharmacokinetics 64
distal radioulnar joint, intra-articular injections 266
distraction, unsuitability for chronic patients 135, 136
dorsal column stimulation see spinal cord stimulation
dorsal root ganglion (cervical), radiofrequency lesioning 334–335
  adverse effects 335
  contraindication 334
  efficacy of treatment 335
  indication 334
  technique 334–335
    cannula introduction 335, 336
    diagnostic root blocks 334–335
    electrode position 335, 336
    "tunnel-vision" projection 335, 335
dorsal root ganglion (lumbar), radiofrequency lesioning 337–338
  contraindication 337
  efficacy of treatment 338
  indication 337
  technique 337–338
    diagnostic root blocks 337
    electrode positioning 338
drug interactions, effect on opioid pharmacokinetics/
  pharmacodynamics 64, **65**
dural puncture
  epidural steroid injection complication 423
  intrathecal catheterization technique 290
    adverse effects 300–301
dural tap, spinal cord stimulation complication 388
dynamic pain, relief with epidural analgesia 409

education, patient see patient(s), education
ejaculatory failure, lumbar sympathetic block complication 243
elbow
  intra-articular injections 264–265
    lateral epicondyle 264–265, 265
    medial epicondyle 265
    posterior approach 264, 265
  nerve blocks 210–213
    anatomical aspects 211
    indications 210
    see also individual types
elderly, pain intensity assessment 21
electrical-evoked potentials 34–35
electrical muscle stimulation (EMS) 186
electrical stimulation 185–186
electromagnetic fields 186

electromyograph-assisted relaxation 124–125
electrotherapeutic techniques 185–186
emotion, pain measure 5
endorphins, release during acupuncture 356
enriched enrollment study designs, in cancer pain clinical
  trials 474
epidural analgesia 409–416
  abdominoperineal surgery 415
  alternative mixtures 415
  in children 442–443
    administration 433
    caudal approach 442
    drug doses and infusion rates 443, **443**
    lumbar and thoracic approach 442–443
    urine retention 443
  closed delivery system *413*
  dynamic pain relief 409
  epinephrine
    effectiveness increase 412
    importance in efficacy/safety of postoperative
      analgesia 413
    no decrease in spinal cord blood flow 412–413
    safety increase 412
  local anesthetics 409, 410
    complications 410
  lower limb surgery 415
  monitoring 413–414
  necessary requirements for successful management
    program 414
  optimizing efficacy and safety 410–411, *411*
  outcome 413–414
  patient-controlled, for postoperative pain relief 413–414
  prescription for safe and effective delivery 413–414
  for refractory pain *see* epidural treatment of refractory pain
  risks to patient 410
  steroid addition *see* epidural steroid injections
  thoracic or lumbar catheter choice 409–410
epidural opioids
  adverse effects 312–313
    hypotension 313
    nausea and vomiting 313
    pruritus 313
    respiratory depression 312–313
    see also opioids, adverse effects
  algorithm for instituting therapy **310,** *311*
  complications 410
  doses and regimens **312**
epidural space scarring, spinal cord stimulation
  contraindication 382
epidural steroid injections 417–427
  anatomical aspects 417–418
  complications 423–424, **424**
    additives in preparation 423
    incidence 424
    local anesthesia induced 423
    mechanical aspects 423
    misplacement of drugs 424
    steroid induced 423
  contraindications 419
  drugs used 422–423
    injectate 422
    local anesthetics 422
    steroid preparations 422
  evidence for particular therapy or drug 424–425
    meta-analyses 424–425
    RCTs 424–425
  historical aspects 417
  imaging techniques 422

indications 418–419
  sciatica 418
number and frequency of injections 419
preparation 419–420
  of equipment 420
  of patient 419–420
technique 420–422
  caudal approach 418, 421
  general 421
  lumbar approach 417–418, 421
  monitoring 421
  perineural and periradicular injections 421
epidural treatment of refractory pain 307–317
  advantages and disadvantages **308**
  adverse effects 311–313
    infections 311–312
    mechanical problems 311–312, **312**
    pharmacological 312–313
      see also epidural opioids, adverse effects
  algorithm for instituting opioid therapy **310,** *311*
  catheter and pump selection 313–315
  clinical settings 308–310
    cancer pain 308
    nonmalignant pain 308–310
  contraindications 310–311
    to epidural catheter 310
    to running an infusion 311
  doses and regimens 311, **312**
  drugs used **307**
  efficacy 316
  indications for long-term therapy 308, 310
    in nonmalignant pain **309**
  indications for medium-term therapy **310**
  intrathecal comparison **308,** 316
  patient selection 310
  practical tips 315
    advice to patients with implantable pumps 315
    gas-driven pumps 315
  pump classification 313–315
    delivery system classification 313–315
  role of intraspinal pumps **309**
  techniques
    implanted pumps 315, *315*
    insertion of tunneled catheter *314*
    Port-A-Cath ports 314
    totally implanted systems 314–315
epinephrine
  epidural, spinal cord blood flow not decreased 412–413
  increased effectiveness of epidural infusion *411,* 412
    potentiation of epidural analgesia by fentanyl *411*
    potentiation of epidural analgesia from bupivacaine and
      fentanyl *411*
  increased efficacy/safety of prolonged postoperative epidural
    analgesia 413
  increased safety of bupivacaine and fentanyl epidural
    analgesia 412
ethical issues
  cancer pain clinical trials *see* cancer pain clinical trials
  clinical experimental pharmacological protocols 491
ethical review board (ERB), experimental protocol review 491
E-TRANS® **402**
evidence-based medicine *495,* 495–496
expert medicolegal report 509–516
  conclusion and opinion 515–516
    predicted work time loss after injury **516**
  examination 515
    musculoskeletal system 515
    neurological 515

history 514–515
    previous behavior 514
    sickness record 514
    social impact of injury **514**
    source information for medical reports **514**
    preparation 514
    see also medicolegal aspects
explanatory studies 449–450, **450**

faces pain scale *19*
    child pain assessment 432, *433*
facet joints *see* zygapophyseal joints
facet joint syndrome 269
fascia iliaca compartment block, in children 440
    anatomical aspects 440
    local anesthetic solution 440
    method 440
fear, pain-related *see* pain-related fear
Fear-Avoidance Beliefs Questionnaire 166
Fear of Pain Questionnaire 165
femoral nerve block 221–222
    anatomical aspects 221
    complications 222
    indications 221
    landmarks and practical steps 221–222, *222*
fentanyl 67
    in children
        analgesia for patients over 6 months 436
        intravenous infusion protocols **437**
    oral *see* oral transmucosal fentanyl citrate (OTFC)
    pharmacokinetics 67
    potentiation of epidural analgesia by epinephrine *411*
    potentiation of epidural analgesia from bupivacaine and
        epinephrine *411*
    transdermal, patient-controlled analgesia (PCA) 402
    transmucosal delivery in PCA 403
fibromyalgia, exaggerated reaction to muscle stimulation 35
foot, intra-articular injections 261–262
    metatarsophalangeal joint of hallux 261–262
forearm, nerve block *see individual nerve blocks*

gabapentin
    adverse effects 107
    contraindications 105
    dosing schedule and pretreatment safety measures **106,** 107
ganglion impar block 252–253
    anatomical aspects 235, 252
    technique 253
        needle placement *253*
Gasserian ganglion, radiofrequency lesioning 330–331
    adverse effects 331
    anatomical aspects 330
    complications and incidence 331
    discomfort to patient 331
    historical aspects 330
    indication 330
    results 331
    technique 330
        electrical stimulation 330
        general anesthesia administration 330
        needle insertion 330, *331*
        projection of needle-electrode 330, *331*
gastrointestinal tract
    opioids' pharmacological effects 62–63
    patient-controlled analgesia (PCA) route 402
gate control theory
    descending inhibition of pain 114

role in TENS development 343
gender, effect on pain perception 16
genitofemoral nerve *244*
    block 218
        anatomical aspects 218
        complications 218
        indications 218
        landmarks and practical steps 218, *219*
    neuralgia, lumbar sympathetic block complication 243
genitourinary system, opioids' pharmacological effects 63
Gillette test 190
glenohumeral joint, intra-articular injections 263
    anterior approach 263, *264*
    posterior approach 263, *263*
    RCTs 255
Graseby syringe drivers *87*
guanethidine, intravenous regional sympathetic block 243–244,
    245
    duration 244

hand, intra-articular injections 266–267
    metacarpophalangeal joint 266–267, *267*
    proximal interphalangeal joint 267
headaches
    biofeedback 130, 158
    cluster, radiofrequency lesioning indication 331
    tension type, improvement rates from meta-analyses **131**
head and neck peripheral nerve blocks 200–203
    see also individual types
health care resources, pain measures 8
heat
    pain condition 356
    physiotherapy agent 185
heat stimulation, abnormal sensory disturbances *33*
hematoma, cervical, stellate ganglion block complication 239
hepatic disease, effect on opioid pharmacokinetics 64
high-velocity, low-amplitude thrust 191
hip, unloading effect on *184*
historical control study designs, in cancer pain clinical trials 472–
    473
hoarseness, stellate ganglion block complication 239
Horner syndrome, stellate ganglion block complication 239
hydrocodone, in children
    analgesia for patients over 6 months 434–435
    doses **435**
hydromorphone 66
    analgesia for children over 6 months 436
hyperalgesia 28
hyperesthesia, postsympathectomy, lumbar sympathetic block
    complication 243
hyperventilation, diaphragmatic breathing in children 150
hypervigilance 164
hypnoanalgesia 151–152
    see also hypnosis
hypnosis 115–116
    in children 116, 150–155
        emergency situations 152
        goal 151
        hypnoanalgesia 151–152
        intramuscular injections positions 153
        limitations 159–160
        mechanisms of change 160–161
        pain switch technique 151
        potential nonspecific pain control mechanisms 161
        potential specific pain control mechanisms 160–161
        preschool patients 152–153
        school-age and adolescents 153–154
        self-regulatory techniques as aid in diagnosis 154–155

training 161
trance 151
components of pain treatment utilizing self-hypnosis **115**
mechanisms 115, 116
    controlled dissociation 115
    cortical effects 116
    imaging and metaphors 115
    muscle relaxation 115
    perceptual alteration 115
process *152*
of self *see* self-hypnosis
hypogastric plexus, superior 251
    block *see* superior hypogastric plexus block
hypotension
    opioid-induced 62
        epidural infusion 313
    orthostatic
        celiac plexus block complications 249, 250
        intravenous regional sympathetic block complication 245

ibuprofen, in children, doses **435**
iliohypogastric/ilioinguinal nerve block 218
    anatomical aspects 218
    in children 440
        anatomical aspects 440
        complications 440
        local anesthetic solution 440
        method 440
    complications 218
    indications 218
    landmarks and practical steps 218, *219*
ilioinguinal nerve block *see* iliohypogastric/ilioinguinal nerve
    block *(above)*
imagery, biofeedback component 126
imipramine, treatment schedule *103*
infants, pain intensity assessment 21
infections
    bacterial, epidural steroid injection complication 423
    intra-articular injection complications 259
    intrathecal catheterization adverse effects 301–302
    spinal cord stimulation complication 388
    systemic, spinal cord stimulation contraindication 381
inflammatory pain, randomized controlled trials in acute
    pain 487–488
informed consent 511
    in cancer pain clinical trials 479
    in dental pain clinical trials 463
    lack of 511–512
    in opioid therapy 80–81
infraclavicular block 208
    landmarks and practical steps 208, *209*
infraorbital nerve block 201
    in children 440–441
        anatomical aspects 440–441
        local anesthetic solution 441
        method 441
    landmarks and practical steps 201
inhalation administration of drugs
    in children 433–434
    patient-controlled analgesia route 401–402
intercostal nerve block 216
    anatomical aspects 216
        branches **216**
    in children 441–442
        anatomical aspects 441
        catheter techniques 441
        local anesthetic solution 442
        method 441–442

paravertebral block 441
subcostal block 441
complications 216
cryoanalgesia for post-thoracotomy 322–323
indications 216
    local anesthetic and steroid block 216
    local anesthetic block 216
    neurolytic block 216
landmarks and practical steps 216, *217*
    anterior approach 216
    midaxillary approach 216
    posterior approach 216
interference, pain measure 8
interferential therapy 344
internal consistency, pain measure 9
interphalangeal joint, proximal, intra-articular injections 267
interpleural analgesia (IPA) 247
interpleural block 216–218
    anatomical aspects 217
    complications 217–218
    contraindications 217
    indications 216–217
        cancer pain 217
        chronic pain 216
        postsurgical analgesia 216
    landmarks and practical steps 217, *218*
interpleural phenol blocks 247–248
    complications 248
    drugs and dosing 247–248
    efficacy 248
    technique 248
interrater reliability, pain measure 9–10
interscalene block 206–207
    landmarks and practical steps 206, *207*
interventional techniques, persistent cancer pain 477
intra-articular blocks 227–229
    cervical zygapophyseal (facet) joints 272–273
    complications 229
    indications 227
    landmarks and practical steps 227–229, *228*
    lumbar zygapophyseal (facet) joints 272
intra-articular injections 255–268
    in children, evidence for use 256
    complications 259
    contraindications 258–259
    drugs 259–260
    equipment 259
    evidence for effectiveness 255–256
        in children 256
        glenohumeral joint RCTs 255
        lateral epicondyle elbow pain RCTs 256
        osteoarthritis RCTs 256
        subacromial injection RCTs 255–256
    general principles 256–257
        aseptic technique 256
        counseling of patient 256–257
        mechanisms of action 256
    historical aspects 255
    indications 258
    joint injection methods 260–267
        ankle 261, *262*
        see also individual joints
    technique 257–258
        correct placement 257, **258**
        delivery methods 257, **258**
        frequency 257
        preparation 257
intra-articular sepsis, intra-articular injection

contraindication 258
intracisternal treatment, of refractory pain 285–305
    advantages 303
    adverse effects 302–303
    anatomical aspects 286, *287*
    bupivacaine test 295
    bupivacaine treatment 295
    care of patient and infusion system 298, 300
        dressing tunnel exit 298
        exchanging bacterial filter 298
        exchanging infusion container 300
        taking a shower 300
    clinical results **299**
    historical aspects 286
    indications 288
        malignant pain 288
        nonmalignant pain 288
    insertion complications **297**
    limitations 288
    solutions 295, 297
        bupivacaine 295
        buprenorphine 297
        mixtures of opioid/bupivacaine 297
        morphine 295, 297
    technique 295
        catheter direction 295
        catheter endpoint 295, *296*
        insertion site 295, *296*
intramuscular administration of drugs
    in children 433
    opioids, acute pain management 70
intranasal patient-controlled analgesia (PCINA) *403*, 403–404
    system characteristics **404**
intraspinal analgesia 307
    opioids, cancer pain management 71
    role of pumps in pain management **309**
    see also entries beginning with epidural and intrathecal
intrathecal treatment, of refractory pain 285–305
    advantages 303, **308**
    advantages of external versus internal catheters/pumps 303–304
        large reservoir volumes 303–304
        lower costs 304
        PCA option 304
        reduced complications 303
        reduced technical failures 303
        simplicity 304
    adverse effects 300–302
        from bupivacaine 300
        from catheterization 300–302
        equipment related 302
        from morphine 300
    anatomical aspects 286, *286*
    care of patient and infusion system 298, 300
        dressing tunnel exit 293, *294*, 298
        exchanging bacterial filter 298
        exchanging infusion container 300
        taking a shower 300
    clinical results **299**
    disadvantages 304, **308**
        epidural comparison 304
        external versus internal catheters/pumps 304
    efficacy 304–305
        epidural comparison 304
        external versus internal catheters/pumps 304–305
    epidural comparison 304, **308**, 316
    guidelines for adjustment 297–298
    high cervical bupivacaine test 295

    high cervical catheterization technique 295
        adverse effects 302–303
        catheter direction 295
        catheter endpoint 295
        insertion site 295
    historical aspects 285–286
    indications 286–288
        malignant pain 287
        nonmalignant pain 287
    insertion complications **297**
    limitations 288
        malignant pain 288
        nonmalignant pain 288
    solutions 295, 297
        bupivacaine 295
        buprenorphine 297
        mixtures of opioid/bupivacaine 297
        morphine 295, 297
    technique 288–295
        anesthesia 290
        connecting infusion pump 293
        connecting Millipore filter 293, *294*
        dressing incisions and tunnel exit 293, *294*, 298
        dural puncture 290
        equipment 288–289
        fixing catheter to skin 293, *294*
        imaging/location technique 289
        insertion of catheter 291
        instructing patient and next of kin 293, 295
        instructing ward personnel 293, 295
        landmarks and insertion sites 289–290
        location for catheterization procedure 289
        monitoring 289
        patient preparation 288
        Portex tunneling device 291, *292*
        position of patient and operator 289, *290*
        postcatheterization care 295
        preparation of operation site 289
        skin incision at insertion site 291, *292*
        substituting for spilt cerebrospinal fluid 293
        testing catheter patency 291, *291, 293*
        tunneling catheter 291–292, *292*
intravenous administration of drugs
    in children 432
    patient-controlled analgesia (PCA) 395
    randomized controlled trials in acute pain 487–488
intravenous alfentanyl, doses and paradigms 45
intravenous opioids 44–45
    acute pain management 70
    adverse effects 45
    background 44–45
    contraindication 45
    doses and paradigms 45
    indication 45
    practical tips 45
intravenous regional sympathetic block 243–245
    adverse effects 245
    guanethidine 245
        duration 244
    technique 245
ischemic pain
    adenosine effect on allodynia development and pain scores **487**
    TENS 352
IsoMed implantable pump *315*

joints
    complications of intra-articular injections 259

manipulation with anesthesia (MUJA) 192
    sepsis, intra-articular injection contraindication 258
    see also individual joints

ketamine
    analgesia for children over 6 months 437–438
        protocol for morphine combined infusions **438**
    intravenous 43–44
        adverse effects 44
        background 43
        contraindications 44
        doses and paradigms 44
        indications 43–44
        pharmaceutical considerations 44
        practical tips 44
    subcutaneous infusions in cancer pain control 92
ketobemidone 68
    pharmacokinetics 68
ketorolac
    in children, doses **435**
    subcutaneous infusions in cancer pain control 91
kidney disease, effect on opioid pharmacokinetics 64
kinesiophobia 163
knee
    intra-articular injections 260–261
        anterior approach 260–261, *261*
        medial and lateral approaches 260, *261*
        RCTs 256
    nerve blocks 227–229
        anatomical aspects 227
        indications 227
        see also individual types

Labat method of nerve block *see* cervical plexus block, deep
L'Abbé plots 498–499, *499*
labor pain, TENS 351
lamotrigine
    adverse effects 107
    contraindications 105
    dosing schedule and pretreatment safety measures **106,** 107
large intestine, opioids' pharmacological effects 62
laser-evoked potentials 35
laser therapy 186
    low-level (LLLT) 186
lateral cutaneous nerve
    forearm blockade 212
        landmarks and practical steps 212
    thigh blockade 223
        anatomical aspects 223
        complications 223
        indications 223
        landmarks and practical steps 223, *224*
lateral epicondyle, intra-articular injections 264–265, *265*
    RCTs 256
legs *see* lower limbs
levobupivacaine, peripheral nerve block agent 198
levorphanol 67
lidocaine 108
    intravenous 40–42, 108
        adverse effects 41, 109
        background 40
        bolus regimen 40
        contraindications 40
        doses and paradigms 40–41
        dosing and treatment schedule 108, **109**
        evidence for efficacy 41–42
        four-hour infusion 41
        indications 40

    pharmaceutical considerations 41
    practical tips 41
    pretreatment safety measures **109**
    short infusion regimen 40–41
    peripheral nerve block agent 197
    systemic 108
        actions 53
        contraindications 108
limb nerve blocks 219–230
    lower 219–230
    upper 204–214
    see also individual types
liver disease, effect on opioid pharmacokinetics 64
local anesthetics
    blocks *see* peripheral nerve blocks
    in children *see* children, local anesthetic techniques
    epidural analgesia 409, 410
    in epidural steroid injections 422
    joint manipulation (MUJA) 192
    lumbar sympathetic block dose 242
    sympathetic blockade 237
low back pain
    chronic, pain-related fear 164
        see also pain-related fear
    radiofrequency lesioning indication 336
lower limbs
    diffuse pain, radiofrequency lesioning indication 338
    epidural analgesia after surgery 415
    leg length difference 190–191
    peripheral nerve blocks 219–230
        see also individual types
low-level laser therapy (LLLT) 186
lumbar analgesia
    in children 442–443
    epidural steroid injections 417–418, 421
lumbar plexus block 219–220
    anatomical aspects 219
    complications 220
    indications 219
    landmarks and practical steps 219–220, *220*
        distal technique 220
        paravertebral technique 220
        psoas compartment technique 220
lumbar spine, radiofrequency lesioning 336
lumbar sympathetic block *241,* 241–243
    agents 243
    complications 243
    continuous 242
    local anesthesia dose 242
    neurolytic block 243
    single needle injection 243
    technique 241–242, *242,* 243
lumbar zygapophyseal (facet) joints
    blocks 272
        evidence for use of 274–275
        intra-articular blocks 272
        medial branch blocks 272
        needle positioning *273*
        positioning of C-arm *273*
    denervation with radiofrequency lesioning 336–337
        adverse effects 337
        efficacy of treatment 337
        indication 336
        technique 336–337, *337*
    dysfunction 190
    pain 270
lumbosacral plexus, peripheral branches blockade 221–227
    femoral branch *see* femoral nerve block

lateral cutaneous nerve of thigh *see* lateral cutaneous nerve, thigh blockade
  obturator branch *see* obturator nerve block
  posterior cutaneous nerve of thigh 227
  sciatic branch *see* sciatic nerve block

McGill pain questionnaire 18–21, *20–21*
  construct validity 21
  predictive validity 19, 21
  present pain intensity (PPI) ratings 19
  short form 21, *22*
  strengths 21
  test–retest reliability 21
  weaknesses 21
malingering (false claims) 512
manipulation 191
  of joints with anesthesia (MUJA) 192
manual medicine 183, 189–193
  complications 192
  imaging studies 191
  management 191–192
    articular procedures 191
    high-velocity, low-amplitude thrust 191
    muscle energy technique 191
    myofascial release 192
    soft-tissue techniques 191
  manipulation of joints with anesthesia (MUJA) 192
  results 192
  structural diagnosis of syndromes 189–191
    cervical zygapophyseal (facet) joint dysfunction 190
    lumbar zygapophyseal (facet) joint dysfunction 190
    sacroiliac joint dysfunction 190–191
    thoracic zygapophyseal (facet) and rib dysfunction 190
    see also individual syndromes
manual therapy (MT) *see* manual medicine
massage 185
medial cutaneous nerve, forearm blockade 212
  landmarks and practical steps 212
medial epicondyle, intra-articular injections 265
median nerve block
  at elbow 212
    landmarks and practical steps 212, *212*
  at wrist 213
    landmarks and practical steps 213, *214*
medical exercise therapy (MET) 183
  shoulder rotator device *183*
medical products agency (MPA), experimental protocol review 491
medicolegal aspects 509–516
  clinical governance 512
    best practice 512
    clinical guidelines 512
    complaints procedure 512
  concerns to expert 510–512
    competence or otherwise of clinician 511
    informed consent 511
    lack of consent 511–512
    malingering (false claims) 512
    nature of incident or complication 511
    personal loss and suffering 510–511
    standards of care 510
    suitability of treatment 511
  expert report *see* expert medicolegal report
  legal standing 512–514
    Bolam 513
    Woolf recommendations 513–514
  litigation
    context of complaints 510

    potential sources **509**
    reasons for complaints 510
    types **510**
  see also expert medicolegal report
meningitis, intrathecal catheterization adverse effect 302
mental nerve block 200
  landmarks and practical steps 200
meperidine (pethidine) 67
  acute pain management 69
  adverse effects 67
  analgesia for children over 6 months 436
  pharmacokinetics 67
  transmucosal delivery in PCA 403
meta-analysis 457, 498–501
  in biofeedback 131, **131**
  data analysis 498–501
    confidence intervals 500–501
    heterogeneity 500
    intervention effectiveness 500
    intervention safety 501
    L'Abbé plots 498–499, *499*
    number needed to harm (NNH) 501
    number needed to treat (NNT) 500
      see also number needed to treat (NNT)
    statistical significance 499–500
  epidural steroid injections 424–425
  quality control 498
    Oxford Quality Rating Scale **498, 499**
  see also systematic reviews
metacarpophalangeal joint, intra-articular injections 266–267, *267*
metatarsophalangeal joint of hallux, intra-articular injections 261–262
methadone 67
  analgesia for children over 6 months 436
  equianalgesic dose ratio 472
  pharmacokinetics 67
mexiletine 108
  adverse effects 109
  contraindications 108
  dosing and treatment schedule 108, **109**
  pretreatment safety measures **109**
microneurography 35
migraine
  antidepressants indication 101
  antiepileptic indication 107
  biofeedback 158
  improvement rates from separate meta-analyses **131**
mindfulness-based stress reduction 117
minimal effective analgesic concentration (MEAC) of opioids 66
mobilization 191
molars, surgical removal of impacted third molar 461, *461*
  indications **463**
  see also dental pain model
mood alterations, opioid induced 62
mood disorders and pain 114
  see also anxiety; depression
morphine 66
  acute pain management 69
  alternative epidural analgesia 415
  in children
    analgesia for patients 6 months or younger 439, **439**
    analgesia for patients over 6 months 435
    intravenous administration protocols **437**
    monitoring for patients on systemic infusions 437
    protocol for ketamine combined infusions **438**
  intrathecal administration, adverse effects 300
  intravenous

administration protocols in children **437**
    doses and paradigms 45
pharmacokinetics 66
pharmacological effects 62–63
    skin 63
postoperative analgesia RCTs 488
preparations 66
synthetic derivatives 66–67
    see also diamorphine; hydromorphone; oxymorphone
muscle discrimination training
    biofeedback psychophysiological assessment 123–124
    progressive muscle relaxation training addition 129
muscle energy technique 191
muscle pain 29
    experimental methods and models 29
muscle relaxation, in children 150
    progressive training *see* progressive muscle relaxation training
muscle scanning, biofeedback psychophysiological
    assessment 123
musculoskeletal pain
    physiotherapy 181
    TENS indication 344
        experimental evidence 351
musculoskeletal system, examination for expert medicolegal
    report 515
Myobloc (BTX-B) 277
    dosing guidelines for spasticity treatment **281**
    preparation 278, **279**
myofascial pain, TENS indication 344
    experimental evidence 351
myofascial release 192

nalbuphine 68
naloxone 68
    pharmacokinetics 68
naltrexone 68
narcosis, opioid-induced 90
nasal administration of drugs
    opioids
        acute pain management 70
        cancer pain management 71
    patient-controlled analgesia transmucosal route 401
nausea
    opioid induced 62, 437
        epidural infusion 313
    PCA induced, management 398
    TENS reduction in postoperative expulsions 350–351
neck peripheral nerve blocks 200–203
    see also individual types
needle phobia 149
needle shock 357–358
nerve blocks, pain diagnosis 49–56
    difficulties with use 49
    historical aspects 49
    patient selection and preparation 50–51
    procedural guidelines 51, **51**
        block validation 51
        imaging assistance 51
    prognostic interpretation 55
    response assessments and outcome monitoring 51
        pain scores 51
        physiological measures 51
    response interpretation 54–55
        common misconceptions **54**
        "straight line" concept of pain 54
    response patterns 52–54
        aberrant solution spread 53–54
        abnormal conduction pathways 54

"bag of tricks" 52
        desired block if successful 52–53
        neuronal desensitization 54
        operator variability 54
        patient misrepresentation 54
        placebo responses 53
        procedural failure 54
        systemic actions of lidocaine 53
    scope 50, **50**
    sites **50**
nerve blocks, therapeutic *see* peripheral nerve blocks;
    sympathetic blocks; *individual blocks*
neuritis, postprocedural complication of zygapophyseal
    blocks 274
Neurobloc (BTX-B) 277
    dosing guidelines for spasticity treatment **281**
    preparation 278, **279**
neuroendocrine system, opioids' pharmacological effects 62
neurography 34
neurological examination, for expert medicolegal report 515
neurolytic blocks 198–199, 247–254
    agents 198
        alcohol 198
        phenol 198
    complications 237
    of lumbar sympathetic ganglia 243
    of stellate ganglion 240
    techniques 198–199
        cryoanalgesia 198–199
        pulsed radiofrequency 199
    verification of blocking solution 237
    see also peripheral nerve blocks; *individual types*
neuropathic pain 29–30
    antidepressants indication 101
    characteristics **30**
    diagnosis 27, 30
    intravenous lidocaine indication 40
    opioids, treatment protocols for chronic pain 77
    sensory abnormalities 27, 30, **30**
    tactile sensibility reduction 31
    TENS indication 344
        experimental evidence 351
    transient postsympathectomy, lumbar sympathetic block
        complication 243
    types 29–30
neurophysiological techniques 27–38
    conventional 34–35
        neurography 34
        sensory-evoked potentials 34–35
    microneurography 35
    see also sensory testing
nitrous oxide
    in cryoanalgesia 321
    inhalation in children 433–434
nociceptive pain 29
    in cervical area, radiofrequency lesioning indication 334
    nociceptor sensitization 28, 29
    opioids, treatment protocols for chronic pain 77
nociceptors
    activation in pain 27
    sensitization 28, 29
    silent 27–28
nonmalignant pain
    chronic *see* chronic pain
    epidural treatment of refractory pain 308–310
        indications **309**
    treatment protocols for opioids *see* opioids, in chronic
        nonmalignant pain (protocols)

non-neoplastic pain, treatment indications for opioids in chronic
  pain 78
nonsteroidal anti-inflammatory drugs (NSAIDs)
  in children
    analgesia for patients 6 months or younger 438
    analgesia for patients over 6 months 434
    rectal administration 432
  subcutaneous infusions in cancer pain control 91
    toxicity 91–92
normeperidine, acute pain management 69
number needed to treat (NNT) 500
  calculation 500
  limitations 501
  systematic review examples **501**
numerical rating scale (NRS) 17
  dental pain assessment 463
nurse-controlled analgesia (NCA), analgesia for children over 6
  months 436

obturator nerve block 222
  anatomical aspects 222
  complications 222
  indications 222
  landmarks and practical steps 222, *223*
occipital nerve block 200
  anatomical aspects 200
  complications 200
  indications 200
  landmarks and practical steps 200, *201*
opioids 59–76, **72–73**
  acute pain management 69–70
    administration routes 70
    choice of agent 69
    dosage/schedule 69–70
  addiction (psychological dependence) 65, 80
  administration routes
    acute pain management 70
    cancer pain management 70–71
  adverse effects 63, 80–81, 436–437
    breakthrough pain 80
    central nervous system 62, 63
    constipation 63
    drug treatment **438**
    of epidural analgesia *see* epidural opioids, adverse effects
    nausea and vomiting 62, 437
    pruritus 63
    respiratory depression 80, 437
  cancer pain management 70–71, 74
    administration guidelines 71, 74
    administration routes 70–71
    choice of agent 70
    WHO analgesic ladder 70, *71*
  in children 74–75
    analgesia for patients 6 months or younger 439
    analgesia for patients over 6 months 435–436
    dosage and administration routes **436**
    dosing guidelines 74–75
    guidelines 74
    monitoring for patients on systemic infusions 437, **438**
    patient-controlled analgesia (PCA) 435–436
    tolerance 74
  in chronic nonmalignant pain *see* opioids, in chronic
    nonmalignant pain (protocols)
  chronic pain management 74
    aberrant drug-related behavior monitoring **75**
    guidelines 74
  classification systems 59, **60**
  clinical applications 69–75

epidural *see* epidural opioids
indications
  intrathecal administration for refractory pain 286–288
  for long-term use in chronic non-neoplastic pain 78
intravenous *see* intravenous opioids
mechanism of action 59–62
in percutaneous cervical cordotomy 330
pharmacodynamics 66
  drug- or age-induced alterations **65**
pharmacokinetics **65,** 65–66
  drug- or age-induced alterations **65**
  factors influencing 64
pharmacological effects 62–63
  cardiovascular system 62
  central nervous system 62
  gastrointestinal system 62–63
  genitourinary system 63
  respiratory system 63
  skin 63
pharmacology 66–68
  agonist–antagonist drugs 67
  antagonists 67
  naturally occurring alkaloids 66
  synthetic compounds 67
  synthetic derivatives of codeine 67
  synthetic derivatives of morphine 66–67
physical dependence 64–65, 80
pseudoaddiction 80
receptors 59–62, **61**
  delta (δ) 60
  epsilon (ε) 60
  kappa (κ) 60
  mu (μ) 60
  opioid-like receptors (OLR) 61
  presynaptic *61*
  sigma (σ) 60
reduced consumption effect on patient outcome 251
subcutaneous infusions in cancer pain control **89**
  opioid-naive subjects 90
  opioid switching 88–90
  prescribing 88–90
  unresponsiveness 91
switching, in cancer pain management 90
terminology 59
tolerance 64, 80
  management 64
toxicity 90–91
  management 91
transdermal PCA delivery 402
transmucosal PCA delivery 402–404
vulnerability of patients to compliance problems 78–79
withdrawal syndrome 64–65, 80
  clinical manifestations 64
  management 65
see also individual drugs
opioids, in chronic nonmalignant pain (protocols) 77–83
  acute pain episode treatment 81–82
    case history 81–82
    comments 82
  complications 80–81
    see also under opioids
  drug-related behaviors causing concern 81
  evidence base 79
    assessment of opioid response 79
    guidelines 79–80
    justification for maintenance of opioid therapy 79
    maintenance opioid therapy 79–80
  indications for long-term use in non-neoplastic pain 78

neuropathic pain 77
nociceptive pain 77
patient information and consent 80–81
selection of patients, implementation and follow-up 78–79
   determination of improvements in pain and quality of life 78
   vulnerability to compliance problems 78–79
opiophobia, in cancer patients 477
oral administration of drugs
   in children 432
   opioids
      acute pain management 70
      cancer pain management 70
   patient-controlled analgesia (PCA) 402
      bedside delivery 404
      transmucosal delivery route 401
oral transmucosal fentanyl citrate (OTFC) 404, *404*
   breakthrough pain management 470
orthoses 184
orthostatic hypotension *see* hypotension, orthostatic
osteoarthritis, intra-articular injections, RCTs 256
outcome
   botulinum toxin injections 280
   clinical trials 457
   effect of reduced opioid consumption 251
   epidural analgesia 413–414
   monitoring in nerve blocks in pain diagnosis 51
   pain treatment trials 455
   patient(s), effect of reduced opioid consumption 251
oxcarbazepine
   adverse effects 107
   contraindications 105
   dosing schedule and pretreatment safety measures 105, **106,** 107
Oxford Quality Rating Scale **498**
   scoring of items **499**
oxycodone 67
   in children
      analgesia for patients over 6 months 434–435
      doses **435**
oxymorphone 66

pacemaker
   spinal cord stimulation contraindication 382
   TENS contraindication 345
pain
   attention to 114
      regulation in chronic pain patients *see* attention regulation in chronic pain
   behavioral responses 163
   blood stagnation 355–356
   categories 28, 469
      see also individual types
   cold condition 356
   conditions 28–29
   cortical modulation 113–114
   damp condition 356
   diagnosis, nerve blocks for *see* nerve blocks, pain diagnosis
   heat condition 356
   meaning of 114
      differences in analgesia requirements 114
   memory of 16
   mood disorders and 114
      see also anxiety; depression
   neurophysiological mechanisms 27–28
   somatosensory evaluation 28
Pain and Impairment Relationship Scale (PAIRS) 165
Pain Anxiety Symptoms Scale (PASS) 165

pain assessment
   in children 431–432
      behavioral measures 432, *433*
      self-reporting 432, *433*
      somatosensory evaluation 28
pain behavior 6
pain catastrophizing 163–164
pain experience 4, 113, 147, *471*
   reconceptualization 136
      see also attention regulation in chronic pain
pain intensity *451*
   clinically important reduction 455
   measurements 15–26, 455
      assessment at extremes of age 21, 23
      cancer pain 23
      chronic pain 23
      difference (PID) calculation **24**
      faces pain scale *19*
      memory of pain 16
      nonverbal patients 21
      results, interpretation and handling 24–25
      scales 16–18
         see also individual types
      serial measures of pain 23–24
      total pain relief (TOTPAR) calculation **24**
      visual analog toy *19*
      see also McGill pain questionnaire
   summed differences (SPID) *451,* 456
pain intensity differences (PID) 23, *456*
   calculation **24**
pain measures 3–14
   behavior and activity 6–8
      compound measures 6, 8
      health care resources 8
      interference 8
      pain behavior 6
      quality of life *see* quality of life
      satisfaction 8
      third-party-defined outcomes 8
   biomedical domains 4–5
      see also pain experience; pain relief
   content 3–8
   outcome domains 3, 4–8
   estimating change or difference 11–13
      clinical significance 11
      example 12–13
      raw data plots *12*
      type I errors 11
      type II errors 11
   fear of pain
      movement/(re)injury and pain catastrophizing *172*
      severity *172*
   of function and disability **7**
   histogram of score change with treatment *12*
   nonoutcome variables 8
   psychometric qualities and interpretation of output 3, 9–13
   psychosocial domains 5–6
      affect or emotion 5
      cognitive measures 5–6
      coping 6
   reliability 9–10
      internal consistency 9
      interrater 9–10
      test–retest 9
   scatterplot of pretreatment and post-treatment scores *12*
   selection and application 3–14
      considerations 3–8
      method of measurement 4

sensitivity to change 10–11
  validity 10
    concurrent 10
    cut-off points 10
    divergent 10
pain perception 114
  factors affecting 15–16
    anxiety 15–16
    childhood experiences 15
    circadian variation 16
    climatic conditions 16
    depression 16
  somatic 114
pain-related fear 163–176
  attention 164
  characteristics 163–164
    escape/avoidance behaviors 164
    kinesiophobia 163
    pain catastrophizing 163–164
  cognitive–behavioral assessment 165–168, *167*
    behavioral tests 168
    determining treatment goals 167–168
    graded hierarchies 168
    interview **166,** 166–168
    specific questionnaires 165–166
      see also individual scales
  disconfirmation of harm beliefs 164–165
    match/mismatch model 164
  education 169
  effectiveness 173–174
    crossover design studies 173
    daily measures of fears and pain catastrophizing *173*
  graded exposure *in vivo* 169–172
    behavioral experiments 169
    case illustrations 169–171
    complicating factors 171–172
    daily measures of fear of pain severity *172*
    example dialogue in behavior experiment **171**
    exposure 169, 172
    graded activity comparison 165
    maintenance of change 172
    systemic desensitization 169
  graded hierarchies 168
    example patients **170**
  pathways for acquisition of excessive pain 169–171
    case illustrations 169–171, **170**
pain relief 4–5
  cold application *see* cryoanalgesia
  postoperative, with patient-controlled epidural analgesia
    (PCEA) 413–414
  total (TOTPAR), calculation **24**
pain schools 182
pain switch technique 151
paracervical block 231–232
  anatomical aspects 231
  complications 232
  indications 231
  landmarks and practical steps *231,* 231–232
paracetamol *see* acetaminophen (paracetamol)
paresthesia, stellate ganglion block complication 239
parallel studies *see under* clinical trials
paraplegia, celiac plexus block complications 250
parents, involvement in biofeedback in children 156
patient(s)
  education
    in biofeedback 125
    in cryoanalgesia 324
    in pain-related fear 169

    in PCA 394
  epidural analgesia risks 410
  information on dental pain clinical trials 463
  outcome, effect of reduced opioid consumption 251
  physiotherapy demands 186
  vulnerability to opioid compliance problems 78–79
patient-controlled analgesia (PCA) 393–399
  alternative delivery systems 401–405, **402**
    applied anatomy 401–404
    contraindications and limitations 404, **404**
  analgesia for children over 6 months 435–436
  background 393–394
  buccal and sublingual delivery systems 404
  equipment and drugs 394
  gastrointestinal route 402
  guidelines 394
  inhalation route 401–402
  intranasal (PCINA) devices *403,* 403–404
    system characteristics **404**
  intravenous 395
    advantages 395
    disadvantages 395
  management of adverse effects 398
    nausea and vomiting 398
    pruritus 398
    respiratory depression 398
    sedation 398
  monitoring 395–398
    chart *396–397,* 397–398
    regular observations 397–398
  nasal transmucosal route 401
  oral route 402
    bedside delivery 404
    transmucosal delivery 401
  patient information 394
  practical points and protocols 393–399
  relative potency decision 453
  safety criteria 393–394
  setting up 394–395
    antiemetic inclusion 394–395
    background infusions 394
  staffing and training 394
  subcutaneous 395
    advantages 395
    disadvantages 395
  transdermal route 401
    ideal drug properties **403**
    iontophoretic systems **402**
    opioid delivery 402
  transmucosal opioid delivery 402–404
    ideal drug properties **403**
    oral and nasal routes 401
patient-controlled epidural analgesia (PCEA), postoperative pain
  relief 413–414
patient-controlled intranasal analgesia (PCINA) devices *403,* 403–
  404
  system characteristics **404**
pediatric pain management *see* children
pelvic peripheral nerve blocks 230–232
  see also individual types
penile dorsal nerve blocks, in children 440
  anatomical aspects 440
  complications 440
  local anesthetic solution 440
  method 440
pentazocine 68
  pharmacokinetics 68
percutaneous cervical cordotomy 328–330

adverse effects 329
anatomical aspects 328
complications and incidence 329
discomfort to patient 329–330
historical aspects 327, 328
indications 328
limitations 328
results 329
technique 328–329
electrode guiding needle 328–329, *329*
visible three lines 328, *329*
peri-articular sepsis, intra-articular injection
contraindication 258
perineal visceral pain, ganglion impar block 252–253
see also ganglion impar block
perioperative pain, RCTs in acute pain 488
peripheral nerve blocks 197–232
agents and techniques 197–200
aseptic technique 199
general principles 199–200
insulated or noninsulated needles 199
local anesthetics 197–198
see also individual agents
needles 199–200
nerve location by peripheral nerve stimulation 199
neurolysis 198–199
see also neurolytic blocks
resuscitation equipment 199
in children **439,** 440–442
see also individual types
diagnostic *see* nerve blocks, pain diagnosis
head and neck blocks 200–203
lower limb blocks 219–230
pelvic blocks 230–232
thorax and abdomen blocks 215–218
upper limb blocks 204–214
see also individual types
peripheral nerve stimulation
historical aspects 343
nerve location 199
insulated or noninsulated needles 199
peroneal nerve block
at ankle 230
landmarks and practical steps *229,* 230
at knee 227
landmarks and practical steps 227, *228*
pethidine *see* meperidine
pharmacological diagnostic tests 39–47
intravenous drug challenges 39
advantages 39
disadvantages 39–40
quantitative sensory testing (QST) combination 39
see also individual intravenous drugs
phenol
interpleural blocks *see* interpleural phenol blocks
lumbar sympathetic block agent 243
neurolytic agent 198
cryoanalgesia comparison 324–325
phentolamine, intravenous 42–43
adverse effects 43
background 42
contraindications 42
doses and paradigms 42–43
efficacy 43
indications 42
pharmaceutical considerations 43
practical tips 43
phenytoin

adverse effects 107
contraindications 105
dosing schedule and pretreatment safety measures 105, **106**
Photograph Series of Daily Activities (PHODA) 168, *168*
physical dependence, in opioid therapy 80
physical therapies 182–183
McKenzie approach 183
medical exercise therapy (MET) 183
shoulder rotator device *183*
physicians, physiotherapists cooperation 186
physiotherapy 179–187
causal treatment 181–184
cognitive interventions 181–182
ergonomic advice 182
manual therapy 183
see also manual medicine
physical training 182–183
see also physical therapies
psychomotor physiotherapy 184
relationship to pain and tissue capacity *182*
examination 180–181
clinical findings 181
clinical history 181
interdisciplinary cooperation 186
demands on patient 186
with physician 186
pain and 179–180
acute and chronic differentiation 180
communication 179–180
symptomatic treatment 184–186
massage 185
physical agents 185–186
unloading 184, *184*
treatment process 179, *180*
placebo blocks
medial branch blocks 271
zygapophyseal joints injections 271
placebo responses, nerve blocks for pain diagnosis 53
placebo trials *see* clinical trials
pneumothorax, stellate ganglion block complication 240
polyneuropathy, antiepileptic indication 105
polypharmacy, problem in cancer pain clinical trials 471–472
popliteal fossa block 227
complications 227
landmarks and practical steps 227, *228*
Port-A-Cath ports 314
Portex tunneling device 291, *292*
posterior cutaneous nerve
forearm blockade 212–213
complications 213
thigh blockade 227
postherniorrhaphy pain
diagnostic nerve block 50
ilioinguinal nerve block 322
postoperative pain management
cryoanalgesia 322–323
ilioinguinal nerve block 322
intercostal nerve block 322
open technique 323
randomized controlled trials in acute pain 488
postsympathectomy hyperesthesia, lumbar sympathetic block
complication 243
post-thoracotomy pain
diagnostic nerve block 50
intercostal nerve block 322–323
postural hypotension *see* hypotension, orthostatic
pragmatic 450, **450**
pregnancy, TENS contraindication 345

prescribing errors, subcutaneous infusions 97–98
pressure threshold, determination with algometer 32
prilocaine, peripheral nerve block agent 197–198
progressive muscle relaxation training 127–130, **128**
    abbreviated muscle groups **129**
    in children 150
    initial muscle groups and procedures for testing 127, 129,
        129
    muscle discrimination training addition 129
    number of sessions 129
    practice 129
    relaxation-induced anxiety 130
propoxyphene 67
propranolol, adverse effects 43
proximal interphalangeal joint, intra-articular injections 267
pruritus
    opioid-induced 63
        epidural infusions 313
    PCA-induced, management 398
pseudoaddiction, in opioid therapy 80
psychological dependence, in opioid therapy 80
psychomotor physiotherapy 184
psychophysiologic profile in biofeedback see biofeedback
pudendal nerve block 230–231
    anatomical aspects 230
    complications 231
    indications 230
    landmarks and practical steps 230, 230–231
pulsed radiofrequency 199
pupils, opioid-induced 62

qi (energy) see acupuncture
quality of life 6
    assessment 457
    determination of improvements with opioid therapy 78
quantitative sensory testing (QST) 31
    pharmacological diagnostic test combination 39

radial nerve block
    at elbow 212
        landmarks and practical steps 212, 212
    at wrist 213
        complications 213
        landmarks and practical steps 213, 214
radicular pain, radiofrequency lesioning indication 337
radiocarpal joint, intra-articular injections 265–266, 266
radiofrequency lesioning 327–340
    in cervical area 333
    clinical application in pain 327–328
    contraindications **328**
    equipment **328**
    of Gasserian ganglion see Gasserian ganglion
    historical aspects 327
    in lumbar area 336
        dorsal root ganglia see dorsal root ganglion (lumbar)
        sympathetic ganglia see sympathetic ganglia (lumbar)
    opioid administration 330
    percutaneous
        cervical cordotomy see percutaneous cervical cordotomy
        of cervical dorsal root ganglia see dorsal root ganglion
            (cervical)
        cervical zygapophyseal joint denervation see under cervical
            zygapophyseal (facet) joints
        lumbar zygapophyseal joint denervation see under lumbar
            zygapophyseal (facet) joints
    of sphenopalatine ganglion see sphenopalatine ganglion
    theoretical aspects 327
    tissue heating 327

vertebrogenic pain treatment see vertebrogenic pain
radiofrequency neurolysis, cryoanalgesia comparison 325
radioulnar joint, distal, intra-articular injections 266
Raggedy Ann, relaxation technique in children 150
Raj nerve block technique see infraclavicular block
randomized controlled trials (RCTs)
    acute pain 487–488
    in cancer pain clinical trials 473
    chronic pain 489
    epidural steroid injections 424–425
    intra-articular injections 255–256
rectal administration of drugs
    in children 432
    opioids, acute pain management 70
refractory pain (malignant and nonmalignant)
    cancer pain clinical trials 477–478
    epidural treatment see epidural treatment of refractory pain
    intracisternal catheterization see intracisternal treatment, of
        refractory pain
    intrathecal catheterization see intrathecal treatment, of
        refractory pain
regulatory issues, clinical experimental pharmacological
    protocols 491
relative potency assay 452, 452–453
relaxation
    anxiety induction 130
    biofeedback aid see biofeedback, relaxation aid
    in children 150
        muscle relaxation 150
        progressive relaxation 150
        Raggedy Ann 150
    electromyograph assisted 124–125
    skin conductance assisted 125
    skin temperature assisted 125
reliability, psychometric pain measure 9–10
remifentanil 68
    pharmacokinetics 68
renal disease, effect on opioid pharmacokinetics 64
respiratory arrest, TENS complication 349
respiratory depression
    opioid induced 45, 63, 80, 437, 439
        epidural infusion 312–313
    PCA-induced, management 398
respiratory disease, effect on opioid pharmacokinetics 64
respiratory system, opioids' pharmacological effects 63
responsiveness, in cancer pain management 470
retinal hemorrhage, epidural steroid injection complication 423
retroperitoneal hemorrhage, celiac plexus block
    complications 250
rib and thoracic zygapophyseal (facet) dysfunction 190
ropivacaine
    alternative epidural analgesia 415
    peripheral nerve block agent 198

sacral plexus block 220–221
    anatomical aspects 220–221
    complications 221
    indications 220
    landmarks and practical steps 221, 221
sacroiliac joint dysfunction 190–191
    Gillette test 190
    leg length difference 190–191
    shear dysfunction 191
saphenous nerve block
    at ankle 229
        landmarks and practical steps 229, 229
    at knee 227
        complications 227

landmarks and practical steps 227, *228*
satisfaction, pain measure 8
sciatica 418
    epidural steroid injection *see* epidural steroid injections
sciatic nerve block 223–226
    anatomical aspects 224
    anterior approach 225–226
        landmarks and practical steps 225–226, *226*
    complications 226
    indications 224
    lateral approach 226
        landmarks and practical steps 226, *226*
    lithotomy approach 225
        landmarks and practical steps 225, *225*
    posterior approach 224
        landmarks and practical steps 224, *225*
sedation, PCA induced, management 398
sedatives, subcutaneous infusions in cancer pain control **89,** 92
selective serotonin reuptake inhibitors (SSRIs) 101
    adverse effects 104
    contraindication 102
    dosing and treatment schedules 102, **103**
    pretreatment safety measures **103**
self-hypnosis **115,** 116
    analgesia comparison with PCA 116
    frequency 116
self-regulation skills training **148**
    in adolescents
        benefits 148–149
        hypnosis 153–154
    in adults 113–119
        attention to pain 114
        managing expectancy 117
        meaning of pain 114
        mindfulness-based stress reduction 117
        mood disorders and pain 114
        "rehabilitation" model 117
    in children 147–162
        aid to hypnosis in diagnosis 154–155
        anxiety, fear, and pain 149
        benefits 148–149
        bubble blowing 150
        common features 161
        conditions suitable for aid **148**
        diaphragmatic breathing 149–150
        mechanisms of change 160–161
        procedures for which approaches are helpful **148**
        theoretical rationale 160–161
    see also biofeedback; hypnosis; relaxation; self-hypnosis
sensory-evoked potentials 34–35
sensory qualities 30
sensory testing 27–38
    abnormal temporal summation testing 34
    basis 30–31
    evaluation of pain 28
    future perspectives in advanced testing 35–37
        combination with patient history and examination 35
        semiconductor lasers *36,* 37
        thermode stimulators based on heat-foil technology 36, *36*
    goal 30
    pressure threshold determination with algometer 32
    tactile sensibility estimation with von Frey filaments 31
    thermotest *see* thermotest
    vibratory threshold determination with vibrameter 31–32
    see also neurophysiological techniques
sepsis
    in joints, intra-articular injection contraindication 258

spinal cord stimulation contraindication 381
sequential trials, in cancer pain clinical trials 473
serotonergic syndrome 102
serotonin and norepinephrine reuptake inhibitors (SNRIs) 101
    adverse effects 104
    contraindication 102
    dosing and treatment schedules 102, **103**
    pretreatment safety measures **103**
shear dysfunction 191
short therapy (ST) 186
shoulder
    intra-articular injections 262–263
        glenohumeral joint *see* glenohumeral joint
        subacromial bursa *262,* 262–263
    rotator device *183*
skin
    burn, TENS complication 348
    irritation, TENS complication 348
    opioids' pharmacological effects 63
skin conductance-assisted relaxation 125
skin temperature-assisted relaxation 125
small intestine, opioids' pharmacological effects 62
sodium valproate
    adverse effects 107
    contraindications 105
    dosing schedule and pretreatment safety measures **106,** 107
spasticity
    botulinum toxin injections dosing guidelines **281**
    epidural treatment of refractory pain 309
    TENS indication 344
sphenopalatine ganglion, radiofrequency lesioning 331–332
    anatomical aspects 331
    complications and incidence 332
    efficacy of treatment 332
    historical aspects 331
    indications 331
    results 332
    technique 331–332
        anesthesia administration 331
        electrode projection 331–332, *332*
        projection of sphenopalatine fossa 331, *332*
spinal accessory nerve block 202–203
    anatomical aspects 202
    complications 203
    indications 202
    landmarks and practical steps 202, *202*
spinal cord
    analgesia 410
        see also epidural analgesia
    blood flow not decreased with epinephrine 412–413
    physiotherapy McKenzie approach 183
spinal cord stimulation 381–389
    anatomical aspects 381
    complications 388
    contraindications 381–382
    electrodes *382*
        flat plate *382*
        insertion 381, 385
    implantation of system 384–388
        first stage 384–387
        identifying desired level of entry 384–385
        patient positioning 384
        performing test stimulation 386
        permanent implantation 387–388
        screening trial 386–387
        second stage 387–388
        sedation 385
    indications 382

limitations 382
  patient selection 382
preparation 382–384
  equipment 382–384
  patient 384
programming 388
radiofrequency (RF)-coupled system 383
  external transmitter unit *383*
  radioreceiver *383*
totally implantable system 382–383
  implantable pulse generator (IPG) 382–383, *383*
spinal nerve root pain 417
  diagnosis 418
stellate ganglion block 237–240
  complications 239–240
    less dramatic 239–240
    life-threatening 239
  neurolytic 240
  signs 239
  technique 238–239
  see also sympathetic blocks
steroids, in epidural steroid injections 422
stimulation-induced analgesia
  action potential stimulation therapy 344
  cutaneous field stimulation 186, 344
  electrical muscle stimulation (EMS) 186
  electrical stimulation 185–186
  interferential therapy 344
  of spinal cord *see* spinal cord stimulation
stomach, opioids' pharmacological effects 62
stress, mindfulness-based reduction 117
subacromial bursa, intra-articular injections *262,* 262–263
  RCTs 255–256
subarachnoid space 286, *286*
subclavian perivascular nerve block technique *see* supraclavicular
  block
subcutaneous administration of drugs 85–86
  advantages 85–86
  cancer pain management *see* cancer pain, subcutaneous
    infusions
  in children 432–433
  patient-controlled analgesia (PCA) 395
subdural hematoma, spinal cord stimulation complication 388
subdural space 286
sublingual administration of drugs
  opioids, acute pain management 70
  patient-controlled analgesia delivery route 404
sufentanil 68
  alternative epidural analgesia 415
  transmucosal delivery in PCA 402
summed pain intensity differences (SPID) *451,* 456
superior hypogastric plexus block 251–252
  anatomical aspects 251
  complications 252
  efficacy 252
  technique 251–252
    needle placement and contrast medium spread *252*
supraclavicular block 207–208
  landmarks and practical steps *207,* 208
supraorbital nerve block 202
  complications 202
  landmarks and practical steps 202
suprascapular nerve block 210
  anatomical aspects 210
  complications 210
  indications 210
    local anesthetic and depot steroid blocks 210
    local anesthetic block 210

  neurolytic block 210
  landmarks and practical steps 210, *211*
supratrochlear nerve block 202
  complications 202
  landmarks and practical steps 202
sural nerve block 229
  landmarks and practical steps 229, *229*
Survey of Pain Attitudes (SOPA) 166
sympathectomies, indications 233
sympathetic axis, neurolysis 247
  see also individual nerve blocks
sympathetic blocks 233–246
  contraindications 237
  image intensifier and contrast enhancement 237
  indications 233, 235–236
    acute pain 235
    chronic pain 235–236
  intravenous regional *see* intravenous regional sympathetic
    block
  local anesthetics 237
  lumbar *see* lumbar sympathetic block
  stellate ganglion *see* stellate ganglion block
  tests
    blood flow 236
    for completeness 236
    of function 236
    of pain 236
    pain assessment 237
    skin conductance response 237
    skin temperature 236–237
    of sympathetic function 236
  thoracic *see* thoracic sympathetic block
  verification of blocking solution 237
sympathetic chain 233, 235
  cervicothoracic 237, *238*
    block *see* stellate ganglion block
sympathetic ganglia (lumbar), radiofrequency lesioning 338–339
  adverse effects 339
  complications 339
  contraindication 338
  efficacy of treatment 339
  indication 338
  technique 338–339
sympathetic nervous system 233
  anatomy 233–235, *234*
  nerve endings and receptors *236*
  nerve supply to blood vessels *234*
SynchroMed externally programmable pump *315*
syringe drivers 85
  administration rates 87–88
    PCA 87
    reasons to prefer fixed rate to variable rate 87
  choice 87
    differing volume syringes *87*
    Graseby models *87*
  connecting tubing *88*
  types 88
  use 86–88
systematic reviews 495–505
  definition 495
  evidence accumulation 496–497
    sensitive search strategies 497, **497**
    trials to include 496–497
  evidence appraisal 497–498
  evidence-based medicine *495,* 495–496
  hierarchy of evidence **496**
  qualitative 501–503
    efficacy assessment 502–503

evidence appraisal 501–503
    quality control 501–502
    validity assessment 502–503, **503**
  quantitative *see* meta-analysis
  review process *496*
  review question 496, **497**
systemic infection, spinal cord stimulation contraindication 381

tachycardia, meperidine-induced 62
tactile sensibility, estimation with von Frey filaments 31
Tampa Scale for Kinesiophobia (TSK) 166
temperature, opioid induced 62
temporal summation, testing of abnormal findings 34
TENS *see* transcutaneous electrical nerve stimulation (TENS)
tension-type headache, improvement rates from meta-
    analyses **131**
test–retest reliability, pain measure 9
thermal thresholds, measurements with thermotest *32*
thermotest 32–34
  abnormal sensory disturbances to heat stimulation *33*
  choice of skin area tested 33
  execution 34
  indications 34
  method of limits 33
  normal thermal thresholds measured *32*
  potential influences of results 33
  two-alternative forced choice method 32–33
  typical findings 34
thigh
  lateral cutaneous nerve block *see* lateral cutaneous nerve,
    thigh blockade
  posterior cutaneous nerve block 227
third-party-defined outcomes, pain measures 8
thoracic epidural anesthesia (TEA), in children 442–443
thoracic paravertebral block 215
  anatomical aspects 215
  complications 215
  indications 215
    local anesthetic and steroid block 215
    local anesthetic block 215
    neurolytic block 215
  landmarks and practical steps 215, *215*
thoracic sympathetic block *240*, 240–241
  complications 241
  indications 240
  technique 241
thoracic zygapophyseal (facet) and rib dysfunction 190
thoracotomy, intercostal nerve block cryoanalgesia 322–323
thorax peripheral nerve blocks 215–218
  see also individual types
tibial nerve block
  at ankle 230
    landmarks and practical steps *229, 230*
  at knee 227
    landmarks and practical steps 227, *228*
tolerance
  in cancer pain management 470
  in opioid therapy 64, 80
    management 64
  TENS complication 348–349
total pain relief (TOTPAR) calculation **24**
tourniquet method, adenosine effect on
  allodynia development **487**
  pain scores in ischemia-induced pain **487**
traction 184
tramadol 67
  in children
    analgesia for patients over 6 months 435

    doses **435**
transcutaneous electrical nerve stimulation (TENS) 185–186,
    343–354
  adverse effects 349
  application site 347–348
  applied anatomy 344
  caution 345
  complications 348–349
  contraindications 345
  electrodes 346
    carbon–rubber 346
    positioning 346, *347*
    self-adhesive 346
  equipment 346
    connection to stimulator 346
    failure 348
  experimental evidence for use 349–352
    acute pain 350–351
    efficacy comparison of continuous and pulsed
      modalities *350*
    frequency 349–350
    pain reduction over time *350*
  frequency of therapy 345
  historical aspects 401–402
  indications 344–345
    acute pain 344
    chronic pain 344–345
  limitations 345
  mechanism of action 344
  stimulation characteristics **349**
  stimulation types 347
  stimulator setting 348
    acupuncture-like TENS 348
    choice of stimulation modality 348
    continuous (conventional) stimulation 348
    pulsed (burst) stimulation 348
    sequential stimulation 348
  trial 348
transdermal administration of drugs
  opioids, cancer pain management 70–71
  patient-controlled analgesia (PCA) 401
    ideal drug properties **403**
    iontophoretic systems **402**
    opioid delivery 402
TRANSFENTA® **402**
transient motor paralysis, celiac plexus block complications 250
transient postsympathectomy neuropathic pain, lumbar
    sympathetic block complication 243
transmucosal patient-controlled analgesia (PCA)
  ideal drug properties **403**
  opioid delivery 402–404
  oral and nasal routes 401
treatment protocols for opioids *see* opioids, in chronic
    nonmalignant pain
tricyclic antidepressants (TCAs) 101
  adverse effects 103–104
  contraindications 102
  dosing and treatment schedule 102, **103**
    if contraindications are present 102, *104*
    if no contraindications 102, *103*
  pretreatment safety measures **103**
trigeminal nerve, peripheral branches blockade 200–202
  anatomical aspects 200, *201*
  indications **202**
  infraorbital block *see* infraorbital nerve block
  mental branch *see* mental nerve block
  supraorbital branch *see* supraorbital nerve block
  supratrochlear branch *see* supratrochlear nerve block

trigeminal neuralgia
    antiepileptic indication 104–105, 105, 107
    resistance to drugs, radiofrequency lesioning indication 330
Tuohy needle, in spinal cord stimulation 381, 385

ulnar nerve block
    at elbow 211–212
        landmarks and practical steps 211–212, 212
    at wrist (medial approach) 213
        landmarks and practical steps 213, 214
ultrasound (US) therapy 186
upper limb peripheral nerve blocks 204–214
    see also individual types
ureter
    lumbar sympathetic block complications 243
    opioids' pharmacological effects 63
urinary retention, epidural analgesic-induced in children 443
uterus, opioids' pharmacological effects 63

validity, pain measures 10
verbal rating scale (VRS) 17, 455
vertebrogenic pain, radiofrequency lesioning 332–333
    anatomical aspects of spine 332–333
        dorsal compartment 332–333
        ventral compartment 333
vibrameter, vibratory threshold determination 31–32
vibratory threshold, determination with vibrameter 31–32
visceral pain, TENS indication 345
    experimental evidence 351
vision disturbance, epidural steroid injection complication 423
visual analog scale (VAS) 17–18, 18
    advantages 18
    dental pain assessment 463
    disadvantages 18
    pain measurement by pictures and toys 18, 19
vomiting
    opioid-induced 62, 437
        epidural infusion 313

PCA-induced, management 398
TENS reduction in postoperative expulsions 350–351
von Frey filaments 31
    tactile sensibility estimation 31

windup 28
withdrawal syndrome, in opioid therapy see under opioids
World Health Organization (WHO) analgesic ladder 70, 71
wrist
    intra-articular injections 265–266
        distal radioulnar joint 266
        radiocarpal joint 265–266, 266
    nerve blocks 213–214
        anatomical aspects 213
        indications 213
        see also individual types

yin and yang 355

zygapophyseal joints
    anatomy 269–270, 270
    cervical see cervical zygapophyseal (facet) joints
    injections and medial branch blocks 269–276
        complications 274
        contraindications 271
        evidence for use of 274–275
        gauge needles 271–272
        indications 270–271
        limitations of treatment 271
        monitoring 272
        preparation 271–274
        repeat and placebo blocks 271
        screening of needle insertions 271
    lumbar see lumbar zygapophyseal (facet) joints
    pain features 270

Cumulative index to Clinical Pain Management

Page numbers in **bold** refer to tables and boxes; page numbers in *italic* refer to figures. Page numbers are prefixed by a code indicating the volume in which the index entry is to be found. The codes are as follows:

A   Acute Pain
Ca   Cancer Pain
Ch   Chronic Pain
P   Practical Applications and Procedures

This index contains the complete list of topics for all four volumes of *Clinical Pain Management*. As there are individual volumes on acute pain, chronic pain, and cancer pain, subentries have been kept to a minimum under these entries, particularly with respect to acute pain and chronic pain. Readers are advised to seek more specific subjects.

Abbreviations

CBT   cognitive–behavioral therapy
CNS   central nervous system
CPRP   comprehensive pain rehabilitation programs
CRPSs complex regional pain syndromes
CT   computed tomography
EMLA   eutectic mixture of local anesthetics
ICU   intensive care unit

IOC   International Olympic Committee
MRI   magnetic resonance imaging
NSAIDs nonsteroidal anti-inflammatory drugs
PCA   patient-controlled analgesia
PCEA   patient-controlled epidural analgesia
PHN   postherpetic neuralgia
RCTs   randomized controlled trials
TENS   transcutaneous electrical nerve stimulation
TMJ   temporomandibular joint
WHO   World Health Organization

abdomen peripheral nerve blocks P215–P218
   see also individual types
abdominal angina Ch580
abdominal aortic dissection, celiac plexus block
   complications P250
abdominal gynecological surgery, timing of administration of
   local anesthetics A120
abdominal migraine Ch582
abdominal (flexion) muscles Ch524
abdominal nerve entrapment, in pregnancy A377
abdominal pain A373–A376
   in AIDS patients *see under* AIDS
   functional, children Ch640
   management
      analgesia A374
      laparoscopy role A374
   recurrent *see under* children
   red flag potentials **A373**
   sites for indication of neurolytic celiac plexus block
      use **Ca239**
   visceral Ch567–Ch586
      anatomical aspects *Ch569*
      archetype disorders Ch570–Ch578
      evaluation Ch569–Ch570
      general painful disorders Ch578
      inflammation Ch569
      somatic pain comparison A373–A374
      sources **Ch568**
      stimuli Ch567–Ch569
      see also pelvic pain
   of wall A376
   yellow flag psychosocial potentials **A373**
   see also individual conditions

abdominal rectopexy, postsurgical pain syndromes Ch421
abdominal trauma
   nerve block administration A270–A271
   pain management A353–A354
abdominoperineal surgery, postoperative epidural
   analgesia P415
aberrant behavior, opioid trials Ch209, **Ch209**
ablative surgery *see under* neurosurgical modalities/techniques
abnormal temporal summation, testing P34
accountability Ch35–Ch36
acetaminophen (paracetamol) A63, Ca33–Ca35, Ca129, Ca184–
   Ca186, Ch233–Ch236
   administration Ch233
   adverse effects Ca34, Ca185, Ch234–Ch235, Ch262
      gastric complications Ch234
      hepatic complications Ch234
      hepatotoxicity A441, Ca34, Ch234
      liver disease Ch235
      nephrotoxicity Ca34
      renal complications Ch234
   analgesia provision in ICU A342
   ceiling effect Ca184
   in children A441, Ca338
      administration and pharmacokinetics A441
      analgesia for patients 6 months or younger P438
      analgesia for patients over 6 months P434
      doses **P435**
      indications A441
      rectal administration P432
      toxicity A441
   clinical trials Ch232–Ch233, Ch235
   combinations **Ch234**
      codeine Ch233–Ch234

contraindications Ca185
cyclo-oxygenase (COX) inhibitor Ca184–Ca186
cytochrome P$_{450}$ Ch235
dose recommendations Ca35, Ca185, Ch233
    with respect to age **Ca185**
drug interactions Ca34
efficacy Ch235
    arthritic pain Ch235
    chronic back pain Ch235
    evidence for Ca185–Ca186
    headache Ch235
in elderly A473, Ca355, Ch653–Ch654
    codeine combination Ca357
    dextropropoxyphene combination Ca357
indications Ca184–Ca185
mechanism of action Ca33, Ch233
metabolism Ch233, Ch235
in neonates *see under* neonatal pain management
number needed to treat (NNT) A62
pain control after discharge home A334–A335
pharmaceutical issues Ch235
pharmacokinetics Ca33–Ca34, Ca185
practical tips Ca185
presentations Ca35
toxicity A63
treatment (of)
    chronic back pain Ch526–Ch527
    fibromyalgia Ch235
    low back pain A410
    osteoarthritis Ch233, Ch235
    rheumatoid arthritis Ch235
    sweating Ca309
    tension-type headache Ch473, Ch639
acetic acids A65–A66
acetylcholine, in inflammatory pain A24
acetylsalicylic acid *see* aspirin
Achilles bursitis Ch547
Achilles tendinitis Ch547
aciclovir *see* acyclovir
acquired tolerance Ca48
action potentials
    generation in central sensitization A29
    generation in peripheral sensitization A18
    stimulation therapy P344
active intervention studies, false placebos Ch274–Ch275
Activities of Daily Living (ADL) Ch653
acuesthesia, definition **Ch404**
acupressure Ca271
acupuncture Ca270–Ca272, Ch339, Ch340–Ch343, P355–P379
    abbreviations to identify meridians **P373**
    administration frequency Ca271
    adverse effects Ca272, Ch342
        contact dermatitis Ch342
        syncope Ch342
    audits Ca271
    for cancer symptoms other than pain Ca272
    complications P357–P358
        needle shock P357–P358
    complications and contraindications Ca272
    cun P357
        lengths *P362–P363*
    duration Ch341
    efficacy Ch343
        assessment in systematic review *P503*
    electrical stimulation Ch341, *Ch342*
    endorsements in medicine P356
    energy (qi) P355
        channels P355

deficiency P355
excess P355
frequency Ch341
history Ca270–Ca272, Ch340–Ch341
management (of)
    acute herpes zoster pain Ch445
    back pain Ch343, Ch531–Ch532
    childbirth pain A432
    CRPS Ch395
    dysesthetic vulvodynia Ch604
    headache Ch343
    low back pain A413
    migraine Ch343
    nausea Ca272
    neurologic disease Ch362
    osteoarthritis Ch343
    pelvic pain Ch603
    peripheral neuropathy Ch378
    phantom pain Ch434
mechanism of action Ca272, P344
needles Ch341, P357
neurohumoral response P356
pain clinics **Ch159**
pain management in pregnancy A378
points *see* acupuncture points *(below)*
scientific basis Ch342–Ch343
    endogenous opioid production Ch342
    neurochemical production Ch342–Ch343
stimulation characteristics **P349**
techniques Ch341–Ch342
theory Ch340
treatment P356–P357
    frequency of sessions P356
    methods Ca270–Ca271
    needle insertion P356, P357
    patient assessment P356
    prescriptions **P379**
    stimulation of needles P356
    symptom worsening after P356
    test period P356
trigger/traditional points Ca270
yin and yang P355
acupuncture points Ch341–Ch342, **P374–P378**
ankle *P372, P373*
anterior view of whole body *P359*
arm *P368*
elbow *P368*
face/head *P364*
    anterior view *P364*
    lateral view *P366*
    posterior view *P365*
    top of *P365*
foot *P372, P373*
hand *P370*
hip *P372*
knee *P370, P371, P372*
lateral view of whole body *P361*
leg *P370, P371, P372*
location P357
neck *P365*
posterior view of whole body *P360*
scapula *P369*
shoulder *P368, P369*
spine *P367*
thigh *P371*
upper body *P367*
acute aseptic meningitis, in AIDS patients Ca377
acute herpes zoster pain Ch437–Ch449

clinical manifestations Ch438–Ch439
   complications Ch438–Ch439
   dermatomes affected Ch438
   rash Ch438
clinical suggestions Ch446
   immunocompetent patients Ch446
   immunosuppressed patients Ch446
diagnosis Ch439
epidemiology Ch438
   age **Ch438**
management A370–A372, *A372,* Ch439–Ch446
   acupuncture Ch445
   analgesics Ch440–Ch441
   anticonvulsants A371, Ch440
   antidepressants A371, Ch440
   anti-inflammatory agents Ch440
   antiviral therapy A370, Ch439–Ch440
   capsaicin Ch218
   corticosteroids A371, Ch440
   cost-effectiveness of antiviral agents A371
   cranial ganglionic blocks Ch444–Ch445
   cranial nerve blocks Ch444–Ch445
   epidural analgesia/anesthesia Ch442
   laser Ch445
   lumbar sympathetic block Ch444
   nerve blocks Ch442–Ch443
   neuroleptics Ch440
   nonopioid analgesia Ch441
   opioids A371, Ch441
   stellate ganglion block Ch443
   sympathetic nerve block A371–A372, Ch443
   TENS Ch445
   thoracic sympathetic block Ch443–Ch444
   topical local anesthesia Ch441–Ch442
   tricyclic antidepressants Ch440
   vaccination A372
   see also individual drugs
   pathophysiology Ch437
   risk factors Ch438
acute inflammatory polyneuropathy Ch358
acutely painful medical conditions management A369–A391
   see also individual disorders
acute pain
   clinical RCTs P487–P488
      see also clinical experimental pharmacological protocols
   neurophysiological mechanisms P27–P28
      nociceptor activation P27
      sensitization of C-nociceptors P28
   opioids *see* opioids, acute pain management
   TENS indications P344
      experimental evidence P350–P351
   see also individual causes of pain and management modalities
acute pain service (APS) A183–A202
   aims A184
   assessment A190
      of pain intensity A190–A191
      pain scores A190, **A190**
      scales *A191*
      see also pain assessment
   delivery A188–A191
      communication A189
      equipment A189–A190
      errors A196
      follow-up A189
      referral pattern A188–A189
   development issues A197–A198
      cost of not providing service A197
      economic considerations A197

implementing change A198, *A199*
      indirect economic benefits A197–A198
      initiating a service A197, **A197**
      optimization A198
   documentation A192–A198
      bedside evaluation check list **A189**
      bedside pain management flow chart A193, **A196**
      epidural chart from Royal Adelaide Hospital (RAH) **A194–A195**
      policies or protocols A193
      quality improvement A193, A196
      standardized prescriptions and orders A192, **A193**
      teaching A196–A197
   guidelines A184, *A184*
   models of provision A184–A185
      doctor-led A185
      nurse-led A185
   monitoring and safety A191–A192
      Bromage scale **A192**
      hypotension A192
      motor blockade A192
      respiratory depression A191
      sedation score **A192**
   organization A183–A202
   responsibility of supervision A183
   structure **A185,** A185–A188
      analgesia methods A186–A187, **A188**
      information A183, A187–A188, **A188,** A196–A197
      patient factors A187–A188
      personnel A183, A185–A186
      preparation of patient A188
      selection of patients A187
acute pancreatitis, in AIDS patients Ca389
acute rehabilitation of sports injuries *see* sports injury
   rehabilitation
acyclovir
   acute herpes zoster pain management Ch439
   HSV infection treatment in AIDS Ca380
   postherpetic neuralgia prevention Ch455
   varicella-zoster virus infection treatment in AIDS Ca380
adaptation Ca74
   biofeedback psychophysiological assessment P122
   mechanisms Ca80
addiction Ca49
   in children Ca344
   definition Ch208, Ch633
   management, acupuncture Ch343
   misconceptions among physicians Ch32
   in opioid therapy A51, Ca49, Ca131–Ca132, Ca177, Ca404,
      Ch633, P65, P80
   psychiatric diagnosis Ch633–Ch634
   see also pseudoaddiction; substance abuse
adenosine
   in experimental protocols P485–P486
      acute tissue damage P485–P486
      analogs P483–P484
      animal data P483–P484
      combinations with other analgesics P484
      effect on allodynia development and pain scores **P487**
      inflammatory pain RCTs P487–P488
      intrathecal administration RCTs P488, P489
      intravenous administration RCTs P487–P488, P489
      normal state P485
      pain-reducing effects **P487**
      perioperative pain RCTs P488
      safety perspectives P485
   pharmacology P484
adenosine receptors

antagonists Ch264–Ch265
  adverse effects Ch265
    neuropathic pain treatment Ch265
    refractory angina pectoris treatment Ch557–Ch558
    studies Ch265
  mechanism of action Ch264
adenosine triphosphate (ATP), in inflammatory pain A24
adequate disclosure Ch176–Ch179
adhesiolysis Ch589–Ch590
adhesions (pelvic) Ch589–Ch590
  diagnosis Ch589
  incidence Ch589
  management Ch589–Ch590
  prevention Ch590
  symptoms/signs Ch589
  see also pelvic pain
adjudicator/claims manager, disability evaluation (USA) Ch43–Ch44
adjunct therapies Ca126, Ca134–Ca136, Ca209–Ca234
  in analgesic ladder Ca126, Ca134
  back pain management Ch527–Ch528
  in children see children, adjuvant analgesics
  definition Ca209
  in elderly see elderly, adjuvant analgesics
  in ICU see under intensive care unit (ICU)
  opioid adverse effects management Ca169
  see also individual drugs
administration routes, analgesics A205–A218, Ca128–Ca129, Ch262
  see also individual drugs/routes
adrenaline see epinephrine
adrenal suppression, epidural steroid injection complication P423
α_2-adrenergic agonists Ch265
  as adjuvant analgesic Ca210–Ca211
  mechanism of action Ch265
  in multimodal anesthesia A323
  pain management in ICU A344–A345
  studies Ch265
  treatment (of)
    central pain syndromes Ch409
    CRPS Ch391
  see also clonidine
advance statements Ca119
aerobic activity, physical therapy Ch316
affect, pain measure P5
aftersensations Ch116–Ch117, **Ch121**
age, effect on opioid pharmacokinetics P64
Agency for Health Care Policy and Research (AHCPR) A164
  guidelines A164
aging Ch649
  effect on local anesthesia pharmacokinetics A80–A81
  effect on residual limb pain Ch429
  increased analgesic effects of opioids Ca357
  physiological changes A464–A466, **A465**
  see also elderly
agitated behavior, mistreatment as pain Ca68
agranulocytosis, NSAIDs adverse effects Ch231
AIDS Ca367–Ca390
  abdominal pain Ca387–Ca389
    acute pancreatitis Ca389
    causes by location of pain Ca388
    colitis Ca389
    cramp Ca389
    hepatic disease Ca388
    investigation Ca387
    lower or diffuse Ca389
    presentation Ca387

    right iliac fossa pain Ca388
    right upper quadrant pain Ca388
    treatment Ca387–Ca388
    upper Ca388–Ca389
    urolithiasis Ca389
  anal pain Ca382–Ca383
    anorectal ulceration Ca383
    squamous cell carcinoma Ca383
  antiretroviral treatments Ca367–Ca371, **Ca368**
    adverse effects Ca367
    drug interactions Ca367
    see also individual drugs
  chest pain Ca385–Ca386
    frequency **Ca386**
    lung involvement Ca385
    opportunistic infections Ca386
    Pneumocystis cysts Ca386
    pneumonia Ca386
  cutaneous pain Ca382
    bed sores Ca382
    causes **Ca383**
    Kaposi's sarcoma nasal lesion Ca382
    toxic epidermal neurolysis Ca383
  joint/rheumatic pain Ca384–Ca385
    arthralgia Ca385
    causes **Ca385**
    fibromyalgia syndrome Ca385
    myositis Ca385
    osteonecrosis Ca385
    septic arthritis Ca385
  lung involvement Ca386
    Kaposi's sarcoma Ca386
  neurological pain syndromes Ca374–Ca378
    headache see headaches, in AIDS patients
    neuropathies Ca374–Ca376, **Ca376**
    relationship of complications to CD4 count Ca375
  neuropathy see HIV-associated neuropathy
  ocular manifestations Ca383–Ca384, **Ca384**
    Kaposi's sarcoma Ca384
  odynophagia (painful swallowing) Ca386–Ca387
    causes **Ca387**
    esophageal candidiasis Ca386
    herpes simplex esophagitis Ca386
    ulcerations of esophagus Ca387
  opportunistic infections Ca367
  oral pain Ca378–Ca382
    causes **Ca379**
    Kaposi's sarcoma Ca381, Ca381
    see also individual disorders
  pain Ca367, Ca403
    assessment Ca373
    comparison with cancer pain **Ca372,** Ca372–Ca373
    factors influencing the nature and presentation **Ca371**
    literature Ca371–Ca374
    prevalence Ca371–Ca372
    syndromes Ca374, **Ca375**
  pain management Ca373–Ca374
    education Ca373
    investigation of barriers Ca373
    pharmacological Ca374
    physical and psychological therapies Ca374
    principal reasons for undertreatment **Ca373**
    underdiagnosis and undertreatment Ca373
  somatic pain Ca378–Ca385
  stigma associated with infection
  visceral pain Ca385–Ca387
    etiology and pathophysiology Ca385–Ca386
airway obstruction, management Ca294

alcohol
    as neurolytic agent Ca236–Ca237, **Ca238,** P198
        concentration effect on nerve cell destruction **Ca237**
        mechanism of action Ca236
        painful spasticity management Ch463
        peripheral neuropathies management Ch372
        trigeminal neuralgia management **Ch496**
    restrictions according to IOC medical code A500
alcoholic neuropathy A372
    management A372
Alcohol Use Disorders Identification Consumption Test (AUDIT-C) Ch71
alfentanil A49, P67–P68
    epidural, in PCEA **A247**
    intravenous, doses and paradigms P45
    pain management in ICU A343
    pharmacokinetics **A346,** P68
    procedural pain management Ca326
algometer
    pressure threshold determination P32
algorithm
    neuropathic pain management *Ch80–Ch81*
alkaloids, toxic neuropathy Ch372
allachesthesia, definition **Ch404**
allergic reactions
    to esters A82
    to local anesthesia A82
    to NSAIDs A59, A62, Ch261
    TENS complication P348
allodynia A360, Ch115–Ch116, P28
    animal models Ch190
    changes in stimulus intensity *A17*
    in CRPS Ch383–Ch384
    definition Ch115, **Ch404**
    in Guillain–Barré syndrome Ch115
    mechanism Ch115
    in peripheral neuropathies Ch368
    quantification Ch115–Ch116
    in sciatica Ch115
almotriptan, migraine management Ch471
alternative medicine *see* complementary and alternative medicine
amantadine, CRPS management Ch394
ambulatory infusion of opioids, cancer pain management P71
ambulatory surgery, intraspinal opioids A248
    lipophilic advantage over local anesthetic for spinal block **A248**
American Academy of Pain Medicine, opioid use Ch166–Ch167
American Botanical Council (ABC) Ch346
American College of Rheumatology (ACR)
    acetaminophen recommendations Ch235
    fibromyalgia diagnosis Ch640–Ch641
American Herbal Products Association (AHPA) Ch346
American Medical Association (AMA)
    disability evaluation guidelines Ch40
    impairment guidelines Ch49–Ch50
    pain rating guidelines Ch184–Ch185
American Pain Society (APS)
    guidelines A166
    opioid use Ch166–Ch167
    sickle cell pain management guidelines Ch643
American Society of Addiction Medicine, opioid use Ch167
amethocaine, structure, physiochemical properties and clinical profile **A84**
amides
    metabolism A80
    structure, physiochemical properties and clinical profile **A84–A85**

α-amino-3-hydroxy-5-methyl-4-isoxazole propionic acid receptors
    see AMPA receptors
aminoamides A83, A86–A87
γ-aminobutyric acid *see* GABA
aminoesters A83
amitriptyline
    adjuvant analgesic in elderly Ca358
    clinical trials Ch252
    dose titrations Ch244–Ch245
    in elderly A473
    mechanism of action Ch239–Ch240
    pain management in ICU A344
    pharmacokinetics Ca217
    pharmacology **Ch240**
    serum concentration–effect relations *Ch245*
    structure *Ch240*
    therapeutic index Ch245
    therapeutic window Ch245
    treatment (of)
        acute herpes zoster pain Ch440
        central pain syndrome Ch409, **Ch409**
        chronic back pain Ch528
        dysesthetic vulvodynia Ch604
        fibromyalgia Ch625
        migraine Ch475
        neuropathic pain Ch242, Ch376–Ch377
        painful spasticity **Ch461**
        postherpetic neuralgia Ch452–Ch453
        postsurgical pain syndrome Ch423
        tension-type headache Ch475
        TMJ pain **Ch486**
    treatment schedule *P103*
ammonium compounds, neurolytic agents Ca237
amoxicillin, maxillary sinusitis management Ch487
AMPA receptors **A25**
    excitatory postsynaptic potentials A8, *A32*
amphetamines, opioid-induced sedation management Ca170
amprenavir, in AIDS pain management Ca371
amputation
    CRPS management Ch395
    pain after *see* phantom limb pain; postamputation pain; residual limb pain
    postsurgical pain syndromes Ch421
amyloidosis, primary, autoimmune neuropathy Ch373
anabolic agents, prohibitions in IOC medical code A499 A
    examples A501 A
anal candidiasis *Ca384*
analgesia
    adjuvant *see* adjunct therapies
    administration routes A205–A218, Ca128–Ca129, Ch262
        see also individual routes
    adverse effects Ch441
    balanced A175–A176
        in pain management in children A440
    caudal *see* caudal analgesia
    in cryotherapy *see* cryoanalgesia
    demand as measure of pain A107
    development of novel drug from compound *P488*
    drug use during breast-feeding A379–A380, **A384–A385**
    economics Ch10
    in elderly A469–A477
        see also under elderly
    epidural *see* epidural analgesia/anesthesia
    in ICU *see under* intensive care unit (ICU)
    improvements in pulmonary outcome measures **A171**
    intra-articular *see* intra-articular analgesia
    intrapleural, postoperative pain management A319–A320
    intraspinal *see* intraspinal analgesia

intrathecal *see* intrathecal analgesia
intravenous *see* intravenous analgesia
lumbar *see* lumbar analgesia
mechanism of action Ch3–Ch4
nonopioid *see* nonopioid analgesia
oral *see* oral analgesic therapy
preemptive *see* preemptive analgesia
preventive *see* preventive analgesia
principles Ca125–Ca128
    by the analgesic ladder Ca126
       see also World Health Organization (WHO) analgesic
          ladder
    attention to detail Ca128
    by the clock Ca126
    for the individual Ca126–Ca127
    by mouth Ca125
       see also oral analgesic therapy
regional *see* regional analgesia
sites of action A176
stimulation-induced *see* stimulation-induced analgesia
subcutaneous infusions **P89**
systemic *see* systemic analgesics
topical *see* topical analgesia
treatment combinations in perioperative period A115
see also pain relief; *individual drugs and treatment modalities*
analgesic ladder *see* World Health Organization (WHO) analgesic
   ladder
anal pain, in AIDS patients *see under* AIDS
anandamide, in inflammatory pain A23–A24
anemia, aplastic *see* aplastic anemia
anesthesia
   central pain syndromes management Ch409
   definition **Ch404**
   epidural *see* epidural analgesia/anesthesia
   general *see* general anesthesia
   infiltration A88
      pain management in pregnancy A380
   intrathecal catheterization P290
   local *see* local anesthesia
   postherpetic neuralgia management Ch453
anesthesia dolorosa, definition **Ch404**
anesthesiologists
   pain units Ch156
   role in acute pain service A183, A185
aneurysms, central pain syndromes Ch403
anger Ch165
   assessment Ch105–Ch106
   behavioral comorbidities Ch73
   coping mechanism Ca80
angina, abdominal Ch580
angina pectoris Ch554–Ch555
   cardiocardiac reflex Ch555, *Ch555*
   character Ch554
   clinical considerations Ch554–Ch555
   duration Ch554
   esophageal pain comparison **Ch559**
   history Ch554
   localization Ch554
   management Ch555
      angioplasty Ch555
      CBT Ch555
      coronary artery surgery (CABG) Ch555, **Ch555**
      internal mammary (IMA) ligation Ch555
      TENS *see below*
   provoking/relieving factors Ch554
   psychological aspects Ch554–Ch555
   refractory *see* angina pectoris, refractory *(below)*
   severity Ch554

symptoms Ch554
TENS A279, P345
   electrode positioning P348
   experimental evidence P351–P352
angina pectoris, refractory Ch555–Ch557
   assessment Ch555–Ch556
      differential diagnosis Ch555–Ch556
   management Ch556, **Ch556,** Ch556–Ch557
      angiogenesis Ch557
      anti-ischemic medication Ch556
      endoscopic thoracic sympathectomy Ch557
      enhanced external counterpulsation (EECP) Ch557
      gene therapy Ch557
      intermittent urokinase therapy Ch557
      left stellate ganglion injection Ch557
      myocardial revascularization Ch557
      pain beliefs Ch556
      psychological distress Ch556
      rehabilitation program Ch556
      spinal cord stimulation Ch556–Ch557
      TENS Ch556
      thoracic epidural anesthesia Ch557
   prevalence Ch555
angiogenesis
   refractory angina pectoris management Ch557
   role in tissue repair A487
angiography
   femoral, postoperative relaxation exercises A290
   uterine fibroids *A505*
angioplasty
   angina pectoris management Ch555
   pain relief in interventional radiology A503–A504
angiotensin-converting enzyme (ACE) inhibitors, NSAIDs
   interaction A57–A58
angor animi Ch554
anhedonia Ch165
animal models Ch189–Ch199, **Ch194**
   central pain Ch191–Ch192
      ischemic spinal cord injury Ch191–Ch192
   clinical experimental pharmacological protocols P483–P484
   ethical considerations Ch189–Ch190
   experimental allergic neuritis Ch191
   pain management development Ch193–Ch194
      cholecystokinin (CCK) antagonists Ch194
      drug screening Ch193
      NMDA receptor antagonists Ch194
      opioids Ch193–Ch194
   pathophysiology Ch192–Ch193
   peripheral neuropathic pain Ch190–Ch191
      complete nerve injury Ch190
      partial nerve injury Ch190–Ch191
   results Ch192–Ch193
   variability Ch192
      age Ch192
      endogenous opioid systems Ch192
      environment Ch192
      genetics Ch192
   see also individual diseases/disorders
ankle
   intra-articular injections P261, *P262*
   nerve blocks P229–P230
      anatomical aspects P229
      complications P230
      indications P229
      landmarks and practical steps *P229*
      see also individual types
   pain A402–A403, Ch547
      investigations/management A402–A403

ankylosing spondylitis A408
    management, apazone Ch228
    neck pain Ch508
annulus fibrosis, intervertebral disk *Ch522*
anorectal ulceration, in AIDS patients Ca383, *Ca384*
anorexia–cachexia syndrome Ca304–Ca307
    clinical findings and investigations Ca305
    management Ca305–Ca307
        corticosteroids Ca306
        progestogens Ca306
    pathophysiology **Ca307**
anserine bursitis Ch547
anterior commissure–posterior commissure (AC–PC),
    neurosurgical techniques Ch297–Ch298
anterior longitudinal ligaments *Ch522*
anterior superior iliac spine (ASIS), local anesthetic infiltration
    into cavity A269
anterolateral cordotomy (ACC) Ca263–Ca264
antiarrhythmics P108–P109
    as adjuvant analgesics Ca135, Ca211–Ca213
        adverse effects Ca212
        classification Ca211
        contraindications Ca212
        doses and treatment paradigms Ca212
        evidence for efficacy Ca213
        indications Ca212
        oral Ca212
        pharmacokinetics Ca212–Ca213
        practical tips Ca213
        see also individual drugs
    adverse effects P109
    clinical trials Ch255–Ch257
    contraindications P108
    dosing and treatment schedule P108, **P109**
    efficacy, antidepressants comparison Ch246–Ch247, *Ch247*
    mechanism of action Ch255
    pretreatment safety measures **P109**
    treatment (of)
        CRPS Ch394
        peripheral neuropathy Ch377
    see also individual drugs
antibiotics
    maxillary sinusitis management Ch487
    urethral syndrome management Ch595
anticoagulant drugs, epidural analgesia and A476
anticonvulsants (antiepileptics) P104–P108
    as adjuvant analgesics Ca134–Ca135, Ca213–Ca215
        adverse effects Ca214
        in children Ca342
        contraindications Ca214
        doses and treatment paradigms Ca214
        drug interactions Ca214
        in elderly Ca358–Ca359
        evidence for efficacy Ca215
        indications Ca213
        mechanism of action Ca213
        pharmacokinetics Ca214–Ca215
        practical tips Ca215
        see also individual drugs
    adverse effects Ch253, Ch254, **Ch255, Ch461,** Ch493–Ch494,
        P107–P108
        central nervous system Ch254
        communication Ch253
        evidence Ch253
    clinical trials Ch252–Ch253
    contraindications P105
    dose range **Ch461**
    dosing and treatment schedules P105–P107, **P106**

efficacy, antidepressants comparison Ch246, *Ch247*
    in elderly A473, Ch655
    history Ch251
    indications P104–P105
    mechanism of action Ch251–Ch252
    practical use Ch253–Ch254
        combination therapy Ch254
        indications Ch253
        response Ch254
    pretreatment safety measures **P106**
    safety aspects Ch254–Ch255
        compliance Ch255
        serum monitoring Ch254–Ch255
    treatment (of)
        acute herpes zoster pain A371, Ch440
        central pain syndromes Ch409
        chronic back pain Ch528
        CRPS Ch394
        migraine Ch253
        neurologic disease Ch361
        neuropathic pain Ch253, **Ch254**
        painful spasticity **Ch461,** Ch461–Ch462
        pelvic pain Ch599–Ch600
        peripheral neuropathy Ch377
        phantom limb pain Ch642
        postherpetic neuralgia Ch453
        postsurgical pain syndrome Ch423
        trigeminal neuralgia Ch253, Ch493–Ch494
    see also individual drugs
anticytokine therapies, anorexia–cachexia syndrome
    management Ca307
antidepressants Ch239–Ch249, P101–P104
    as adjuvant analgesics Ca215–Ca218
        adverse effects Ca216–Ca217
        in children Ca342
        contraindications Ca216
        doses and treatment paradigms Ca216
        drug interactions Ca217
        in elderly Ca358
        evidence for efficacy Ca217
        indications Ca216
        neuropathic pain treatment Ca215–Ca216
        pharmacokinetics Ca217
        practical tips Ca217
        see also individual drugs
    adverse effects Ch243–Ch244, **Ch244,** P103–P104
        cardiac Ch243
        dry mouth Ch243–Ch244
    animal trials Ch241
    clinical trials Ch241–Ch242, Ch246
    contraindications P102
    dosing and treatment schedule Ch244–Ch245, P102
        dose–effect relations Ch244
        individual tailoring Ch244
        serum concentration–effect relations Ch244–Ch245, *Ch245*
        titrations Ch244–Ch245
    drug choice Ch245–Ch246, **Ch246**
    efficacy Ch242–Ch243, Ch246–Ch247
        antiarrhythmics comparison Ch246–Ch247, *Ch247*
        anticonvulsants comparison Ch246, *Ch247*
        numbers needed to treat (NNT) figures Ch242–Ch243,
            Ch243
        opioid comparison Ch246, *Ch247*
    in elderly Ch243
    indications P101
    in management **Ch243**
    mechanism of action Ch241–Ch242
    pain management in ICU A344

pharmacokinetics Ch241, *Ch241*
pharmacology Ch239–Ch241, **Ch240, Ch242**
   hepatic metabolism Ch241
treatment (of)
   acute herpes zoster pain A371, Ch440
   central pain syndromes Ch409, **Ch409**
   chronic back pain Ch528
   CRPS Ch394
   migraine Ch243
   nerve pain **Ch243**
   neurologic disease Ch361
   neuropathic pain Ca215–Ca216, Ch242–Ch243
   nociceptive pain Ch243
   pelvic pain Ch599–Ch600
   peripheral neuropathy Ch376–Ch377
   postherpetic neuralgia **Ch243,** Ch244–Ch245, Ch452–
     Ch453
   rheumatoid arthritis Ch539
   TMJ pain **Ch486**
see also individual types
antiemetics Ca299–Ca300
   adjuvant analgesics Ca136
   adverse effects in AIDS patients Ca372
   agents
     droperidol A233
     5-hydroxytryptamine 3 (5-HT$_3$) antagonists A233
     hyoscine A233
     nalmefene A233
     promethazine A233
     propofol A233
   classification **Ca302**
   inclusion in PCA solution P394–P395
   nausea and vomiting treatment A257
   subcutaneous infusions **P89**
antiepileptics *see* anticonvulsants (antiepileptics)
antifungals, vulvar pain syndrome management Ch606
antihistamines
   interstitial cystitis management Ch596
   pruritus management Ca308
   vulvar pain syndrome management Ch606
anti-inflammatory agents
   topical, acute herpes zoster pain Ch440
   treatment (of)
     acute herpes zoster pain Ch440
     dental pain Ch483–Ch484
     refractory cancer pain Ca152
     TMJ pain **Ch486**
   see also nonsteroidal anti-inflammatory drugs (NSAIDs)
anti-ischemic medication, refractory angina pectoris
   management Ch556
antioxidant therapy, chronic pancreatitis management Ch574
antireflux valves, incorrect use of, or failure to use in PCA A230
antiretroviral treatments, in AIDS *see under* AIDS
antisecretory drugs Ca296, Ca312
   subcutaneous infusions **P90**
antispasmodics
   subcutaneous infusions in cancer pain control P92
antiviral agents, treatment (of)
   acute herpes zoster pain A371, Ch439–Ch440
   antiretroviral agents *see under* AIDS
   peripheral neuropathies Ch372–Ch373
   vulvar pain syndrome Ch605–Ch606
anxiety Ca81–Ca82, Ca310
   cognitive theory P164
   disorders Ch69, Ch71, Ch632
     assessment Ch71, **Ch71,** Ch105
     pain association Ch149–Ch150, Ch632
   effect on pain perception P15–P16, P114

   in children P149
   etiology Ca310
   management Ca310
   maternal, influence on childbirth pain A429–A430
   pain measure P5
   in patient-controlled analgesia (PCA) A226
   predisposing factors Ca82
   prevalence Ca310
   psychological therapies Ca310
   relaxation-induced P130
   risk assessment Ca81–Ca82
anxiety reduction theory Ch278–Ch279
anxiety relief theory Ch276–Ch277
anxiolytics
   adjuvant analgesics Ca135
   breathlessness management Ca295
   subcutaneous infusions in cancer pain control P92
aorta dissection, celiac plexus block complications P250
apazone
   characteristics **Ch229**
   treatment (of)
     ankylosing spondylitis Ch228
     rheumatoid arthritis Ch228
aphthous ulceration, oral pain in AIDS patients Ca381–Ca382,
   Ca382
aplastic anemia
   anticonvulsant-induced Ch254
   NSAID induced Ch231
arachidonic acid metabolism *Ca36*
arachnoiditis Ch523
   causes Ch523
aromatherapy Ca276, Ch339
arrhythmias, drugs for *see* antiarrhythmics
arsenical polyneuropathy Ch372
arterial flow, CRPS diagnosis Ch388–Ch389
arteriovenous malformation (AVM) A505
   central pain syndromes Ch403
   embolization A505
   selective catheterization A505, *A506*
arthralgia
   in AIDS patients Ca385
   see also joint pain
arthritis
   apatite-associated destructive Ch543
   bacterial A396–A397
   crystal *see* crystal arthritis
   gouty A397
   inflammatory, NSAIDs Ch228
   management
     acetaminophen Ch235
     NSAIDs Ch232–Ch233
     topical capsaicin Ch220, Ch221
     topical NSAIDs Ch216, Ch217
   rheumatoid *see* rheumatoid arthritis
   septic A396–A397
     in AIDS patients Ca385
Arthritis Impact Measurement Scale Ch103–Ch104
Arthritis Self-Efficacy Scale (AES) Ch74, Ch148
arthropathy
   exacerbation by intra-articular injections P259
   pelvic, in pregnancy A377–A378
arthroscopic surgery
   knee pain
     intra-articular analgesia A333
     local anesthetic infiltration into cavity A269
   shoulder, postsurgical pain syndromes Ch420
articular cartilage
   deterioration by intra-articular injections P259

artificial disk replacement, chronic back pain
   management Ch529
aspartate, role in nociceptive signaling in dorsal horn A8
aspirin A64, Ca129–Ca130, Ca191–Ca192
   adverse effects Ca186–Ca187, Ca191–Ca192
      hepatotoxicity Ca191
      hypersensitivity Ca191–Ca192
   characteristics **Ch229**
   in children Ca338
   contraindications Ca191
   cyclo-oxygenase (COX) inhibitor Ca191–Ca192
   doses and treatment protocols Ca191
   in elderly Ca355
   evidence for efficacy Ca190
   historical aspects Ca183
   indications Ca191
   L'Abbé plot *P499*
   mechanism of action Ca36
   pharmacokinetics Ca191
   treatment (of)
      acute herpes zoster pain Ch439–Ch440
      tension-type headache Ch473
assessment *see* pain assessment
asthma, NSAID induced A59, A62, Ca37, Ca190
ATP, in inflammatory pain A24
attention regulation in chronic pain P135–P146
   clinical case example P144–P146
      development of purposeful attention P145–P146
   phase I – reconceptualizing pain experience P136
      acknowledging pain P137–P138
      complications P139
      context P138–P139
      establishing rationale for self-management P138
      giving difficult messages P138
      reconceptualizing pain experience P138
      understanding patient's expectations and pain
         experience P138
   phase II – developing awareness through objective
      observation P136
      clinical tools **P141**
      complications P140
      delivery stages P139
      practical tips P139
   phase III – reengagement of attention to ability P136
      clinical tools **P142**
      complications P140–P141
      delivery stages P140
      practical tips P139, P140
   phase IV – development of purposeful attention P136–P137
      clinical tools **P142**
      complications P143–P144
      delivery process P143
      practical tips P141, P143
   phase V – generalization and maintenance P137
      clinical tools **P143**
      complications P144
      delivery process P144
      practical tips P144
   treatment phases P136–P137
      application P137–P144
attention span Ch101
atypical facial pain *see* facial pain, atypical
atypical odontalgia *see under* facial pain
augmentative surgical procedures Ca262, Ch297
auriculoacupuncture Ca271
autoimmune neuropathy *see* neuropathies, autoimmune
autonomic nervous system (ANS)
   activation in pain A285

   effect on gastrointestinal mobility A170, *A171*
avascular bone necrosis **Ca14,** Ca16
   MRI scan *Ca16*
avoidance
   comorbidities Ch76, Ch78
   pain response P163
axillary block P208–P210
   in children A446, P441
      anatomical aspects P441
      local anesthetic solution P441
      method P441
   landmarks and practical steps P208–P210, *P209, P211*
axonotmesis Ch418
axotomy Ch190
azithromycin, maxillary sinusitis management Ch487

background pain, burns A360–A361
back pain Ch521–Ch536
   arachnoiditis Ch523
      causes Ch523
   bone pain Ch521
   celiac plexus block complications P250
   in children *see under* children
   clinical presentation Ch524
   diagnosis Ch137–Ch140
      algorithm Ch137–Ch140, *Ch139*
      CT Ch139–Ch140
      MRI Ch137–Ch138, Ch139
      nerve blocks Ch132, Ch138–Ch139
      pain location Ch138
   differential diagnosis **Ch525**
   disability assessment Ch524–Ch525
      abnormal illness behavior Ch525
      psychosocial risk factors Ch525
   diskogenic pain Ch137, Ch522
      disk herniation Ch522
      internal disk disruption (IDD) Ch522
      prevalence Ch522
   epidemiology Ch23, Ch137, Ch524
      lifetime prevalence Ch524
   epidural steroid injection *see* epidural steroid injections
   etiology/pathophysiology Ch23, Ch521–Ch523
   low *see* low back pain
   management Ch526–Ch533
      acetaminophen Ch235
      acupuncture Ch531–Ch532
      adjuvant medication Ch527–Ch528
      alternative/complementary medicine Ch531–Ch532
      analgesics Ch526–Ch527
         see also analgesia
      bisphosphonates Ch528
      botulinum toxins Ch530
      CBT Ch532
      epidural injections Ch530
      evidence-based evaluation **Ch527**
      facet injections Ch530
      massage Ch532
      nerve root injections Ch530
      neuromodulation Ch531
      NSAIDs Ch232, Ch527
      percutaneous electrical nerve stimulation (PENS) Ch531
      psychophysiological (respondent) therapy Ch532–Ch533
      relaxation Ch532
      spa therapy Ch532
      spinal cord stimulation Ch531
      TENS Ch531
      tricyclic antidepressants (TCAs) Ch527–Ch528
   meningeal carcinomatosis feature Ca9

nerve root pain Ch523, Ch524
   causes Ch523
   occurrence Ch23
   physical management Ch528–Ch529
      back schools Ch528–Ch529
      exercise Ch528
      functional restoration Ch528
      spinal manipulation Ch528
      traction Ch528
   in pregnancy A376–A377
   radiological investigations Ch525–Ch526
      bone scans Ch526
      cross-sectional imaging Ch526
      CT Ch526
      MRI Ch526
      radiographs Ch525–Ch526
   recovery Ch23
   risk factors **Ch526**
   sacroiliac joint pain Ch521–Ch522
   serious spinal pathology Ch524
      risk factors **Ch524**
   surgical management Ch529–Ch530
      artificial disk replacement Ch529
      chemonucleolysis Ch529
      decompression/fusion Ch529
      diskectomy Ch529
      gene transfer therapy Ch529–Ch530
      intradiskal electrothermy (IDET) Ch529
      rate Ch23
   zygapophyseal (facet) joint pain Ch521
   see also low back pain
back schools, chronic back pain management Ch528–Ch529
baclofen Ca219
   adverse effects Ca220
   clinical trials Ch257
   doses and pharmacokinetics Ca220
   intrathecal Ch257
   mechanism of action Ch257
   treatment (of)
      neurologic disease Ch361, Ch362
      painful spasticity **Ch462**
      trigeminal neuralgia Ch257, Ch494, **Ch494–Ch495**
bacterial arthritis A396–A397
bacterial infections
   epidural steroid injection complication P423
   oral problem Ca298
balanced analgesia A175–A176
   in pain management in children A440
barbotage, neurologic disease management Ch363
barriers to pain management **Ca89**
   in AIDS patients Ca373
   in elderly patients Ca359–Ca360
   nurses' role in elimination Ca87, Ca89
Barthel Index, painful spasticity assessment Ch460
Beck Depression Inventory (BDI) Ch71, Ch105, Ch150
bed rest P184
   low back pain management A411
bed sores, in AIDS patient *Ca382*
behavioral comorbidities *see* comorbidities, behavioral
behavioral measures/assessment A102
   child pain assessment P432, *P433*
   in pain-related fear *see under* pain-related fear
behavioral rating scale Ch65
behavioral therapies
   in children Ca334
   see also cognitive–behavioral therapy (CBT)
Bennet and Xie model Ch190
benzocaine

structure, physiochemical properties and clinical profile **A84**
   topical A87
Benzodiazepine Dependence Questionnaire Ch71
benzodiazepines
   delirium medication Ca311
      opioid-induced cases Ca172
   pain relief in interventional radiology A510
   substance abuse Ch633–Ch634
   treatment (of)
      breathlessness Ca295, Ca312
      myofascial pain (MFP) Ch625
      neurologic disease Ch361
      painful spasticity **Ch462**
benztropine, clinical trial Ch204
bereavement, in AIDS patients Ca373
β-blockers
   migraine prophylaxis management Ch475
   NSAIDs interaction A57–A58
   refractory angina pectoris management Ch557
   restrictions according to IOC medical code A500
      examples A501
Bier block A88
bilateral cordotomies Ca264
biliary colic A376
   management A376
biliary spasm, opioid-induced Ca177
biliary tract
   opioids' pharmacological effects P63
biobehavioral, definition A286
biofeedback A289, P117, P121–P133
   in children P155–P160
      components of training P155–P156
      discern–control–generalize P156–P157
      integrated approaches P157–P159
      limitations P159–P160
      parental involvement P156
      physiological modality P156
      potential nonspecific pain control mechanisms P161
      potential specific pain control mechanisms P160–P161
      practice P155–P156
      psychophysiologic profile P157
      schedule P155
      technique P156
      training and professional certification P161
   definition P121
   evidence-based reviews P131–P132
   general approach P121–P122
      assumptions P121–P122
   indirect approaches P124
   meta-analyses P131
      average improvement rates **P131**
   modalities and abbreviations **P155**
   operations P121
   psychophysiological assessment P122
      adaptation P122
      baseline P122
      components P122–P124, **P123**
      muscle discrimination P123–P124
      muscle scanning P123
      reactivity P122–P123
      recommendations **P124**
      recovery P123
   relaxation aid P124–P125
      electromyograph-assisted relaxation P124–P125
      skin conductance-assisted relaxation P125
      skin temperature-assisted relaxation P125
   select treatment considerations P125–P130
      autogenic training P127

coaching model P125–P126
components of session P126
diaphragmatic breathing P127
education of patient P125
goals P126
imagery P126
learning and practicing skills P126
progressive muscle relaxation training P127–P130, **P128**
see also progressive muscle relaxation (PMR)
specific approaches P122–P124, P130
headaches P130
biopsies, peripheral neuropathies Ch370
birth pain *see* childbirth pain
bisphosphonates Ca222–Ca224
adjuvant analgesics Ca135
adverse effects Ca223
efficacy Ca223
practical tips Ca223
treatment (of)
bone pain Ca288–Ca289
chronic back pain Ch528
hypercalcemia Ca300
see also clodronate; pamidronate
bladder
opioids' pharmacological effects P63
phantom pain Ca13
spasms Ca13
causes **Ca13**
bleeding disorders
spinal cord stimulation contraindication P382
bleeding diverticula Ch580
blepharospasm, botulinum toxin injections Ch464
blood count
low back pain investigations A409
musculoskeletal pain diagnosis
articular A395
nonarticular A396
blood doping, prohibited method in IOC medical code A499
blood tests, peripheral neuropathies Ch370
body fat, physiological changes with age A466
Bolam v. Friern Hospital Management Committee, medical
liability Ch177
bone
harvesting, postsurgical pain syndromes Ch421
pain *see* bone pain
response to injury A488–A489
fracture management A489
healing stages A489
scans *see* bone scans
secondary tumors *see* bone metastases
sporting injuries A488–A489
avulsion injuries A489
epiphyseal injuries A489
overuse injuries A489
bone marrow aspiration *Ca320*
bone metastases
chemosensitivity of primary tumors **Ca287**
incidence **Ca282**
MRI scan of vertebral column *Ca5*
pain due to Ca281
see also bone pain
radiotherapy in elderly Ca359
bone pain Ca281–Ca292
avascular bone necrosis **Ca14**, Ca16
MRI scan *Ca16*
causes **Ca282**
chemotherapy Ca287–Ca288
breast cancer metastasis Ca287

multiple myeloma metastases Ca288
nonsmall-cell lung cancer metastasis Ca287
small-cell lung cancer metastasis Ca287
chronic back pain Ch521
chronic chest pain Ch558–Ch559
clinical presentation Ca281
diagnosis Ch135
criteria Ca282
etiology and pathophysiology Ca281
hormone treatment Ca288
breast cancer Ca288
endometrial cancer Ca288
prostate cancer Ca288
renal cancer Ca288
indication for NSAIDs Ca169, Ca186
management
evidence-based evaluation Ca282–Ca290
overview *Ca290*
pharmacological management Ca282–Ca283
bisphosphonates Ca288–Ca289
NSAIDs Ca130, Ca282–Ca283
opioids Ca283
prognosis Ca290
survival curves *Ca289*
radioisotope therapy Ca285–Ca287
phosphorus Ca287
radioiodine Ca286–Ca287
rhenium Ca287
samarium Ca286
strontium Ca286
radiotherapy Ca283–Ca287
bone pain in multiple sites Ca285
localized bone pain Ca283–Ca284
radiation dose and bone pain Ca284–Ca285
rate of onset of pain relief after administration *Ca284*
trials assessing effect of single-fraction therapy **Ca284**
wide-field irradiation *see* wide-field irradiation
surgery Ca289–Ca290
bone scans Ch129
applications Ch129
chronic back pain Ch526
CRPS diagnosis Ch129
mechanism Ch129
stress fractures diagnosis Ch129
botanical therapy Ch345–Ch346
applications Ch346
classification Ch346, **Ch347, Ch348**
history Ch345–Ch346
migraine treatment **Ch347**
prevalence Ch346
safety Ch346, **Ch348**
Botox (BTX-A) P277
dosing guidelines for spasticity treatment **P281**
preparation P278, **P279**
botulinum toxin injections P277–P283
additional treatments and outcomes P280
BTX-A Botox *see* Botox (BTX-A)
BTX-B Myobloc P277
contraindications **P279**
dose selection P280
dosing guidelines for spasticity treatment **P281**
duration of benefit P280
equipment and patient considerations P278–P279
adverse effects P279, **P279**
explanation of injections P279
requirements for EMG-guided injections **P279**
topical anesthetic creams P278–P279
historical aspects P277

mechanism of action Ch464, P277–P278, *P278*
  neuromuscular conduction inhibition P278
preparation P278, **P279**
suboptimal response or treatment failure P280, P282
  causes P280
    guidelines for reducing resistance risk **P282**
    neutralizing antibody formation P280, P282
    serological tests P282
    test dose injections P282, *P282*
techniques P279–P280
  EMG guidance P279–P280
  nontarget muscle testing P280
  steps to ensure correct needle placement **P280**
treatment (of)
  chronic back pain Ch530
  neurologic disease Ch363
  painful spasticity Ch463–Ch464, **Ch465**
  tension-type headache Ch475
bowel function, PCA adverse effects A234
brachial plexopathy Ca9–Ca10, Ca16–Ca17
  pain characteristics **Ca17**
brachial plexus block A271, P204–P210
  anatomical aspects P205–P206, *P206*
  in children P441
  complications **P211**
  indications P205
  in musculoskeletal injuries A355
  postoperative pain management A320
  testing of four main peripheral nerves **P207**
  see also individual types
brachial plexus neuropathies Ch374
  malignancy Ch374
  neuralgic amyotrophy Ch374
  postsurgical pain syndromes Ch419
  radiation therapy Ch374
  traumatic lesions Ch374
bradycardia
  opioid-induced P62
bradykinin
  CRPS pathogenesis Ch387
  receptors A22
  synthesis in inflammation A22, *A23*
brain
  imaging, central pain examination Ch406
  metastases Ca254
  radiotherapy for tumors Ca254
  stimulation-induced analgesia *see* brain stimulation
  symptoms and signs caused by meningeal carcinomatosis **Ca8**
  tumors, headache diagnosis Ch470
brain-derived neurotrophic factor (BDNF), in inflammatory
  pain A34
brain stimulation Ch293–Ch294, Ch302
  central pain syndromes management Ch410
  complications Ch302
  deep Ca249
    adverse effects Ca249
    efficacy Ca249
    sites for use Ca249
  indications Ch302
  mechanism of action Ch293
  motor cortex stimulation Ch294
  outcomes Ch302
  periventricular gray stimulation Ch293, Ch302
  sensory thalamic stimulation Ch294
breakthrough pain Ca152
  burns A360–A361
  in cancer patients P470
  childbirth pain A431

management
  morphine Ca133
  oral transmucosal fentanyl citrate (OTFC) Ca54
  in opioid therapy P80
  oral transmucosal fentanyl citrate (OTFC) P470
  prevention in children Ca341
  see also incident pain
breast cancer
  bone metastasis
    chemotherapy Ca287
    hormone treatment Ca288
  hypophysectomy Ch299
  radiotherapy Ca255–Ca256
breast-feeding, analgesia use A379–A380, **A384–A385**
breast surgery pain Ch420
  epidemiology Ch22
breathing techniques
  advantages and disadvantages A293
  diaphragmatic *see* diaphragmatic breathing
  in muscle relaxation A288
breathlessness (dyspnea) Ca293–Ca296
  history and examination Ca293–Ca294
  investigations Ca294
  management Ca294–Ca295
    acupuncture Ca272
  palliative therapies Ca295–Ca296
    anxiolytics Ca295
    nebulized drugs Ca296
    opioids Ca295, Ca312
    oxygen Ca295
    retention of secretions Ca296, Ca312
  pathophysiology Ca293
Brief Pain Inventory (BPI) of Wisconsin Ch120
Bromage scale **A192**
bronchial carcinoma
  radiotherapy Ca253–Ca254
  unilateral facial pain Ca9
BTX-A *see* Botox (BTX-A)
BTX-B *see* Myobloc (BTX-B)
bubble blowing
  in children P150
  role in distraction techniques A288
buccal administration of drugs A205–A206
  opioids A210–A211
  patient-controlled analgesia (PCA) P404
bupivacaine A86
  alternative epidural analgesia P415
  cardiotoxicity A86
  childbirth pain treatment A431
  in children A444
    adverse effects and toxicity A444
    indications A444
    major surgery A448
  epidural *see* epidural bupivacaine
  intra-articular administration A333
  intracisternal infusion, indications for refractory pain P288
  intrathecal administration
    adverse effects P300
    indications for refractory pain P286–P288
  peripheral nerve block agent P198
  pH and pK_a graph *A78*
  pharmacokinetics **A346**
  physiochemical properties and clinical profile **A79, A85**
  potentiation of epidural analgesia by epinephrine *P411*
  potentiation of epidural analgesia by fentanyl *P411*
  preemptive effect A332
  structure **A85**
buprenorphine A49–A50, Ca55, Ca134, P68

administration A210
ceiling effect Ca134
pharmacokinetics Ca55
burning mouth syndrome **Ch482,** Ch488–Ch489
clinical history Ch488
diagnosis **Ch488,** Ch488–Ch489
differential diagnosis Ch489
epidemiology Ch488
etiology/pathophysiology Ch488, **Ch489**
management Ch489
prognosis Ch489
xerostomia Ch488
burns A359–A367
assessment of pain A361
central pain Ch407
depth A359
evolution of pain A361
general anesthesia A363–A364
management A360, A361–A364
nonopioid analgesia A363
nonpharmacological approaches A364
NSAIDs A363
pain characteristics after injury A360
central mechanisms A360
consciousness influence A360
nociceptive and neuropathic pain A360
peripheral mechanisms A360
pain mechanisms A359–A361
background, breakthrough and procedural A360–A361
burn injury A359–A360
pain relief in practice A364
psychological factors effect on pain A361
wound dressing A364
bursitis A396–A397
buspirone, breathlessness management Ca295
butorphanol P68
administration A212
transmucosal delivery in PCA P403
treatment of intraspinal opioid adverse effects A258
butorpharol tartrate, malpractice claims Ch179–Ch180
butyl-aminobenzoate (BAB) A88–A89

cachexia see anorexia–cachexia syndrome
caffeine A68
calcitonin Ca222–Ca224
adjuvant analgesics Ca135
adverse effects Ca223
hypercalcemia treatment Ca300
practical tips Ca223
calcium
effect of increased intracellular concentration A26
second messenger role **A20**
calcium channel blockers Ca224–Ca225, Ch267
adverse effects Ca224
classes Ca224
contraindications Ca224
doses and treatment paradigms Ca224
efficacy Ca224
indications Ca224
mechanism of action Ch267
pharmacokinetics Ca224
practical tips Ca224
treatment (of)
central pain syndromes Ch409–Ch410
refractory angina pectoris Ch557
ziconotide Ch267
calcium channels, voltage-gated, anticonvulsants Ch251
calcium crystal arthropathies A397

calcium metabolism-associated drugs Ca222–Ca224
adverse effects Ca223
contraindications Ca223
doses and treatment paradigms Ca223
evidence for efficacy Ca223
indications Ca223
pharmacokinetics Ca223
practical tips Ca223
Canadian Centre on Substance Abuse Act, opioids legal
controls Ch175
cancer pain
AIDS pain comparison **Ca372,** Ca372–Ca373
analgesia requirements P469–P470
responsiveness P470
tolerance P470
variability P469–P470
classification Ca124, **Ca124**
clinical trials see cancer pain clinical trials (below)
diagnosis Ch134
epidemiology see epidemiology (cancer pain)
epidural treatment of refractory pain P308
see also epidural treatment of refractory pain
etiology **Ca124**
instability P470
intrapelvic Ca12–Ca13
sites of Ca12–Ca13, **Ca13**
management
alternative/complementary therapy Ch348–Ch349
lidocaine, intravenous Ch256
opioids see opioids, cancer pain management
organizations of interest **Ca92**
pain intensity measurements P23
for patients with persistent pain P23
persistent P477–P478
refractory see refractory cancer pain
subcutaneous infusions P85–P99
advantages P85
analgesia choice P88
assumptions P86
complications P96–P98
drug reactions P97
equipment malfunction P96
prescribing errors P97–P98
reactions at injection site P96–P97
contraindications P86
drug combinations P92, **P93–P94**
drugs administered P88, **P89–P90**
drugs to be mixed with normal saline **P92**
indications P86, **P86**
initiation P95
managerial issues P98–P99
guidelines P98
policies P98
procedures P98
protocols P98
standards P98–P99
monitoring P95–P96
nonopioid analgesics P91–P92
opioids see opioids, subcutaneous infusions in cancer pain
control
preparation of infusion P95
prescribing P95
priming and siting P95
syringe drivers P85
see also syringe drivers
suicide risk see suicide, cancer-related
syndromes Ca3–Ca19
characterization **Ca65,** Ca65–Ca66

prevalence of pain **Ca3**
refractory *see* refractory cancer pain
   see also individual conditions/diseases
temporal aspects P470
types **Ca124**
visceral, neurolytic blocks P247–P253
   see also individual types
see also individual cancers and management modalities
cancer pain clinical trials P92, P95, P469–P481
anticonvulsants Ch253
comparison groups P472
ethical issues P478–P479
   individual versus collective ethics P478
   patient information and consent P479
   placebo treatment P478–P479
factors difficult to control P476–P477
   incidence of adverse effects P476
   patient compliance P476–P477
   patient withdrawals P477
   supplementary treatment P477
inclusion criteria and accretion of patients P475
   organ dysfunction patient exclusion P475
   problems P475
   terminal patient exclusion P475
pain assessment P471
   animal experiments P471
   evaluation instruments P471
   pain categories P469, P471
   pain experience *P471*
   terminology P471
pain instability P470
polypharmacy as problem P471–P472
   adjuvant analgesics P471–P472
   drug interactions P472
requirements P472
selection and stratification of patients P474–P475
   heterogeneity reduction strategies P475
   staging system P475
size and duration of study P475–P476
   factors causing decreased accrual rate P476
   factors influencing number of subjects required P476
specific problems P477–P478
   assessment of analgesic cost P478
   methodological P92, P95
   persistent/intractable cancer pain P477–P478
study design issues P472–P474
   cluster-randomized trials P474
   crossover designs P473–P474, *P474*
   enriched enrollment study designs P474
   historical control study designs P472–P473
   parallel designs P473, *P474*
   randomized controlled trials P473
   sequential trials P473
variability in analgesic requirements P469–P470
candidiasis
anal *Ca384*
corticosteroid induced Ca219
esophageal *see* esophageal candidiasis
oral *see* oral candidiasis
see also pseudomembranous candidiasis (thrush)
cannabinoid receptor agonists Ch266
adverse effects Ch266
mechanism of action Ch266
cannabinoids
antinociceptive action A12
endogenous, in inflammatory hyperalgesia A29
marijuana restrictions according to IOC medical code A500
receptors A12, A29

cannulation, clinical trials of EMLA **Ca324**
capsaicin Ca225
adverse effects Ca225
contraindications Ca225
doses and treatment paradigms Ca225
efficacy Ca225
indications Ca225
practical tips Ca225
topical *see* topical capsaicin
treatment (of)
   acute herpes zoster pain Ch218
   osteoarthritis Ch218, **Ch219**
   peripheral neuropathies Ch377
   postherpetic neuralgia **Ch219**
   pruritus Ca308
carbamazepine
adjuvant analgesic in elderly Ca358
adverse effects Ca214, Ch493, P107
clinical trials Ch252
contraindications P105
doses and treatment paradigms Ca214, P105, **P106**
   pretreatment safety measures P105, **P106**
in elderly Ch655
pharmacokinetics Ca214
structure *Ch240*
treatment (of)
   central pain syndrome Ch409
   CRPS Ch394
   Guillain–Barré syndrome A372
   multiple sclerosis A372
   neuropathic pain Ca215
   painful spasticity **Ch461**
   peripheral neuropathy Ch377
   postherpetic neuralgia Ch453
   postsurgical pain syndrome Ch423
   trigeminal neuralgia Ch493, **Ch494–Ch495**
cardiac arrhythmia, drugs for *see* antiarrhythmics
cardiac complications
abdominal pain due to cardiac failure Ch582
antidepressant-induced Ch243
arrhythmia, intravenous regional sympathetic block complication P245
management in ICU A347
NSAID induced Ca189, Ch231
in postoperative period A166–A168, A311–A312
cardiac output
determinant of local anesthesia absorption A79
general anesthesia effect **A169**
physiological changes with age A464
postoperative pain management and outcome measures A166–A168
   effect of anesthesia and analgesia **A169**
   intraspinal opioid effects A251
cardiocardiac reflex, angina pectoris Ch555, *Ch555*
cardiovascular fitness, fibromyalgia/myofascial pain management Ch624
cardiovascular system
opioids' pharmacological effects P62
carers
demographics Ca353
knowledge and experience in elderly care Ca353–Ca354
psychological evaluation Ca76
carpal tunnel syndrome
disability assessment, case history Ch53–Ch54
in pregnancy A377
release, postsurgical pain Ch420
Cartesian approach, to pain assessment Ch89
case–control studies, definition Ch18–Ch19

catecholamines
    increased release during childbirth A427
    in inflammatory pain A24
catheters, epidural, placement and removal complications A174
cauda equina syndrome A408, Ca6
    intraspinal opioid complication A250–A251
    local anesthesia complication A81
caudal analgesia
    in children P442
    delayed respiratory depression after administration A447
    epidural steroid injections P418, P421
    ketamine A447–A448
    morphine A447
    opioids A447
caudal blocks
    complications A447
        delayed urine passage A447
    in pediatric surgery A446–A448
        pharmacokinetics A446–A447
        volume versus height of block **A446**
causalgia *see* complex regional pain syndrome II (CRPS-II)
cavity administration of drugs A207–A208
    nonsteroidal anti-inflammatory drugs A210
    opioids A212–A213
cefalexin, maxillary sinusitis management Ch487
celecoxib A67, Ca200–Ca201
    adverse effects Ca200–Ca201, Ch230
    characteristics **Ch229**
    clinical trials Ch232
    contraindications Ca187, Ca200
    doses and treatment protocols Ca200
    drug interactions **Ca201**
    elderly pain management Ch654
    evidence for efficacy Ca201
    indications Ca186–Ca187
    pharmacokinetics Ca201, **Ca201**
celiac plexus block P248–P251
    anatomical aspects P248
    complications P249–P250
        abdominal aortic dissection P250
        backache P250
        diarrhea P249, P250
        malposition of needle P250
        orthostatic hypotension P249, P250
        paraplegia and transient motor paralysis P250
        retroperitoneal hemorrhage P250
    drugs and dosing P249
    efficacy P250–P251
    indications P248
    neurolytic Ca238–Ca239
        complications Ca239
        controversies **Ca239**
        efficacy Ca239
        evidence for efficacy **Ca239**
        indications Ca238–Ca239, **Ca239**
        procedure Ca239
    new perspectives P251
    persistent cancer pain P477–P478
    refractory cancer pain management Ca152
    technique P248–P249
        needle placement and contrast medium spread *P249*
Center for Epidemiologic Studies – Depression (CES-D) Ch150
central hypogastric pain Ca12–Ca13
central lesions, painful spasticity Ch460
central nervous system (CNS)
    anticonvulsant adverse effects Ch254
    CRPS pathogenesis Ch387
    depressants interactions with local anesthesia A83

NSAIDs adverse effects A59, Ca190
opioids' pharmacological effects Ca46–Ca47, P62, P63
pain management of injuries in ICU A345
plasticity concept Ca146
stimulation *see* brain stimulation; spinal cord stimulation
    (SCS)
systems primarily affected by opioids Ca40
tumors, in children Ca333
central pain syndromes Ch403–Ch416
    ablative management Ch410–Ch411
        brain Ch411
        brainstem Ch411
        conclusions **Ch411**
        nerves Ch410
        spinal cord Ch410–Ch411
        see also individual procedures
    animal models *see* animal models
    clinical presentation Ch407–Ch408
        examination Ch408
        history Ch407
        pain descriptors Ch407
    definition Ch403
    diagnosis Ch408
        associated disorders Ch408
        brainstem criteria Ch408
        spinal cord criteria Ch408
        suprathalamic criteria Ch408
        thalamic criteria Ch408
    epidemiology Ch406–Ch407, **Ch407**
        associated conditions Ch406
        family impact Ch406
        magnitude Ch406
        stroke Ch406
    etiology Ch403–Ch405
        iatrogenic lesions Ch404
        lesion types Ch403–Ch404
        spinal cord lesions Ch404
    management Ch408–Ch411, Ch409–Ch410
        central nervous system stimulation Ch410
        evidence evaluation Ch408–Ch409
        intracerebral stimulation Ch410
        ketamine Ch264
        peripheral nerve stimulation Ch410
        physical therapy Ch317, Ch411
        posterior column stimulation Ch410
        stepwise approach Ch411–Ch412, **Ch412**
        TENS Ch410
    pathophysiology Ch405–Ch406
        denervation supersensitivity Ch405
        disinhibition Ch405
        hemispheric dominance Ch405
        maladaptive reorganization Ch406
        nociceptive feedback control Ch405
        spinothalamic tract (STT) involvement Ch405
    pharmacological management
        adrenergic agents Ch409
        anesthetics Ch409
        anticonvulsants Ch409
        antidepressants Ch409, **Ch409**
        opioids Ch409
    prognosis Ch412
        partially reversible lesions Ch412
        reversible lesions Ch412
    supraspinal Ch404–Ch405
    terms **Ch404**
central sensitization A29–A36, Ca146, P28
    attenuation with NMDA receptor blockers Ca221
    clinical features **A314**

decreased inhibitory input to dorsal horn neurons A34–A35
experimental models illustrating P486–P487, **P487**
increased excitatory input to dorsal horn neurons A32–A34
from primary afferent neurons A32–A34
from supraspinal centers A34
intracellular events leading to *A33*
long-term depression (LTD) A29, *A30–A31*
long-term potentiation (LTP) A29, *A30–A31*
synaptic reorganization A35
transcriptional and post-translational changes in dorsal
horn A35–A36
windup A29, *A30*
see also peripheral sensitization
cerebellar stimulation, painful spasticity management **Ch463**
cerebral metastases, radiotherapy Ca254
cerebrospinal fluid (CSF)
examination, peripheral neuropathies Ch370
opioid instillation in neurosurgical procedures Ca262
adverse effects Ca262
production and loss P286
cervical dilation, childbirth pain A424–A425, *A425*
cervical diskography Ch132, Ch137
cervical dystonia, management, botulinum toxin
injections Ch464
cervical hematoma, stellate ganglion block complication P239
cervical osteoarthritis, neck pain Ch508
cervical plexus block P203
anatomical aspects *P204*
deep P203
anatomical aspects P203
complications P203
landmarks and practical steps P203, *P205*
indications P203
superficial P203
anatomical aspects *P204*
landmarks and practical steps P203, *P204*
cervical posterior rhizotomy, painful spasticity
management **Ch463**
cervical spine
damage during whiplash Ch509
radiofrequency lesioning P333
referred pain Ch505–Ch506, *Ch506*
cervical spondylosis
headache diagnosis Ch470
neck pain Ch508
plain radiography Ch510–Ch511
cervical zygapophyseal (facet) joints
blocks P272–P274
evidence for use of P274–P275
intra-articular blocks P272–P273
medial branch blocks P273–P274
needle positioning *P275*
positioning of C-arm *P274*
denervation with radiofrequency lesioning P333–P334
adverse effects P334
indications P333
results P334
technique P333–P334, *P334*
dysfunction P190
accompanying myofascial pain P190
etiology P190
referred pain P190
pain P270
cervicothoracic sympathetic chain P237, *P238*
block *see* stellate ganglion block
Cesarean section, timing of administration of local
anesthetics A120
chamomile, botanical therapy **Ch347**

Chappel v. Hart, medical liability Ch178
chemical hyperalgesia Ch119, **Ch121**
chemical manipulation, prohibited method in IOC medical
code A499–A500
chemodenervation, painful spasticity management Ch463–
Ch464, **Ch464**
chemonucleolysis, chronic back pain management Ch529
chemotherapy
bone pain management *see under* bone pain
intrathecal administration *Ca320*
chest pain Ch553–Ch565
in AIDS patients *see under* AIDS
angina pectoris *see* angina pectoris
assessment Ch553–Ch556
multiple syndromes Ch553–Ch554
psychological predispositions Ch554, **Ch554**
specific syndromes Ch553
bone pain Ch558–Ch559
cardiac related Ch556–Ch558
differential diagnosis Ch554
epidemiology Ch553
etiology Ch553
gastroesophageal reflux disorder *see* gastroesophageal reflux
disorder (GERD)
indication for radiotherapy Ca253–Ca254
joints Ch559
costochondral pain Ch559
manubriosternal pain Ch559
Tietze syndrome Ch559
twelfth rib syndrome Ch559
left internal mammary artery pain syndrome Ch560
management Ch554
guidelines **Ch561**
musculoskeletal syndromes Ch558, **Ch559**
myofascial pains Ch559–Ch560
noncardiac Ch558–Ch560
postsurgical Ch560, **Ch560**
assessment Ch560, **Ch561**
management Ch560, **Ch561**
psychological aspects Ch560–Ch561
screening Ch560–Ch561, **Ch561**
radicular pain Ch560
referred pain Ch560
refractory angina pectoris *see* angina pectoris, refractory
slipping rib syndrome Ch560
syndrome X *see* syndrome X
wall rigidity, opioid-induced P63
chest trauma
analgesic techniques A352–A353, **A354**
complications A352
chest wall rigidity, opioid induced P63
childbirth pain A423–A435
anatomy A424–A426
course of normal childbirth A424–A425
pain of dysfunctional labor A425–A426, *A426*
somatic pain A425
visceral pain A425
breakthrough pain A431
clinical presentation A429
educational preparation A291
factors influencing A429–A430
maternal characteristics A430
obstetrics A430
psychological and social A429–A430
magnitude A424
severity *A425*
management A431–A432
epidural analgesia A244, A430, A431

intrathecal opioids A249, A431
investigations of methods A430–A431
neuraxial A431
non-neuraxial A431–A432
nonpharmacological methods A432
pharmacological methods A431–A432
TENS A278–A279, P351
measurement A427–A429
descriptive measurement tools A428
scalar measurement tools A428
surrogate tools A428–A429
neurological transmission A426
sympathetic efferent nerves *A427*
physiological responses A426–A427
relationship to stage of labor A424–A425, **A425**
stimulus A424–A425
variations A423, *A424*
childbirth preparatory techniques, influence on childbirth
pain A429
children Ca333–Ca347, Ch637–Ch647
abdominal pain, recurrent Ch639–Ch640
associated syndromes Ch640
CBT Ch640
classification Ch640
dietary fiber Ch640
epidemiology Ch640
management Ch640
psychiatric disorders Ch640
stress Ch640
acetaminophen *see under* acetaminophen (paracetamol)
addiction Ca344
adjuvant analgesics Ca342–Ca344
anticonvulsants Ca342
antidepressants Ca342
corticosteroids Ca342
neuroleptics Ca343–Ca344
psychostimulants Ca342
radionucleotides Ca342–Ca343
analgesia for patients 6 months or younger P438–P439
systemic analgesia P438–P439
see also individual drugs
analgesia routes P432–P434
epidural P433
inhalation P433–P434
intramuscular cA340, P433
intravenous Ca340, P432
oral Ca340, P432
rectal Ca340–Ca341, P432
subcutaneous Ca340, P432–P433
topical Ca340
analgesia studies **Ca335–Ca337**
aspirin Ca338
back pain Ch641
associated conditions Ch641
diagnostic criteria Ch641
epidemiology Ch641
management Ch641
prevalence Ch641
see also back pain
biofeedback *see* biofeedback, in children
bubble blowing A288, P150
cognitive–behavioral therapy (CBT) Ca334
CRPS-I Ch386, Ch642
etiology Ch642
management Ch642
prevalence Ch642
see also complex regional pain syndrome I (CRPS-I)
developmental issues P147–P148

development of nociception/response to pain A437–A438
peripheral and central mechanisms A438
sensory processing differences in adults A438
diaphragmatic breathing P149–P150
distraction A288, Ca275
epidemiology of cancer pain Ca333–Ca334
treatment-related pain Ca333–Ca334
tumor-related pain Ca333–Ca334
epidemiology of chronic pain Ch20–Ch21
gender-specific pain Ch20–Ch21
puberty Ch21
epidural analgesia *see* epidural analgesia/anesthesia, in
children
fibromyalgia Ch640–Ch641
age-of-onset Ch641
CBT Ch641
etiology Ch641
management Ch641
prevalence Ch641
prognosis Ch641
see also fibromyalgia
headaches Ch637–Ch639
diagnostic criteria Ch637
gender bias Ch637
prevalence Ch637
tension-type *see* children, tension-type headaches *(below)*
see also headaches
hypnosis *see* hypnosis, in children
imagery technique A289
intra-articular injections, evidence for use P256
irritable bowel syndrome (IBS) Ch640
local anesthetic techniques A80–A81, A444–A448, P439–P443
EMLA Ca340
epidural A448
major surgery A448
in patients 6 months or younger P439–P443
peripheral nerve blocks **P439,** P440–P442
postoperative pain management A444–A448
see also individual blocks
management access Ch643
migraine Ch638–Ch639
genetics Ch638
management Ch638–Ch639
prevalence Ch638
symptoms Ch638
see also migraine
modeling Ch643
musculoskeletal pain Ch640–Ch641
neurological diseases Ca403
neuropathic pain Ch641–Ch642
nitrous oxide inhalation P433–P434
nonopioid analgesics Ca338
nonpharmacological management Ca334
NSAIDs *see under* nonsteroidal anti-inflammatory drugs
(NSAIDs)
opioid analgesia *see* opioids, in children
pain assessment P431–P432
behavioral measures P432, *P433*
self-reporting P432, *P433*
pain behavior reinforcement Ch643
pain disability Ch643–Ch644
pain intensity assessment P21
pain measurement *see under* pain measurement
pain score–pain management action plan **P434**
pain studies A437
PCA *see under* patient-controlled analgesia (PCA)
peripheral nerve blocks **P439,** P440–P442
see also individual blocks

phantom limb pain Ch642
   anticonvulsants Ch642
   description Ch642
   management Ch642
   sample sizes Ch642
   see also phantom limb
pharmacological management A440–A444, Ca334–Ca344
   administration routes and methods Ca340–Ca341
   agents and guideline doses for analgesia in ICU **A343**
   see also individual drugs
physical dependence Ca344
postoperative pain management A444–A450, A448–A449
   complex local blocks for major surgery A448–A449
   local anesthesia A444–A448
   systemic analgesia A449–A450
      see also systemic analgesics
principles and organization of pain management A440
   balanced analgesia A440
   information and protocols A440, **A440**
   multispecialist teams A440
   parental role A440
procedural pain management A451–A452
   hypnosis Ca274
   nitrous oxide A452
   psychological and complementary therapies A452
   topical local anesthesia A452
procedures for pain management P431–P445
   developmental level P431
   general considerations P431–P434
   pain assessment P431–P432
      see also children, pain assessment
   planning P431
psychogenic explanations Ch644
psychological evaluation Ca78–Ca79
psychological therapies A287–A293
   see also psychological therapies
psychosocial contexts Ch644
relaxation *see* relaxation, in children
self-regulation skills *see* self-regulation skills training, in
   children
self-reporting of pain A105–A106, P432, *P433*
separation anxiety Ch643
sickle cell pain Ch642–Ch643
   see also sickle cell disease
surgery
   axillary nerve block A446
   caudal blocks *see under* caudal blocks
   ilioinguinal nerve block A445
   infraorbital nerve block A446
   intercostal nerve blocks A448
   intrapleural block A448
   lumbar plexus block A448–A449
   paravertebral nerve blocks A448
   penile nerve block A445–A446
   simple nerve blocks A445–A448
   thoracic paravertebral blocks A448–A449
   wound infiltration of local anesthesia A445, **A445**
systemic analgesia A441–A442, A449–A450
   nausea and vomiting A450
   parenteral opioid infusion A449
   rectal administration A449
   timing and route of analgesia A449
systemic analgesia for patients over 6 months P433–P438
   adverse effects of opioid analgesia P436–P437
      see also opioids, adverse effects
   alternative drugs for moderate to severe pain P437–P438
   analgesics for mild to moderate pain P433–P435, **P435**
   analgesics for moderate to severe pain P435–P436

   monitoring for patients on systemic opioid
      infusions P437, **P438**
   see also individual drugs
tension-type headaches Ch639
   criteria Ch639
   etiology Ch639
   management Ch639
   persistence Ch639
   prevalence Ch639
   see also tension-type headaches
tolerance Ca344
trauma
   caution with analgesic techniques A356
   musculoskeletal injuries A356
   see also neonatal pain management
Chinese herbs Ca273
Chinese medicine Ch339
chiropractic therapy Ch344–Ch345
   adverse effects Ch345
   efficacy Ch345
   history Ch344
   scope Ch344–Ch345
   theory Ch344–Ch345
      innate intelligence Ch344
      long-lever adjustments Ch345
      recoil adjustments Ch345
      subluxation complex Ch344–Ch345
   treatment (of)
      back pain Ch345
      headache Ch345
      pelvic pain Ch603
   value Ch345
chloroprocaine A83
   structure, physiochemical properties and clinical profile **A84**
chlorpromazine, central pain syndrome management Ch409
chlorprothixene, postherpetic neuralgia management Ch453
cholangitis, sclerosing, abdominal pain cause in AIDS
   patients Ca388
cholecystokinin (CCK)
   antagonist development Ch194
   modulation of nociceptive messages A13
choline magnesium trisalicylate A64
   characteristics **Ch229**
   in children Ca338
chondromalacia patella Ch547
chondroprotective agents, osteoarthritis management Ch544
chronic back and leg pain (CBLP)
   periventricular gray stimulation Ch290–Ch293
   spinal cord stimulation Ch290–Ch293
chronic fatigue and immune dysfunction syndrome (CFIDS),
   fibromyalgia Ch623
chronic inflammatory demyelinating neuropathy (CIDP), in AIDS
   patients Ca376
chronic intractable benign pain (CIBP), associated
   syndromes Ch65, Ch66
   see also comorbidities
chronic mesenteric ischemia Ch579–Ch580
chronic pain
   analgesia **Ca160–Ca161**
   attention regulation *see* attention regulation in chronic pain,
     phase I
   clinical pattern P135–P136
   clinical RCTs P489
      see also clinical experimental pharmacological protocols
   cryoanalgesia P323–P325
      duration of pain P325
      limitations P323
      patient education P324

patient selection P323–P324
percutaneous technique P324
risks P323
distraction unsuitability for patients P135, P136
epidemiology *see* epidemiology (chronic pain)
opioids *see* opioids, chronic pain management
pain intensity measurements P23
postoperative neuropathic *see* postoperative neuropathic
pain, chronic
regular around-the-clock medication Ca126
TENS indications P344–P345
experimental evidence P351
treatment protocols *see* opioids, in chronic nonmalignant
pain (protocols)
see also individual causes of pain and management modalities
Chronic Pain Self-Efficacy Scale (CPSS) Ch148
chronic pain syndrome Ch634–Ch635
diagnosis **Ch78,** Ch634
Chung model Ch190–Ch191
Churg–Strauss syndrome, autoimmune neuropathy Ch373
cinchocaine, structure, physiochemical properties and clinical
profile **A85**
cingulotomy Ca265, Ch302–Ch303
complications Ch303
indications Ch302–Ch303
management (of), central pain syndromes Ch411
technique Ch303
circadian variation
effect on pain perception P16
circumcision, penile nerve block A446
cisplatin, toxic neuropathy Ch372
cisterna magna P286, *P287*
citalopram Ca217
pharmacology **Ch240**
tension-type headache management Ch475
civil justice system P513
areas of concern P513
changes to speed up process P513
see also medicolegal aspects
class actions, malpractice claims Ch180
see also medicolegal aspects
classification of cancer pain Ca124, **Ca124**
cleft lip, infraorbital nerve block A446
climatic conditions
effect on pain perception P16
clinical assessment Ch89–Ch100
Cartesian approach Ch89
communication with physician Ch90
complications Ch93
evaluation questions Ch91–Ch92, **Ch96**
formats Ch92–Ch94
interviews Ch92–Ch93, Ch96–Ch97
pain interpretation Ch92
patients perspective **Ch93**
targets covered **Ch92**
multiaxial Ch97–Ch98
outcome *see* outcome measures
pain diaries Ch94, Ch97
psychological Ch94–Ch97
overt expressions of pain Ch96–Ch97
psychiatric diagnoses Ch95
psychometric assessments Ch95–Ch96
purposes Ch91
referrals Ch96
self-report Ch93–Ch94
functional activities Ch94
rating scales *Ch94*
see also diagnostic procedures; pain assessment; pain history/

examination
clinical experimental pharmacological protocols P483–P493
acute pain studies P487–P488
inflammatory pain P487–P488
intrathecal administration P488
intravenous administration P487–P488
perioperative pain P488
postoperative analgesia P488
adenosine P485–P486
see also adenosine
animal data P483–P484
adenosine and adenosine analogs P483–P484
adenosine combinations with other analgesics P484
general interpretation P484
background P485
research P483
central sensitization models P486–P487, **P487**
chronic pain studies P488
intrathecal administration P488
intravenous administration P488
correlation between animal models and clinical
problem P487
development of novel drugs from compound to
analgesic *P488*
ethical, regulatory and financial considerations P491
flow chart for evaluation of RCTs *P491*
interpreting data P490–P491
pharmacology of substances P484
pitfalls in results P490–P491
qualitative and quantitative sensory assessments **P486**
safety perspectives P484–P485
study design techniques and considerations P489–P490, *P490*
basics P489
gender aspects P489–P490
parallel groups or crossover *P490*
substances *P491*
see also clinical trials
clinical governance *see under* medicolegal aspects
clinical history *see* pain history/examination
clinical neurophysiology *see* neurophysiological techniques
clinical pharmacology Ca33–Ca63
see also individual drugs
Clinical Standards Advisory Group (CSAG), pain clinics Ch158,
Ch161
clinical trials P449–P459
analgesia onset P456–P457
assay sensitivity P450
blinding and unblinding of treatment P454
cancer pain *see* cancer pain clinical trials
crossover designs P454–P455, P473–P474, *P474*
four-group complete **P455**
problems P454–P455
three-group complete **P455**
typical two-treatment **P455,** *P474*
dental pain P462–P463
see also dental pain model
evoked pain P457
nature of mechanical stimulus and proposed research
tools **P458**
explanatory and pragmatic studies P449–P450, **P450**
global assessment P457
inclusion of patients P454
long-term trials P457
outcomes for use in meta-analysis P457
outcomes of pain treatment trials P455
meaningful endpoints P455
pain intensity *P451,* P455
clinically important reduction P455

difference (PID) *P456*
  summed difference (SPID) *P451*, P456
parallel design P454–P455, P473
  three-treatment assessment *P474*
placebo
  active P454
  essentiality of knowing response P453
  treatment ethicality P454
primary efficacy variable choice P450
publishing P458
purpose of study P450
quality of life assessment P457
randomization P454
  see also randomized controlled trials (RCTs)
remedication time P457
repeated measurements P456
rescue analgesia consumption P456
  difference in pain intensity and morphine
    consumption *P456*
result possibilities **P458**
statistical issues P458
study design P450
  balanced design P455
  parallel or crossover studies P455–P456, *P490*
treatments and controls choice P450–P453
  additive effects P453
  equivalence trials P452
  isobologram *P453*
  relative potency *P452*, P452–P453
  superiority studies *P451*, P452
  synergy P453
uncontrolled, placebos Ch274
see also clinical experimental pharmacological protocols
clinicians
  accountability Ch35–Ch36
  pain diagnosis failure Ch30–Ch31
clodronate
  bone pain management Ca288–Ca289
  doses and treatment paradigms Ca223
  pharmacokinetics Ca223
clomipramine
  mechanism of action Ch239–Ch240
  pharmacology **Ch240**
  treatment (of)
    neuropathic pain Ch242
    peripheral neuropathy Ch376
    postherpetic neuralgia Ch453
clonazepam
  adverse effects Ca214
  clinical trials Ch253
  doses and treatment paradigms Ca214
  pharmacokinetics Ca215
  treatment (of)
    central pain syndrome Ch409
    myofascial pain (MFP) Ch625
    painful spasticity **Ch462**
    peripheral neuropathy Ch377
    postsurgical pain syndrome Ch423
    trigeminal neuralgia Ch494, **Ch494–Ch495**
clonidine Ca210–Ca211
  adjuvant to local anesthetic for nerve blockade A271
  adverse effects Ca211
  in children A443, A448
    administration A443
    adverse effects and toxicity A443
    analgesia for patients over 6 months P438
    pharmacology and indications A443
  contraindications Ca210–Ca211

doses and treatment paradigms Ca211
evidence for efficacy Ca211
indications Ca210
pain management in ICU A344–A345
pharmacokinetics Ca211
practical tips Ca211
topical Ch222
  evidence Ch222
treatment (of)
  burn pain A363
  CRPS Ch391
  facial pain Ch222
  migraine Ch475
  neurologic disease Ch362
  neuropathic pain Ca210, Ch222
  painful spasticity **Ch462**
  see also α_2-adrenergic agonists
clorazepate, painful spasticity management **Ch462**
closed kinetic chain exercise, definition **Ch316**
cluster headaches **Ch482, Ch499**
  radiofrequency lesioning indication P331
cluster-randomized trials
  in cancer pain clinical trials P474
CMR1 A19–A20
coagulation, postoperative pain management and outcome
  measures A170–A171
coanalgesics *see* adjunct therapies
cocaine A83
  historical aspects A73
  structure, physiochemical properties and clinical profile **A84**
Cochrane Back Review Group, low back pain guidelines **A415**
Cochrane Collaboration A164, A176, P509
codeine A48, Ca52, Ca131, Ch207, P66
  acetaminophen combinations Ch233–Ch234
    in elderly Ca357
  adverse effects Ca131
  in children A442, Ca338
    administration A442
    adverse effects and toxicity A442
    analgesia for patients 6 months or younger P439
    analgesia for patients over 6 months P434
    doses **P435**
    indications A442
  elderly pain management Ch653–Ch654
  pain control after discharge home A335
  pharmacokinetics Ca52
  for refractory cancer pain Ca144–Ca145
  synthetic derivatives P67
  see also oxycodone; tramadol
cognitive–behavioral therapy (CBT) Ch325–Ch333
  assessment of pain-related fear *see under* pain-related fear
  in children Ca334
  components Ch327–Ch329
    attention management Ch328
    behavioral change Ch328
    cognitive restructuring Ch328–Ch329
    education Ch328
    exercise and fitness training Ch328
    generalization and maintenance strategies Ch329
    goal setting Ch328
    problem solving Ch329
    relaxation Ch328
  definition A286
  efficacy Ch331–Ch333
    outcome identification Ch332–Ch333
    risks Ch332
  evidence based Ch329–Ch331
    active management comparison *Ch332*

assumptions/exclusions Ch330
  problems Ch330
  systematic review process Ch329–Ch330
  waiting list control comparison *Ch331*
general principles Ch327
  behavioral experiment Ch327
  consulting teaching style Ch327
  empathic discussion Ch327
  integration and synergy Ch327
  limitation recognition Ch327
  practicing skills Ch327
  qualified staff Ch327
imagery techniques in children A289
management aims Ch326–Ch327
sources of development Ch325
treatment (of)
  angina pectoris Ch555
  anxiety Ca310
  burning mouth syndrome Ch489
  chronic back pain Ch532
  CPRP Ch166, Ch320
  depression Ca309
  fibromyalgia Ch641
  irritable bowel syndrome (IBS) Ch578
  migraine Ch638–Ch639, **Ch639**
  myofascial pain (MFP) Ch626
  pelvic pain Ch603
  procedural pain Ca322
  procedural pain in children A452
  recurrent abdominal pain Ch640
  TMJ pain **Ch486**
  vulvar pain syndrome Ch607
cognitive impairment A469
  assessment in elderly A106, A469
  assessment tools Ca64–Ca65
  interference in patient assessment Ca64
  opioid-induced A472, Ca46, Ca132, Ca170–Ca171, Ch206
    clinical presentation and findings Ca170
    definition Ca170
    evidence-based evaluation of management Ca171
cognitive measures of pain P5–P6
cohort studies, definition Ch18, Ch19
cold
  pain condition P356
  physiotherapy agent P185
cold allodynia, anticonvulsant therapy Ch254
cold- and menthol-sensitive receptor 1 (CMR1) A19–A20
cold hyperalgesia Ch115, **Ch121**
cold hypersensitivity, CRPS Ch384
cold I-T injection, neurologic disease management Ch363
cold packs, in cryotherapy A493
collagen, role in tissue repair A487–A488
colonic diverticula Ch580
colorectal cancer, radiotherapy Ca255
combination therapies Ch262
  dosages Ch262
  efficacy Ch262
  multiple mechanisms Ch262
combined spinal–epidural (CSE)
  childbirth pain treatment A244, A431
  suggested drug doses and mixtures **A245**
Commission on Accreditation of Rehabilitation Facilities
  (CARF) Ch168, Ch169–Ch170
commissural myelotomy Ca264
communication
  difficulties
    delirious and demented patients Ca67
    in elderly patients Ca359–Ca360

importance Ca77
in neurosurgical modalities Ca261
in physiotherapy P179–P180
comorbidities Ch74–Ch78
  avoidance behavior Ch76, Ch78
  behavioral Ch71–Ch74
    anger Ch73
    effects on spouse Ch74
    fear of pain Ch73–Ch74
    measurement Ch72, **Ch72**
    stress Ch71–Ch72
    unrealistic expectations Ch73
    workers' compensation *see* medicolegal aspects; workers'
      compensation
  concentration loss Ch75
  definition Ch68
  disability perception Ch75
  fatigue Ch74–Ch75
  malingering Ch78
  management effects **Ch77**
  memory problems Ch75
  neuropathic pain *see* neuropathic pain
  perception discrepancy Ch76
  psychiatric Ch68–Ch71
    burning mouth syndrome Ch488
    classification **Ch69**
    impact Ch70–Ch71
    management decisions *Ch82,* Ch82–Ch83
    measurement **Ch71**
    type I Ch68–Ch69
    type II Ch69
    type III Ch69
    type IV Ch69
    type V Ch70
    type VI Ch70–Ch71
      false information groups Ch70
    see also psychological effects, assessment; *individual types*
  secondary gain expectations Ch76, Ch78
  sexual dysfunction Ch74
  sleep disorders Ch74
  somatization *see* somatization disorders
  suicidal tendencies Ch76
complementary and alternative medicine Ca269–Ca280, Ch335–
  Ch351
  acupuncture *see* acupuncture
  aromatherapy Ca276, Ch339
  case examples Ch346, Ch348–Ch349
  centers of research (USA) **Ch338**
  Chinese medicine Ch339
    herbs Ca273
  chiropractic management *see* chiropractic therapy
  classification *Ch339,* Ch339–Ch340, *Ch340*
  cost Ch336
  definitions Ch335, Ch337–Ch338
  distraction *see* distraction
  in elderly Ca359
  healing/therapeutic touch Ca276
  health care professionals' attitudes Ca270
  herbal medicine, vitamins and food supplements Ca273
  homeopathy *see* homeopathy
  hypnosis *see* hypnosis
  massage *see* massage
  movement-based Ch339–Ch340
  physician attitudes Ch336–Ch337
    discipline Ch337
  placebos Ch282
  see also placebos
  popularity Ch335–Ch336

management discomfort Ch336
physician–patient relationship Ch336
prevalence Ch336
   Canada Ch336
   Europe Ch336
   by type **Ch337**
   USA Ch336
reasons for increased use Ca269–Ca270
relaxation *see* relaxation
treatment (of)
   cancer pain Ch348–Ch349
   chronic back pain Ch531–Ch532
   low back pain A413
   migraine Ch346
   pelvic pain Ch603
   procedural pain management in children A452
visualization Ca275–Ca276
complete blood count (CBC), pelvic pain diagnosis Ch599
complex regional pain syndrome(s) (CRPSs) Ch374, Ch383–Ch401
   clinical features Ch383–Ch386
      allodynia Ch383–Ch384
      cold hypersensitivity Ch384
      hyperalgesia Ch383–Ch384
      hyperpathia Ch384
      impaired coordination Ch385
      motor abnormality Ch385–Ch386
      myoclonus Ch385
      pain Ch383
      sensory function Ch384
      symptom spread Ch385
      tenderness Ch383
      tremor Ch385
      trophic changes Ch385
      vasomotor/sudomotor changes Ch384–Ch385
      weakness Ch385
   complications Ch385
   diagnosis **Ch384,** Ch388–Ch391
      bone scans Ch129
      electrodiagnostic techniques Ch388
      microneurography (MCNG) Ch390
      MRI Ch390
      quantitative sudomotor axon reflex test (QSART) Ch390–Ch391, *Ch392*
      radiographic findings Ch389
      radionuclide studies Ch389–Ch390
      resting sweat output Ch391
      revision **Ch384**
      scoring system Ch391, **Ch393**
      sympathetic nerve blocks Ch131
      sympathetic skin response Ch391
      thermography Ch130–Ch131
   intravenous phentolamine indication P42
   management Ch391–Ch395
      acupuncture Ch395
      amputation Ch395
      antiarrhythmics Ch394
      anticonvulsants Ch394
      antidepressants Ch394
      capsaicin, topical **Ch219,** Ch221, Ch393
      hydrotherapy Ch395
      massage Ch395
      NSAIDs Ch392–Ch393
      opioids Ch394
      physical therapy Ch317, Ch391, Ch395
      psychological therapy Ch395
      spinal cord stimulation (SCS) Ch395
      steroids Ch392–Ch393
      TENS Ch394–Ch395

topical agents Ch393
pathogenesis Ch386–Ch388
   central nervous system (CNS) Ch387
   dorsal root ganglion (DRG) Ch387
   ectopic discharges Ch386
   nerve damage Ch386
   neurotransmitters Ch387
   predisposition Ch388
   primary afferent neurons (PAN) Ch386–Ch387
   primary hyperalgesia Ch387
   spinal cord Ch387
   stress response Ch386
   sympathetic postganglionic neurons (SPGNs) Ch387–Ch388
postsurgical pain syndromes Ch418
sympathetically maintained pain (SMP) Ch387
   diagnosis **Ch384**
sympathetic block indication P235–P236
sympathetic hyperactivity Ch122
vascular diagnosis Ch388–Ch389
   arterial flow Ch388–Ch389
   lactate levels Ch389
   skin blood-flow Doppler probes Ch389
   venous oxygen Ch389
   whole-body heating/cooling Ch389
see also complex regional pain syndrome I (CRPS-I); complex regional pain syndrome II (CRPS-II)
complex regional pain syndrome I (CRPS-I)
   in children *see* children, CRPS-I
   clinical features
      motor abnormality Ch385
      sensory function Ch384
   diagnosis **Ch384**
      radionuclide studies Ch389–Ch390
      recommendations **Ch393**
   gender difference Ch386
   human leukocyte antigen (HLA) involvement Ch386
   incidence Ch384
   management, spinal cord stimulation (SCS) Ch289–Ch290
   pathogenesis Ch386–Ch387
   see also complex regional pain syndromes (CRPSs)
complex regional pain syndrome II (CRPS-II)
   clinical features
      motor abnormality Ch385
      sensory function Ch384
   diagnosis **Ch384**
   incidence Ch385
   management, peripheral nerve stimulation (PNS) Ch287
   see also complex regional pain syndromes (CRPSs)
comprehensive pain rehabilitation programs (CPRP) Ch163–Ch171, Ch318–Ch322
   accreditation Ch168–Ch170
      Commission on Accreditation of Rehabilitation Facilities (CARF) Ch168
      components Ch169
      National Advisory Committees (NAC) Ch168
      revision Ch168–Ch169
   behavioral adjustment Ch166
      maladaptive abnormal illness attitudes Ch166
   benefits **Ch321**
   CBT Ch166, Ch320
   clinical trials Ch321
   efficacy Ch320–Ch322
      patient satisfaction Ch322
      quality of life Ch322
      reinjury rates Ch322
      spinal motion range Ch321
   family issues Ch167

financial issues Ch167
goals Ch170
history Ch163–Ch165
  active components Ch164
  customization Ch164
  detoxification Ch164
  fee for service Ch163
  Johns Hopkins Hospital Ch163–Ch164
  result durability Ch164–Ch165
  return to work Ch164
information systems Ch169
  analysis Ch169
  patient Ch169
  program level Ch169
leadership Ch169
legal issues Ch168
  see also medicolegal aspects
management systems Ch169
measurable criteria Ch170
medical utilization Ch168
  reduction Ch168
  reimbursement Ch168
medication issues Ch166–Ch167
  opioid contracts Ch167
  opioids Ch166–Ch167
  substance abuse Ch167
  see also opioids
net benefit Ch165
operant conditioning techniques Ch319
outcome measurements *see* outcome measures
pain behavior Ch320
pain reduction Ch321
patient evaluation Ch320
performance improvement Ch169
physical reconditioning Ch165
progressive goals Ch320
psychological reconditioning Ch165–Ch166
  anger Ch165
  anhedonia Ch165
  guilt Ch165–Ch166
  libido loss Ch165
psychology Ch318–Ch319
referral Ch322
  guidelines **Ch322**
steps Ch320
team Ch319, **Ch319**
  nurses Ch320
  patient Ch320
  physical therapists Ch319–Ch320
  physician Ch319
  psychologist Ch320
team components Ch170
work issues Ch167
  payments Ch167
  return to work Ch167
see also physical therapies
compression, sport injury management A491
computed tomography (CT) Ch128
  ablation guidance Ca265
  advantage Ch128
  investigations/diagnosis into
    chronic back pain Ch139–Ch140, Ch526
    maxillary sinusitis Ch487
    neck pain Ch511
    ovarian remnant syndrome Ch593
    pelvic pain Ch599
  mechanism Ch128
  neurosurgical techniques Ch297, Ch298

validity Ch128
concentration loss Ch101
  comorbidities Ch75
concentric strain, definition **Ch316**
concept validity, definition Ch125
concurrent validity, pain measure P10
conditioning, emotional, placebos Ch278
conditioning theory, placebos Ch276
confrontation, pain response P163
Confusional Assessment Method (CAM), delirium diagnosis Ca172
congenital insensitivity to pain, peripheral neuropathies Ch375
congestive cardiac failure (CCF), NSAID induced Ch231
consciousness, influence on burn pain A360
conscious sedation A509
  procedural pain management *see under* procedural pain
  see also sedation
constipation Ca17, Ca303–Ca304
  in AIDS patients Ca388
  clinical findings Ca303
  functional Ch640
  investigations Ca303
  management Ca303–Ca304
    see also laxatives
  opioid-induced Ca47, Ca174–Ca176, Ca357, Ch206, P63
    clinical presentation and findings Ca175
    definition Ca174–Ca175
    diagnostic criteria and evaluation of investigations Ca175
    epidemiology Ca175
    etiology and pathophysiology Ca175
    evidence-based evaluation of management Ca175–Ca176
    notes on unevaluated treatments Ca176
    prevention Ca176
  pathophysiology Ca303
construct validity, definition Ch126
contact dermatitis, acupuncture-induced Ch342
contingency tables, definition **Ch126**
contrast ventriculography, neurosurgical techniques Ch297
controlled substances Ch173
  see also opioids
Controlled Substances Act (CSA), opioid legal controls Ch174
convulsions, opioid-induced P62
coping strategies Ca74, Ch314
  assessment of skills Ch106
  mechanisms Ca80
  pain measure P6
Coping Strategies Questionnaire (CSQ) Ch74, Ch106, Ch148–Ch149
cordectomy, central pain syndromes management Ch411
cordotomy Ch304–Ch305
  bilateral Ca264
  complications Ch305
  indications Ch304
  open surgical technique Ch305
  outcomes Ch304–Ch305
  percutaneous technique Ch305
    cervical *see* percutaneous cervical cordotomy
    electrode placement *Ch298*
  refractory cancer pain management Ca153
coronary artery surgery (CABG), angina pectoris
  management Ch555, **Ch555**
cortical pain modulation P113–P114
  inhibition of pain response P114
cortical spreading depression, migraine pathophysiology Ch469
corticosteroids
  adjuvant analgesics Ca218–Ca219
    adverse effects Ca218–Ca219
    in children Ca342
    contraindications Ca218

doses and treatment paradigms Ca218
evidence for efficacy Ca219
indications Ca218
pharmacokinetics Ca219
practical tips Ca219
see also individual drugs
adverse effects Ch262
caution of use in AIDS patients Ca372
epidural injections *see* epidural steroid injections
historical aspects P255
injections A496
intra-articular administration *see* intra-articular injections
local anesthesia combination A496
NSAIDs interaction A57
postherpetic neuralgia prevention Ch455
restrictions according to IOC medical code A500
subcutaneous infusions in cancer pain control **P90**, P92
transdermal administration A496
treatment (of)
acute herpes zoster pain A371, Ch440
anorexia–cachexia syndrome Ca306
herpes zoster acute pain A371
osteoarthritis Ch543–Ch544
rheumatoid arthritis Ch539
sickle cell disease A383
sport injury A495–A496
cost-effectiveness A174
costochondral pain, chronic chest pain Ch559
cough Ca296–Ca297
history and examination Ca296
opioid-induced P62
treatment Ca296–Ca297
COX-2-selective inhibitors A66–A67, Ca200–Ca202
see also celecoxib; rofecoxib
coxibs Ca200–Ca201
drug interactions **Ca201**
pharmacokinetics **Ca201**
see also celecoxib; rofecoxib
cracked tooth syndrome Ch481, **Ch482, Ch483**
cranial nerve blocks, acute herpes zoster pain Ch444–Ch445
cranial nerves
disorders Ca6
foramina on skull base *Ca6*
symptoms and signs caused by meningeal carcinomatosis **Ca8**
cranial neuropathy Ch371
see also neuropathies, peripheral
cranial vessel dilation, migraine pathophysiology Ch469
critical care, pain assessment A106
critical limb ischemia (CLI) A504
Crohn's disease A375, Ch579
crossover studies *see under* clinical trials
cross-sectional studies, definition Ch18
cross-tolerance Ca48
in opioid therapy Ca48–Ca49
cryoanalgesia P185, P198–P199, P319–P326
administration techniques A493
chronic pain management *see under* chronic pain
clinical applications P322
cold packs A493
comparisons P324–P325
phenol neurolysis P324–P325
radiofrequency neurolysis P325
duration of freeze P320
historical aspects P319
ice massage A493
lesion size P320
machinery P320–P322
see also cryoprobes
muscle response to A492–A493

neurolytic blocks physical agents Ca241
percutaneous technique P324
physics and physiology of freezing P319–P320
cryolesioning P320
ice ball formation P319–P320
ice crystal formation P319
nerve regeneration P320
postsurgical *see under* postoperative pain management
sport injury management A492–A493
contraindications A493
physiological effects A492–A493
possible therapeutic uses A493
trigeminal neuralgia management **Ch496**
cryohypophysectomy, stereotactic Ch300
cryoneurolysis Ca241, P322
advantages and disadvantages **Ca242**
cryoprobes P320–P322
change of phase type P320, *P321*
gas expansion type P320–P322, *P321*
characteristics **P322**
ice ball shapes *P321*
tip geometry P321–P322
crystal arthritis A397
calcium crystal arthropathies A397
gout A397
cumulative prevalence, definition Ch16
curative model Ch28
characteristics **Ch28**
inherent assumptions/attitudes Ch31
cutaneous field stimulation P186, P344
cutaneous nerve blocks
lateral *see* lateral cutaneous nerve
medial *see* medial cutaneous nerve
posterior *see* posterior cutaneous nerve
cutaneous pain, in AIDS patients *see under* AIDS
cyanosis, prilocaine adverse effect A86
cyclobenzaprine, myofascial pain (MFP) management Ch625
cyclo-oxygenase (COX) A56, A472–A473, Ca35
inhibitors A324, A331
elderly pain management Ch654
myofascial pain (MFP) management Ch625
NSAIDs A56, A331, A351, Ca184, Ca186–Ca190, Ch227–Ch228
isoforms A56, Ca184
COX-1 Ch227–Ch228
COX-2 Ch228
nonselective inhibitors acting primarily in CNS Ca184–Ca186
see also acetaminophen (paracetamol)
nonselective inhibitors in CNS and periphery Ca186–Ca190
in elderly Ca355
see also nonsteroidal anti-inflammatory drugs (NSAIDs)
nonselective inhibitors of COX-1 and COX-2 Ca191–Ca197
see also individual drugs
preferential inhibitors of COX-2 over COX-1 Ca198–Ca200
pharmacokinetics **Ca194**
see also individual drugs
receptors *Ca184*
specific inhibitors of COX-2 A66–A67, Ca200–Ca202
see also COX-2-selective inhibitors; coxibs
cyproheptadine
anorexia–cachexia syndrome management Ca306
painful spasticity management **Ch462**
cysts, pelvic pain Ch593–Ch594
cytochrome P_{450}, acetaminophen Ch235
cytokines, in inflammatory pain A24
cytomegalovirus, in AIDS patients Ca376
colitis Ca389
cytostatic drugs, peripheral neuropathies Ch37

Dallas Pain Questionnaire Ch65
dampness, pain condition P356
dantrolene Ca219
    adverse effects Ca221
    doses and pharmacokinetics Ca220
    treatment (of)
        neurologic disease Ch361
        painful spasticity **Ch462**
day surgery *see under* postoperative pain management
deafferentation pain Ca261
death
    acceptance Ca106
    place of Ca107–Ca108, Ca350
        home or hospital Ca107–Ca108
        hospice of palliative care unit Ca108
    see also home care; palliative care
decompression/fusion, chronic back pain management Ch529
deep vein thrombosis (DVT), postoperative pain
    management A170–A171
Dejerine–Roussy syndrome
    central pain Ch403, Ch408
    symptoms **Ch403**
delirium A469, Ca310–Ca311
    assessment tools Ca64–Ca65
    causes of confusion in terminally ill patients Ca310–Ca311
    clinical features Ca310
    communication problems Ca67
    elderly patients Ch658
        assessment A469
    management Ca311
    medication Ca311
    opioid-induced Ca171–Ca172
        clinical presentation Ca171–Ca172
        definition Ca171
        epidemiology Ca171
        etiology and pathophysiology Ca171
        evidence-based evaluation of management Ca172
        examination and diagnostic criteria Ca172
        prognosis Ca172
Delirium Rating Scale (DRS) Ca64–Ca65
dementia
    communication problems Ca67
    elderly patients Ch657–Ch658
    prevalence rates Ch657–Ch658
demyelinating myelopathy, multiple sclerosis Ch357
denervation supersensitivity, central pain syndromes Ch405
denial, coping mechanism Ca80
Denny–Brown syndrome Ch374
dental pain Ch419–Ch420, Ch481–Ch484
    abscess Ch481
    clinical presentation Ch483, **Ch483**
        tooth appearance **Ch483**
    cracked tooth syndrome Ch481, **Ch482, Ch483**
    definitions Ch481
    dentinal pain Ch482, **Ch483**
    dentinoenamel defects Ch481
    diagnosis Ch133–Ch134, Ch483
        pulp testing Ch483
        radiographs Ch483
    epidemiology Ch482–Ch483
        age related Ch21
    etiology/pathophysiology Ch482
    gingival pain Ch482
    management Ch483–Ch484
    model *see* dental pain model
    periapical periodontitis Ch481
    periodontal pain Ch482, **Ch483**
    pulpal pain Ch482, **Ch482, Ch483**

pulpitis Ch481
    surgery, wound infiltration in pediatric surgery A445
dental pain model P461
    advantages P462
    clinical trials P461–P468
        baseline pain intensity as confounding factor P465, *P465*
        downside assay sensitivity P465
        exclusion criteria P464
        improving and documenting assay sensitivity P464
        inclusion criteria P464
        operative procedures P463
        pain intensity rating comparisons between
            analgesics *P466*
        patient compliance with protocol P463
        patient information, consent and monitoring P463
        patient understanding of instructions P463
        placebo control P466
        practical tips P467
        protocol and good trial practice P462–P463
        rescue analgesic drug P466
        upside assay sensitivity P465–P466
    crossover design P461–P462
    limitations P462
    parallel group design P462
    surgical removal of impacted third molars P461, *P461*
        indications **P463**
dentinal pain Ch482, **Ch483**
dentinoenamel defects Ch481
dentistry, postsurgical pain syndromes Ch419–Ch420
depression Ca80–Ca81, Ca309–Ca310, Ch68–Ch69, Ch103
    assessment Ch105
    diagnosis/screening Ca81, Ca309, **Ch71**
        Endicott substitution criteria **Ca309**
    effect on pain perception P16, P114
    elderly patients Ch658
    management Ca309
    pain association Ch95–Ch96, Ch149–Ch150, Ch326
        measurements Ch150, P5
    painful spasticity Ch460
    pelvic pain Ch598
    predisposing factors Ca81
    prevalence Ca309
    psychological therapies Ca309
    risk assessment Ca80–Ca81
    suicide risk Ca310, Ch634
dermatitis, topical NSAID induced Ch215
dermatomes, herpes zoster infection A370, Ch437, Ch438
descriptive studies *see* epidemiology of pain
descriptor/differential scale Ch65
desipramine
    pharmacology **Ch240**
    treatment (of)
        central pain syndrome **Ch409**
        neuropathic pain Ch242
        postherpetic neuralgia Ch453
desmoid rectal pain Ca13
detoxification, CPRP Ch164
Detoxification Feat Survey Schedule (DFSS) Ch71
dexamethasone Ca218
dexmedetomidine, pain management in ICU A345
dextrans, local anesthesia addition A78
dextroamphetamine, adjuvant analgesic in children Ca342
dextromethorphan
    timing of treatment studies A122–A123, **A148–A151**
    treatment (of)
        CRPS Ch394
        neuropathic pain Ch264
dextromoramide Ca134

procedural pain management Ca326
dextropropoxyphene Ca52, Ca131
    acetaminophen combination in elderly Ca357
    pharmacokinetics Ca52
dextroproxyphene Ch207
dextrorphan Ch263
diabetes mellitus, animal models Ch191
diabetic neuropathies Ch370–Ch371
    acute Ch371
    asymmetric Ch371–Ch372
    clinical trials Ch241–Ch242, Ch252
    cranial neuropathy Ch371
    diagnosis, nerve conduction studies Ch130
    distal symmetric sensorimotor polyneuropathy Ch371
    lower limb asymmetric motor neuropathy Ch371–Ch372
    management
        anticonvulsants Ch253
        antidepressants **Ch243,** Ch244–Ch245
        capsaicin Ch218, **Ch219**
        neurokinin 1 (NK1) antagonists Ch267
        topical capsaicin Ch219–Ch220, *Ch220,* Ch221
    management induced Ch371
    peripheral nerves Ch371
    radiculopathy Ch371–Ch372
    small-fiber neuropathy Ch371
    thoracoabdominal radiculopathy Ch371
diagnosis-related groups (DRGs) Ch168
Diagnostic and Statistical Manual of Mental Disorders (DSM-IV) Ch631
    axis I disorders Ch68–Ch71
    axis II disorders Ch69
    psychological assessment of pain patients Ch95, Ch631
diagnostic confidence, definition Ch126–Ch127
diagnostic epidural blocks *see* epidural nerve blocks, diagnostic
diagnostic procedures Ch125–Ch144
    applications Ch133–Ch140
        visceral pain Ch133, **Ch133**
    concept validity Ch125
    construct validity Ch126
    contingency tables **Ch126**
    diagnostic confidence Ch126–Ch127
    face validity Ch125
    false-negative result Ch126, **Ch126**
    false-positive result Ch126, **Ch126**
    nerve blocks *see* nerve blocks in pain diagnosis
    objectives Ch125
    pharmacological *see* pharmacological diagnostic tests
    positive likelihood ratio Ch126
    prevalence association Ch127
    principles Ch125–Ch127
    properties Ch127
    reliable test Ch125
    sensitivity Ch126
    specificity Ch126
    true-negative result Ch126, **Ch126**
    true-positive result Ch126, **Ch126**
    validity Ch125–Ch126
    see also clinical assessment; pain history/examination;
        individual procedures
diamorphine A47–A48, Ca55, P66–P67
    alternative epidural analgesia P415
    epidural, characteristics **A243**
    pharmacokinetics P67
diaphragmatic breathing
    biofeedback component P127
    in children P149–P150
diarrhea Ca304
    celiac plexus block complications P249, P250

clinical findings Ca304
    investigations Ca304
    management Ca304
        specific antidiarrheal therapies **Ca306**
        symptomatic treatments **Ca306**
    pathophysiology Ca304
diathesis Ch326
diazepam Ca219
    adverse effects Ca220
    doses Ca220
    pharmacokinetics **A346,** Ca220
    treatment (of)
        myofascial pain (MFP) Ch625
        painful spasticity **Ch462**
dibucaine, topical A87
diclofenac A66, Ca192
    administration A209
    adverse effects Ca187–Ca190
    characteristics **Ch229**
    in children, doses **P435**
    cyclo-oxygenase (COX) inhibitor Ca192
    dose and treatment protocols Ca192
    evidence for efficacy Ca192
    indications and contraindications Ca186–Ca187
    number needed to treat (NNT) A62
    pharmacokinetics Ca192
    practical tips Ca192
didanosine
    nucleoside analog in AIDS pain management Ca368
    toxic neuropathy Ch372
dietary fiber, recurrent abdominal pain Ch640
diet modifications in pain management
    interstitial cystitis **Ch596**
    irritable bowel syndrome (IBS) Ch578
    rheumatoid arthritis Ch542
    vulvar pain syndrome Ch607
diflunisal A64, Ca192–Ca193
    adverse effects Ca187–Ca190
    cyclo-oxygenase (COX) inhibitor Ca192–Ca193
    doses and treatment protocols Ca192
    evidence for efficacy Ca190, Ca193
    indications and contraindications Ca10, Ca186–Ca187
    pharmacokinetics Ca192
    practical tips Ca192–Ca193
dihydrocodeine Ca52, Ca131
dihydroergotamine, migraine prophylaxis Ch475
dimethylsulfoxide (DMSO)
    interstitial cystitis Ch596
    topical Ch222
        evidence Ch223
diphenhydramine, central pain syndromes management Ch410
diphenylhydantoin, CRPS management Ch394
dipyrone Ca129
disability Ch149, Ch325–Ch326
    assessment Ch107
        see also disability evaluation (USA)
    conceptual models Ch44–Ch45
        objective findings Ch44
        transparency Ch44
        veracity Ch44–Ch45
    definition Ch42–Ch43
    economic loss Ch46
    impairment linkage Ch43
    perception Ch75
        measurement **Ch75,** Ch76
    physical therapy *Ch315*
    red flags Ch46–Ch47
    social status Ch41

types **Ch42**
disability evaluation (USA) Ch39–Ch61
  ability to work Ch51
  adjudicator/claims manager Ch43–Ch44
  administrative model Ch40–Ch41
  agencies Ch41–Ch42
    impact Ch41
  case histories Ch53–Ch60
  causation Ch48
  diagnosis Ch47–Ch48
  eligibility criteria Ch42
  ethical considerations Ch40–Ch41
    patient advocates Ch40
    patient–physician relationship Ch40
  form (example) *Ch45*
  general principles Ch51–Ch52
    context Ch51–Ch52
    flexibility Ch51
    form Ch52
    key issues Ch52
    legal help Ch52
    length of disability Ch52
    patient consultation Ch52
    physician's opinion Ch52–Ch53
  impairment
    classification Ch48–Ch49
    judgment Ch43
    from pain Ch50
    quantification Ch49
    severity Ch43
  knowledge deficits Ch40
  legislation Ch40
  management need Ch48
  mechanics Ch43–Ch44, **Ch47**
  participants Ch43–Ch44, **Ch44**
  physician's role expectations Ch39–Ch41, **Ch41,** Ch43–Ch44
  preparation Ch46–Ch47
    management options Ch46–Ch47
    physician's attitudes Ch46
  problems Ch39–Ch40
  severity Ch43
  Social Security Administration (SSA) Ch39
  Social Security Disability Income (SSDI) Ch39, Ch41
  Supplemental Security Income (SSI) Ch39
  workers' compensation systems Ch40
  see also disability; medicolegal aspects
disability syndrome Ch46
Discomfort Scale for Dementia of Alzheimer's Type (DS-DAT) A106
disease interactions
  effect on opioid pharmacokinetics P64
disease-modifying antirheumatic drugs, rheumatoid arthritis management Ch539, **Ch540–Ch541**
disk derangement, myofascial pain association Ch616
diskectomy A412
  chronic back pain management Ch529
diskogenic pain *see under* back pain
diskography Ch132
  mechanism Ch132
disk stimulation Ch511
  neck pain investigations Ch511–Ch512
distal radioulnar joint, intra-articular injections P266
distal symmetrical axonal neuropathy, in AIDS patients Ca375–Ca376
distal symmetric sensorimotor polyneuropathy, diabetic neuropathy Ch371
distraction A288–A289, Ca275–Ca276
  bubble blowing A288, P150

in children A288, Ca275
  parental role A288
  procedural pain management Ca322
  unsuitability for chronic patients P135, P136
district hospitals, pain clinics (UK) Ch159
disuse syndrome Ch102
diuretics
  NSAIDs interaction A57
  prohibited substances in IOC medical code A499 A
    examples A501 A
divergent validity, pain measure P10
diverticular disease Ch580
doctors
  role in acute pain service (APS) A185
  role in elderly care
    attitudes towards cancer pain Ca351–Ca352
    knowledge and experience Ca353–Ca354
  see also general practitioners
doctrine of double effect Ca116–Ca117
  conditions to justify action Ca116–Ca117
  euthanasia not justified by rule Ca118
  use Ca117
doctrine of similars, homeopathic theory Ch343
dorsal column stimulation *see* spinal cord stimulation (SCS)
dorsal horn neurons
  in central sensitization A29
    decreased inhibitory input from supraspinal nuclei A34–A35
    increased excitatory input A32–A34
    synaptic reorganization A35
    transcriptional and post-translational changes A35–A36
  classification A6–A7
  modulation of nociceptive messages *A13,* A13–A14, Ca146
  terminations A6, *A7*
dorsal root entry zone (DREZ) lesions Ch305–Ch306
  complications Ch305
  indications Ch305
  location *Ch300*
  mechanism of action Ch305
  outcomes Ch305
  technique Ch305–Ch306
    electrode placement *Ch299*
  treatment (of)
    central pain syndromes Ch410–Ch411
    postherpetic neuralgia Ch454
dorsal root ganglion (DRG)
  animal model results Ch192–Ch193
  CRPS pathogenesis Ch387
  in peripheral sensitization A19, *A28*
  radiofrequency lesioning of cervical cells P334–P335
    adverse effects P335
    contraindication P334
    efficacy of treatment P335
    indication P334
    technique P334–P335
      cannula introduction P335, *P336*
      diagnostic root blocks P334–P335
      electrode position P335, *P336*
      "tunnel-vision" projection P335, *P335*
  radiofrequency lesioning of lumbar cells P337–P338
    contraindication P337
    efficacy of treatment P338
    indication P337
    technique P337–P338
      diagnostic root blocks P337
      electrode positioning *P338*
dorsal root ganglionitis Ch374
dothiepin, TMJ pain management **Ch486**

doxepin, central pain syndrome management Ch409, **Ch409**
doxycycline, maxillary sinusitis management Ch487
droperidol
  antiemetic A233
  epidural, nausea and vomiting treatment A257
Drug Abuse Screening Test (DAST) Ch71
drug interactions
  acetaminophen Ca34
  anticonvulsans Ca214
  antidepressants Ca217
  antiretrovirals Ca367
  celecoxib **Ca201**
  effect on opioid pharmacokinetics/pharmacodynamics P64, **P65**
  ibuprofen Ca193
  local anesthetics A82–A83
    with CNS depressants A83
  NSAIDs A57, Ca37, **Ca41**
  nucleoside analogs **Ca368**
  protease inhibitors Ca369
  rofecoxib **Ca201**
drug screening, animal models Ch193
dry mouth see xerostomia
duodenal ulcers, NSAID induced Ca188, Ch230
duodenum, ulceration Ch582
dural puncture
  epidural steroid injection complication P423
  intrathecal catheterization technique P290
    adverse effects P300–P301
dural tap
  spinal cord stimulation complication P388
Dyadic Adjustment Scale Ch108
dyclonine hydrochloride, topical A87
dynamic hyperalgesia Ch115, **Ch121**
dynamic lumbar stabilization Ch318
  clinical studies Ch318
  definition Ch318
  goals Ch318
dynamic pain
  relief with epidural analgesia P409
dynamic stabilization exercise, definition **Ch316**
dysesthesiae Ch116
  central pain Ch407–Ch408
  definition **Ch404**
  peripheral neuropathies Ch368
dysesthetic vulvodynia Ch604
dysfunctional labor pain A425–A426
  risk factor relationship to epidural analgesia *A426*
dyskinesia Ch358–Ch359
dysmenorrhea
  endometriosis Ch591
  management
    NSAIDs Ch228
    TENS A279
  primary Ch594
  secondary Ch594
dyspareunia Ch633
  endometriosis Ch591
dyspepsia, children Ch640
dysphagia Ca298–Ca299
  clinical findings Ca298–Ca299
  etiology Ca298
  investigation Ca299
  management Ca299
dyspnea see breathlessness (dyspnea)

ear acupuncture Ca271
eccentric strain, definition **Ch316**

echinacea, botanical therapy **Ch347**
ectopic discharges, CRPS pathogenesis Ch386
edema, NSAID induced Ca356
Edmonton Symptom Assessment System (ESAS) Ca66, **Ca68**
education
  AIDS management Ca373
  CBT component Ch328
  elderly pain management Ch656
  of family in elderly care Ca353
  osteoarthritis management Ch544
  pain-related fear P169
  preparation for pain A291–A292
    evidence supporting effectiveness A292
  of staff
    in acute pain service (APS) A196–A197
    in PCA A224
  see also patient(s), education
eicosanoids in inflammatory pain A23
  see also prostaglandins
eicosapentaenoic acid, anorexia–cachexia syndrome
  management Ca306–Ca307
ejaculatory failure, lumbar sympathetic block complication P243
elbow
  intra-articular injections P264–P265
    lateral epicondyle P264–P265, *P265*
    medial epicondyle P265
    posterior approach P264, *P265*
  nerve blocks P210–P213
    anatomical aspects P211
    indications P210
    see also individual types
  pain A400–A401
    investigations A400
    management A400–A401
elderly A463–A483, Ca349–Ca365, Ch649–Ch660
  adjuvant analgesics Ca358–Ca359, Ch654–Ch655
    anticonvulsants Ca358–Ca359
    antidepressants Ca358
  aged care medicine Ch649–Ch650
  analgesic drugs A469–A473, Ch653–Ch655
    anticonvulsants A473, Ch655
    antidepressants Ch243
    epidural analgesia A475–A476
    epidural local anesthetic A475
    local anesthetics A472
    NSAIDs A472–A473, Ca355–Ca356, Ch227, Ch228, Ch233, Ch261, Ch654
    opioids see opioids, in elderly patients
    simple see elderly, simple analgesics
    techniques A473–A477
    topical preparations Ch655
    tramadol A473
    tricyclic antidepressants (TCAs) A473, Ch654
  assessments Ch652–Ch653
    behavioral indicators Ch652
    functional indicators Ch652
  carer knowledge and experience Ca353–Ca354
    family members Ca353
    nurses Ca353–Ca354
  complementary and alternative medicine Ca359
  death in hospitals Ca350
  decreased reporting of pain Ch651
  delirious patients Ch658
    assessment A469
  dementia patients Ch657–Ch658
  dose responses A463
    opioids A470–A471
  epidemiology Ch650–Ch651

of cancer pain Ca349
of chronic pain *see* epidemiology (chronic pain), in elderly
functional impairment Ch650
health care professionals' attitudes Ca351–Ca352
    doctors Ca351–Ca352
    nurses Ca352
misconceptions about analgesics Ca352
monitoring patients on epidural analgesia A476
multidisciplinary management Ch656–Ch657
    clinic exclusion Ch656–Ch657
    outcome studies Ch657
    special considerations Ch657
    specialized clinicians Ch657
nonpharmacological management Ca359, Ch655–Ch656
    massage Ca359
    physical therapies Ch655–Ch656
    psychological therapies Ch656
    radiotherapy Ca359
    TENS Ca359, Ch655–Ch656
opioids *see* opioids, in elderly patients
pain assessment A106, A468–A469, Ca350–Ca351, Ch652
    cognitive impairment A106, A469
    delirium A469
    reporting of pain A469
pain control Ca351
pain experience compared with youth Ca350
    altered tolerance from various stimuli Ca350
    analgesia provision Ca350
pain intensity assessment P21
pain measurements A469, Ca351
pain perception changes A468
pain physiology Ch651–Ch652
    absence in certain visceral diseases Ch651
    nerve fiber transmissions Ch651
    nociceptive pathway changes Ch651–Ch652
pain prevalence variations Ch650–Ch651
    reasons Ch650–Ch651
patient-controlled analgesia (PCA) A228, A474
    management A474–A475, **A475**
patient knowledge and experience Ca354
patients' attitudes Ca351
pharmacodynamics A466, Ca355
pharmacokinetic changes A464–A466, **A465**
    physiological A464–A466, **A465**
    systemic A464
pharmacokinetics Ca354–Ca355
    distribution Ca354–Ca355
physiological changes A464–A466, **A465**
quality of life issues Ca352–Ca353
    suicide risk Ca352–Ca353
self-reporting of pain Ca351
simple analgesics Ca355–Ca356, Ch653–Ch654
    acetaminophen Ca355
    aspirin Ca355
    cyclo-oxygenase (COX) inhibitors Ca355
    nonsteroidal anti-inflammatory drugs (NSAIDs) Ca355–
        Ca356
    proton pump inhibitors Ca356
simulations of consequences of aging A466–A468
    fentanyl administration *A467, A468*
specific problems of later life Ca359–Ca360
    dealing with nonverbal patients Ca359–Ca360
    nursing/residential home patients Ca360
electrical-evoked potentials P34–P35
electrical muscle stimulation (EMS) P186
electrical stimulation P185–P186
    acupuncture Ch341, *Ch342*
    percutaneous *see* percutaneous electrical nerve stimulation
      (PENS)

electroacupuncture Ca270
electromagnetic fields P186
electromyograph-assisted relaxation P124–P125
electromyography (EMG)
    myofascial pain (MFP) Ch616
    peripheral neuropathies Ch369
electrophysiology, animal model results Ch192–Ch193
electrotherapeutic techniques P185–P186
    sport injury management A496
eletriptan, migraine therapy, efficacy in RCT Ch471
elevation, sport injury management A491–A492
Ellis v. Wallsend District Hospital, medical liability Ch177
emergency room
    pain assessment A103–A104
    self-reporting of pain A104
EMLA *see* eutectic mixture of local anesthetics (EMLA)
emotion, pain measure P5
emotional distress, psychometric assessment Ch95–Ch96
encephalotomy, stereotactic, painful spasticity
    management **Ch463**
Endicott substitution criteria for depression **Ca309**
end of life care Ca311–Ca312
    causes of nonpeaceful death **Ca110**
    frequency of symptoms **Ca110**
    home patients Ca311
    interventions Ca109–Ca110
      simplifying treatment Ca109
      terminal cancer syndrome Ca109
    symptom control Ca311–Ca312
      antisecretory drugs Ca312
      opioids Ca312
      sedatives Ca312
      when death is near Ca109–Ca110
    see also home care; palliative care
endogenous ligands, opioid receptor action A44
endogenous opioids Ca40
    in inflammatory hyperalgesia A29
    modulation of nociceptive messages A11
    preferred receptor and actions upon activation **Ca42**
    production
      acupuncture Ch342
      animal model variability Ch192
endometrial cancer, bone metastasis hormone treatment Ca288
endometriosis Ch590–Ch591
    bowel complications Ch594–Ch595
    diagnosis Ch591
    etiology Ch590–Ch591
    incidence Ch590
    management Ch591, **Ch592**
    outcome Ch591
    symptoms/signs Ch591
    see also pelvic pain
endorphins, release during acupuncture P356
endoscopic retrograde cholangiopancreatography (ERCP), chronic
    pancreatitis management Ch572
endoscopic thoracic sympathectomy, refractory angina pectoris
    management Ch557
endoscopy, maxillary sinusitis Ch487
enhanced external counterpulsation (EECP), refractory angina
    pectoris management Ch557
enriched enrollment study designs, in cancer pain clinical
    trials P474
enteral administration of drugs A205–A206
    nonsteroidal anti-inflammatory drugs A208–A209
    opioids A210–A211
Entonox *see* nitrous oxide
epicondylitis Ch546
    lateral Ch317
      physical therapy Ch317

medial Ch546
    physical therapy Ch317
epicritic pain, definition **Ch404**
epidemiology (cancer pain) Ca21–Ca32
    in children Ca333–Ca334
    in elderly Ca349
    future challenges Ca29
    pain measurement Ca21–Ca22
    prevalence Ca22
        in advanced/terminal disease Ca22, **Ca26–Ca27**
        assessment Ca21
        in early disease Ca22, **Ca23–Ca25**
        effect of metastatic disease Ca22
        by primary tumor site Ca22, **Ca28**
    relationships with other factors Ca22, Ca29
    uniqueness Ca73–Ca74
epidemiology (chronic pain) Ch15–Ch26
    analytical studies Ch17, Ch18–Ch19
        case–control studies Ch18–Ch19
        cohort studies Ch18, Ch19
    cross-cultural factors Ch20
    descriptive studies Ch17–Ch18
        cross-sectional Ch18
        longitudinal population studies Ch18
        simple Ch18
    disease definition Ch16
    disease etiology Ch17
        factor identification Ch17
    disease frequency Ch15
    disease management Ch17
    disease occurrence Ch16–Ch17
    disease outcome Ch17
    disease prevention Ch15–Ch16
    in elderly Ch21–Ch22
        biological factors Ch22
        diseases/disorders Ch21–Ch22
        error sources Ch22
        impact Ch21
        prevalence Ch21
    gender differences Ch19–Ch20
        biology Ch19–Ch20
        disease definition Ch19
        experiences Ch20
        experimenter gender Ch19
        population selection Ch19
        prevalence Ch19
        psychological/sociological factors Ch20
    incidence Ch16
    medical service provision Ch15
    methodology Ch17–Ch19
        study design Ch17–Ch19
    pain triangle Ch17, *Ch17*
    pediatric pain Ch20–Ch21
        gender-specific pain Ch20–Ch21
        puberty Ch21
    prevalence Ch16–Ch17
    role Ch15–Ch16
epidemiology of pain
    acute herpes zoster pain Ch438
    back pain Ch23, Ch137, Ch524
    breast surgery pain Ch22
    burning mouth syndrome Ch488
    cancer pain *see* epidemiology (cancer pain) *above*
    central pain syndromes *see under* central pain syndromes
    chest pain Ch553
    chronic pain *see* epidemiology (chronic pain) *above*
    dental pain Ch482–Ch483
    facial pain Ch481

headaches Ch21
herpes zoster A369
low back pain A406–A407
lower limb pain Ch546–Ch547
maxillary sinusitis Ch487
migraine *see under* migraine
multiple sclerosis Ch356–Ch357
neck pain Ch507
osteoarthritis Ch542
postherpetic neuralgia (PHN) *see under* postherpetic neuralgia
    (PHN)
rheumatoid arthritis Ch538
shoulder pain Ch545
stomach pain Ch21
temporomandibular joint (TMJ) pain Ch485
tension-type headache *see under* tension-type headaches
thoracotomy pain Ch22
vasectomy pain Ch22
vulvar pain syndrome Ch604
vulvar vestibulitis Ch605
epidural alfentanil, in PCEA **A247**
epidural analgesia/anesthesia P409–P416
    abdominoperineal surgery P415
    administration A207–A208
        onset A208
        site A207–A208
    adverse effects A174
    alternative mixtures P415
    anticoagulant drugs and A476
    in children A448–A449, P442–P443
        administration P433
        caudal approach P442
        drug doses and infusion rates P443, **P443**
        indications A448
        insertion, management and complications A449
        local anesthetic A448
        lumbar and thoracic approach P442–P443
        opioid–local anesthetic A448–A449
        urine retention P443
    closed delivery system *P413*
    cost-effectiveness A174
    dynamic pain relief P409
    in elderly A475–A476
        monitoring A476
    epinephrine
        effectiveness increase P412
        importance in efficacy/safety of postoperative
            analgesia P413
        no decrease in spinal cord blood flow P412–P413
        safety increase P412
    failure A320, A322
        responsible factors **A322**
        technical rates **A322**
    local anesthetics *see* epidural local anesthesia
    lower limb surgery P415
    monitoring P413–P414
        of elderly patients A476
    necessary requirements for successful management
        program P414
    optimizing efficacy and safety P410–P411, *P411*
    outcome P413–P414
    pain clinics **Ch159**
    patient-controlled *see* patient-controlled epidural analgesia
        (PCEA)
    postoperative pain improvements A307, A320–A322
        cardiac outcomes A168, **A169**
        evidence **A175**
        gastrointestinal recovery, comparison with systemic

analgesia **A172**
graft occlusion rates following administration in vascular
bypass surgery **A173**
ileus treatment A170
pulmonary outcomes A168, **A171**
prescription for safe and effective delivery P413–P414
relationship to dysfunctional labor risk factors *A426*
risks to patient P410
severe pain relief technique **A188**
standardized prescriptions' important elements **A193**
steroid addition *see* epidural steroid injections
thoracic or lumbar catheter choice P409–P410
treatment (of)
acute herpes zoster pain Ch442
acute just postamputation pain Ch427
chest trauma A353
childbirth pain A244, A430, A431
chronic back pain Ch530
refractory pain *see* epidural treatment of refractory pain
sickle cell disease A383
see also individual agents
epidural bupivacaine
adverse effects A245
labor pain analgesia A244
epidural catheters, placement and removal complications A174
epidural diamorphine, lipid solubility, doses, onset and analgesia
duration **A243**
epidural droperidol, nausea and vomiting treatment A257
epidural fentanyl
labor pain analgesia A244
lipid solubility, doses, onset and analgesia duration **A243**
in PCEA **A247**
epidural hematoma
following epidural anesthesia and analgesia
administration A174
risk for development A174, A476
epidural hydromorphone, lipid solubility, doses, onset and
analgesia duration **A243**
epidural local anesthesia P409, P410
adverse effects **A173**
in children A448
complications P410
effect on pulmonary sequelae of pain A311
in elderly A475
in multimodal anesthesia A323
nerve blocks *see* peripheral nerve blocks
opioid combination *see* epidural opioids, local anesthetic
combinations
pain management in ICU A343
postoperative improvements
cardiac outcomes **A169**
pulmonary outcomes A168, **A171**
thoracic, cardiac outcome management A167
wound infiltration A332
see also epidural analgesia/anesthesia
epidural meperidine
lipid solubility, doses, onset and analgesia duration **A243**
in PCEA **A247**
epidural methadone, lipid solubility, doses, onset, and analgesia
duration **A243**
epidural morphine
administration A213
after surgery **A476**
analgesic effects A242
lipid solubility, doses, onset, and analgesia duration **A243**
in PCEA **A247**
respiratory depression risk A243, A255
epidural nerve blocks

acute herpes zoster pain Ch442–Ch443
complications Ch442–Ch443
diagnostic Ch132–Ch133
advantages Ch133
limitations Ch133
mechanism Ch132–Ch133
neuropathic pain Ch132
nociceptive pain Ch132
see also peripheral nerve blocks
epidural neurolytic blockade Ca240
epidural opioids Ca51
administration A213
barriers A242
frequency **A242**
adverse effects A173, **A173**, A252–A257, P312–P313
hypotension P313
nausea and vomiting P313
pruritus P313
respiratory depression *see* respiratory depression, epidural
opioid induced
treatment and prophylaxis A257–A258
see also opioids, adverse effects
algorithm for instituting therapy **P310**, *P311*
complications P410
doses and regimens **P312**
effect on pulmonary sequelae of pain A311
in elderly A475, **A476**
lipid solubility, doses, onset and analgesia duration **A243**
local anesthetic combinations A244–A246, A476
age-based infusion rates **A476**
in children A448–A449
infusion rates A245–A246
problems A245–A246
respiratory depression induction incidence **A257**
sites of actions A244
timing of treatment studies A124–A125, **A152–A154**
mechanisms of action A243
in multimodal anesthesia A323
pain management in ICU A343
postoperative pain management A241–A242
pulmonary outcome improvements A168, **A171**
selection from hydrophilic and lipophilic opioids A242–A244
choices in Europe **A242**
timing of treatment studies A120–A121, **A144–A147**
see also epidural morphine; intrathecal opioids
epidural space scarring, spinal cord stimulation
contraindication P382
epidural steroid injections P417–P427
anatomical aspects P417–P418
complications P423–P424, **P424**
additives in preparation P423
incidence P424
local anesthesia induced P423
mechanical aspects P423
misplacement of drugs P424
steroid induced P423
contraindications P419
drugs used P422–P423
injectate P422
local anesthetics P422
steroid preparations P422
evidence for particular therapy or drug P424–P425
meta-analyses P424–P425
RCTs P424–P425
historical aspects P417
imaging techniques P422
indications P418–P419
sciatica P418

number and frequency of injections P419
preparation P419–P420
  of equipment P420
  of patient P419–P420
technique P420–P422
  caudal approach P418, P421
  general P421
  lumbar approach P417–P418, P421
  monitoring P421
  perineural and periradicular injections P421
epidural steroids
injections *see* epidural steroid injections
low back pain treatment A412
epidural sufentanil
lipid solubility, doses, onset and analgesia duration **A243**
in PCEA **A247**
epidural treatment of refractory pain P307–P317
advantages and disadvantages **P308**
adverse effects P311–P313
  infections P311–P312
  mechanical problems P311–P312, **P312**
  pharmacological P312–P313
    see also epidural opioids, adverse effects
algorithm for instituting opioid therapy **P310**, *P311*
catheter and pump selection P313–P315
clinical settings P308–P310
  cancer pain P308
  nonmalignant pain P308–P310
contraindications P310–P311
  to epidural catheter P310
  to running an infusion P311
doses and regimens P311, **P312**
drugs used **P307**
efficacy P316
indications for long-term therapy P308, P310
  in nonmalignant pain **P309**
indications for medium-term therapy **P310**
intrathecal comparison **P308**, P316
patient selection P310
practical tips P315
  advice to patients with implantable pumps P315
  gas-driven pumps P315
pump classification P313–P315
  delivery system classification P313–P315
role of intraspinal pumps **P309**
techniques
  implanted pumps P315, *P315*
  insertion of tunneled catheter *P314*
  Port-A-Cath ports P314
  totally implanted systems P314–P315
epilepsy, central pain Ch406
epileptiform seizures, multiple sclerosis Ch357
epinephrine
epidural, spinal cord blood flow not decreased P412–P413
increased effectiveness of epidural infusion *P411*, P412
  potentiation of epidural analgesia by fentanyl *P411*
  potentiation of epidural analgesia from bupivacaine and
    fentanyl *P411*
increased efficacy/safety of prolonged postoperative epidural
  analgesia P413
increased safety of bupivacaine and fentanyl epidural
  analgesia P412
local anesthesia addition A77–A78
erector spinae (sacrospinalis) muscle Ch523
ergotamine, migraine management Ch471
erythema
capsaicin adverse effects Ch219
topical NSAIDs adverse effects Ch215

erythrocyte sedimentation rate (ESR)
low back pain investigations A409
maxillary sinusitis diagnosis Ch487
esophageal candidiasis Ca298
odynophagia cause in AIDS Ca386
treatment Ca298
Essaic Ca273
esters
allergic reactions A82
metabolism A80
structure, physiochemical properties and clinical profile **A84–
  A85**
estrogen in pain management
burning mouth syndrome Ch489
syndrome X Ch558
vulvar pain syndrome Ch606
ethical issues Ca113–Ca119, Ch27–Ch38
conflict between obligation to relieve suffering and to
    prolong life Ca115–Ca118, **Ca119**
  balance of benefit to harm and risk in dying
    patient Ca116
  distinction between intended and foreseen effects Ca117
  doctrine or rule of double effect *see* doctrine of double
    effect
  euthanasia unjustified by doctrine of double effect Ca118
  importance of clear thinking and integrity Ca117
  legal/moral prohibition against causing death of
    another Ca115–Ca116
  life-shortening consequences of analgesia Ca116
  need to alleviate pain Ca116
  praiseworthy and blameworthy actions Ca118
  problem of what causes death Ca117
control of psychosocial aspects of pain Ca114–Ca115
decision-making for competent patients Ca118
decision-making for incompetent patients Ca118–Ca119
  advance statements/living wills Ca119
  differences between countries Ca118
  disagreements Ca119
goals of medicine Ch29
informed consent and honesty in pain control Ca113–Ca114
  information on adverse effects Ca114
  withheld knowledge of diagnosis Ca113–Ca114
limitations to pain relief Ch30–Ch36
  accountability Ch35–Ch36
  insufficient knowledge Ch32–Ch33
  opioid regulation Ch33–Ch34
  pain identification failure Ch30–Ch31
"myth of two pains" Ch28
obligation not to harm patients Ca115
pain control
  moral balances Ca115
  moral basis **Ca116**
  as moral obligation Ca113
physician's duty to relief suffering Ch28–Ch29
suffering and semantic points Ch27–Ch28
undertreated pain Ch10–Ch11, Ch29–Ch30
ethical review board (ERB), experimental protocol review P491
etidocaine A86
structure, physiochemical properties and clinical profile **A85**
etiology of cancer pain **Ca124**
etodolac A66, Ca199–Ca200
adverse effects Ca200
characteristics **Ch229**
cyclo-oxygenase (COX) inhibitor Ca199–Ca200
doses and treatment protocols Ca200
evidence for efficacy Ca200
indications and contraindications Ca186–Ca187
pharmacokinetics Ca200

practical tip Ca200
E-TRANS® **P402**
European Organization for Research and Treatment of Cancer
  (EORTC) Ca351
European Scientific Cooperative of Phytotherapy (ESCOP) Ch346
eutectic mixture of local anesthetics (EMLA) A87, Ca322
    adverse effects Ca225
    in children Ca340
        procedural pain management A452
    clinical trials for venepuncture/cannulation **Ca324**
    patch *Ca323*
    practical tips Ca225
euthanasia Ca108–Ca109, Ch176
    requests Ca108–Ca109
        group A (afraid) Ca109
        group B (burn-out) Ca109
        group C (control-oriented) Ca109
        group D (depressed) Ca109
        group E (extreme) Ca109
    unjustified by doctrine of double effect Ca118
evidence-based medicine A315, *P495,* P495–P496
    postoperative pain *see under* postoperative pain management
examination *see* pain assessment; pain history/examination;
    patient(s), assessment
exercise
    CBT component Ch328
    chronic back pain management Ch528
    osteoarthritis management Ch544
expectancy/cognitive theory, placebos Ch277
    definition Ch277
experimental allergic neuritis Ch191
experimental models *see* animal models
expert medicolegal report P509–P516
    conclusion and opinion P515–P516
        predicted work time loss after injury **P516**
    examination P515
        musculoskeletal system P515
        neurological P515
    history P514–P515
        previous behavior P514
        sickness record P514
        social impact of injury **P514**
        source information for medical reports **P514**
    preparation P514
    see also medicolegal aspects
explanatory studies P449–P450, **P450**
extracellular matrix, deposition in tissue repair A487
eye, manifestations in AIDS patients Ca383–Ca384, **Ca384**

Fabry's disease, hereditary neuropathy Ch373
Faces Pain Scale (FPS) A105, *P19*
    child pain assessment P432, *P433*
facet joints *see* zygapophyseal joints
facet joint syndrome P269
face validity, definition Ch125
facial arthromyalgia (FAM) *see* temporomandibular joint (TMJ)
    pain
facial pain Ch481–Ch504
    accurate diagnosis Ch481
    atypical **Ch482,** Ch489–Ch490
        diagnosis Ch490, **Ch490**
        epidemiology Ch490
        etiology/pathophysiology Ch490
        management **Ch490**
    atypical odontalgia **Ch482,** Ch490–Ch491
        diagnosis Ch490–Ch491
        epidemiology Ch490
        etiology/pathophysiology Ch490

        management Ch491
        vasodilation Ch490
    burning mouth syndrome *see* burning mouth syndrome
    cluster headaches **Ch482, Ch499**
    cracked tooth syndrome Ch481, **Ch482, Ch483**
    dental pain *see* dental pain
    epidemiology Ch481
    etiology **Ch482**
    geniculate neuralgia **Ch482,** Ch485
    giant cell arteritis **Ch482, Ch499**
    glossopharyngeal neuralgia **Ch482, Ch499**
    management
        capsaicin **Ch219**
        capsaicin, topical Ch221
        clonidine Ch222
    maxillary sinusitis *see* maxillary sinusitis
    nervus intermedius neuralgia Ch500
    ophthalmic postherpetic neuralgia **Ch482,** Ch494
    otitis externa **Ch482**
    periodontal pain Ch482, **Ch482, Ch483**
    pretrigeminal neuralgia **Ch482, Ch499**
    pulpal pain Ch482, **Ch482, Ch483**
    Raeder syndrome **Ch482,** Ch485
    short-lasting unilateral neuralgiform pain with conjunctival
        injection and tearing (SUNCT) Ch485
    TMJ pain *see* temporomandibular joint (TMJ) pain
    Tolosa–Hunt syndrome **Ch482,** Ch485
        diagnosis Ch133
    trigeminal neuralgia *see* trigeminal neuralgia
    unilateral, in bronchial cancer Ca9
factitious disorder Ch632
    diagnosis Ch632
    etiology Ch632
    medical background Ch632
    by proxy Ch632
factor VIII therapy, hemophilia management A380
failed back surgery syndrome (FBSS), spinal cord
    stimulation Ch291, **Ch292**
false claims *see* malingering (false claims)
false-negative result, definition Ch126
false placebos *see* placebos, false
false-positive result, definition Ch126
famciclovir
    acute herpes zoster pain Ch440
    varicella-zoster virus infection treatment in AIDS
        patient Ca380
familial Mediterranean fever Ch580
    management Ch580
    source of pain **Ch568**
family
    burden of caring Ca77
    care for members Ca110
    elderly care
        education Ca353
        knowledge and experience Ca353
    impact on central pain syndromes Ch406
    importance Ca77–Ca78
    needs Ca77
        letting go Ca110
        presence at death Ca110
    predisposing factors to emotional risk Ca78
    psychological evaluation *see* psychological evaluation of
        patients and family
Family Environment Scale Ch108
fascia iliaca compartment block, in children P440
    anatomical aspects P440
    local anesthetic solution P440
    method P440

in pediatric surgery A446
fatigue Ch74–Ch75
    fibromyalgia association Ch616
    measurement Ch75, **Ch75**
    painful spasticity Ch460
fear
    pain related *see* pain-related fear
Fear Avoidance Beliefs Questionnaire (FABQ) Ch73, P166
Fear of Pain Questionnaire Ch105, P165
Federal Food, Drug and Cosmetic Act (FFDCA), opioid legal
    controls Ch174
Feldene "Melt" A208
femoral angiography, postoperative relaxation exercises A290
femoral nerve block A269–A270, P221–P222
    anatomical aspects P221
    complications P222
    indications P221
    landmarks and practical steps P221–P222, *P222*
    in pediatric surgery A446
    postoperative pain management A320
fenamates A66
fenbufen, characteristics **Ch229**
fenoprofen, characteristics **Ch229**
fentanyl A48–A49, A330, Ca54, P67
    administration A210, A213
    aerosolized A212
    in children A443, Ca339–Ca340
        administration A443
        adverse effects and toxicity A443
        analgesia for patients over 6 months P436
        intravenous infusion protocols **P437**
        pharmacology and indications A443
        starting dose **Ca339**
    epidural *see* epidural fentanyl
    oral *see* oral transmucosal fentanyl citrate (OTFC)
    pain management in ICU A343
    pharmacokinetics **A346**, Ca54, P67
        in elderly A464
    potentiation of epidural analgesia by epinephrine *P411*
    potentiation of epidural analgesia from bupivacaine and
        epinephrine *P411*
    procedural pain management Ca326
    simulations of consequences of aging A467, *A467, A468*
    transdermal therapeutic system (TTS) A211–A212, Ca51, Ca54,
        Ca147, Ca162
        in elderly Ca358
        indications for use Ca162
        patches Ca51, Ca54, Ca128
        patient-controlled analgesia (PCA) P402
        pharmacokinetics Ca162
    transmucosal
        delivery in PCA P403
        refractory cancer pain management Ca152
    trauma pain management A350
    use in early postoperative period A334
fetus, drug categorization according to risk **A380**
feverfew, botanical therapy **Ch347**
fibroblasts, role in tissue repair A487
fibromyalgia
    in AIDS patients Ca385
    in children *see under* children
    chronic fatigue and immune dysfunction syndrome
        (CFIDS) Ch623
    contributing factors Ch620
        muscle health Ch620
        posture Ch620
        psychologic symptoms Ch620
        tension-producing habits Ch620

diagnosis Ch616
    American College of Rheumatology (ACR) Ch640–Ch641
    associated symptoms Ch616
    characteristics Ch616, **Ch618**
etiology/pathophysiology Ch620–Ch623
    central nociceptive input modification Ch622–Ch623
    motor endplate Ch621–Ch622
    muscle fiber type I injury Ch620–Ch621
    muscle nociceptor activation Ch622
    pain transmission Ch622
exaggerated reaction to muscle stimulation P35
jump sign Ch618–Ch619
management Ch623–Ch627
    acetaminophen Ch235
    behavioral factors Ch626
    cardiovascular fitness Ch624
    contributing factor control Ch625–Ch626
    difficulties Ch261
    holistic approach Ch623, **Ch623**
    ketamine Ch264
    long-term pain control Ch623
    mandibular opening Ch624
    massage Ch624
    muscle evaluation Ch624
    muscle exercises Ch623–Ch624
    muscle therapy Ch624–Ch625
    NSAIDs Ch232–Ch233, Ch625
    opioids Ch625
    pain clinic teams Ch626–Ch627
    pharmacotherapy Ch625
    physical conditioning Ch624
    postural corrections Ch625–Ch626
    postural exercises Ch624
    selective serotonin reuptake inhibitors (SSRIs) Ch625
    spray and stretch techniques Ch624–Ch625
    tricyclic antidepressants Ch625
muscle pain disorder relationship Ch619
myofascial pain (MFP) comparison **Ch620**
pain description Ch619
pain history/examination Ch65, Ch68
prevalence Ch616
    age relation Ch616
tender points (TePs) Ch618
    locations Ch618
    palpation Ch618–Ch619
see also myofascial pain (MFP)
fibromyalgia syndrome, in AIDS patients Ca385
Fitness Arthritis and Seniors Trial (FAST), osteoarthritis
    management Ch317
flecainide Ca212
    adverse effects Ca212
    CRPS management Ch394
    peripheral neuropathy management Ch377
    pharmacokinetics Ca212–Ca213
fluconazole, oral candidiasis treatment in AIDS patients Ca379
flunarizine
    clinical trials Ch253
    migraine prophylaxis Ch475
fluoxetine
    central pain syndrome management **Ch409**
    chronic back pain management Ch528
    pharmacology **Ch240**
    postherpetic neuralgia management Ch453
    TMJ pain management **Ch486**
fluphenazine
    central pain syndrome management Ch409
    postherpetic neuralgia management Ch453
flurbiprofen Ca193

adverse effects Ca187–Ca190
    cyclo-oxygenase (COX) inhibitor Ca193
    doses and treatment protocols Ca193
    indications and contraindications Ca186–Ca187, Ca193
    pharmacokinetics Ca193
Food and Drug Administration (FDA)
    herbal medicines Ch346
    topical NSAIDs Ch214
food supplements Ca273
foot, intra-articular injections P261–P262
    metatarsophalangeal joint of hallux P261–P262
foot pain A402–A403
    investigations/management A402–A403
forearm
    nerve blocks *see individual nerve blocks*
    soft-tissue disorders Ch545–Ch546
        diagnosis Ch545–Ch546
        epidemiology Ch545–Ch546
        management Ch546
fractures, CRPS Ch386
friends, psychological evaluation Ca76
frontal leukotomy, central pain syndromes management Ch411
Functional Assessment Screening Questionnaire (FASQ) Ch76
Functional Capacity Evaluation (FCE) Ch146
Functional Independence Measure (FIM), painful spasticity
    assessment Ch460
functional residual capacity (FRC), reduction in postoperative
    period A310

G-protein receptors *see* G-protein-coupled receptors (GPCRs)
GABA **A34**
    agonists, neurologic disease management Ch361
    modulation of nociceptive messages A11–A12
GABA$_B$ receptor activation, spinal cord stimulation (SCS) Ch288
GABA-mediated inhibition, deficiencies Ch405
gabapentin
    adverse effects Ca214, P107
    clinical trials Ch252
    contraindications P105
    doses and treatment paradigms Ca214, **P106,** P107
    mechanism of action Ca213, Ch251
    pharmacokinetics Ca215
    pretreatment safety measures **P106,** P107
    treatment (of)
        acute herpes zoster pain Ch440
        central pain syndromes Ch410
        elderly pain Ch655
        neuropathic pain Ca376
        painful spasticity **Ch461**
        peripheral neuropathy Ch377
        trigeminal neuralgia Ch494, **Ch494–Ch495**
galanin, modulation of nociceptive messages A13
gallbladder, pain after removal Ch581
gamma (γ)-aminobutyric acid *see* GABA
Gamma knife Ch300
    trigeminal neuralgia management Ch493, **Ch497**
ganglion impar block P252–P253
    anatomical aspects P235, P252
    technique P253
        needle placement *P253*
garlic, botanical therapy **Ch347**
Gasserian ganglion, radiofrequency lesioning P330–P331
    adverse effects P331
    anatomical aspects P330
    complications and incidence P331
    discomfort to patient P331
    historical aspects P330
    indication P330

results P331
    technique P330
        electrical stimulation P330
        general anesthesia administration P330
        needle insertion P330, *P331*
        projection of needle–electrode P330, *P331*
Gasserian ganglion block
    acute herpes zoster pain Ch444
    complications Ch444
gastric complications
    acetaminophen-induced Ch234
    ibuprofen-induced Ch230
    NSAID induced Ch230–Ch231, Ch261
    ulcers Ch230
        NSAID induced Ca187–Ca188
gastric emptying, delayed A254
    effect of intraspinal opioids A254
gastroesophageal reflux disorder (GERD) Ch558
    angina comparison **Ch559**
    assessment Ch558
    diagnosis Ch558, **Ch559**
    management Ch558, **Ch559**
gastrointestinal tract
    effect of autonomic innervation A170, *A171*
    NSAIDs adverse effects A58, A171, A173, A495, Ca37, Ca130,
        Ca187–Ca188
        risk factors **Ca189**
    obstruction in advanced cancer Ca301–Ca303
        clinical features Ca301–Ca302
        incidence Ca301
        management Ca302–Ca303
        pathophysiology Ca301
        results Ca303
    opioids' adverse effects Ca47, Ca175, P62–P63
        intraspinal infusions A254
    patient-controlled analgesia (PCA) route P402
    postoperative pain management and outcome
        measures A168, A170
        epidural analgesia *versus* systemic analgesia **A172**
    problems Ca297–Ca304
        functional pains Ca17–Ca18
        see also individual disorders
gate control theory *A13,* A13–A14, Ch285
    descending inhibition of pain P114
    opioids' sites of action *A14*
    role in TENS development P343
    supraspinal/descending control A14, *A14*
gender, effect on pain perception P16
    see also epidemiology (chronic pain), gender differences
general anesthesia
    burn pain treatment A363–A364
    effect on postoperative cardiac outcomes **A169**
    effect on postoperative pain A330
    Gasserian ganglion radiofrequency lesioning P330
    graft occlusion rates following administration in vascular
        bypass surgery **A173**
general practitioners
    home care Ca108
    pain clinics (UK) Ch156
    see also doctors
gene therapy
    chronic back pain management Ch529–Ch530
    refractory angina pectoris management Ch557
geniculate neuralgia **Ch482,** Ch485
genitofemoral nerve *P244*
    block P218
        anatomical aspects P218
        complications P218

indications P218
landmarks and practical steps P218, *P219*
neuralgia, lumbar sympathetic block complication P243
genitourinary system, opioids' pharmacological effects P63
giant cell arteritis **Ch482, Ch499**
Gillette test P190
ginger, botanical therapy **Ch347**
gingival pain Ch482
gingivitis, oral pain in AIDS patients Ca381
ginkgo, botanical therapy **Ch347**
glenohumeral joint, intra-articular injections P263
anterior approach P263, *P264*
posterior approach P263, *P263*
RCTs P255
glial cells, role in inflammatory pain A36
glossopharyngeal neuralgia **Ch482, Ch499**
glucosamine sulfate, osteoarthritis management Ch544
glutamate
in inflammatory pain A24, A32
receptors **A25**
activation A32
ionotropic *see* ionotropic glutamate receptors
metabotropic *see* metabotropic glutamate receptors
(mGluR)
role in nociceptive signaling in dorsal horn A8
glycerol
neurolytic agent Ca237, **Ca238**
trigeminal neuralgia management **Ch497**
glyceryl trinitrate, adverse effects Ca221
glycine **A34**
modulation of nociceptive messages A11–A12
glycoprotein hormones, prohibited substances in IOC medical
code A499 A
golfer's elbow Ch546
gouty arthritis A397
G-protein-coupled receptors (GPCRs) **A20**
in inflammatory pain A25–A26
phosphorylation A27
graft occlusion, rates following peripheral vascular bypass
surgery **A173**
grapeseed extract, botanical therapy **Ch347**
Graseby syringe drivers *P87*
groin pain *see* abdominal pain, visceral
guanethidine
CRPS management Ch391
intravenous regional sympathetic block P243–P244, P245
duration P244
Guidelines for the Assessment of Herbal Medicines Ch346
Guillain–Barré syndrome A372, Ch358
in AIDS patients Ca376
allodynia Ch115
animal models Ch191
autoimmune neuropathy Ch373
management A372
capsaicin **Ch219**
guilt Ch165–Ch166
gut, localized pain *A97*
gyrectomy, postcentral, central pain syndromes
management Ch411

Haemophilus influenzae, maxillary sinusitis Ch485
haloperidol
delirium medication Ca311
opioid-induced delirium management Ca172
hand
intra-articular injections P266–P267
metacarpophalangeal joint P266–P267, *P267*
proximal interphalangeal joint P267

soft-tissue disorders Ch545–Ch546
diagnosis Ch545–Ch546
epidemiology Ch545–Ch546
management Ch546
hard tissues, sport injury classification A486
headaches Ch467–Ch479
in AIDS patients Ca377–Ca378
acute aseptic meningitis Ca377
causes **Ca377**
frequency **Ca378**
late stage Ca377–Ca378
opportunistic infections and tumors Ca378
biofeedback P130, P158
in children *see under* children
cluster **Ch482, Ch499**
radiofrequency lesioning indication P331
differential diagnosis Ch470
drug induced Ch470
epidemiology, age related Ch21
fibromyalgia association Ch616
indication for radiotherapy Ca254
management Ch471–Ch475
acetaminophen Ch235
acupuncture Ch343
chiropractic management Ch345
topical capsaicin Ch221
meningeal carcinomatosis feature Ca9
patient information/teaching A292
in pregnancy A377
psychological therapies A291
tension-type *see* tension-type headaches
see also migraine
head and neck peripheral nerve blocks P200–P203
see also individual types
head trauma A352
healing Ca276
Health Authorities, pain clinics (UK) Ch155
health care institutions, failure to hold clinicians accountable for
pain relief Ch35–Ch36
health care resources, pain measures P8
health maintenance organizations (HMO) Ch168
Health Status of Older People Ch22
Health Status Questionnaire (HSQ) Ch150
heart *see entries beginning cardiac*
heart attack, intraspinal opioid reduction in postoperative
risk A252
heat
pain condition P356
pain management in pregnancy A378
physiotherapy agent P185
stimulation, abnormal sensory disturbances *P33*
heat hyperalgesia Ch115, **Ch121**
heat hyperalgesia, anticonvulsant therapy Ch254
Helicobacter pylori, role in NSAID-induced peptic ulcers Ca188
hemarthrosis A399
hematological disorders A380, A382–A383
radiotherapy Ca255
see also hemophilia; sickle cell disease
hematoma
cervical, stellate ganglion block complication P239
epidural *see* epidural hematoma
hematopoiesis, NSAID induced Ca37
hematostasis, NSAID induced Ca37
hemibody radiotherapy *see* wide-field irradiation
hemifacial spasm, botulinum toxin injections Ch464
hemispheric dominance, central pain syndromes Ch405
hemodialysis-related pruritus, management, capsaicin **Ch219**
hemophilia A380

management A380
pain features A380
hemoptysis Ca297
history and examination Ca297
treatment Ca297
hemorrhage
central pain syndromes Ch403
retinal, epidural steroid injection complication P423
retroperitoneal, celiac plexus block complications P250
hemorrhoidectomy, treatment A336
hemostasis impairment, NSAIDs adverse effects A58–A59
heparin
epidural hematoma risk A476
low-molecular-weight (LMWH), altered coagulation A174
hepatic complications
acetaminophen-induced Ch234
NSAID induced Ca37, Ca189–Ca190, Ch231
toxicity see hepatotoxicity
hepatic disease
acetaminophen induced Ch235
in AIDS patients Ca388
effect on opioid pharmacokinetics P64
influence on opioid pharmacokinetics Ca45
hepatic metastases, radiotherapy Ca254–Ca255
hepatic pain Ca12
indication for radiotherapy Ca254–Ca255
hepatobiliary system, pain relief and sedation in interventional
radiology A505–A507
hepatomegaly
pain origins **Ca12**
right hypochondrial pain **Ca12**
hepatotoxicity
acetaminophen induced A441, Ca34, Ch234
aspirin induced Ca191
NSAID induced A58, Ca37, Ca189–Ca190, Ch231
herbal medicine Ca273
adverse effects Ca273
see also botanical therapy
hereditary coproporphyria Ch580
hereditary neuropathy Ch373
hereditary sensory and autonomic neuropathy (HSAN),
peripheral neuropathies Ch375
hernia, pelvic pain Ch595
hernioplasty, postsurgical pain syndromes Ch22, Ch420–Ch421
herniorrhaphy
ilioinguinal nerve block A445
wound infiltration in pediatric surgery A445
heroin A47–A48
herpes simple virus (HSV) infection
anal infection in AIDS patient Ca384
esophagitis, odynophagia cause in AIDS Ca386
oral pain in AIDS patient Ca379–Ca380
oral ulcerations Ca381
treatment Ca380
herpes zoster A369–A372, Ch437
acute pain see acute herpes zoster pain
in AIDS patients Ca380, Ca381
clinical features A370
dermatomes involved A370
nature of pain A370
epidemiology A369
investigation A370
pathophysiology A369–A370
varicella-zoster virus reactivation A369
progression to postherpetic neuralgia A369
prevention strategies A371
risk factors A370, **A370**
see also postherpetic neuralgia (PHN)

herpetic infections, oral problem Ca298
high cervical bupivacaine test, intrathecal treatment of refractory
pain P295
high cervical catheterization technique see under intrathecal
treatment of refractory pain
high-threshold (HT) neurons, response to distension A6
high-velocity, low-amplitude thrust P191
hip
pain A401, Ch546–Ch547
clinical features A401
investigations/management A401
unloading effect on P184
histamine, in inflammatory pain A24
historical control study designs
in cancer pain clinical trials P472–P473
history-taking, pain see pain history/examination
HIV-associated neuropathy A373, Ch373
etiology **A373**
management A373
capsaicin **Ch219**
mexiletine clinical trials Ch256
peripheral neuropathies Ch373
hoarseness, stellate ganglion block complication P239
holistic medicine Ch338
approach to psychological assessment Ca75
fibromyalgia management Ch623–Ch627
myofascial pain (MFP) management Ch623
see also complementary and alternative medicine
home care Ca107–Ca108, Ca311
by general practitioners Ca108
reasons for discontinuation Ca107–Ca108
reasons for increase in popularity Ca107
see also end of life care; palliative care
homeopathy Ca273, Ch343–Ch344
adverse effects Ch344
history Ch343–Ch344
migraine management Ch344
research Ch344
theory Ch343
doctrine of similars Ch343
potentization by dilution Ch343
hormone treatment, bone pain management see under bone pain
Horner syndrome
stellate ganglion block complication P239
hospices
palliative care Ch35
place of dying Ca108
Hospital Anxiety and Depression Scale (HADS) Ca81, Ch105
hospitals
feedback to health care policies A164–A165
inpatients, postoperative pain management see postoperative
pain management
place of dying Ca107–Ca108
hot flushes, reduction with acupuncture Ca272
human immunodeficiency virus (HIV), pain Ca367
see also AIDS
human leukocyte antigen (HLA)
CRPS-I Ch386
postherpetic neuralgia Ch374
human papillomavirus (HPV), pelvic pain Ch603–Ch604
Hunner's ulcers Ch575
hyaline articular cartilage, response to injuries A489
hyaluronan, osteoarthritis management Ch544
hyaluronidase, local anesthesia addition A78
hydrazine sulfate, anorexia–cachexia syndrome
management Ca306
hydrocodone A48
in children A442

analgesia for patients over 6 months P434–P435
doses **P435**
pain control after discharge home A335
hydromorphone Ca55, Ca134, P66
in children Ca339
analgesia for children over 6 months P436
starting dose **Ca339**
in elderly Ca357–Ca358
epidural, characteristics **A243**
hydrophilic opioids
selection A242–A244
see also epidural opioids
hydrotherapy
CRPS management Ch395
elderly pain management Ch655
5-hydroxytryptamine (5-HT) *see* serotonin (5-HT)
5-hydroxytryptamine 3 (5-HT$_3$) antagonists, as antiemetic A233
hyoscine butylbromide Ca220
adverse effects Ca221
doses and pharmacokinetics Ca220
hyoscine hydrobromide
as antiemetic A233
breathlessness management Ca296
hyperalgesia A17, A360, Ch115–Ch116, P28
animal models Ch190
changes in stimulus intensity *A17*
chemical Ch119, **Ch121**
cold Ch115, **Ch121**
CRPS Ch383–Ch384
definition Ch115, **Ch404**
dynamic Ch115, **Ch121**
endogenous attenuation of inflammation A29
heat Ch115, **Ch121**
inducers A21–A25
nerve growth factor (NGF) A21–A22, *A23*
opioid induced Ca174
definition Ca174
diagnostic criteria Ca174
epidemiology and clinical presentation Ca174
etiology and pathophysiology Ca174
evidence-based evaluation of management Ca174
notes on unevaluated treatments Ca174
peripheral neuropathies Ch368
primary, CRPS pathogenesis Ch387
provoked Ch115–Ch116
punctate Ch115, **Ch121**
quantification Ch115–Ch116
static Ch115, **Ch121**
stimulus-dependent pain Ch115
see also peripheral sensitization
hyperalgesia, definition **Ch404**
hypercalcemia
management Ca300
suitable patients Ca300
in nausea and vomiting Ca300–Ca301
hypercoagulation, postoperative pain management A170
hyperesthesia
central pain Ch407–Ch408
definition **Ch404**
postherpetic neuralgia Ch452
postsympathectomy, lumbar sympathetic block
complication P243
hypericum perforatum, botanical therapy **Ch347**
hyperkinetic disorders Ch359–Ch360
classification **Ch360**
pain Ch360
hyperpathia Ch116
CRPS Ch384

definition **Ch404**
hyperplastic candidiasis, in AIDS patient Ca378
hypersensitivity reactions, NSAID induced Ch231
hypertension, NSAID induced Ca356
hyperthermia Ca241
hypertonic solutions, neurolytic agents Ca238
hyperventilation, diaphragmatic breathing in children P150
hypervigilance P164
hypnoanalgesia P151–P152
see also hypnosis
hypnosis A289–A290, Ca273–Ca275, P115–P116
adverse effects Ca275
in children P116, P150–P155
emergency situations P152
goal P151
hypnoanalgesia P151–P152
intramuscular injections positions P153
limitations P159–P160
mechanisms of change P160–P161
pain switch technique P151
potential nonspecific pain control mechanisms P161
potential specific pain control mechanisms P160–P161
preschool patients P152–P153
procedural pain management Ca274
school-age and adolescents P153–P154
self-regulatory techniques as aid in diagnosis P154–P155
training P161
trance P151
components of pain treatment utilizing self-hypnosis **P115**
mechanisms Ca275, P115, P116
controlled dissociation P115
cortical effects P116
imaging and metaphors P115
muscle relaxation P115
perceptual alteration P115
nausea management Ca275
pain clinics **Ch159**
posthypnotic suggestion Ca274
process *P152*
of self *see* self-hypnosis
techniques to diminish/abolish pain Ca274
treatment (of)
burn pain A364
childbirth pain A432
pelvic pain Ch603
procedural pain Ca322
hypocarbia, maternal, response to childbirth pain A426
hypochondria Ch567
hypochondrial pain, right, in hepatomegaly patients **Ca12**
hypoesthesia, definition **Ch404**
hypogastric plexus, superior P251
block *see* superior hypogastric plexus block
hypophysectomy Ca265, Ch299–Ch300
central pain syndromes management Ch411
chemical Ch299–Ch300
complications Ch300
indications Ch299
mechanism of action Ch300
hypothalamus Ch300
neurotransmitter release Ch300
mortality Ch300
outcome Ch300
stereotactic radiofrequency Ch300
technique Ch300
hypotension
epidural analgesia-induced A192
opioid-induced P62
epidural infusion P313

orthostatic
    celiac plexus block complications P249, P250
    intravenous regional sympathetic block
        complication P245
hypothalamotomy Ch303–Ch304
    indications Ch303
    mechanism of action Ch303–Ch304
    outcomes Ch303
hypothalamus, hypophysectomy Ch300
hypothermia Ca241
hypothyroid neuropathy Ch371
hypotonic solutions, neurolytic agents Ca238
hypoxemia A191, A310
    causes **A310**
    indicator of respiratory depression A232
    maternal and fetal, response to childbirth pain A426
    opioid-induced A471–A472
hysterectomy Ch601–Ch602
    adverse effects Ch601
    contraindications Ch601
    efficacy Ch601–Ch602
    indications Ch601

iatrogenic drugs
    addiction, malpractice claims Ch179–Ch180
    substance abuse Ch633
iatrogenic lesions, central pain syndromes Ch404
iatrogenic pain, multiple sclerosis Ch358
ibuprofen A65, Ca193
    administration and absorption A208, A209
    adverse effects Ca37, Ca187–Ca190
        gastric complications Ch230
    characteristics **Ch229**
    in children, doses **P435**
    cyclo-oxygenase (COX) inhibitor Ca193
    doses and treatment protocols Ca193
    drug interactions Ca193
    evidence for efficacy Ca190, Ca193
    indications and contraindications Ca186–Ca187, Ca193
    number needed to treat (NNT) A62
    pharmacokinetics Ca193
    practical tips Ca193
    treatment (of)
        anorexia–cachexia syndrome Ca306
        hemophilia A382
        tension-type headache Ch639
ice massage, in cryotherapy A493
ice packs, in cryotherapy A493
idiopathic neuropathy Ch375
    see also neuropathies, peripheral
ileus A168
    postoperative pain management A168, A170
iliac fossa pain Ca13
    right, in AIDS patients Ca388
iliohypogastric/ilioinguinal nerve block P218
    anatomical aspects P218
    in children P440
        anatomical aspects P440
        complications P440
        local anesthetic solution P440
        method P440
        pediatric surgery A445
    complications P218
    indications P218
    landmarks and practical steps P218, *P219*
ilioinguinal nerve block see iliohypogastric/ilioinguinal nerve
    block *(above)*
Illness Behavior Questionnaire, chronic back pain Ch525

imagery technique A289, Ca275–Ca276
    advantages and disadvantages A293
    biofeedback component P126
    in children A289
imaging
    articular musculoskeletal pain diagnosis A395–A396
    nonarticular musculoskeletal pain diagnosis A396
    of pain A107
imipramine
    dose titrations Ch244–Ch245, *Ch245*
    mechanism of action Ch239–Ch240
    pharmacokinetics *Ch241*
    pharmacology **Ch240**
    structure *Ch240*
    therapeutic index Ch245
    treatment (of)
        central pain syndrome management **Ch409**
        neuropathic pain Ch242
        peripheral neuropathy Ch376–Ch377
    treatment schedule *P103*
immobilization
    sport injury management A492
    in trauma A350, **A355**
immune system
    abnormalities, myofascial pain (MFP) Ch623
    NSAIDs adverse effects Ca37
immunization, sucrose administration for pain relief in
    infants A297
impairment
    definitions Ch42
        American Medical Association (AMA) Ch49–Ch50
        World Health Organization (WHO) Ch183
    disability linkage Ch43
    see also disability; disability evaluation (USA)
impairment ratings Ch48–Ch49
incidence, definition Ch16
incident pain Ca152
    morphine rescue analgesia Ca133
    see also breakthrough pain
inclinometry Ch146
index of suspicion, opioid trials Ch207
indinavir, in AIDS pain management Ca369–Ca370
    pharmacokinetics **Ca369**
    toxicities **Ca370**
    urolithiasis induction Ca389
indomethacin A65, Ca194
    characteristics **Ch229**
    cyclo-oxygenase (COX) inhibitor Ca194
    doses and treatment protocols Ca194
    evidence for efficacy Ca190
    indications and contraindications Ca186–Ca187, Ca194
    pharmacokinetics Ca190, Ca194
    practical tips Ca194
infants
    breast-feeding
        analgesia use in A379–A380, **A384–A385**
        drug exposure during A379–A380
    immunization pain relief with sucrose A297
    local anesthesia A81
    pain assessment A104–A105
    pain intensity assessment P21
    physical strategies *see under* physical therapies
infections Ca13–Ca14
    bacterial *see* bacterial infections
    intra-articular injection complications P259
    intrathecal catheterization adverse effects P301–P302
    in multiple sclerosis Ch358
    opportunistic, in AIDS Ca367

oral problems Ca297–Ca298
  bacterial Ca298
  candidiasis Ca297–Ca298
    see also oral candidiasis
  herpetic Ca298
  spinal cord stimulation complication P388
  systemic, spinal cord stimulation contraindication P381
infective parotitis, oral problem Ca298
inferior alveolar nerves, postsurgical pain syndromes Ch419
infiltration anesthesia A88
  pain management in pregnancy A379
inflammatory arthritis, NSAIDs Ch228
inflammatory bowel disease A375, Ch579
  management Ch579
  sources of pain **Ch568**
inflammatory bowel disorders A375
inflammatory joint pain
  exacerbations of chronic diseases A397
  interpretation as acute musculoskeletal pain A393–A404
    see also musculoskeletal injuries/pain
  NSAIDs Ch228
inflammatory neuritis, animal models Ch191
inflammatory pain A17–A41
  allodynia *see* allodynia
  applied physiology A17–A41
    see also central sensitization; peripheral sensitization
  definitions A17–A18
  glial cell role A36
  hyperalgesia *see* hyperalgesia
  in joints *see* inflammatory joint pain
  management A396–A397
  musculoskeletal *see* musculoskeletal injuries/pain
  randomized controlled trials in acute pain P487–P488
informed consent P511
  in cancer pain clinical trials P479
  in dental pain clinical trials P463
  lack of P511–P512
  in opioid therapy Ch208, P80–P81
infraclavicular block P208
  landmarks and practical steps P208, *P209*
infraorbital nerve block P201
  in children P440–P441
    anatomical aspects P440–P441
    local anesthetic solution P441
    method P441
    pediatric surgery A446
  landmarks and practical steps P201
inguinal hernia repair, timing of administration of local
  anesthetics A119
inguinal perivascular femoral nerve block, in musculoskeletal
  injuries A355
inhalation of drugs A207
  analgesia provision in trauma A350, **A350**
  anesthesia in burn pain treatment A363
  in children P433–P434
  opioids A212, A319
  patient-controlled analgesia route P401–P402
inhibitory amino acids, and receptors **A34**
injection techniques
  low back pain A412–A413
  noninflammatory joint pain management A398
  pelvic pain management Ch600
injuries *see* trauma
innate intelligence, chiropractic theory Ch344
insoles, osteoarthritis management Ch544
integrative medicine, definition Ch338
  see also complementary and alternative medicine
intensive care unit (ICU) A341–A348

adjuvant analgesia A344–A345
  α_2-adrenergic agonists A344–A345
  antidepressants A344
  sedatives A344
analgesia methods A342–A344
  local anesthetics A343–A344
  nonopioid analgesics A342–A343, **A343**
  nonpharmacological A342
  opioids A343
indications for pain relief A341
limitations of analgesia use A341–A342
management goals A341
multiple organ failure patients A345–A347
  cardiac failure A347
  central nervous system injury A345
  liver failure A347
  pharmacokinetics of analgesics and sedatives **A346**
  renal failure A347
  respiratory failure A345, A347
pain assessment A342
intensivists, role in acute pain service A185
intercostal nerve blocks A270–A271, P216
  anatomical aspects P216
    branches **P216**
  chest trauma management A353
  in children P441–P442
    anatomical aspects P441
    catheter techniques P441
    local anesthetic solution P442
    method P441–P442
    paravertebral block P441
    pediatric surgery A448
    subcostal block P441
  complications P216
  cryoanalgesia for post-thoracotomy P322–P323
  effect on pulmonary sequelae of pain A311
  improvements in pulmonary outcome measures A168, **A171**
  indications P216
    local anesthetic and steroid block P216
    local anesthetic block P216
    neurolytic block P216
  landmarks and practical steps P216, *P217*
    anterior approach P216
    midaxillary approach P216
    posterior approach P216
  pain management in ICU A344
intercostal rib resection, postsurgical pain syndromes Ch420
intercostobrachial nerve, damage in breast surgery *Ca15*
interference, pain measure P8
interferential therapy P344
intermediate column (longissimus) muscle Ch523
intermittent acute porphyria (IAP) Ch580
intermittent urokinase therapy, refractory angina pectoris
  management Ch557
internal carotid artery dissection
  headache Ch508
  neck pain Ch508
internal consistency, pain measure P9
internal mammary (IMA) ligation, angina pectoris
  management Ch555
International Association for the Study of Pain (IASP)
  animal model guidelines Ch189–Ch190
  central pain syndromes definition Ch403
  CRPS definition Ch383
  maxillary sinusitis definition Ch487
  pain classifications Ch16
  Task Force on Epidemiology Ch15
  trigeminal neuralgia definition Ch491

International Headache Society (IHS)
    atypical facial pain definition Ch489
    classification
        headaches, tension-type Ch639
        migraine Ch638
    trigeminal neuralgia diagnosis Ch492
International Narcotics Control Board (INCB) Ch30
    opioid legal control Ch173
International Olympic Committee (IOC) medical code A498–A502
    amendments to IOC list A501–A502
    prohibited classes of substances A498–A499
        anabolic agents A499
        diuretics A499
        examples A501
        narcotics A499
        peptide and glycoprotein hormones and analogs A499
        stimulants A498
    prohibited methods A499–A500
        blood doping A499
        pharmaceutical, chemical, and physical
            manipulation A499–A500
    regulations for drugs needing physician written
        notification A500
    restricted drugs A500
        alcohol A500
        β-blockers A500
        corticosteroids A500
        local anesthetics A500
        marijuana A500
    urinary limits for drug concentrations A500
Interpersonal Adjective Test List, placebo response Ch281
interphalangeal joint, proximal, intra-articular injections P267
interpleural analgesia (IPA) P247
interpleural block A270–A271, P216–P218
    anatomical aspects P217
    complications P217–P218
    contraindications P217
    indications P216–P217
        cancer pain P217
        chronic pain P216
        postsurgical analgesia P216
    landmarks and practical steps P217, P218
interpleural phenol blocks P247–P248
    complications P248
    drugs and dosing P247–P248
    efficacy P248
    technique P248
interrater reliability, pain measure P9–P10
interscalene block P206–P207
    landmarks and practical steps P206, P207
interspinous ligaments Ch522, Ch523
interstitial cystitis Ch575–Ch577, Ch595–Ch596
    clinical features Ch575
    diagnosis Ch576, Ch596
    diseases associations Ch575
    etiology Ch596
    management Ch575–Ch577, Ch576, Ch596
        diet Ch596
    symptoms/signs Ch596
interstitial radiation Ch300
interventional radiology, pain relief and sedation A503–A512
    endovascular procedures A503–A505
        blood flow improvements A503–A504
        blood flow reductions A504–A505
    hepatobiliary system A505–A507
    intravenous sedation and analgesia A509–A510
        drugs A510
        monitoring A509–A510

        principles A509
        sedation scale A510
    provision of relief A509–A511
        general requirements A509
        regional analgesia A510–A511
            advantages and disadvantages A511
            techniques for common painful procedures A512
        see also individual techniques
interventional techniques, persistent cancer pain P477
intervertebral disks see under spine
intra-articular analgesia A333
    administration A207
        opioids A212–A213
    knee pain A333
    nonsteroidal anti-inflammatory drugs A210
    osteoarthritis management Ch543–Ch544
intra-articular blocks P227–P229
    cervical zygapophyseal (facet) joints P272–P273
    complications P229
    indications P227
    landmarks and practical steps P227–P229, P228
    lumbar zygapophyseal (facet) joints P272
intra-articular injections P255–P268
    in children, evidence for use P256
    complications P259
    contraindications P258–P259
    drugs P259–P260
    equipment P259
    evidence for effectiveness P255–P256
        in children P256
        glenohumeral joint RCTs P255
        lateral epicondyle elbow pain RCTs P256
        osteoarthritis RCTs P256
        subacromial injection RCTs P255–P256
    general principles P256–P257
        aseptic technique P256
        counseling of patient P256–P257
        mechanisms of action P256
    historical aspects P255
    indications P258
    joint injection methods P260–P267
        ankle P261, P262
        see also other individual joints
    osteoarthritis management Ch543–Ch544
    technique P257–P258
        correct placement P257, P258
        delivery methods P257, P258
        frequency P257
        preparation P257
intra-articular sepsis, intra-articular injection
    contraindication P258
intracerebral stimulation, central pain syndromes
    management Ch410
intracisternal treatment of refractory pain P285–P305
    advantages P303
    adverse effects P302–P303
    anatomical aspects P286, P287
    bupivacaine test P295
    bupivacaine treatment P295
    care of patient and infusion system P298, P300
        dressing tunnel exit P298
        exchanging bacterial filter P298
        exchanging infusion container P300
        taking a shower P300
    clinical results P299
    historical aspects P286
    indications P288
        malignant pain P288

nonmalignant pain P288
insertion complications **P297**
limitations P288
solutions P295, P297
bupivacaine P295
buprenorphine P297
mixtures of opioid/bupivacaine P297
morphine P295, P297
technique P295
catheter direction P295
catheter endpoint P295, *P296*
insertion site P295, *P296*
intracranial pressure, headache diagnosis Ch470
intractable pain Ch28
in cancer *see* refractory cancer pain
Intractable Pain Management Act, opioid legal controls Ch174–Ch175
intradiskal electrothermy (IDET), chronic back pain management Ch529
intramuscular administration of drugs A206
in children Ca340, P433
development A220
opioids A211, A316–A317, A473–A474, Ca51
acute pain management P70
disadvantages **A317**
intranasal administration of drugs A207
opioids A212, A318
intranasal patient-controlled analgesia (PCINA) A227, *P403*, P403–P404
system characteristics **P404**
intrapelvic cancer Ca12–Ca13
pain Ca12–Ca13
sites of Ca12–Ca13, **Ca13**
intraperitoneal infiltration, of local anesthesia A332
intrapleural analgesia, postoperative pain management A319–A320
intrapleural blocks
acute herpes zoster pain management Ch444
pain management in ICU A344
in pediatric surgery A448
intrapleural technique (IPA), chest trauma management A353
intraspinal analgesia P307
role of pumps in pain management **P309**
see also entries beginning with epidural and intrathecal
intraspinal opioids A241–A258
adverse effects A252–A257
monitoring routines A256–A257
safety of lipophilic drug A255–A256
safety of parenteral route A256
treatment and prophylaxis A257–A258
in ambulatory surgery A248
lipophilic advantage over local anesthetic for spinal block **A248**
cancer pain management P71
delivery systems **Ca263**
dose escalation Ca262–Ca263
epidural *see* epidural opioids
intrathecal *see* intrathecal opioids
myoclonus induction Ca173
in neurosurgical procedures Ca262
neurotoxicity risk association A250–A251
outcome A251–A252
reduced cardiac problems A251
reduced postoperative morbidity A251
reduced postoperative myocardial infarctions A252
reduced pulmonary problems A251
in refractory cancer pain Ca148
route choice A248–A250

therapeutic applications **A241,** A241–A242
intrathecal administration of drugs
bupivacaine
adverse effects P300
indications for refractory pain P286–P288
chemotherapy *Ca320*
morphine A249
adverse effects P300
opioids A213, Ca51, Ca91
intrathecal analgesia A248–A250
painful spasticity management Ch463, **Ch464**
postoperative pain management A320, A322
risk associations A249–A250
intrathecal baclofen Ch257
intrathecal morphine A249
administration A249
adverse effects P300
adverse effects A250
intrathecal neurolysis Ca239–Ca240
clinical considerations Ca239–Ca240
complications Ca240, **Ca241**
indications **Ca240**
outcomes Ca240
technique Ca240
intrathecal opioids A213, A477
administration A213, Ca51, Ca91
adverse effects A252–A257
treatment and prophylaxis A257–A258
in ambulatory surgery A248
childbirth pain treatment A249, A431
in neurosurgical procedures Ca262
pain management in ICU A343
severe pain relief technique **A188**
see also epidural opioids
intrathecal sufentanil A249
adverse effects A250
intrathecal treatment of refractory pain P285–P305
advantages P303, **P308**
advantages of external *versus* internal catheters/pumps P303–P304
large reservoir volumes P303–P304
lower costs P304
PCA option P304
reduced complications P303
reduced technical failures P303
simplicity P304
adverse effects P300–P302
from bupivacaine P300
from catheterization P300–P302
equipment related P302
from morphine P300
anatomical aspects P286, *P286*
care of patient and infusion system P298, P300
dressing tunnel exit P293, *P294*, P298
exchanging bacterial filter P298
exchanging infusion container P300
taking a shower P300
clinical results **P299**
disadvantages P304, **P308**
epidural comparison P304
external versus internal catheters/pumps P304
efficacy P304–P305
epidural comparison P304
external versus internal catheters/pumps P304–P305
epidural comparison P304, **P308,** P316
guidelines for adjustment P297–P298
high cervical bupivacaine test P295
high cervical catheterization technique P295

adverse effects P302–P303
  catheter direction P295
  catheter endpoint P295
  insertion site P295
historical aspects P285–P286
indications P286–P288
  malignant pain P287
  nonmalignant pain P287
insertion complications **P297**
limitations P288
  malignant pain P288
  nonmalignant pain P288
solutions P295, P297
  bupivacaine P295
  buprenorphine P297
  mixtures of opioid/bupivacaine P297
  morphine P295, P297
technique P288–P295
  anesthesia P290
  connecting infusion pump P293
  connecting Millipore filter P293, *P294*
  dressing incisions and tunnel exit P293, *P294,* P298
  dural puncture P290
  equipment P288–P289
  fixing catheter to skin P293, *P294*
  imaging/location technique P289
  insertion of catheter P291
  instructing ward personnel, patient and next of kin P293, P295
  landmarks and insertion sites P289–P290
  location for catheterization procedure P289
  monitoring P289
  patient preparation P288
  Portex tunneling device P291, *P292*
  position of patient and operator P289, *P290*
  postcatheterization care P295
  preparation of operation site P289
  skin incision at insertion site P291, *P292*
  substituting for spilt cerebrospinal fluid P293
  testing catheter patency P291, *P291, P293*
  tunneling catheter P291–P292, *P292*
intravenous administration of drugs A206–A207
  in children Ca340, P432
  conscious sedation for procedural pain Ca323, Ca325
  development A220
  infusions A206–A207
  opioids A211, A317, **A318,** A474, Ca51
  patient-controlled analgesia (PCA) P395
  randomized controlled trials in acute pain P487–P488
intravenous alfentanyl, doses and paradigms P45
intravenous analgesia A509–A510
  drugs A510
  monitoring A509–A510
  principles A509
intravenous opioids P44–P45
  acute pain management P70
  administration A211, A317, **A318,** A474, Ca51
  advantages and disadvantages **A318**
  adverse effects P45
  background P44–P45
  contraindication P45
  doses and paradigms P45
  indication P45
  practical tips P45
  timing of treatment studies A120–A121, **A144–A147**
  see also individual drugs
intravenous regional anesthesia A88
intravenous regional sympathetic block P243–P245

adverse effects P245
  guanethidine P245
    duration P244
  technique P245
intravenous sedation A509–A510
  assessment scale **A510**
  drugs A510
  monitoring A509–A510
  principles A509
intraventricular infusion, opioids
  clearance rate Ch301
  indications Ch301
  lipophilic opioids Ch301–Ch302
  morphine sulfate Ch301
intraventricular opioids Ch301–Ch302
  delivery systems **Ca263**
    see also intraventricular infusion, opioids
  in neurosurgical procedures Ca262
invasive management, neurologic disease Ch362
ionotropic glutamate receptors **A25**
  activation A32
  excitatory postsynaptic potentials (EPSPs) A32, *A32*
  phosphorylation in inflammation A27
iontophoresis A207
  opioids Ca51
irritable bowel syndrome (IBS) A374, Ca17–Ca18, Ch577–Ch578
  in AIDS patients Ca388
  in children Ch640
  clinical presentations Ch577
  diagnosis **Ch577**
  etiology Ch577
  fibromyalgia association Ch616
  management Ch577–Ch578, **Ch578**
    CBT Ch578
    dietary modifications Ch578
  Rome I and II criteria comparison **A375**
  visceral hyperalgesia A374
ischemic brainstem injury, central pain syndrome Ch408
ischemic colitis Ch579–Ch580
ischemic heart disease, pain Ca403
ischemic pain
  animal models Ch191
  effect of adenosine on allodynia development and pain scores **P487**
  management
    capsaicin **Ch219**
    spinal cord stimulation (SCS) Ch289, Ch290
    TENS P352
ischemic spinal cord injury, animal models Ch191–Ch192
isokinetic strain, definition **Ch316**
IsoMed implantable pump *P315*
isometric exercises, physical therapy Ch316
isometric strain, definition **Ch316**
isothermognosis, definition **Ch404**
isotonic exercises, physical therapy Ch316
isotonic strain, definition **Ch316**

Janus kinase, role in inflammatory pain A27
jaundice, obstructive, percutaneous biliary stenting A507
Johns Hopkins Hospital, CPRP Ch163–Ch164
Joint Commission for the Accreditation of Healthcare Organizations (JCAHO) A107–A108
  standards of pain management Ch36
joint pain Ch537–Ch551
  in AIDS patients *see under* AIDS
  assessment Ch537–Ch538
    GALS screening Ch537–Ch538
  classification of rheumatic diseases **Ch537**

complications of intra-articular injections P259
facet, radiofrequency lesioning Ca242
inflammatory *see* inflammatory joint pain
intra-articular pain relief *see* intra-articular analgesia
manipulation with anesthesia (MUJA) P192
mechanical pain A399
noninflammatory pain *see* noninflammatory joint pain
sepsis, intra-articular injection contraindication P258
see also musculoskeletal injuries/pain; *individual joints*
jump sign, fibromyalgia/myofascial pain Ch618–Ch619

kangaroo care infant pain management A295
    evidence supporting effectiveness A296
Kaposi's sarcoma, in AIDS
    cutaneous lesions *Ca382*
    ocular manifestations *Ca384*
    oral pain Ca381, *Ca381*
    pulmonary involvement Ca386
Katz Activities of Daily Living score Ca351
KDS-15 questionnaire Ch74
ketamine Ca221, Ch263
    addition to opioids in PCA A228
    advantages Ca326
    adverse effects A351, Ca222
    analgesia provision in trauma A351
    caudal analgesia A447–A448
    in children A443–A444
        administration A443–A444
        adverse effects and toxicity A444
        analgesia for patients over 6 months P437–P438
        pharmacology and indications A443
        protocol for morphine combined infusions **P438**
    clinical studies Ch263–Ch264
    doses and treatment paradigms Ca222
    experimental studies Ch263
    intravenous P43–P44
        adverse effects P44
        background P43
        contraindications P44
        doses and paradigms P44
        indications P43–P44
        pharmaceutical considerations P44
        practical tips P44
    pharmacokinetics Ca222
    subcutaneous infusions in cancer pain control P92
    timing of treatment studies A122, **A148–A151**
    treatment (of)
        burn pain A363, A364
        central pain syndrome Ch264
        CRPS Ch394
        fibromyalgia Ch264
        neuropathic pain Ch264
        postamputation pain Ch264
        postherpetic neuralgia Ch264
        procedural pain Ca326
        refractory cancer pain Ca146
ketazolam, painful spasticity management **Ch462**
ketobemidone P68
    pharmacokinetics P68
ketoprofen A65, Ca194
    administration A209
    adverse effects Ca187–Ca190
    characteristics **Ch229**
    cyclo-oxygenase (COX) inhibitor Ca194
    doses and treatment protocols Ca194
    indications and contraindications Ca186–Ca187
    pharmacokinetics Ca194
    rectal A208

ketorolac A65–A66, A331, Ca194–Ca195
    adverse effects A173, Ca187–Ca190, Ca195
    characteristics **Ch229**
    in children, doses **P435**
    contraindications Ca187
    CRPS management Ch391
    cyclo-oxygenase (COX) inhibitor Ca194–Ca195
    doses and treatment protocols Ca195, **Ca195**
    evidence for efficacy Ca195
    indications Ca195
    pharmacokinetics Ca195
    practical tips Ca195
    subcutaneous infusions in cancer pain control P91
kidney disease, effect on opioid pharmacokinetics P64
kidneys
    acetaminophen adverse effects Ch234
    clearance rates, physiological changes with age A466
    NSAIDs adverse effects A59, A173, Ca188–Ca189, Ca356,
        Ch231, Ch261
    opioids adverse effects Ca357
    see also entries beginning with renal
kinesiophobia P163
knee pain A401–A402, Ch547
    arthroscopic surgery
        intra-articular analgesia A333
        local anesthetic infiltration into cavity A269
    clinical features A402
    intra-articular injections P260–P261
        anterior approach P260–P261, *P261*
        medial and lateral approaches P260, *P261*
        RCTs P256
    investigations/management A402
    nerve blocks P227–P229
        anatomical aspects P227
        indications P227
        see also individual types
    replacement surgery, analgesia provision A244
    sporting injuries A489–A490

Labat method of nerve block *see* cervical plexus block, deep
L'Abbé plots P498–P499, *P499*
labor pain *see* childbirth pain
lactate levels, CRPS diagnosis Ch389
lactation, NSAIDs use during Ca36
Lamaze technique in childbirth A429, A432
lamotrigine
    adverse effects Ca214, Ch493, P107
    clinical trials Ch252, Ch253
    contraindications P105
    doses and treatment paradigms Ca214, **P106,** P107
    mechanism of action Ca213, Ch251
    pharmacokinetics Ca215
    pretreatment safety measures **P106,** P107
    treatment (of)
        central pain syndromes Ch410
        CRPS Ch394
        peripheral neuropathy Ch377
        trigeminal neuralgia Ch493, **Ch494–Ch495**
laparoscopic surgery
    in abdominal pain management A374
    postoperative pain A336
        local anesthetic infiltration A268
    timing of administration of local anesthetics A117, A119
laparoscopic uterine nerve ablation (LUNA) Ch206
laparoscopy Ch600–Ch601
    adverse effects Ch601
    contraindications Ch601
    efficacy Ch601

endometriosis diagnosis and management Ch591
    indications Ch600–Ch601
    pelvic congestion diagnosis Ch592
laparotomy
    endometriosis diagnosis and management Ch591
    ovarian remnant syndrome management Ch593
large intestine, opioids' pharmacological effects P62
large myelinated (Aβ) fibers
    stimulation in peripheral nerve stimulation (PNS) Ca248
    stimulation in TENS Ca245–Ca246
laser-evoked potentials P35
laser therapy Ca242, Ca271, P186
    acute herpes zoster pain Ch445
    low level (LLLT) P186
lateral column (iliocostalis) muscle Ch523
lateral cutaneous nerve
    forearm blockade P212
        landmarks and practical steps P212
    thigh blockade P223
        anatomical aspects P223
        complications P223
        indications P223
        landmarks and practical steps P223, *P224*
lateral epicondyle, intra-articular injections P264–P265, *P265*
    RCTs P256
lateral epicondylitis
    physical therapies Ch317
    topical NSAIDs Ch216–Ch217
lateral medullary syndrome, central pain syndrome Ch408
law of negligence Ch176–Ch177
laxatives **Ca304**
    adjuvant analgesics Ca136
    combination with opioids Ca132
    constipation management Ca303–Ca304
        opioid-induced cases Ca176
    methods of action **Ca304**
learned pain behavior, personal injury claims Ch182
learned tolerance Ca48
left internal mammary artery pain syndrome, chronic chest
    pain Ch560
left stellate ganglion injection, refractory angina pectoris
    management Ch557
legal action *see* medicolegal aspects
legs, length difference P190–P191
    see also lower limb pain
leprosy, peripheral neuropathies Ch375
lesions, thalamic Ch406
leukotomy, frontal, central pain syndromes management Ch411
leukotrienes, in inflammatory pain A23
levobupivacaine A86
    peripheral nerve block agent P198
levomepromazine, nausea and vomiting management Ca299–
    Ca300
levorphanol Ca55, Ca134, P67
Lewis hunting reaction A492
Lhermitte's sign, multiple sclerosis Ch357
liability, medicolegal *see* medicolegal aspects
libido loss Ch165
Lickert rating scale Ch120
lidocaine A83, Ca211–Ca212, P108
    clinical trial Ch205
    complications A81
    contraindications Ca212
    doses and treatment paradigms Ca212
    historical aspects A73
    indications Ca212
    intravenous P40–P42, P108
        adverse effects P41, P109

        background P40
        bolus regimen P40
        cancer pain management Ch256
        clinical trials Ch256–Ch257
        contraindications P40
        doses and paradigms P40–P41
        dosing and treatment schedule P108, **P109**
        evidence for efficacy P41–P42
        four-hour infusion P41
        indications P40
        nerve pain management Ch256
        neuropathic pain management Ch256
        pharmaceutical considerations P41
        practical tips P41
        pretreatment safety measures **P109**
        short infusion regimen P40–P41
    mechanism of action Ch255
    metabolism A80, *A80*
    peripheral nerve block agent P197
    pH and pK_a graph *A78*
    pharmacokinetics **A346**
    physiochemical properties and clinical profile **A79, A84**
    structural formula *A77*, **A84**
    systemic P108
        actions P53
        contraindications P108
    topical Ch257
    treatment (of)
        burn pain A363
        central pain syndrome Ch409
        CRPS Ch391
        postherpetic neuralgia Ch256
ligaments
    response to injury A490
    spinal *see* spine (vertebral column), ligaments
ligand-gated ion channels, in inflammatory pain A25
lignocaine *see* lidocaine
limb amputations, local anesthetic infusions A269
limb nerve blocks P219–P230
    lower P219–P230
    upper P204–P214
    see also individual types
limb pain *see* lower limb pain; upper limb pain
limited myelotomy Ca264
lingual nerves, postsurgical pain syndromes Ch419
lipophilic opioids
    in ambulatory surgery A248
        advantage over local anesthetics for spinal block A248
    safety A255–A256
    selection A242–A244
    see also epidural opioids
listening skills Ch9–Ch10
lithium, NSAIDs interaction A57
liver
    acetaminophen adverse effects Ch234
    clearance, physiological changes with age A464, A466
    metastases, radiotherapy Ca254–Ca255
    NSAIDs adverse effects A58, Ca37, Ca189–Ca190, Ch231
    pain Ca12
        indication for radiotherapy Ca254–Ca255
liver disease *see* hepatic disease
liver failure, pain management in ICU A347
living wills Ca119
local anesthesia A73–A91, **A332**, A332–A334
    additives A77–A78
    agents A83–A87
        see also individual drugs
    alkalinization A78

in ambulatory surgery A248
blocks *see* peripheral nerve blocks
cellular electrophysiology A73–A74
    action potential characteristics A74, **A74**
    myelinated fiber transmission A74
in children *see* children, local anesthetic techniques
clinical uses A87–A89
    contraindications A87, **A87**
    indications A87
    infiltration anesthesia A88
    intravenous regional anesthesia (Bier block) A88
    ophthalmologic anesthesia A88
    topical anesthesia A87
combinations A78
    corticosteroids A496
complications **A81**, A81–A83
    allergic reactions A82
    cauda equina syndrome A81
    differential diagnosis of collapse **A82,** A83
    drug interactions A82–A83
    local A81
    miscellaneous systemic effects A83
    systemic A81–A83
    toxicity clinical presentation **A82**
    toxicity treatment **A82**
diffusion A76
drug additions for peripheral nerve blockades A271
in elderly A472
epidural *see* epidural analgesia/anesthesia; epidural local
    anesthesia
in epidural steroid injections P422
eutectic mixture *see* eutectic mixture of local anesthetics
    (EMLA)
future directions A88–A89
    butyl-aminobenzoate (BAB) A88–A89
    drug alterations A88
    modification into prolonged-release preparations A88
history **A73,** A73–A74
in infants A81
iontophoresis administration A319
joint manipulation (MUJA) P192
local infiltration A267–A269
    clinical tips Ca322
    intraperitoneal infiltration A332
    pain management in ICU A343
    procedural pain management Ca322
    in proximity to peripheral nerve sheaths A269
    subcutaneous infiltration A268
    into surgical cavities A269
    wound infiltration *see* wound infiltration of local
        anesthesia
lumbar sympathetic block dose P242
mechanism of action A74–A78
    decremental block A76
    differential sensitivity A76, **A76**
    effect of pH A77
    effect on action potential transmission A74
    frequency- and voltage-dependent actions A75–A76
    modulated-receptor hypothesis A75–A76
    pattern of onset and recovery of blockade A76
    penetration in base form into nerve axon **A78**
    site of action A74–A75
    sodium channel interactions A74–A75
in neonates *see under* neonatal pain management
nerve/nerve plexus infusions A269–A271
pain management
    in ICU A343–A344
    new concepts A333–A334

pharmacokinetics A78–A81
    absorption A79
    distribution A79–A80
    effect of age A80
    elimination A80
    factors affecting plasma concentration after injection *A80*
    metabolism A80
    in neonatal pain management A451
    protein binding A79
physiochemical properties and clinical profile **A79, A84–A85**
restrictions according to IOC medical code A500
structure A77, **A84–A85**
    subunits A77
sympathetic blockade P237
timing of treatment studies A116–A120, **A136–A143, A161–
    A162**
topical *see* topical local anesthesia
treatment (of)
    burn pain A363
    musculoskeletal nonarticular pain A396
    musculoskeletal trauma A355
    myofascial pain (MFP) Ch625
    neurologic disease Ch362
    phantom pain Ch434
    postoperative pain **A332,** A332–A334
    treatment combinations in perioperative period *A115*
Locke–Wallace Marital Adjustment Test Ch108
lofepramaine, TMJ pain management **Ch486**
loin pain, indication for radiotherapy Ca255
longitudinal myelotomy, painful spasticity management **Ch463**
longitudinal population studies, definition Ch18
    see also epidemiology of pain
long-lever adjustments, chiropractic theory Ch345
long-term depression (LTD) A29, *A30–A31*
long-term potentiation (LTP) A29, *A30–A31*
lopinavir, in AIDS pain management Ca371
lorazepam Ca325
low back pain A405–A422
    chronic, pain-related fear P164
        see also pain-related fear
    clinical findings A408–A409
    clinical presentation A407–A408, Ch524
    diagnosis Ch317
        criteria A406
        nerve blocks Ch132
        psychiatric Ch631
    disability assessment, case history Ch54–Ch60
    epidemiology A406–A407
        age-related factors Ch21
        cultural factors Ch20
    etiology and pathophysiology A405–A406, Ch317
    evaluation of investigations A409
    evidence-based medicine A416–A418
    examination framework **A98**
    gastroduodenal ulcer treatment A410
    guidelines A416–A418
        Cochrane Back Review Group **A415**
        New Zealand guide *A417,* A416–A418
    history A407–A408
    management A409–A414
        acupuncture Ch343
        chiropractic management Ch345
        complementary and alternative medicine A413, Ch348
        efficacy Ch317–Ch318
        evaluation A409–A410
        injection techniques A412–A413
        NSAIDs A410, Ch232
        physical therapy A411, Ch317–Ch318

psychological therapy A413–A414
surgery A411–A412
multiple sclerosis Ch358
nonspecific A406–A407
prevalence A406
prognosis A4154–A416
psychosocial predictors of outcome **A414**
return-to-work statistics A415–A416
radiofrequency lesioning indication P336
recurrence A414
red flags A407, **A407,** A416
specific syndromes **A407**
surgery A411–A412
yellow flags **A408,** A416–A417
see also back pain
lower limb pain Ch546–Ch547
asymmetric motor neuropathy, diabetic neuropathy Ch371–Ch372
diffuse, radiofrequency lesioning indication P338
epidemiology and diagnosis Ch546–Ch547
examination framework **A98**
management Ch547
epidural analgesia after surgery P415
peripheral nerve blocks P219–P230
see also individual types
low-level laser therapy (LLLT) P186
low-threshold (LT) neurons A7
response to distension *A6*
lumbar analgesia
in children P442–P443
epidural steroid injections P417–P418, P421
lumbar diskography Ch132
lumbar disk pain, radiofrequency lesioning Ca242
lumbar plexus block A269–A270, P219–P220
anatomical aspects P219
complications P220
indications P219
landmarks and practical steps P219–P220, *P220*
distal technique P220
paravertebral technique P220
psoas compartment technique P220
in musculoskeletal injuries A355
in pediatric surgery A448–A449
lumbar spine
dynamic stabilization Ch318
clinical studies Ch318
definition Ch318
goals Ch318
radiofrequency lesioning P336
lumbar sympathetic block *P241,* P241–P243
acute herpes zoster pain management Ch444
agents P243
complications P243
continuous P242
local anesthesia dose P242
neurolytic block P243
single needle injection P243
technique P241–P242, *P242,* P243
lumbar zygapophyseal (facet) joints
blocks P272
evidence for use of P274–P275
intra-articular blocks P272
medial branch blocks P272
needle positioning *P273*
positioning of C-arm *P273*
denervation with radiofrequency lesioning P336–P337
adverse effects P337
efficacy of treatment P337

indication P336
technique P336–P337, *P337*
dysfunction P190
pain P270
lumbosacral plexopathy Ca10
clinical features Ca10
etiology Ca10
malignant psoas syndrome Ca10
pain Ca10, Ca13
renal bed recurrence Ca10
lumbosacral plexus, peripheral branches blockade P221–P227
femoral branch *see* femoral nerve block
lateral cutaneous nerve of thigh *see* lateral cutaneous nerve, thigh blockade
obturator branch *see* obturator nerve block
posterior cutaneous nerve of thigh P227
sciatic branch *see* sciatic nerve block
lung cancer
hemoptysis Ca297
see also hemoptysis
nonsmall cell, bone metastasis chemotherapy Ca287
radiotherapy Ca255–Ca256
small cell, bone metastasis chemotherapy Ca287
lungs
local anesthesia passage A79
postoperative complications *see* pulmonary complications
Lyme disease, motor function Ch368
lymphangitis carcinomatosis, management Ca294–Ca295
lymph node biopsy, postsurgical pain syndromes Ch420

McGill Pain Questionnaire A361, Ca66, Ch65, Ch94, Ch104, Ch120, Ch147, Ch252, P18–P21, *P20–P21*
childbirth pain measurement A428
construct validity P21
in elderly Ca351
long form A101
predictive validity P19, P21
present pain intensity (PPI) ratings P19
short form A101–A102, A428, P21, *P22*
strengths P21
test–retest reliability P21
trigeminal neuralgia Ch492
weaknesses P21
McKenzie physiotherapy exercises, low back pain management A411
magnetic resonance imaging (MRI) Ch128
advantages Ch128
investigations/diagnosis into
chronic back pain Ch137–Ch138, Ch526
CRPS Ch390
neck pain Ch511
ovarian remnant syndrome Ch593
pelvic congestion Ch592
pelvic pain Ch599
TMJ pain Ch485
trigeminal neuralgia Ch491, Ch492
limitations Ch128
mechanism Ch128
neurosurgical techniques Ch298
sensitivity Ch128
validity Ch128
magnetic resonance tomographic angiography (MRTA), trigeminal neuralgia diagnosis Ch491, Ch492
maladaptive reorganization, central pain syndromes Ch406
malingering (false claims) Ch78, Ch97, Ch632–Ch633, P512
diagnosis Ch632
financial benefits Ch633
measurement **Ch75**

personal injury claims Ch183
malocclusion, TMJ pain Ch484
mammary artery pain syndrome, left internal, chronic chest
    pain Ch560
mandibular nerve block, acute herpes zoster pain Ch444
mandibular opening, fibromyalgia/myofascial pain
    management Ch624
manipulation P191
    of joints with anesthesia (MUJA) P192
    low back pain management A411
manual medicine P183, P189–P193
    complications P192
    imaging studies P191
    management P191–P192
        articular procedures P191
        high-velocity, low-amplitude thrust P191
        muscle energy technique P191
        myofascial release P192
        soft-tissue techniques P191
    manipulation of joints with anesthesia (MUJA) P192
    neck pain management Ch512–Ch514
    results P192
    structural diagnosis of syndromes P189–P191
        cervical zygapophyseal (facet) joint dysfunction P190
        lumbar zygapophyseal (facet) joint dysfunction P190
        sacroiliac joint dysfunction P190–P191
        thoracic zygapophyseal (facet) and rib dysfunction P190
        see also individual syndromes
manual therapy (MT) see manual medicine
manubriosternal pain, chronic chest pain Ch559
maprotiline
    neuropathic pain management Ch242
    pharmacology **Ch240**
Marañón's Myoclonus Assessment Scale (MMAS) **Ca174**
marijuana, restrictions according to IOC medical code A500
masking agents, prohibited substances in IOC medical code A501
massage A290, Ca276, P185
    chronic back pain management Ch532
    CRPS management Ch395
    in elderly Ca359
    fibromyalgia/myofascial pain management Ch624
    mechanisms of action Ca276
    physical effects Ca276
mastalgia, benign, topical NSAIDs Ch217
maternal anxiety, influence on childbirth pain A429–A430
maternal hypocarbia, response to childbirth pain A426
Maudsley Obsessional Compulsive Inventory (MOCI) Ch71
maxillary nerve block, acute herpes zoster pain Ch444
maxillary sinusitis **Ch482,** Ch485, Ch487–Ch488
    diagnosis Ch133–Ch134, Ch487, **Ch487**
    epidemiology Ch487
    etiology/pathophysiology Ch485
    examination Ch487
    investigations Ch487
    management Ch487–Ch488
    predisposing factors **Ch487**
    prognosis Ch488
mechanism-based approach Ch262–Ch263
medial column (spinalis) muscle Ch524
medial cutaneous nerve, forearm blockade P212
    landmarks and practical steps P212
medial epicondyle, intra-articular injections P265
medial epicondylitis, physical therapies Ch317
median nerve block
    at elbow P212
        landmarks and practical steps P212, *P212*
    at wrist P213
        landmarks and practical steps P213, *P214*

median nerve compression *see* carpal tunnel syndrome
medical exercise therapy (MET) P183
    shoulder rotator device *P183*
medical products agency (MPA)
    experimental protocol review P491
medical service provision, epidemiology Ch15
medical therapy, neck pain management Ch514
medicolegal aspects Ch27–Ch38, Ch173–Ch188, P509–P516
    adequate disclosure Ch176–Ch179
    clinical governance P512
        best practice P512
        clinical guidelines P512
        complaints procedure P512
    concerns to expert P510–P512
        competence or otherwise of clinician P511
        informed consent P511
        lack of consent P511–P512
        malingering (false claims) P512
        nature of incident or complication P511
        personal loss and suffering P510–P511
        standards of care P510
        suitability of treatment P511
    court action Ch36–Ch37
        physician-assisted suicide Ch36
        undermanagement of terminal illnesses Ch36
    euthanasia Ch176
    expert report *see* expert medicolegal report
    law of negligence Ch176–Ch177
    legal standing P512–P514
        Bolam P513
        Woolf recommendations P513–P514
    liability Ch175–Ch181
        Bolam v. Friern Hospital Management Committee Ch177
        Chappel v. Hart Ch178
        complications Ch177
        Ellis v. Wallsend District Hospital Ch177
        Reibl v. Hughes Ch178
        Rogers v. Whitaker Ch177
        Sidaway Case Ch177
    litigation
        context of complaints P510
        potential sources **P509**
        reasons for complaints P510
        types **P510**
    malingering *see* malingering (false claims)
    malpractice claims Ch179–Ch181
        butorpharol tartrate Ch179–Ch180
        class actions Ch180
        drug-specific liability issues Ch180–Ch181
        failure to provide adequate pain relief Ch180
        iatrogenic narcotic addiction Ch179–Ch180
        meperidine Ch181
        Regina v. Adams Ch180
        Smith v. Royal Melbourne Hospital Ch180
    material risk Ch178
    opioids *see* opioids, legal controls
    personal injury claims Ch181–Ch185
        clinical opinion Ch182–Ch183
        compensation effects Ch183
        disability determination Ch182
        fraudulent claims Ch183
        impairment ratings Ch183–Ch185
        learned pain behavior Ch182
        malingering Ch183
        medical terminology Ch183
        organic causes Ch182
        pain evaluation Ch182–Ch183, Ch184
        pain underestimation Ch183

postsurgical pain syndromes Ch421
    workers' compensation Ch181–Ch182
physician's duty Ch28–Ch29
substance abuse patients Ca401
undertreated pain Ch10–Ch11, Ch29–Ch30
valid consent to management Ch176–Ch179
    purpose Ch176
    written consent Ch179
see also disability evaluation (USA); expert medicolegal report
medroxyprogesterone acetate (MPA), pelvic congestion
    management Ch593
mefenamic acid A66, Ca195–Ca196
    adverse effects Ca195
    characteristics **Ch229**
    cyclo-oxygenase (COX) inhibitor Ca195–Ca196
    doses and treatment protocols Ca195
    evidence for efficacy Ca190
    indications and contraindications Ca186–Ca187, Ca195
    pharmacokinetics Ca195
    practical tips Ca196
megesterol acetate, anorexia–cachexia syndrome
    management Ca306
meloxicam A66, Ca198
    adverse effects Ca198, Ch230
    characteristics **Ch229**
    cyclo-oxygenase (COX) inhibitor Ca198
    doses and treatment protocols Ca198
    evidence for efficacy Ca198
    indications and contraindications Ca186–Ca187, Ca198
    pharmacokinetics **Ca194,** Ca198
memantine Ch263
    postherpetic neuralgia management Ch264
membrane stabilizers as adjuvant analgesics Ca134–Ca135
    see also individual drugs
Memorial Delirium Assessment Scale (MDAS) Ca64, Ca172
Memorial Pain Assessment Card Ca66
Memorial Symptom Assessment Scale 10-18 (MSAS 10-18) Ca333
memory problems Ch75, Ch101
meningeal carcinomatosis Ca8–Ca9
    MRI scan of cauda equina infiltration *Ca9*
    pain syndromes caused by **Ca4, Ca7**
    symptoms and signs Ca8–Ca9
        cerebral **Ca8**
        cranial nerve **Ca8**
        spinal **Ca8**
meningitis
    acute aseptic, in AIDS patients Ca377
    intrathecal catheterization adverse effect P302
menstrual pain, epidemiology, age-related factors Ch20–Ch21
mental nerve block P200
    landmarks and practical steps P200
meperidine A50, Ca55, Ca134, P67
    adverse effects A432, P67
    in children Ca340
        analgesia for children over 6 months P436
        starting dose **Ca339**
    epidural
        lipid solubility, doses, onset, and analgesia duration **A243**
        in PCEA **A247**
    malpractice claims Ch181
    pharmacokinetics P67
        in elderly A464
    suggested starting doses **A317**
    transmucosal delivery in PCA P403
    treatment (of)
        acute pain P69
        childbirth pain A431–A432
        procedural pain Ca325

mepivacaine A83, A86
    structure, physiochemical properties and clinical profile **A85**
meralgia paresthetica, management, capsaicin **Ch219**
mercury poisoning, peripheral neuropathies Ch372
Merkel's diverticulum Ch580
mesencephalic tractomy *see* mesencephalotomy
mesencephalotomy Ch303
    complications Ch303
    indications Ch303
    outcomes Ch303
    stereotactic, central pain syndromes management Ch411
    technique Ch303
meta-analysis P457, P498–P501
    in biofeedback P131, **P131**
    data analysis P498–P501
        confidence intervals P500–P501
        heterogeneity P500
        intervention effectiveness P500
        intervention safety P501
        L'Abbé plots P498–P499, *P499*
        number needed to harm (NNH) P501
        number needed to treat (NNT) P500
            see also number needed to treat (NNT)
        statistical significance P499–P500
    epidural steroid injections P424–P425
    quality control P498
        Oxford Quality Rating Scale **P498, P499**
    see also systematic reviews
metabolic neuropathies Ch370–Ch371
    see also diabetic neuropathies
metabotropic glutamate receptors (mGluR) **A25**
    activation A33
metacarpophalangeal joint, intra-articular injections P266–P267,
    P267
metastases
    bone *see* bone metastases
    brain Ca254
    central pain syndromes Ch403
    hepatic, radiotherapy Ca254–Ca255
    rib Ca5
    skull *see* skull base metastases
    vertebral *see* vertebral metastases
metatarsophalangeal joint of hallux
    intra-articular injections P261–P262
methadone A49, Ca53–Ca54, Ca133–Ca134, Ch206–Ch207, P67
    burn pain treatment A362
    in children **Ca339,** Ca340
        analgesia for patients over 6 months P436
    dose Ch207
    epidural, characteristics **A243**
    equianalgesic dose ratio P472
    half-life Ca162
    mechanism of action Ch207
    neuropathic pain treatment Ca134
    pharmacokinetics Ca53–Ca54, P67
    rotation Ca133
    selection as alternative to morphine Ca159, Ca162
    in substance abuse patients Ca399–Ca400
    toxicity Ch207
methotrexate, NSAIDs interaction A57
methotrimeprazine
    adjuvant analgesic in children Ca343–Ca344
    central pain syndrome management Ch409
N-methyl-D-aspartate receptors *see* NMDA receptors
methylphenidate
    adjuvant analgesic in children Ca342
    opioid-induced cognitive impairment management Ca171
methysergide, migraine prophylaxis Ch475

mexiletine Ca212, P108
    adverse effects Ca212, Ch256, P109
    central pain syndrome management Ch409
    clinical trials Ch256
    contraindications P108
    CRPS management Ch394
    dosing and treatment schedule P108, **P109**
    peripheral neuropathy management Ch377
    pharmacokinetics Ca212
    pretreatment safety measures **P109**
mianserin, pharmacology **Ch240**
Michigan Alcoholism Screening Test (MAST) Ch71
microcompression, trigeminal neuralgia management **Ch497**
microneurography P35
    CRPS diagnosis Ch390
microvascular decompression, trigeminal neuralgia
    management Ch493, **Ch497**
midazolam Ca325
    pharmacokinetics **A346**
midbrain tractotomy Ca264
    complications Ca264–Ca265
midline myelotomy Ch306–Ch307
    indications Ch306
    mechanism of action Ch306–Ch307
    outcomes Ch306
    radiofrequency techniques Ch307
migraine
    abdominal Ch582
    anticonvulsant clinical trials Ch253
    antidepressants indication P101
    antiepileptic indication P107
    associated symptoms Ch468, Ch638
    biofeedback P158
    in children *see under* children
    classification Ch467
    clinical features Ch468
    diagnosis Ch470
        recall bias Ch470
    epidemiology Ch467–Ch468
        age-of-onset Ch468
        gender difference Ch467
        prevalence Ch467–Ch468
    improvement rates from separate meta-analyses **P131**
    International Headache Society (IHS) classification Ch638
    management Ch471–Ch473, Ch638–Ch639
        acupuncture Ch343
        alternative/complementary therapy Ch346, Ch348
        analgesics Ch471, Ch638
        anticonvulsants Ch253
        antidepressants Ch243
        botanical therapy **Ch347**
        CBT Ch638–Ch639, **Ch639**
        ergotamine Ch471, Ch472–Ch473
        homeopathy Ch344
        NSAIDs Ch471
        sumatriptan *see* sumatriptan
        triptans *see* triptans
    nausea Ch468
    pain description Ch468
    pathophysiology Ch468–Ch469
        cortical spreading depression Ch469
        cranial vessel dilation Ch469
        genetics Ch468
        neurogenic inflammation Ch469
        precipitating factors Ch468, Ch638
        trigeminal system activation Ch469
        visual symptoms Ch468–Ch469
    in pregnancy A377

prophylactic management **Ch470,** Ch475
    adverse effects **Ch470,** Ch475
    β-blockers Ch475
    clinical efficacy **Ch470**
milk thistle, botanical therapy **Ch347**
Million Scale Ch65
milnacipran, pharmacology **Ch240**
mind–body Ca275–Ca276
    definition A286
mindfulness-based stress reduction P117
Mini-Mental State Exam (MMSE), delirium diagnosis Ca64, Ca172
minimum effective analgesic concentration (MEAC) A223
    opioids A206, **A206,** P66
Minnesota Multiphasic Personality Inventory (MMPI) Ch74, Ch95,
    Ch106, Ch149
    placebo response Ch281
misoprostol
    in elderly Ca356
    NSAIDs combination Ch231
mistletoe Ca273
Misuse of Drugs Act, opioid legal controls Ch175
mitempfindung, definition **Ch404**
mixed pain syndromes, spinal cord stimulation (SCS) Ch290–
    Ch293
mobilization P191
moclobemide, mechanism of action Ch240
modulation, pain signal A3
molars, surgical removal of impacted third molar P461, *P461*
    indications **P463**
    see also dental pain model
monoamine oxidase inhibitor antidepressants, mechanism of
    action Ch240
mood alterations, opioid-induced P62
mood disorders and pain P114
    see also anxiety; depression
morbidity, NSAIDs adverse effect Ch261
morphine A47, Ca53, Ca132–Ca133, P66
    adjuvant to local anesthetic for nerve blockade A271
    administration routes A47, Ca128, Ch441
        intra-articular A212–A213, A319, A333
        intrathecal A249
        rectal Ca128
        transdermal A212
    adverse effects Ca46
    aerosolized A212
    alternative epidural analgesia P415
    buccal A210–A211
    caudal analgesia A447
    in children A442–A443, Ca338–Ca339
        administration A443
        adverse effects and toxicity A443
        analgesia for patients 6 months or younger P439, **P439**
        analgesia for patients over 6 months P435
        intravenous administration protocols **P437**
        monitoring for patients on systemic infusions P437
        pharmacology and indications A442–A443
        protocol for ketamine combined infusions **P438**
        starting dose Ca338, **Ca339**
    chronic pain analgesia **Ca160–Ca161**
    clinical trial Ch205
    controlled-release preparations Ca53, Ca133
        dosages Ca133
    in elderly Ca356–Ca357
    epidural *see* epidural morphine
    evidence for selection of alternative Ca159, Ca162
    immediate-release preparations Ca132–Ca133
    intraspinal, in refractory cancer pain Ca148
    intrathecal *see* intrathecal morphine

intravenous
    administration protocols in children **P437**
    doses and paradigms P45
  metabolites A47, Ca53
  Minnesota Multiphasic Personality Inventory (MMPI)
    acute just postamputation pain Ch427
    chronic back pain Ch527
  neonatal sensitivity to A343
  oral A210, Ca53
    clinical trial Ch204
    potency **A211**
  pain management in ICU A343
  parenteral formulations Ca53
  patient-controlled analgesia (PCA)
    abdominal pain management A374
    dose A222
    ketorolac addition in cardiac pain management A167
  pharmacodynamics A45
  pharmacokinetics **A346,** Ca53, P66
    in elderly A464
  pharmacological effects P62–P63
    skin P63
  political and social acceptance Ca123, Ca144
  postoperative analgesia RCTs P488
  preparations P66
  rescue medication Ca133
  starting doses Ca132
  suggested starting doses **A317**
  suppositories A211
  synthetic derivatives P66–P67
    see also diamorphine; hydromorphone; oxymorphone
  treatment (of)
    acute pain P69
    breakthrough pain Ca133
    breathlessness Ca295
    burn pain A362
    refractory cancer pain Ca152
  use in early postoperative period A334
morphine sulfate, intraventricular infusion Ch301
mortality, NSAIDs adverse effects Ch261
motor blockade A192
  Bromage scale **A192**
motor cortex stimulation Ch294
motor nerve block, definition Ch463
motor neuron disease (MND) pain Ca403
motor point block, definition Ch463
movement disorders Ch358–Ch359
  neuropathic pain Ch358
  pain Ch358
  related terms Ch358–Ch359
MS-Contin™ Ca133
mucositis **Ca14,** Ca15
  oral problem Ca298
multiaxial assessment of pain (MAP) Ch97–Ch98
Multidimensional Pain Inventory (MPI) Ch75, Ch98, Ch103–Ch104, Ch107, Ch149
multidisciplinary pain management, pelvic pain management Ch603
multifidi muscle dysfunction, deconditioning Ch314
multimodal anesthesia
  postoperative pain management A322–A323
    treatment options **A323**
  timing of treatment studies A125, **A161–A162**
multiparous parturients, childbirth pain A424
multiple analgesic A333–A334
multiple myeloma, bone metastasis chemotherapy Ca288
multiple organ failure patients *see under* intensive care unit (ICU)
multiple sclerosis A372, Ch356–Ch358

  anticonvulsant clinical trials Ch253
  central pain syndrome Ch406, Ch408
  clinical features Ch356
  epidemiology Ch356–Ch357
  management A372
    capsaicin **Ch219**
  nature of disease Ch356
  pain classification **Ch357**
  pain presentation patterns Ca403, Ch357–Ch358
    miscellaneous Ch358
    neuropathic pain Ch358
    nociceptive musculoskeletal pain Ch357–Ch358
    pains of primary neurogenic origin Ch357
Münchausen syndrome Ch632
muscle(s)
  energy technique P191
  examination for expert medicolegal report P515
  health in fibromyalgia/myofascial pain Ch620
  pain P29
    experimental methods and models P29
    see also musculoskeletal injuries/pain
  physiological changes with age A466
  recruitment patterns, deconditioning Ch314–Ch315
  reflex contractions A285
  relaxation techniques A288
    agents *see* muscle relaxants
    breathing techniques A288
    in children P150
    mechanisms of action A288
    progressive *see* progressive muscle relaxation (PMR)
  response to cryotherapy A492–A493
  response to injury A490
  scanning, biofeedback psychophysiological assessment P123
  spasticity in multiple sclerosis Ch357–Ch358
  therapy, fibromyalgia/myofascial pain management Ch623–Ch624, Ch624–Ch625
muscle discrimination training
  biofeedback psychophysiological assessment P123–P124
  progressive muscle relaxation training addition P129
muscle fibers
  type I
    characteristics Ch620–Ch621, **Ch621**
    injury, fibromyalgia Ch620–Ch621
  type II, characteristics Ch621, **Ch621**
muscle relaxants
  as adjuvant analgesics Ca219–Ca221
    adverse effects Ca220–Ca221
    contraindications Ca220
    doses and treatment paradigms Ca220
    evidence for efficacy Ca221
    indications Ca220
    practical tips Ca221
    see also individual drugs
  low back pain management A410
muscle therapy
  fibromyalgia management Ch624–Ch625
  myofascial pain (MFP) management Ch623–Ch624
musculoskeletal injuries/pain A393–A404
  back pain in pregnancy A376–A377
  in children Ch640–Ch641
  cingulotomy Ca265
  clinical assessment A395
    presentation and evaluation A395
  diagnostic tests A395–A396
    articular pain A395–A396
    nonarticular pain A396
  epidemiology, age-related Ch21
  functional taxonomy A394

management A355–A356
    ketamine use A351
    local anesthetic techniques A355
    nonarticular syndromes A399–A403
    NSAIDs A355–A356, Ch228, Ch232
    pharmacological methods A355–A356
    physiotherapy P181
nociceptive, multiple sclerosis Ch357–Ch358
outcome measures Ch146
pathophysiology A394
presenting symptoms Ch537
TENS indication P344
    experimental evidence P351
trauma A355–A356
    pediatric A356
    see also trauma
music therapy A290, Ca275
    advantages and disadvantages A293
    postoperative pain management A291
myelography Ch128–Ch129
    mechanism Ch128
Myobloc (BTX-B) P277
    dosing guidelines for spasticity treatment **P281**
    preparation P278, **P279**
myocardial infarction, intraspinal opioid reduction in
    postoperative risk A252
myocardial revascularization, refractory angina pectoris
    management Ch557
myoclonus
    CRPS Ch385
    opioid-induced Ca46, Ca173–Ca174
        clinical presentation and findings Ca173
        definition Ca173
        diagnostic criteria Ca173
        epidemiology Ca173
        etiology and pathophysiology Ca173
        evidence-based evaluation of management Ca174
        notes on unevaluated treatments Ca174
myofascial pain (MFP)
    affected muscles Ch615
    contributing factors Ch620
        muscle health Ch620
        posture Ch620
        psychologic symptoms Ch620
        tension-producing habits Ch620
    diagnosis Ch615–Ch616, **Ch616**
        accompanying signs Ch616
        associated disorders Ch616
        electromyographic studies Ch616
    etiology/pathophysiology Ch620–Ch623
        central nociceptive input modification Ch622–Ch623
        motor endplate Ch621–Ch622
        muscle fiber type I injury Ch620–Ch621
        muscle nociceptor activation Ch622
        pain transmission Ch622
    fibromyalgia comparison **Ch620**
    frequency Ch615
    immune system abnormalities Ch623
    jump sign Ch618–Ch619
    management Ch623–Ch627
        benzodiazepine Ch625
        cardiovascular fitness Ch624
        CBT Ch626
        contributing factor control Ch625–Ch626
        holistic approach Ch623, **Ch623**
        local anesthesia Ch625
        long-term pain control Ch623
        mandibular opening Ch624

        massage Ch624
        muscle evaluation Ch624
        muscle therapy Ch623–Ch624, Ch624–Ch625
        NSAIDs Ch625
        pain clinic teams Ch626–Ch627
        pharmacotherapy Ch625
        physical conditioning Ch624
        postural corrections Ch625–Ch626
        postural exercises Ch624
        spray and stretch techniques Ch624–Ch625
        tricyclic antidepressants (TCAs) Ch625
    muscle pain disorder relationship Ch619
    pain description Ch619
    pain history/examination Ch65, Ch68
    pelvic pain Ch596–Ch597
        management Ch597
        pathophysiology Ch596–Ch597
        symptoms/signs Ch597
    TENS indication P344
        experimental evidence P351
    trigger points (TrPs) Ch618
        definition Ch615
        positions *Ch617*
    zone of reference, definition Ch615
    see also fibromyalgia
myofascial release P192
myopathy, corticosteroid induced Ca218
myositis, in AIDS patients Ca385

nabumetone A66, Ca196
    adverse effects Ca196
    characteristics **Ch229**
    cyclo-oxygenase (COX) inhibitor Ca196
    doses and treatment protocols Ca196
    evidence for efficacy Ca196
    indications and contraindications Ca186–Ca187
    pharmacokinetics Ca196
nalbuphine Ca55–Ca56, P68
    pharmacokinetics Ca56
    treatment of intraspinal opioid adverse effects A258
nalmefene Ca56
    antiemetic agent A233
naloxone Ca56, P68
    central pain syndromes management Ch409
    clinical trials Ch241
    opioid-induced pruritus management A252–A253
    opioid-induced respiratory depression management Ca47,
        Ca56
    opioid-induced urinary retention management A253
    pharmacokinetics P68
    treatment of intraspinal opioid adverse effects A257, A258
naltrexone Ca56, P68
naproxen A65, Ca196–Ca197
    adverse effects Ca187–Ca190
    characteristics **Ch229**
    clinical trials Ch204, Ch233
    contraindications Ca187
    cyclo-oxygenase (COX) inhibitor Ca196–Ca197
    doses and treatment protocols Ca196
    in elderly Ca356
    evidence for efficacy Ca196–Ca197
    indications Ca186–Ca187, Ca196
    osteoarthritis management Ch233
    pharmacokinetics Ca196
    practical tips Ca196
naratriptan, migraine management Ch471
    efficacy in RCT Ch471
    therapeutic use Ch473

narcosis, opioid induced P90
narcotic prohibitions in IOC medical code A499
    examples A501
nasal administration of drugs
    opioids
        acute pain management P70
        cancer pain management P71
        patient-controlled analgesia transmucosal route P401
nasogastric administration of opioids Ca50
National Advisory Committees (NAC), CPRP Ch168
National Health Service (NHS) Trusts, pain clinics (UK) Ch156
natural medicine, definition Ch338–Ch339
    see also complementary and alternative medicine
nausea Ca299–Ca301
    clinical findings Ca299
    etiology **Ca300**
    hypercalcemia Ca300–Ca301
    management Ca299–Ca300, *Ca300*
        acupuncture Ca272
        antiemetics A257
            see also antiemetics
        drug classification **Ca302**
        hypnosis Ca275
        opioids Ch206
    migraine Ch468
    opioid-induced A253–A254, A472, Ca47, Ca132, Ca176,
        Ch206, P62, P437
        epidemiology Ca176
        epidural infusion P313
        etiology and pathophysiology Ca176
        evidence-based evaluation of management Ca176
    PCA induced A233
        management P398
    systemic analgesia complication in children A450
    TENS reduction in postoperative expulsions P350–P351
nebulized drugs, breathlessness management Ca296
neck carcinoma, trigeminal tractotomy Ch300–Ch301
neck fractures Ch508
    due to whiplash Ch508–Ch509
neck pain Ch505–Ch519
    anterior Ch505
    clinical assessment **Ch509,** Ch509–Ch510
        red flag diagnosis **Ch509,** Ch509–Ch510
    definition Ch505
    diagnosis Ch135–Ch137
        algorithm Ch136–Ch137, *Ch137*
        nerve blocks Ch136–Ch137
        pain maps Ch135–Ch137, *Ch138*
        radiographs Ch136
    epidemiology Ch507
    etiology Ch135–Ch136, Ch507–Ch508, **Ch508**
        cervical zygapophysial joint damage Ch136
        ligament damage Ch135–Ch136
        synovial joint damage Ch136
    invasive techniques Ch511–Ch512
        disk stimulation Ch511–Ch512
        zygapophysial joint blocks Ch512
    investigations Ch510–Ch511
        CT Ch511
        MRI Ch511
        plain radiography Ch510–Ch511
        single-photon emission computed tomography
            (SPECT) Ch511
    management Ch512–Ch515
        after whiplash Ch513–Ch514
        chiropractic management Ch345
        medical therapy Ch514
        physical and manual therapy Ch512–Ch514

        recommendations Ch514–Ch515
        surgical therapy Ch514
        whiplash independent Ch512–Ch513
    natural history Ch507
    patterns Ch506
    physical examination Ch510
    posterior Ch505
    referred pain Ch505–Ch506, *Ch506*
    risk factors Ch507
neck peripheral nerve blocks P200–P203
    see also individual types
needle phobia P149
needle shock P357–P358
nefasodone, postherpetic neuralgia management Ch453
nelfinavir, in AIDS pain management Ca370
nefopam Ca35
    adverse effects Ca35
    dose recommendations Ca35
    pharmacokinetics Ca35
    presentations Ca35
Neonatal Facial Coding System (NFCS) A105
neonatal pain management A450–A451
    acetaminophen A450–A451
        dosage, administration, and indications A451
        pharmacokinetics and metabolism A451
    agents and guideline doses for analgesia in ICU **A343**
    assessment A104–A105
    local anesthesia A451
        pharmacokinetics A451
        toxicity A451
    opioids A450
        pharmacokinetics A450
        respiratory depression A450
    see also children
neostigmine A333
    intra-articular administration A333
nephrotoxicity
    acetaminophen-induced Ca34
    NSAID induced A442, Ca37
nerve blocks, therapeutic see peripheral nerve blocks;
    sympathetic blocks; *specific nerve blocks*
nerve blocks in pain diagnosis Ch131–Ch132, P49–P56
    difficulties with use P49
    epidural see epidural nerve blocks, diagnostic
    false placebos Ch275
    historical aspects P49
    mechanism Ch131
    neck pain diagnosis Ch136–Ch137
    neuropathic pain diagnosis Ch131–Ch132
    patient selection and preparation P50–P51
    procedural guidelines P51, **P51**
        block validation P51
        imaging assistance P51
    prognostic interpretation P55
    response assessments and outcome monitoring P51
        pain scores P51
        physiological measures P51
    response interpretation P54–P55
        common misconceptions **P54**
        "straight line" concept of pain P54
    response patterns P52–P54
        aberrant solution spread P53–P54
        abnormal conduction pathways P54
        "bag of tricks" *P52*
        desired block if successful P52–P53
        neuronal desensitization P54
        operator variability P54
        patient misrepresentation P54

placebo responses P53
procedural failure P54
systemic actions of lidocaine P53
scope P50, **P50**
sites **P50**
zygapophysial joints Ch132
nerve conduction studies (NCS) Ch130
carpal tunnel syndrome diagnosis Ch130
diabetic neuropathy diagnosis Ch130
false-positive rate Ch130, **Ch131**
mechanism Ch130
peripheral neuropathy diagnosis Ch369
postsurgical pain syndromes diagnosis Ch422
sensitivity Ch130, **Ch131**
specificity Ch130, **Ch131**
nerve entrapment
pelvic pain Ch597
management Ch597
pathophysiology Ch597
symptoms/signs Ch597
postsurgical pain syndromes diagnosis Ch422
nerve fibers
action potential transmissions A74
herpes zoster infection Ch437
large myelinated *see* large myelinated (Aβ) fibres
local anesthesia penetration in base form into axon **A78**
susceptibility to local anesthetics A76, **A76**
nerve growth factor (NGF) Ch266
inflammatory hyperalgesia induction A21–A22, *A23*
mechanism of action Ch266
nerve injury
classification Ch418
axonotmesis Ch418
neurapraxia Ch418
neurotmesis Ch418
CRPS Ch386
nerve pain
indications for radiotherapy Ca255–Ca256
pelvic pain Ca255
upper limb pain Ca255–Ca256
management
antidepressant **Ch243**
lidocaine, intravenous Ch256
nerve root injections, chronic back pain management Ch530
nerve root pain Ch523, Ch524
causes Ch523
nervus intermedius neuralgia Ch500
neural administration of drugs A207
nonsteroidal anti-inflammatory drugs A210
opioids A213
neuralgia
definition **Ch404**
postherpetic *see* postherpetic neuralgia (PHN)
pretrigeminal **Ch482, Ch499**
trigeminal, opioid management Ch205
neuralgic amyotrophy, brachial plexus neuropathies Ch374
neurapraxia Ch418
neurectomy
painful spasticity management **Ch463**
trigeminal neuralgia management **Ch496**
neuritis, postprocedural complication of zygapophyseal
blocks P274
neuroaugmentative techniques Ch285–Ch296
developments Ch285
historical perspective Ch285
mechanism of action Ch285
see also individual stimulation techniques
neuroaxial blockade A324

childbirth pain treatment A431
Neurobloc (BTX-B) P277
dosing guidelines for spasticity treatment **P281**
preparation P278, **P279**
neurochemical production, acupuncture Ch342–Ch343
neuroendocrine system, opioids' pharmacological effects P62
neurogenic inflammation, migraine pathophysiology Ch469
neurogenic pain
definition **Ch404**
spinal cord stimulation Ch289–Ch290
TENS Ca246
neurography P34
neurokinin 1 (NK1) antagonists Ch266–Ch267
diabetic neuropathy management Ch267
osteoarthritis management Ch267
see also substance P
neurokinin receptors **A25**
neuroleptics
acute herpes zoster pain management Ch440
adjuvant analgesic in children Ca343–Ca344
neurologic disease management Ch361
neurological disease/disorders A369–A373, Ch355–Ch365
alcoholic neuropathy A372
in children Ca403
classification **Ch356**
epidural catheter placement complication A174
Guillain–Barré syndrome *see* Guillain–Barré syndrome
herpes zoster *see* herpes zoster
HIV-associated neuropathy *see* HIV-associated neuropathy
management Ch360–Ch364, *Ch363*
general considerations Ch360
invasive management Ch362
pharmacological Ch360–Ch361
physical therapies Ch362
psychological management Ch364
surgery Ch363–Ch364
TENS Ch362
see also individual drugs
multiple sclerosis *see* multiple sclerosis
nutritional neuropathies A372
pain management in ICU A345
neurological examination, for expert medicolegal report P515
neurological status, relationship to cancer pain Ca29
neurological transmission, childbirth pain A426
neurolytic blocks Ca235–Ca244, P198–P199, P247–P254
chemical agents **Ca235,** Ca235–Ca241, **Ca238,** P198
alcohol *see* alcohol
ammonium compounds Ca237–Ca238
clinical applications Ca238–Ca241
see also individual nerve blocks
glycerol Ca237
history **Ca236**
hypertonic and hypotonic solutions Ca238
phenol Ca237, **Ca238,** P198
complications P237
epidural blockade Ca240
of lumbar sympathetic ganglia P243
pathophysiology Ca236, **Ca237**
physical agents **Ca235,** Ca241–Ca243
cryoanalgesia Ca241
hyperthermia Ca241
hypothermia Ca241
lasers Ca242
radiofrequency lesioning Ca242
see also radiofrequency lesioning
selective Ca236
of stellate ganglion P240
surgical sectioning comparison **Ca236**

techniques P198–P199
    cryoanalgesia P198–P199
    pulsed radiofrequency P199
treatment (of)
    central pain syndromes Ch410
    interstitial cystitis Ch576
    neurologic disease Ch362–Ch363
verification of blocking solution P237
see also peripheral nerve blocks; *individual types*
neurolytic celiac plexus block (NCPB), pancreatic cancer
    management Ch571, Ch574
neuroma, cause of residual limb pain Ch428
neuronal modulation, pelvic pain Ch588–Ch589
neurons, classification **A4**
    see also individual types
neuropathic pain Ca65, Ca259, Ca260–Ca261, Ch76, Ch113–
    Ch122, Ch355, P29–P30
    aftersensations Ch116–Ch117, **Ch121**
    in AIDS patients Ca374–Ca376, **Ca376**
        treatment Ca375–Ca376
    allodynia *see* allodynia
    animal models *see* animal models
    antidepressants indication P101
    applied physiology *see* animal models
    assessment *see* neuropathic pain assessment
    central origin
        anticonvulsant clinical trials Ch252
        diagnosis, epidural blocks Ch132
        management difficulties Ch261
    characteristics **P30**
    children Ch641–Ch642
    classification Ch113–Ch114
        by mechanism Ch114, **Ch114**
        by symptoms Ch114, Ch117
    clinical features **A97, A314**
    definition Ch113, **Ch404**
    diagnosis P27, P30
        see also neuropathic pain assessment
    dysesthesiae *see* dysesthesiae
    evoked Ch114–Ch115
    heterogeneity Ch113
    hyperalgesia *see* hyperalgesia
    hyperkinetic disorders Ch360
    hyperpathia *see* hyperpathia
    intravenous lidocaine indication P40
    lesion sites Ch113
    management **A314,** Ch120
        algorithm *Ch80–Ch81*
        amitriptyline Ch242, Ch376–Ch377
        anticonvulsants Ch253, **Ch254**
        antidepressants Ca215–Ca216, Ch242–Ch243
        carbamazepine Ca215
        clinical trials Ch252–Ch253
        clomipramine Ch242
        clonidine Ca210, Ch222
        desipramine Ch242
        dextromethorphan Ch264
        imipramine Ch242
        ketamine Ch264
        lidocaine, intravenous Ch256
        maprotiline Ch242
        methadone Ca134
        neurosurgical techniques Ch297
        nortriptyline Ch242
        NSAIDs Ch233
        opioids Ca262, Ch205
        selective serotonin reuptake inhibitors (SSRIs) Ch242–
            Ch243

surgery Ca261
        topical capsaicin Ch119
        topical NSAIDs Ch217–Ch218
        tricyclic antidepressants (TCAs) Ch242–Ch243
    movement disorders Ch358
    multiple sclerosis Ch358
    nervous system changes Ch113
    ongoing Ch114–Ch115
    opioids Ca262, Ch205
        responsiveness Ca158
        treatment protocols for chronic pain P77
    pain radiation Ch116
    paresthesiae *see* paresthesiae
    Parkinson's disease Ch359
    paroxysms Ch116
    peripheral origin, management
        adenosine receptor antagonists Ch265
        clinical trials Ch252
        difficulties Ch261
    postoperative *see* postoperative neuropathic pain, chronic
    in postoperative period A314
    referred pain *see* referred pain
    refractory cancer pain *see under* refractory cancer pain
    in refractory cancer pain *see under* refractory cancer pain
    sensory abnormalities P27, P30, **P30**
    sensory deficit Ch115
    stimulus dependent **Ch114,** Ch115
    stimulus independent Ch114, **Ch114**
    sympathetic **Ch121**
    syndromes in malignancy **Ca260**
    tactile sensibility reduction P31
    TENS indication P344
        experimental evidence P351
    transient postsympathectomy, lumbar sympathetic block
        complication P243
    types **Ca124,** P29–P30
    underdiagnosis and undertreatment A198–A199
    windup-like pain Ch116–Ch117, **Ch121**
    see also neuropathic pain, central origin; neuropathic pain,
        peripheral origin
neuropathic pain assessment **Ch75,** Ch104, Ch117–Ch122
    chemical stimuli Ch119, **Ch121**
    clinical examination Ch117–Ch118
        classification Ch117–Ch118
        cold/warm sensations Ch117
        pinprick sensations Ch117
        sensory modalities Ch117
        vibration Ch117
    clinical pain measures Ch120
        differentiation Ch120
        evoked pain Ch120
        ongoing pain Ch120
    diagnostic nerve blocks Ch131–Ch132
    history Ch117
        patient pain descriptors Ch117
    laboratory/experimental examination Ch118–Ch119
        equipment *Ch118*
    mechanical stimuli Ch118
        von Frey hairs Ch118, *Ch118*
    mechanism link Ch122
    outcome measures Ch119–Ch121
        functional improvement Ch119, Ch120
        quality of life Ch119, Ch120
    pain map Ch117
    paradoxical sensitivity Ch119
    spatial/temporal changes Ch119
    stimulus/response measures **Ch119**
    sympathetic activity assessment Ch119

diagnostic nerve blocks Ch119
sweating Ch119
thermal stimuli Ch118
Neuropathic Pain Scale Ch76
neuropathies
autoimmune Ch373
Churg–Strauss syndrome Ch373
Guillain–Barré syndrome Ch373
Wegener's granulomatosis Ch373
brachial plexus see brachial plexus neuropathies
definition **Ch404**
hereditary Ch373
Fabry's disease Ch373
nutritional A373
peripheral see neuropathies, peripheral
polyneuropathies Ch367–Ch368
acute inflammatory Ch358
antiepileptic indication P105
toxic Ch372–Ch373
alcohol Ch372
antiretroviral drugs Ch372–Ch373
arsenical polyneuropathy Ch372
cisplatin Ch372
cytostatic drugs Ch372
didanosine Ch372
mercury poisoning Ch372
stavudine Ch373
taxols Ch372
thallium poisoning Ch372
vinca alkaloids Ch372
zalcitabine Ch372–Ch373
neuropathies, peripheral Ca10, **Ca14,** Ch367–Ch381
clinical descriptions Ch367–Ch368
motor function Ch368
polyneuropathies Ch367–Ch368
sensory loss Ch368
tendon reflexes Ch368
complex regional pain syndrome see complex regional pain
syndromes (CRPSs)
deficiency states Ch371–Ch372
niacin Ch372
vitamin B$_1$ (thiamine) Ch371–Ch372
vitamin B$_6$ (pyridoxine) Ch372
diagnosis Ch133, Ch367
etiological classification Ch369–Ch370, **Ch369–Ch370**
biopsies Ch370
blood tests Ch370
cerebrospinal fluid examination Ch370
electromyography (EMG) Ch369
nerve conduction studies (NCS) Ch369
quantitative sensory and autonomic testing (QST) Ch370
management Ch375–Ch378, **Ch376**
acupuncture Ch378
antiarrhythmics Ch377
anticonvulsants Ch377
antidepressants Ch376–Ch377
capsaicin Ch377
opioids Ch377
specific therapy Ch375–Ch376
spinal cord stimulation Ch378
symptomatic therapy Ch376–Ch378
TENS Ch377–Ch378
tramadol Ch377
mechanisms Ch368–Ch369
ectopic discharges Ch368–Ch369
potassium channels Ch369
sodium channels Ch368–Ch369
nerve invasion Ca10

painless
congenital insensitivity to pain Ch375
hereditary sensory and autonomic neuropathy
(HSAN) Ch375
leprosy Ch375
Tangier syndrome Ch375
positive symptoms Ch368
allodynia Ch368
dysesthesiae Ch368
hyperalgesia Ch368
paresthesiae Ch368
types Ch370–Ch375
autoimmune see neuropathies, autoimmune
brachial plexus see brachial plexus neuropathies
cranial Ch371
hereditary see neuropathies, hereditary
HIV-associated neuropathy see HIV-associated neuropathy
hypothyroid Ch371
idiopathic Ch375
metabolic Ch370–Ch371
see also diabetic neuropathies
paraneoplastic Ch374–Ch375
postherpetic neuralgia see postherpetic neuralgia (PHN)
toxins see neuropathies, toxic
see also neuropathic pain, peripheral origin
neuropeptides, role in nociceptive signaling in dorsal horn A8–
A9
neurophysiological techniques P27–P38
conventional P34–P35
neurography P34
sensory-evoked potentials P34–P35
microneurography P35
see also sensory testing
neurosurgical modalities/techniques Ca259–Ca267, **Ca263,**
Ch297–Ch308
ablative procedures Ca262, **Ca262,** Ca263–Ca266, Ch297
bilateral, midline and pelvic–perineal pain Ca264
central pain syndrome management see under central pain
syndromes
CT-guided ablations Ca265
pain above C5 Ca264–Ca265
unilateral lower extremity and torso pain Ca263–Ca264
anterior commisure–posterior commissure (AC–PC) Ch297–
Ch298
augmentative procedures Ca262, Ch297
cingulotomy see cingulotomy
clinical assessment Ca260–Ca261
contrast ventriculography Ch297
CT Ch297, Ch298
hypophysectomy see hypophysectomy
hypothalmotomy see hypothalamotomy
intracranial procedures Ch298–Ch304
advantage Ch297
combined Ch304
intraventricular infusion see intraventricular infusion
mesencephalotomy see mesencephalotomy
MRI Ch298
noninvasive Ch298
opioid therapy Ca262
pain recurrence Ch297, Ch298
patients suited for surgery Ca261
pulvinotomy see pulvinotomy
radiosurgery Ch298
ablative sites Ch297
spinal procedures Ch304–Ch307
see also cordotomy; midline myelotomy
stereotaxis Ch298
surgical approaches **Ca262,** Ca262–Ca263

thalamotomy *see* thalamotomy
timing and communication Ca261
treatment (of)
  neuropathic pain Ch297
  nociceptive pain Ch297
treatment failure Ca261
trigeminal tractotomy *see* trigeminal tractotomy
neurotmesis Ch418
neurotomy, central pain syndromes management Ch410
neurotoxicity
  intraspinal opioid induced A250–A251
  local anesthesia complication A81
neurotransmitters
  animal model results Ch192
  CRPS pathogenesis Ch387
  fibromyalgia/myofascial pain Ch622
  release, hypophysectomy Ch300
neurotransmitter systems
  in central sensitization A32–A34
  in dorsal horn A7–A9, **A8**
neurotrophins **A22**
niacin deficiency, peripheral neuropathies Ch372
nifedipine Ca224–Ca225
  adverse effects Ca224
  contraindications Ca224
  doses and treatment paradigms Ca224
  efficacy Ca225
  indications Ca224
  pharmacokinetics Ca224
nimesulide A67, Ca198–Ca199
  adverse effects Ca199
  characteristics **Ch229**
  contraindications Ca199
  cyclo-oxygenase (COX) inhibitor Ca198–Ca199
  dose and treatment protocols Ca199
  evidence for efficacy Ca199
  indications Ca186–Ca187, Ca198–Ca199
  pharmacokinetics **Ca194,** Ca199
  practical tips Ca199
nimodipine Ca224–Ca225
  adverse effects Ca224
  contraindications Ca224
  doses and treatment paradigms Ca224
  efficacy Ca225
  indications Ca224
  pharmacokinetics Ca224
nitric oxide
  in inflammatory pain A24
  modulation of nociceptive messages A12–A13
nitric oxide synthase, animal model results Ch192
nitroglycerin Ca220
  doses and pharmacokinetics Ca220
nitrous oxide
  in cryoanalgesia P321
  inhalation in children P433–P434
  procedural pain management in children A452
nitrous oxide (Entonox) A350
  advantages and disadvantages Ca326
  burn pain treatment A362
  childbirth pain treatment A432
  procedural pain management Ca326
  provision in trauma **A350**
NMDA receptors **A25**
  activation in pain Ca146
  antagonists Ca221–Ca222, Ch263–Ch264
    administration timing studies A121–A123, **A148–A151**
    adverse effects Ca222
    antidepressants Ch240, Ch242

central sensitization attenuation Ca221
contraindications Ca221
development Ch194
doses and treatment paradigms Ca222
evidence for efficacy Ca222
human clinical studies Ch263–Ch264
human experimental studies Ch263
indications Ca221
limiting factors Ch263
neurologic disease management Ch361
pharmacokinetics Ca222
practical tips Ca222
windup Ca221
central pain involvement Ch263, Ch405
excitatory postsynaptic potentials A8, *A32*
structure Ch405
N-methyl-ᴅ-aspartate receptors *see* NMDA receptors
nociceptin A44
nociception A3–A16
  applied physiology A3–A16
  in brain A9–A11
    functional roles of cortical areas **A11**
    pain processing relation to circuitry A10–A11
  development in children A437–A438
    peripheral and central mechanisms A438
    sensory processing differences in adults A438
  modulation of nociceptive messages A11–A13
    in dorsal horn *A13,* A13–A14, Ca146
    "pain pathway" A11
    segmental (spinal) control A11–A13, *A12*
  peripheral aspects A3–A5
  somatic versus visceral A5, **A6**
  in spinal cord A5–A9
    anatomical aspects A6–A7, *A7*
    neurotransmitters in dorsal horn A7–A9, **A8**
    referred pain mechanisms A9, *A10*
    terminations of neurons in dorsal horn A6, *A7*
  spinal cord to brain A9
    ascending pathways A9
  transmission A3
nociceptive feedback control, central pain syndromes Ch405
nociceptive pain Ca65, Ca260, Ch90, Ch355, P29
  anticonvulsant clinical trials Ch253
  in cervical area, radiofrequency lesioning indication P334
  diagnosis, epidural blocks Ch132
  hyperkinetic disorders Ch360
  management Ca260
    antidepressants Ch243
    neurosurgical techniques Ch297
    opioids for chronic pain P77
    TENS Ca246
  movement disorders Ch358
  nociceptor sensitization P28, P29
  subtypes Ca65, **Ca124**
  see also somatic pain; visceral pain
nociceptive-specific cells (NS) A7
nociceptors A3, **A5,** A360
  activation in pain P27
  classification A3–A5, *A4*
  C polymodal A4–A5
  neuropeptide synthesis A33
  postsynaptic inhibition A35
  presynaptic inhibition A34–A35
  receptors A21–A26
  role in burn pain A360
  role in childbirth pain A426
  sensitization A18–A29, P28, P29
    increased intracellular calcium concentration A26

morphological changes A19
neurochemical changes A18–A19
physiological changes A18, *A18*
transducers' role A19, A21
see also peripheral sensitization
silent P27–P28
stimuli A4–A5, **A5**
nonacetylated salicylates A64
noninflammatory joint pain
general considerations A397–A398
management A397–A399
nonmalignant advanced diseases Ca403–Ca404
controversy concerning opioid use Ca404–Ca405, **Ca405**
management guidelines Ca405
pain Ca403–Ca407
nonmalignant pain
chronic *see* chronic pain
epidural treatment of refractory pain P308–P310
indications **P309**
treatment protocols for opioids *see* opioids, in chronic
nonmalignant pain
non-neoplastic pain, treatment indications for opioids in chronic
pain P78
non-neuroaxial blockade
childbirth pain treatment A431–A432
non-nucleoside reverse transcriptase inhibitors, AIDS pain
treatment Ca368–Ca369
non-nutritive sucking (NNS), infant pain management A295
evidence supporting effectiveness A296–A297
nonopioid analgesia Ca33–Ca40, Ca129–Ca130, Ca183–Ca207,
Ca208
adverse effects Ch441
in analgesic ladder Ca126, Ca129
ceiling effect Ca126
in children Ca338
combination with opioids Ca129
in elderly Ca355–Ca356
mechanism of action Ca183–Ca184
treatment (of)
acute herpes zoster pain Ch441
burn pain A363
opioids' adverse effects Ca169
pain in ICU A342–A343, **A343**
use in early postoperative period A334
see also individual drugs
nonoral administration of drugs Ca147–Ca148
see also individual methods
nonparoxysmal central pain, multiple sclerosis Ch357
nonpharmacological pain management
burns A364
childbirth pain A432
in children Ca334
definition A286
in elderly *see under* elderly
ICU analgesia methods A342
nurses role Ca91, Ca93
osteoarthritis Ch544–Ch545
postoperative pain A323
pregnancy pain A378
in procedural pain *see under* procedural pain
rheumatoid arthritis Ch539, Ch542
nonsmall cell lung cancer, bone metastasis chemotherapy Ca287
nonsteroidal anti-inflammatory drugs (NSAIDs) A55–A72, A331,
Ca35–Ca40, Ca129–Ca130, Ch227–Ch233
absorption A208
adjuvant analgesia A68, Ca169
combination with opioids Ca130
to local anesthetic for nerve blockade A271

administration A62–A63, A208–A210, Ch228–Ch229
analgesic efficacy of different routes **A210**
cavity A210
in children A441
enteral routes A208–A209
oral A208
parenteral A209
rectal A208–A209
surface A209–A210
transdermal A209, A495, Ca197–Ca198
adverse effects A58–A59, A62, **A62**, A331, **A331**, A351, A495,
Ca37, Ca187–Ca190, **Ca189,** Ca355–Ca356, Ch227, Ch229–
Ch231, **Ch230,** Ch261, Ch654
allergies A59, A62, Ch261
asthma A59, A62, Ca37, Ca190
cardiac complications Ca189, Ch231
CNS effects A59, Ca190
consequences for use in elderly Ca355–Ca356
gastric complications Ch230–Ch231, Ch261
gastrointestinal toxicity A58, A171, A173, A495, Ca37,
Ca130, Ca187–Ca188
guidelines to avoid renal toxicity **A62**
hematostasis and hematopoiesis Ca37
hemostasis impairment A58–A59
hepatic complications Ca37, Ca189–Ca190, Ch231
hepatotoxicity A58
immune system Ca37
limitations Ch213–Ch214
morbidity Ch261
mortality Ch261
nephrotoxicity Ca37
platelet complications Ch231
renal complications A59, A173, Ca188–Ca189, Ca356,
Ch231, Ch261
respiratory Ch231
risk factors for gastrointestinal toxicity **Ca189**
urinary Ca188–Ca189
analgesia provision
in ICU A342–A343
in interventional radiology A510
in trauma A351
avoidance of use in infants and neonates A442
"ceiling effect" A331
chemical classes **Ca38–Ca39**
in children A441–A442, Ca338
administration A441
adverse effects and toxicity A441–A442
analgesia for patients 6 months or younger P438
analgesia for patients over 6 months P434
indications A441
rectal administration P432
choice Ca37, Ca40, Ca130, Ca186
classification **A63, Ca183,** Ca184
clinical trials Ch232–Ch233
contraindications A57, Ca187, Ch228, **Ch228**
cyclo-oxygenase (COX) inhibition A56, A331, A351, Ca184,
Ca186–Ca190, Ch227–Ch228
prostaglandin production limitation A22–A23, *A494*
doses and treatment paradigms A58, **A60–A61,** Ch228–Ch229
drug interactions A57, Ca37, **Ca41**
opioid combination A55
efficacy **Ch232,** Ch232–Ch233
arthritic pain Ch232–Ch233
evidence for Ca190
musculoskeletal pain Ch232
in elderly A472–A473, Ca355–Ca356, Ch227, Ch228, Ch233,
Ch261, Ch654
evidence for particular therapy or drug A62–A63

number needed to treat (NNT) A62
gastroprotective agent combination Ch230–Ch231
historical aspects Ca183
indications Ca186–Ca187, Ch228, **Ch228,** Ch232–Ch233
intra-articular analgesia A210
limitations A331
mechanisms of action A55–A56, Ca35–Ca36, *Ca36,* Ca183–
    Ca184, Ch227–Ch228
in multimodal anesthesia A322, A323
nonefficacy Ch261
patient response Ch228
pharmaceutical considerations A63–A68, Ch231–Ch232
    acetic acids A65–A66
    fenamates A66
    nonacetylated salicylates A64
    oxicams A66
    para-aminophenol derivatives A63–A64
    propionic acids A64–A65
    pyrazoles A64
    salicylates A64
    sulfones/sulfonamides A66–A67
pharmacokinetic and toxicological profiles **A60–A61, A209**
pharmacokinetics A56–A57, Ca36, **Ca38–Ca39, Ca188**
    absorption A56
    distribution A56
    metabolism and elimination A56–A57
    pregnancy and lactation Ca36
    properties **A56**
    protein binding A56
postoperative pain management A322
    evidence classified according to level **A323**
    premedication A329–A330
practical tips Ca190
renal syndrome associations A410
risk–benefit assessment Ch227
selection for pain management A67–A68, **A68**
subcutaneous infusions in cancer pain control P91
    toxicity P91–P92
timing of treatment studies A123–A124, **A152–A154, A161–
    A162**
topical *see* nonsteroidal anti-inflammatory drugs, topical (T/
    NSAIDs) *(above)*
treatment (of)
    back pain Ch232, Ch527
    bone pain Ca130, Ca282–Ca283
    burn pain A363
    CRPS Ch392–Ch393
    fibromyalgia Ch232–Ch233, Ch625
    inflammatory arthritis Ch228
    low back pain A410, Ch232
    migraine Ch471
    musculoskeletal trauma A355–A356, Ch228, Ch232
    myofascial pain (MFP) Ch625
    neuropathic pain Ch233
    noninflammatory joint pain A398
    osteoarthritis Ch228, Ch232–Ch233, Ch543
    pelvic pain Ch599–Ch600, Ch603
    procedural pain Ca323
    rheumatoid arthritis Ch232, Ch539
    sickle cell disease A383
    sport injuries A494–A495
    sweating Ca309
    tension-type headache Ch473
    TMJ pain **Ch486**
usage Ch227
see also aspirin; *individual drugs as on Ch229; individual types*
nonsteroidal anti-inflammatory drugs, topical (T/NSAIDs) Ch213–
    Ch218

adverse effects Ch214–Ch215
    incidence Ch214
    local Ch215
    systemic Ch214, Ch215
clinical trials Ch215–Ch216
contraindications Ch214
dosage Ch214
    clinical effect duration Ch214
    precision Ch214
    preparation type Ch214
efficacy Ch215–Ch216, Ch217–Ch218, *Ch218*
indications Ch214, **Ch215**
    anatomical sites Ch214
    at-risk populations Ch216
market value Ch214
nomenclature **Ch215**
pharmaceutical considerations Ch215
    concentration gradient Ch215, **Ch217**
    mechanism of action Ch215
treatment (of) Ch214
    arthritis Ch216, Ch217
    lateral epicondylitis Ch216–Ch217
    mastalgia, benign Ch217
    neuropathic pain Ch217–Ch218
    postherpetic neuralgia Ch217
    soft-tissue injuries Ch216–Ch217, Ch217
    tendinitis Ch216
noradrenaline *see* norepinephrine
norepinephrine
    CRPS pathogenesis Ch387, Ch388
    in inflammatory pain A24
    role in descending control of pain A14
normeperidine Ca55
    acute pain management P69
nortriptyline
    mechanism of action Ch239–Ch240
    pharmacology **Ch240**
    treatment (of)
        central pain syndrome **Ch409**
        chronic back pain Ch527–Ch528
        fibromyalgia Ch625
        neuropathic pain Ch242
        painful spasticity **Ch461**
        postherpetic neuralgia Ch453
        TMJ pain **Ch486**
notalgia paresthetica, management, capsaicin **Ch219**
novel agents Ch261–Ch271
NSAIDs *see* nonsteroidal anti-inflammatory drugs (NSAIDs)
nucleoside analogs, AIDS pain treatment Ca368
    adverse effects **Ca368**
    drug interactions **Ca368**
nucleotide analogs, AIDS pain treatment Ca368
nucleotractotomy, stereotactic Ca265
nucleus pulposus, intervertebral disk *Ch522*
number needed to treat (NNT) P500
    calculation P500
    definition Ch120
    limitations P501
    systematic review examples **P501**
number of words chosen (NWC) A101
numerical rating scale (NRS) A99–A100, *A100,* Ch65, Ch104,
    Ch147, P17
    advantages and disadvantages A99–A100
    dental pain assessment P463
nurse-controlled analgesia (NCA) in pediatric care A228, A450
    analgesia for children over 6 months P436
nurses
    in CPRP Ch320

role in acute pain service (APS) A185–A186
   key elements of job description **A187**
role in elderly care
   attitudes toward cancer pain Ca352
   knowledge and experience Ca353–Ca354
roles in pain management Ca87–Ca94, *Ca88*
   elimination of barriers to pain relief **Ca89**
   multidimensional approach Ca87
   nondrug pain management Ca91, Ca93
   organizations and websites of interest in pain
      management **Ca92**
   pain assessment Ca89–Ca90
   patient education Ca87, Ca89, Ca90–Ca91
   pharmacological pain management Ca90
   quality improvement in pain management Ca93
nursing homes, problems for elderly patients Ca360
nutritional neuropathies A372
nystagmus, central pain syndrome Ch408

obese patients, patient-controlled analgesia (PCA) A228–A229
obsessive–compulsive disorder (OCD), measurement Ch71
obstructive jaundice, percutaneous biliary stenting A507
obstructive sleep apnea (OSA), patient-controlled analgesia
   (PCA) A228–A229
obturator nerve block P222
   anatomical aspects P222
   complications P222
   indications P222
   landmarks and practical steps P222, *P223*
occipital nerve block P200
   anatomical aspects P200
   complications P200
   indications P200
   landmarks and practical steps P200, *P201*
occipital neuralgia, peripheral nerve stimulation (PNS) Ch287
occipital pain Ch506
   referred pain patterns Ch506, *Ch507*
occiput-posterior (OP) position, influence on childbirth
   pain A430
occupational therapy, osteoarthritis management Ch544–Ch545
odynophagia (painful swallowing), in AIDS patients *see under* AIDS
omeprazole
   in elderly Ca356
   NSAIDs combination Ch231
open kinetic chain exercise, definition **Ch316**
operant conditioning techniques, CPRP Ch319
operant conditioning theory, placebos Ch277
ophthalmic nerve block, acute herpes zoster pain Ch444
ophthalmic postherpetic neuralgia **Ch482,** Ch494
ophthalmologic anesthesia A88
opioid-irrelevant pain Ca125
opioids A43–A53, Ca40–Ca56, P59–P76, **P72–P73**
   abuse Ch633
      potential **Ch79,** Ch81, Ch179
   acute pain management P69–P70
      administration routes P70
      choice of agent P69
      dosage/schedule P69–P70
   addiction A51, Ca49, Ca131–Ca132, Ca177, Ca404, Ch633,
      P65, P80
   adjuvant analgesia Ca158
      combination with laxatives Ca132
      combination with nonopioids Ca129
      to local anesthetic for nerve blockade A271
      NSAIDs combination A55
   administration A210–A213, A473–A477, Ca50–Ca51, **Ca163**
      in acute pain management P70
      in cancer pain management P70–P71

      cavity A212–A213
      in children A449–A450, **P436**
      continuous infusions A474
      enteral routes A210–A211
      epidural A213, **A242**
      inhaled A212, A319
      intramuscular A211, A316–A317, **A317,** A473–A474, Ca51
      intranasal A212, A318
      intrathecal A213, Ca51, Ca91
      intravenous A211, A317, **A318,** A474, Ca51
      iontophoresis Ca51
      nasogastric tube Ca50
      neural A213
      oral A210, A316, **A316,** A474, Ca50
      oral to parenteral potency ratios **Ca50**
      parenteral A211
      patient-controlled analgesia (PCA) A211, A317–A318,
         A318, A474
      in postoperative period A241–A242
      rectal A211, A319, **A319,** Ca51
      subcutaneous A211, A317, A474, Ca51
      sublingual A210–A211, A318, Ca50
      surface A211–A212
      switch Ca162
      traditional regimens A473–A474
      transdermal A211–A212, A319, Ca51
      transmucosal A210–A211, A318–A319, Ca50–Ca51
   adverse effects A171, A232–A234, A471–A472, Ca46–Ca47,
      Ca158, **Ca168,** Ch261–Ch262, P63, P80–P81, P436–P437
      breakthrough pain P80
      central nervous system effects Ca46–Ca47, P62, P63
      in children Ca342, **Ca343,** P436–P437
      cognitive impairment *see* cognitive impairment, opioid-
         induced
      constipation *see* constipation, opioid induced
      delirium *see* delirium, opioid induced
      drug treatment **P438**
      in elderly Ca356–Ca357
      epidemiology Ca167–Ca168
      of epidural analgesia *see* epidural opioids, adverse effects
      etiology and pathophysiology Ca167
      gastrointestinal effects Ca47, Ca175, P62–P63
      hyperalgesia *see* hyperalgesia, opioid-induced
      hypoxemia A471–A472
      with long-term use Ca47–Ca49
      management Ca167–Ca182, **Ca343**
      myoclonus *see* myoclonus, opioid-induced
      nausea *see* nausea, opioid-induced
      organic hallucinosis *see* organic hallucinosis, opioid-
         induced
      in PCA *see under* patient-controlled analgesia (PCA)
      prevalence **Ca168**
      pruritus *see* pruritus, opioid-induced
      renal impairment Ca357
      respiratory depression A173, A309–A310, Ca46–Ca47,
         Ca176–Ca177, P45, P63, P80, P437, P439
      sedation *see* sedation, opioid induced
      seizures Ca173–Ca174
      urinary retention A253, Ca177
      vomiting *see* vomiting, opioid induced
      xerostomia *see* xerostomia, opioid induced
   in AIDS patients Ca374
   American Academy of Pain Medicine Ch166–Ch167
   American Pain Society Ch166–Ch167
   American Society of Addiction Medicine Ch167
   analgesia provision in trauma A350–A351, **A351**
   cancer pain management Ch175, P70–P71, P74, P88–P90
      administration guidelines P71, P74

administration routes P70–P71
choice of agent P70
subcutaneous infusions *see* opioids, subcutaneous
infusions in cancer pain control
switching P90
WHO analgesic ladder P70, *P71*
caudal analgesia A447
in children A442, Ca338–Ca340, P74–P75
administration A449–A450, **P436**
adverse effects Ca342, **Ca343,** P436–P437
analgesia for patients 6 months or younger P439
analgesia for patients over 6 months P435–P436
codeine *see* codeine, in children
dose calculation and escalation **Ca341**
dose schedules and guidelines Ca341, P74–P75, **P436**
fentanyl *see* fentanyl, in children
guidelines P74
hydromorphone *see* hydromorphone, in children
meperidine *see* meperidine, in children
methadone **Ca339,** Ca340, P436
monitoring for patients on systemic infusions P437, **P438**
morphine *see* morphine, in children
oxycodone *see* oxycodone, in children
patient-controlled analgesia (PCA) P435–P436
pharmacokinetics **Ca339**
starting doses **Ca339**
switching Ca341–Ca342
tolerance P74
chronic pain management P74
aberrant drug-related behavior monitoring **P75**
guidelines P74
classification A45, **A46,** Ca40, Ca42, Ca157
by action at receptor **Ca43**
systems P59, **P60**
clinical applications P69–P75
controversy over use Ca404–Ca405, **Ca405**
dependence A51, Ch633
development Ch193–Ch194
dose–response curves Ca42, *Ca44*
efficacy and potency Ca157
antidepressants comparison Ch246, *Ch247*
in elderly patients A470–A472, Ca356–Ca358, Ch206, Ch654
administration techniques A473–A477
associated problems Ca356–Ca357
combinations Ca357
concurrent administration A471
dose and dose intervals A470–A471
strong Ca357–Ca358
suitable drugs A470
titration concerns A471
weak Ca356–Ca357
end of life care Ca311–Ca312
see also end of life care
endogenous *see* endogenous opioids
epidural *see* epidural opioids
fear of use (opiophobia) Ca47, Ca130, Ca131–Ca132, Ch29, Ch32
in cancer patients P477
guideline requirements Ch33, **Ch79,** Ch80–Ch81
indications
intrathecal administration for refractory pain P286–P288
for long-term use in chronic non-neoplastic pain P78
in intensive care unit A343
intraoperative analgesic A330
intraspinal *see* intraspinal opioids
intrathecal analgesia A477
intravenous *see* intravenous opioids
intraventricular *see* intraventricular opioids

legal controls Ch33–Ch34, Ch173–Ch175
Canada Ch175
fear Ch33–Ch34
history Ch173–Ch174
International Narcotic Control Board (INCB) Ch173
prescriptions Ch174–Ch175
schedules Ch174
state law Ch174
United Kingdom Ch175
USA Ch174–Ch175
lipophilic *see* lipophilic opioids
mechanism of action Ca40, Ca42, P59–P62
CNS systems primarily affected Ca40
metabolites A470
minimum effective analgesic concentration (MEAC) A206, **A206**
monitoring guidelines **Ch179**
in neonates *see under* neonatal pain management
in neurosurgical modalities/techniques Ca262
nonefficacy Ch261
pain clinics **Ch159**
pain control after discharge home A335
pain relief in interventional radiology A510
pain transmission sites of action *A14*
in percutaneous cervical cordotomy P330
pharmacodynamics A45–A46, **A46,** P66
CNS effects A45
drug- or age-induced alterations **P65**
efficacy and potency A43–A44
gastrointestinal system effects A46
histamine release A46
muscular effects A46
respiratory effects A45
variability A47
pharmacokinetics A46–A47, Ca42, Ca44–Ca46, **P65,** P65–P66
absorption Ca42
bioavailability A46–A47, **A47,** Ca44
calculation of dose regimen Ca44–Ca45
clearance Ca44
drug- or age-induced alterations **P65**
elimination half-life Ca44
factors influencing P64
first-pass clearance Ca44
half-life and volume of distribution A47, **A48**
influencing factors Ca45
in neonatal pain management A450
variability A47
volume of distribution Ca44
pharmacological effects P62–P63
cardiovascular system P62
central nervous system P62
gastrointestinal system P62–P63
genitourinary system P63
respiratory system P63
skin P63
pharmacology A47–A50, Ca158–Ca159, **Ca160–Ca161,** P66–P68
agonist–antagonist drugs P67
analgesia for chronic pain **Ca160–Ca161**
analgesia for mild to moderate pain Ca52–Ca53
analgesia for moderate to severe pain Ca53–Ca56
antagonists Ca56, P67
concepts relevant to opioid switching Ca157–Ca158
full agonists A47–A49, Ca53–Ca55
mixed agonist–antagonists A50, Ca55–Ca56
naturally occurring alkaloids P66
partial agonists A49–A50, Ca55
synthetic compounds P67

synthetic derivatives of codeine P67
synthetic derivatives of morphine P66–P67
physical dependence Ca49, Ca131, Ca177, Ca404, P64–P65, P80
premedication in postoperative pain management A329
pseudoaddiction Ca49, Ca404, P80
psychological dependence A51, Ca49, Ca131–Ca132, Ca177, Ca404, P65, P80
receptors A44–A45, Ca40, P59–P62, **P61**
    delta (δ) P60
    endogenous ligands A44
    epsilon (ε) P60
    kappa (κ) P60
    location A44
    mechanism of action A44
    modulation of nociceptive messages A11
    mu (μ) P60
    opioid-like receptors (OLR) P61
    orphan (ORL1) A44–A45
    presynaptic *P61*
    reclassification A44, A45
    response on activation and preferred opioid peptide **Ca42**
    sigma (σ) P60
reduced consumption effect on patient outcome P251
responsiveness Ca158
rotation *see* opioid switching and rotation
sedation scale **A471**
sites of action in gate control theory *A14*
strong Ca131–Ca134, Ch441
    in analgesic ladder Ca126
    risk of drug diversion Ca132
subcutaneous infusions in cancer pain control **P89**
    opioid-naive subjects P90
    opioid switching P88–P90
    prescribing P88–P90
    unresponsiveness P91
in substance abuse patients *see under* substance abuse patients
switching *see* opioid switching and rotation
systemic, in multimodal anesthesia A322
terminology A43, Ca40, P59
timing of treatment studies A120–A121, **A144–A147, A161–A162**
tolerance A50, Ca48–Ca49, Ca131, Ca177, Ca404, Ch206, Ch209, P64, P80
    management P64
    oral opioids Ch206, Ch209
topical Ch222
    administration A211–A212
    evidence Ch222
    procedural pain management Ca323
toxicity Ca167, P90–P91
    epidemiology Ca167–Ca168
    etiology and pathophysiology Ca167
    management P91
transdermal PCA delivery P402
transmucosal PCA delivery P402–P404
treatment (of)
    abdominal pain A374
    acute herpes zoster pain A371, Ch441
    acute pain *see* opioids, acute pain management
    bone pain Ca283
    breathlessness Ca295
    burn pain A362
    cancer pain *see* opioids, cancer pain management
    central pain syndromes Ch409
    chest trauma A353
    childbirth pain A431–A432

chronic pain *see* opioids, chronic pain management
chronic pancreatitis Ch574
cough Ca296
CPRP Ch166–Ch167
CRPS Ch394
fibromyalgia Ch625
nausea Ch206
neurologic disease Ch360–Ch361
neuropathic pain Ca262, Ch205
nociceptive pain P77
noninflammatory joint pain A398
peripheral neuropathy Ch377
postherpetic neuralgia Ch205, Ch453
procedural pain Ca325–Ca326
sickle cell disease A383
substance abuse patients *see under* substance abuse
TMJ pain **Ch486**
traumatic brain injury (TBI) A352
treatment protocols for chronic nonmalignant pain *see*
    opioids, in chronic nonmalignant pain *(below)*
vulnerability of patients to compliance problems P78–P79
weak Ca130–Ca131, Ch441
    in analgesic ladder Ca126, Ca130–Ca131
withdrawal syndrome P64–P65, P80
    clinical manifestations P64
    management P65
see also individual drugs
opioids, in chronic nonmalignant pain (protocols) P77–P83
    acute pain episode treatment P81–P82
        case history P81–P82
        comments P82
    complications P80–P81
        see also under opioids
    drug-related behaviors causing concern P81
    evidence base P79
        assessment of opioid response P79
        guidelines P79–P80
        justification for maintenance of opioid therapy P79
        maintenance opioid therapy P79–P80
    indications for long-term use in non-neoplastic pain P78
    neuropathic pain P77
    nociceptive pain P77
    patient information and consent P80–P81
    selection of patients, implementation and follow-up P78–P79
        determination of improvements in pain and quality of life P78
        vulnerability to compliance problems P78–P79
opioids, oral Ch203–Ch211
    administration A210, A316, **A316,** A474, Ca50
    adverse effects Ch206
        cognitive dysfunction Ch206
        constipation Ch206
        nausea Ch206
        sedation Ch206
        sensitivity Ch206
        tolerance Ch206, Ch209
    clinical trials Ch203–Ch204
    consent Ch208
        informed Ch208
        verbal Ch208
    contraindications Ch205–Ch206
        substance abuse Ch205, Ch207
    efficacy evidence Ch203–Ch204
    mechanism of action Ch203
    monitoring Ch209
        aberrant behavior Ch209, **Ch209**
        reviews Ch209
        tolerance Ch209

patient selection Ch204–Ch205, **Ch210**
conditions Ch205
neuropathic pain Ch205
pain etiology Ch205
previous management Ch205
psychological assessment Ch205
pharmaceutical considerations Ch206–Ch207
methadone Ch206–Ch207
sustained-release preparations Ch206
practical administration Ch207
index of suspicion Ch207
trial guidelines Ch208–Ch209
dose changes Ch208
expectations Ch209
goal definitions Ch208
review Ch208
see also opioids
opioid switching and rotation Ca157–Ca165
in cancer pain management P90
in children Ca341–Ca342
clinical evidence of benefits Ca159
evidence for selection of alternative to morphine Ca159, Ca162
opioid responsiveness Ca158
pharmacological relevant concepts Ca157–Ca158
preclinical evidence for different responses Ca159
rationale Ca158
in refractory cancer pain Ca145
route switch Ca162
in toxicity management Ca168
opioid-tolerant patients, patient-controlled analgesia (PCA) A229
opiophobia Ca47, Ca130, Ca131–Ca132, Ch29, Ch32
in cancer patients P477
opium
history and development A219–A220
laws Ch173
oral administration of drugs A205
in children Ca340, P432
conscious sedation for procedural pain Ca323, Ca325
contraindications in palliative care practice **Ca147**
nonsteroidal anti-inflammatory drugs A208
opioids A210, A316, **A316,** A473, Ca50
acute pain management P70
cancer pain management P70
patient-controlled analgesia (PCA) P402
bedside delivery P404
transmucosal delivery route P401
preference in WHO analgesia ladder Ca143
oral analgesic therapy Ca123–Ca142
contraindications Ca125
evaluation of efficacy Ca128
painful spasticity management **Ch461,** Ch461–Ch463, **Ch462**
pharmacological management Ca129–Ca136
see also individual drugs
principles Ca123–Ca142
oral candidiasis Ca297–Ca298
in AIDS patients Ca378–Ca379
hyperplastic Ca378
oral hairy leukoplakia Ca378, *Ca379*
pseudomembranous (thrush) Ca378, *Ca379*
treatment Ca379, **Ca380**
risk factors Ca297–Ca298
oral hairy leukoplakia, in AIDS patients Ca378, *Ca379*
oral problems Ca297–Ca298
in AIDS *see under* AIDS
dry mouth *see* xerostomia
infections Ca297–Ca298
bacterial Ca298

candidiasis *see* oral candidiasis
herpetic Ca298
oral transmucosal fentanyl citrate (OTFC) A211, A222, Ca51, Ca54–Ca55, Ca326, P404, *P404*
breakthrough pain management Ca54, P470
in children Ca340
procedural pain management Ca326
orchialgia Ch581
management Ch581
organic hallucinosis, opioid-induced Ca171
clinical presentation and findings Ca171
definition Ca171
evidence-based evaluation of management Ca171
organization, of pain service *see* acute pain service (APS)
organizations of interest **Ca92**
orofacial pain *see* facial pain
orthopedic abnormalities, painful spasticity Ch460
orthoses P184
orthostatic hypotension *see* hypotension
osteoarthritis A398–A399, Ch542–Ch545
clinical features Ch543
definition Ch542
diagnosis, radiographs Ch127
epidemiology Ch542
erosive Ch543
etiology **Ch543**
intra-articular injections, RCTs P256
investigations Ch543
management Ch316–Ch317, Ch543–Ch545
acetaminophen Ch233, Ch235
acupuncture Ch343
capsaicin Ch218, **Ch219**
Fitness Arthritis and Seniors Trial (FAST) Ch317
intra-articular injections Ch543–Ch544
naproxen Ch233
neurokinin 1 (NK1) antagonists Ch267
nonpharmacological therapies Ch544–Ch545
NSAIDs Ch228, Ch232–Ch233, Ch543
pharmacological therapies Ch543–Ch544
physical therapy Ch316–Ch317, Ch544
surgical Ch545
topical analgesia Ch543
topical capsaicin *Ch220,* Ch543
myofascial pain association Ch616
osteonecrosis A399
in AIDS patients Ca385
osteoporosis
chronic back pain Ch521
management, physical therapy Ch317
Oswestry Low Back Pain Questionnaire (OLBPQ) Ch107, Ch149
otitis externa **Ch482**
Oucher Scale A106
outcome measures A163–A181, Ch104, Ch145–Ch153
botulinum toxin injections P280
clinical trials P457
cost-effectiveness A174
CPRP Ch164
disability from pain Ch149
effect of reduced opioid consumption P251
epidural analgesia P413–P414
factors leading to increased emphasis on A163
financial constraints Ch150
future trends in improving perioperative outcomes A175–A176
accelerated recovery programs A176
balanced analgesia A175–A176
monitoring in nerve blocks in pain diagnosis P51
outcome movement and evidence-based medicine A163–

A165
    genesis of movement A163–A164
    health care policy and pain management A164–A165
pain measurement A165–A166
    see also pain measurement
pain treatment trials P455
patient(s), effect of reduced opioid consumption P251
physical capacity Ch146–Ch147
    functional capacity Ch146–Ch147
    lifting capacity Ch146
    range of motion Ch146
    strength Ch146
postoperative pain management A166–A175
    cardiac outcome A166–A168
    coagulation A170–A171
    gastrointestinal function A168, A170
    pulmonary outcomes A168
psychological functioning Ch147–Ch150
    general Ch149–Ch150
    pain intensity Ch147–Ch148
    pain-specific measures Ch148–Ch149
    psychosocial impact Ch148
risks and complications A171, A173–A174
targets Ch145
timing Ch145
variables Ch150
see also clinical assessment; individual techniques
ovarian cancer, radiotherapy Ca255
ovarian remnant syndrome Ch593
    diagnosis Ch593
    management Ch593
    pathophysiology Ch593
    symptoms/signs Ch593
    see also pelvic pain
oxaprozin A65
    characteristics **Ch229**
oxcarbazepine
    adverse effects P107
    contraindications P105
    dosing schedule and pretreatment safety measures P105,
        P106, P107
    painful spasticity management **Ch461**
    trigeminal neuralgia management Ch494, **Ch494–Ch495**
Oxford Quality Rating Scale **P498**
    scoring of items **P499**
oxicams A66
oxybutynin Ca220
    adverse effects Ca221
    doses and pharmacokinetics Ca220
oxycodone A48, Ca53, Ca134, Ch207, P67
    in children A442, Ca338
        analgesia for patients over 6 months P434–P435
        doses **P435**
        starting dose **Ca339**
    chronic back pain management Ch527
    clinical trial Ch204
    in elderly Ca358
    pain control after discharge home A335
oxygen
    breathlessness management Ca295
    consumption, increase during childbirth A426
oxymorphone Ca55, P66
oxyphenbutazone A64

P_2X_3 receptor antagonists Ch266
    mechanism of action Ch266
pacemaker
    spinal cord stimulation contraindication P382

TENS contraindication Ca246, P345
pain
    assessment see pain assessment
    attention to P114
        regulation in chronic pain patients see attention regulation
            in chronic pain
    behavioral responses P163
    behaviors Ch76, Ch91, Ch96, P6
        frequency Ch97
        measurement **Ch75,** Ch76
    beliefs Ch8
        assessment Ch107
        diagnostic uncertainty Ch314
        expectations Ch314
        Pain and Impairment Relationship Scale (PAIRS) Ch315
    blood stagnation P355–P356
    categories P28, P469
        see also individual types
    cellular level Ch3
    classification Ca124, **Ca124**
    clinics see pain clinics
    cold condition P356
    components Ca75
        in two different patients Ca67
    compositional levels Ch90–Ch91
    conditions P28–P29
    conscious interpretation Ch8
    cortical activation Ch3
    cortical modulation P113–P114
    cultural differences Ch7–Ch8
    damp condition P356
    definition A305, Ca21, Ch3, Ch5
        subjective Ch16
    definition (IASP) Ch4–Ch5
        Cartesian definition Ch4–Ch5
        circularity Ch5
        ethical concerns Ch5
        objections Ch4–Ch5
    differing types Ch6–Ch7
    dual function of brain Ch7
    ethical considerations Ch8–Ch10
    etiology **Ca4**
    experience see pain experience
    fear of see pain-related fear
    gender differences Ch7
    heat condition P356
    history see pain history/examination
    impact Ch90–Ch91, Ch149
        on quality of life *Ca88*
    integration with other symptoms Ca69
    intensity see pain intensity
    meaning of P114
        differences in analgesia requirements P114
    measurements see clinical assessment; diagnostic procedures;
        pain history/examination; pain measurement
    measures see pain measures
    memory of P16
    mood disorders and P114
        see also anxiety; depression
    narrative-based medicine Ch8–Ch9
    neurophysiological mechanisms P27–P28
    perception see pain perception
    phenomenology Ca259–Ca260
    prevalence **Ca3,** Ch4
    psychosocial factors see psychological effects
    relief see pain relief
    schools P182
    somatosensory evaluation P28

staging Ca68
symptoms **Ch164**
syndrome response Ch7
syndromes *see* cancer pain, syndromes
treatment principles Ca124–Ca125
    control after discharge home A334–A335
    control in early postoperative period A334
    goals Ca127
    plan Ca124–Ca125
undertreatment *see* undertreatment of pain
see also individual diseases/disorders
Pain and Impairment Relationship Scale (PAIRS) Ch76, Ch315, P165
  pain belief Ch315
Pain Anxiety Symptoms Scale (PASS) Ch74, Ch105, P165
pain assessment A93–A111, Ca21, Ca63–Ca71, Ca260–Ca261
  in acute pain service (APS) A190
  in AIDS patients Ca373
  burns A361
  characterization of cancer pain syndrome **Ca65,** Ca65–Ca66
  in children *see under* children
  clinical research A106–A107
    analgesia demand A107
    imaging pain A107
    repeated measurements over time A107
    retrospective measurements A107
  clinical standards A107
  description A95–A97
    localized pain in gut *A97*
    location body maps *A96*
    neuropathic pain clinical features **A97**
  in elderly *see under* elderly
  goals A94
  influencing factors A93–A94
  integration of pain with other symptoms Ca69
  intensity evaluation Ca66–Ca67
    graphic display of results Ca67
    instruments used **Ca66**
    see also individual tools
  multidimensional Ca67–Ca68
  musculoskeletal A395
  nonverbal patients Ca67
    elderly Ca359–Ca360
  nurses' role Ca89–Ca90
  pain scores A190, **A190**
    value **A190**
  physical examination A98
    additional investigations A98
    framework **A98**
  picture scales *A101,* A101
  in postoperative period A102–A103, *A104,* A308–A310
  process A94–A98
  somatosensory evaluation P28
  special situations A102–A108
    cognitively impaired A106
    critical care A106
    elderly *see* elderly, pain assessment
    emergency room A103–A104
    intensive care unit (ICU) A342
    pediatrics A104–A106
      see also pain measurement, in children
  staging of pain Ca68
  substance abuse history Ca67
  in trauma A349
  see also clinical assessment; pain history/examination; pain
    measurement; patient(s), assessment
pain avoidance, physical therapy Ch314
Pain Beliefs and Perception Inventory (PBPI) Ch72, Ch74

pain catastrophizing P163–P164
pain clinics Ch155–Ch161, Ch326
  background Ch155
  clinical activity Ch158, **Ch159**
    variation Ch158
    work patterns Ch158
  Clinical Standards Advisory Group (CSAG) Ch158, Ch161
  district hospital Ch159
    staffing Ch159
  expenditures Ch157
    running costs **Ch158**
    salaries Ch157, **Ch157**
  income Ch160–Ch161
    contract negotiation Ch160–Ch161
  indications **Ch78**
  management Ch158
  organization Ch155–Ch156
    general practitioner Ch156
    health authorities Ch155
    NHS trusts Ch156
    primary assessment Ch156
  provision Ch156
  staffing Ch156–Ch157
  teaching hospitals Ch159–Ch160
    clinical activity Ch160
    staffing Ch159–Ch160
  teams, fibromyalgia/myofascial pain management Ch626–Ch627
pain control
  after discharge home A334–A335
  in early postoperative pain period A334
  for radiological procedures *see* interventional radiology, pain
    relief and sedation
Pain Disability Index (PDI) Ch76, Ch107, Ch149
pain experience P4, P113, P147, *P471*
  reconceptualization P136
    see also attention regulation in chronic pain, phase I
painful procedures Ca319–Ca329, **Ca321**
  background Ca319
    analgesia provision Ca319
    incidence of pain Ca319
  future directions Ca326
  see also procedural pain
pain history/examination A94–A97, Ca260, Ch63–Ch88
  in acute pain service (APS) A187
  assessment in postoperative period A102–A103, A308–A310
  classification problems Ch68
  diagnostic algorithm *Ch64*
  diagnostic significance **Ch66–Ch67**
  factors relevant to treatment A97–A98
  fibromyalgia/myofascial pain Ch65, Ch68
  framework for assessment **A95,** *A309*
  functional and medical aspects A97
  internal pain scale Ch65
  nonspecific pain Ch63–Ch65
  pain measurement Ch64–Ch65
    see also individual tests
  patient evaluation Ca63–Ca65, **Ca64**
  problems Ch79
  questions **Ch66–Ch67**
  sexual Ca79–Ca80
  style Ch63
  see also clinical assessment; diagnostic procedures; pain
    assessment; pain measurement
Pain Information and Beliefs Questionnaire (PIBQ) Ch148
pain intensity *P451*
  assessment in children P21
  assessment in elderly P21

clinically important reduction P455
measurements P15–P26, P455
    assessment at extremes of age P21, P23
    cancer pain P23
    chronic pain P23
    difference (PID) calculation **P24**
    faces pain scale *P19*
    memory of pain P16
    nonverbal patients P21
    results, interpretation and handling P24–P25
    scales P16–P18
        see also individual types
    serial measures of pain P23–P24
    total pain relief (TOTPAR) calculation **P24**
    visual analog toy *P19*
    see also McGill pain questionnaire
summed differences (SPID) *P451,* P456
pain intensity differences (PID) P23, *P456*
    calculation **P24**
pain maps
    neck pain diagnosis Ch135–Ch137, *Ch138*
    neuropathic pain assessment Ch117
pain measurement A98–A102, A165–A166, Ca21–Ca22, Ca63–Ca71
    in children A104–A106, A438–A439
        assessment tools A104–A105, **A439**
        behavioral or observational A439, **A439**
        multidimensional assessment A439
        physiological A439
        proxy/observer reports A105
        self-report A105–A106, A438–A439
    effectiveness as quality of care measure A166
    in elderly A469, Ca351
    ideal assessment tool characteristics **A99**
    multiple-dimension scales Ch65
    self-reporting *see* self-reporting of pain
    single-dimension scales Ch65
    temporal factors Ch65
    unidimensional tools A99–A102
        categorical scales A99
        numerical *see* numerical rating scale (NRS)
        picture scales *A101,* A101
        verbal *see* verbal rating scale (VRS)
        visual *see* visual analog scale (VAS)
    variables and techniques **A102**
    see also pain assessment; pain history/examination
pain measures P3–P14
    behavior and activity P6–P8
        compound measures P6, P8
        health care resources P8
        interference P8
        pain behavior P6
        quality of life *see* quality of life (QoL)
        satisfaction P8
        third-party-defined outcomes P8
    biomedical domains P4–P5
        see also pain experience; pain relief
    content P3–P8
        outcome domains P3, P4–P8
    estimating change or difference P11–P13
        clinical significance P11
        example P12–P13
        raw data plots *P12*
        type I errors P11
        type II errors P11
    fear of pain
        movement/(re)injury and pain catastrophizing *P172*
        severity *P172*

of function and disability **P7**
histogram of score change with treatment *P12*
of intensity *see* pain intensity, measurements
nonoutcome variables P8
psychometric qualities and interpretation of output P3, P9–P13
psychosocial domains P5–P6
    affect or emotion P5
    cognitive measures P5–P6
    coping P6
reliability P9–P10
    internal consistency P9
    interrater P9–P10
    test–retest P9
scatterplot of pretreatment and post-treatment scores *P12*
selection and application P3–P14
    considerations P3–P8
    method of measurement P4
sensitivity to change P10–P11
validity P10
    concurrent P10
    cut-off points P10
    divergent P10
pain narratives Ch8–Ch10
pain perception A3, Ca21, P114
    changes in elderly A468
    factors affecting P15–P16
        anxiety P15–P16
        childhood experiences P15
        circadian variation P16
        climatic conditions P16
        depression P16
    placebos Ch281–Ch282
    somatic P114
    see also nociception
pain radiation, neuropathic pain Ch116
Pain Rating Index (PRI) A101
pain rehabilitation *see* comprehensive pain rehabilitation programs (CPRP)
pain-related fear P163–P176
    attention P164
    characteristics P163–P164
        escape/avoidance behaviors P164
        kinesiophobia P163
        pain catastrophizing P163–P164
    cognitive–behavioral assessment P165–P168, *P167*
        behavioral tests P168
        determining treatment goals P167–P168
        graded hierarchies P168
        interview **P166,** P166–P168
        specific questionnaires P165–P166
            see also individual scales
    disconfirmation of harm beliefs P164–P165
        match/mismatch model P164
    education P169
    effectiveness P173–P174
        crossover design studies P173
        daily measures of fears and pain catastrophizing *P173*
    graded exposure *in vivo* P169–P172
        behavioral experiments P169
        case illustrations P169–P171
        complicating factors P171–P172
        daily measures of fear of pain severity *P172*
        example dialogue in behavior experiment **P171**
        exposure P169, P172
        graded activity comparison P165
        maintenance of change P172
        systemic desensitization P169

graded hierarchies P168
   example patients **P170**
pathways for acquisition of excessive pain P169–P171
   case illustrations P169–P171, **P170**
pain relief P4–P5
   cold application *see* cryoanalgesia
   postoperative, with patient-controlled epidural analgesia
     (PCEA) P413–P414
   scale Ch65
   total (TOTPAR), calculation **P24**
   see also analgesia
Pain Relief Act, opioid legal controls Ch175
Pain Resource Nurse (PRN) Program Ca89
pain schools P182
Pain Self-Efficacy Scale Ch107
pain service, acute *see* acute pain service (APS)
Pain Society Ch155
pain switch technique P151
pain transmission A175–A176, *A176*
pain triangle Ch17, *Ch17*
palfium *see* dextromoramide
palliative care Ca105–Ca111, Ch28, Ch31
   acceptance of death Ca106
   aims Ca106
   anticipation of patients' needs Ca105–Ca106
     apparent needs Ca105–Ca106
     deeply hidden needs Ca106
     subconscious needs Ca105
   care for family members Ca110
   characteristics **Ch28**
   dealing with euthanasia requests Ca108–Ca109
     see also euthanasia
   definition Ca105
   ethical issues Ch10–Ch11
   place of dying Ca107–Ca108
     home or hospital Ca107–Ca108
     hospice of palliative care unit Ca108
   total pain concept Ca106–Ca107
     see also total pain
   see also end of life care; home care
pamidronate
   bone pain management Ca288–Ca289
   doses and treatment paradigms Ca223
   pharmacokinetics Ca223
Pancoast tumor, radiotherapy Ca255–Ca256
pancreatic cancer Ch570–Ch571
   management Ch570–Ch571, **Ch571**
   pain Ca12
     sites of **Ca12**
     syndromes **Ch570**
pancreatic pseudocysts Ch574
   management Ch574
pancreatitis A376
   acute, in AIDS patients Ca389
   chronic Ch571–Ch575
     alcoholic Ch572, Ch574
     antioxidant management Ch574
     management and evaluation of pain **Ch572**, *Ch573*
     opioids Ch574
     oral pancreatic enzymes Ch574
panic attacks Ch632
papaveretum A49, Ca55
para-aminophenol derivatives A63–A64
   see also acetaminophen (paracetamol); propacetamol
para-aortic lymphadenopathy, indication for radiotherapy Ca255
paracervical block P231–P232
   anatomical aspects P231
   childbirth pain treatment A432

complications P232
indications P231
landmarks and practical steps *P231*, P231–P232
paracetamol *see* acetaminophen (paracetamol)
paraesthesia, stellate ganglion block complication P239
parallel studies *see under* clinical trials
paraneoplastic neuropathies Ch374–Ch375
paraplegia
   celiac plexus block complications P250
   management, dorsal root entry zone lesions Ch305
parasympathetic nerves, sacral, pelvis enervation Ch587–Ch588
paravertebral nerve blocks A270–A271
   acute herpes zoster pain management Ch443
   complications Ch443
   in pediatric surgery A448
parenteral administration of drugs A206–A207
   nonsteroidal anti-inflammatory drugs A209
   opioids A211
     in children A449–A450
   safety A256
parents
   help to talk to children Ca79
   involvement in biofeedback in children P156
   role in distraction technique A288
   role in pain management in children A440, Ca334
paresthesiae Ch116
   central pain Ch407–Ch408
   definition **Ch404**
   fibromyalgia association Ch616
   peripheral neuropathies Ch368
Parkinson's disease Ch358, Ch359
   causes **Ch359**
   central pain Ch406
   management Ch359
     thalamotomy Ch298
   nature of disease Ch359
   pain Ch359, **Ch360**
paroxetine Ca217
   pharmacology **Ch240**
paroxysmal pain, multiple sclerosis Ch357
paroxysms, neuropathic pain Ch116
passive modalities, physical therapy Ch315
patient(s)
   assessment Ca63–Ca65
     investigations Ca65
     medical history Ca63–Ca65, **Ca64**
     of needs **Ca321**
     of opioid responsiveness Ca158
     physical examination Ca65
     review of previous treatments Ca63, Ca66
     of substance abusers Ca64, Ca396–Ca397, **Ca397**
     see also pain assessment; psychological evaluation of
       patients and family
   attitudes of elderly Ca351
   comparison with AIDS patients **Ca372**, Ca372–Ca373
   decision-making by relatives and health professionals Ca118–
     Ca119
     see also ethical issues
   education
     in acute pain service (APS) A196–A197
     in AIDS management Ca373
     in biofeedback P125
     childbirth pain preparation A291
     in cryoanalgesia P324
     in elderly care Ca353–Ca354
     nurses' role Ca87, Ca89, Ca90–Ca91
     in pain-related fear P169
     in PCA A224, P394

program content **Ca90**
teaching principles **Ca91**
TENS Ch286
emotional problems Ch326
epidural analgesia risks P410
information on dental pain clinical trials P463
knowledge and experience in elderly care Ca354
outcome, effect of reduced opioid consumption P251
physiotherapy demands P186
preparation and procedural explanations Ca320
psychological evaluation *see* psychological evaluation of
patients and family
reliance of medical support Ch325–Ch326
subgroups Ch98
substance abusers *see* substance abuse patients
substandard medical care Ch35
vulnerability to opioid compliance problems P78–P79
patient advocates, disability evaluation (USA) Ch40
patient-controlled analgesia (PCA) A206–A207, A219–A239,
A306–A307, A335, P393–P399
adjustable analgesic parameters A222–A223
background infusion A223
bolus dose A222–A223
dose limit A223
loading dose A223
lockout interval A223
advantages and disadvantages **A220**
adverse effects
management P398
nausea A233
pruritus A233
respiratory depression A232–A233
urinary retention A234
vomiting A233
background P393–P394
basic principles A220–A221, *A221*
in children A228, Ca341
analgesia for patients over 6 months P435–P436
bolus dose A222
systemic analgesia A449–A450
contraindications A224
cost-effectiveness A174
delivery systems
alternative P401–P405, **P402**
applied anatomy P401–P404
contraindications and limitations P404, **P404**
buccal and sublingual P404
epidural versus intravenous **A321**
gastrointestinal route P402
inhalation route P401–P402
intranasal (PCINA) devices *P403*, P403–P404
system characteristics **P404**
intravenous P395
advantages P395
disadvantages P395
nasal transmucosal route P401
oral route P402
bedside delivery P404
transmucosal delivery P401
subcutaneous route (SC-PCA) A335, P395
advantages P395
disadvantages P395
transdermal route P401
ideal drug properties **P403**
iontophoretic systems **P402**
opioid delivery P402
transmucosal opioid delivery P402–P404
ideal drug properties **P403**

oral and nasal routes P401
drugs P394
efficacy A226–A228
analgesic A226
cost comparisons A227
of nonopioids added to regimens A228
of opioids used with parenteral PCA A228
patient satisfaction A226–A227
significance of patient's beliefs and attitudes A307, *A307*
via other nonintravenous routes A227
in elderly A228, A474
management A474–A475, **A475**
equipment A221–A222, P394
disposable pumps A221–A222
programmable pumps A221
transdermal devices A222
transmucosal devices A222
guidelines P394
history and development A219–A220
indications A223–A224
monitoring P395–P398
chart *P396–P397*, P397–P398
regular observations P397–P398
in morbidly obese patients A228–A229
in obstructive sleep apnea (OSA) patients A228–A229
opioids administration A211, A317–A318, A474
advantages over conventional analgesia **A318**
in opioid-tolerant patients A229
pain management in ICU A343
patient information P394
potential hazards/complications A229–A234, **A230**
mechanical errors A232
damaged or malfunctioning infusion
components A232
failure of pump to deliver set volume A232
"run-away" pump A232
operator errors A229–A231
inappropriate patient selection A231
inappropriate use of concurrent medications A231
incorrect placement or damage of syringe/
cartridge A230–A231
incorrect use of, or failure to use, antireflux
valves A230
programming errors A229–A230
opioid adverse effects A232–A234
bowel function A234
nausea and vomiting A233
pruritus A233
respiratory depression A232–A233
urinary retention A234
patient-related errors A231–A232
assisted PCA A231
failure to understand PCA A231
tampering with machines A231–A232
practical points and protocols P393–P399
preparation A224–A225
monitoring requirements A225
patient education A224, P394
staff education A224
standard orders and nursing procedure protocols A224–
A225
psychological factors A225–A226
anxiety A226
responsibility of producing side-effects A226
satisfaction A226
relative potency decision P453
safety criteria P393–P394
setting up P394–P395

antiemetic inclusion P394–P395
background infusions P394
severe pain relief technique **A188**
side-effect influence on "feedback" loop A221, *A221*
staffing and training P394
standardized prescriptions' important elements **A193**
stopping PCA and subsequent analgesia A225
treatment (of)
    acute just postamputation pain Ch427
    burn pain A362
    postoperative pain A306–A307, P413–P414
patient-controlled epidural analgesia (PCEA) A208, A246–A248
cost A247
drug choice A227
efficacy A227
infusion rates, doses, and lockout intervals **A247**
postoperative pain relief P413–P414
problems A246–A247
patient-controlled intranasal analgesia (PCINA) devices *P403,*
  P403–P404
system characteristics **P404**
patient–physician relationship, disability evaluation (USA) Ch40
pediatric pain management *see* children
pelvic arthropathy, in pregnancy A377
pelvic congestion Ch592–Ch593
diagnosis Ch592–Ch593
management Ch593
pathophysiology Ch592
symptoms/signs Ch592
see also pelvic pain
pelvic disease, ureteric stent placement A507
pelvic pain Ch587–Ch613
adhesions *see* adhesions (pelvic)
clinical findings Ch599
    examination Ch599
clinical presentation Ch598–Ch599
    history Ch598–Ch599
cyclic Ch594
    diagnosis Ch594
    management Ch594
    pathophysiology Ch594
    symptoms/signs Ch594
diagnosis Ch599
endometriosis *see* endometriosis
epidemiology Ch587
etiology/pathophysiology Ch587–Ch598, **Ch590**
    hernia Ch595
    neuronal modulation Ch588–Ch589
    somatic pain Ch588
    visceral pain Ch588
gastroenterologic causes Ch594–Ch595
indication for radiotherapy Ca255
management Ch599–Ch603
    after trauma A353–A354
    alternative/complementary medicine Ch603
    injection therapy Ch600
    multidisciplinary pain management Ch603
    nerve blocks Ch600, P230–P232
        see also individual types
    physical therapy Ch600
    psychological therapies Ch602–Ch603
nerve entrapment Ch597
    management Ch597
    pathophysiology Ch597
    symptoms/signs Ch597
neurologic/musculoskeletal Ch596–Ch597
    see also myofascial pain (MFP), pelvic pain
no obvious cause Ch597

ovarian remnant syndrome *see* ovarian remnant syndrome
pelvic congestion *see* pelvic congestion
pharmacological management Ch599–Ch600
prognosis Ch603
psychological factors Ch597–Ch598
    depression Ch598
    personality profile Ch598
    sexual/physical abuse Ch598
    see also comorbidities, psychiatric
salpingo-oophoritis Ch593–Ch594
surgical management Ch600–Ch603
    hysterectomy *see* hysterectomy
    laparoscopy *see* laparoscopy
    presacral neurectomy *see* presacral neurectomy (PSN)
tumors/cysts Ch593–Ch594
urological causes Ch595–Ch596
    differential diagnosis Ch595
    interstitial cystitis *see* interstitial cystitis
    pathophysiology Ch595
    recurrent infectious cystitis Ch595
    urethral syndrome *see* urethral syndrome
see also abdominal pain, visceral; vulvar pain syndrome
pelvic trauma, pain management A353–A354
pelvis, enervation Ch587–Ch588, **Ch588**
penciclovir, acute herpes zoster pain Ch440
penicillin, maxillary sinusitis management Ch487
penile nerve blocks
complications A446
dorsal, in children P440
    anatomical aspects P440
    complications P440
    local anesthetic solution P440
    method P440
in pediatric surgery A445–A446
pentazocine Ca55, P68
pharmacokinetics Ca55, P68
pentosan polysulfate sodium (PPS), interstitial cystitis
  management Ch596
pentoxifylline, anorexia–cachexia syndrome management Ca306
peppermint oil, botanical therapy **Ch347**
peptic ulcer, NSAID induced A58
Helicobacter pylori role Ca188
peptide hormone prohibitions in IOC medical code A499
examples A501
perception A3
perception discrepancy Ch76
percutaneous biliary stenting A507
percutaneous cervical cordotomy P328–P330
adverse effects P329
anatomical aspects P328
complications and incidence P329
discomfort to patient P329–P330
historical aspects P327, P328
indications P328
limitations P328
results P329
technique P328–P329
    electrode guiding needle P328–P329, *P329*
    visible three lines P328, *P329*
percutaneous electrical nerve stimulation (PENS)
acute herpes zoster pain management Ch445
chronic back pain management Ch531
percutaneous laser revascularization (PMLR) Ch557
percutaneous stereotactic commissurotomy Ca264
percutaneous transluminal angioplasty (PTA), pain relief in
  interventional radiology A503–A504
percutaneous vertebroplasty (PVP) A507–A508, *A508*
complications A508

CT image after needle withdrawal *A508*
periapical periodontitis Ch481
periarticular sepsis, intra-articular injection
    contraindication P258
pericranial muscles, tension-type headache Ch469–Ch470
perineal visceral pain, ganglion impar block P252–P253
    see also ganglion impar block
perineoplasty, vulvar pain syndrome management Ch606–Ch607
perineum, innervation *A427*
periodontal disease, oral pain in AIDS patients Ca381
periodontal pain Ch482, **Ch482, Ch483**
periodontitis, periapical Ch481
period prevalence, definition Ch16
perioperative pain, RCTs in acute pain P488
periosteal irritation, chronic back pain Ch521
peripheral artery disease, spinal cord stimulation (SCS) Ch289
peripheral nerve blocks A267–A274, A332–A333, A352, P197–
    P232
    additions to local anesthetics A271
    administration
        local infiltration *see under* local anesthesia
        nerve/nerve plexus infusions A269–A271
    agents and techniques P197–P200
        aseptic technique P199
        general principles P199–P200
        insulated or noninsulated needles P199
        local anesthetics P197–P198
            see also individual agents
        needles P199–P200
        nerve location by peripheral nerve stimulation P199
        neurolysis P198–P199
            see also neurolytic blocks
        resuscitation equipment P199
    in children **P439,** P440–P442
        see also individual types
    complex A448–A449
    diagnostic *see* nerve blocks in pain diagnosis
    epidural *see* epidural nerve blocks
    general principles A267
    head and neck blocks P200–P203
    intrapleural *see* intrapleural blocks
    lower limb blocks P219–P230
    in multimodal anesthesia A323
    neurolytic *see* neurolytic blocks
    pain clinics **Ch159**
    pain management in ICU A344
    paravertebral, acute herpes zoster pain management Ch443
    pelvic blocks Ch600, P230–P232
    simple, in pediatric surgery A445–A448
        efficacy **A445**
    sympathetic Ch131
        acute herpes zoster pain Ch443
        CRPS diagnosis Ch131
        mechanism Ch131
        phantom pain Ch431
        placebo effect Ch131
        validity Ch131
    thorax and abdomen blocks P215–P218
    treatment (of)
        acute herpes zoster pain Ch442–Ch443
        nerve entrapment Ch597
        neurologic disease Ch362
        pain in pregnancy A379
        pelvic pain Ch600
        postherpetic neuralgia Ch454
    trigeminal, acute herpes zoster pain Ch444
    upper limb blocks P204–P214
    see also individual types

peripheral nerves
    injury, painful spasticity Ch460
    neurolysis Ca240–Ca241
        see also peripheral nerve blocks
    tumors, radiation induced Ca17
peripheral nerve stimulation (PNS) Ca248, Ch287
    central pain syndromes management Ch410
    efficacy Ch287
    historical aspects P343
    indications Ch287
    nerve location P199
        insulated or noninsulated needles P199
peripheral neuropathies *see* neuropathies, peripheral
peripheral polyneuropathic pain, spinal cord stimulation Ch290
peripheral sensitization A18–A29
    endogenous attenuation A29
    increased intracellular calcium concentration A26
    intracellular events leading to *A21*
    plastic changes A18–A19
        induction A19, *A21,* A21–A27
        nociceptor morphology A19
        nociceptor neurochemistry A18–A19
        nociceptor physiology A18, *A18*
    receptors A21–A26
        chemical activators A21–A25
        G-protein-coupled receptors (GPCRs) **A20,** A25–A26
        ligand-gated ion channels A25
        tyrosine kinase receptors **A20, A22,** A26
    second messenger systems **A20**
    sensory neuronal role in development of inflammation A27
    transcriptional and post-translational changes A26–A27
        effects on transcriptional machinery A27
        phosphorylation A27, *A28*
    transducers A19, A21
    voltage-gated ion channels **A19**
    see also central sensitization
peritoneal pain *see* abdominal pain, visceral
periventricular gray stimulation Ch293, Ch302
peroneal nerve block
    at ankle P230
        landmarks and practical steps *P229,* P230
    at knee P227
        landmarks and practical steps P227, *P228*
persistent pain states A313–A314
    cancer pain P477–P478
    causes **A314**
personal injury claims *see* medicolegal aspects
personality
    disorders Ch69, Ch634
    placebos Ch280
    profiles, pelvic pain Ch598
    psychometric assessment Ch95–Ch96
        see also psychological effects, assessment
pethidine *see* meperidine
pH, effect on local anesthetics A77
phantom bladder pain Ca13
phantom breast pain Ca15
phantom limb pain Ca15, Ch429, Ch434
    burning Ch433
    in children *see under* children
    cramping Ch433
    management and evaluation Ch430–Ch434
        biofeedback and relaxation techniques Ch432
        dorsal root entry zone lesions Ch305
        history of attempts Ch430–Ch431
        invasive interventions Ch431
        rational/background Ch432–Ch433
        recommended procedure Ch510–Ch512

short-term follow-up Ch433
TENS Ch430
mental status fears Ch430
red flags Ch431
sensations Ch429
see also postamputation pain
pharmaceutical manipulation prohibition in IOC medical
code A499–A500
pharmacodynamics
aging changes A466, Ca355
morphine A45
opioids *see under* opioids
pharmacodynamic tolerance Ca48
pharmacokinetics
acetaminophen Ca33–Ca34, Ca185
in children A441
in neonatal pain management A451
aging changes A464–A466, **A465**
physiological A464–A466, **A465**
systemic A464
alfentanil **A346**
amitriptyline Ca217
antiarrhythmic agents Ca212–Ca213
anticonvulsants Ca214–Ca215
antidepressants Ca217, Ch241, *Ch241*
aspirin Ca191
baclofen Ca220
bupivacaine **A346**
buprenorphine Ca55
calcium channel blockers Ca224
calcium metabolism-associated drugs Ca223
carbamazepine Ca214
caudal blocks in pediatric surgery A446–A447
celecoxib Ca201, **Ca201**
in children, opioid analgesics **Ca339**
citalopram Ca217
clodronate Ca223
clonazepam Ca215
clonidine Ca211
codeine Ca52
corticosteroids Ca219
coxibs **Ca201**
cyclo-oxygenase preferential inhibitors of COX-2 over COX-
1 **Ca194**
dantrolene Ca220
dextropropoxyphene Ca52
diazepam **A346,** Ca220
diclofenac Ca192
diflunisal Ca192
in elderly Ca354–Ca355
etodolac Ca200
fentanyl **A346,** Ca54
in elderly A464
transdermal Ca162
flecainide Ca212–Ca213
flurbiprofen Ca193
gabapentin Ca215
hyoscine butylbromide Ca220
ibuprofen Ca193
imipramine *Ch241*
indinavir **Ca369**
indomethacin Ca190, Ca194
ketamine Ca222
ketoprofen Ca194
ketorolac Ca195
lamotrigine Ca215
lidocaine **A346**
local anesthesia *see* local anesthesia, pharmacokinetics

mefenamic acid Ca195
meloxicam **Ca194,** Ca198
meperidine, in elderly A464
methadone Ca53–Ca54
mexiletine Ca212
midazolam **A346**
morphine **A346,** Ca53
in elderly A464
nabumetone Ca196
nalbuphine Ca56
naproxen Ca196
nefopam Ca35
nifedipine Ca224
nimesulide **Ca194,** Ca199
NSAIDs **A60–A61, A209,** Ca36, **Ca38–Ca39, Ca188**
opioids *see under* opioids
oxybutynin Ca220
pamidronate Ca223
paroxetine Ca217
pentazocine Ca55
piroxicam Ca197
prednisolone Ca219
propofol **A346**
quinine Ca220
rofecoxib Ca202
saquinavir **Ca369**
sodium valproate Ca214
terminology Ca42, Ca44
absorption Ca42
bioavailability Ca44
clearance Ca44
elimination half-life Ca44
first-pass clearance Ca44
volume of distribution Ca44
tramadol Ca52–Ca53
transdermal fentanyl Ca162
vigabatrin Ca215
pharmacokinetic tolerance Ca48
pharmacological diagnostic tests P39–P47
intravenous drug challenges P39
advantages P39
disadvantages P39–P40
quantitative sensory testing (QST) combination P39
see also diagnostic procedures
pharmacological management Ca90
AIDS Ca374
analgesia provision in trauma A350–A351
anxiety Ca310
bone pain Ca282–Ca283
central pain syndromes *see under* central pain syndromes
childbirth pain treatment A431–A432
in children *see under* children
depression Ca309
low back pain A409–A410
musculoskeletal pain management A355–A356
nurses' role Ca90
oral analgesic therapy Ca129–Ca136
osteoarthritis Ch543–Ch544
pelvic pain Ch599–Ch600
pregnancy acute pain management A378–A380, **A380**
procedural pain *see under* procedural pain
sport injury rehabilitation management A493–A495
vulvar pain *see under* vulvar pain syndrome
pharmacotherapy, myofascial pain (MFP) management Ch625
phenobarbital, CRPS management Ch394
phenol
interpleural block *see* interpleural phenol blocks
lumbar sympathetic block agent P243

neurolytic agent Ca237, **Ca238,** P198
   cryoanalgesia comparison P324–P325
   painful spasticity management Ch463
phenomenology of cancer pain Ca259–Ca260
phenothiazines
   central pain syndromes management Ch410
   postherpetic neuralgia management Ch453
phenoxybenzamine, CRPS management Ch392
phentolamine
   CRPS management Ch391
   intravenous P42–P43
      adverse effects P43
      background P42
      contraindications P42
      doses and paradigms P42–P43
      efficacy P43
      indications P42
      pharmaceutical considerations P43
      practical tips P43
phenylazine, mechanism of action Ch240
phenylbutazone A64
   characteristics **Ch229**
   clinical use Ch228
phenytoin
   adjuvant analgesic in elderly Ca358
   adverse effects P107
   clinical trials Ch252, Ch253
   contraindications P105
   dosing schedule and pretreatment safety measures P105,
      P106
   mechanism of action Ch251
   treatment (of)
      central pain syndrome Ch409
      painful spasticity **Ch461**
      peripheral neuropathy Ch377
      postherpetic neuralgia Ch453
      trigeminal neuralgia Ch494, **Ch494–Ch495**
phonophobia, migraine Ch468
phosphorus, metastatic bone pain treatment Ca287
Photograph Series of Daily Activities (PHODA) P168, *P168*
photophobia, migraine Ch468
physical abuse, pelvic pain Ch598
physical conditioning, fibromyalgia/myofascial pain
   management Ch624
physical dependence Ca49
   in children Ca344
   definition Ch208
   in opioid therapy Ca49, Ca131, Ca177, Ca404, P64–P65, P80
      substance abuse patients Ca396
physical examination Ca65
   see also patient(s), assessment
physical manipulation prohibition in IOC medical code A499–
   A500 A
physical resources, assessment of Ca76
physical therapies Ch313–Ch324, P182–P183
   approaches Ch315–Ch316
      aerobic activity Ch316
      isometric exercises Ch316
      isotonic exercises Ch316
      motion Ch316
      passive modalities Ch315
      static strengthening Ch316
      templates Ch315–Ch316
   in children Ca334
   coping strategies Ch314
   CPRP *see* comprehensive pain rehabilitation programs (CPRP)
   deconditioning Ch314–Ch315
      multifidi muscle dysfunction Ch314

muscle recruitment patterns Ch314–Ch315
   definition A286
   disability *Ch315*
   dynamic lumbar stabilization Ch318
      clinical studies Ch318
      definition Ch318
      goals Ch318
   goals Ch313
   McKenzie approach P183
   medical exercise therapy (MET) P183
      shoulder rotator device *P183*
   Pain and Impairment Relationship Scale (PAIRS) Ch315
   pain avoidance Ch314
   pain beliefs Ch313–Ch314
   pain clinics **Ch159**
   spine rehabilitation programs Ch318
      flexion exercises Ch318
      primary extension exercises Ch318
   treatment (of)
      central pain syndromes Ch317, Ch411
      CRPS Ch317, Ch391, Ch395
      dysesthetic vulvodynia Ch604
      elderly pain Ch655–Ch656
      infant pain A293–A297
      lateral epicondylitis Ch317
      low back pain A411, Ch317–Ch318
      medial epicondylitis Ch317
      neck pain Ch512–Ch514
      neurologic disease Ch362
      osteoarthritis Ch316–Ch317, Ch544
      osteoporosis Ch317
      painful spasticity Ch461
      pelvic pain Ch600
      rheumatoid arthritis Ch539, Ch542
   types **Ch314**
   see also physiotherapy
physical therapists, CPRP Ch319–Ch320
physical training P182–183
physicians
   CPRP Ch319
   disciplinary actions Ch33–Ch34
   duty Ch28–Ch29
   insufficient knowledge Ch32–Ch33
   physiotherapists cooperation P186
physiotherapy P179–P187
   causal treatment P181–P184
      cognitive interventions P181–P182
      ergonomic advice P182
      manual therapy P183
         see also manual medicine
      physical training P182–P183
         see also physical therapies
      psychomotor physiotherapy P184
      relationship to pain and tissue capacity *P182*
   examination P180–P181
      clinical findings P181
      clinical history P181
   hemophilia management A382
   interdisciplinary cooperation P186
      demands on patient P186
      with physician P186
   McKenzie exercises for low back pain A411
   pain and P179–P180
      acute and chronic differentiation P180
      communication P179–P180
   pain management in pregnancy A378
   symptomatic treatment P184–P186
      massage P185

physical agents P185–P186
    unloading P184, *P184*
treatment process P179, *P180*
see also physical therapies
phytotherapy *see* botanical therapy
picture scales in pain assessments *A101,* A101
pimozide
    clinical trials Ch252
    trigeminal neuralgia management Ch493, **Ch494–Ch495**
pinprick test, postherpetic neuralgia Ch452
piroxicam A66, Ca197
    adverse effects Ca187–Ca190, Ca197
    characteristics **Ch229**
    cyclo-oxygenase (COX) inhibitor Ca197
    evidence for efficacy Ca197
    indications and contraindications Ca186–Ca187
    pharmacokinetics Ca197
    practical tips Ca197
Pittsburgh Sleep Quality Index Ch74
pituitary ablation Ca256
pizotifen, migraine prophylaxis Ch475
placebos Ch273–Ch284
    alternative/complementary therapies Ch282
    anxiety relief theory Ch276–Ch277
    biological basis Ch280–Ch281
        nonopioid-mediated effects Ch280
        opioid-mediated effects Ch280
    conditioning theory Ch276
    definition Ch273, Ch276
    expectancy/cognitive theory Ch277
        definition Ch277
    experimental use Ch273–Ch274
    false Ch274–Ch276
        active intervention studies Ch274–Ch275
        diagnostic nerve blocks Ch275
        disease progression/remission Ch275
        environmental effects Ch275
        experimental recorder bias Ch275
        patient bias Ch276
        physiological variables Ch275
        publication bias Ch276
        statistical errors Ch274, Ch276
        statistical regression to the mean Ch276
    mind–body connections Ch274
    noncebo response Ch273
    personality Ch280
    problems Ch281–Ch282
        data interpretation Ch281
        pain perception Ch281–Ch282
    psychological behaviorism (PB) theory Ch277–Ch280
        anxiety reduction Ch278–Ch279
        conditioning Ch278
        emotional conditioning Ch278
        emotional states Ch277
        expectancy Ch279
        language conditioning Ch279–Ch280
        language process Ch279
        negative emotional response Ch277
        operant conditioning Ch277
        personality Ch278, Ch279
        positive emotional response Ch277–Ch278
        positive reinforcement Ch277
        psychosocial conditioning Ch279–Ch280
        suggestion principle Ch278
        vocabulary Ch278
    suggestion Ch274
    therapeutic use Ch273–Ch274
    uncontrolled clinical trials Ch274

unified theory Ch280
see also clinical trials
plain radiography, neck pain investigations Ch510–Ch511
plantar fasciitis Ch547
platelet-activating factors, in inflammatory pain A24
platelets, NSAIDs adverse effects Ch231
pleural disease, radiotherapy Ca254
pneumonia, in AIDS patients Ca386
    Pneumocystis cysts *Ca386*
pneumothorax, stellate ganglion block complication P240
point prevalence, definition Ch16
polyneuropathies Ch367–Ch368
    acute inflammatory Ch358
    antiepileptic indication P105
polypharmacy, problem in cancer pain clinical trials P471–P472
popliteal fossa block P227
    complications P227
    landmarks and practical steps P227, *P228*
porphyria Ch580–Ch581
    management Ch580–Ch581
    source of pain **Ch568**
    subgroups Ch580
Port-A-Cath ports P314
Portex tunneling device P291, *P292*
positioning in infant pain management A295
    evidence supporting effectiveness A295–A296
positive likelihood ratio, definition Ch126
positron emission tomography (PET), central pain
    examinations Ch405
postamputation pain **Ca14,** Ca15, Ch427–Ch435
    acute just Ch427–Ch428
        management Ch427–Ch428, Ch434
        nerve desensitization Ch428
        pain sensation magnification Ch427
        preventive actions Ch428
        residual limb pain Ch427
    chronic residual limb pain Ch428–Ch429
        aging effects Ch429
        bone spurs Ch428
        management Ch431
        neuroma growth Ch428
    management
        ketamine Ch264
        topical capsaicin Ch221
    phantom pain *see* phantom limb pain
    phantom sensations Ch429
postanesthesia discharge scoring system (PADSS) **A510**
postaxillary dissection pain Ca15, *Ca15*
postcentral cordectomy, central pain syndromes
    management Ch411
postcentral gyrectomy, central pain syndromes
    management Ch411
postcholecystectomy syndrome Ch581
posterior arch *Ch522*
posterior column stimulation, central pain syndromes
    management Ch410
posterior cutaneous nerve
    forearm blockade P212–P213
        complications P213
    thigh blockade P227
posterior longitudinal ligaments *Ch522*
postherniorrhaphy pain
    diagnostic nerve block P50
    ilioinguinal nerve block P322
postherpetic neuralgia (PHN) A369, Ch374, Ch451–Ch458
    anticonvulsant clinical trials Ch252
    clinical presentation
        examination Ch452

history Ch452
epidemiology Ch452
age relation Ch452
gender Ch452
severity Ch452
etiology/pathophysiology Ch451–Ch452
herpes zoster virus (HZV) Ch437
human leukocyte antigen (HLA) involvement Ch374
management Ch452–Ch454
anesthetics Ch453
anticonvulsants Ch253, Ch453
antidepressants **Ch243,** Ch244–Ch245, Ch452–Ch453
capsaicin **Ch219**
ketamine Ch264
lidocaine Ch256
memantine Ch264
nerve blocks Ch454
opioids Ch205, Ch453
surgery Ch454
TENS Ch454
topical agents Ch453–Ch454
topical capsaicin Ch220, *Ch220,* Ch221, Ch453–Ch454
topical NSAIDs Ch217
ophthalmic **Ch482,** Ch494
prevention Ch454–Ch455
acyclovir Ch455
corticosteroids Ch455
varicella vaccine Ch455
prognosis Ch455
progression from herpes zoster A369
prevention strategies *A371*
risk factors A370, **A370**
postlaminectomy syndrome, opioid management Ch205
postmastectomy pain **Ca14,** Ca15
scar pain Ca15
postoperative neuropathic pain, chronic **Ca14,** Ca14–Ca15
postamputation pain Ca15
postmastectomy pain Ca15
postradical neck dissection pain Ca15
post-thoracotomy pain Ca14
postoperative pain management A329–A340
addendum A324
cyclo-oxygenase 2 inhibitors A324, A331
neuroaxial blockade A324
aggressive control of pain A344
assessment of pain and pain history A102–A103, A308–A310
monitoring A309–A310
nursing observation sheet *A104*
respiratory depression A309–A310
in children *see under* children
cryoanalgesia A323, P322–P323
ilioinguinal nerve block P322
intercostal nerve block P322
open technique P323
day surgery A329–A340
anesthetic technique effects A330
consequences of inadequate management **A329**
future developments A335–A336
inadequate A329
local anesthetic techniques **A332,** A332–A334
new concepts A333–A334
pain control after discharge home A334–A335
pain control in early postoperative period A334
preoperative considerations A329–A330
surgical considerations A336
epidural analgesia *see under* epidural analgesia/anesthesia
evidence-based treatment A314–A323
levels of clinical evidence A315

modalities of treatment A315–A319, **A316**
multimodal anesthesia A322–A323
nonsteroidal anti-inflammatory drugs A322
regional techniques A319–A322
scientific evidence A315
general anesthesia A330
immediate postoperative period A306–A307
epidural analgesia A307
patient-controlled analgesia (PCA) A306–A307
incidence of pain A305–A306
studies **A306**
inpatient A305–A328
recommendations A305–A306
see also specific subentries above/below
intermediate postoperative period A307–A308
bridging the analgesia gap **A308**
intrathecal analgesia A320
late postoperative period A308
nonpharmacological methods A323
opioid administration A241–A242, A315–A319
outcome measures *see under* outcome measures
pain sequelae and influence of surgery/analgesic
regimens A310–A314
cardiac complications A311–A312
neuroendocrine response to surgery A312–A313
neuropathic pain A314
pulmonary complications A310–A311
psychological therapies A323
randomized controlled trials in acute pain P488
relaxation and music therapy A291
TENS A277–A278, A323
transition from acute to chronic pain A308, A313–A314
persistent pain states A313–A314, **A314**
see also specific drugs
postradical neck dissection pain **Ca14,** Ca15
poststroke pain Ch406
anticonvulsant clinical trials Ch252–Ch253
antidepressant management **Ch243,** Ch244
central, intravenous lidocaine Ch256
motor cortex stimulation Ch294
see also stroke pain
postsurgical pain syndromes Ch417–Ch425
chest *see* chest pain, postsurgical
CRPS Ch418
diagnosis Ch422
nerve conduction studies Ch422
nerve entrapment Ch422
quantitative sensory testing (QST) Ch422
differential diagnosis Ch417
epidemiology Ch22–Ch23
frequency Ch419
iatrogenic injury Ch418, Ch421–Ch422
incidence Ch418–Ch419
management Ch422–Ch423
conservative management Ch423
pharmacology Ch423
surgery Ch422–Ch423
topical capsaicin *Ch220,* Ch220–Ch221, Ch221
nerves at risk Ch418–Ch419
ilioinguinal nerve Ch420
inferior alveolar nerves Ch419
lingual nerves Ch419
non-neurologic causes Ch417–Ch418
nontraumatic cause Ch418
residual pain Ch417
surgical interventions Ch419–Ch421
abdominal rectopexy Ch421
amputation Ch421

bone harvesting Ch421
brachial plexus injury Ch419
breast surgery Ch420
carpal tunnel release Ch420
dentistry Ch419–Ch420
hernioplasty Ch420–Ch421
intercostal rib resection Ch420
lymph node biopsy Ch420
shoulder arthroscopy Ch420
thoracotomy Ch420
postsympathectomy hyperesthesia, lumbar sympathetic block
complication P243
post-thoracotomy pain Ca14, **Ca14**
diagnostic nerve block P50
intercostal nerve block P322–P323
post-traumatic pain management, TENS A280
postural hypotension *see* hypotension, orthostatic
posture, fibromyalgia/myofascial pain due to Ch620
corrections Ch625–Ch626
exercises Ch624
potentization by dilution, homeopathic theory Ch343
pragmatic P450, **P450**
prednisolone, pharmacokinetics Ca219
prednisone, pharmacokinetics Ca219
preemptive analgesia A113–A162
definition A114–A116
history and recent progress A114
targets A114
timing of treatment A115
see also preventive analgesia; timing of treatment
pregnancy
abdominal nerve entrapment A377
acupuncture A378
acute pain management A376–A380
nonpharmacological options A378
pharmacological options A379, **A380**
back pain A376–A377
carpal tunnel syndrome A377
hand symptoms A377
headache A377
NSAIDs contraindication Ca36
opioid-induced pruritus risk A252
pain problems frequently encountered A376
pelvic arthropathy A377
TENS contraindication Ca246, P345
ureteric obstruction A377
see also childbirth pain
prepatellar bursitis Ch547
presacral neurectomy (PSN) Ch602
adverse effects Ch602
contraindications Ch602
efficacy Ch602
indications Ch602
prescribing errors, subcutaneous infusions P97–P98
Present Pain Intensity Scale (PPIS) A101
pressure threshold, determination with algometer P32
pretrigeminal neuralgia **Ch482, Ch499**
prevalence, definition Ch16
preventive analgesia A113–A162
definition A114–A116
targets A114
timing of treatment A115
see also preemptive analgesia; timing of treatment
prilocaine A86
adverse effects A86
peripheral nerve block agent P197–P198
physiochemical properties and clinical profile **A79, A84–A85**
structure **A84–A85**

primary afferent neurons
central sensitization A29–A36
increased excitatory input to dorsal horn neurons A32–
A34
characteristics *A4*
CRPS pathogenesis Ch386–Ch387
low- and high-threshold response to distension *A6*
nociceptive *see* nociceptors
peripheral sensitization *A18*, A18–A29
primary amyloidosis, autoimmune neuropathy Ch373
primary hyperalgesia, CRPS pathogenesis Ch387
primary prevention, definition Ch15–Ch16
primiparous parturients, childbirth pain A424
procaine A83
structure, physiochemical properties and clinical profile **A84**
procedural pain Ca319–Ca326
burns A360–A361
conscious sedation Ca323, Ca325–Ca326
administration routes Ca325–Ca326
monitoring precautions **Ca325**
sedative drugs Ca325
efficacy of sucrose A297
future directions Ca326
incidence Ca319
management in children *see under* children
management plan development Ca319–Ca320, **Ca321**
assessment of individual patient Ca320, **Ca321**
patient preparation and procedural explanations Ca320
nonpharmacological interventions Ca320, Ca322
cognitive–behavioral therapy (CBT) Ca322
distraction Ca322
hypnosis Ca322
psychological therapies A452
relaxation Ca322
TENS A279–A280
pharmacological management
Entonox Ca326
ketamine Ca326
local anesthetic infiltration Ca322
nonsteroidal anti-inflammatory drugs Ca323
strong opioids Ca325–Ca326
topical local anesthesia Ca322–Ca323
topical opioids Ca323
proctalgia fugax Ch582
proctitis A209
progesterone, burning mouth syndrome management Ch489
progestogens, anorexia–cachexia syndrome management Ca306
Progressive Isoinertial Lifting Evaluation (PILE) Ch146
progressive muscle relaxation (PMR) A288, P127–P130, **P128**
abbreviated muscle groups **P129**
advantages and disadvantages A293
in children P150
initial muscle groups and procedures for testing (18
steps) P127, P129, **P129**
muscle discrimination training addition P129
number of sessions P129
practice P129
relaxation-induced anxiety P130
promethazine, as antiemetic A233
propacetamol A63–A64
in children A441
toxicity A441
neonatal pain management A451
proparcaine, trigeminal neuralgia management Ch494, **Ch494–**
Ch495
propionic acids A64–A65
propofol Ca325
antiemetic A233

pain management in ICU A344
    pharmacokinetics **A346**
propoxyphene P67
propranolol
    adverse effects P43
    central pain syndrome management Ch409
    clinical trials Ch253
prospective studies *see* epidemiology of pain
prostadynia Ch581
    management Ch581
prostaglandin E, CRPS pathogenesis Ch387
prostaglandins, synthesis in inflammation A22, *A24*
    limitation with NSAIDs administration A22, *A24*
prostate cancer
    bone metastasis hormone treatment Ca288
    hypophysectomy Ch299
prostate pain Ch581
prosthetic joints, infection A396–A397
protease inhibitors, AIDS pain treatment Ca369–Ca371
    drug interactions Ca369
    toxicities Ca369
    see also individual drugs
proteinases, modulation of nociceptive messages A13
protein binding
    in local anesthetics A79
    physiological changes with age A466
proton pump inhibitors, gastroesophageal reflux disorder (GERD)
    management Ch558
protons, in inflammatory pain A22
protopathic pain, definition **Ch404**
provoked hyperalgesia Ch115–Ch116
proximal interphalangeal joint, intra-articular injections P267
proxy/observer reports, pain assessment A105
pruritus Ca307–Ca308
    clinical findings Ca307–Ca308
    investigations Ca308
    management Ca308
        general measures **Ca308**
        systemic treatments Ca308
        TENS Ca308
        topical treatments Ca308
    opioid-induced A252–A253, A472, Ca46, Ca177, P63
        epidural infusions P313
        management A252–A253
    pathology Ca307
    PCA induced A233
        management P398
pseudoaddiction Ca49, Ch31
    in opioid therapy Ca49, Ca404, P80
    in substance abuse patients Ca397
    see also addiction
pseudomembranous candidiasis (thrush) Ca298
    in AIDS patient Ca378, *Ca379*
    see also oral candidiasis
psoas syndrome, malignant Ca10
    clinical features Ca10
    CT scan *Ca11*
    plain radiograph *Ca11*
psoriasis, management, topical capsaicin **Ch219**, *Ch220*
psychiatric comorbidities *see* comorbidities, psychiatric
psychiatric disorders Ca309–Ca311
    in AIDS patients Ca373
    see also anxiety; delirium; depression
psychological behaviorism (PB) theory *see under* placebos
psychological dependence *see* addiction
psychological disorders Ca309–Ca311
    see also anxiety; delirium; depression
psychological effects Ch101–Ch104, *Ch102*

assessment *see* psychological effects, assessment *(below)*
    attention span Ch101
    concentration Ch101
    direct Ch101–Ch102
    disuse syndrome Ch102
    fibromyalgia/myofascial pain Ch620
    memory Ch101
    see also individual diseases/disorders
psychological effects, assessment Ch101–Ch111, Ch631–Ch635
    addiction Ch633–Ch634
    anxiety disorders Ch632
        disease association Ch632
    chronic pain syndrome Ch634–Ch635
        diagnostic criteria Ch634
    coping skills Ch106
    Diagnostic and Statistical Manual of Mental Disorders Ch95,
        Ch631
    disability *see* disability
    factitious disorder Ch632
        diagnosis Ch632
        etiology Ch632
        medical background Ch632
        by proxy Ch632
    family influences Ch108
    formats **Ch103,** Ch103–Ch104
        self-report questionnaires Ch103
    health care resources Ch108
    interpretations Ch631
    low back pain Ch631
    malingering Ch632–Ch633
        diagnosis Ch632
        financial benefits Ch633
    mood Ch105–Ch106
    Münchausen syndrome Ch632
    panic attacks Ch632
    panic disorders Ch632
    personality Ch106
    personality disorders Ch634
    primary domains **Ch104**
    psychometric Ch95–Ch96, Ch104
    self-injury Ch634
    sexual pain disorders Ch633
        dyspareunia Ch633
        vaginismus Ch633
    sleep disorders Ch634
    somatization disorder Ch632–Ch633
        diagnosis Ch632
        etiology Ch632–Ch633
        secondary medical problems Ch632
    substance abuse Ch633–Ch634
    substance dependence Ch633–Ch634
    suicide Ch634
        depression link Ch634
        evaluation Ch634
    see also comorbidities, psychiatric
psychological evaluation of patients and family Ca73–Ca85
    assessment Ca74, Ca76–Ca77
        family, friends and carers Ca76, Ca78
        patient Ca76
        physical resources Ca76
        social resources Ca76–Ca77
        see also patient(s), assessment
    children Ca78–Ca79
    coping mechanisms Ca80
        anger Ca80
        denial Ca80
    holistic assessment *Ca75*
    importance of communication Ca77

importance of family Ca77–Ca78
parental advice on talking to children Ca79
risk assessment for depression, suicide and anxiety Ca80–Ca82
sexuality and intimacy Ca79–Ca80
taking sexual history Ca79–Ca80
psychological factors
effect on pain after burns A361
influencing childbirth pain A429–A430
in patient-controlled analgesia *see under* patient-controlled analgesia (PCA)
in pelvic pain *see under* pelvic pain
relationship to cancer pain Ca29, Ca73
psychological therapies A285–A302, Ch325
child and adult techniques A287–A293
advantages and disadvantages A292–A293, **A294**
patient information/teaching A291–A292
relaxation *see* relaxation
evidence supporting effectiveness of techniques
patient information/teaching A292
relaxation A290–A291
infant techniques A293
mechanisms of action A285–A286
misbeliefs A287
physiological benefits A286
terminology A286–A287
treatment (of)
anxiety Ca310
chronic back pain Ch532–Ch533
CRPS management Ch395
depression Ca309
elderly pain Ch656
low back pain A413–A414
neurologic disease Ch364
pelvic pain Ch602–Ch603
postoperative pain A323
procedural pain in children A452
trauma pain A352
see also physical therapies
psychologists, CPRP Ch320
psychometric assessment Ch104
psychomotor physiotherapy P184
psychophysiological assessment *see under* biofeedback
psychoprophylactic techniques of Lamaze, role in childbirth A429, A432
psychosis, anticonvulsants adverse effects Ch254
psychosocial factors Ch8
assessment A97
control in painful conditions Ca114–Ca115
in low back pain A407, A414
relationship to cancer pain Ca74
psychosocial support, substance abuse patients Ca399
psychosocial therapy, pain management in pregnancy A379
psychostimulants
adjuvant analgesic in children Ca342
adverse effects Ca170
opioid-induced sedation management Ca170
pudendal nerve block P230–P231
anatomical aspects P230
childbirth pain treatment A432
complications P231
indications P230
landmarks and practical steps *P230,* P230–P231
pulmonary complications, in postoperative period A168
effect of different analgesia regimens A311
hypoxemia *see* hypoxemia
intraspinal opioid reduction in risk A251
management A168

outcome improvements associated with analgesic therapies **A171**
outcome measures A168
proposed mechanisms *A170*
reduced functional residual capacity (FRC) A310
reduced lung volume A310
pulmonary embolism, postoperative pain management A171
pulpal pain Ch482, **Ch482, Ch483**
pulpitis Ch481
pulp testing, dental pain diagnosis Ch483
pulsed radiofrequency P199
pulvinotomy Ch304
indicators Ch304
outcomes Ch304
technique Ch304
punctate hyperalgesia Ch115, **Ch121**
punctate midline myelotomy Ca264
pupils, opioids adverse effects P62
purines, in inflammatory pain A24
pygeum, botanical therapy **Ch347**
pyrazoles A64
pyridoxine deficiency, peripheral neuropathies Ch372

qi (energy) *see under* acupuncture
quality assurance (QA) A166
quality improvements (QI) A166, Ca93
monitoring Ca93
strategies Ca93
quality of life (QoL) P6
assessment P457
determination of improvements with opioid therapy P78
elderly issues Ca352–Ca353
impact of pain *Ca88*
maintenance in palliative care Ca106
quantitative sensory testing (QST) P31
CRPS Ch384
peripheral neuropathy diagnosis Ch370
pharmacological diagnostic test combination P39
postsurgical pain syndromes diagnosis Ch422
quantitative sudomotor axon reflex test (QSART), CRPS diagnosis Ch390–Ch391, *Ch392*
quinine Ca219–Ca220
adverse effects Ca221
doses and pharmacokinetics Ca220

radial nerve block
at elbow P212
landmarks and practical steps P212, *P212*
at wrist P213
complications P213
landmarks and practical steps P213, *P214*
radiation myelopathy **Ca14,** Ca17
radiation plexopathy **Ca14,** Ca16–Ca17
radiation therapy *see* radiotherapy
radicular pain Ch505, Ch506
management, dorsal root entry zone lesions Ch305
radiofrequency lesioning indication P337
radiculopathy, diabetic neuropathy Ch371–Ch372
radiocarpal joint, intra-articular injections P265–P266, *P266*
radiofrequency hypophysectomy, stereotactic Ch300
radiofrequency lesioning Ca242, P327–P340
advantages and disadvantages **Ca242**
in cervical area P333
clinical applications Ca242–Ca243, P327–P328
facet joint pain Ca242
lumbar disk pain Ca242
sympathetic chain Ca242–Ca243
trigeminal neuralgia Ca242

contraindications **P328**
equipment **P328**
of Gasserian ganglion *see* Gasserian ganglion
historical aspects P327
in lumbar area P336
    dorsal root ganglia *see under* dorsal root ganglion (DRG)
    sympathetic ganglia *see* sympathetic ganglia (lumbar)
opioid administration P330
percutaneous
    cervical cordotomy *see* percutaneous cervical cordotomy
    of cervical dorsal root ganglia *see under* dorsal root ganglion (DRG)
    cervical zygapophyseal joint denervation *see under* cervical zygapophyseal (facet) joints
    lumbar zygapophyseal joint denervation *see under* lumbar zygapophyseal (facet) joints
of sphenopalatine ganglion *see* sphenopalatine ganglion
theoretical aspects P327
tissue heating P327
vertebrogenic pain treatment *see* vertebrogenic pain
radiofrequency neurolysis, cryoanalgesia comparison P325
radiofrequency thermocoagulation, trigeminal neuralgia
    management **Ch496**
radiographs Ch127
dental pain diagnosis Ch483
limitations Ch127
neck pain diagnosis Ch136
osteoarthritis diagnosis Ch127
sensitivity Ch127
validity Ch127
radioiodine, metastatic bone pain treatment Ca286–Ca287
radioisotope therapy, bone pain management Ca285–Ca287
radiology, interventional, pain relief *see* interventional radiology
radionucleotides, adjuvant analgesic in children Ca342–Ca343
radionuclide studies, CRPSs diagnosis Ch389–Ch390
radiosurgery, neurosurgical techniques Ch298
ablative sites *Ch297*
radiotherapy Ca253–Ca257
bone pain management *see under* bone pain
brachial plexus neuropathies Ch374
in elderly Ca359
pain relief Ca253
pituitary ablation Ca256
specific indications Ca253–Ca256
    nerve pain **Ca254,** Ca255–Ca256
        see also nerve pain
    soft-tissue pain Ca253–Ca255, **Ca254**
        see also soft-tissue injuries/pain
tumor shrinkage Ca253
radioulnar joint, distal, intra-articular injections P266
Raeder syndrome **Ch482,** Ch485
Raggedy Ann, relaxation technique in children P150
Raj nerve block technique *see* infraclavicular block
Ramsay Hunt syndrome A370
Ramsay score, pain assessment in ICU **A342**
randomized controlled trials (RCTs)
acute pain P487–P488
in cancer pain clinical trials P473
chronic pain P489
epidural steroid injections P424–P425
intra-articular injections P255–P256
see also clinical trials
ranitidine, NSAIDs combination Ch231
Raynaud's phenomena, fibromyalgia association Ch616
recoil adjustments, chiropractic theory Ch345
rectal administration of drugs A206
in children Ca340–Ca341, P432
    systemic analgesia A449

morphine Ca128
nonsteroidal anti-inflammatory drugs A208–A209
opioids A211, A319, Ca51
    acute pain management P70
    advantages and disadvantages **A319**
rectal pain Ca13
anorectal ulceration in AIDS patients Ca383, *Ca384*
desmoid pain Ca13
recurrent infectious cystitis, pelvic pain Ch595
red flags
abdominal pain potentials **A373**
disability Ch46–Ch47
low back pain A407, **A407,** A416
neck pain Ch509–Ch510
phantom pain Ch431
spinal injuries A407, **A407**
referred pain Ch116, Ch505
cervical Ch505–Ch506, *Ch506*
cervical zygapophyseal (facet) joints P190
chest pain Ch506
mechanisms A9, *A10*
neck pain Ch505–Ch506, *Ch506*
occipital Ch506, *Ch507*
somatic Ch506
wide dynamic range (WDR) neurons Ch116
reflex sympathetic dystrophy *see* complex regional pain syndrome I (CRPS-I)
refractory cancer pain Ca143–Ca155
analgesic resistance Ca146
classification **Ca149**
mechanistic approach to management Ca148–Ca153
    interventions Ca148
    three-level approach Ca148, *Ca150*
    see also World Health Organization (WHO) analgesic ladder
neuropathic pain Ca152–Ca153
    clinical characteristics **Ca149**
    interventions *Ca151*
    management Ca148, Ca152–Ca153
    mixed – tumor associated Ca152–Ca153
    pure – nontumor associated Ca153
nonoral administration routes Ca147–Ca148
    intraspinal Ca148
    subcutaneous Ca147
    transdermal Ca147
potential mechanisms Ca146–Ca147
somatic pain Ca150–Ca152
    clinical characteristics **Ca149**
    deep Ca152
    interventions *Ca150*
    management Ca148, Ca151–Ca152
    superficial Ca151–Ca152
visceral pain Ca152
    clinical characteristics **Ca149**
    interventions *Ca151*
    management Ca148, Ca152
refractory pain
epidural treatment *see* epidural treatment of refractory pain
intracisternal catheterization *see* intracisternal treatment of refractory pain
intrathecal catheterization *see* intrathecal treatment of refractory pain
malignant *see* refractory cancer pain
Refsum syndrome, motor function Ch368
Regina v. Adams, malpractice claims Ch180
regional analgesia A510–A511
advantages and disadvantages **A511**
techniques for interventional radiology **A512**
regional anesthesia techniques

complications A330, A352
    effect on postoperative pain A330
    intravenous (Bier block) A88
    trauma pain management A352
rehabilitation
    after sports injuries *see* sports injury rehabilitation
    pain programs *see* comprehensive pain rehabilitation
        programs (CPRP)
Reibl v. Hughes, medical liability Ch178
reinjury rates, CPRP Ch322
relative potency assay *P452*, P452–P453
relaxation A287–A290, Ca275–Ca276
    advantages and disadvantages A293
    anxiety induction P130
    biofeedback aid *see* biofeedback, relaxation aid
    CBT component Ch328
    in children P150
        muscle relaxation P150
        progressive relaxation P150
        Raggedy Ann P150
    cognitive methods A288–A289
        see also distraction; imagery technique
    electromyograph assisted P124–P125
    evidence supporting effectiveness A290–A291
    massage *see* massage
    of muscle *see* muscle(s), relaxation techniques
    music *see* music therapy
    skin conductance assisted P125
    skin temperature assisted P125
    treatment (of)
        chronic back pain Ch532
        postoperative pain A291
        procedural pain Ca322
        tension-type headache Ch639
    see also complementary and alternative medicine
reliability, psychometric pain measure P9–P10
reliable test, definition Ch125
remifentanil A49, A350, P68
    pain management in ICU A343
    pharmacokinetics P68
remote pain, definition **Ch404**
renal cancer
    bone metastasis hormone treatment Ca288
    radiotherapy Ca255
    recurrence Ca10
renal colic A376
    management A376
renal complications/impairment
    acetaminophen induced Ch234
    influence on opioid pharmacokinetics Ca45–Ca46
    NSAID induced A59, A173, Ca188–Ca189, Ca356, Ch231,
        Ch261
    opioid induced Ca357
renal disease, effect on opioid pharmacokinetics P64
renal failure
    NSAID induced A59, A472
    pain management in ICU A347
reoperation, spinal cord stimulation comparison Ch291
reorientation, in intensive care unit (ICU) A342
reserpine, CRPS management Ch391
residential homes, problems for elderly patients Ca360
residual limb pain Ch428–Ch429
    acute just postamputation pain Ch427
    chronic *see under* postamputation pain
Resource-based Relative Value Scale (RBRVS) Ch168
respiratory arrest, TENS complication P349
respiratory complications, NSAIDs adverse effects Ch231
respiratory depression A191

delayed
    caudal analgesia induced A447
    epidural opioid induced A255
    epidural local anesthesia–opioid combination incidence **A257**
    epidural opioid-induced A173, A243, A254–A255, P312–P313
        incidence **A257**
        predisposing factors **A255**
        treatment and prophylaxis A258
    misconceptions among physicians Ch32
    in neonates A450
    opioid induced A173, A309–A310, Ca46–Ca47, Ca176–Ca177,
        P45, P63, P80, P437, P439
    PCA induced A232–A233
        management P398
        monitoring A225
respiratory disease, effect on opioid pharmacokinetics P64
respiratory distress, detection in elderly A471
respiratory failure, pain management in ICU A345, A347
respiratory symptoms Ca293–Ca297
    see also breathlessness (dyspnea); cough; hemoptysis
respiratory system, opioids' pharmacological effects P63
responsiveness, in cancer pain management P470
rest, sport injury management A491
    see also bed rest
resting sweat output, CRPS diagnosis Ch391
retinal hemorrhage, epidural steroid injection
    complication P423
retroperitoneal hemorrhage, celiac plexus block
    complications P250
retroperitoneal sarcoma, radiotherapy Ca255
Rexed's laminae A6–A7, *A7*
Reye's syndrome, aspirin induced Ca191
rhenium, metastatic bone pain treatment Ca287
rheumatic diseases Ch537
    classification **Ch537**
    disease-modifying antirheumatic drugs Ch539, **Ch540–Ch541**
    see also joint pain
rheumatoid arthritis Ch538–Ch542
    clinical features and investigations Ch538
    definition Ch538
    epidemiology Ch538
    laboratory features **Ch539**
    management Ch538–Ch542
        acetaminophen Ch235
        antidepressants Ch243
        apazone Ch228
        capsaicin **Ch219**
        diet modifications Ch542
        nonpharmacological therapy Ch539, Ch542
        NSAIDs Ch232, Ch539
        pharmacological therapy Ch539
        physical therapies Ch539, Ch542
    neck pain Ch508
    prognosis Ch542
        indicators of poor outcome **Ch542**
rheumatological pain, as acute musculoskeletal pain A393–A404
    see also musculoskeletal injuries/pain
rhizotomies Ca265
    central pain syndromes management Ch410
rib and thoracic zygapophyseal (facet) dysfunction P190
rib metastases Ca5
right hypochondrial pain, in hepatomegaly patients **Ca12**
right iliac fossa pain, in AIDS patients Ca388
right upper quadrant pain, in AIDS patients Ca388
rigidity Ch358
Riley–Day syndrome, motor function Ch368
ritonavir, in AIDS pain management Ca370
    potential drug contraindications **Ca370**

toxicities **Ca370**
rizatriptan, migraine management
efficacy in RCT Ch471
therapeutic use Ch473
rocking, infant pain management A295
evidence supporting effectiveness A296
rofecoxib A67, Ca201–Ca202
adverse effects Ca202, Ch230
characteristics **Ch229**
doses and treatment protocols Ca201
drug interactions **Ca201**
elderly pain management Ch654
evidence for efficacy Ca202
indications and contraindications Ca186–Ca187
pharmacokinetics Ca202
practical tips Ca202
Rogers v. Whitaker, medical liability Ch177
Roland–Morris Disability Scale Ch107
ropivacaine A86–A87, A334
alternative epidural analgesia P415
in pediatric surgery A448
peripheral nerve block agent P198
structure, physiochemical properties and clinical profile **A85**
routes of analgesia administration A205–A218, Ca128–Ca129,
Ch262
see also individual drugs/routes
roxithromycin, maxillary sinusitis management Ch487
Royal Adelaide Hospital (RAH) epidural chart **A194–A195**
Royal College of Anaesthetists Ch155
ryodoraku Ca271

sacral parasympathetic nerves, pelvis enervation Ch587–Ch588
sacral plexus block P220–P221
anatomical aspects P220–P221
complications P221
indications P220
landmarks and practical steps P221, *P221*
sacroiliac joint dysfunction P190–P191
chronic back pain Ch521–Ch522
Gillette test P190
leg length difference P190–P191
shear dysfunction P191
saddle block spinal, refractory cancer pain management Ca153
salicylates A64, Ca183
adverse effects Ca191
salicylic acid Ca183
salivary flow, increased with acupuncture Ca272
salpingo-oophoritis, pelvic pain Ch593–Ch594
samarium, metastatic bone pain treatment Ca286
gamma camera pictures *Ca287*
saphenous nerve block
at ankle P229
landmarks and practical steps P229, *P229*
at knee P227
complications P227
landmarks and practical steps P227, *P228*
saquinavir, in AIDS pain management Ca369
pharmacokinetics **Ca369**
toxicities **Ca369**
sarcoplasmic reticulum, damage, fibromyalgia/myofascial
pain Ch622
satisfaction, pain measure P8
saw palmetto, botanical therapy **Ch347**
saxitoxin, sodium channel interaction A75
Schober technique Ch146
sciatica A412, P418
allodynia Ch115
epidural steroid injection *see* epidural steroid injections

sciatic nerve block A269, P223–P226
anatomical aspects P224
anterior approach P225–P226
landmarks and practical steps P225–P226, *P226*
complications P226
indications P224
lateral approach P226
landmarks and practical steps P226, *P226*
lithotomy approach P225
landmarks and practical steps P225, *P225*
posterior approach P224
landmarks and practical steps P224, *P225*
sclerosing cholangitis, abdominal pain cause in AIDS
patients Ca388
scoliosis, chronic back pain Ch521
screening
animal model drugs Ch193
chest pain Ch560–Ch561, **Ch561**
depression diagnosis Ca81, Ca309
Endicott substitution criteria **Ca309**
spinal cord stimulation trial P386–P387
substance abuse patients Ca397, Ca400–Ca401, **Ca401**
zygapophyseal joint injections P271
secondary prevention, definition Ch16
second messenger systems **A20**
transcriptional and post-translational changes A26–A27
sedation
assessment scale **A192, A510**
conscious, in procedural pain management *see under*
procedural pain
end of life care Ca312
intravenous *see* intravenous sedation
opioid induced Ca46, Ca132, Ca169–Ca170, Ch206
clinical presentation Ca169
epidemiology Ca169
etiology and pathophysiology Ca169
evidence-based evaluation of management Ca169–Ca170
opioids Ch206
pain management in ICU A344
PCA induced, management P398
procedural pain management Ca325
for radiological procedures *see* interventional radiology
subcutaneous infusions in cancer pain control **P89**, P92
seizures, opioid induced Ca173–Ca174
selective serotonin reuptake inhibitors (SSRIs) Ca215, P101
adverse effects Ca217, Ch244, **Ch244,** P104
antidepressant drug choice Ch246
contraindications Ca216, **Ch486,** P102
dosing and treatment schedules P102, **P103**
mechanism of action Ch240
pharmacology **Ch240**
practical tips Ca217
pretreatment safety measures **P103**
treatment (of)
depression Ca309
elderly pain Ch654
fibromyalgia Ch625
neuropathic pain Ch242–Ch243
pelvic pain Ch599–Ch600
TMJ pain **Ch486**
see also antidepressants
self-hypnosis A289–A290, Ca274, **P115,** P116
analgesia comparison with PCA P116
frequency P116
pain management in pregnancy A379
self-injury Ch634
experimental animals Ch190
self-regulation skills training **P148**

in adolescents
    benefits P148–P149
    hypnosis P153–P154
  in adults P113–P119
    attention to pain P114
    managing expectancy P117
    meaning of pain P114
    mindfulness-based stress reduction P117
    mood disorders and pain P114
    "rehabilitation" model P117
  in children P147–P162
    aid to hypnosis in diagnosis P154–P155
    anxiety, fear, and pain P149
    benefits P148–P149
    bubble blowing P150
    common features P161
    conditions suitable for aid **P148**
    diaphragmatic breathing P149–P150
    mechanisms of change P160–P161
    procedures for which approaches are helpful **P148**
    theoretical rationale P160–P161
  see also biofeedback; hypnosis; relaxation; self-hypnosis
self-reporting of pain A469
  in children A105–A106, A438–A439, P432, *P433*
  in elderly Ca351
  in emergency rooms A104
Seltzer model Ch190–Ch191
sensation information A292
sensitivity
  definition Ch126
  opioid induced Ch206
sensory-evoked potentials P34–P35
sensory qualities P30
sensory testing P27–P38
  abnormal temporal summation testing P34
  basis P30–P31
  evaluation of pain P28
  future perspectives in advanced testing P35–P37
    combination with patient history and examination P35
    semiconductor lasers *P36,* P37
    thermode stimulators based on heat-foil technology P36, *P36*
  goal P30
  pressure threshold determination with algometer P32
  tactile sensibility estimation with von Frey filaments P31
  thermotest *see* thermotest
  vibratory threshold determination with vibrameter P31–P32
  see also neurophysiological techniques
sensory thalamic stimulation Ch294
sepsis
  in joints, intra-articular injection contraindication P258
  management A396
  spinal cord stimulation contraindication P381
septic arthritis A396–A397
  in AIDS patients Ca385
sequential trials, in cancer pain clinical trials P473
serotonergic syndrome Ca217, P102
serotonin (5-HT)
  5-HT$_3$ antagonists, as antiemetic A233
  CRPS pathogenesis Ch387
  fibromyalgia/myofascial pain Ch622
  in inflammatory pain A24
  role in descending control of pain A14
serotonin and norepinephrine reuptake inhibitors (SNRIs) P101
  adverse effects **Ch244,** P104
  contraindication P102
  dosing and treatment schedules P102, **P103**
  pharmacology **Ch240**

pretreatment safety measures **P103**
  see also antidepressants
serotonin syndrome Ca217, P102
sertraline, central pain syndrome management **Ch409**
sexual dysfunction Ch74
  assessment Ch633
  libido loss Ch165
  measurement Ch74, **Ch75**
sexuality
  history assessment Ca79–Ca80
  importance in relationships Ca79–Ca80
  potential problems Ca79
sexual/physical abuse, pelvic pain Ch598
shear dysfunction P191
shiatsu acupressure Ca271
shiatsu massage Ca276
shingles *see* herpes zoster
short-lasting unilateral neuralgiform pain with conjunctival injection and tearing (SUNCT) Ch485
short therapy (ST) P186
shoulder
  intra-articular injections P262–P263
    glenohumeral joint *see* glenohumeral joint
    subacromial bursa *P262,* P262–P263
  pain A399–A400, Ch545
    clinical features A399
    epidemiology and diagnosis Ch545
    investigations/management A399–A400
    management Ch545
  rotator device *P183*
  surgery
    arthroscopy, postsurgical pain syndromes Ch420
    nerve blocks A271, A333
shoulder–hand syndrome, CRPS Ch386
sickle cell disease A382, Ch642–Ch643
  crises A280
  diagnosis Ch642
  management A383, Ch643
    American Pain Society Ch643
    corticosteroids A383
    epidural analgesia A383
    nonsteroidal anti-inflammatory drugs A383
    opioids A383
  pain Ca403
    in children Ch642–Ch643
    features A382–A383
  precipitating mechanisms Ch643
  prevalence Ch642–Ch643
Sickness Impact Profile (SIP) Ch76, Ch103–Ch104, Ch150, Ch653
Sidaway Case, medical liability Ch177
simple analgesics, in elderly *see under* elderly
simple nerve blocks, in pediatric surgery A445–A448
  efficacy **A445**
simple studies, definition Ch18
single-photon emission computed tomography (SPECT) Ch130
  neck pain investigations Ch511
sinusitis, headache diagnosis Ch470
SIP-Roland Ch149
SIP-Roland (pain questionnaire) Ch149
Sjögren syndrome, motor function Ch368
skin
  blood-flow Doppler probes, CRPS diagnosis Ch389
  burn, TENS complication P348
  irritation, TENS complication Ca247, P348
  opioids' pharmacological effects P63
skin conductance-assisted relaxation P125
skin temperature-assisted relaxation P125
skin-to-skin contact with parent, infant pain management A295

evidence supporting effectiveness A296
skull base metastases Ca5–Ca6
    clinical features Ca5–Ca6
    CT scan *Ca7*
    foramina of cranial nerves *Ca6*
sleep apnea, patient-controlled analgesia (PCA) A228–A229
sleep disorders Ch74, Ch634
    fibromyalgia association Ch616
    measurement Ch74, **Ch75**
slippery elm, botanical therapy **Ch347**
slipping rib syndrome, chronic chest pain Ch560
small-cell lung cancer, bone metastasis chemotherapy Ca287
small-fiber neuropathy, diabetic neuropathy Ch371
small intestine, opioids' pharmacological effects P62
Smith v. Royal Melbourne Hospital, malpractice claims Ch180
social factors, influencing childbirth pain A429–A430
    see also psychosocial factors
social resources, assessment Ca76–Ca77
Social Security Administration (SSA)
    disability definition Ch42
    disability evaluation (USA) Ch39
Social Security Disability Income (SSDI), disability evaluation
    (USA) Ch39, Ch41
    case history Ch53–Ch60
sodium channels
    antagonists
        antiarrhythmics Ch255
        neurologic disease management Ch361
    local anesthesia interaction A74–A75
    structure and function A74, *A75*
sodium valproate
    adverse effects Ca214, P107
    clinical trials Ch253
    contraindications P105
    doses and treatment paradigms Ca214, **P106**, P107
    mechanism of action Ch252
    pharmacokinetics Ca214
    pretreatment safety measures **P106**, P107
    treatment (of)
        central pain syndrome Ch409
        CRPS Ch394
        migraine Ch475
        painful spasticity **Ch461**
        peripheral neuropathy Ch377
        tension-type headache Ch475
soft-tissue injuries/pain Ch545–Ch547
    classification Ch545
    indications for radiotherapy Ca253–Ca255, **Ca254**
        chest pain Ca253–Ca254
        headache Ca254
        liver pain Ca254–Ca255
        loin pain Ca255
        para-aortic lymphadenopathy Ca255
        pelvic pain Ca255
        splenic pain Ca255
    management, topical NSAIDs Ch216–Ch217, Ch217
    sport injury classification A486
Somatic Amplification Scale Ch76
somatic pain A5, A96, Ca65, Ca260
    in AIDS patients Ca378–Ca385
    childbirth pain A425
    pelvic pain Ch588
    referred Ch506
    in refractory cancer pain *see under* refractory cancer pain
    visceral pain comparison **A6**
        in abdominal pain A373–A374
somatization, poor prognostic factor Ca67
somatization disorders Ch69, Ch71, Ch75, Ch632–Ch633

diagnosis **Ch71,** Ch632
etiology Ch632–Ch633
measurement Ch71, Ch75, **Ch75**
secondary medical problems Ch632
somatostatin, role in nociceptive signaling in dorsal horn A9
sorivudine, acute herpes zoster pain Ch439
spasticity, painful Ch358, Ch459–Ch466
    assessment techniques Ch460, **Ch461**
    causes **Ch459**
    central lesions Ch460
    clinical outcomes Ch464–Ch465
    depression Ch460
    epidural treatment of refractory pain P309
    focal muscle activity Ch460
        external stimuli Ch460
        noxious stimuli Ch460
        overuse/fatigue Ch460
    management Ch461–Ch464
        botulinum toxin injections Ch463–Ch464
            dosing guidelines **P281**
        chemodenervation Ch463–Ch464, **Ch464**
        intrathecal medications Ch463, **Ch464**
        oral medications **Ch461,** Ch461–Ch463, **Ch462**
        phenol/alcohol neurolysis Ch463
        physical therapy Ch461
        surgery Ch463, **Ch463**
    orthopedic abnormalities Ch460
    pathophysiology Ch459–Ch460
    peripheral nerve injury Ch460
    spinal cord injury Ch460
    TENS indication P344
spa therapy, chronic back pain management Ch532
specificity, definition Ch126
sphenopalatine ganglion, radiofrequency lesioning P331–P332
    anatomical aspects P331
    complications and incidence P332
    efficacy of treatment P332
    historical aspects P331
    indications P331
    results P332
    technique P331–P332
        anesthesia administration P331
        electrode projection P331–P332, *P332*
        projection of sphenopalatine fossa P331, *P332*
sphincter dyssynergia, management, botulinum toxin
    injections Ch464
Spielberger State–Trait Anxiety Inventory Ch105
spinal accessory nerve block P202–P203
    anatomical aspects P202
    complications P203
    indications P202
    landmarks and practical steps P202, *P202*
spinal cord
    analgesia P410
        intraspinal opioids *see* intraspinal opioids
        see also epidural analgesia/anesthesia; intrathecal
            analgesia
    blood flow not decreased with epinephrine P412–P413
    compression *see* spinal cord compression
    damage due to intraspinal opioids A250–A251
    injury *see* spinal cord injury
    modulation of nociceptive activity A11–A13, *A12*
    nociception *see* nociception, in spinal cord
    physiotherapy McKenzie approach P183
    stimulation *see* spinal cord stimulation (SCS)
    symptoms and signs caused by meningeal carcinomatosis **Ca8**
    yellow flags of injuries **A408**
spinal cord compression Ca6, Ca8

associated cancers Ca6
imaging Ca6, Ca8
MRI scan *Ca8*
pain Ca6
pain syndromes caused by **Ca4, Ca7**
spinal cord injury
central pain Ch406
central pain syndromes Ch404
CRPS pathogenesis Ch387
management, lidocaine, intravenous Ch256
painful spasticity Ch460
spinal cord stimulation (SCS) Ca248–Ca249, Ch287–Ch293, P381–
P389
anatomical aspects P381
complications Ca248, P388
contraindications P381–P382
efficacy Ca249
clinical Ch556
electrodes *P382*
flat plate *P382*
insertion P381, P385
implantation of system P384–P388
first stage P384–P387
identifying desired level of entry P384–P385
patient positioning P384
performing test stimulation P386
permanent implantation P387–P388
screening trial P386–P387
second stage P387–P388
sedation P385
inclusion/exclusion criteria Ch289
indications Ch289–Ch293, P382
see also individual disorders
limitations P382
patient selection P382
mechanism of action Ca248, Ch556
ischemic pain states Ch289
neurochemical mechanisms Ch288
neurophysiological mechanisms Ch288
pain clinics **Ch159**
practical issues Ca248
electrode positioning Ca248
trial stimulation period Ca248
preparation P382–P384
equipment P382–P384
patient P384
programming P388
radiofrequency (RF)-coupled system P383
external transmitter unit *P383*
radioreceiver *P383*
reoperation comparisons Ch291
safety Ch556
totally implantable system P382–P383
implantable pulse generator (IPG) P382–P383, *P383*
treatment (of)
chronic back pain Ch531
CRPS Ch395
peripheral neuropathy Ch378
refractory angina pectoris Ch556–Ch557
syndrome X Ch558
spinal drugs, neurologic disease management Ch362
spinal manipulation
chronic back pain management Ch528
low back pain management A411
spinal nerve root pain P417
diagnosis P418
spine (vertebral column)
cervical *see* cervical spine

enervation **Ch523,** Ch523–Ch524
functional spinal unit Ch523
facet joint *Ch522*
intervertebral disks Ch522
anatomy *Ch522*
annulus fibrosis *Ch522*
damage Ch137–Ch140
nucleus pulposus *Ch522*
ligaments Ch523
anatomy *Ch522*
anterior longitudinal *Ch522*
interspinous *Ch522,* Ch523
posterior longitudinal *Ch522*
supraspinous *Ch522*
lumbar *see* lumbar spine
muscles Ch523
nerve roots Ch522–Ch523
pain
diagnosis Ch134, Ch135
differential diagnosis Ch135
red flags Ch431
see also back pain
vertebrae Ch521
anatomy *Ch522*
posterior arch *Ch522*
spinous processes *Ch522*
superior articular facets *Ch522*
trabeculae Ch521
transverse processes *Ch522*
vertebral body *Ch522*
vertebral end plate *Ch522*
spine rehabilitation programs Ch318
flexion exercises Ch318
primary extension exercises Ch318
spinomesencephalic pathway A9
spinoreticular pathway A9
spinothalamic tract (STT) A9
central pain syndromes Ch405
spinous processes *Ch522*
spiritual pain Ca107
splenic pain, indication for radiotherapy Ca255
splints, osteoarthritis management Ch544
sports injury rehabilitation A485–A496
classification of injuries A485–A486
according to tissue involved A486
acute A485
overuse A485
secondary A485–A486
clinical presentation A490–A491
acute injuries A490
overuse injuries A490–A491
investigations A491
imaging A491
management A491–A496
corticosteroids A495–A496
cryotherapy *see under* cryoanalgesia
electrotherapeutic modalities A496
immobilization A492
initial treatment A491–A492
pharmacological therapy A493–A495
superficial heat therapy A493
pathophysiology of tissue injury and repair A486–A490
see also tissue response to injury
prognosis A496–A497
Spouse Response Scale Ch108
spray and stretch techniques, fibromyalgia/myofascial pain
management Ch624–Ch625
squamous cell carcinoma, in AIDS patients

anal pain Ca383
oral pain Ca381
squint surgery, wound infiltration in pediatric surgery A445
SSRIs *see* selective serotonin reuptake inhibitors (SSRIs)
Staphylococcus aureus, pathogen in AIDS cutaneous pain Ca382
State–Trait Anxiety Inventory Ch71, Ch105–Ch106
static hyperalgesia Ch115, **Ch121**
static strengthening, physical therapy Ch316
stavudine, toxic neuropathy Ch373
stellate ganglion block Ch131, P237–P240
    acute herpes zoster pain Ch443
    complications Ch443, P239–P240
        less dramatic P239–P240
        life-threatening P239
    neurolytic P240
    signs P239
    technique P238–P239
    see also sympathetic blocks
stellate ganglion injection, left, refractory angina pectoris
    management Ch557
stenting
    pain relief in interventional radiology A503–A504
    percutaneous biliary A507
stereoisomers A86
    of lactic acid *A86*
stereotactic cryohypophysectomy Ch300
stereotactic encephalotomy, painful spasticity
    management **Ch463**
stereotactic medial thalamotomy Ca265–Ca266
stereotactic mesencephalic tractomy, central pain syndromes
    management Ch411
stereotactic nucleotractotomy Ca265
stereotactic radiofrequency hypophysectomy Ch300
stereotaxis, neurosurgical techniques Ch298
steroid pseudorheumatism **Ca14,** Ca15–Ca16
steroids
    adjuvant analgesics Ca135
    adverse effects Ca135
    CRPS management Ch392–Ch393
    epidural, low back pain treatment A412
    in epidural steroid injections P422
    refractory cancer pain management Ca152
    TMJ pain management **Ch486**
    see also corticosteroids
Stevens–Johnson syndrome, anticonvulsants adverse
    effects Ch254
stiffness, fibromyalgia association Ch616
stimulants prohibited in IOC medical code A498
    examples A501 A
stimulation-induced analgesia A14, Ca245–Ca251
    action potential stimulation therapy P344
    of brain *see* brain stimulation
    cutaneous field stimulation P186, P344
    electrical muscle stimulation (EMS) P186
    electrical stimulation P185–P186
    historical aspects Ca245
    interferential therapy P344
    peripheral nerve stimulation *see* peripheral nerve stimulation
        (PNS)
    pragmatic approach Ca249–Ca250
    of spinal cord *see* spinal cord stimulation (SCS)
    TENS *see* transcutaneous electrical nerve stimulation (TENS)
St John's wort, botanical therapy **Ch347**
stomach
    complications *see* gastric complications
    delayed emptying A254
    opioids' pharmacological effects P62
stomach pain

chronic ulceration Ch582
    epidemiology, age related Ch21
    ulcers, NSAID induced Ca187–Ca188
strabismus surgery, wound infiltration in pediatric surgery A445
Streptococcus pneumoniae, maxillary sinusitis Ch485
stress Ch326
    mindfulness-based reduction P117
    recurrent abdominal pain Ch640
stress fractures, diagnosis, bone scans Ch129
stress response, CRPS pathogenesis Ch386
stress response hormones, increased release during
    childbirth A427
stroke pain Ca403
    central pain syndromes Ch406
    see also poststroke pain
strontium, metastatic bone pain treatment Ca286
subacromial bursa, intra-articular injections *P262,* P262–P263
    RCTs P255–P256
subacromial space, local anesthetic infiltration into cavity A269
subarachnoid administration of drugs A208
subarachnoid analgesia *see* intrathecal analgesia
subarachnoid space P286, *P286*
subclavian perivascular nerve block technique *see* supraclavicular
    block
subcutaneous administration of drugs A206, P85–P86
    advantages P85–P86
    cancer pain management *see* cancer pain, subcutaneous
        infusions
    in children Ca340, P432–P433
    infiltration of local anesthesia A268
    opioids A211, A317, A474, Ca51
    patient-controlled analgesia (PCA) A227, P395
    in refractory cancer pain Ca147
subdural hematoma, spinal cord stimulation complication P388
subdural space P286
subintimal angioplasty, pain relief in interventional
    radiology A504
sublingual administration of drugs A205–A206, Ca128
    opioids A210–A211, A318, Ca50
        acute pain management P70
    patient-controlled analgesia delivery route P404
subluxation complex
    chiropractic theory Ch344–Ch345
    myofascial pain association Ch616
substance abuse Ch69, Ch70–Ch71, Ch71
    behavioral patterns **Ch71**
    benzodiazepines Ch633–Ch634
    CPRP Ch167
    definition Ch633
    diagnosis **Ch71**
        psychiatric Ch633–Ch634
    iatrogenic drugs Ch633
    laboratory findings **Ch71**
    measurement Ch71
    opioids Ca395, Ca399–Ca400, Ch205, Ch207, Ch633
        methadone Ca399–Ca400
        physical dependence Ca396
        underprescribing Ca396
    patients *see* substance abuse patients
    physical findings **Ch71**
    pseudoaddiction Ca397
    research Ca401
    spectrum of clinical problems **Ca397**
    undertreatment of pain Ca396
    see also addiction
substance abuse patients Ca395–Ca402
    assessment Ca64, Ca396–Ca397, **Ca397**
    care team workers **Ca397**

case example Ca401
drug testing Ca400–Ca401
body fluid screening Ca400–Ca401, **Ca401**
substance detection Ca400–Ca401
impact of abuse on pain management Ca396, **Ca397**
effect on outcome of treatment Ca398
management guidelines Ca397–Ca398
case series **Ca398**
contraindications to opioid therapy Ca398
multidisciplinary program Ca397, **Ca398**
screening procedures Ca397
medicolegal issues Ca401
psychosocial support groups Ca399
pilot program structure **Ca399**
written care agreements Ca399
outcomes **Ca399**
sample content *Ca400*
suggested criteria **Ca399**
substance dependence *see* addiction
substance P
central pain involvement Ch406
in inflammatory pain A27, A33–A34
see also neurokinin 1 (NK1) antagonists
sucrose, infant pain management A295
evidence supporting effectiveness A297
sufentanil A49, P68
alternative epidural analgesia P415
epidural
lipid solubility, doses, onset and analgesia duration **A243**
in PCEA **A247**
intrathecal A249
adverse effects A250
procedural pain management Ca326
transmucosal delivery in PCA P402
suffering Ch91
definition Ch5–Ch6
clinical Ch6
cultural conditioning Ch6
medical discussion Ch5–Ch6
pain synonym Ch5
suggestion principle, placebos Ch274, Ch278
suicide Ch634
cancer-related Ca29, Ca81
in depressive patients Ca310
in elderly Ca352–Ca353
risk assessment Ca81
depression link Ca310, Ch634
evaluation Ch634
sulfonamides A66–A67
sulfones A66–A67
sulindac A65
characteristics **Ch229**
sumatriptan, migraine management Ch471
children Ch638
efficacy in RCT Ch471
therapeutic use Ch473
summed pain intensity differences (SPID) *P451*, P456
superficial heat therapy, sport injury management A493
superior articular facets *Ch522*
superior hypogastric plexus block P251–P252
anatomical aspects P251
complications P252
efficacy P252
technique P251–P252
needle placement and contrast medium spread *P252*
superior vena caval syndrome (SVCS), management Ca294
Supplemental Security Income (SSI), disability evaluation
(USA) Ch39

supplements, food Ca273
support groups, trigeminal neuralgia Ch493–Ch494
supraclavicular block P207–P208
landmarks and practical steps *P207*, P208
supraorbital nerve block P202
complications P202
landmarks and practical steps P202
suprascapular nerve block P210
anatomical aspects P210
complications P210
indications P210
local anesthetic and depot steroid blocks P210
local anesthetic block P210
neurolytic block P210
landmarks and practical steps P210, *P211*
supraspinous ligaments *Ch522*
supratrochlear nerve block P202
complications P202
landmarks and practical steps P202
sural nerve block P229
landmarks and practical steps P229, *P229*
suramin Ch266
surface administration of drugs A207
nonsteroidal anti-inflammatory drugs A209–A210
opioids A211–A212
surgeons, role in acute pain service A183, A185
surgery
abdominal gynecological, timing of administration of local
anesthetics A120
ablative *see under* neurosurgical modalities/techniques
ambulatory, intraspinal opioids A248, **A248**
arthroscopic *see* arthroscopic surgery
in children *see under* children
considerations A336
day case, pain management *see under* postoperative pain
management
dental, wound infiltration in pediatric surgery A445
laparoscopic *see* laparoscopic surgery
limiting factors A329
metabolic response **A313**
neural pathways activated in response to *A167*
neuroendocrine response *A167*, A312–A313, **A313**
effect of different analgesic regimens A312–A313
postoperative pain causes **A314**
postsurgical pain *see* postsurgical pain syndromes
treatment (of)
neck pain management Ch514
neurologic disease Ch363–Ch364
neuropathic pain Ca261
osteoarthritis Ch545
painful spasticity Ch463, **Ch463**
postherpetic neuralgia Ch454
treatment options in perioperative period *A115*
see also individual conditions, procedures
surgical sectioning of nerves, neurolysis comparison **Ca236**
Survey of Pain Attitudes (SOPA) Ch107, Ch148, P166
swaddling, infant pain management A295
evidence supporting effectiveness A295–A296
swallowing, painful, in AIDS patients *see* AIDS, odynophagia
(painful swallowing)
sweating Ca308–Ca309
clinical findings and investigations Ca308
management Ca308–Ca309
pathology Ca308
resting output, CRPS diagnosis Ch391
sympathectomy
central pain syndromes management Ch410
indications P233

phantom pain management Ch431
sympathetic activity A167
    neural pathways activated in response to surgery *A167*
sympathetically maintained pain (SMP) Ch387
    diagnosis **Ch384**
sympathetic axis, neurolysis P247
    see also individual nerve blocks
sympathetic blocks Ch131, P233–P246
    acute herpes zoster pain management A371–A372, Ch443
    contraindications P237
    CRPS diagnosis Ch131
    image intensifier and contrast enhancement P237
    indications P233, P235–P236
        acute pain P235
        chronic pain P235–P236
    intravenous regional *see* intravenous regional sympathetic
        block
    local anesthetics P237
    lumbar *see* lumbar sympathetic block
    mechanism Ch131
    phantom pain Ch431
    placebo effect Ch131
    stellate ganglion *see* stellate ganglion block
    tests
        blood flow P236
        for completeness P236
        of function P236
        of pain P236
        pain assessment P237
        skin conductance response P237
        skin temperature P236–P237
        of sympathetic function P236
    thoracic *see* thoracic sympathetic block
    validity Ch131
    verification of blocking solution P237
sympathetic chain P233, P235
    cervicothoracic P237, *P238*
        block *see* stellate ganglion block
    neurolytic nerve blocks Ca240
    radiofrequency lesioning Ca242–Ca243
sympathetic ganglia (lumbar)
    neurolytic blocks P243
    radiofrequency lesioning P338–P339
        adverse effects P339
        complications P339
        contraindication P338
        efficacy of treatment P339
        indication P338
        technique P338–P339
sympathetic hyperactivity, CRPS Ch122
sympathetic nervous system P233
    anatomy P233–P235, *P234*
    nerve endings and receptors *P236*
    nerve supply to blood vessels *P234*
sympathetic postganglionic neurons (SPGNs), CRPS
    pathogenesis Ch387–Ch388
sympathetic skin response, CRPS diagnosis Ch391
sympatholytic drugs A330
symptomatic osteoarthrosis A398–A399
Symptom Checklist 90-Revised (SCL 90-R) Ch75, Ch106, Ch149
syncope
    acupuncture induced Ch342
    local anesthesia adverse effect A83
SynchroMed externally programmable pump *P315*
syndrome X Ch557–Ch558
    assessment Ch557–Ch558
    clinical considerations Ch557
    management Ch557–Ch558, **Ch558**

synesthesalgesia, definition **Ch404**
synovial fluid aspiration, articular musculoskeletal pain
    diagnosis A395
synovial joints, response to injuries A489–A490
syringe drivers P85
    administration rates P87–P88
        PCA P87
        reasons to prefer fixed rate to variable rate P87
    choice P87
        differing volume syringes *P87*
        Graseby models *P87*
    connecting tubing *P88*
    types P88
    use P86–P88
syringomyelia, diagnosis Ch133
systematic reviews P495–P505
    definition P495
    evidence accumulation P496–P497
        sensitive search strategies P497, **P497**
        trials to include P496–P497
    evidence appraisal P497–P498
    evidence-based medicine *P495,* P495–P496
    hierarchy of evidence **P496**
    qualitative P501–P503
        efficacy assessment P502–P503
        evidence appraisal P501–P503
        quality control P501–P502
        validity assessment P502–P503, **P503**
    quantitative *see* meta-analysis
    review process *P496*
    review question P496, **P497**
systemic analgesics
    in children *see under* children
    effect on pulmonary sequelae of pain A311
    gastrointestinal recovery, comparison with epidural
        analgesia **A172**
    pain management in pregnancy A379
        analgesia ladder *A378*
        drugs not frequently used **A382**
        drugs used **A381**
    see also individual drugs
systemic infection
    spinal cord stimulation contraindication P381
systemic opioids, in multimodal anesthesia A322
systemic toxicity
    clinical presentation **A82**
    local anesthesia complication A81
systemic treatments, pruritus management Ca308

tachycardia, meperidine induced P62
tachykinins **A25**
    CRPS pathogenesis Ch387
    in inflammatory pain A24–A25
    synthesis in nociceptors A33
tactile sensibility, estimation with von Frey filaments P31
tamoxifen, breast cancer treatment Ca288
Tampa Scale for Kinesiophobia (TSK) Ch74, Ch105, P166
Tangier syndrome Ch375
    motor function Ch368
taste alterations Ca298
taxols, toxic neuropathy Ch372
teaching hospitals, pain clinics (UK) Ch159–Ch160
teamworking Ca95–Ca104
    downside and potential ways of failure Ca98–Ca100
        absent planning and maintenance Ca100
        conflict and communication breakdown Ca98–Ca99
        problems with power, status, and communication Ca99–
            Ca100

time Ca98
experienced team Ca96–Ca97
    review Ca102
factors contributing to success Ca98, **Ca99**
    clarity Ca98
    support and peer supervision Ca98
    time Ca98
    variety of members Ca98, **Ca99**
inexperienced team Ca95–Ca96
    review Ca101–Ca102
management strategies *Ca103*
planning and developing a team Ca100–Ca101, **Ca101**
    natural stages **Ca101**
    organizational development (OD) Ca100–Ca101
requirement in cancer management Ca97
    issues for clinician Ca97
    issues for patient Ca97
review of scenarios Ca101–Ca102
setting the scene Ca95–Ca97
team definition Ca97
temperature changes, opioid induced P62
temporal summation, testing of abnormal findings P34
temporomandibular joint (TMJ) pain **Ch482**, Ch484–Ch485
    anticonvulsant clinical trials Ch253
    clinical presentation Ch485
    definitions Ch484
    diagnosis Ch135, Ch484, Ch485, **Ch485**
    epidemiology Ch485
    etiology/pathophysiology Ch484–Ch485
        occlusal factors Ch484
        psychological factors Ch484
        traumatic factors (meniscal displacement) Ch484–Ch485
    management **Ch486**
        capsaicin **Ch219**
tenderness, CRPS Ch383
tender points (TePs)
    fibromyalgia Ch618
    locations Ch618
    palpation Ch618–Ch619
tendinitis, management, topical NSAIDs Ch216
tendonopathy, diagnosis, ultrasound Ch129
tendons
    lengthening, painful spasticity management **Ch463**
    reflexes in peripheral neuropathies Ch368
    response to injury A490
tennis elbow Ch546
tenovir disoproxil fumarate, AIDS pain treatment Ca368
tenoxicam, characteristics **Ch229**
TENS *see* transcutaneous electrical nerve stimulation (TENS)
tension-type headaches
    in children *see under* children
    classification Ch467
    clinical features Ch468
    diagnosis Ch470
    epidemiology Ch468
        frequency Ch468
        gender differences Ch468
        prevalence Ch468
    improvement rates from meta-analyses **P131**
    improvement rates from separate meta-analyses **P131**
    International Headache Society (IHS) classification Ch639
    location Ch468
    management Ch473
        acetaminophen Ch473, Ch639
        acupuncture Ch343
        antidepressants Ch243
        aspirin Ch473
        ibuprofen Ch639

nonpharmaceutical Ch473, Ch475, Ch639
        NSAIDs Ch473
        relaxation techniques Ch639
        tricyclic antidepressants (TCAs) Ch475
    pain description Ch468
    pathophysiology Ch469–Ch470
        initiating factors Ch470
        pain sensitivity Ch470
        pericranial muscles Ch469–Ch470
        stress Ch469
    in pregnancy A377
    prophylactic management Ch475
        botulinum toxin Ch475
        tricyclic antidepressants Ch475
terminal cancer syndrome Ca109
tertiary prevention, definition Ch16
testes, pain Ch581
test–retest reliability
    pain measure P9
tetracaine A83
tetracyclic antidepressants
    osteoarthritis management Ch544
    pharmacology **Ch240**
Δ9-tetra-hydrocannabinol (THC), anorexia–cachexia syndrome
    management Ca306
tetrodotoxin, sodium channel interaction A75
thalamotomy Ch298–Ch299
    complications Ch298
    implanted electrodes Ch299
    indications Ch298–Ch299
    intraoperative physiological testing Ch299
    macrostimulation Ch299
    microelectrode recording Ch299
    nociceptive pain management Ch298
    stereotactic medial Ca265–Ca266
    targets Ch298
thalamotomy, central pain syndromes management Ch411
thalamus, fibromyalgia/myofascial pain Ch622
thalidomide, aphthous ulceration treatment in AIDS
    patients Ca382
thallium poisoning, peripheral neuropathies Ch372
therapeutic dependence Ca49
therapeutic touch Ca276
thermal grill Ch405
thermal thresholds, measurements with thermotest *P32*
thermocoagulation, radiofrequency, trigeminal neuralgia
    management **Ch496**
thermography Ch130–Ch131
    CRPS diagnosis Ch130–Ch131
    mechanism Ch130
    validity Ch131
thermotest P32–P34
    abnormal sensory disturbances to heat stimulation *P33*
    choice of skin area tested P33
    execution P34
    indications P34
    method of limits P33
    normal thermal thresholds measured *P32*
    potential influences of results P33
    two-alternative forced choice method P32–P33
    typical findings P34
thiamine deficiency, peripheral neuropathies Ch371–Ch372
thigh
    lateral cutaneous nerve block *see* lateral cutaneous nerve,
        thigh blockade
    posterior cutaneous nerve block P227
third-party-defined outcomes, pain measures P8
thoracic epidural anesthesia (TEA)

cardiac outcome management A167
in children P442–P443
refractory angina pectoris management Ch557
thoracic paravertebral block A270, P215
anatomical aspects P215
chest trauma management A353
complications P215
indications P215
local anesthetic and steroid block P215
local anesthetic block P215
neurolytic block P215
landmarks and practical steps P215, *P215*
in pediatric surgery A448–A449
thoracic sympathetic block *P240*, P240–P241
acute herpes zoster pain Ch443–Ch444
complications P241
indications P240
technique P241
thoracic trauma, epidural analgesia A343–A344
thoracic zygapophyseal (facet) and rib dysfunction P190
thoracoabdominal radiculopathy, diabetic neuropathy Ch371
thoracolumbar sympathetic nerves, pelvis enervation Ch587–
Ch588
thoracotomy
intercostal nerve block cryoanalgesia P322–P323
postoperative pain
assessment *A105*
epidemiology Ch22
relief A244
postsurgical pain syndromes Ch420
thorax peripheral nerve blocks P215–P218
see also individual types
thrombolysis, pain relief in interventional radiology A503–A504
thrush *see* pseudomembranous candidiasis (thrush)
tibial nerve block
at ankle P230
landmarks and practical steps *P229,* P230
at knee P227
landmarks and practical steps P227, *P228*
Tietze syndrome, chronic chest pain Ch559
timing of treatment A113–A162
definitions and terminology A114–A116
future research recommendations A125–A127
analgesia consumption measures A126–A127
improving quality of studies A126
pain measures A126
preexisting pain and analgesia relationship A125
preventive opioid analgesia A125–A126
literature review A116–A125
local anesthesia administration A116–A120, **A136–A143,
A161–A162**
multimodal analgesia administration A125, **A161–A162**
NMDA receptor antagonist administration A121–A123,
A148–A151
NSAIDs administration A123–A124, **A152–A154, A161–
A162**
opioid administration A120–A121, **A144–A147, A161–
A162**
opioid–local anesthesia combination A124–A125
opioid–local anesthesia combination
administration **A155–A160**
studies
according to target agent administered **A119**
criteria for including studies A116
excluded experiments **A117**
search strategies A116
variety and frequency of designs **A118**
targets of preemptive and preventive analgesia A114

treatment options in perioperative period *A115*
see also preemptive analgesia; preventive analgesia
tissue response to injury A486–A490
acute inflammatory response A486–A487, *A487*
chemical mediator release A486–A487
classical local signs A486
individual reactions of tissues A488–A490
remodeling and maturation phase A487–A488
pathophysiology and treatment of injuries A488, *A488*
repair and regeneration phase A487
scar tissue formation A487
see also individual tissues
tizanidine
clinical trials Ch252
treatment (of)
CRPS Ch391
neurologic disease Ch361
painful spasticity **Ch462**
trigeminal neuralgia Ch493, **Ch494–Ch495**
tocainide
clinical trials Ch252
treatment (of)
central pain syndrome Ch409
trigeminal neuralgia Ch493, **Ch494–Ch495**
tolerance Ca48
acquired Ca48
in cancer pain management P470
in children Ca344
cross-tolerance Ca48
definition Ch208
in elderly Ca350
fear of Ca48
learned Ca48
in opioid therapy A50, Ca48–Ca49, Ca131, Ca177, Ca404,
Ch206, Ch209, P64, P80
cross-tolerance Ca48–Ca49
management P64
pharmacodynamic Ca48
pharmacokinetic Ca48
TENS complication Ca247, P348–P349
tolmetin A66
characteristics **Ch229**
Tolosa–Hunt syndrome **Ch482,** Ch485
diagnosis Ch133
tonsillectomy
timing of administration of local anesthetics A117
wound infiltration in pediatric surgery A445
tooth appearance, dental pain **Ch483**
topical administration of drugs A87, A207
in children Ca340
opioids A211–A212
pruritus management Ca308
see also transdermal administration of drugs
topical analgesia Ch213–Ch226
anti-inflammatory agents, acute herpes zoster pain Ch440
benzocaine A87
dibucaine A87
lidocaine Ch257
NSAIDs *see* nonsteroidal anti-inflammatory drugs, topical (T/
NSAIDs)
opioids *see* opioids, topical
transcutaneous delivery Ch213
dosing Ch213
treatment (of)
acute herpes zoster pain Ch441–Ch442
CRPS Ch393
elderly pain Ch655
osteoarthritis Ch543

postherpetic neuralgia Ch453–Ch454
pruritus Ca308
trigeminal neuralgia Ch494
see also individual drugs
topical anesthesia A87
local *see* topical local anesthesia
procedural pain management in children A452
topical capsaicin Ch218–Ch221, Ch265–Ch266
adverse effects Ch219
erythema Ch219
noncompliance Ch219
clinical studies Ch266
contraindications Ch218
definition Ch218
doses Ch218–Ch219
amount Ch218
application Ch218
co-management Ch218–Ch219
frequency Ch218
efficacy Ch219, Ch221
indications Ch218, *Ch219*
management paradigms Ch218–Ch219
mechanism of action Ch218
treatment (of)
arthritis Ch220, Ch221
CRPS **Ch219,** Ch221, Ch393
diabetic neuropathy Ch219–Ch220, *Ch220,* Ch221
dysesthetic vulvodynia Ch604
facial pain Ch221
headache Ch221
neuropathic pain Ch119
osteoarthritis *Ch220,* Ch543
peripheral neuropathy Ch377
postamputation pain Ch221
postherpetic neuralgia Ch220, *Ch220,* Ch221, Ch453–
Ch454
postsurgical pain syndromes Ch220, *Ch220,* Ch221,
Ch453–Ch454
psoriasis **Ch219,** *Ch220*
trigeminal neuralgia **Ch494–Ch495**
vulvar pain syndrome Ch606
topical local anesthesia Ch221–Ch222
acute herpes zoster pain Ch441–Ch442
clinical tips Ca323
clinical trials Ch222
evidence Ch222–Ch223
preparations Ca322–Ca323
procedural pain management Ca322–Ca323
in children A452
topiramate
mechanism of action Ch251
treatment (of)
CRPS Ch394
painful spasticity **Ch461**
total body irradiation (TBI), bone pain management Ca285,
Ca286
total pain Ca21, Ca74, Ca106–Ca107, Ca114–Ca115, Ca124
elements *Ca75,* Ca106–Ca107
total pain relief (TOTPAR) calculation **P24**
tourniquet method, adenosine effect on
allodynia development **P487**
pain scores in ischemia-induced pain **P487**
toxic epidermal necrolysis, in AIDS patients *Ca383*
toxic neuropathy *see* neuropathies, toxic
toxoplasmosis, central pain syndromes Ch403
trabeculae Ch521
traction P184
traction, chronic back pain management Ch528

traditional Chinese acupuncture Ca270
see also acupuncture
tramadol A50, A335, Ca52–Ca53, Ca131, Ch207, P67
adverse effects Ca53
in children A442
analgesia for patients over 6 months P435
doses **P435**
pharmacology and indications A442
in elderly A473
pharmacokinetics Ca52–Ca53
treatment (of)
chronic back pain Ch527
fibromyalgia Ch625
musculoskeletal trauma A356
peripheral neuropathy Ch377
transcutaneous electrical nerve stimulation (TENS) A275–A283,
Ca245–Ca248, Ch286–Ch287, P185–P186, P343–P354
adverse effects Ch287, P349
allergic reaction P348
applications A277–A280
acute postoperative pain A277–A278
angina A279
dysmenorrhea A279
labor pain A278–A279, A432
pain management in pregnancy A378
postoperative pain management A323
post-traumatic pain A280
procedural pain A279–A280
sickle cell crisis A280
site P347–P348
applied anatomy P344
caution P345
childbirth pain treatment A278–A279, P351
clinical experience Ch286
contraindications A275, Ca246, Ch287, P345
efficacy Ch286, Ch556
electrodes A276, P346
carbon-rubber P346
positioning Ca246–Ca247, P346, *P347*
self-adhesive P346
equipment A276, Ca246, P346
connection to stimulator P346
failure P348
stimulator A276
evidence for efficacy Ca247–Ca248
evidence for therapy A277
experimental evidence for use P349–P352
acute pain P350–P351
efficacy comparison of continuous and pulsed
modalities *P350*
frequency P349–P350
pain reduction over time *P350*
forms A276
frequency of therapy P345
historical aspects P401–P402
indications A275, Ca246, Ch286–Ch287, P344–P345
acute pain P344
chronic pain P344–P345
limitations P345
mechanism of action A275, Ca245–Ca246, Ch556, P344
modes of stimulation **Ca247**
obstacles/difficulties in research A277
pain clinics **Ch159**
patient education Ch286
practical issues Ca246
preparation A276
problems with use A277, Ca247, Ch445, P348–P349
skin irritation Ca247

tolerance Ca247
stimulation characteristics **P349**
stimulation types P347
stimulator setting P348
    acupuncture-like TENS P348
    choice of stimulation modality P348
    continuous (conventional) stimulation P348
    pulsed (burst) stimulation P348
    sequential stimulation P348
technique A276–A277
treatment (of)
    acute herpes zoster pain Ch445
    central pain syndromes Ch410
    chronic back pain Ch531
    CRPS Ch394–Ch395
    dysesthetic vulvodynia Ch604
    elderly pain Ca359, Ch655–Ch656
    interstitial cystitis Ch596
    neurologic disease Ch362
    nociceptive pain Ca246
    osteoarthritis Ch544
    peripheral neuropathy Ch377–Ch378
    phantom pain Ch430
    postherpetic neuralgia Ch454
    postoperative pain A277–A278
    pruritus Ca308
    refractory angina pectoris Ch556
    syndrome X Ch558
trial stimulation period Ca247, P348
transdermal administration of drugs A207
corticosteroids A496
fentanyl *see* fentanyl, transdermal therapeutic system (TTS)
NSAIDs A209, A495, Ca197–Ca198
opioids A211–A212, A319, Ca51
    cancer pain management P70–P71
patient-controlled analgesia (PCA) P401
    ideal drug properties **P403**
    iontophoretic systems **P402**
    opioid delivery P402
in refractory cancer pain Ca147
see also entries beginning topical
transduction (nociceptor activation) A3
TRANSFENTA® **P402**
transient motor paralysis, celiac plexus block complications P250
transient neurological symptoms (TNSs), reduction in ambulatory
    surgery A248
transient postsympathectomy neuropathic pain, lumbar
    sympathetic block complication P243
transient radicular irritation (TRI), local anesthesia
    complication A81
transient receptor potential M8 (TRPM8) A19–A20
transjugular intrahepatic portosystemic shunt (TIPS) A506–A507
balloon dilation A506
direct portal venogram of shunt *A507*
indications A506
portography *A506*
regional techniques A507
transmission (in nociception) A3
transmucosal administration of drugs A205–A206
    fentanyl, refractory cancer pain management Ca152
    opioids A210–A211, A318–A319, Ca50–Ca51
transmucosal patient-controlled analgesia (PCA)
    ideal drug properties **P403**
    opioid delivery P402–P404
    oral and nasal routes P401
transmyocardial laser revascularization (TMLR) Ch557
transuterine venogram, pelvic congestion diagnosis Ch592
transverse processes *Ch522*

trauma A349–A358
abdominal *see* abdominal trauma
analgesia methods of provision **A349,** A350–A352
    inhalation methods A350, **A350**
    pharmacological methods A350–A351
    physical methods A350
    psychological methods A352
    regional anesthesia A352
        see also regional anesthesia techniques
assessment A349
central pain syndromes Ch403
of chest *see* chest trauma
head injury A352
immobilization A350, **A355**
musculoskeletal injuries A355–A356
nitrous oxide provision **A350**
pelvic A353–A354
traumatic brain injury (TBI), management A352
traumatic lesions, brachial plexus neuropathies Ch374
trazodone
    central pain syndrome management Ch409, **Ch409**
    postherpetic neuralgia management Ch453
treatment protocols for opioids in chronic nonmalignant pain *see*
    opioids, in chronic nonmalignant pain (protocols)
treatment-related pain syndromes **Ca14,** Ca14–Ca17
    avascular bone necrosis Ca16
        MRI scan *Ca16*
    chronic postoperative neuropathic pain Ca14–Ca15
        see also postoperative neuropathic pain, chronic
    mucositis Ca15
        oral problem Ca298
    radiation-induced peripheral nerve tumors Ca17
    radiation myelopathy Ca17
    radiation plexopathy Ca16–Ca17
    steroid pseudorheumatism Ca15–Ca16
tremor, CRPS Ch385
tricyclic antidepressants (TCAs) P101
    adjuvant analgesics Ca135
        in children Ca342
        in elderly Ca358
    adverse effects Ca216–Ca217, **Ch244,** Ch377, Ch440, **Ch461,**
        Ch654, P103–P104
    contraindications Ca216, Ch244, **Ch486,** P102
    dosage range **Ch461**
    dosing and treatment schedule Ca216, P102, **P103**
        if contraindications are present P102, *P104*
        if no contraindications P102, *P103*
    drug choice Ch246
    in elderly A473
    mechanism of action Ch239–Ch240
    nomenclature Ch239
    pain management in ICU A344
    pharmacology **Ch240**
    practical tips Ca217
    pretreatment safety measures **P103**
    treatment (of)
        acute herpes zoster pain Ch440
        chronic back pain Ch527–Ch528
        CRPS Ch394
        depression Ca309
        dysesthetic vulvodynia Ch604
        elderly pain A473, Ch654
        fibromyalgia/myofascial pain Ch625
        interstitial cystitis Ch596
        neurologic disease Ch361
        neuropathic pain Ch242–Ch243
        painful spasticity **Ch461**
        pelvic pain Ch603

peripheral neuropathy Ch376
postsurgical pain syndrome Ch423
syndrome X Ch558
tension-type headache Ch475
TMJ pain **Ch486**
vulvar pain syndrome Ch606
see also antidepressants; *individual drugs*
trigeminal nerve, peripheral branches blockade P200–P202
anatomical aspects P200, *P201*
indications **P202**
infraorbital block *see* infraorbital nerve block
mental branch *see* mental nerve block
supraorbital branch *see* supraorbital nerve block
supratrochlear branch *see* supratrochlear nerve block
trigeminal nerve block, acute herpes zoster pain Ch444
trigeminal neuralgia **Ch482,** Ch491–Ch494
antiepileptic indication P104–P105, P105, P107
clinical presentation Ch491–Ch492
bilateral cases Ch492
clinical trials Ch252
definition Ch491
diagnosis Ch492, **Ch492**
epidemiology Ch491
etiology/pathophysiology Ch491
neurovascular contact Ch491
investigations Ch492
management **Ch498**
anticonvulsants Ch253, Ch493–Ch494
baclofen Ch257, Ch494, **Ch494–Ch495**
pharmacology Ch492–Ch493, **Ch494–Ch495**
multiple sclerosis Ch357
prognosis Ch494
radiofrequency lesioning Ca242
resistance to drugs, radiofrequency lesioning indication P330
support groups Ch493–Ch494
surgical management Ch493–Ch494, **Ch496–Ch497**
mortality Ch493
recurrence rates Ch493
Trigeminal Neuralgia Association Support Group Ch493–Ch494
trigeminal neuropathy, motor cortex stimulation Ch294
trigeminal system activation
fibromyalgia/myofascial pain Ch622
migraine pathophysiology Ch469
trigeminal tractotomy Ch300–Ch301
complications Ch301
indications Ch300–Ch301
lesion location Ch301
open surgery technique Ch301
outcomes Ch301
percutaneous technique Ch301
trigger points (TrPs)
definition Ch615
myofascial pain (MFP) Ch618
positions *Ch617*
triptans, migraine management **Ch467,** Ch471–Ch472, Ch638
abuse Ch473
adverse effects **Ch469**
children Ch638
comparison with other drugs Ch472–Ch473
contraindications **Ch469,** Ch473
doses **Ch469**
efficacy in RCT **Ch468, Ch469,** Ch471–Ch473
mechanism of action Ch471
therapeutic use **Ch469,** Ch473
trochanteric bursitis Ch546–Ch547
TRPM8 A19–A20
true-negative result, definition Ch126
true-positive result, definition Ch126

tuberculosis, central pain syndromes Ch403
tumors
embolization of blood supply A504–A505
pelvic pain Ch593–Ch594
Tuohy needle, in spinal cord stimulation P381, *P385*
twelfth rib syndrome, chronic chest pain Ch559
21-point scale Ch65
tyrosine kinase receptors (trk) **A20, A22**
in inflammatory pain A26

UAB Pain Behavior Scale Ch76
ulcerative colitis A375, Ch579
ulnar nerve block
at elbow P211–P212
landmarks and practical steps P211–P212, *P212*
at wrist (medial approach) P213
landmarks and practical steps P213, *P214*
ultrasound Ch129, P186
limitations Ch129
mechanism Ch129
pelvic pain diagnosis Ch599
reliability Ch129
sensitivity Ch129
specificity Ch129
tendonopathy diagnosis Ch129
transvaginal, pelvic congestion diagnosis Ch592
validity Ch129
undertreatment of pain Ch10–Ch11, Ch29–Ch30
in AIDS Ca373
principal reasons **Ca373**
reasons Ca123
in substance abuse patients Ca396
unstable cancer pain *see* refractory cancer pain
upper limb pain Ch545–Ch546
aching pain Ch506
diagnosis for disorders **Ch546**
indications for radiotherapy Ca255–Ca256
peripheral nerve blocks P204–P214
see also individual types
see also forearm; shoulder
upper motor neuron lesions Ch459
features **Ch459**
upper quadrant pain, right, in AIDS patients Ca388
ureter
lumbar sympathetic block complications P243
opioids' pharmacological effects P63
ureteric obstruction, in pregnancy A377–A378
ureteric stent placement A507
urethral syndrome Ch595
diagnosis Ch595
etiology Ch595
management Ch595
symptoms/signs Ch595
urinary retention
epidural analgesia induced in children P443
opioid induced A253, Ca177
PCA induced A234
urinary tract, NSAIDs adverse effects Ca188–Ca189
urolithiasis, in AIDS patients Ca389
uterine artery embolization (UAE), uterine fibroid pain
relief A504–A505
therapeutic plan **A511**
uterine cancer, radiotherapy Ca255
uterine fibroids A504
angiogram following bilateral selective catheterization *A505*
pain relief A504–A505
reduced vascularity after embolization *A505*
uterosacral transection Ch602

see also presacral neurectomy (PSN)
uterus
    contractions causing childbirth pain A424–A425
    innervation A427
    opioids' pharmacological effects P63

vaccination, acute herpes zoster pain management A372
vaginismus Ch633
valaciclovir, acute herpes zoster pain Ch439
valerian, botanical therapy **Ch347**
validity Ch125–Ch126
    concept Ch125
    construct Ch126
    definition Ch125–Ch126
    determination Ch126
    divergent, pain measure P10
    face Ch125
    pain measure see under pain measures
    of procedures
        computed tomography (CT) Ch128
        diagnostic Ch125–Ch126
        magnetic resonance imaging (MRI) Ch128
        radiographs Ch127
        sympathetic nerve blocks Ch131
        thermography Ch131
        ultrasound Ch129
valproic acid
    postherpetic neuralgia management Ch453
    trigeminal neuralgia management Ch494, **Ch494–Ch495**
Vanderbilt Pain Management Inventory Ch106
vanilloid receptor see topical capsaicin
varicella vaccine, postherpetic neuralgia prevention Ch455
varicella-zoster virus (VZV) Ch437
    chickenpox-causing agent A369
    herpes zoster-causing agent A369
    oral pain in AIDS patients Ca380, Ca381
variegate porphyria Ch580
vascular bypass surgery, graft occlusion rates **A173**
vascular stents, pain relief in interventional radiology A503–
    A504
vasculitis, in AIDS patients Ca376
vasectomy pain, epidemiology Ch22
vasodilation, atypical odontalgia Ch490
venepuncture, clinical trials of EMLA **Ca324**
venlafaxine
    central pain syndrome management **Ch409**
    pharmacology **Ch240**
ventilation, increase during childbirth A426
ventroposteromedialis (VPM) stimulation, postherpetic neuralgia
    management Ch454
verapamil, migraine prophylaxis Ch475
verbal consent, opioid trials Ch208
verbal descriptor rating scale (VDRS) A190–A191, Ch65
verbal numerical rating score (VNRS) A191, A309
verbal rating scale (VRS) A99, Ch147, P17, P455
    advantages and disadvantages A99
    childbirth pain measurement A428
vertebral artery dissection, neck pain Ch508
vertebral body Ch522
vertebral column see spine (vertebral column)
vertebral end plate Ch522
vertebral metastases Ca4–Ca5
    MRI scan Ca5
    pain syndromes caused by **Ca4, Ca7**
vertebrogenic pain, radiofrequency lesioning P332–P333
    anatomical aspects of spine P332–P333
        dorsal compartment P332–P333
        ventral compartment P333

vestibular papillomatosis, vulvar pain syndrome Ch603
vibrameter, vibratory threshold determination P31–P32
vibratory threshold, determination with vibrameter P31–P32
vigabatrin
    CRPS management Ch394
    mechanism of action Ca213
    pharmacokinetics Ca215
vinca alkaloids, toxic neuropathy Ch372
viscera
    cancers Ch578–Ch579
        sources of pain **Ch568**
    hyperalgesia, irritable bowel syndrome (IBS) Ch577
    inflammation Ch569
    nerve supply Ch569
visceral pain A5, A97, Ca65, Ca260, Ch567–Ch569
    in AIDS patients Ca385–Ca387
        etiology and pathophysiology Ca385–Ca386
    childbirth pain A425
    diagnosis, nerve blocks Ch132
    gut localized pain A97
    pelvic pain Ch588
    in refractory cancer pain see under refractory cancer pain
    somatic pain comparison **A6**
        in abdominal pain A373–A374
    TENS indication P345
        experimental evidence P351
    see also abdominal pain, visceral
vision disturbance, epidural steroid injection complication P423
visual analog scale (VAS) A100, A100–A101, A191, Ch65, Ch68,
    Ch104, Ch120, Ch147, P17–P18, P18
    advantages A100, P18
    childbirth pain measurement A428
    comparison with numerical and visual rating scales A101
    dental pain assessment P463
    disadvantages A100, P18
    opioid clinical trials Ch203–Ch204
    pain measurement by pictures and toys P18, P19
    pain measurement in children A438
    postoperative pain measurement A308–A309
    variations A100
visualization Ca275–Ca276
vitamin B₁ (thiamine) deficiency, peripheral
    neuropathies Ch371–Ch372
vitamin B₆ (pyridoxine) deficiency, peripheral
    neuropathies Ch372
vitamins Ca273
voltage-gated ion channels **A19**
    phosphorylation A27
vomiting Ca299–Ca301
    clinical findings Ca299
    etiology **Ca300**
    hypercalcemia Ca300–Ca301
    management Ca299–Ca300, Ca300
        antiemetics A257
            see also antiemetics
        drug classification **Ca302**
        hypnosis Ca275
    opioid induced A253–A254, A472, Ca47, Ca132, Ca176, P62,
        P437
        epidemiology Ca176
        epidural infusion P313
        etiology and pathophysiology Ca176
        evidence-based evaluation of management Ca176
    PCA induced A233
        management P398
    systemic analgesia complication in children A450
    TENS reduction in postoperative expulsions P350–P351
von Frey hairs P31

neuropathic pain assessment Ch118, *Ch118*
tactile sensibility estimation P31
vulvar dermatoses, vulvar pain syndrome Ch603
vulvar pain syndrome Ch603–Ch607
  clinical presentation
    examinations Ch604
    history Ch604
  definition Ch603–Ch604
  dermatoses Ch603
  dysesthetic vulvodynia Ch604
  epidemiology Ch604
  etiology Ch604, **Ch604,** *Ch605*
  management Ch605–Ch607
    biofeedback Ch607
    CBT Ch607
    diet modification Ch607
  pharmacological management Ch605–Ch606
    antifungals Ch606
    antihistamines Ch606
    antivirals Ch605–Ch606
    estrogen Ch606
    topical capsaicin Ch606
    tricyclic antidepressants (TCAs) Ch606
  prognosis Ch607
  surgical management Ch606–Ch607
    lasers Ch607
    perineoplasty Ch606–Ch607
  vestibular papillomatosis Ch603
  vulvovaginitis Ch603
  see also pelvic pain
vulvar vestibulitis Ch603, Ch605
  characterization Ch605
  epidemiology Ch605
  etiology Ch605
  management Ch605
vulvodynia *see* vulvar pain syndrome
vulvovaginitis, vulvar pain syndrome Ch603

waiting lists Ch156
Wallenberg syndrome, central pain syndrome Ch408
Wallerian degeneration Ca236
warfarin, epidural hematoma risk A476
websites of interest **Ca92**
Wegener's granulomatosis, autoimmune neuropathy Ch373
Western medical acupuncture Ca270
Western Ontario and McMaster Osteoarthritis Index Ch65
West Haven–Yale Multidimensional Pain Inventory Ch65
whiplash Ch136, Ch508–Ch509
  incidence Ch508
  injuries due to Ch508–Ch509
  zygapophysial joint pain Ch512
  see also neck pain
wide dynamic range (WDR) neurons A7
  in inflammatory pain A32–A33
  referred pain Ch116
wide-field irradiation, bone pain management Ca285
  radiation fields *Ca286*
  toxicity **Ca287**
windup A29, *A30,* A360, Ca146, P28
  NMDA receptor blocker association Ca221
windup-like pain, neuropathic pain Ch116–Ch117, **Ch121**
Wisconsin Brief Pain Questionnaire Ch65
withdrawal syndrome, in opioid therapy *see under* opioids
workers' compensation systems Ch72–Ch73
  disability evaluation (USA) Ch40
  involuntary job loss Ch73
  negligence perceptions Ch73
  preinjury job stress Ch73

World Health Organization (WHO)
  impairment definitions Ch183
  opioid use guidelines Ch175
World Health Organization (WHO) analgesic ladder Ca126, *Ca127,* Ca143–Ca155, *Ca144,* P70, *P71*
  background Ca143–Ca144
  failure Ca143, Ca147
  limitations Ca144–Ca147
    advances in understanding of pain pathophysiology Ca146–Ca147
    assessing and categorizing pain intensity and response Ca145–Ca146
    opioid drug class Ca144–Ca145
    other interventions Ca146
    pain mechanism Ca145
    political and social acceptance of morphine Ca144
  nonoral administration routes Ca147–Ca148
  oral administration routes
    contraindications **Ca147**
    preference Ca143, Ca147
  sequential use of analgesic medication Ca126
  three-level approach Ca126, Ca143
    to refractory cancer pain management Ca148, *Ca150*
wound infiltration of local anesthesia A267–A268, A332
  in pediatric surgery A445
    efficacy **A445**
  postoperative pain management A320
wrist
  intra-articular injections P265–P266
    distal radioulnar joint P266
    radiocarpal joint P265–P266, *P266*
  nerve blocks P213–P214
    anatomical aspects P213
    indications P213
    see also individual types
  pain A401
    investigations/management A401

xerostomia Ca297
  antidepressant-induced Ch243–Ch244
  burning mouth syndrome Ch488
  causes **Ca298**
  opioid induced Ca177
    definition Ca177
    epidemiology Ca177
    etiology and pathophysiology Ca177
    evidence-based evaluation of management Ca177

yellow flags
  abdominal pain psychosocial potentials **A373**
  low back pain **A408,** A416–A417
  spinal injuries **A408**
yin and yang P355

zalcitabine, toxic neuropathy Ch372–Ch373
ziconotide Ch267
zidovudine, nucleoside analog in AIDS pain management Ca368
zimelidine, postherpetic neuralgia management Ch453
zolmitriptan, migraine therapy
  efficacy in RCT Ch471
  therapeutic use Ch473
zone of reference, definition Ch615
zonisamide, painful spasticity management **Ch461**
zoster-associated pain A369
zygapophyseal joints
  anatomy P269–P270, *P270*
  blocks Ch512
    controls Ch512

neck pain investigations Ch512
cervical *see* cervical zygapophyseal (facet) joints
injections and medial branch blocks P269–P276
    chronic back pain management Ch530
    complications P274
    contraindications P271
    evidence for use of P274–P275
    gauge needles P271–P272
    indications P270–P271

    limitations of treatment P271
    monitoring P272
    preparation P271–P274
    repeat and placebo blocks P271
    screening of needle insertions P271
lumbar *see* lumbar zygapophyseal (facet) joints
pain P270
    radiofrequency lesioning Ca242